Guidelines | Low Art 041-04W

Illustrations | Up Veins 051-05W

Approach Table | Low Veins 061-06W

A-C | Lymph & Hemic 072-07Y

D-E | Eye 080-08X

F-I | Ear, Nose, Sinus 090-09W

J-L | Resp 0B1-0BY

M-O | Mouth & Throat 0C0-0CX

P-Q | Gastro 0D1-0DY

R-Z | Hepato & Pancr 0F1-0FY

Med/Surg 001-0YW | Endo 0G2-0GW

Cen Nerv / Cran Nerves 001-00X | Skin & Breast 0H0-0HX

Periph Nerv 012-01X | Sub Tiss & Fascia 0J0-0JX

Heart & Great Vess 021-02Y | Muscles 0K2-0KX

Up Art 031-03W | Tend 0L2-0LX

Burs & Ligam 0M2-0MX | Admin 302-3E1

Head & Fac Bones 0N2-0NW | Meas & Monit 4A0-4B0

Up Bones 0P2-0PW | System Ass't & Perf 5A0-5A2

Low Bones 0Q2-0QW | Therap 6A0-6AB

Up Joints 0R2-0RW | Osteo 7W0

Low Joints 0S2-0SW | Oth Pxs 8C0-8E0

Urin 0T1-0TY | Chiro 9WB

Fem Repr 0U1-0UY | Imag B00-BY4

Male Repr 0V1-0VX | Nuc Med C01-CW7

Anat Reg, Gen 0W0-0WY | Rad Ther D00-DWY

Anat Reg, Up Extr 0X0-0XY | Rehab & Dx Aud F00-F15

Anat Reg, Low Extr 0Y0-0YW | Ment Health GZ1-GZJ

Ob 102-10Y | Subst Ab Tx HZ2-HZ9

Placem't – Reg 2W0-2W6 | New Tech X2A-XY0

Placem't – Orif 2Y0-2Y5 | Appendixes

D1157483

ICD-10-CM 2019
For Physicians & Hospitals

Find codes faster and master over 500 code changes for 2019 with the **ICD-10-CM for Physicians & Hospitals 2019**—with new and revised ICD-10-CM codes, full code descriptors, the Official ICD-10-CM Guidelines for Coding and Reporting and online tips for each Tabular chapter.

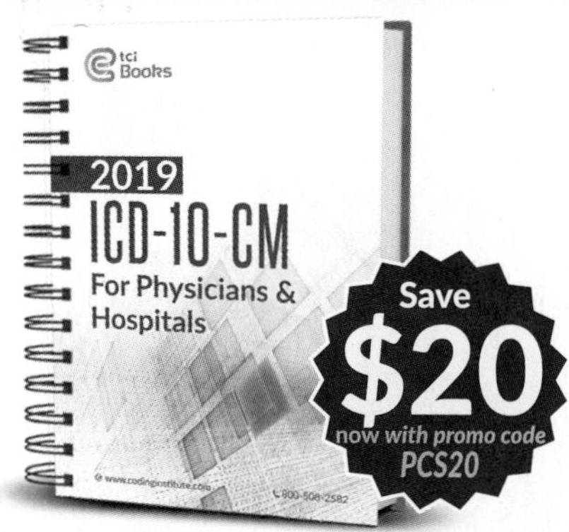
tci Books
2019
ICD-10-CM
For Physicians & Hospitals
Save
$20
now with promo code
PCS20

Avoid unspecified code denials with best-in-class features at your fingertips:

- **Complete 2019 ICD-10-CM code set**, including new code additions, deletions, and revisions
- **Full code descriptors** to conquer new and revised codes
- **Official ICD-10-CM Coding Guidelines & Conventions** to defeat claim denials in the front of the book
- **NEW!** Enhanced and detailed illustrations
- **NEW!** Certification exam prep advice
- **NEW!** More colored symbols for quick code searches
- **NEW!** Coding tips and definitions throughout the Tabular List
  - **NEW!** Chapter on using HCC codes
  - **NEW!** MACRA updates
  - **NEW!** Expanded stick-on tabs
- **Alphabetic Index, Index to External Causes, and Tabular List** to move swiftly and locate essential information
- **Colored vertical lines throughout the Alphabetic Index** to locate subterms and codes to cross reference
- **Table of Drugs and Chemicals and Neoplasm Table**
- **Appendix of Z-codes** for long-term use of drugs
- **Appendix of symbols for 7-character** codes
- **AHA Coding Clinic® references** to negotiate intricate coding scenarios
- **Full-page colored anatomical illustrations** with explanations before Tabular List chapters
- **Colored symbols and highlights throughout Tables** for at-a-glance identification
  - MACRA codes, HCC diagnosis codes, and RxHCC codes
  - New and revised codes, revised code title, and revised text
  - 7th characters
  - Unspecified codes, other specified codes, and manifestation codes
  - Additional 4th, 5th, 6th, and 7th characters throughout the Tabular List
  - Extension "X" alerts
  - Includes notes, and Excludes1 and Excludes2 notes
  - Z codes used as the first-listed diagnosis
  - Medicare Code Edits (MCEs) for gender, primary diagnosis only, questionable admission, unacceptable principal diagnosis, and age—newborn, pediatric, maternity, and adult
  - Complication or comorbidity and major complication or comorbidity
  - Principle diagnosis as its own CC/ Principle diagnosis as its own MCC
  - CC/MCC exclusion
  - HAC alerts
- **Dictionary-style headers and colored bleed tabs** with chapter title, number, and code ranges on every page to save time and effort
- **Notes pages** included after every Tabular List chapter to keep your go-to notes handy

Code accurately and quickly with TCI's **ICD-10-CM for Physicians & Hospitals 2019.**

PRE-ORDER ONLINE or call **1-800-508-2582** today.

Visit https://www.codinginstitute.com/books/icd-10-cm-for-physicians-and-hospitals.html?year=2019.

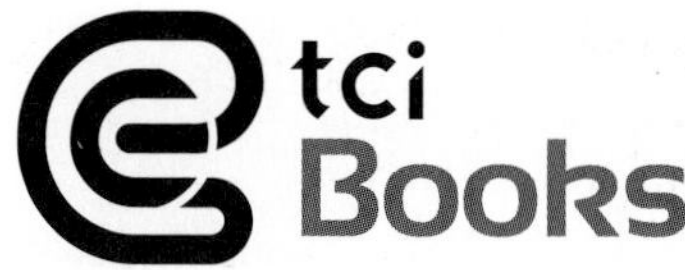
tci
Books

Call us: 800-508-2582 | www.codinginstitute.com

The Coding Institute LLC

2222 Sedwick Road Durham, NC 27713

Coders' Dictionary & Sourcebook 2018

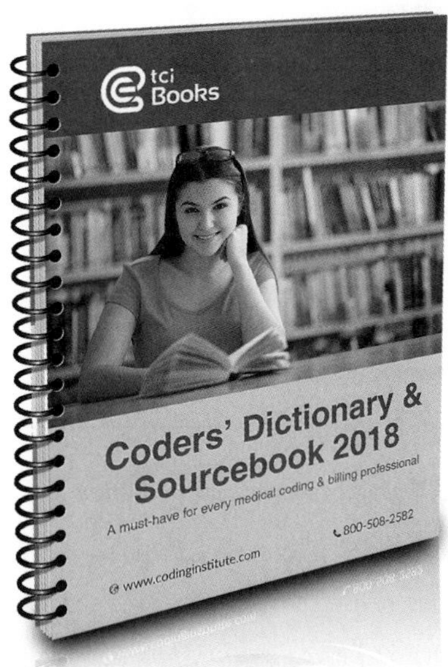
tci Books
Coders' Dictionary & Sourcebook 2018
A must-have for every medical coding & billing professional
800-508-2582
www.codinginstitute.com

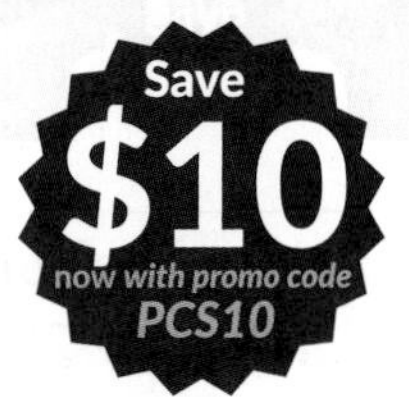
Save
$10
now with promo code
PCS10

A must-have for every medical coding and billing professional!

Say goodbye to all those resources heaped on your desktop and rev up your productivity with the all-new, completely updated **Coders' Dictionary & Sourcebook 2018**, TCI's best-selling, comprehensive look-up guide.

This one-of-a-kind coding resource organizes all the supporting information you rely on in one sourcebook for fast, at-a-glance answers to your questions.

Turbocharge your coding efficiency with swift access to:

- **NEW in 2018: Advice for new, revised, and deleted CPT® codes**
- **Exhaustive list of thousands of medical terms with definitions** in an easy-to-understand language
- **Billing, coding, and reimbursement terms and definitions** to acquaint you with current regulations, requirements, processes, and regulatory agencies
- **How-to guidance for coding procedures from the Surgery section,** with explanations of common terms
- **Evaluation and Management (E/M) Survival Guide** to help you identify the right choice for E/M service levels
- **Anesthesia primer** to distinguish between various types of anesthesia
- **Modifiers and lay descriptions for CPT® and HCPCS modifiers** in plain English to determine when and how to apply modifiers
- **Lists of prefixes, suffixes, abbreviations, and eponyms** frequently used in coding
- **Anatomical illustrations** to enhance your understanding of services and procedures
- **Vital signs and lab values** to identify normal/abnormal signs or test results
- **Place of service** (POS) and type of service (TOS) lists
- **And much more!**

To order the ***Coders' Dictionary & Sourcebook 2018***, call **1-800-508-2582** or visit https://www.codinginstitute.com/books/coders-dictionary-and-sourcebook.html.

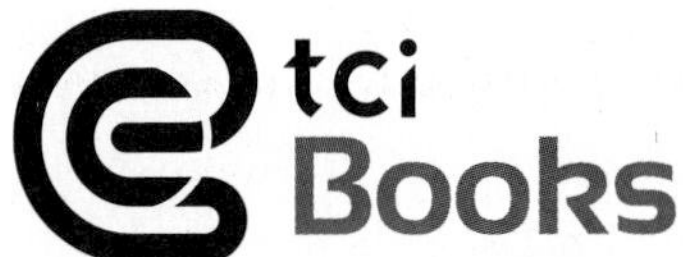
tci
Books

Call us: 800-508-2582 | www.codinginstitute.com
The Coding Institute LLC
2222 Sedwick Road Durham, NC 27713

CPT® is a registered trademark of the American Medical Association

Risk Adjustment Primer 2018

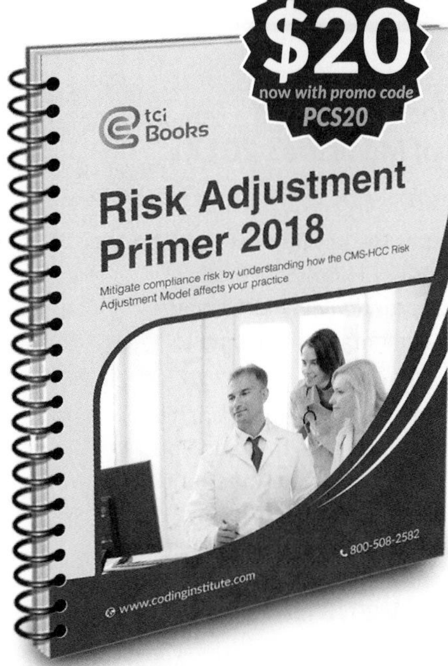

Save
$20
now with promo code
PCS20
tci Books
Risk Adjustment Primer 2018
Mitigate compliance risk by understanding how the CMS-HCC Risk Adjustment Model affects your practice
800-508-2582
www.codinginstitute.com

Ensure you understand the nuts and bolts of the CMS' risk adjustment program.

Are you struggling to get a handle on the CMS risk adjustment programs? We can help.

Bank on TCI's end-to-end **Risk Adjustment Primer 2018** to ensure you grasp the impact of these programs on your organization and equip you to navigate the risk assessment data that factors into patients' risk scores.

Learn how to calculate Hierarchical Condition Category (HCC) diagnostic codes. Rely on essential tools to nail down documentation deficiencies and improve your risk scores. Reduce the impact of the value-based purchasing program, sort out the CMS overpayment rule... and so much more.

Master your risk adjustment regulatory requirement challenges:

- The Nuts and Bolts of Hierarchical Condition Categories (HCCs)
- Get the Lowdown on Risk Adjustment (RA)
- Zip Through HCC Coding Tips
- Identify Your Top HCCs and Master Specificity
- Round up AWOL Revenue with a Solid Clinical Documentation Improvement (CDI) Process
- Power up for Risk Adjustment Data Validation (RADV) Audits
- Tackle Insight on HCCs and MACRA
- When VBP Risk Adjustment Doesn't Compensate Enough
- **Conquer Risk Adjustment with the CMS Toolkit**
  - ✓ Annual Schedule
  - ✓ Risk Adjustment Models – Overview
  - ✓ Calibration of the CMS-HCC Risk Adjustment Models
  - ✓ CMS-HCC Risk Adjustment Model
  - ✓ End Stage Renal Disease (ESRD)
  - ✓ Prescription Drug Hierarchical Condition Categories (RxHCC)
  - ✓ CMS RxHCC Risk Adjustment Model Compared with the CMS-HCC Risk Adjustment Model
  - ✓ Frailty Adjuster
  - ✓ Normalization Factor
  - ✓ MA Coding Adjustment
  - ✓ High-Level Checklist Of All Plan Requirements
  - ✓ Risk Adjustment Process and Payment Operations
  - ✓ Data Collection to Support Risk Adjustment
  - ✓ Submission and Flow of Risk Adjustment Data
  - ✓ Risk Score Verification Tools Glossary of Terms
  - ✓ **And so much more!**

Lessen your compliance risk by understanding how the CMS-HCC Risk Adjustment Model affects your practice.

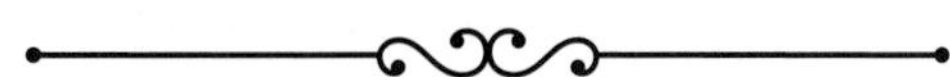

To order the ***Risk Adjustment Primer 2018***, call **1-800-508-2582**
or visit https://www.codinginstitute.com/books/risk-adjustment-primer.html?year=2018.

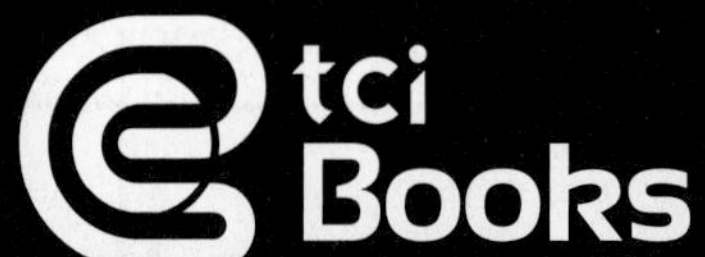

tci
Books

Call us: 800-508-2582 | www.codinginstitute.com
The Coding Institute LLC
2222 Sedwick Road Durham, NC 27713

Clinical Documentation Sourcebook 2018

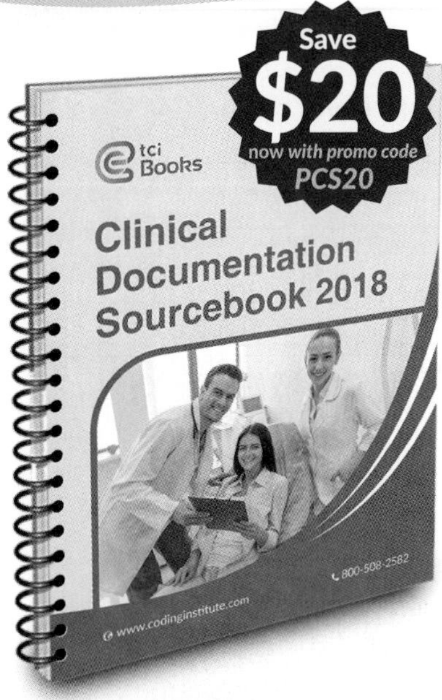
Save
$20
now with promo code
PCS20
tci Books
Clinical Documentation Sourcebook 2018
800-508-2582
www.codinginstitute.com

Did you know that insufficient documentation accounts for a whopping 64.1% of Medicare's 2017 improper payment error rate?

Inadequately documenting ICD-10 codes at the point of care leads to inaccurate reimbursement, clinician/coder EHR dissatisfaction, inefficient clinical workflow, and a loss of productivity—all of which are costly—these are but a few of the documentation hotspots to hurt revenue and invite auditors.

The **Clinical Documentation Sourcebook 2018** is the extensive guide filled with page after page of helpful insights to guide you in developing or expanding the qualities necessary to meet and manage clinical documentation guidelines. If you're struggling to increase revenue, improve the quality of patient care, or develop a stronger data source for healthcare analytics,
TCI's **Clinical Documentation Sourcebook 2018** is for you!

Take a look at the high-impact guidance in this invaluable resource:

- ✓ Get the inside scoop on coding pitfalls and how to avoid them
- ✓ Jumpstart your coding with our Clip & Save CDI Coding Tips for Conditions
- ✓ Learn the essential steps for prepping for an audit—from the auditor's perspective
- ✓ Shore up deficiencies in documentation with our multi-specialty pointers
- ✓ Grasp the ins and outs of documenting to defend medical necessity
- ✓ Master the general principles of documentation from CMS
- ✓ Strengthen communication by detecting documentation issues from a provider's perspective

Broaden your clinical documentation expertise:

- ✓ Coding examples and exercises
- ✓ Real-life documentation scenarios
- ✓ Leverage the ICD-10 CDI Toolkit
- ✓ Capitalize on TCI expert advice
- ✓ Bank on expert answers to frequently asked CDI questions
- ✓ Access documentation guidelines for E/M

Solidify your clinical documentation and collect audit-ready, optimal reimbursement:

- ✓ Grasp the legal aspects of documentation
- ✓ Anticipate and avoid documentation trouble spots
- ✓ Skirt these common documentation faux pas identified by CERT/RAC
- ✓ Don't miss these costly EMR errors
- ✓ Master documentation in the EMR with guidelines and tips
- ✓ Stop compliance issues in their tracks with these pointers
- ✓ Benefit from tips to select the correct diagnosis code from the superbill
- ✓ Capitalize on auditing advice for ICD-10 and CDI
- ✓ Know Medicare eligibility criteria for home care
- ✓ Nail down documentation for E/M coding
- ✓ Conquer CDI time-based coding for E/M
- ✓ Leverage pointers for trauma, infection, and medical conditions documentation
- ✓ Ace coding the initial preventative physical examination for Medicare

And much more!

Master accurate and timely documentation that reflects the scope of services provided.

To order the ***Clinical Documentation Sourcebook 2018***, call **1-800-508-2582**
or visit https://www.codinginstitute.com/books/clinical-documentation-sourcebook.html.

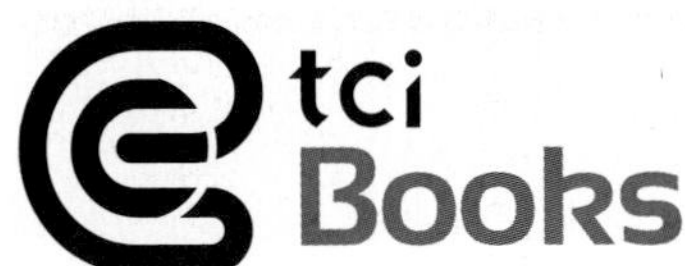
tci
Books

Call us: 800-508-2582 | www.codinginstitute.com
The Coding Institute LLC
2222 Sedwick Road Durham, NC 27713

HIPAA Handbook 2018

Complying with changing HIPAA security regulations is imperative, now more than ever.

HIPAA compliance scrutiny for all practices is high, and rightly so. PHI is more valuable to cyber criminals than credit card numbers, as it contains names, birth dates, social security numbers, insurance policy numbers, and, yes, personal medical records.

Is your HIPAA compliance program and breach reporting up-to-date?

Save your practice from unintentional breaches and penalties with the **HIPAA Handbook 2018**.

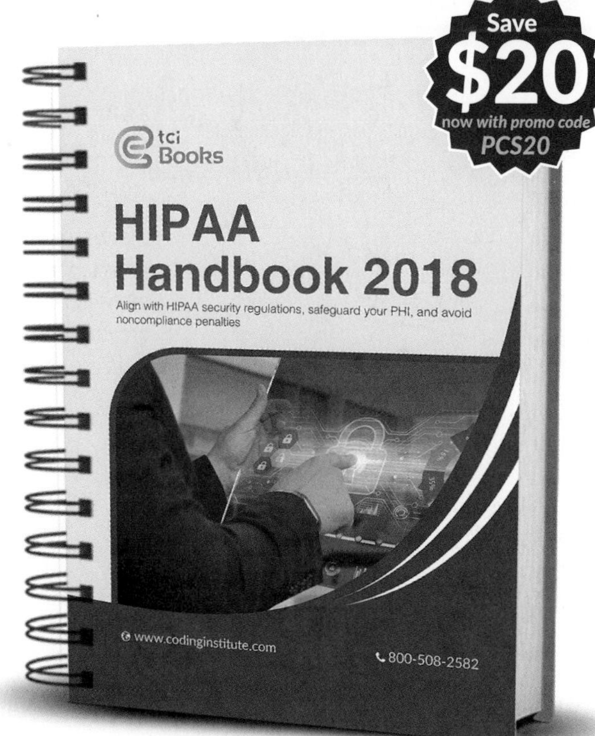
Save
$20
now with promo code
PCS20
tci Books
HIPAA
Handbook 2018
Align with HIPAA security regulations, safeguard your PHI, and avoid noncompliance penalties
www.codinginstitute.com
800-508-2582

Wield proactive measures with expert analysis:

- ✔ Is Your Office HIPAA Plan Up-to-Date?
- ✔ Discover These 3 Common Ways That Practices Violate HIPAA
- ✔ Head Off Potential HIPAA Breaches With These Surefire Strategies
- ✔ Avoid Phishing Schemes With These 7 Pointers
- ✔ Assess, Analyze, and Manage Your EHR Risk
- ✔ Hurricanes Make HIPAA Hard to Follow
- ✔ Are Your Systems Ready for New Medicare Numbers?
- ✔ New Tech Offering From the AMA Assists With Collaboration of Care
- ✔ Help Patients Access Their PHI With a New Form From AHIMA
- ✔ Keep Transactions HIPAA-Compliant With ASETT from CMS
- ✔ Nail Down Email Compliance Basics or Risk Exposure
- ✔ Protect Yourself and Your EHR Before Disaster Strikes
- ✔ Make Sure Your BAAs Are HIPAA-Compliant to Avoid Getting Burned
- ✔ Does Convenience Beat Utilization Cost in Telehealth?
- ✔ Celebrate Cybersecurity Awareness With Tips from the OCR
- ✔ Don't Let These Common HIT Gaffes Impact Your Revenue
- ✔ Avoid a Botched EHR Implementation With This Expert Advice
- ✔ Utilize Practice Analytics to Streamline Day-to-Day Operations
- ✔ Toolkit: Check Out the New HHS-OCR Breach Reporting Tool
- ✔ MACRA Toolkit to Streamline Processes
- ✔ Tackle Violations Head-On With This Quick-Start Training Guide
- ✔ **And so much more!**

The right resource makes all the difference. Identify your practice's risk areas before the OCR does.

To order the ***HIPAA Handbook 2018***, call **1-800-508-2582** or visit https://www.codinginstitute.com/books/hipaa-handbook.html.

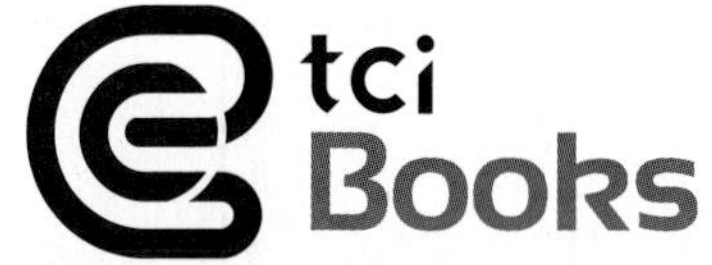
tci
Books

Call us: 800-508-2582 | www.codinginstitute.com

The Coding Institute LLC
2222 Sedwick Road Durham, NC 27713

This page intentionally left blank

2019

ICD-10-PCS

Complete Code Set

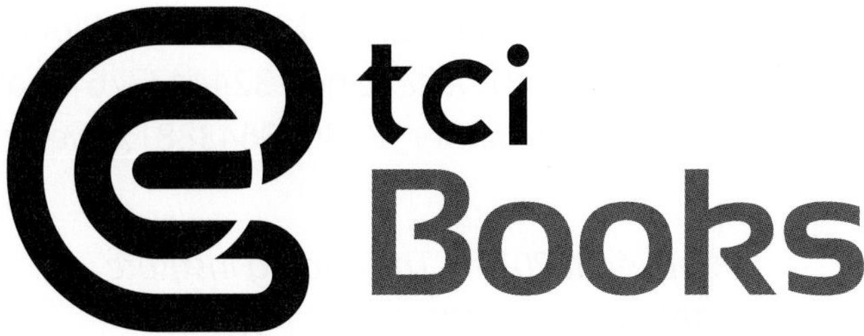
tci
Books

PUBLISHER'S NOTICE

Coding, billing, and reimbursement decisions should not be made based solely upon information within this book. Application of the information in this book does not imply or guarantee claims payment. Inquiries of your local carrier(s)' bulletins, policy announcements, etc., should be made to resolve local billing requirements. Finally, the law, applicable regulations, payers' instructions, interpretations, enforcement, etc., of the codes in this book may change at any time in any particular area. Information in this book is solely based on coding rules and regulations.

Codes in this book are designed to be an accurate and authoritative source regarding coding, and every reasonable effort has been made to ensure accuracy and completeness of content. However, the publisher makes no guarantee, warranty, or representation that this publication is complete, accurate, or without errors. It is understood that the publisher is not rendering any legal or professional services or advice in this code book and bears no liability for any results or consequences arising from use of this book.

THE PUBLISHER'S COMMITMENT TO ACCURACY

The publisher is committed to providing you with accurate and reliable materials. However, codes and the guidelines by which they are applied change or are reinterpreted through the year. This book contains data from Medicare Code Edits (v. 35), MS-DRG v. 35.0 Definitions Manual, and IPPS FY 2019 updates for CMS for symbols and Appendixes, along with the 2019 PCS code set in the tables which was the latest information available at the time of printing. Visit the CMS website at www.cms.gov for further updates. Check www.SuperCoder.com periodically for updates. To report corrections and updates, please contact TCI Customer Service via 1-800-508-2582 or via email to service@codinginstitute.com.

Images/Illustrations by the following artists at shutterstock.com:
stockshoppe - 180896807, 99671552, 180896810, 187162193, 180896855, 180896738, 177790997, 177791516, 180896873 | Blamb - 786347626, 24129706 | Alila Medical Media - 76386163, 72231811, 149230337, 149230217, 228843253, 155445671, 147789479, 228843103, 88094230, 155445686, 101696095, 96426923, 97755608, 147943922, 147943910, 155445662, 147943874, 106263593, 106263560, 125891585, 228843262 | Designua - 430118209, 180938618, 135935735, 165084413 | Suwin - 405537832 | Vecton - 661087531 | Sakurra - 676139677 | stihii - 109588457, 129969767, 124562680, 121824442, 129804629, 225637774, 505306105, 505306069 | DeryaDraws - 557609659 | Naeblys - 650014342 | NatthapongSachan - 416973331, 452997697 | udaix - 502058023, 108531449 | ducu59us- 104022683, 125200733 | BlueRingMedia- 141161404, 141162229, 141161560 | joshya - 261971498 | Della_Liner- 324447776 | snapgalleria - 142194094 | okili77- 156466463 | lotan - 186878060 | Alexander_P - 404964388 | Sylverarts Vectors - 552384124

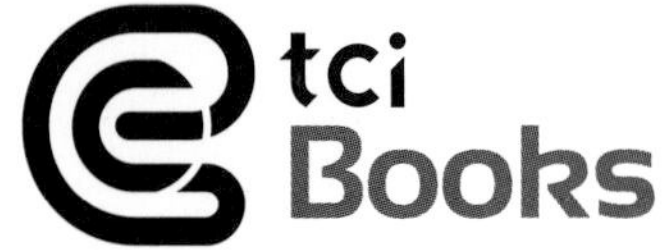
tci
Books

Copyright 2019 © The Coding Institute
ISBN (Print): 978-1-63527-596-4
ISBN (eBook): 978-1-63527-469-1

Table of Contents

Preface 2

Changes for 2019 3

List of Features 4

Using ICD-10-PCS Toward Your Credentialing Examination 5

Official Conventions and Additional Conventions Specific to This ICD-10-PCS Book 7

ICD-10-PCS Official Guidelines for Coding and Reporting 2019 9

Anatomical Illustrations 17

Approach Table 53

ICD-10-PCS Index 55

ICD-10-PCS Tables 169

Medical and Surgical 001-0YW 169

- Central Nervous System and Cranial Nerves 001-00X 169
- Peripheral Nervous System 012-01X 181
- Heart and Great Vessels 021-02Y 191
- Upper Arteries 031-03W 207
- Lower Arteries 041-04W 223
- Upper Veins 051-05W 239
- Lower Veins 061-06W 251
- Lymphatic and Hemic Systems 072-07Y 263
- Eye 080-08X 275
- Ear, Nose, Sinus 090-09W 289
- Respiratory System 0B1-0BY 305
- Mouth and Throat 0C0-0CX 319
- Gastrointestinal System 0D1-0DY 331
- Hepatobiliary System and Pancreas 0F1-0FY 351
- Endocrine System 0G2-0GW 361
- Skin and Breast 0H0-0HX 369
- Subcutaneous Tissue and Fascia 0J0-0JX 383
- Muscles 0K2-0KX 401
- Tendons 0L2-0LX 413
- Bursae and Ligaments 0M2-0MX 425
- Head and Facial Bones 0N2-0NW 441
- Upper Bones 0P2-0PW 453
- Lower Bones 0Q2-0QW 467
- Upper Joints 0R2-0RW 479
- Lower Joints 0S2-0SW 495
- Urinary System 0T1-0TY 511
- Female Reproductive System 0U1-0UY 523
- Male Reproductive System 0V1-0VX 539
- Anatomical Regions, General 0W0-0WY 555
- Anatomical Regions, Upper Extremities 0X0-0XY 567
- Anatomical Regions, Lower Extremities 0Y0-0YW 575

Obstetrics 102-10Y 583

Placement-Anatomical Regions 2W0-2W6 589

Placement-Anatomical Orifices 2Y0-2Y5 597

Administration 302-3E1 599

Measurement and Monitoring 4A0-4B0 615

Extracorporeal or Systemic Assistance and Performance 5A0-5A2 621

Extracorporeal or Systemic Therapies 6A0-6AB 623

Osteopathic 7W0 627

Other Procedures 8C0-8E0 629

Chiropractic 9WB 633

Imaging B00-BY4 635

Nuclear Medicine C01-CW7 677

Radiation Therapy D00-DWY 689

Physical Rehabilitation and Diagnostic Audiology F00-F15 707

Mental Health GZ1-GZJ 725

Substance Abuse Treatment HZ2-HZ9 729

New Technology X2A-XY0 733

- Cardiovascular System X2A-X2R 733
- Skin, Subcutaneous Tissue, Fascia, and Breast XHR 735
- Muscles, Tendons, Bursae, and Ligaments XK0 737
- Bones XNS 739
- Joints XR2-XRG 741
- Male Reproductive System XV5 745
- Anatomical Regions XW0 747
- Extracorporeal XY0 749

Appendix A: Root Operations Definitions 751

Appendix B: Body Part Key 757

Appendix C: Device Key 777

Appendix D: Device Aggregation Table 785

Appendix E: Character Meaning 789

Appendix F: Substance Key 859

Appendix G: Combination Clusters 861

Appendix H: Non-OR Not Affecting MS-DRG Assignment 877

Preface

Thank you for your purchase! We are pleased to offer you the 2019 ICD-10-PCS official code set in this book.

This manual goes beyond the basics to help you code accurately and efficiently. In addition to including the official Alphabetic Index, Tables, and ICD-10-PCS Official Guidelines, we've crafted a select set of bonus features based on requests from coders in the field as well as the recommendations of our core group of veteran coding educators.

Our goal was to apply our unique approach to focusing on the practical application of the codes to this procedure coding manual.

A few of the other features you'll benefit from page after page include the following:

- Updated and enhanced illustrations of body systems and disease processes at the front of the book so you don't have to search the manual for these large color images of body systems
- An Approach Table at the front of the book listing each approach, its definition, and examples
- Medicare Code Edits, including gender edits and edits for limited coverage, noncovered procedures, HAC-associated procedures, combination clusters, and non-OR procedures affecting MS-DRG assignment
- Intuitive color-coded symbols and alerts identify critical coding and reimbursement issues quickly
- List of non-OR procedures NOT affecting MS-DRG assignment
- Full list of adhesive tabs to label your book to quickly and easily find specific sections

See the complete List of Features to learn about everything this manual has to offer.

Rely on Our Combination of Official Sources and Experience

This manual includes the official ICD-10-PCS 2019 Alphabetic Index and Tables. We've also included the 2019 ICD-10-PCS Official Guidelines.

Additionally, our dedicated team drew on their years of experience using coding manuals to develop this manual's user-friendly symbols, color coding, and tabs, all designed to help you find the information you need quickly.

Let Us Know What You Think

Our goal for this manual is to support those involved in the business side of healthcare, helping them to do their jobs well. We'd appreciate your feedback, including your suggestions for what you'd like to see in an ICD-10-PCS resource, so we can be sure our manuals serve your needs. Thank you.

Changes for 2019

FY 2019 Update Summary

Change Summary Table

2018 Total	New Codes	Revised Titles	Deleted Codes	2019 Total
78,705	392	8	216	**78,881**

ICD-10-PCS Code FY 2019 Totals, By Section

Medical and Surgical	68,639
Obstetrics	302
Placement	861
Administration	1,445
Measurement and Monitoring	414
Extracorporeal or Systemic Assistance and Performance	45
Extracorporeal or Systemic Therapies	46
Osteopathic	100
Other Procedures	60
Chiropractic	90
Imaging	2,941
Nuclear Medicine	463
Radiation Therapy	1,939
Physical Rehabilitation and Diagnostic Audiology	1,380
Mental Health	30
Substance Abuse Treatment	59
New Technology	67
Total	**78,881**

List of FY 2019 Files

2019 Official ICD-10-PCS Coding Guidelines

- New Guideline B3.17 added in response to public comment.
- Guidelines A10, B3.7, and B6.1a revised in response to public comment and internal review.
- Downloadable PDF, file name **pcs_guidelines_2019.pdf**

2019 ICD-10-PCS Code Tables and Index (Zip file)

- Code tables for use beginning October 1, 2018.
- Downloadable PDF, file name is **pcs_2019.pdf**
- Downloadable xml files for developers, file names are **icd10pcs_tables_2019.xml, icd10pcs_index_2019.xml, icd10pcs_definitions_2019.xml**
- Accompanying schema for developers, file names are **icd10pcs_tables.xsd, icd10pcs_index.xsd, icd10pcs_definitions.xsd**

2019 ICD-10-PCS Codes File (Zip file)

- ICD-10-PCS Codes file is a simple format for non-technical uses, containing the valid FY 2019 ICD-10-PCS codes and their long titles.
- File is in text file format, file name is **icd10pcs_codes_2019.txt**
- Accompanying documentation for codes file, file name is **icd10pcsCodesFile.pdf**
- Codes file addenda in text format, file name is **codes_addenda_2019.txt**

2019 ICD-10-PCS Order File (Long and Abbreviated Titles) (Zip file)

- ICD-10-PCS order file is for developers, provides a unique five-digit "order number" for each ICD-10-PCS table and code, as well as a long and abbreviated code title.
- ICD-10-PCS order file name is **icd10pcs_order_2019.txt**
- Accompanying documentation for tabular order file, file name is **icd10pcsOrderFile.pdf**
- Tabular order file addenda in text format, file name is **order_addenda_2019.txt**

2019 ICD-10-PCS Final Addenda (Zip file)

- Addenda files in downloadable PDF, file names are **tables_addenda_2019.pdf, index_addenda_2019.pdf, definitions_addenda_2019.pdf**
- Addenda files also in machine readable text format for developers, file names are **tables_addenda_2019.txt, index_addenda_2019.txt, definitions_addenda_2019.txt**

2019 ICD-10-PCS Conversion Table (Zip file)

- ICD-10-PCS code conversion table is provided to assist users in data retrieval, in downloadable Excel spreadsheet, file name is **icd10pcs_conversion_table_2019.xlsx**
- Conversion table also in machine readable text format for developers, file name is **icd10pcs_conversion_table_2019.txt**
- Accompanying documentation for code conversion table, file name is **icd10pcsConversionTable.pdf**

List of Features

ICD-10-PCS is essential to documenting medical necessity for services rendered, and accurate codes mean better outcomes for the patient, your claims, and your facility.

You can count on this manual to help you choose and report the right ICD-10-PCS code. Unique features, intuitive design, and expert features that coders developed assure this manual will keep your coding on target.

This manual includes the ICD-10-PCS Alphabetic Index and ICD-10-PCS Tables for procedures, effective October 1, 2018 (FY 2019 code set).

To help you make the most of this manual, we include the following features:

- ICD-10-PCS Official Conventions and additional conventions and symbols
- ICD-10-PCS Official Guidelines for Coding and Reporting, effective October 1, 2018 (FY 2019)
- Approach Table with each approach, definition, and example listed at the front of the book for quick reference
- Updated and enhanced color illustrations of body systems and disease processes at the front of the book for easy look-up
- Medicare Code Edits symbols, including gender edits and edits for limited coverage, noncovered procedures, hospital acquired conditions (HAC-) associated procedures, combination clusters, and non-OR procedures affecting MS-DRG assignment
- Intuitive color-coded symbols and alerts for quick identification of coding and reimbursement issues
- Adhesive tabs for specific sections of the book to find information more quickly and easily
- Appendices for root operations definitions in alphabetical order by Tables, body part key, device key and aggregation table, character meaning, substance key, combination clusters, and non-OR procedures not affecting MS-DRG assignment
- A user-friendly page design, including dictionary-style headers, colored bleed tabs, and legend keys

Using ICD-10-PCS Toward Your Credentialing Examination

You've made a smart choice to pursue a CIC™ credential in inpatient medical coding from the American Academy of Professional Coders (AAPC).

Preparing for the credentialing examination adds to your knowledge, and receiving it confirms your professional expertise in your field, regardless of your experience.

The ICD-10-PCS is an essential book for the CIC™ certification examination, and you've made another smart choice by purchasing this ICD-10-PCS for your facility's procedure code book. Developed by coders for coders, this edition includes information essential to your successful completion of the examination. Many enhancements to this book aren't found in other publishers' ICD-10-PCS books.

Code books also required for the CIC™ examination include the ICD-10-CM.

Until December 31, 2018, AAPC examinations require the 2018 code books. Beginning January 1, examinees are tested using 2019 codes, descriptions, and guidelines.

AAPC also offers several examination preparation resources, such as distance learning programs, study guides, practice examinations, and Practicode. Check www.aapc.com for the latest information about these and specific book and resource requirements for your credentialing examination.

Studying for Your Examination

AAPC examinations are open book because you will need to look up codes and guidelines to complete most of the questions correctly. Your familiarity with the content and organization of your code books is essential to success.

The best strategy to prepare for the examination is to read your code books cover to cover.

Successful examinees have well-thumbed code books. Become familiar with all parts of your ICD-10-CM and ICD-10-PCS code books, and know how to locate the codes, guidelines, tables, and instructions within them quickly.

This may be the most important tip we can give you: Go through your books to mark them, tab and label them, and make notes in them for easy reference.

You may highlight, circle or "bubble" parts of the page that help you more easily. Some places where this helps are listed below:

Anything with which you feel you might need some extra help is something we would suggest tabbing or marking.

For the examination, you can write helpful notes in your books and tab them for easy reference. You may not glue, tape, staple, or add anything to the books. You also may wish to highlight certain guidelines in your code books. Keep in mind, notes in your code books should be relevant to work performed daily by a coder, although an occasional note of encouragement can make work or the examination a little easier.

Put notes on or near the codes or sections to which they pertain. You may use the notes pages to add notes, as well.

Things You Cannot Put into Your Book

Proctors will examine your books before the examination begins. You won't be able to bring your books into the examination if they find the following:

- Glued, taped, stapled notes or scratch sheets
- Post-It™ notes
- Study guide questions or cases
- Examinations questions
- Notes on full page tabs (eg. in Optum's code books)

While you've received tabs with your books, feel free to add or modify tabs to help you more efficiently and effectively do your work or pass your examination. Some coders use three sides of the pages to help them find office and topic-specific Items.

If you need additional coding practice, AAPC's online practice tests are excellent test simulation tools. The practice tests follow the same format as the CIC™ examination and are developed by AAPC's examination content team. The practice tests are available at www.aapc.com/training/practice-examinations.aspx.

Attend local chapter meetings, and don't be afraid to let your colleagues know your credentialing aspirations. Not only do some local chapters have credentialing classes and workshops, but you can also find study buddies to help you prepare for the exam.

Taking Your Examination

To register for your credentialing examination, you must be a member of AAPC. Start registration by going to the AAPC website and locating the nearest examination site on https://www.aapc.com/certification/locate-examination.aspx.

Once registered, read your code books, even if you have read them before or you work with them daily. Become familiar with the deadlines. You will have 5 hours, 40 minutes to complete the examination. Most credentials have 150 questions in the examination, and you will not have time to research and learn new guidelines or ideas.

Here are some more tips for the days leading up to your examination, once you've received confirmation:

- Confirm what examination materials are allowed during the examination. Gather these items several days prior to the examination (photo ID, member ID, plenty of #2 pencils, and an eraser along with the appropriate coding manuals). Please view our examination instructions at https://www.aapc.com/documents/exm-instructions.pdf to see what code books and supportive material are acceptable for each examination.
- Successful examinees have well-thumbed code books. Become familiar with all parts of your ICD-10 code books. Learn how to quickly locate the codes, guidelines, tables, and instructions within them. This may be the most important tip we can give you.
- Plan to leave your phone in your car. Electronic devices with an on/off switch (cell phones, smart phones, tablets, etc.) aren't allowed into the examination room. Failure to comply with this policy may result in disqualification of your examination.

Gather the following supplies and information the week before your examination:

- Clothing layers in case the room temperature fluctuates.
- Light, quiet snacks to keep you energized during the examination. We recommend hard candy and peppermint. You won't be able to leave for lunch during your examination.
- Cough drops if you are coughing.
- A water bottle.
- Ear plugs in case the noise in the room disturbs you.
- No. 2 pencils with erasers (You'll need the erasers.).
- Verify the start time and examination address at least two days prior to your test date. If you are unfamiliar with the examination site, consider mapping your driving directions in advance from maps.google.com or www.mapquest.com. Factor potential construction, traffic, or possible inclement weather during your commute, and arrive 10 to 15 minutes early.
- Code books and any errata.

Get a good night's sleep before your examination. Cramming the night before or the morning of probably won't help because you are ready. Watch a favorite movie or spend time with your family and friends instead. Relax.

Eat a healthy - but not too heavy - breakfast the next morning. Stick to your morning routine, but make sure you leave for your examination to get there early. *Proctors need time to check your books* before entering.

Here are some recommendations while you're taking your examination:

- Listen carefully while the proctor reads the instructions. Ask questions before the examination begins if you do not understand the instructions given.
- Be especially careful about marking your answer sheet. Be sure to correctly fill in your selected bubble on the test grid. Examinations are machine graded. To ensure an accurate score, bubbles must be filled out as shown on the examination on your test grid.
- Scan the entire test when you are instructed to begin. Answer the easiest, shortest questions first – this gives you the experience of succeeding and stimulates associations.
- Remember to pace yourself. Stay relaxed and do not panic. You will be able to finish.
- Read each question carefully. Note such words in the question as "not, except, most, least and greatest." These words are often crucial in determining the correct answer. However, there are no "trick" questions on the examination, so don't worry about hidden words or meanings.
- Answer every question. If you do not know the right answer, eliminate as many wrong answers as possible, then select among the remaining answers. If you don't have a clue – guess. A guess is better than a blank response.
- If you skip questions, take care that you are putting the answers on the right lines for subsequent questions. Don't forget to put an answer in the lines you've skipped.
- If you finish with some additional time, use that time to go back and review any questions for which you were not fully sure you had the correct answer. Use the code books again to confirm. Do not spend the extra time talking with others who have also finished their exams.
- If you find the examination environment too distracting, you may elect to discontinue testing, but it will be YOUR responsibility to contact AAPC to address your concerns on the first business day after your examination date. AAPC will review your concerns, and if any portion of the examination has been completed, AAPC reserves the right to still grade the examination.

AAPC grades examinations within seven to 10 business days; however, grading may take more than 10 days during particularly busy times of the year or if your examination takes longer than usual to arrive back at AAPC. Keep checking your AAPC web site page and your mail box for your results.

What happens if you fail? It's not the end of the world. You have the chance to take another examination for the same credential within 12 months. And AAPC will let you know what sections to work on before that examination.

However, plan and prepare to pass. A credential is your passport to better jobs, higher salaries, and more opportunities. For questions about the CIC™ exam, visit AAPC's FAQ section at https://www.aapc.com/certification/faq.aspx, or call AAPC at 800-626-2633. We wish you the best of luck on passing your exam!

Official Conventions and Additional Conventions Specific to This ICD-10-PCS Book

This manual includes the procedure code set from the International Classification of Diseases, 10th Revision, Procedure Coding System (ICD-10-PCS). Hospitals and third-party payers use these codes to classify inpatient procedures.

Official Conventions

Index

Refer to the ICD-10-PCS Index to access the Tables in the manual. The Index mirrors the structure of the Tables, so it follows a consistent pattern of organization and use of hierarchies. The Index is organized as an alphabetic lookup.

Two types of main terms are listed in the Index:

- Based on the value of the third character, such as a root operation (excision, insertion)
- Lists common procedure terms

Main Terms

For the Medical and Surgical and related sections, the root operation values are used as main terms in the Index. In other sections, the values representing the general type of procedure performed, such as nuclear medicine or imaging type, are listed as main terms.

For the Medical and Surgical and related sections, values such as Excision, Bypass, and Transplantation are included as main terms in the Index. The applicable body system entries are listed beneath the main term and refer to a specific table. For the ancillary sections, values such as Fluoroscopy and Positron Emission Tomography, are listed as main terms.

To find the code to cross-reference to the Tables, search for the root operation for the procedure in the Index, followed by the subterm for the anatomic site or the subterm that further describes the procedure. Locate the partial code, and cross-reference it to the Table that matches the first three characters of the code.

Tables

The Tables are organized in alphanumeric order in a series by Section, which is the first character of a code. Tables that begin with 0 to 9 are listed first, then tables beginning with B-D, then letters F-X, are listed next.

The same convention is followed within each table for the second through the seventh characters—numeric values in order first, followed by alphabetical values in order.

The Medical and Surgical section (first character 0) is organized by body system values. Each body system subdivision in the Medical and Surgical section contains tables that list the valid root operations for that body system. These are the root operation tables that form the system. These tables provide the valid choices of values available to construct a code.

The root operation tables consist of four columns and a varying number of rows, as in the following example of the root operation Insertion, in the Subcutaneous Tissue and Fascia body system.

The values for characters 1 through 3 are provided at the top of each table.

Character 1:	0: MEDICAL AND SURGICAL (Section)
Character 2:	J: SUBCUTANEOUS TISSUE AND FASCIA (Body System)
Character 3:	H: INSERTION: Putting in a nonbiological appliance that monitors, assists, performs, or prevents a physiological function but does not physically take the place of a body part (Root Operation)

Four columns contain the applicable values for characters 4 through 7, given the values in characters 1 through 3:

Body Part	Approach	Device	Qualifier
Character 4	**Character 5**	**Character 6**	**Character 7**
S Subcutaneous Tissue and Fascia, Head and Neck **V** Subcutaneous Tissue and Fascia, Upper Extremity **W** Subcutaneous Tissue and Fascia, Lower Extremity	**0** Open **3** Percutaneous	**1** Radioactive Element **3** Infusion Device **Y** Other Device	**Z** No Qualifier
T Subcutaneous Tissue and Fascia, Trunk	**0** Open **3** Percutaneous	**1** Radioactive Element **3** Infusion Device **V** Infusion Device, Pump **Y** Other Device	**Z** No Qualifier

A table may be separated into rows to specify the valid choices of values in characters 4 through 7. A code built using values from more than one row of a table is not a valid code.

Refer to the ICD-10-PCS Official Guidelines for Coding and Reporting in this manual for detailed guidance on assigning ICD-10-PCS codes.

See Reference

The See reference directs you to go elsewhere in the Index to find the root operation that you need.

Use Reference

The Use reference directs you to a character value selection as an additional reference.

Additional Conventions

Additional conventions that you will find in the Tables in this manual include Medicare Code Edits - Symbols and colored font.

Medicare Code Edits – Symbols Applied to 4th Characters

LC Limited Coverage

Procedures that are medically complex and serious in nature that incur extraordinary associated costs. Medicare limits coverage to a portion of the cost.

NC Noncovered

Procedures for which Medicare does not typically reimburse.

HAC HAC-associated Procedure

Procedures that are associated with hospital-acquired conditions (HAC).

CC Combination Cluster

The procedure is part of a procedure code combination, or cluster, listed in Appendix G of this manual. Medicare does not typically pay for these procedures unless you report them with other specific procedures.

DRG Non-OR-Affecting MS-DRG Assignment

Non-operating room procedures which affect MS-DRG assignment for claims reporting.

New/Revised Text in **Orange**

Procedure text was new or revised from the last version of the code set. For new codes, orange text will be shown for all characters in the code. New codes may be shown as their own row in a table and characters 4-7 may be shown in a row that is separate from other characters within that table.

♂ Male

Male procedure only

♀ Female

Female procedure only

Code Lists

Codes that are applicable to each type of symbol in the book are listed after each table.

Notes Pages

Notes pages are included between sections within the Tables.

ICD-10-PCS Official Guidelines for Coding and Reporting 2019

The Centers for Medicare and Medicaid Services (CMS) and the National Center for Health Statistics (NCHS), two departments within the U.S. Federal Government's Department of Health and Human Services (DHHS) provide the following guidelines for coding and reporting using the International Classification of Diseases, 10th Revision, Procedure Coding System (ICD-10-PCS). These guidelines should be used as a companion document to the official version of the ICD-10-PCS as published on the CMS website. The ICD-10-PCS is a procedure classification published by the United States for classifying procedures performed in hospital inpatient health care settings.

These guidelines have been approved by the four organizations that make up the Cooperating Parties for the ICD-10-PCS: the American Hospital Association (AHA), the American Health Information Management Association (AHIMA), CMS, and NCHS.

These guidelines are a set of rules that have been developed to accompany and complement the official conventions and instructions provided within the ICD-10-PCS itself. The instructions and conventions of the classification take precedence over guidelines. These guidelines are based on the coding and sequencing instructions in the Tables, Index and Definitions of ICD-10-PCS, but provide additional instruction.

Adherence to these guidelines when assigning ICD-10-PCS procedure codes is required under the Health Insurance Portability and Accountability Act (HIPAA). The procedure codes have been adopted under HIPAA for hospital inpatient healthcare settings. A joint effort between the healthcare provider and the coder is essential to achieve complete and accurate documentation, code assignment, and reporting of diagnoses and procedures.

These guidelines have been developed to assist both the healthcare provider and the coder in identifying those procedures that are to be reported. The importance of consistent, complete documentation in the medical record cannot be overemphasized. Without such documentation accurate coding cannot be achieved.

Table of Contents

A. **Conventions** 10

B. **Medical and Surgical Section Guidelines (Section 0)** 11

- 2. **Body System** 11
- 3. **Root Operation** 11
- 4. **Body Part** 14
- 5. **Approach** 15
- 6. **Device** 15

C. **Obstetric Section Guidelines (Section 1)** 15

D. **New Technology Section Guidelines (Section X)** 16

Selection of Principal Procedure 16

Conventions

A1
ICD-10-PCS codes are composed of seven characters. Each character is an axis of classification that specifies information about the procedure performed. Within a defined code range, a character specifies the same type of information in that axis of classification.

Example: The fifth axis of classification specifies the approach in sections 0 through 4 and 7 through 9 of the system.

A2
One of 34 possible values can be assigned to each axis of classification in the seven- character code: they are the numbers 0 through 9 and the alphabet (except I and O because they are easily confused with the numbers 1 and 0). The number of unique values used in an axis of classification differs as needed.

Example: Where the fifth axis of classification specifies the approach, seven different approach values are currently used to specify the approach.

A3
The valid values for an axis of classification can be added to as needed.

Example: If a significantly distinct type of device is used in a new procedure, a new device value can be added to the system.

A4
As with words in their context, the meaning of any single value is a combination of its axis of classification and any preceding values on which it may be dependent.

Example: The meaning of a body part value in the Medical and Surgical section is always dependent on the body system value. The body part value 0 in the Central Nervous body system specifies Brain and the body part value 0 in the Peripheral Nervous body system specifies Cervical Plexus.

A5
As the system is expanded to become increasingly detailed, over time more values will depend on preceding values for their meaning.

Example: In the Lower Joints body system, the device value 3 in the root operation Insertion specifies Infusion Device and the device value 3 in the root operation Replacement specifies Ceramic Synthetic Substitute.

A6
The purpose of the alphabetic index is to locate the appropriate table that contains all information necessary to construct a procedure code. The PCS Tables should always be consulted to find the most appropriate valid code.

A7
It is not required to consult the index first before proceeding to the tables to complete the code. A valid code may be chosen directly from the tables.

A8
All seven characters must be specified to be a valid code. If the documentation is incomplete for coding purposes, the physician should be queried for the necessary information.

A9
Within a PCS table, valid codes include all combinations of choices in characters 4 through 7 contained in the same row of the table. In the example below, 0JHT3VZ is a valid code, and 0JHW3VZ is *not* a valid code.

A10
"And," when used in a code description, means "and/or," except when used to describe a combination of multiple body parts for which separate values exist for each body part (e.g., Skin and Subcutaneous Tissue used as a qualifier, where there are separate body part values for "Skin" and "Subcutaneous Tissue").

Example: Lower Arm and Wrist Muscle means lower arm and/or wrist muscle.

A11
Many of the terms used to construct PCS codes are defined within the system. It is the coder's responsibility to determine what the documentation in the medical record equates to in the PCS definitions. The physician is not expected to use the terms used in PCS code descriptions, nor is the coder required to query the physician when the correlation between the documentation and the defined PCS terms is clear.

Example: When the physician documents "partial resection" the coder can independently correlate "partial resection" to the root operation Excision without querying the physician for clarification.

Section: 0 Medical and Surgical
Body System: J Subcutaneous Tissue and Fascia
Operation: H Insertion: Putting in a nonbiological appliance that monitors, assists, performs, or prevents a physiological function but does not physically take the place of a body part

Body Part	**Approach**	**Device**	**Qualifier**
S Subcutaneous Tissue and Fascia, Head and Neck V Subcutaneous Tissue and Fascia, Upper Extremity W Subcutaneous Tissue and Fascia, Lower Extremity	0 Open 3 Percutaneous	1 Radioactive Element 3 Infusion Device	Z No Qualifier
T Subcutaneous Tissue and Fascia, Trunk	0 Open 3 Percutaneous	1 Radioactive Element 3 Infusion Device V Infusion Pump	Z No Qualifier

Medical and Surgical Section Guidelines (Section 0)

B2. Body System

General guidelines

B2.1a
The procedure codes in the general anatomical regions body systems can be used when the procedure is performed on an anatomical region rather than a specific body part (e.g., root operations Control and Detachment, Drainage of a body cavity) or on the rare occasion when no information is available to support assignment of a code to a specific body part.

Examples: Control of postoperative hemorrhage is coded to the root operation Control found in the general anatomical regions body systems.

Chest tube drainage of the pleural cavity is coded to the root operation Drainage found in the general anatomical regions body systems. Suture repair of the abdominal wall is coded to the root operation Repair in the general anatomical regions body system.

B2.1b
Where the general body part values "upper" and "lower" are provided as an option in the Upper Arteries, Lower Arteries, Upper Veins, Lower Veins, Muscles and Tendons body systems, "upper" or "lower "specifies body parts located above or below the diaphragm respectively.

Example: Vein body parts above the diaphragm are found in the Upper Veins body system; vein body parts below the diaphragm are found in the Lower Veins body system.

B3. Root Operation

General guidelines

B3.1a
In order to determine the appropriate root operation, the full definition of the root operation as contained in the PCS Tables must be applied.

B3.1b
Components of a procedure specified in the root operation definition and explanation are not coded separately. Procedural steps necessary to reach the operative site and close the operative site, including anastomosis of a tubular body part, are also not coded separately. *Examples*: Resection of a joint as part of a joint replacement procedure is included in the root operation definition of Replacement and is not coded separately.

Laparotomy performed to reach the site of an open liver biopsy is not coded separately. In a resection of sigmoid colon with anastomosis of descending colon to rectum, the anastomosis is not coded separately.

Multiple procedures

B3.2
During the same operative episode, multiple procedures are coded if:

a. The same root operation is performed on different body parts as defined by distinct values of the body part character.

   Examples: Diagnostic excision of liver and pancreas are coded separately.

   Excision of lesion in the ascending colon and excision of lesion in the transverse colon are coded separately.

b. The same root operation is repeated in multiple body parts, and those body parts are separate and distinct body parts classified to a single ICD-10-PCS body part value.

   Examples: Excision of the sartorius muscle and excision of the gracilis muscle are both included in the upper leg muscle body part value, and multiple procedures are coded.

   Extraction of multiple toenails are coded separately.

c. Multiple root operations with distinct objectives are performed on the same body part.

   Example: Destruction of sigmoid lesion and bypass of sigmoid colon are coded separately.

d. The intended root operation is attempted using one approach, but is converted to a different approach.

   Example: Laparoscopic cholecystectomy converted to an open cholecystectomy is coded as percutaneous endoscopic Inspection and open Resection.

Discontinued or incomplete procedures

B3.3
If the intended procedure is discontinued or otherwise not completed, code the procedure to the root operation performed. If a procedure is discontinued before any other root operation is performed, code the root operation Inspection of the body part or anatomical region inspected.

Example: A planned aortic valve replacement procedure is discontinued after the initial thoracotomy and before any incision is made in the heart muscle, when the patient becomes hemodynamically unstable. This procedure is coded as an open Inspection of the mediastinum.

Biopsy procedures

B3.4a
Biopsy procedures are coded using the root operations Excision, Extraction, or Drainage and the qualifier Diagnostic.

Examples: Fine needle aspiration biopsy of fluid in the lung is coded to the root operation Drainage with the qualifier Diagnostic.

Biopsy of bone marrow is coded to the root operation Extraction with the qualifier Diagnostic.

Lymph node sampling for biopsy is coded to the root operation Excision with the qualifier Diagnostic.

Biopsy followed by more definitive treatment

B3.4b
If a diagnostic Excision, Extraction, or Drainage procedure (biopsy) is followed by a more definitive procedure, such as Destruction, Excision or Resection at the same procedure site, both the biopsy and the more definitive treatment are coded.

Example: Biopsy of breast followed by partial mastectomy at the same procedure site, both the biopsy and the partial mastectomy procedure are coded.

Overlapping body layers

B3.5
If the root operations Excision, Repair or Inspection are performed on overlapping layers of the musculoskeletal system, the body part specifying the deepest layer is coded.

Example: Excisional debridement that includes skin and subcutaneous tissue and muscle is coded to the muscle body part.

Bypass procedures

B3.6a
Bypass procedures are coded by identifying the body part bypassed "from" and the body part bypassed "to." The fourth character body part specifies the body part bypassed from, and the qualifier specifies the body part bypassed to.

Example: Bypass from stomach to jejunum, stomach is the body part and jejunum is the qualifier.

B3.6b
Coronary artery bypass procedures are coded differently than other bypass procedures as described in the previous guideline. Rather than identifying the body part bypassed from, the body part identifies the number of coronary arteries bypassed to, and the qualifier specifies the vessel bypassed from.

Example: Aortocoronary artery bypass of the left anterior descending coronary artery and the obtuse marginal coronary artery is classified in the body part axis of classification as two coronary arteries, and the qualifier specifies the aorta as the body part bypassed from.

B3.6c
If multiple coronary arteries are bypassed, a separate procedure is coded for each coronary artery that uses a different device and/or qualifier.

Example: Aortocoronary artery bypass and internal mammary coronary artery bypass are coded separately.

Control vs. more definitive root operations

B3.7
The root operation Control is defined as, "Stopping, or attempting to stop, postprocedural or other acute bleeding." If an attempt to stop postprocedural or other acute bleeding is unsuccessful, and to stop the bleeding requires performing a more definitive root operation, such as Bypass, Detachment, Excision, Extraction, Reposition, Replacement, or Resection, then the more definitive root operation is coded instead of Control.

Example: Resection of spleen to stop bleeding is coded to Resection instead of Control.

Excision vs. Resection

B3.8
PCS contains specific body parts for anatomical subdivisions of a body part, such as lobes of the lungs or liver and regions of the intestine. Resection of the specific body part is coded whenever all of the body part is cut out or off, rather than coding Excision of a less specific body part.

Example: Left upper lung lobectomy is coded to Resection of Upper Lung Lobe, Left rather than Excision of Lung, Left.

Excision for graft

B3.9
If an autograft is obtained from a different procedure site in order to complete the objective of the procedure, a separate procedure is coded.

Example: Coronary bypass with excision of saphenous vein graft, excision of saphenous vein is coded separately.

Fusion procedures of the spine

B3.10a
The body part coded for a spinal vertebral joint(s) rendered immobile by a spinal fusion procedure is classified by the level of the spine (e.g. thoracic). There are distinct body part values for a single vertebral joint and for multiple vertebral joints at each spinal level.

Example: Body part values specify Lumbar Vertebral Joint, Lumbar Vertebral Joints, 2 or More and Lumbosacral Vertebral Joint.

B3.10b
If multiple vertebral joints are fused, a separate procedure is coded for each vertebral joint that uses a different device and/or qualifier.

Example: Fusion of lumbar vertebral joint, posterior approach, anterior column and fusion of lumbar vertebral joint, posterior approach, posterior column are coded separately.

B3.10c
Combinations of devices and materials are often used on a vertebral joint to render the joint immobile. When combinations of devices are used on the same vertebral joint, the device value coded for the procedure is as follows:

- If an interbody fusion device is used to render the joint immobile (alone or containing other material like bone graft), the procedure is coded with the device value Interbody Fusion Device
- If bone graft is the *only* device used to render the joint immobile, the procedure is coded with the device value Nonautologous Tissue Substitute or Autologous Tissue Substitute
- If a mixture of autologous and nonautologous bone graft (with or without biological or synthetic extenders or binders) is used to render the joint immobile, code the procedure with the device value Autologous Tissue Substitute

Examples: Fusion of a vertebral joint using a cage style interbody fusion device containing morsellized bone graft is coded to the device Interbody Fusion Device.

Fusion of a vertebral joint using a bone dowel interbody fusion device made of cadaver bone and packed with a mixture of local morsellized bone and demineralized bone matrix is coded to the device Interbody Fusion Device.

Fusion of a vertebral joint using both autologous bone graft and bone bank bone graft is coded to the device Autologous Tissue Substitute.

Inspection procedures

B3.11a
Inspection of a body part(s) performed in order to achieve the objective of a procedure is not coded separately.

Example: Fiberoptic bronchoscopy performed for irrigation of bronchus, only the irrigation procedure is coded.

B3.11b
If multiple tubular body parts are inspected, the most distal body part (the body part furthest from the starting point of the inspection) is coded. If multiple non-tubular body parts in a region are inspected, the body part that specifies the entire area inspected is coded.

Examples: Cystoureteroscopy with inspection of bladder and ureters is coded to the ureter body part value.

Exploratory laparotomy with general inspection of abdominal contents is coded to the peritoneal cavity body part value.

B3.11c
When both an Inspection procedure and another procedure are performed on the same body part during the same episode, if the Inspection procedure is performed using a different approach than the other procedure, the Inspection procedure is coded separately. *Example*: Endoscopic Inspection of the duodenum is coded separately when open Excision of the duodenum is performed during the same procedural episode.

Occlusion vs. Restriction for vessel embolization procedures

B3.12
If the objective of an embolization procedure is to completely close a vessel, the root operation Occlusion is coded. If the objective of an embolization procedure is to narrow the lumen of a vessel, the root operation Restriction is coded.

Examples: Tumor embolization is coded to the root operation Occlusion, because the objective of the procedure is to cut off the blood supply to the vessel.

Embolization of a cerebral aneurysm is coded to the root operation Restriction, because the objective of the procedure is not to close off the vessel entirely, but to narrow the lumen of the vessel at the site of the aneurysm where it is abnormally wide.

Release procedures

B3.13
In the root operation Release, the body part value coded is the body part being freed and not the tissue being manipulated or cut to free the body part.

Example: Lysis of intestinal adhesions is coded to the specific intestine body part value.

Release vs. Division

B3.14
If the sole objective of the procedure is freeing a body part without cutting the body part, the root operation is Release. If the sole objective of the procedure is separating or transecting a body part, the root operation is Division.

Examples: Freeing a nerve root from surrounding scar tissue to relieve pain is coded to the root operation Release.

Severing a nerve root to relieve pain is coded to the root operation Division.

Reposition for fracture treatment

B3.15
Reduction of a displaced fracture is coded to the root operation Reposition and the application of a cast or splint in conjunction with the Reposition procedure is not coded separately. Treatment of a nondisplaced fracture is coded to the procedure performed. *Examples*: Casting of a nondisplaced fracture is coded to the root operation Immobilization in the Placement section.

Putting a pin in a nondisplaced fracture is coded to the root operation Insertion.

Transplantation vs. Administration

B3.16
Putting in a mature and functioning living body part taken from another individual or animal is coded to the root operation Transplantation. Putting in autologous or nonautologous cells is coded to the Administration section.

Example: Putting in autologous or nonautologous bone marrow, pancreatic islet cells or stem cells is coded to the Administration section.

Transfer procedures using multiple tissue layers

B3.17
The root operation Transfer contains qualifiers that can be used to specify when a transfer flap is composed of more than one tissue layer, such as a musculocutaneous flap. For procedures involving transfer of multiple tissue layers including skin, subcutaneous tissue, fascia or muscle, the procedure is coded to the body part value that describes the deepest tissue layer in the flap, and the qualifier can be used to describe the other tissue layer(s) in the transfer flap.

Example: A musculocutaneous flap transfer is coded to the appropriate body part value in the body system Muscles, and the qualifier is used to describe the additional tissue layer(s) in the transfer flap.

B4. Body Part

General guidelines

B4.1a
If a procedure is performed on a portion of a body part that does not have a separate body part value, code the body part value corresponding to the whole body part.

Example: A procedure performed on the alveolar process of the mandible is coded to the mandible body part.

B4.1b
If the prefix "peri" is combined with a body part to identify the site of the procedure, and the site of the procedure is not further specified, then the procedure is coded to the body part named. This guideline applies only when a more specific body part value is not available.

Examples: A procedure site identified as perirenal is coded to the kidney body part when the site of the procedure is not further specified.

A procedure site described in the documentation as peri-urethral, and the documentation also indicates that it is the vulvar tissue and not the urethral tissue that is the site of the procedure, then the procedure is coded to the vulva body part.

B4.1c
If a procedure is performed on a continuous section of a tubular body part, code the body part value corresponding to the furthest anatomical site from the point of entry.

Example: A procedure performed on a continuous section of artery from the femoral artery to the external iliac artery with the point of entry at the femoral artery is coded to the external iliac body part.

Branches of body parts

B4.2
Where a specific branch of a body part does not have its own body part value in PCS, the body part is typically coded to the closest proximal branch that has a specific body part value. In the cardiovascular body systems, if a general body part is available in the correct root operation table, and coding to a proximal branch would require assigning a code in a different body system, the procedure is coded using the general body part value. *Examples*: A procedure performed on the mandibular branch of the trigeminal nerve is coded to the trigeminal nerve body part value.

Occlusion of the bronchial artery is coded to the body part value Upper Artery in the body system Upper Arteries, and not to the body part value Thoracic Aorta, Descending in the body system Heart and Great Vessels.

Bilateral body part values

B4.3
Bilateral body part values are available for a limited number of body parts. If the identical procedure is performed on contralateral body parts, and a bilateral body part value exists for that body part, a single procedure is coded using the bilateral body part value. If no bilateral body part value exists, each procedure is coded separately using the appropriate body part value.

Examples: The identical procedure performed on both fallopian tubes is coded once using the body part value Fallopian Tube, Bilateral.

The identical procedure performed on both knee joints is coded twice using the body part values Knee Joint, Right and Knee Joint, Left.

Coronary arteries

B4.4
The coronary arteries are classified as a single body part that is further specified by number of arteries treated. One procedure code specifying multiple arteries is used when the same procedure is performed, including the same device and qualifier values.

Examples: Angioplasty of two distinct coronary arteries with placement of two stents is coded as Dilation of Coronary Artery, Two Arteries with Two Intraluminal Devices.

Angioplasty of two distinct coronary arteries, one with stent placed and one without, is coded separately as Dilation of Coronary Artery, One Artery with Intraluminal Device, and Dilation of Coronary Artery, One Artery with no device.

Tendons, ligaments, bursae and fascia near a joint

B4.5
Procedures performed on tendons, ligaments, bursae and fascia supporting a joint are coded to the body part in the respective body system that is the focus of the procedure. Procedures performed on joint structures themselves are coded to the body part in the joint body systems.

Examples: Repair of the anterior cruciate ligament of the knee is coded to the knee bursa and ligament body part in the bursae and ligaments body system.

Knee arthroscopy with shaving of articular cartilage is coded to the knee joint body part in the Lower Joints body system.

Skin, subcutaneous tissue and fascia overlying a joint

B4.6
If a procedure is performed on the skin, subcutaneous tissue or fascia overlying a joint, the procedure is coded to the following body part:

- Shoulder is coded to Upper Arm
- Elbow is coded to Lower Arm
- Wrist is coded to Lower Arm
- Hip is coded to Upper Leg
- Knee is coded to Lower Leg
- Ankle is coded to Foot

Fingers and toes

B4.7
If a body system does not contain a separate body part value for fingers, procedures performed on the fingers are coded to the body part value for the hand. If a body system does not contain a separate body part value for toes, procedures performed on the toes are coded to the body part value for the foot.

Example: Excision of finger muscle is coded to one of the hand muscle body part values in the Muscles body system.

Upper and lower intestinal tract

B4.8
In the Gastrointestinal body system, the general body part values Upper Intestinal Tract and Lower Intestinal Tract are provided as an option for the root operations Change, Inspection, Removal and Revision. Upper Intestinal Tract includes the portion of the gastrointestinal tract from the esophagus down to and including the duodenum, and Lower Intestinal Tract includes the portion of the gastrointestinal tract from the jejunum down to and including the rectum and anus.

Example: In the root operation Change table, change of a device in the jejunum is coded using the body part Lower Intestinal Tract.

B5. Approach

Open approach with percutaneous endoscopic assistance

B5.2
Procedures performed using the open approach with percutaneous endoscopic assistance are coded to the approach Open.

Example: Laparoscopic-assisted sigmoidectomy is coded to the approach Open.

External approach

B5.3a
Procedures performed within an orifice on structures that are visible without the aid of any instrumentation are coded to the approach External.

Example: Resection of tonsils is coded to the approach External.

B5.3b
Procedures performed indirectly by the application of external force through the intervening body layers are coded to the approach External.

Example: Closed reduction of fracture is coded to the approach External.

Percutaneous procedure via device

B5.4
Procedures performed percutaneously via a device placed for the procedure are coded to the approach Percutaneous.

Example: Fragmentation of kidney stone performed via percutaneous nephrostomy is coded to the approach Percutaneous.

B6. Device

General guidelines

B6.1a
A device is coded only if a device remains after the procedure is completed. If no device remains, the device value No Device is coded. In limited root operations, the classification provides the qualifier values Temporary and Intraoperative, for specific procedures involving clinically significant devices, where the purpose of the device is to be utilized for a brief duration during the procedure or current inpatient stay. If a device that is intended to remain after the procedure is completed requires removal before the end of the operative episode in which it was inserted (for example, the device size is inadequate or a complication occurs), both the insertion and removal of the device should be coded.

B6.1b
Materials such as sutures, ligatures, radiological markers and temporary post-operative wound drains are considered integral to the performance of a procedure and are not coded as devices.

B6.1c
Procedures performed on a device only and not on a body part are specified in the root operations Change, Irrigation, Removal and Revision, and are coded to the procedure performed.

Example: Irrigation of percutaneous nephrostomy tube is coded to the root operation Irrigation of indwelling device in the Administration section.

Drainage device

B6.2
A separate procedure to put in a drainage device is coded to the root operation Drainage with the device value Drainage Device.

Obstetric Section Guidelines (Section 1)

C. Obstetrics Section

Products of conception

C1
Procedures performed on the products of conception are coded to the Obstetrics section. Procedures performed on the pregnant female other than the products of conception are coded to the appropriate root operation in the Medical and Surgical section.

Example: Amniocentesis is coded to the products of conception body part in the Obstetrics section. Repair of obstetric urethral laceration is coded to the urethra body part in the Medical and Surgical section.

Procedures following delivery or abortion

C2
Procedures performed following a delivery or abortion for curettage of the endometrium or evacuation of retained products of conception are all coded in the Obstetrics section, to the root operation Extraction and the body part Products of Conception, Retained.

Diagnostic or therapeutic dilation and curettage performed during times other than the postpartum or post-abortion period are all coded in the Medical and Surgical section, to the root operation Extraction and the body part Endometrium.

New Technology Section Guidelines (Section X)

D. New Technology Section

General guidelines

D1

Section X codes are standalone codes. They are not supplemental codes. Section X codes fully represent the specific procedure described in the code title, and do not require any additional codes from other sections of ICD-10-PCS. When section X contains a code title which describes a specific new technology procedure, only that X code is reported for the procedure. There is no need to report a broader, non-specific code in another section of ICD-10-PCS.

Example: XW04321 Introduction of Ceftazidime-Avibactam Anti-infective into Central Vein, Percutaneous Approach, New Technology Group 1, can be coded to indicate that Ceftazidime-Avibactam Anti-infective was administered via a central vein. A separate code from table 3E0 in the Administration section of ICD-10-PCS is not coded in addition to this code.

Selection of Principal Procedure

The following instructions should be applied in the selection of principal procedure and clarification on the importance of the relation to the principal diagnosis when more than one procedure is performed:

1. Procedure performed for definitive treatment of both principal diagnosis and secondary diagnosis
   a. Sequence procedure performed for definitive treatment most related to principal diagnosis as principal procedure.
2. Procedure performed for definitive treatment and diagnostic procedures performed for both principal diagnosis and secondary diagnosis.
   a. Sequence procedure performed for definitive treatment most related to principal diagnosis as principal procedure
3. A diagnostic procedure was performed for the principal diagnosis and a procedure is performed for definitive treatment of a secondary diagnosis.
   a. Sequence diagnostic procedure as principal procedure, since the procedure most related to the principal diagnosis takes precedence.
4. No procedures performed that are related to principal diagnosis; procedures performed for definitive treatment and diagnostic procedures were performed for secondary diagnosis
   a. Sequence procedure performed for definitive treatment of secondary diagnosis as principal procedure, since there are no procedures (definitive or nondefinitive treatment) related to principal diagnosis.

Anatomical Illustrations

Circulatory System — Arteries and Veins

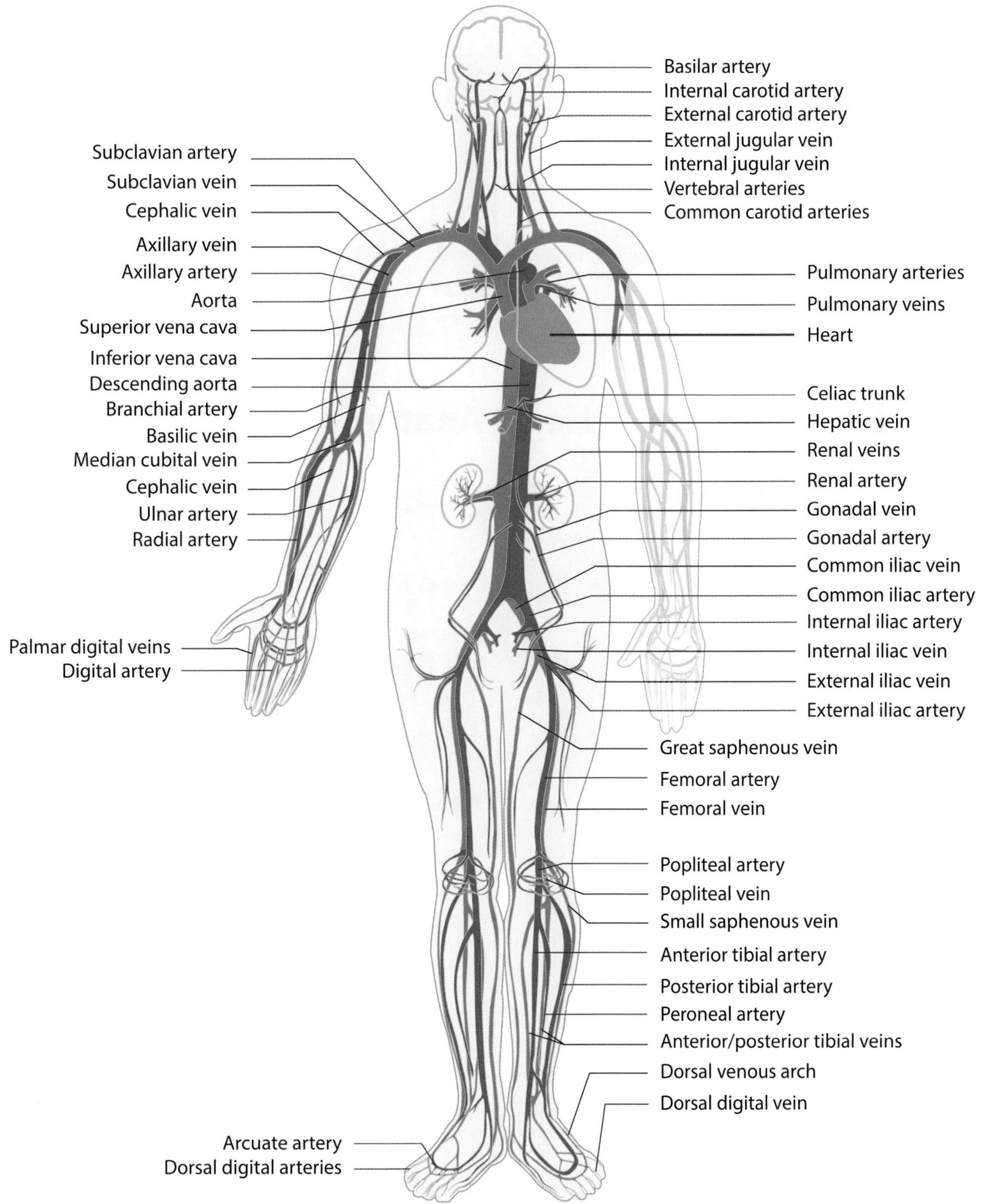
Basilar artery
Internal carotid artery
External carotid artery
External jugular vein
Internal jugular vein
Vertebral arteries
Common carotid arteries
Subclavian artery
Subclavian vein
Cephalic vein
Axillary vein
Axillary artery
Aorta
Superior vena cava
Inferior vena cava
Descending aorta
Branchial artery
Basilic vein
Median cubital vein
Cephalic vein
Ulnar artery
Radial artery
Pulmonary arteries
Pulmonary veins
Heart
Celiac trunk
Hepatic vein
Renal veins
Renal artery
Gonadal vein
Gonadal artery
Common iliac vein
Common iliac artery
Internal iliac artery
Internal iliac vein
External iliac vein
External iliac artery
Palmar digital veins
Digital artery
Great saphenous vein
Femoral artery
Femoral vein
Popliteal artery
Popliteal vein
Small saphenous vein
Anterior tibial artery
Posterior tibial artery
Peroneal artery
Anterior/posterior tibial veins
Dorsal venous arch
Dorsal digital vein
Arcuate artery
Dorsal digital arteries

Title: Circulatory System Labels Biology Diagram, **License:** CC0 Creative Commons (Free for commercial use No attribution required), **URL link:** https://pixabay.com/en/circulatory-system-labels-biology-41523/

Circulatory System — Artery and Vein Anatomy

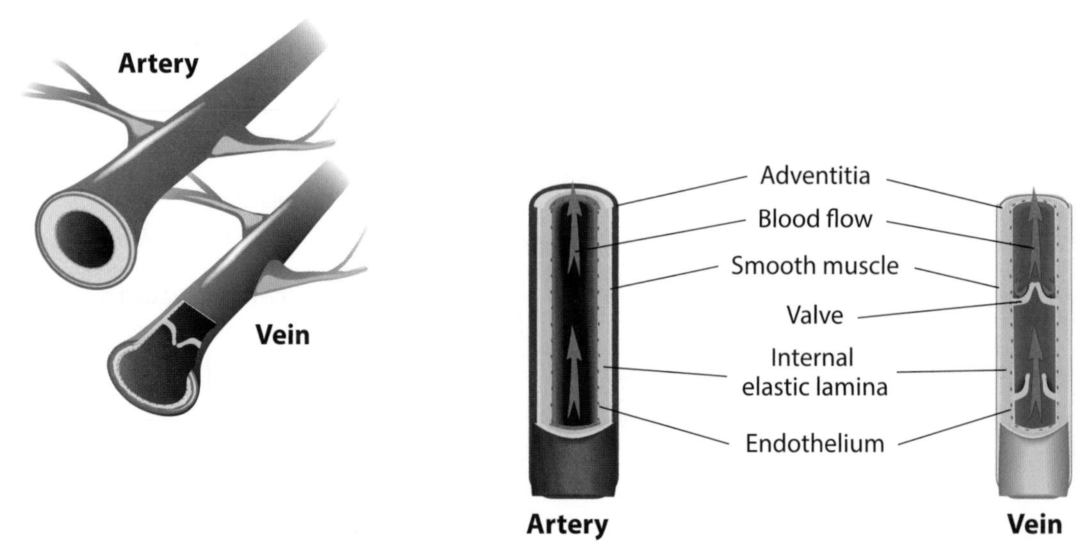
Artery
Vein
Adventitia
Blood flow
Smooth muscle
Valve
Internal elastic lamina
Endothelium
Artery
Vein

Circulatory System — Heart Anatomy and Cardiac Cycle

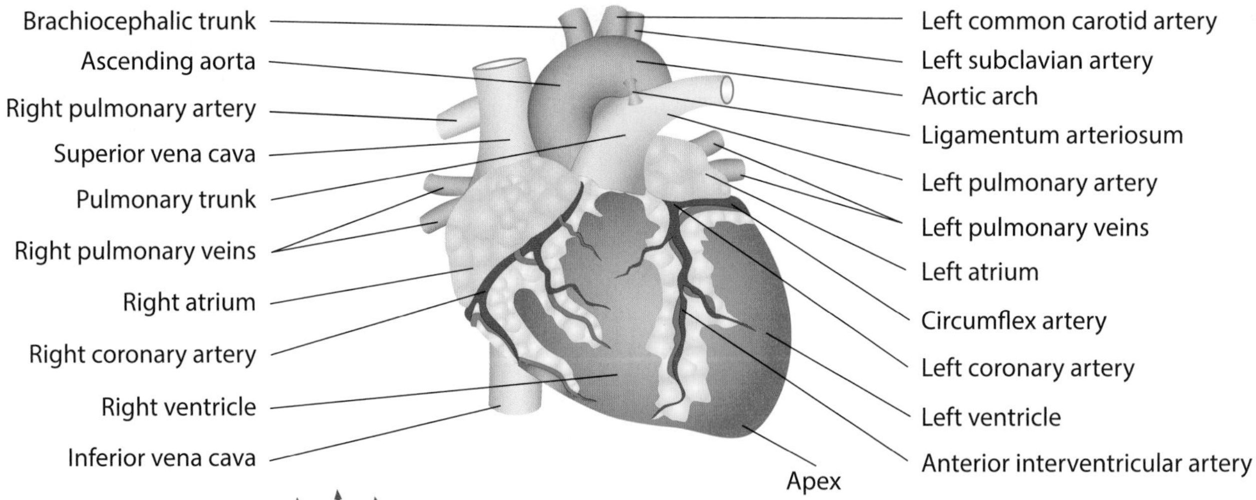

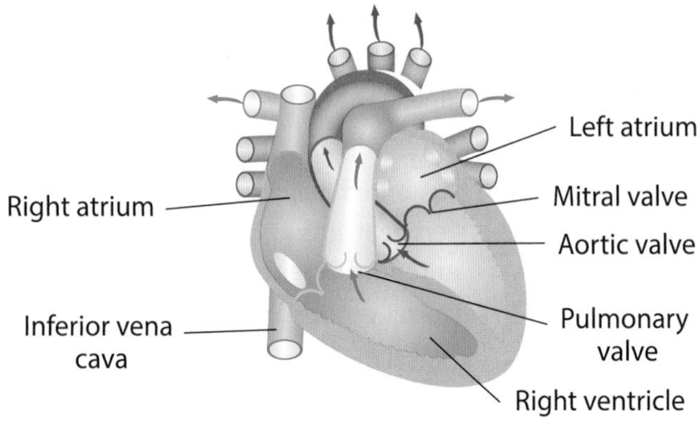

Brachiocephalic trunk
Ascending aorta
Right pulmonary artery
Superior vena cava
Pulmonary trunk
Right pulmonary veins
Right atrium
Right coronary artery
Right ventricle
Inferior vena cava
Apex
Left common carotid artery
Left subclavian artery
Aortic arch
Ligamentum arteriosum
Left pulmonary artery
Left pulmonary veins
Left atrium
Circumflex artery
Left coronary artery
Left ventricle
Anterior interventricular artery

Right atrium
Inferior vena cava
Left atrium
Mitral valve
Aortic valve
Pulmonary valve
Right ventricle

Diastole Ventricular Relaxation and Filling

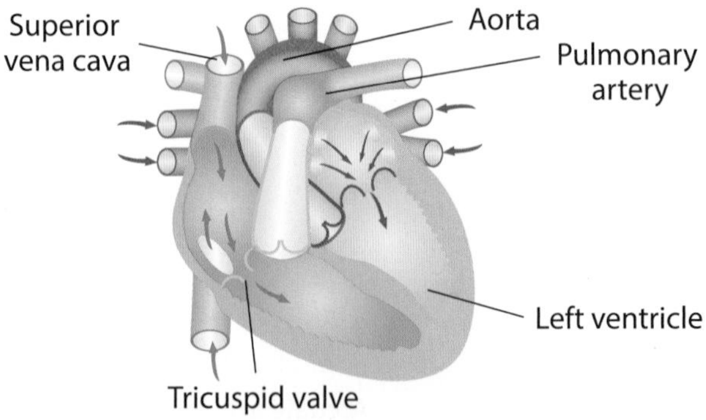

Superior vena cava
Aorta
Pulmonary artery
Left ventricle
Tricuspid valve

Systole Ventricular Contraction and Ejection

Electrical Conducting System of the Heart

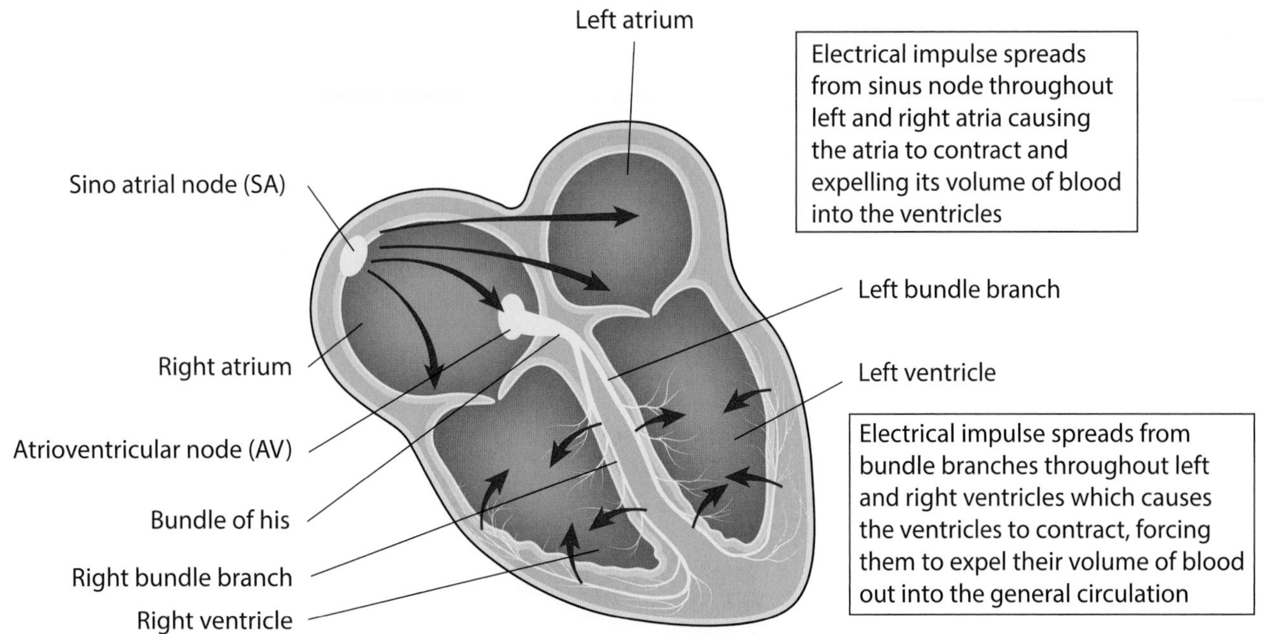
Left atrium
Electrical impulse spreads from sinus node throughout left and right atria causing the atria to contract and expelling its volume of blood into the ventricles
Sino atrial node (SA)
Left bundle branch
Right atrium
Left ventricle
Electrical impulse spreads from bundle branches throughout left and right ventricles which causes the ventricles to contract, forcing them to expel their volume of blood out into the general circulation
Atrioventricular node (AV)
Bundle of his
Right bundle branch
Right ventricle

The Pathway of Blood Flow Through the Heart

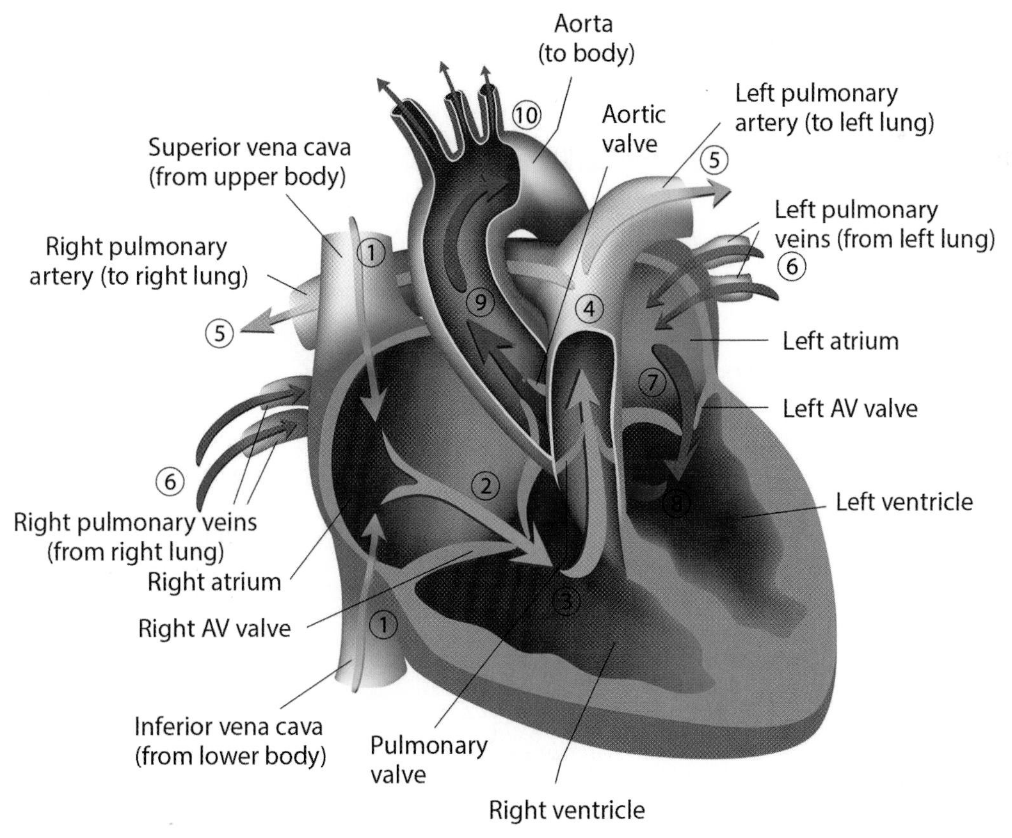
Aorta
(to body)
Left pulmonary
artery (to left lung)
Aortic
valve
Superior vena cava
(from upper body)
Left pulmonary
veins (from left lung)
Right pulmonary
artery (to right lung)
Left atrium
Left AV valve
Left ventricle
Right pulmonary veins
(from right lung)
Right atrium
Right AV valve
Inferior vena cava
(from lower body)
Pulmonary
valve
Right ventricle
1
2
3
4
5
6
7
8
9
10

Digestive System Anatomy

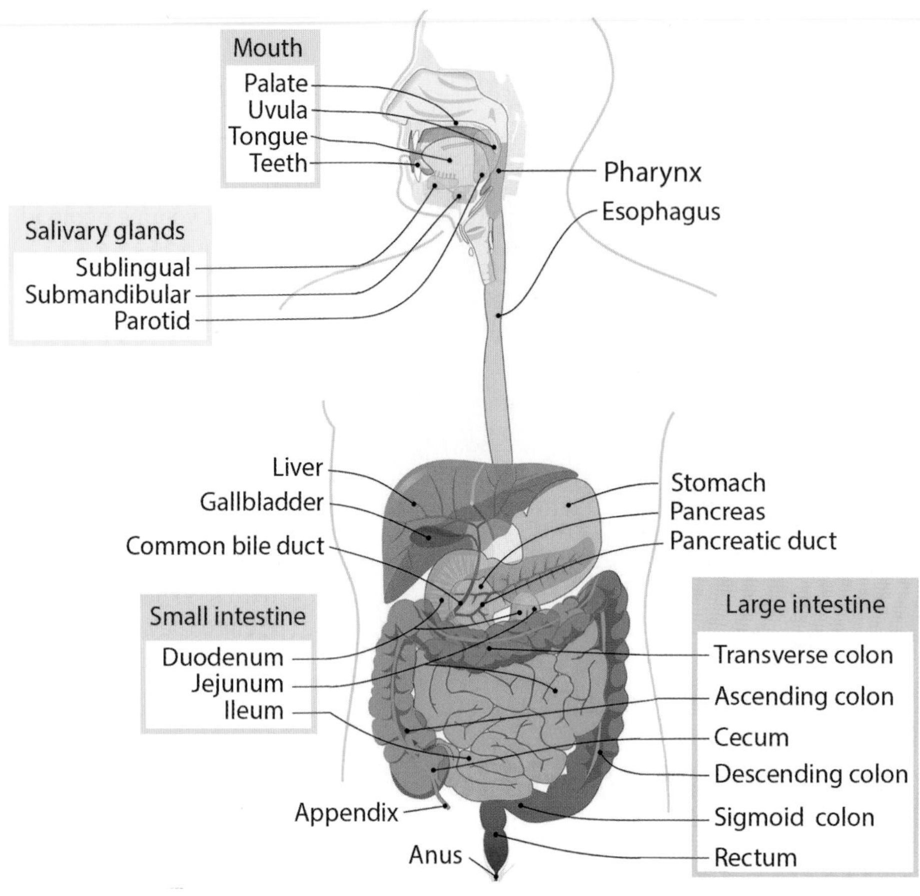
Mouth
Palate
Uvula
Tongue
Teeth
Pharynx
Esophagus
Salivary glands
Sublingual
Submandibular
Parotid
Liver
Gallbladder
Common bile duct
Stomach
Pancreas
Pancreatic duct
Small intestine
Duodenum
Jejunum
Ileum
Large intestine
Transverse colon
Ascending colon
Cecum
Descending colon
Sigmoid colon
Rectum
Appendix
Anus

Title: Diagram of the gastrointestinal tract, **Author:** Mariana Ruiz (Lady of Hats), Jmarchn, **Source:** Own work, **License:** Public domain, **URL link:** https://en.wikiversity.org/wiki/File:Digestive_system_diagram_en.svg

Digestive System — Liver, Gallbladder, Pancreas

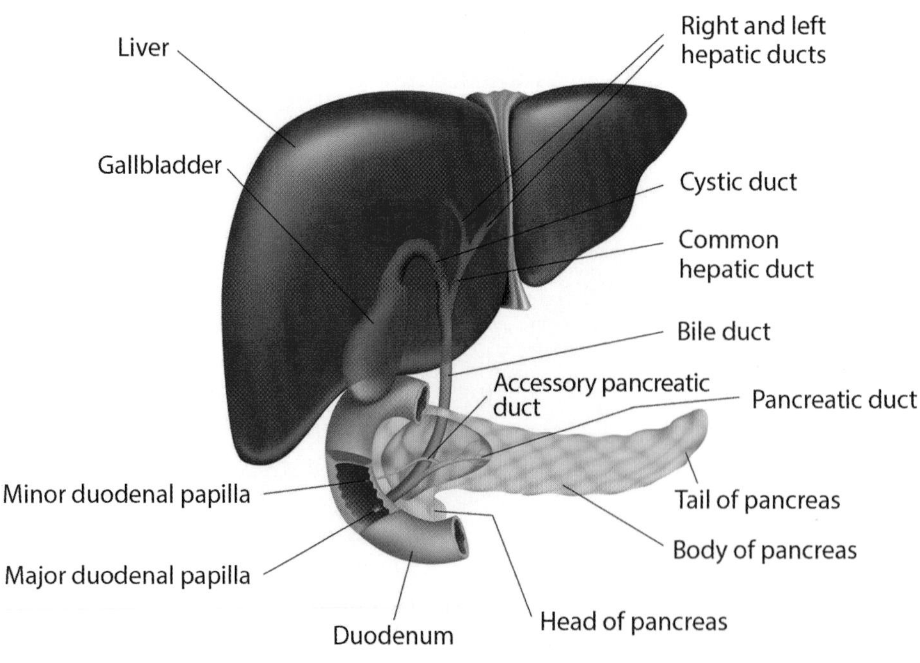
Liver
Right and left hepatic ducts
Gallbladder
Cystic duct
Common hepatic duct
Bile duct
Accessory pancreatic duct
Pancreatic duct
Minor duodenal papilla
Tail of pancreas
Body of pancreas
Major duodenal papilla
Duodenum
Head of pancreas

Digestive System — Mouth Anatomy

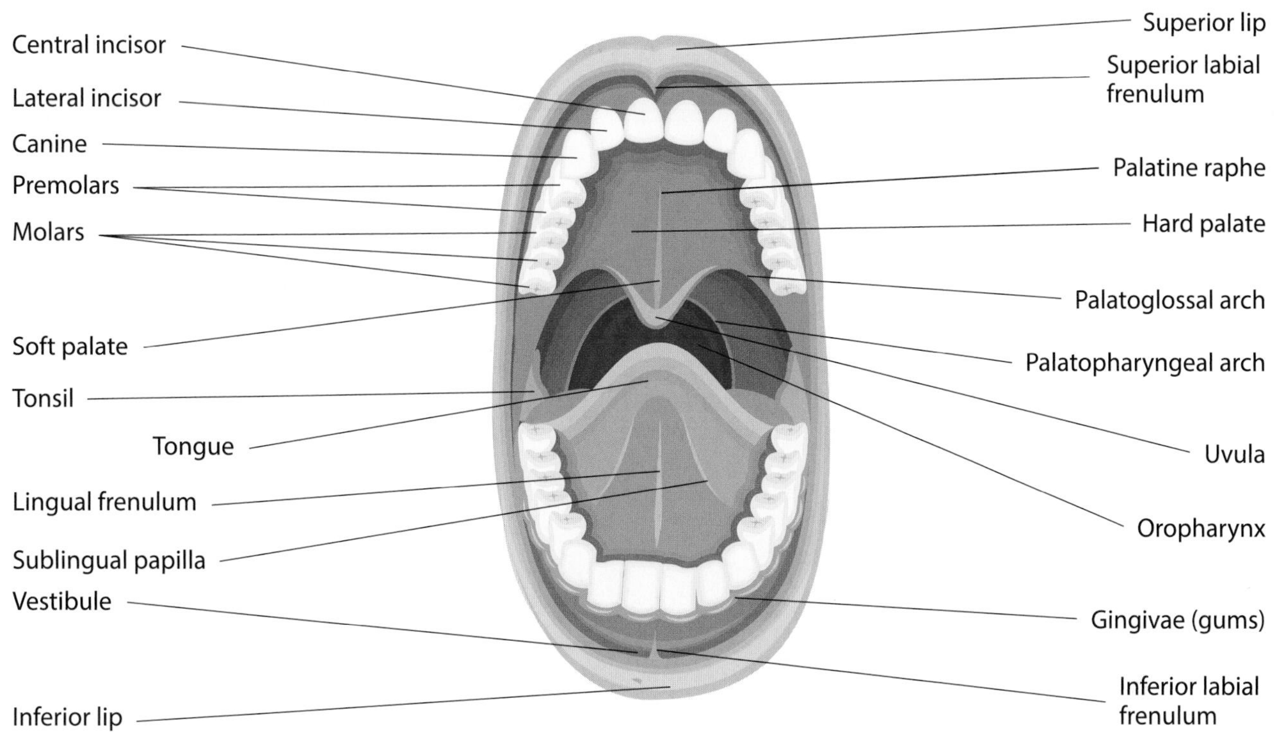
Central incisor
Lateral incisor
Canine
Premolars
Molars
Soft palate
Tonsil
Tongue
Lingual frenulum
Sublingual papilla
Vestibule
Inferior lip
Superior lip
Superior labial frenulum
Palatine raphe
Hard palate
Palatoglossal arch
Palatopharyngeal arch
Uvula
Oropharynx
Gingivae (gums)
Inferior labial frenulum

Digestive System — Tongue Anatomy

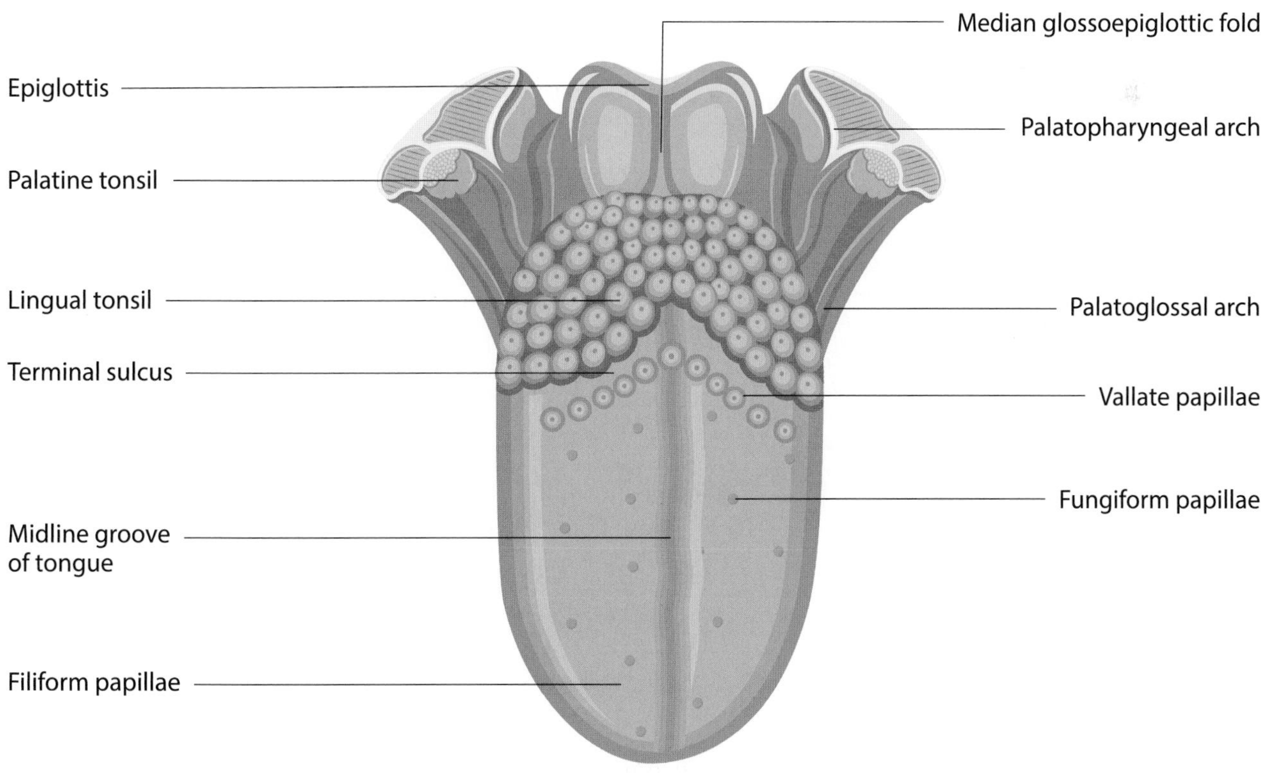
Epiglottis
Palatine tonsil
Lingual tonsil
Terminal sulcus
Midline groove of tongue
Filiform papillae
Median glossoepiglottic fold
Palatopharyngeal arch
Palatoglossal arch
Vallate papillae
Fungiform papillae

Digestive System — Stomach Anatomy

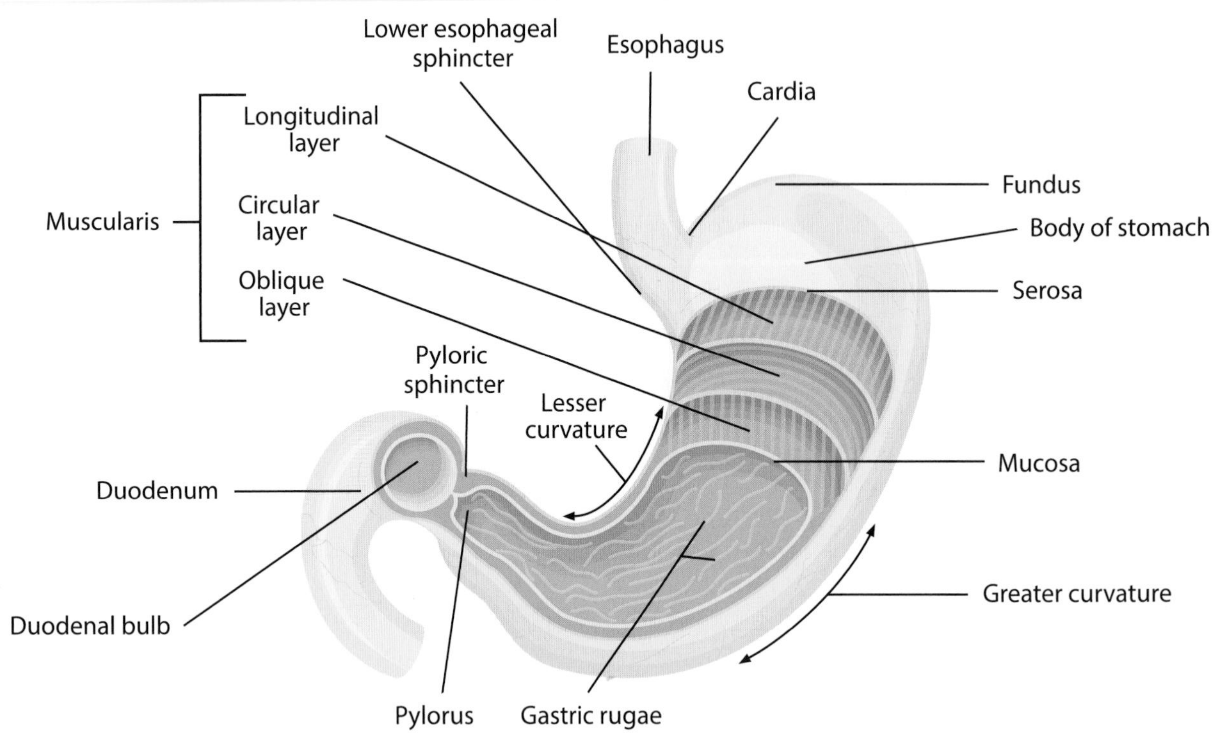
Lower esophageal sphincter
Esophagus
Cardia
Longitudinal layer
Muscularis
Circular layer
Oblique layer
Fundus
Body of stomach
Serosa
Pyloric sphincter
Lesser curvature
Mucosa
Duodenum
Duodenal bulb
Greater curvature
Pylorus
Gastric rugae

Digestive System — Small Intestine Anatomy

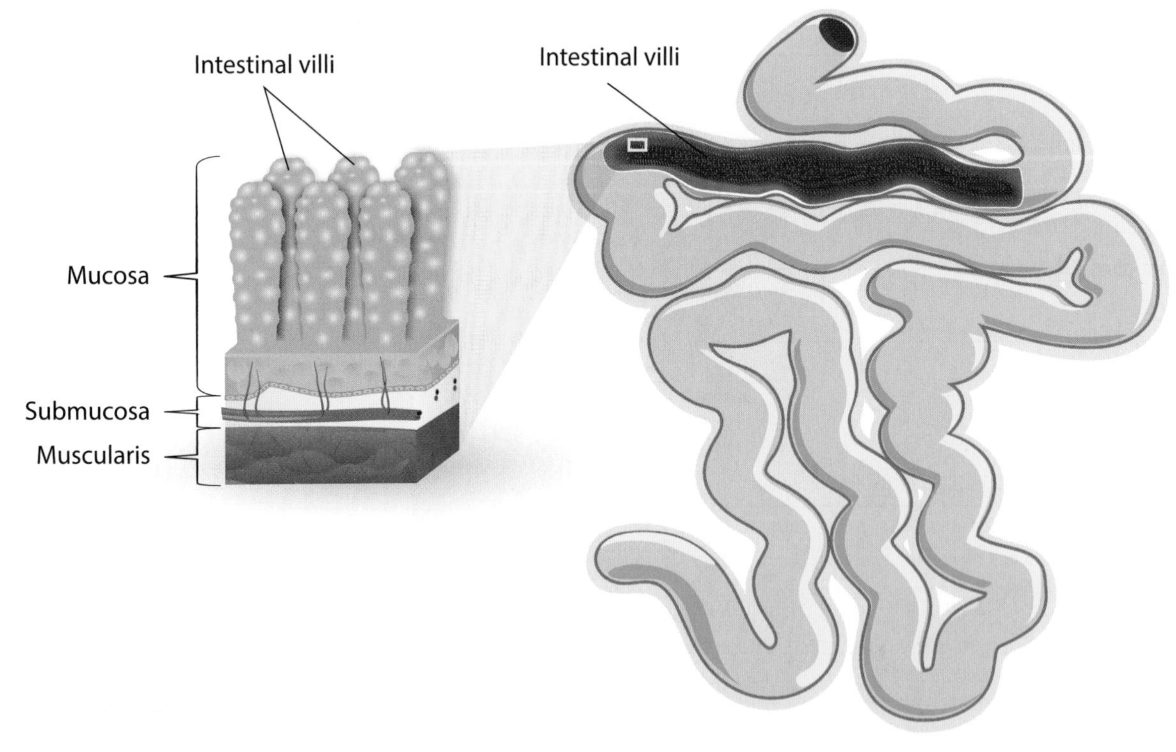
Intestinal villi
Intestinal villi
Mucosa
Submucosa
Muscularis

Digestive System — Large Intestine Anatomy

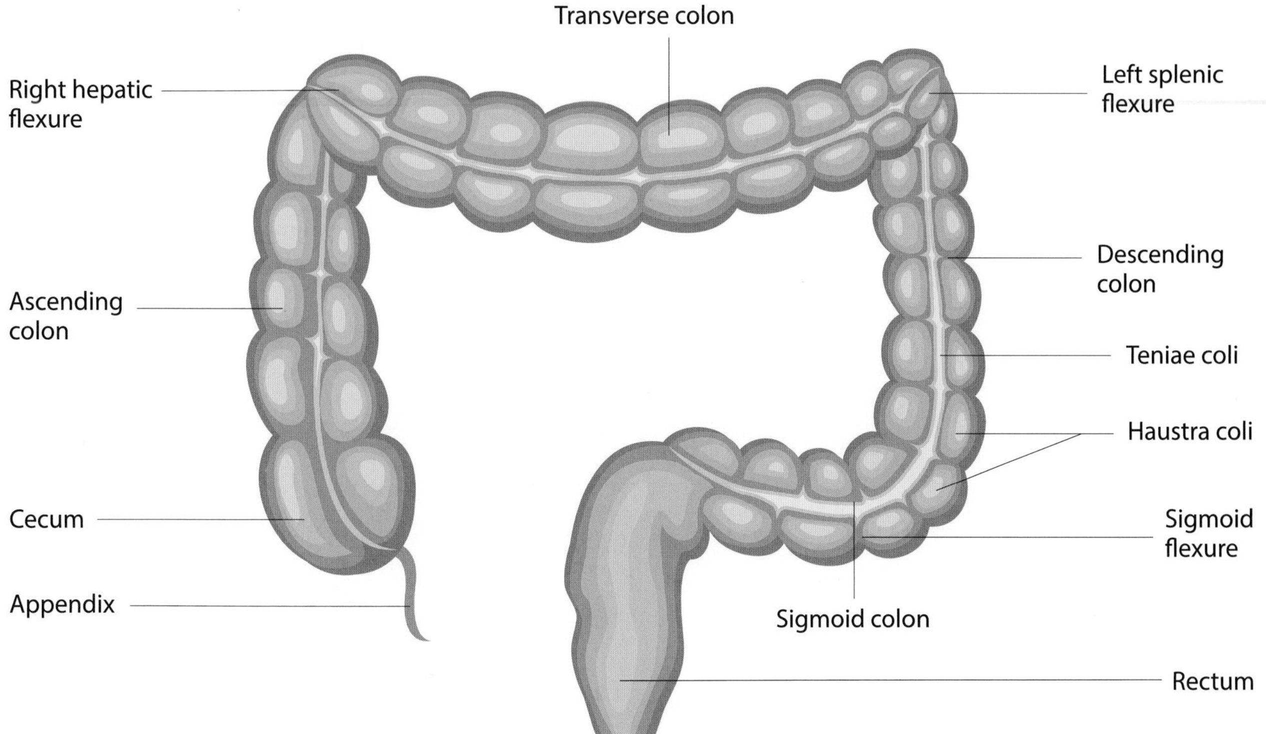
Transverse colon
Right hepatic flexure
Left splenic flexure
Descending colon
Ascending colon
Teniae coli
Haustra coli
Cecum
Sigmoid flexure
Appendix
Sigmoid colon
Rectum

Digestive System — Rectum Anatomy

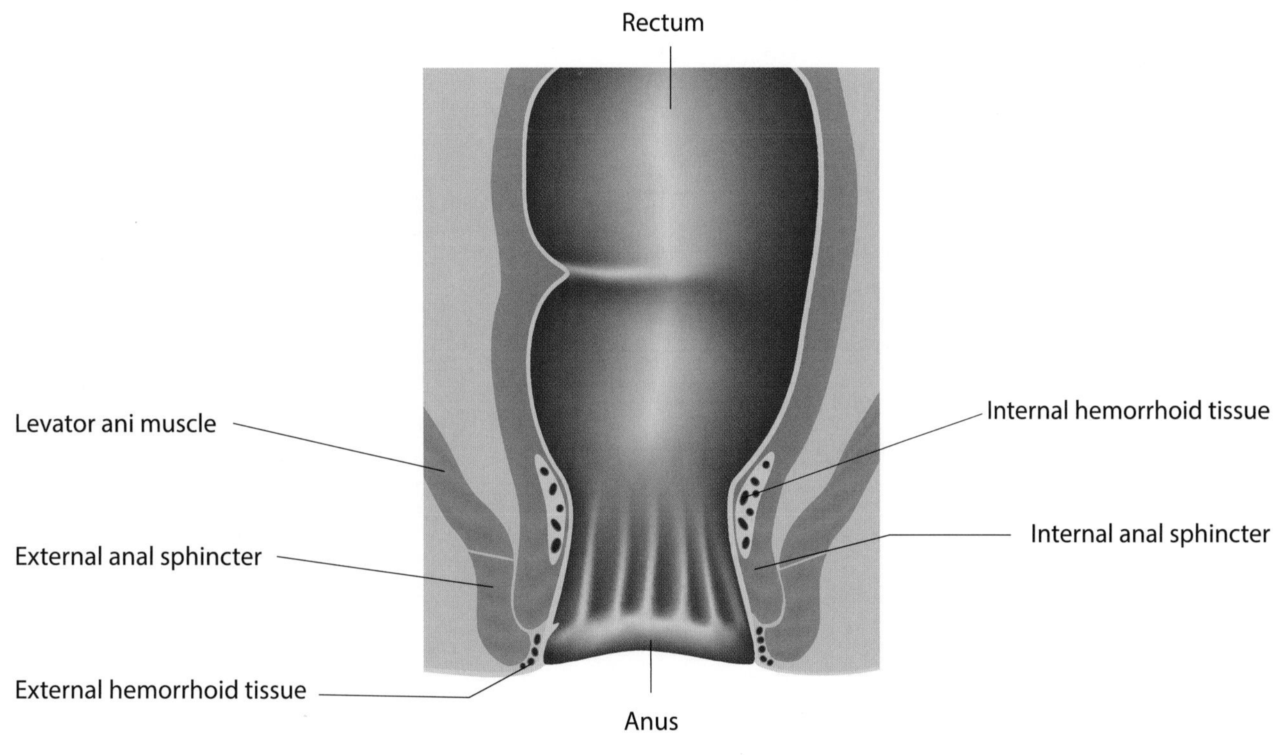
Rectum
Levator ani muscle
Internal hemorrhoid tissue
External anal sphincter
Internal anal sphincter
External hemorrhoid tissue
Anus

Ear Anatomy

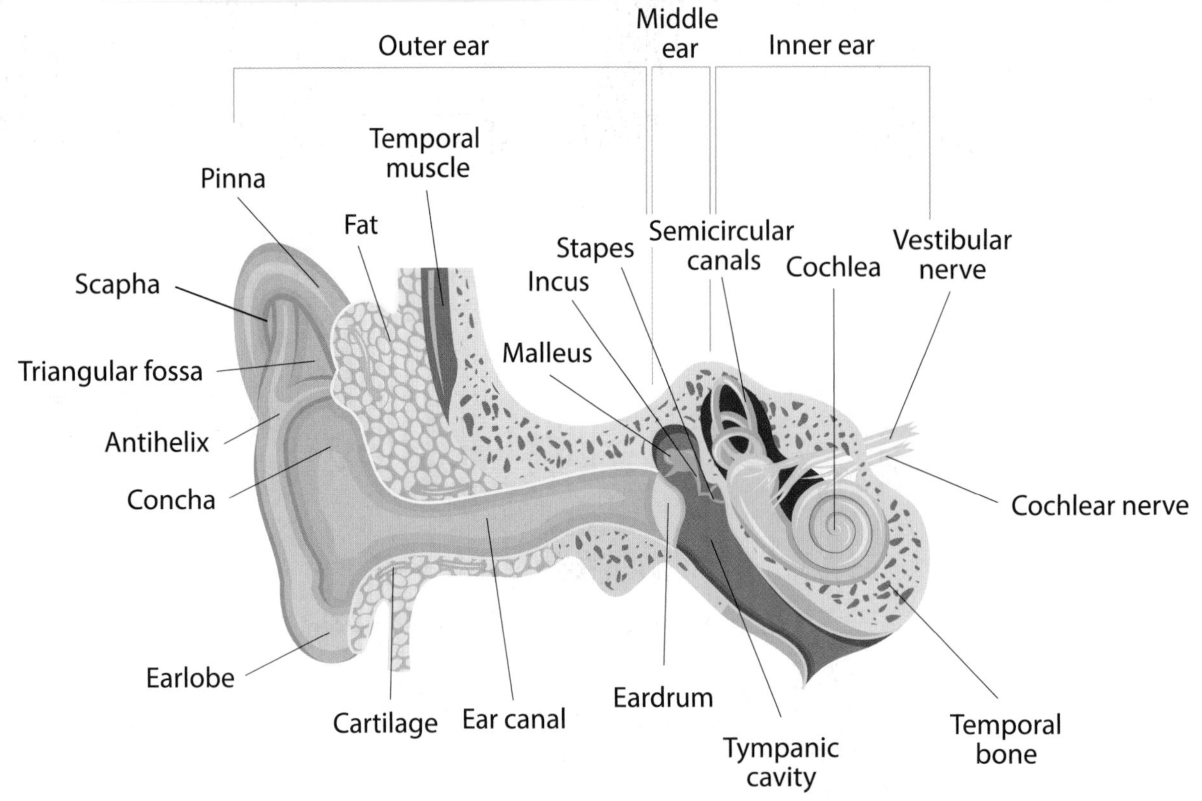
Outer ear
Middle ear
Inner ear
Pinna
Temporal muscle
Fat
Stapes
Semicircular canals
Cochlea
Vestibular nerve
Incus
Scapha
Triangular fossa
Malleus
Antihelix
Concha
Cochlear nerve
Earlobe
Cartilage
Ear canal
Eardrum
Tympanic cavity
Temporal bone

Cochlea Anatomy (Inner Ear)

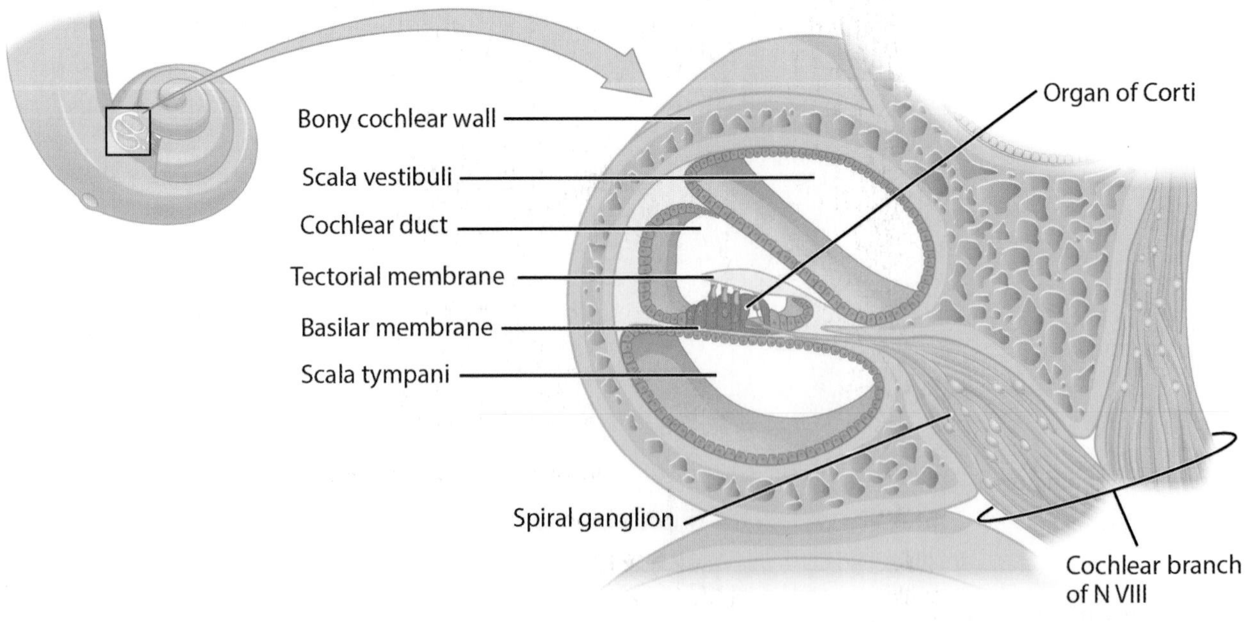
Organ of Corti
Bony cochlear wall
Scala vestibuli
Cochlear duct
Tectorial membrane
Basilar membrane
Scala tympani
Spiral ganglion
Cochlear branch of N VIII

Title: 1406 Cochlea.jpg, **Author:** OpenStax, **Source:** https://cnx.org/contents/FPtK1zmh@8.25:fEI3C8Ot@10/Preface, **License/Permission:** This file is licensed under the Creative Commons Attribution 4.0 International license., **URL link:** https://en.wikiversity.org/wiki/File:1406_Cochlea.jpg

Endocrine System Anatomy and Hormones

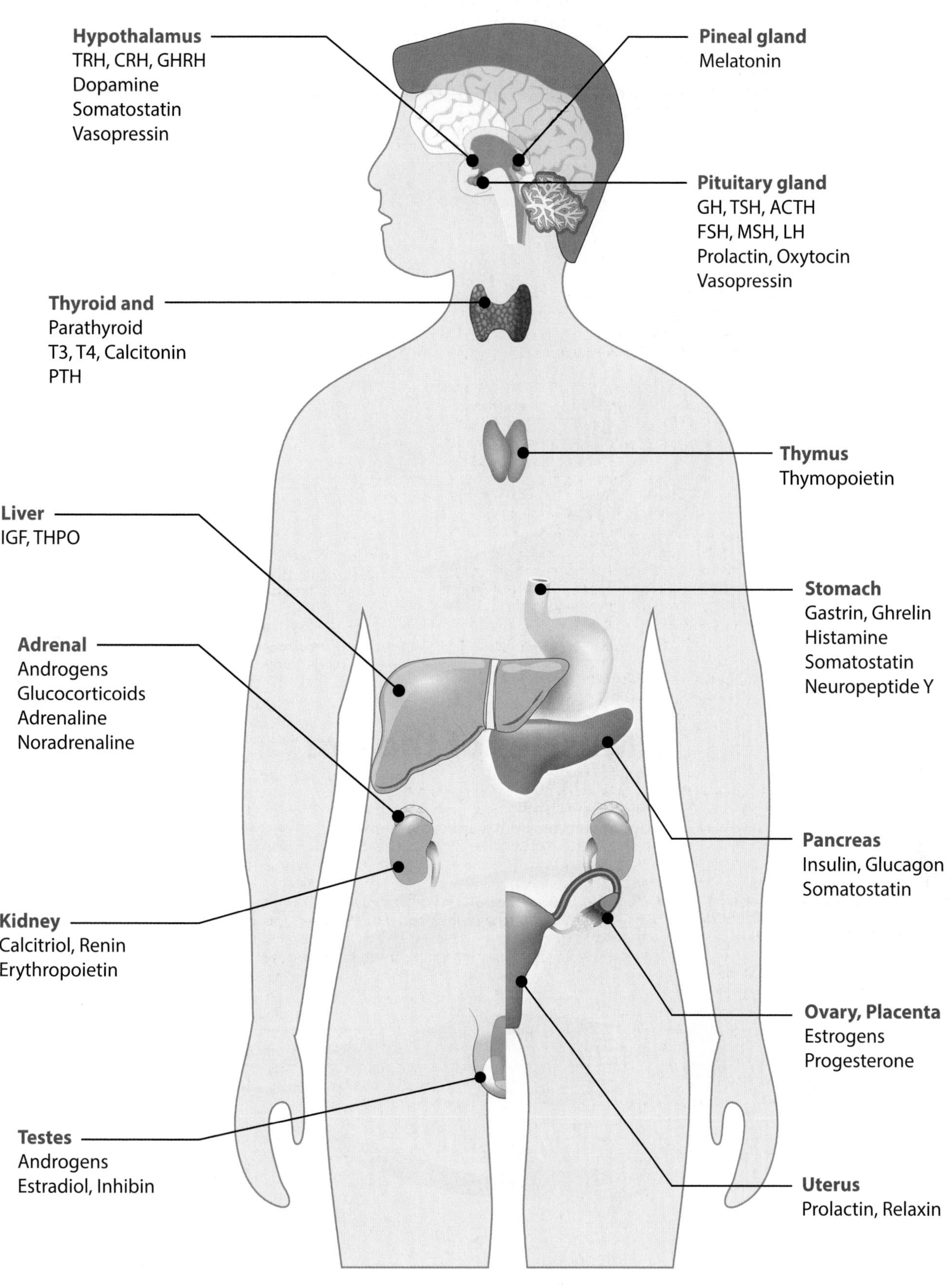
Hypothalamus
TRH, CRH, GHRH
Dopamine
Somatostatin
Vasopressin
Pineal gland
Melatonin
Pituitary gland
GH, TSH, ACTH
FSH, MSH, LH
Prolactin, Oxytocin
Vasopressin
Thyroid and
Parathyroid
T3, T4, Calcitonin
PTH
Thymus
Thymopoietin
Liver
IGF, THPO
Stomach
Gastrin, Ghrelin
Histamine
Somatostatin
Neuropeptide Y
Adrenal
Androgens
Glucocorticoids
Adrenaline
Noradrenaline
Pancreas
Insulin, Glucagon
Somatostatin
Kidney
Calcitriol, Renin
Erythropoietin
Ovary, Placenta
Estrogens
Progesterone
Testes
Androgens
Estradiol, Inhibin
Uterus
Prolactin, Relaxin

Eye Anatomy

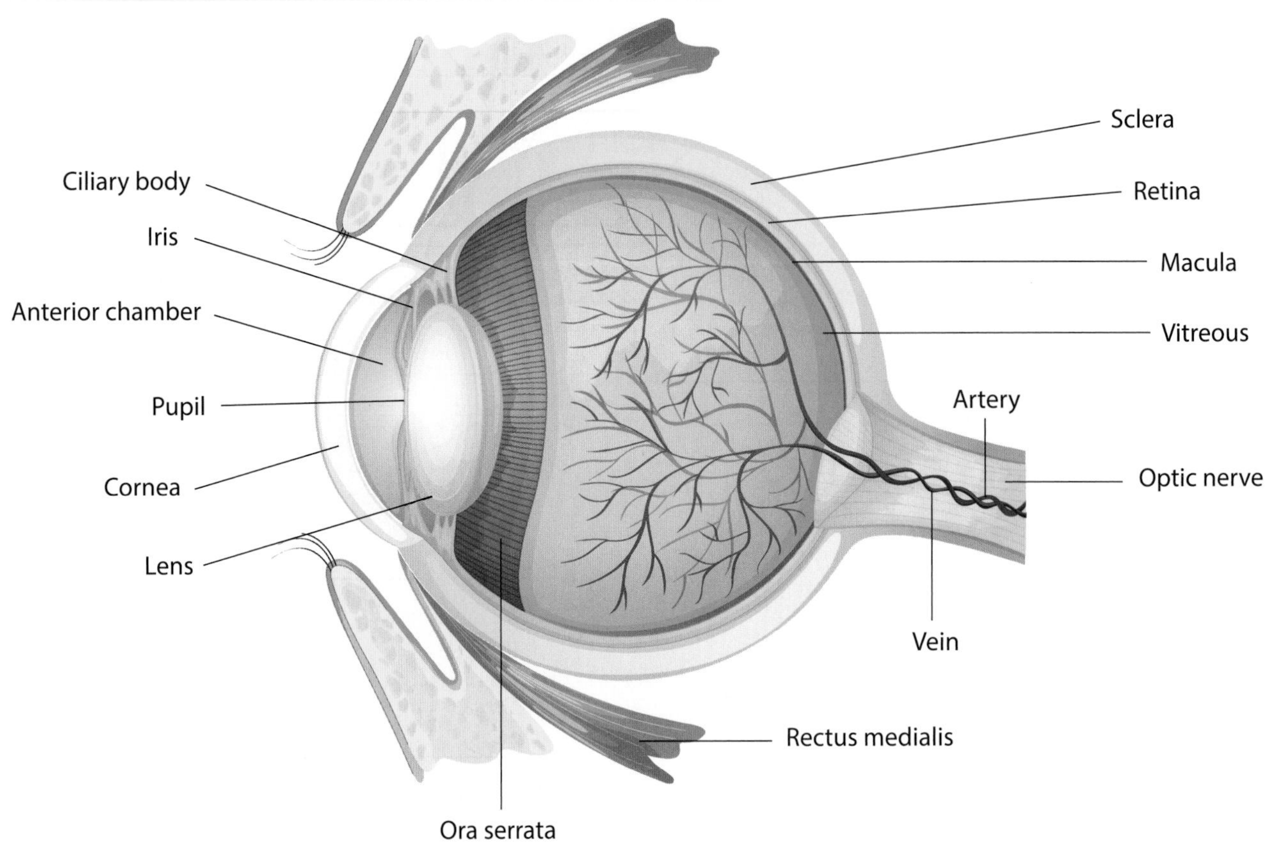
Ciliary body
Iris
Anterior chamber
Pupil
Cornea
Lens
Sclera
Retina
Macula
Vitreous
Artery
Optic nerve
Vein
Rectus medialis
Ora serrata

Muscles of the Eye

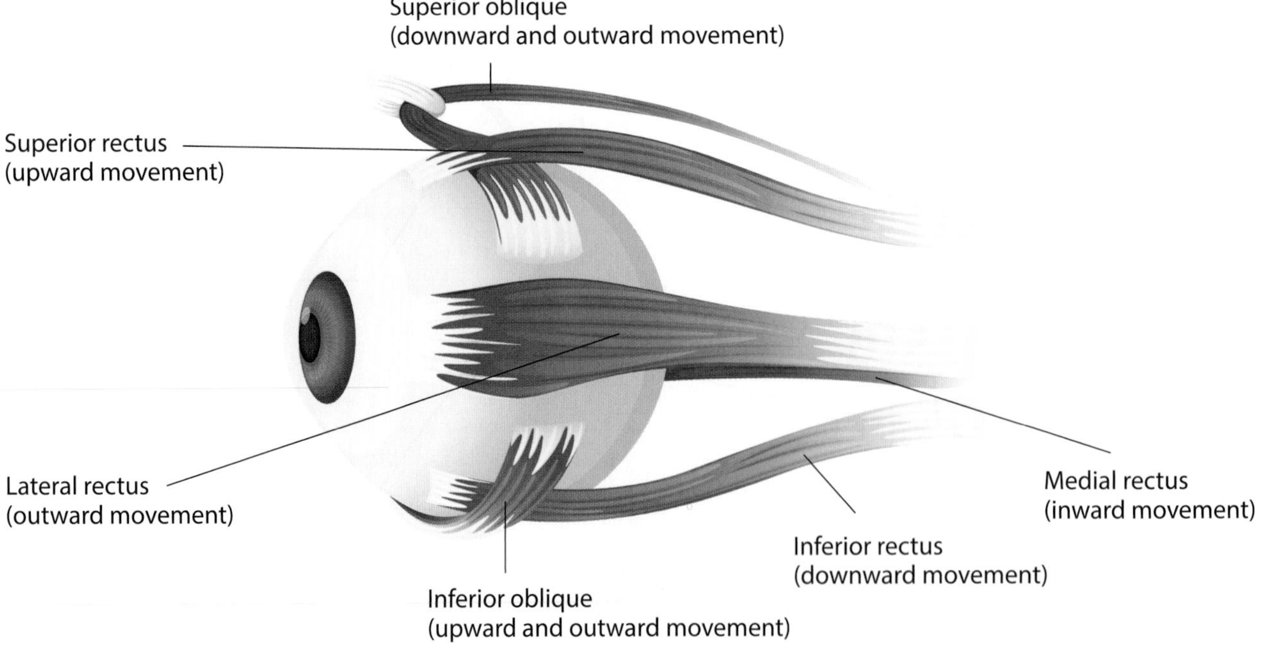
Superior oblique
(downward and outward movement)
Superior rectus
(upward movement)
Lateral rectus
(outward movement)
Medial rectus
(inward movement)
Inferior rectus
(downward movement)
Inferior oblique
(upward and outward movement)

Female Reproductive System — Anatomy

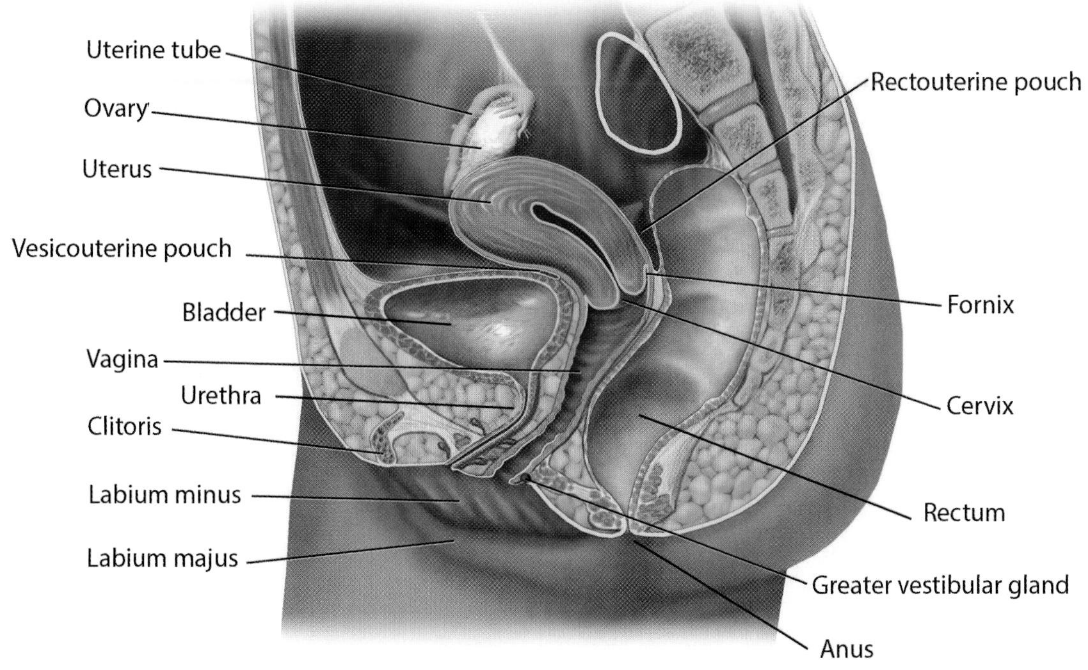
Uterine tube
Ovary
Uterus
Vesicouterine pouch
Bladder
Vagina
Urethra
Clitoris
Labium minus
Labium majus
Rectouterine pouch
Fornix
Cervix
Rectum
Greater vestibular gland
Anus

Title: Blausen 0400 FemaleReproSystem 02b.png, **Author:** BruceBlaus., **Source:** Blausen.com staff (2014). "Medical gallery of Blausen Medical 2014". *WikiJournal of Medicine* **1** (2). DOI:10.15347/wjm/2014.010. ISSN 2002-4436.Modified by User:ArnoldReinhold who released mods under CC0, **License/Permission:** This file is licensed under the Creative Commons Attribution 3.0 Unported license., **URL link:** https://commons.wikimedia.org/wiki/File:Blausen_0400_FemaleReproSystem_02b.png

Female Reproductive System — Uterus and Adnexa Anatomy

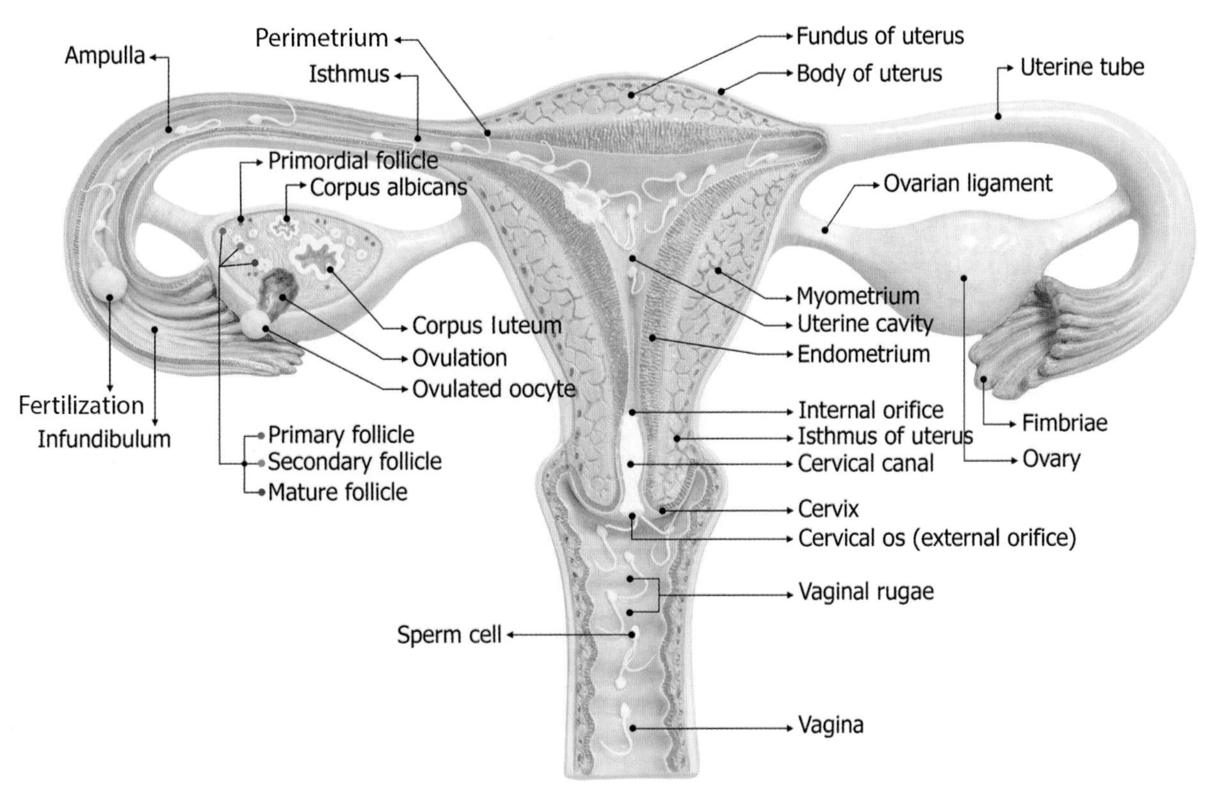
Ampulla
Perimetrium
Isthmus
Fundus of uterus
Body of uterus
Uterine tube
Primordial follicle
Corpus albicans
Ovarian ligament
Myometrium
Uterine cavity
Endometrium
Corpus luteum
Ovulation
Ovulated oocyte
Fertilization
Infundibulum
Primary follicle
Secondary follicle
Mature follicle
Internal orifice
Isthmus of uterus
Cervical canal
Fimbriae
Ovary
Cervix
Cervical os (external orifice)
Vaginal rugae
Sperm cell
Vagina

Female Reproductive System — Breast Anatomy

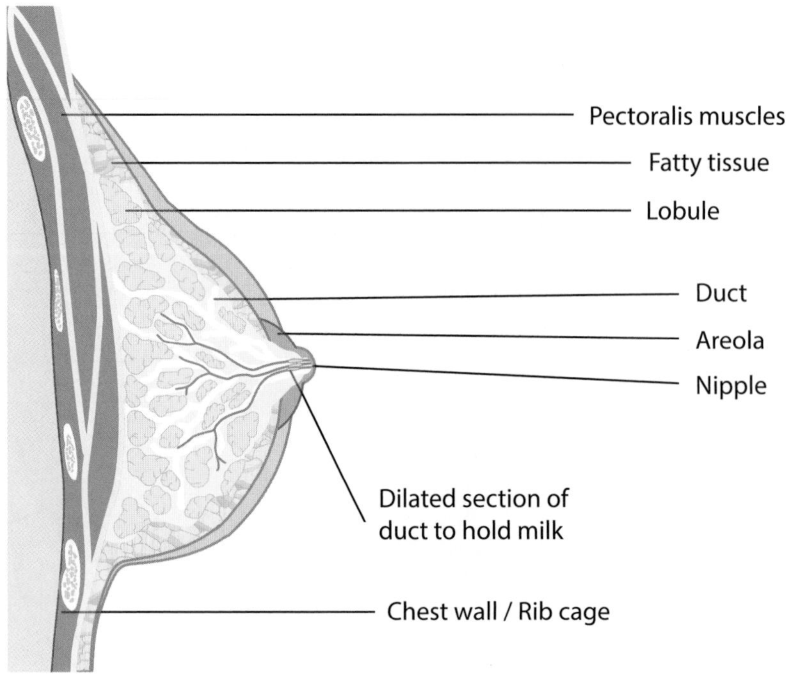
Pectoralis muscles
Fatty tissue
Lobule
Duct
Areola
Nipple
Dilated section of duct to hold milk
Chest wall / Rib cage

Female Reproductive System — Perineum Anatomy

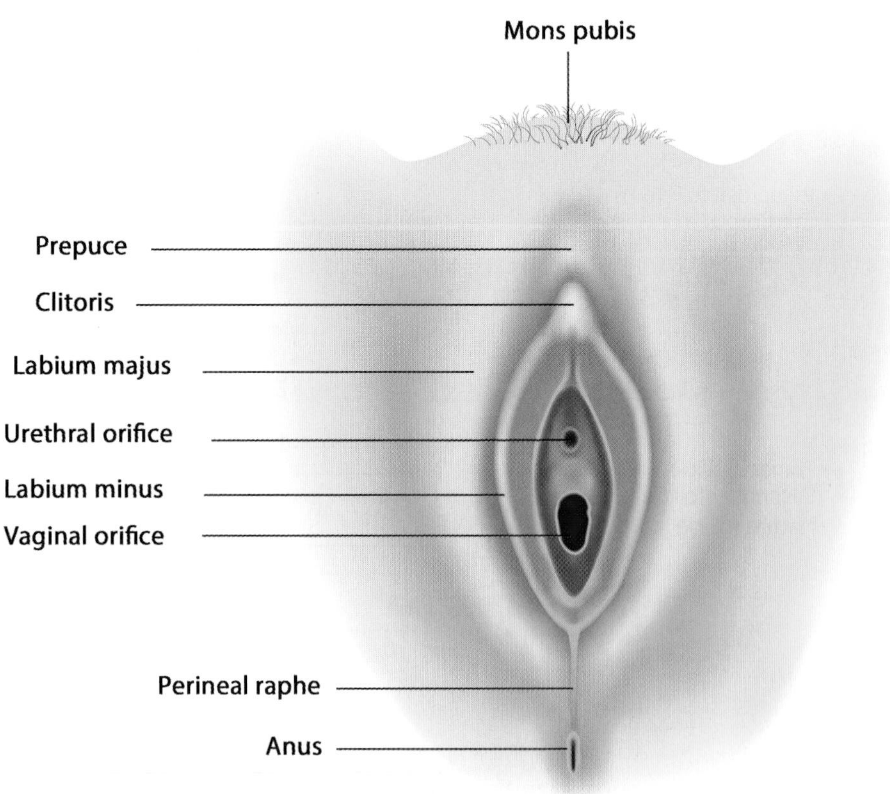
Mons pubis
Prepuce
Clitoris
Labium majus
Urethral orifice
Labium minus
Vaginal orifice
Perineal raphe
Anus

Integumentary System Anatomy

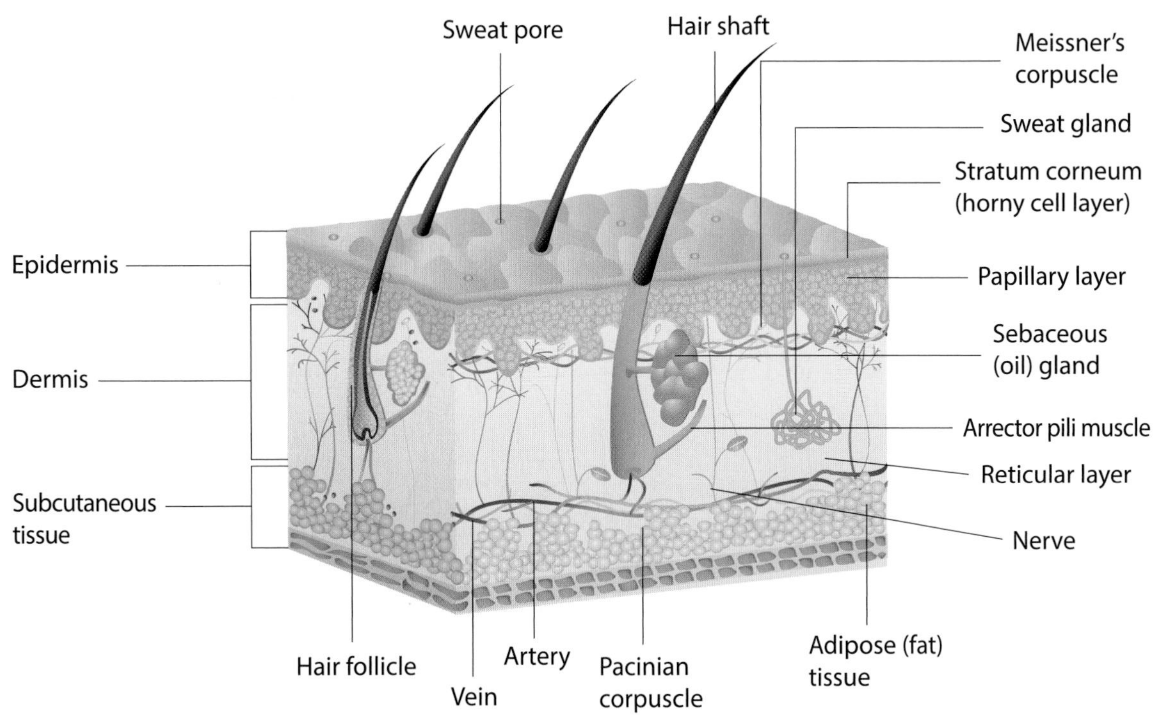
Sweat pore
Hair shaft
Meissner's corpuscle
Sweat gland
Stratum corneum (horny cell layer)
Epidermis
Papillary layer
Dermis
Sebaceous (oil) gland
Arrector pili muscle
Reticular layer
Subcutaneous tissue
Nerve
Hair follicle
Artery
Vein
Pacinian corpuscle
Adipose (fat) tissue

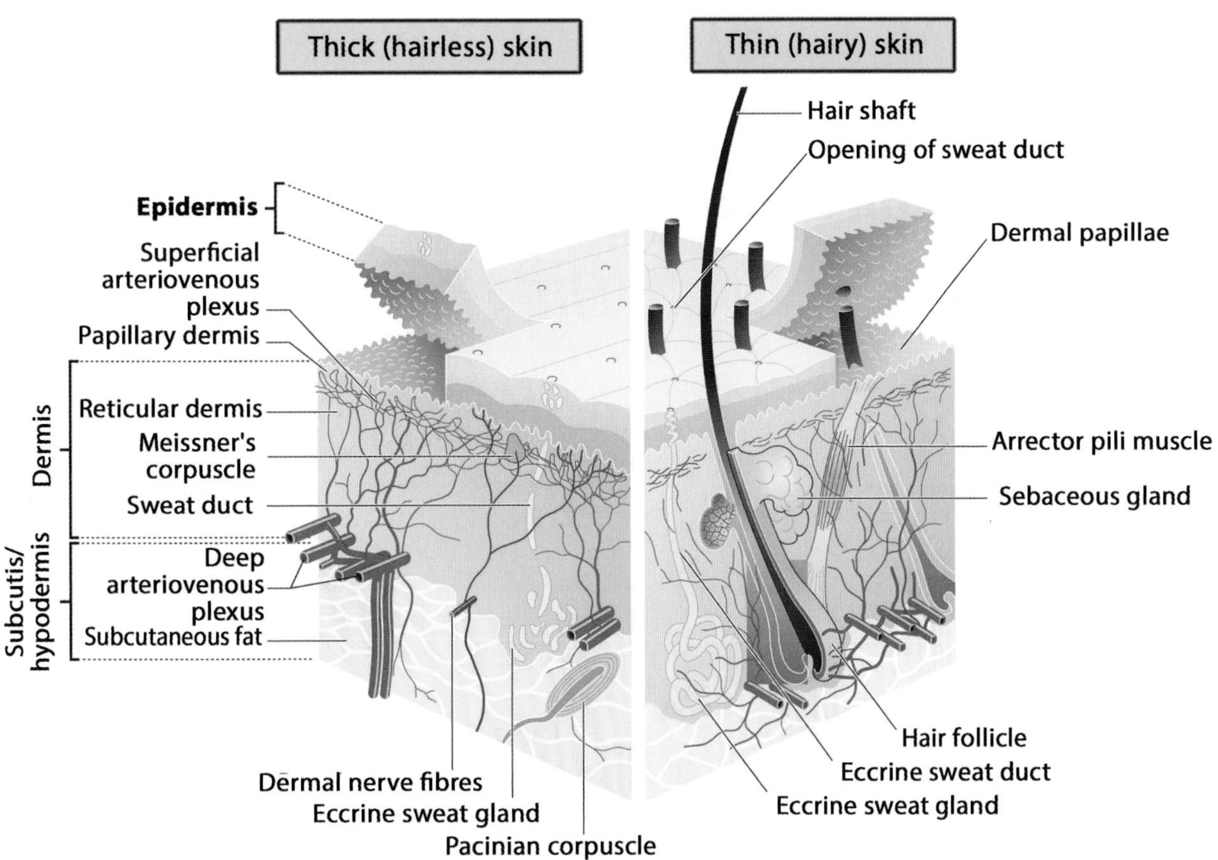
Thick (hairless) skin
Thin (hairy) skin
Hair shaft
Opening of sweat duct
Epidermis
Dermal papillae
Superficial arteriovenous plexus
Papillary dermis
Dermis
Reticular dermis
Meissner's corpuscle
Arrector pili muscle
Sweat duct
Sebaceous gland
Subcutis/ hypodermis
Deep arteriovenous plexus
Subcutaneous fat
Hair follicle
Eccrine sweat duct
Dermal nerve fibres
Eccrine sweat gland
Eccrine sweat gland
Pacinian corpuscle

Title: Skin layers.png, **Author:** Madhero88, **Source:** Own work, **License/Permission:** This file is licensed under the Creative Commons Attribution-Share Alike 3.0 Unported license., **URL link:** https://commons.wikimedia.org/wiki/File:Skin_layers.png,

Lymphatic System Anatomy

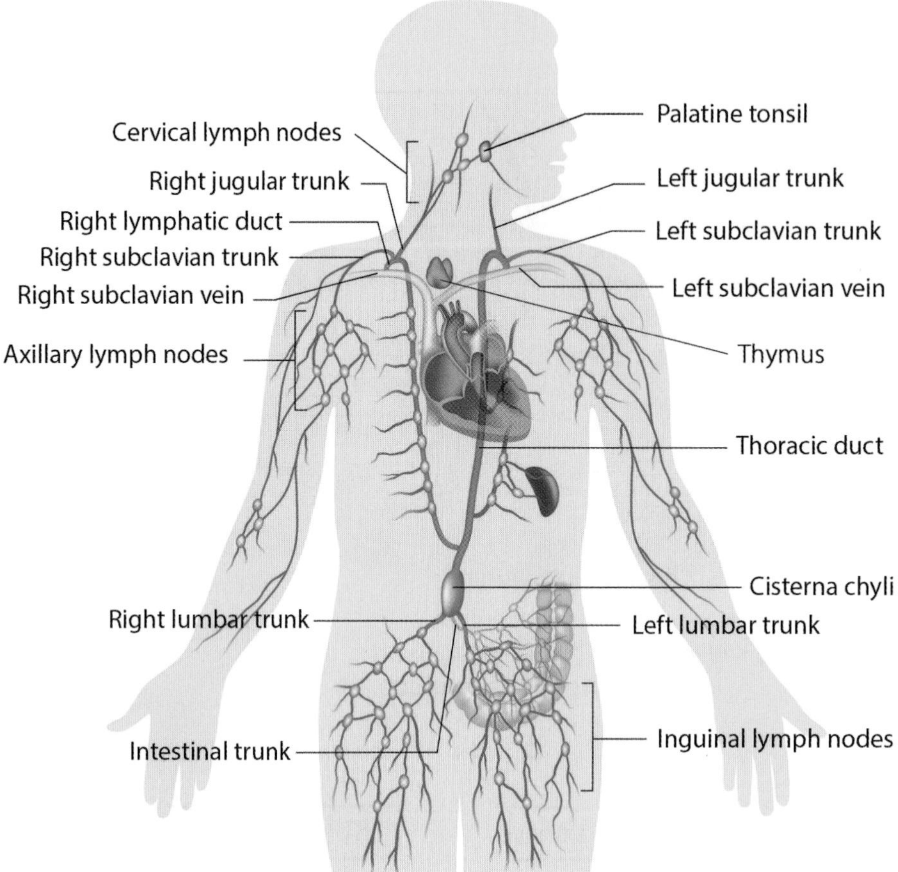
Cervical lymph nodes
Right jugular trunk
Right lymphatic duct
Right subclavian trunk
Right subclavian vein
Axillary lymph nodes
Palatine tonsil
Left jugular trunk
Left subclavian trunk
Left subclavian vein
Thymus
Thoracic duct
Cisterna chyli
Right lumbar trunk
Left lumbar trunk
Inguinal lymph nodes
Intestinal trunk

Lymph Nodes of the Head and Neck

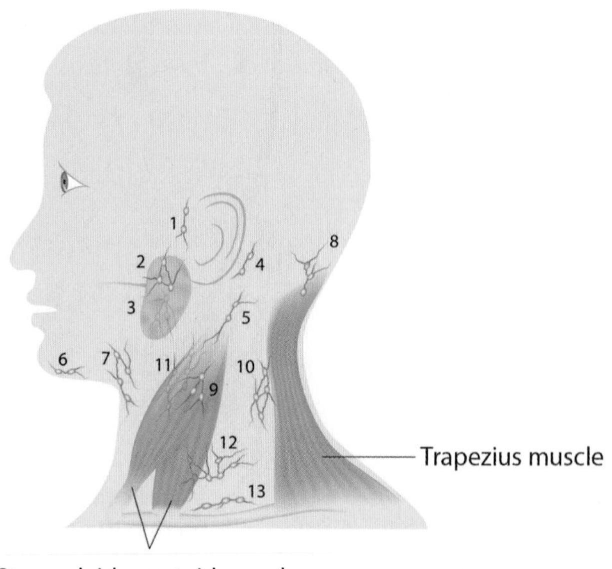
1
2
3
4
5
6
7
8
9
10
11
12
13
Trapezius muscle
Sternocleidomastoid muscle

1. Preauricular
2. Superficial parotid
3. Deep parotid
4. Posterior auricular
5. Mastoid
6. Submental
7. Submandibular
8. Occipital
9. Superficial anterior cervical
10. Superficial posterior cervical
11. Superior deep cervical
12. Inferior deep cervical
13. Supraclavicular

Lymphatic System — Humoral Immunity

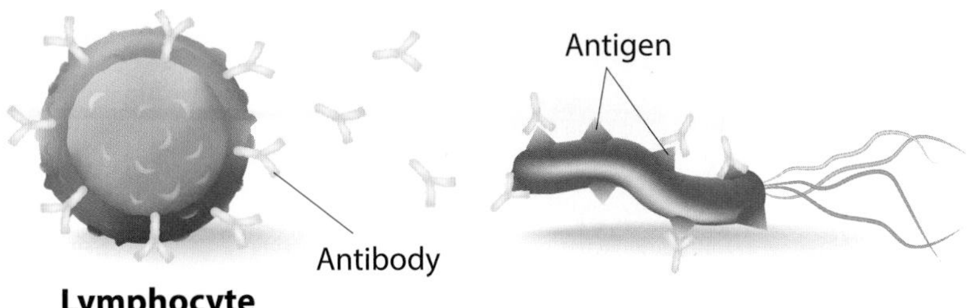
Antigen
Antibody
Lymphocyte

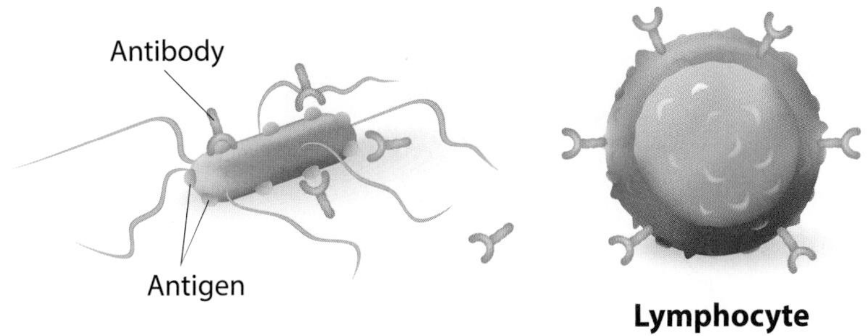
Antibody
Antigen
Lymphocyte

Lymph Node Anatomy

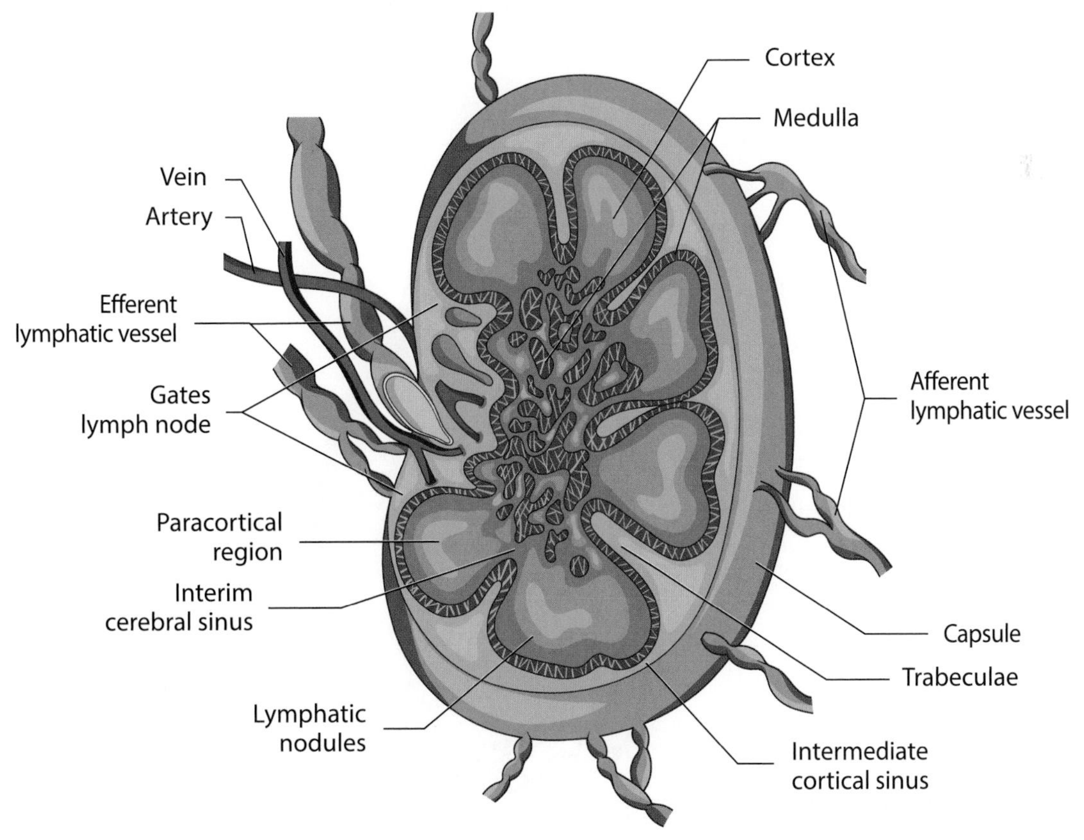
Cortex
Medulla
Vein
Artery
Efferent
lymphatic vessel
Gates
lymph node
Afferent
lymphatic vessel
Paracortical
region
Interim
cerebral sinus
Capsule
Trabeculae
Lymphatic
nodules
Intermediate
cortical sinus

Male Reproductive System Anatomy

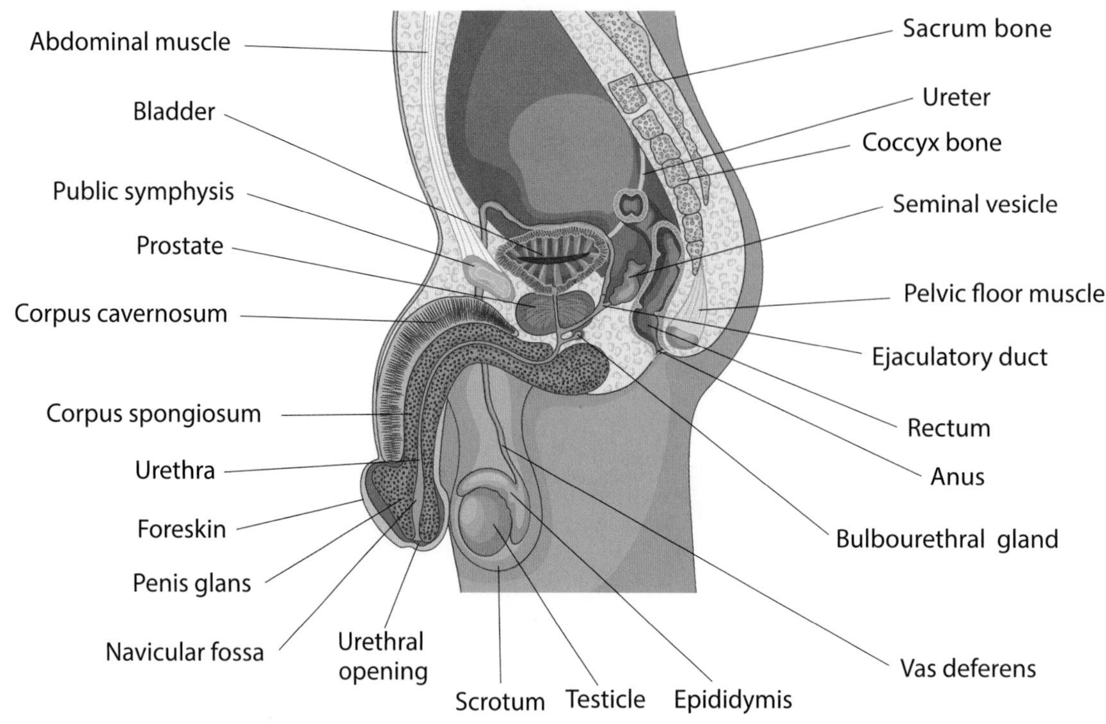
Abdominal muscle
Bladder
Public symphysis
Prostate
Corpus cavernosum
Corpus spongiosum
Urethra
Foreskin
Penis glans
Navicular fossa
Urethral opening
Scrotum
Testicle
Epididymis
Vas deferens
Bulbourethral gland
Anus
Rectum
Ejaculatory duct
Pelvic floor muscle
Seminal vesicle
Coccyx bone
Ureter
Sacrum bone

Male Reproductive System — Testicle

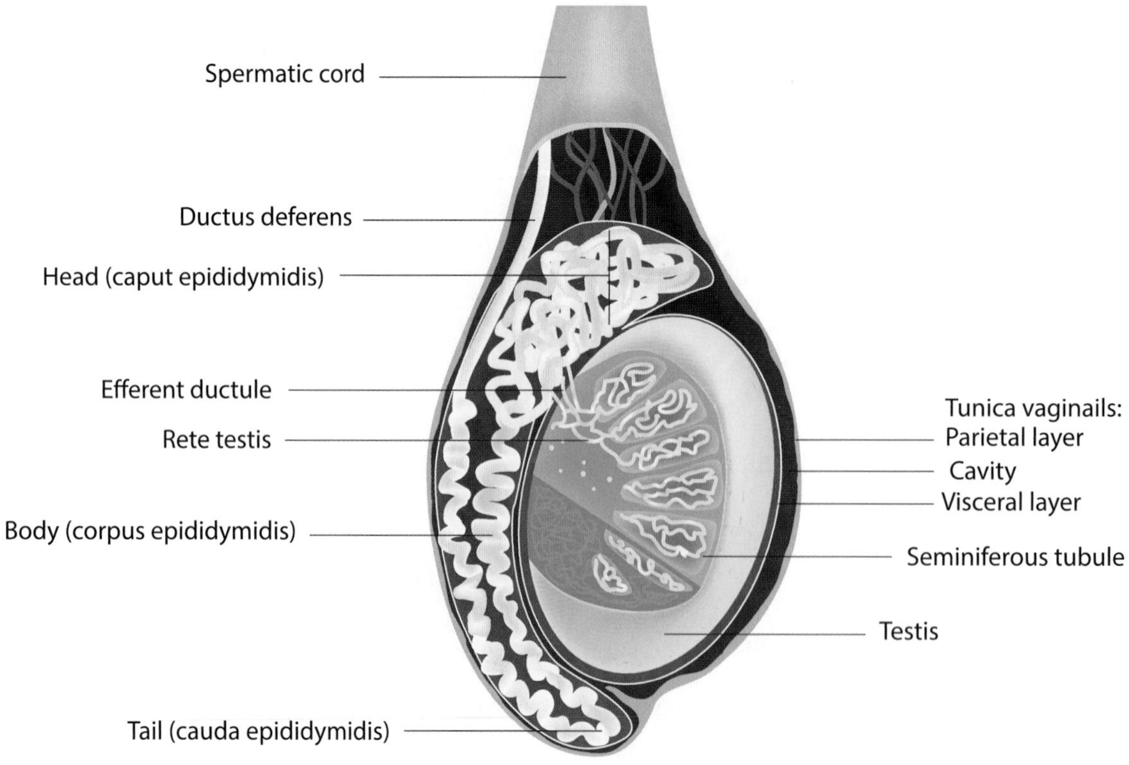
Spermatic cord
Ductus deferens
Head (caput epididymidis)
Efferent ductule
Rete testis
Body (corpus epididymidis)
Tail (cauda epididymidis)
Tunica vaginails:
Parietal layer
Cavity
Visceral layer
Seminiferous tubule
Testis

Male Reproductive System — Penis Anatomy

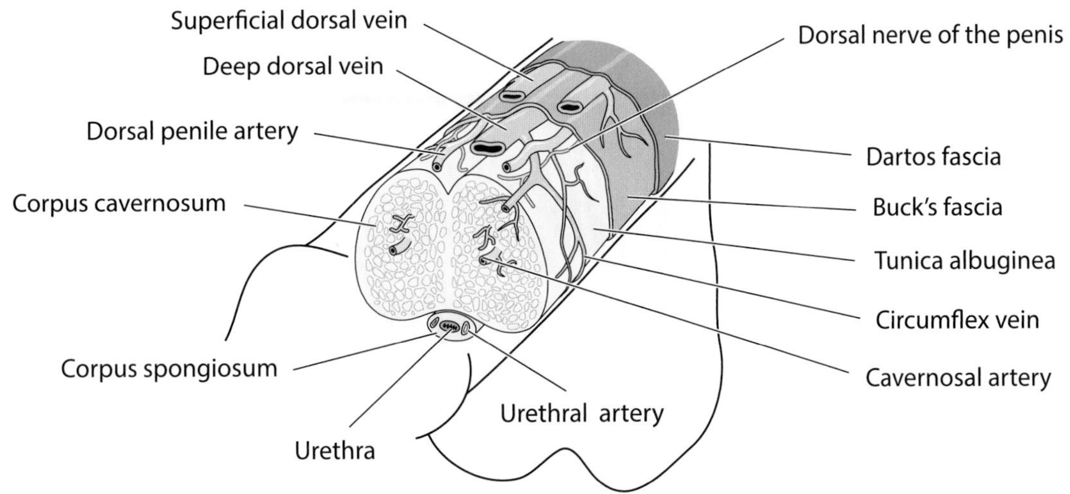
Superficial dorsal vein
Deep dorsal vein
Dorsal penile artery
Corpus cavernosum
Corpus spongiosum
Urethra
Urethral artery
Dorsal nerve of the penis
Dartos fascia
Buck's fascia
Tunica albuginea
Circumflex vein
Cavernosal artery

Muscular System Anatomy

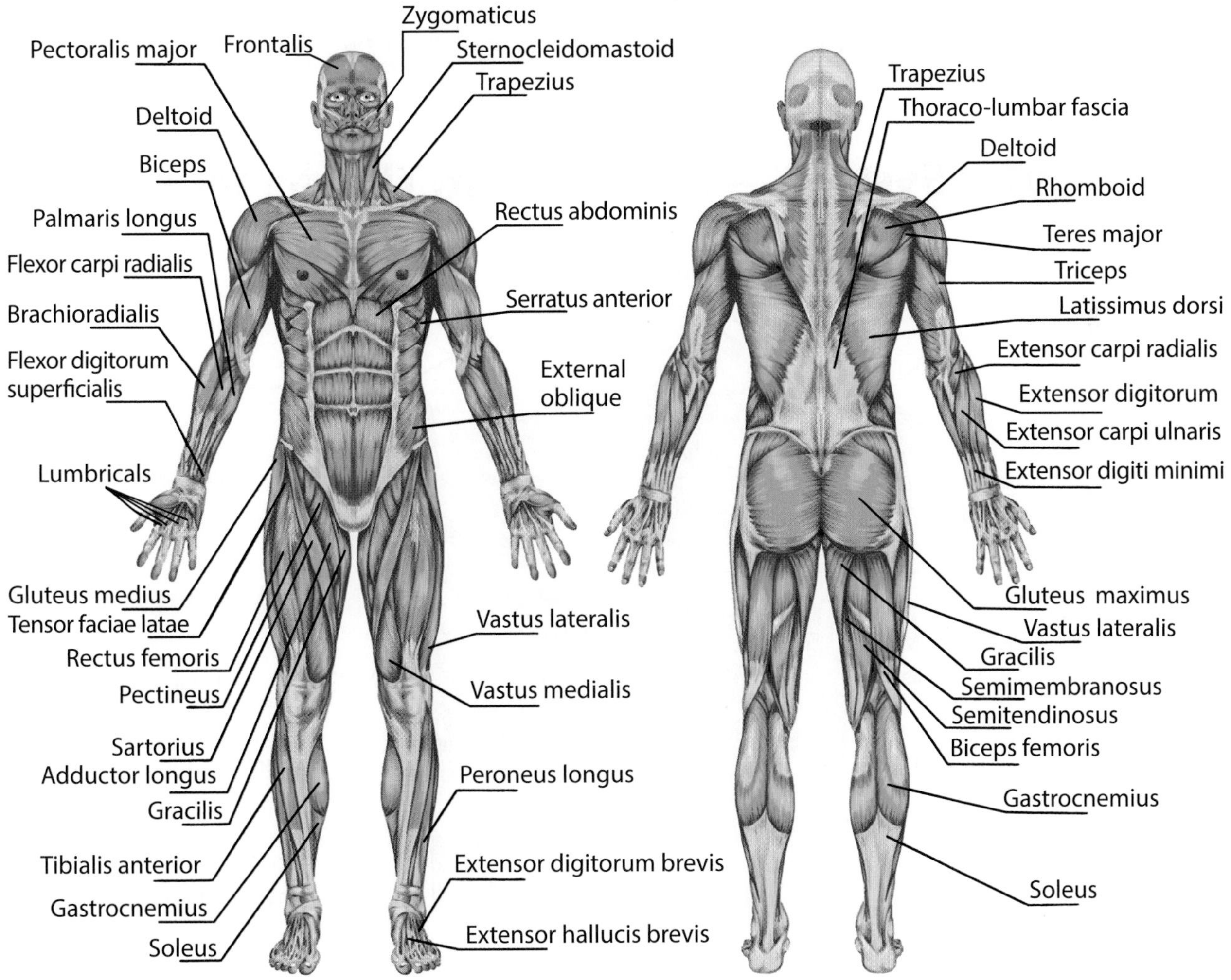

Pectoralis major
Frontalis
Zygomaticus
Sternocleidomastoid
Trapezius
Deltoid
Biceps
Palmaris longus
Flexor carpi radialis
Brachioradialis
Flexor digitorum superficialis
Lumbricals
Rectus abdominis
Serratus anterior
External oblique
Gluteus medius
Tensor faciae latae
Rectus femoris
Pectineus
Sartorius
Adductor longus
Gracilis
Tibialis anterior
Gastrocnemius
Soleus
Vastus lateralis
Vastus medialis
Peroneus longus
Extensor digitorum brevis
Extensor hallucis brevis
Trapezius
Thoraco-lumbar fascia
Deltoid
Rhomboid
Teres major
Triceps
Latissimus dorsi
Extensor carpi radialis
Extensor digitorum
Extensor carpi ulnaris
Extensor digiti minimi
Gluteus maximus
Vastus lateralis
Gracilis
Semimembranosus
Semitendinosus
Biceps femoris
Gastrocnemius
Soleus

Muscular System — Face Muscles

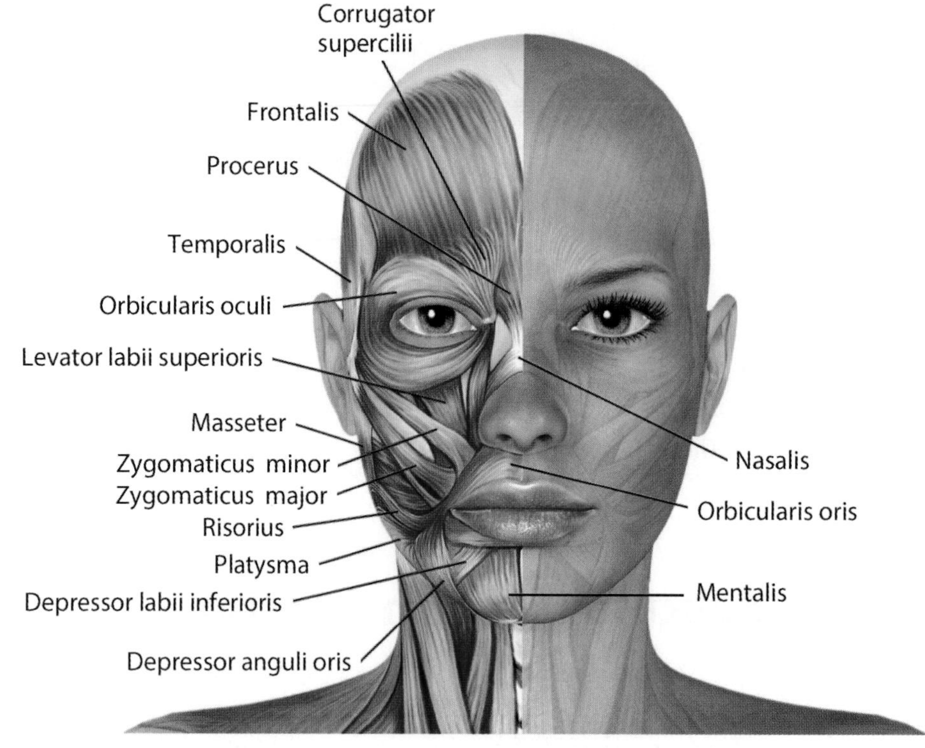
Corrugator supercilii
Frontalis
Procerus
Temporalis
Orbicularis oculi
Levator labii superioris
Masseter
Zygomaticus minor
Zygomaticus major
Risorius
Platysma
Depressor labii inferioris
Depressor anguli oris
Nasalis
Orbicularis oris
Mentalis

Muscular System — Neck, Chest, Thorax Muscles

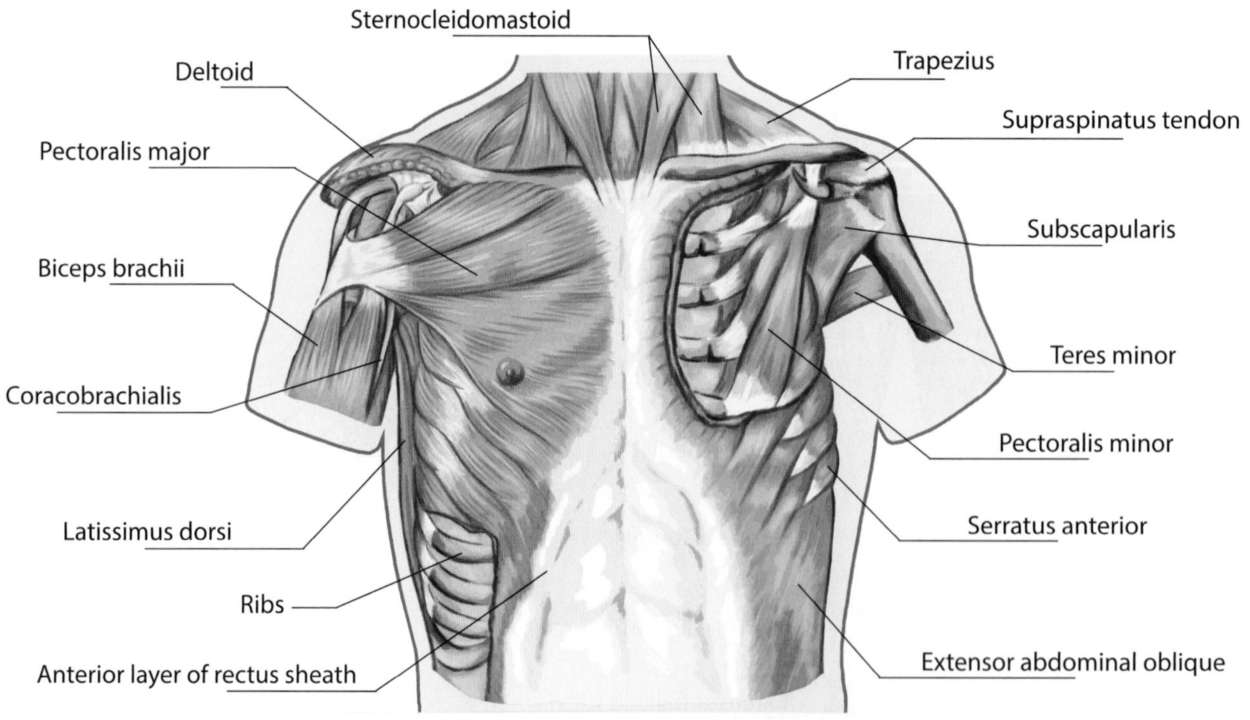
Sternocleidomastoid
Deltoid
Trapezius
Supraspinatus tendon
Pectoralis major
Subscapularis
Biceps brachii
Teres minor
Coracobrachialis
Pectoralis minor
Latissimus dorsi
Serratus anterior
Ribs
Anterior layer of rectus sheath
Extensor abdominal oblique

Muscular System — Shoulder (Rotator Cuff) Muscles

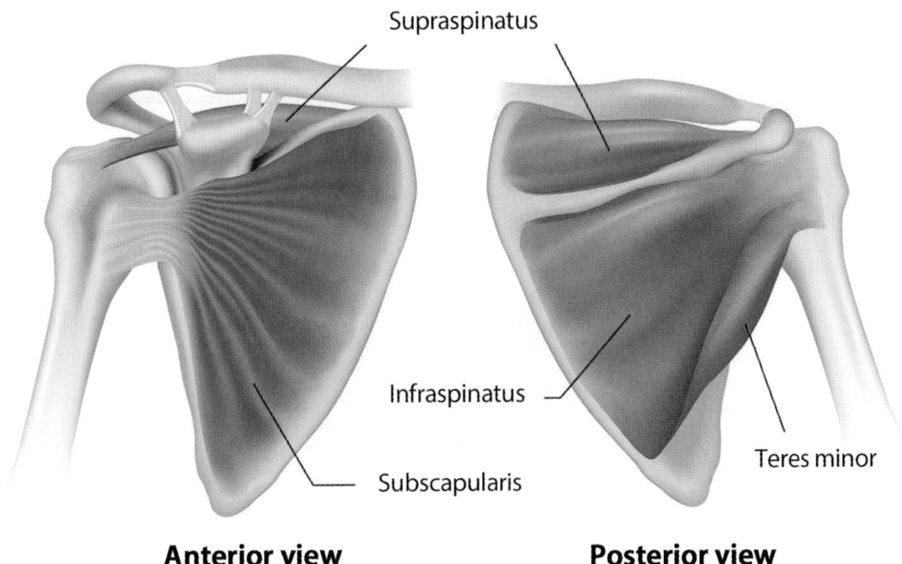
Supraspinatus
Infraspinatus
Subscapularis
Teres minor
Anterior view
Posterior view

Muscular System — Forearm Muscles (Right Arm, Posterior Compartment)

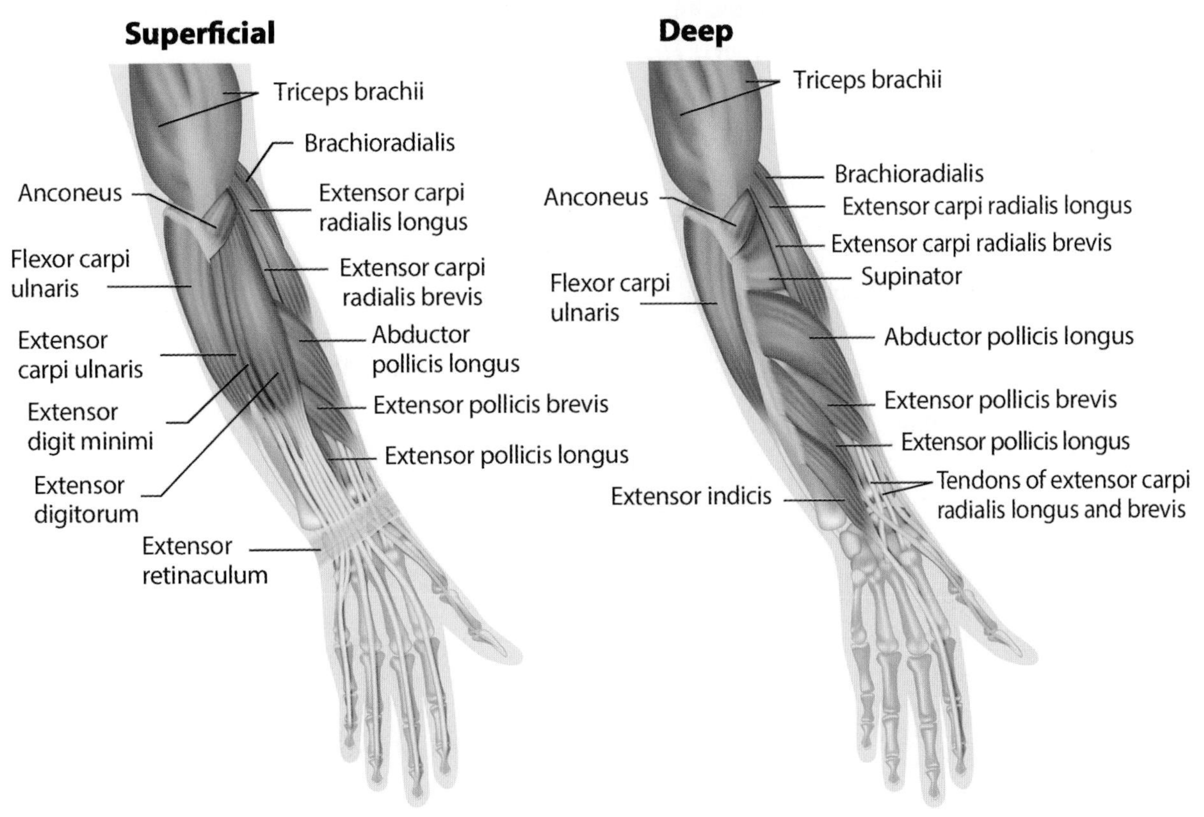
Superficial
Triceps brachii
Brachioradialis
Anconeus
Extensor carpi radialis longus
Flexor carpi ulnaris
Extensor carpi radialis brevis
Extensor carpi ulnaris
Abductor pollicis longus
Extensor digit minimi
Extensor pollicis brevis
Extensor pollicis longus
Extensor digitorum
Extensor retinaculum
Deep
Triceps brachii
Brachioradialis
Anconeus
Extensor carpi radialis longus
Extensor carpi radialis brevis
Supinator
Flexor carpi ulnaris
Abductor pollicis longus
Extensor pollicis brevis
Extensor pollicis longus
Tendons of extensor carpi radialis longus and brevis
Extensor indicis

Muscles of the Hand

(right hand, dorsal view)

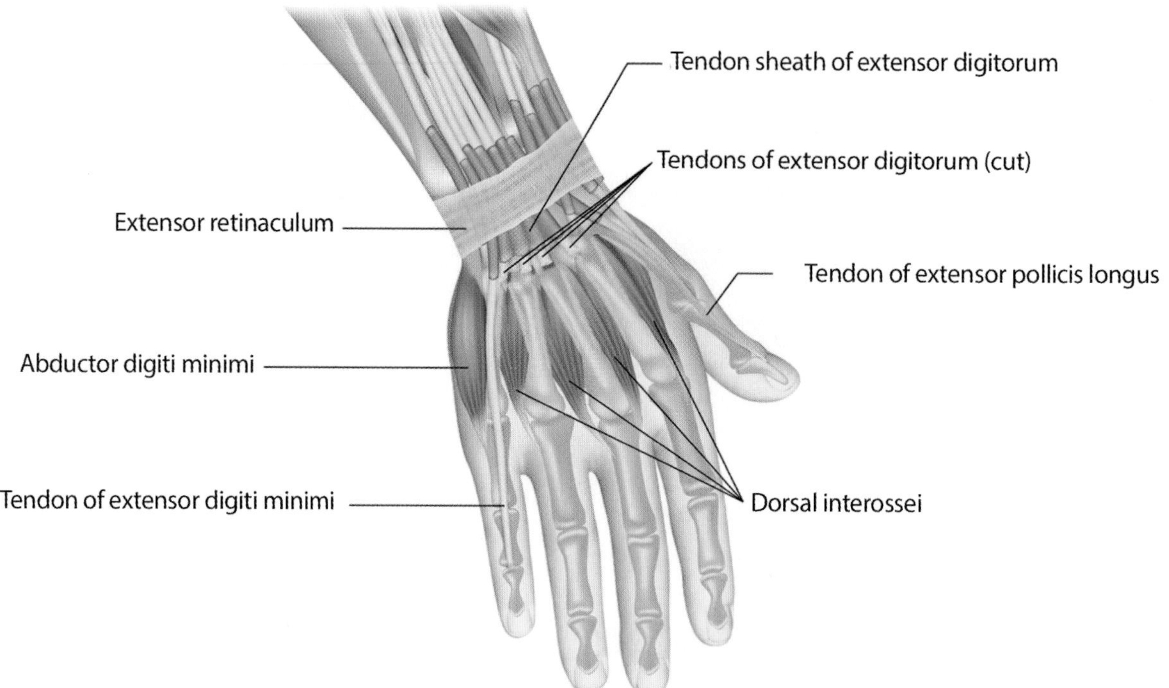
Tendon sheath of extensor digitorum
Tendons of extensor digitorum (cut)
Extensor retinaculum
Tendon of extensor pollicis longus
Abductor digiti minimi
Tendon of extensor digiti minimi
Dorsal interossei

Muscles of the Hand

(right hand, palmar view)

Deep

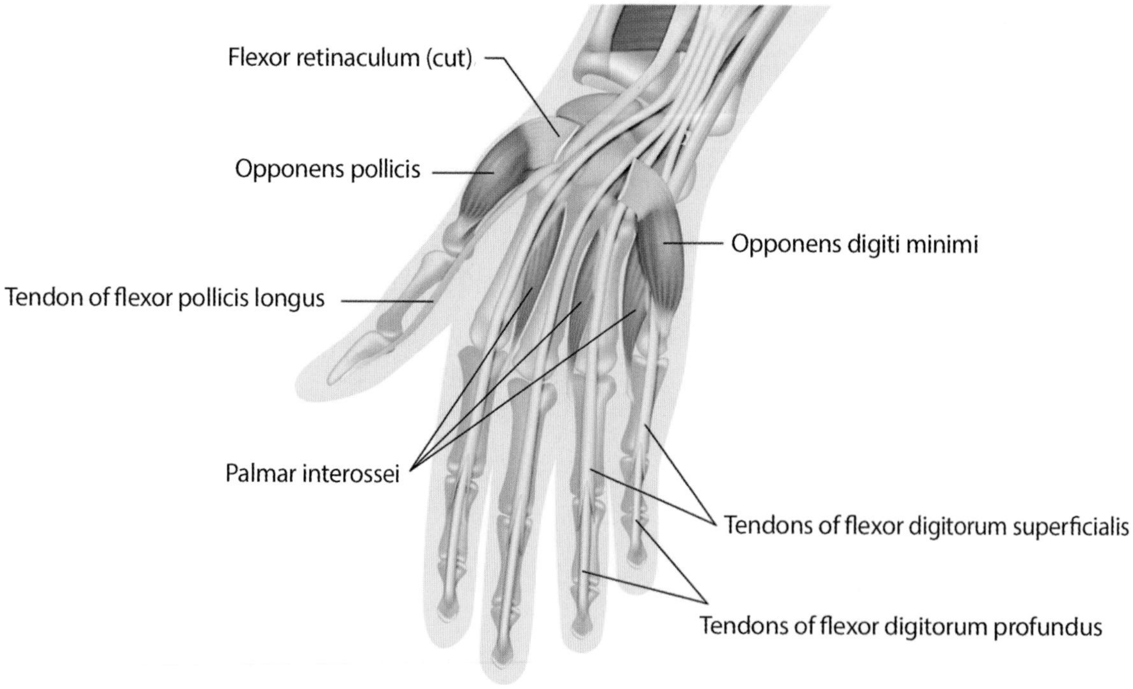

Flexor retinaculum (cut)
Opponens pollicis
Opponens digiti minimi
Tendon of flexor pollicis longus
Palmar interossei
Tendons of flexor digitorum superficialis
Tendons of flexor digitorum profundus

Muscular System — Leg Muscles

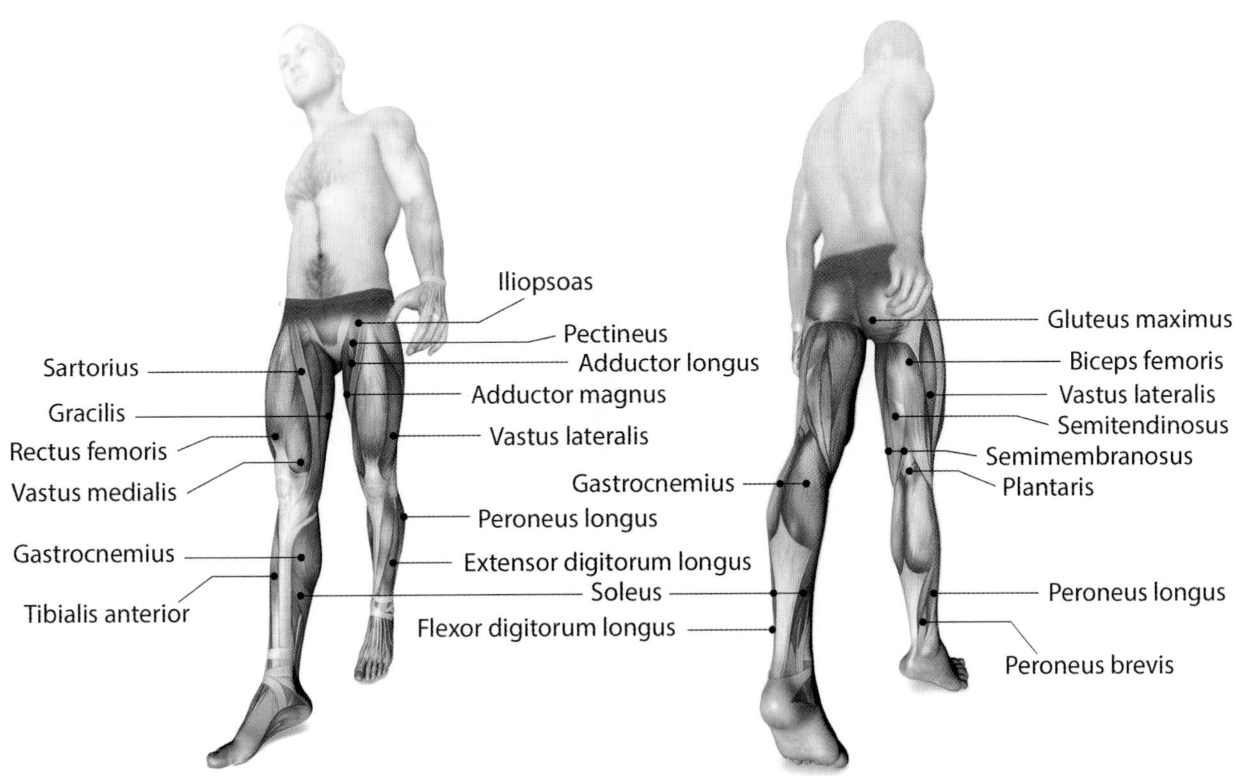
Iliopsoas
Pectineus
Adductor longus
Adductor magnus
Vastus lateralis
Sartorius
Gracilis
Rectus femoris
Vastus medialis
Gastrocnemius
Tibialis anterior
Gastrocnemius
Peroneus longus
Extensor digitorum longus
Soleus
Flexor digitorum longus
Gluteus maximus
Biceps femoris
Vastus lateralis
Semitendinosus
Semimembranosus
Plantaris
Peroneus longus
Peroneus brevis

Muscular System — Knee and Leg

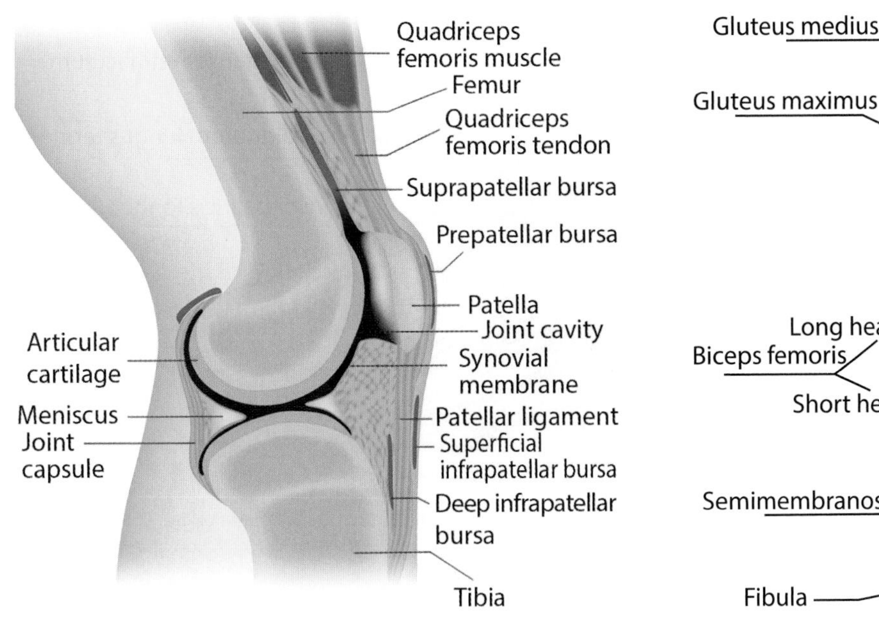
Quadriceps femoris muscle
Femur
Quadriceps femoris tendon
Suprapatellar bursa
Prepatellar bursa
Patella
Joint cavity
Synovial membrane
Patellar ligament
Superficial infrapatellar bursa
Deep infrapatellar bursa
Tibia
Articular cartilage
Meniscus
Joint capsule

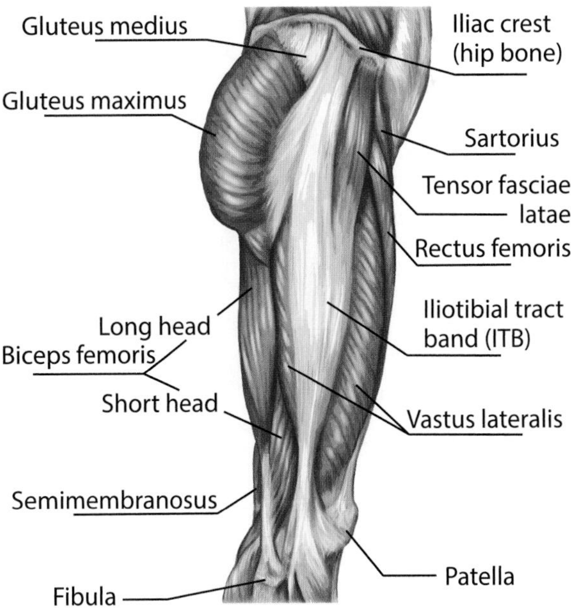
Gluteus medius
Gluteus maximus
Iliac crest (hip bone)
Sartorius
Tensor fasciae latae
Rectus femoris
Iliotibial tract band (ITB)
Long head
Biceps femoris
Short head
Vastus lateralis
Semimembranosus
Patella
Fibula

Muscular System — Foot Muscles

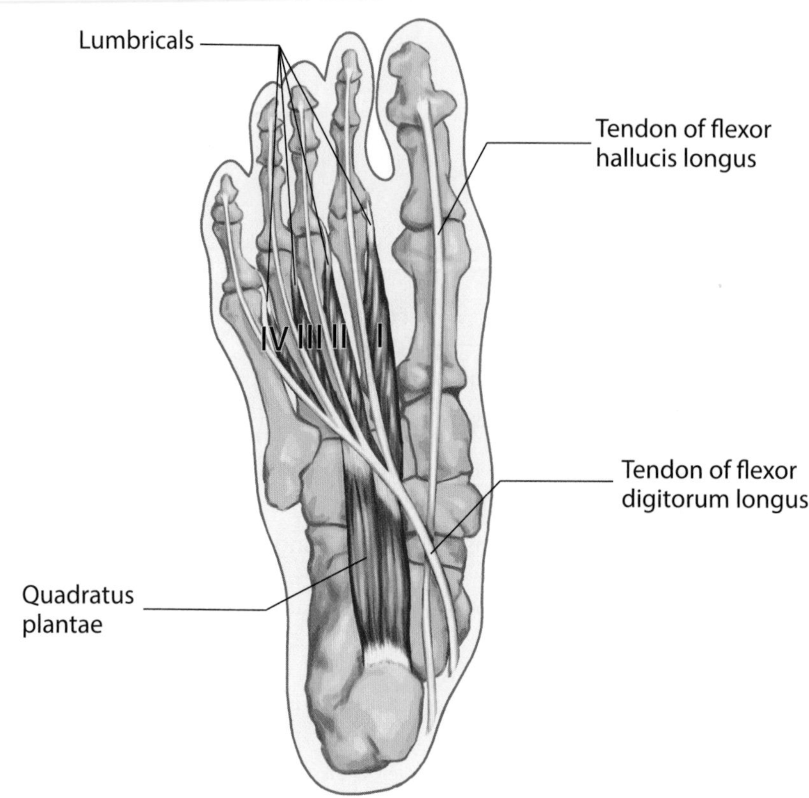
Lumbricals
Tendon of flexor hallucis longus
IV III II I
Tendon of flexor digitorum longus
Quadratus plantae

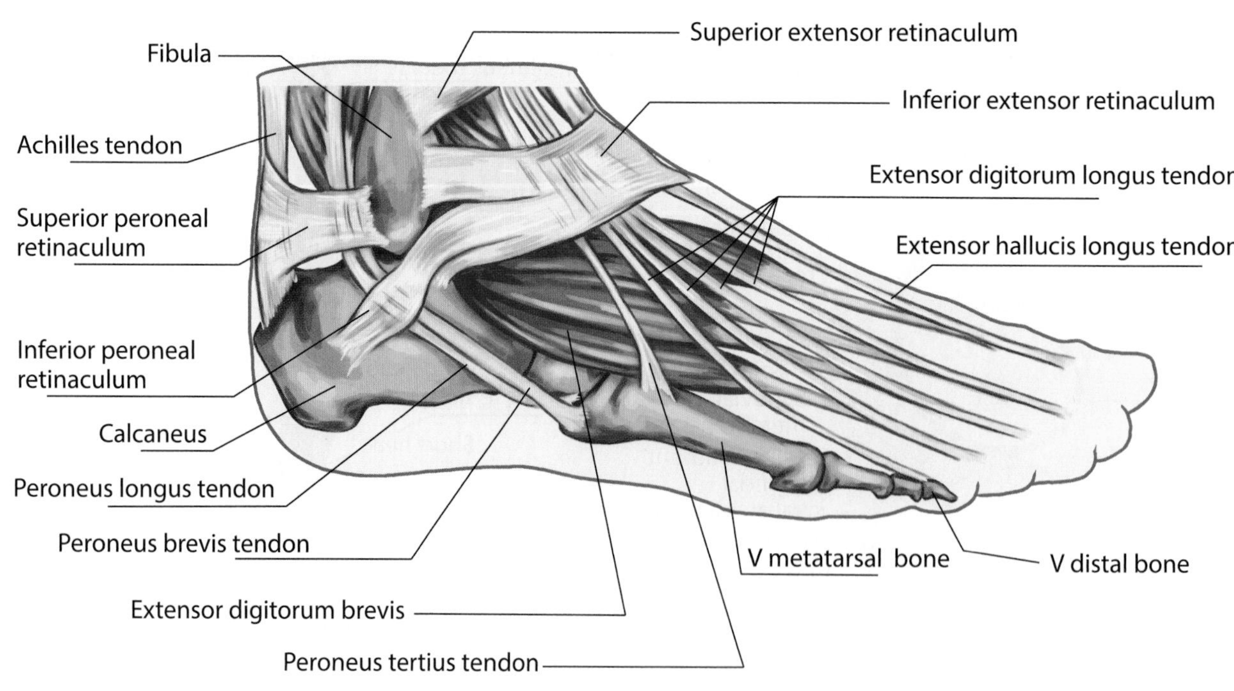
Fibula
Superior extensor retinaculum
Inferior extensor retinaculum
Achilles tendon
Extensor digitorum longus tendon
Superior peroneal retinaculum
Extensor hallucis longus tendon
Inferior peroneal retinaculum
Calcaneus
Peroneus longus tendon
Peroneus brevis tendon
V metatarsal bone
V distal bone
Extensor digitorum brevis
Peroneus tertius tendon

Nervous System Anatomy

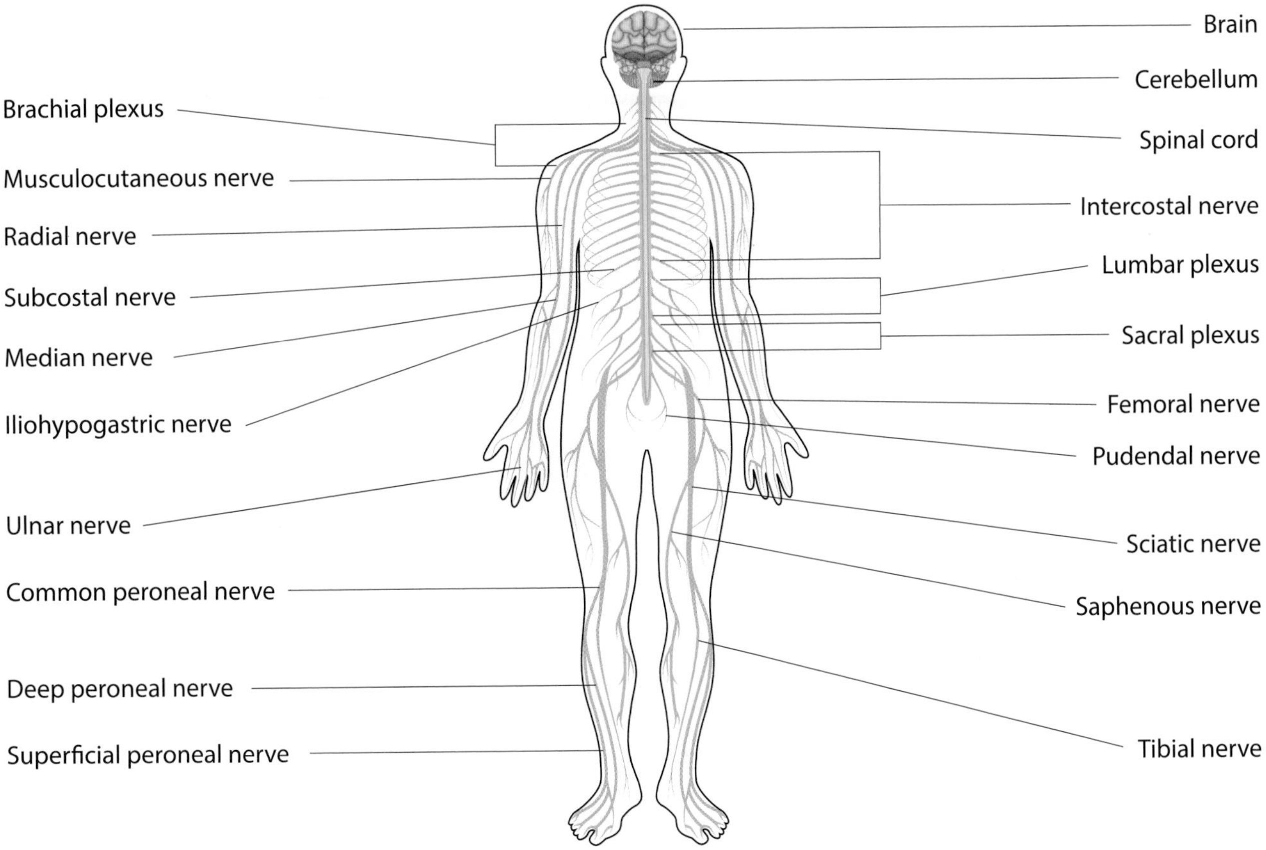

Brain
Cerebellum
Brachial plexus
Spinal cord
Musculocutaneous nerve
Intercostal nerve
Radial nerve
Lumbar plexus
Subcostal nerve
Sacral plexus
Median nerve
Femoral nerve
Iliohypogastric nerve
Pudendal nerve
Ulnar nerve
Sciatic nerve
Common peroneal nerve
Saphenous nerve
Deep peroneal nerve
Tibial nerve
Superficial peroneal nerve

Nervous System — Brain Anatomy

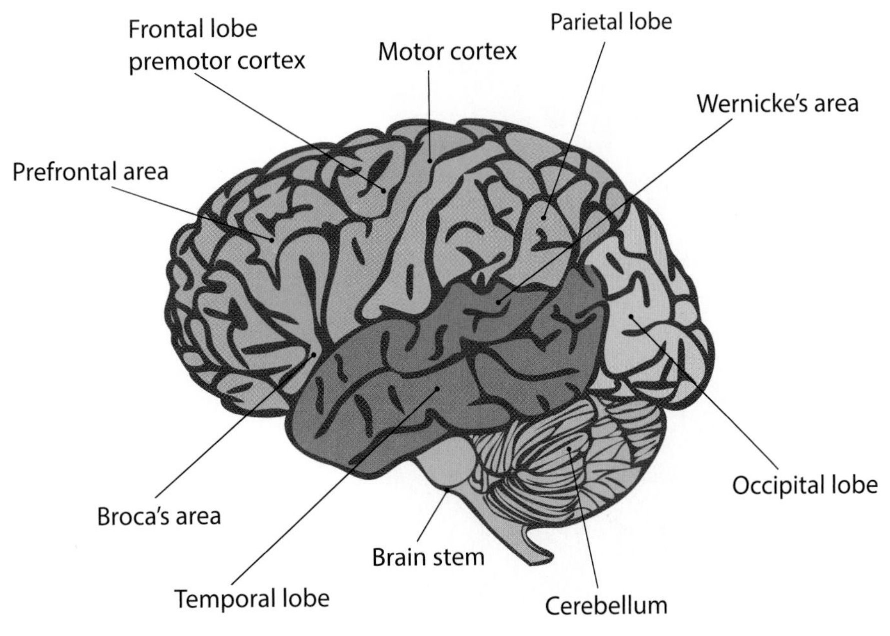
Frontal lobe
premotor cortex
Motor cortex
Parietal lobe
Wernicke's area
Prefrontal area
Occipital lobe
Broca's area
Brain stem
Temporal lobe
Cerebellum

Nervous System — Median Section of the Brain

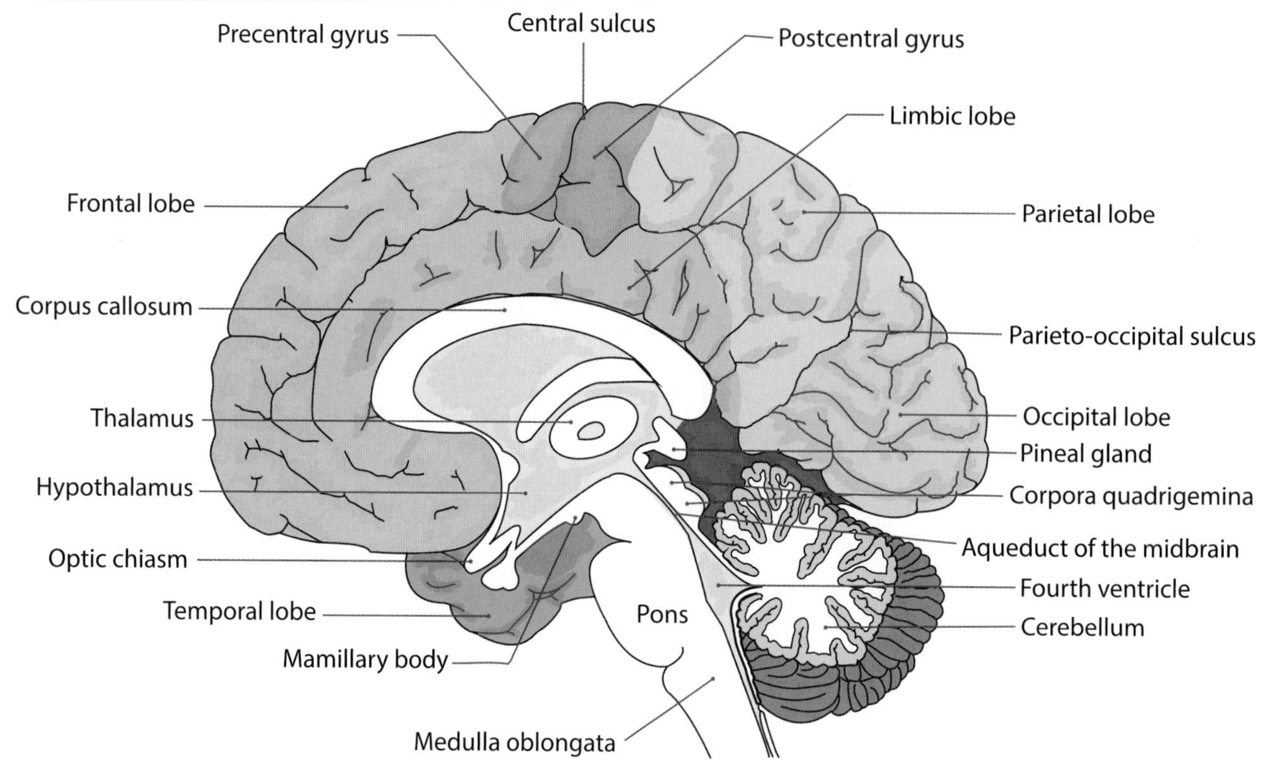
Precentral gyrus
Central sulcus
Postcentral gyrus
Limbic lobe
Frontal lobe
Parietal lobe
Corpus callosum
Parieto-occipital sulcus
Thalamus
Occipital lobe
Pineal gland
Hypothalamus
Corpora quadrigemina
Aqueduct of the midbrain
Optic chiasm
Fourth ventricle
Temporal lobe
Pons
Cerebellum
Mamillary body
Medulla oblongata

Nervous System — Cranial Nerves

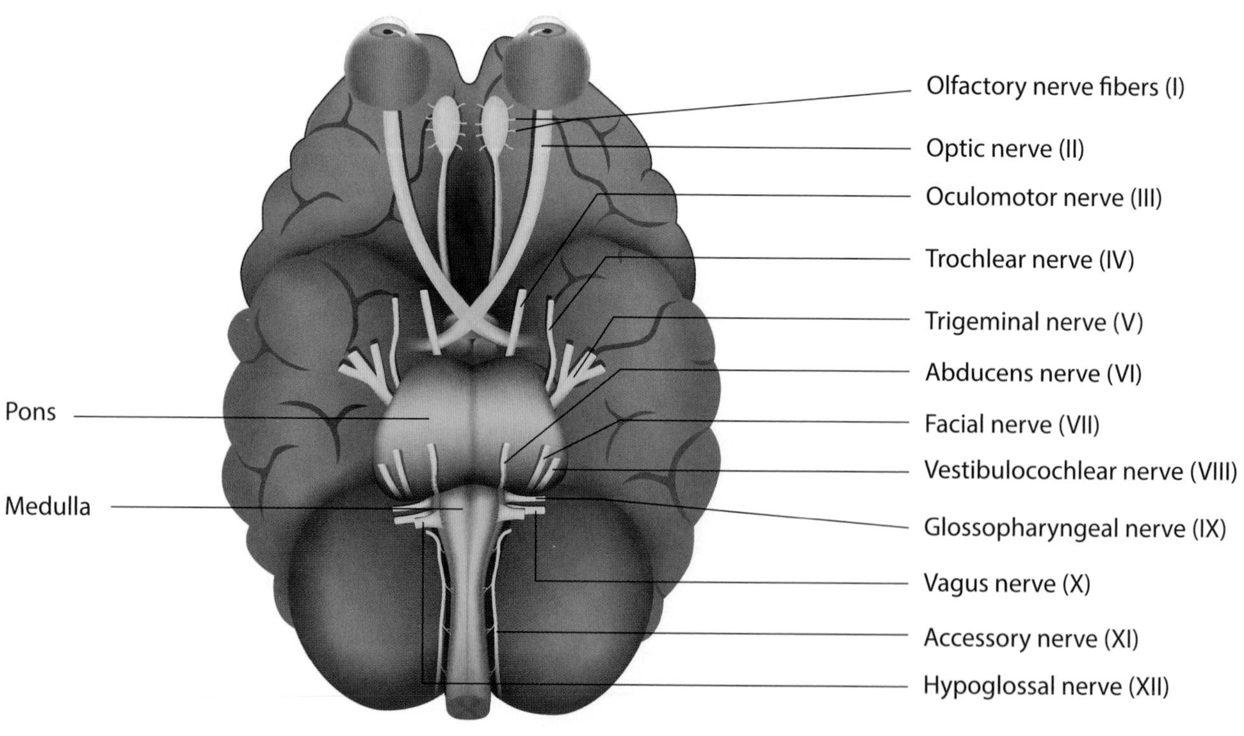
Olfactory nerve fibers (I)
Optic nerve (II)
Oculomotor nerve (III)
Trochlear nerve (IV)
Trigeminal nerve (V)
Abducens nerve (VI)
Pons
Facial nerve (VII)
Vestibulocochlear nerve (VIII)
Medulla
Glossopharyngeal nerve (IX)
Vagus nerve (X)
Accessory nerve (XI)
Hypoglossal nerve (XII)

Nervous System — Nerve Anatomy

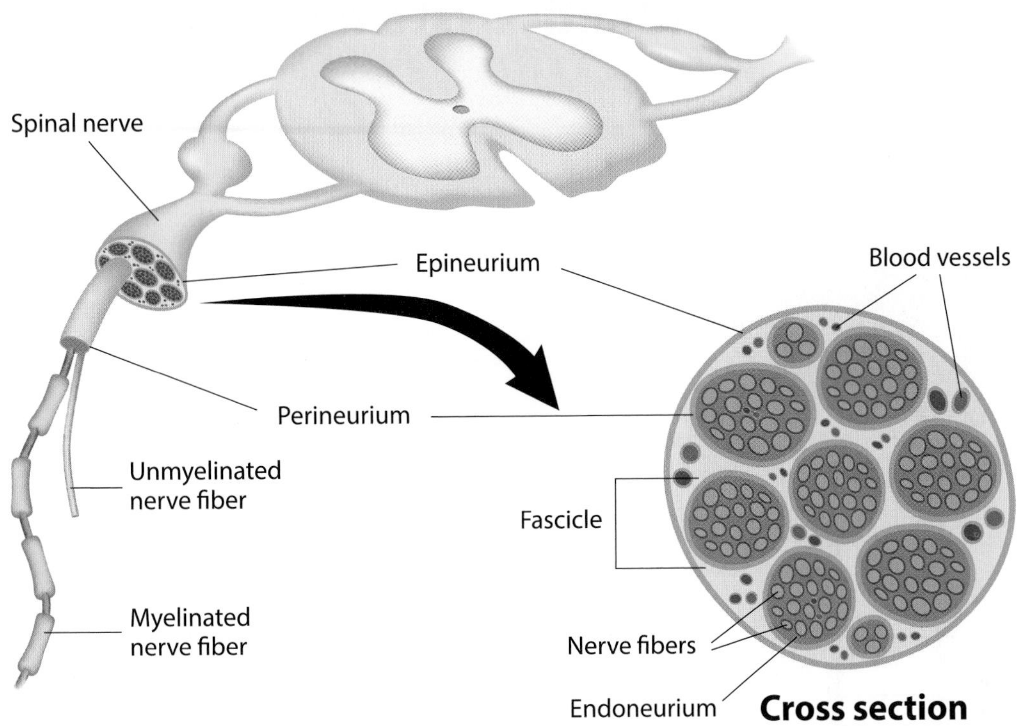
Spinal nerve
Epineurium
Blood vessels
Perineurium
Unmyelinated nerve fiber
Fascicle
Myelinated nerve fiber
Nerve fibers
Endoneurium
Cross section

Nervous System — Parasympathetic System Anatomy

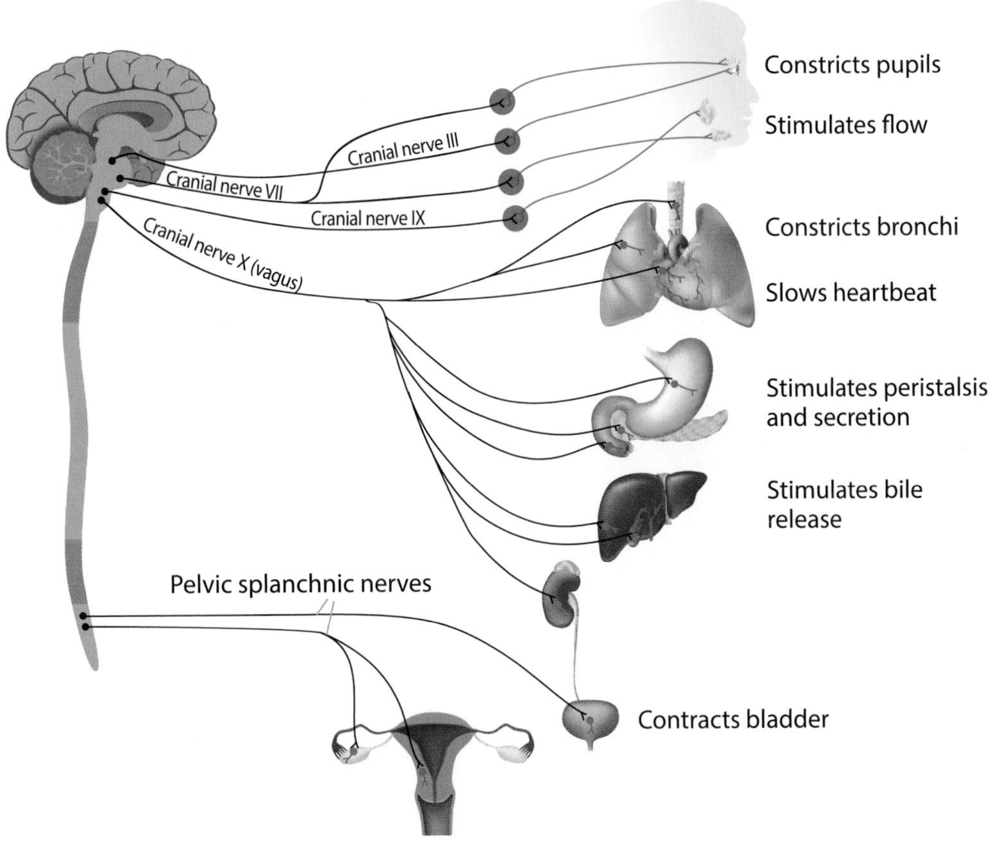
Constricts pupils
Stimulates flow
Cranial nerve III
Cranial nerve VII
Cranial nerve IX
Cranial nerve X (vagus)
Constricts bronchi
Slows heartbeat
Stimulates peristalsis and secretion
Stimulates bile release
Pelvic splanchnic nerves
Contracts bladder

Nervous System — Sympathetic System Anatomy

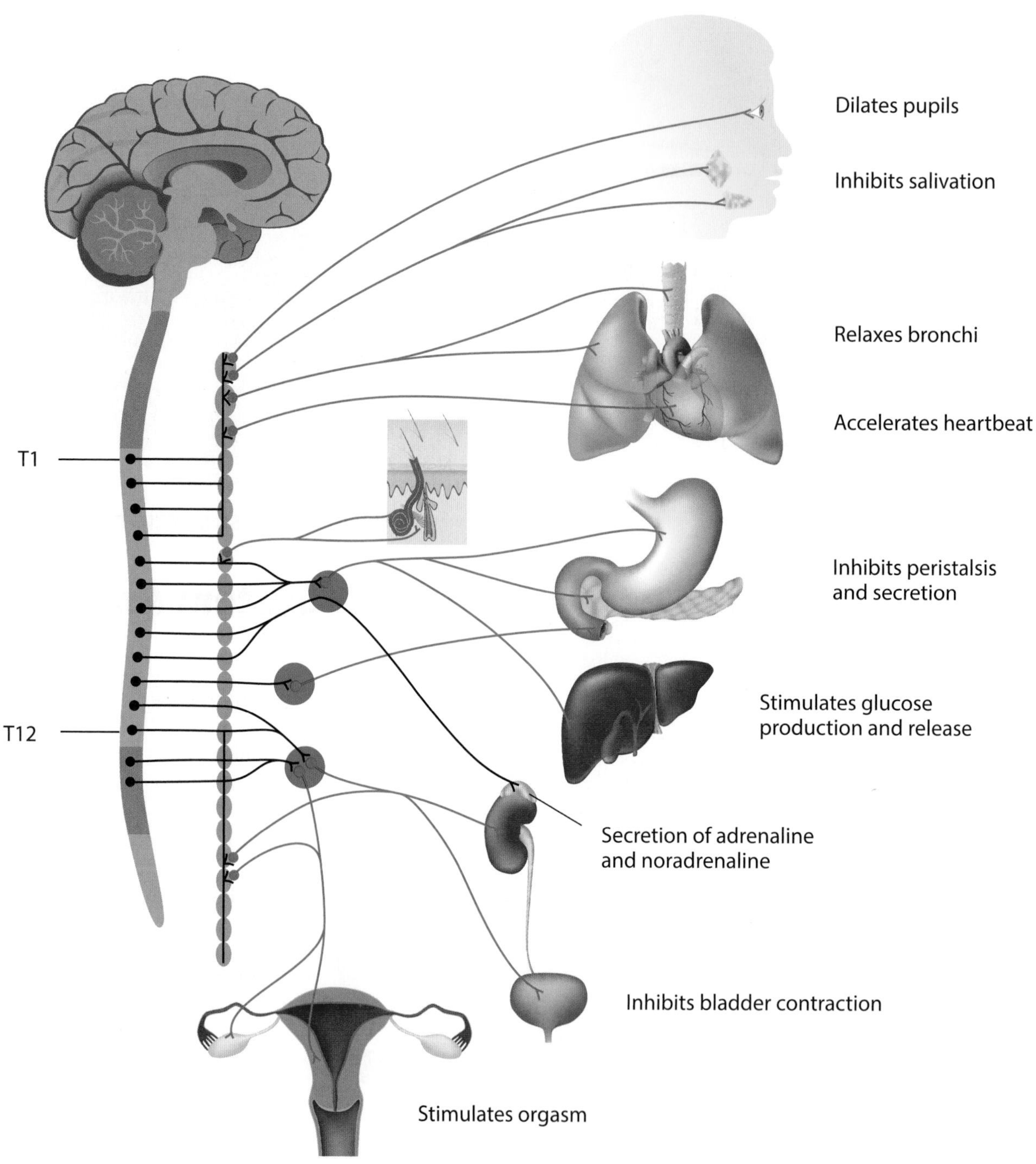
Dilates pupils
Inhibits salivation
Relaxes bronchi
Accelerates heartbeat
T1
Inhibits peristalsis and secretion
Stimulates glucose production and release
T12
Secretion of adrenaline and noradrenaline
Inhibits bladder contraction
Stimulates orgasm

Respiratory System Anatomy

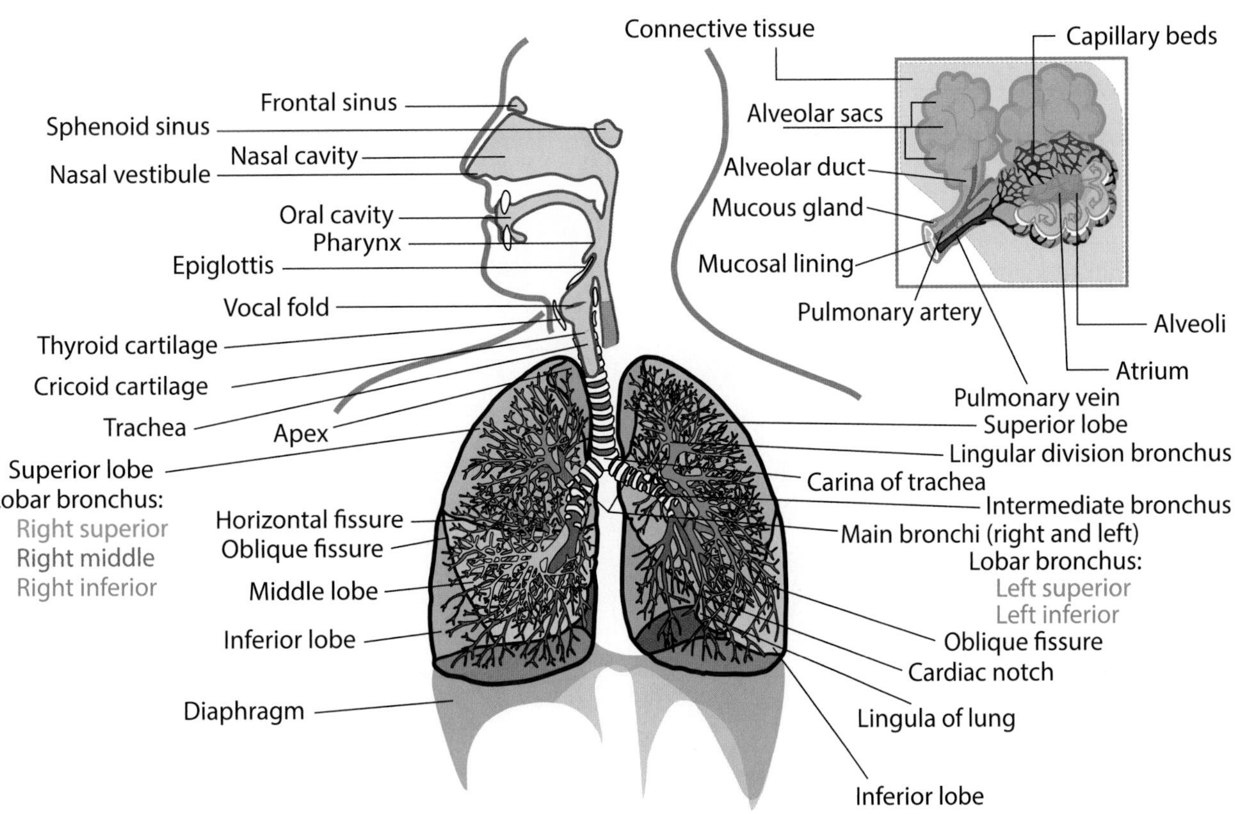
Connective tissue
Capillary beds
Frontal sinus
Sphenoid sinus
Nasal cavity
Nasal vestibule
Alveolar sacs
Alveolar duct
Mucous gland
Mucosal lining
Oral cavity
Pharynx
Epiglottis
Vocal fold
Pulmonary artery
Alveoli
Thyroid cartilage
Atrium
Cricoid cartilage
Pulmonary vein
Trachea
Apex
Superior lobe
Lingular division bronchus
Superior lobe
Carina of trachea
Lobar bronchus:
Right superior
Right middle
Right inferior
Horizontal fissure
Oblique fissure
Intermediate bronchus
Main bronchi (right and left)
Lobar bronchus:
Left superior
Left inferior
Middle lobe
Inferior lobe
Oblique fissure
Cardiac notch
Diaphragm
Lingula of lung
Inferior lobe

Respiratory System — Larynx Anatomy

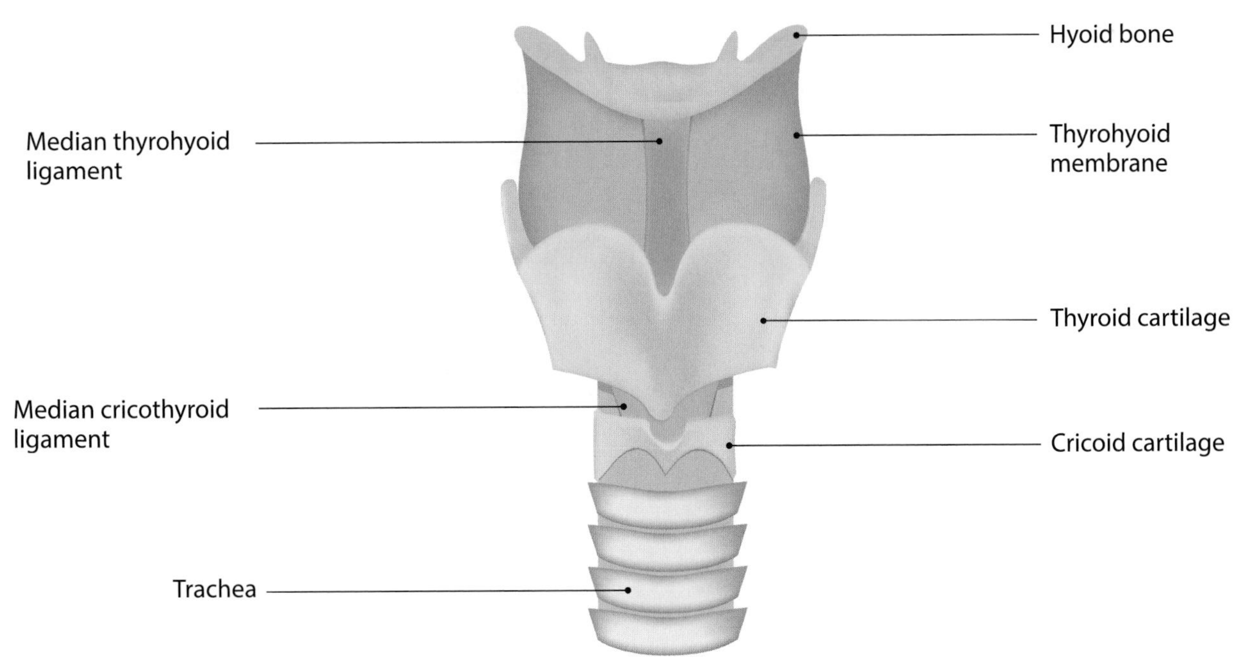
Hyoid bone
Median thyrohyoid ligament
Thyrohyoid membrane
Thyroid cartilage
Median cricothyroid ligament
Cricoid cartilage
Trachea

Respiratory System — Lung Anatomy

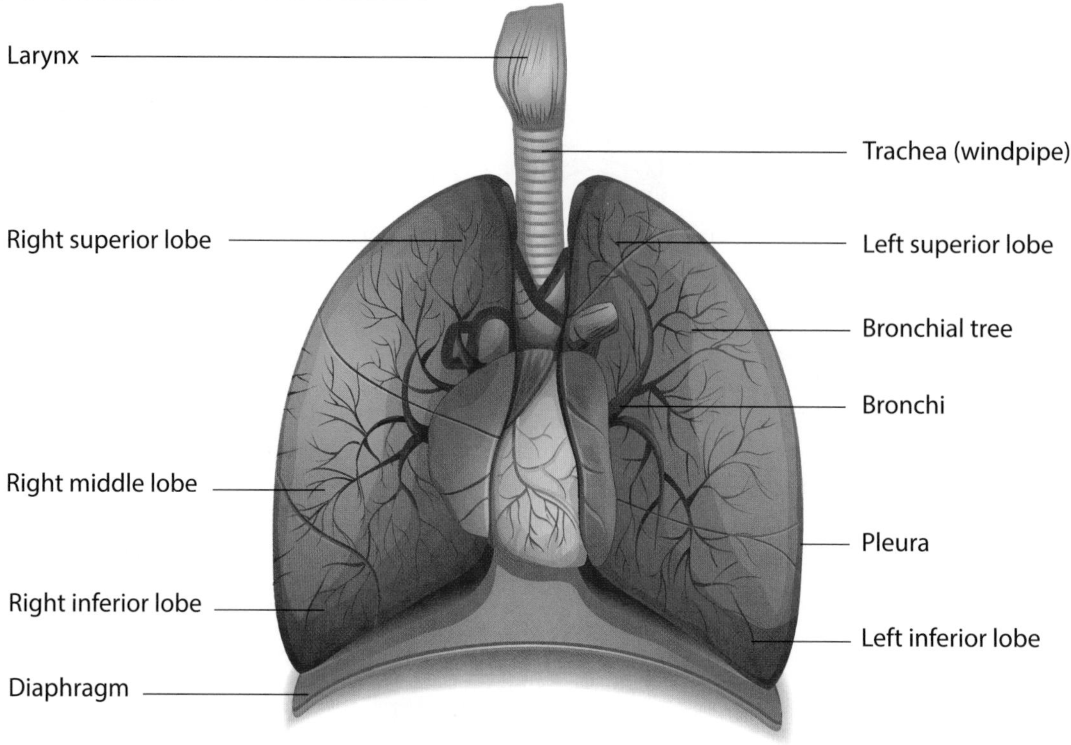
Larynx
Trachea (windpipe)
Right superior lobe
Left superior lobe
Bronchial tree
Bronchi
Right middle lobe
Pleura
Right inferior lobe
Left inferior lobe
Diaphragm

Respiratory System Function

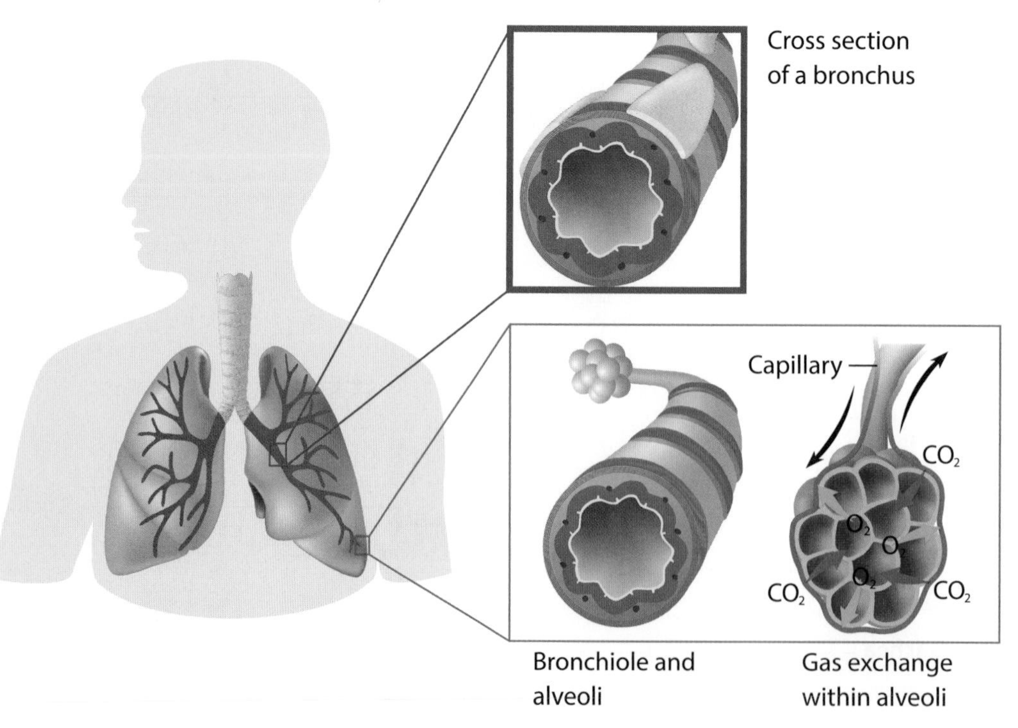
Cross section of a bronchus
Capillary
CO_2
O_2
O_2
O_2
CO_2
CO_2
Bronchiole and alveoli
Gas exchange within alveoli

Respiratory System — Nose Anatomy

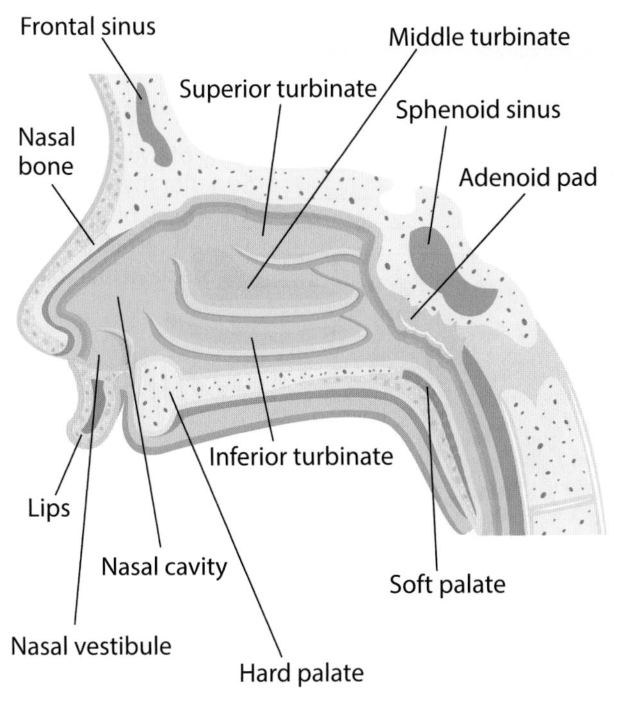
Frontal sinus
Middle turbinate
Superior turbinate
Sphenoid sinus
Nasal bone
Adenoid pad
Inferior turbinate
Lips
Nasal cavity
Soft palate
Nasal vestibule
Hard palate

Respiratory System — Sinus Anatomy

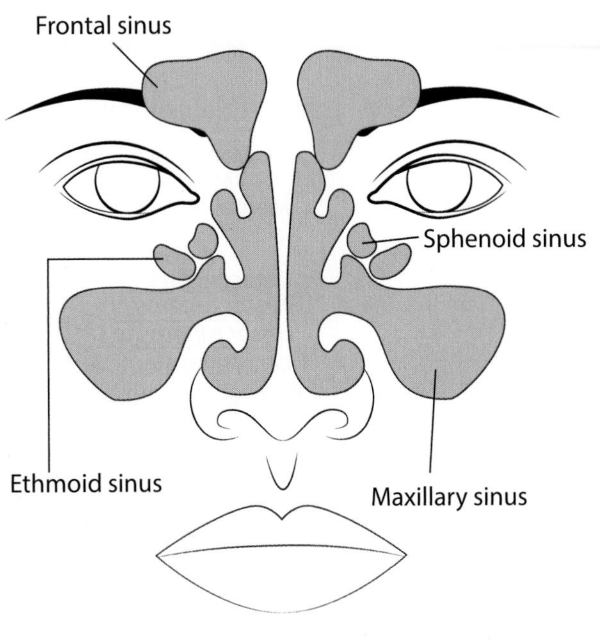
Frontal sinus
Sphenoid sinus
Ethmoid sinus
Maxillary sinus

Respiratory System — Throat Anatomy

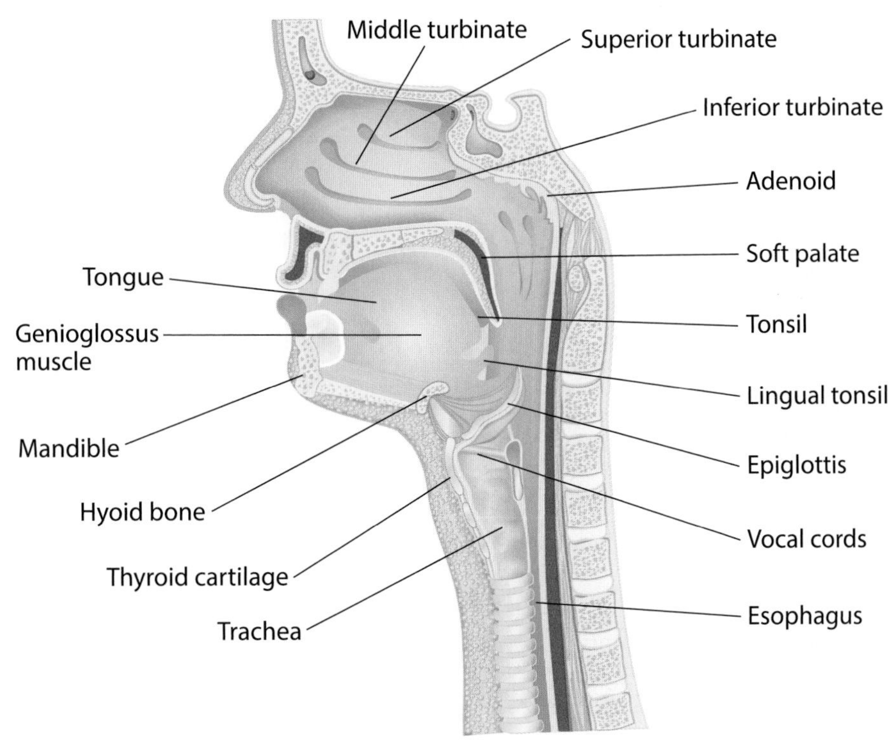
Middle turbinate
Superior turbinate
Inferior turbinate
Adenoid
Soft palate
Tongue
Tonsil
Genioglossus muscle
Lingual tonsil
Mandible
Epiglottis
Hyoid bone
Vocal cords
Thyroid cartilage
Esophagus
Trachea

Skeletal System Anatomy

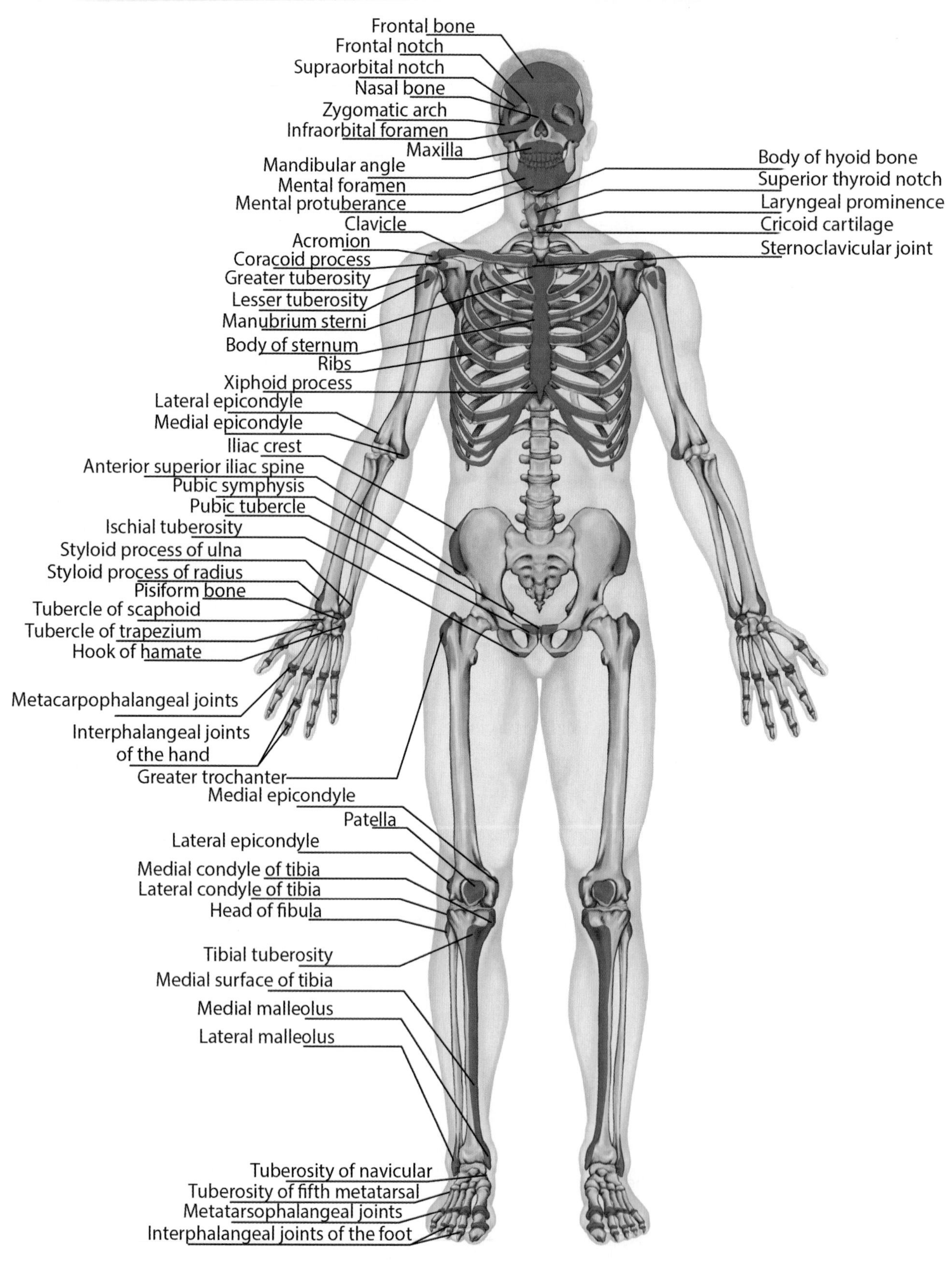
Frontal bone
Frontal notch
Supraorbital notch
Nasal bone
Zygomatic arch
Infraorbital foramen
Maxilla
Mandibular angle
Mental foramen
Mental protuberance
Clavicle
Acromion
Coracoid process
Greater tuberosity
Lesser tuberosity
Manubrium sterni
Body of sternum
Ribs
Xiphoid process
Lateral epicondyle
Medial epicondyle
Iliac crest
Anterior superior iliac spine
Pubic symphysis
Pubic tubercle
Ischial tuberosity
Styloid process of ulna
Styloid process of radius
Pisiform bone
Tubercle of scaphoid
Tubercle of trapezium
Hook of hamate
Metacarpophalangeal joints
Interphalangeal joints of the hand
Greater trochanter
Medial epicondyle
Patella
Lateral epicondyle
Medial condyle of tibia
Lateral condyle of tibia
Head of fibula
Tibial tuberosity
Medial surface of tibia
Medial malleolus
Lateral malleolus
Tuberosity of navicular
Tuberosity of fifth metatarsal
Metatarsophalangeal joints
Interphalangeal joints of the foot
Body of hyoid bone
Superior thyroid notch
Laryngeal prominence
Cricoid cartilage
Sternoclavicular joint

Skeletal System — Bone Structure

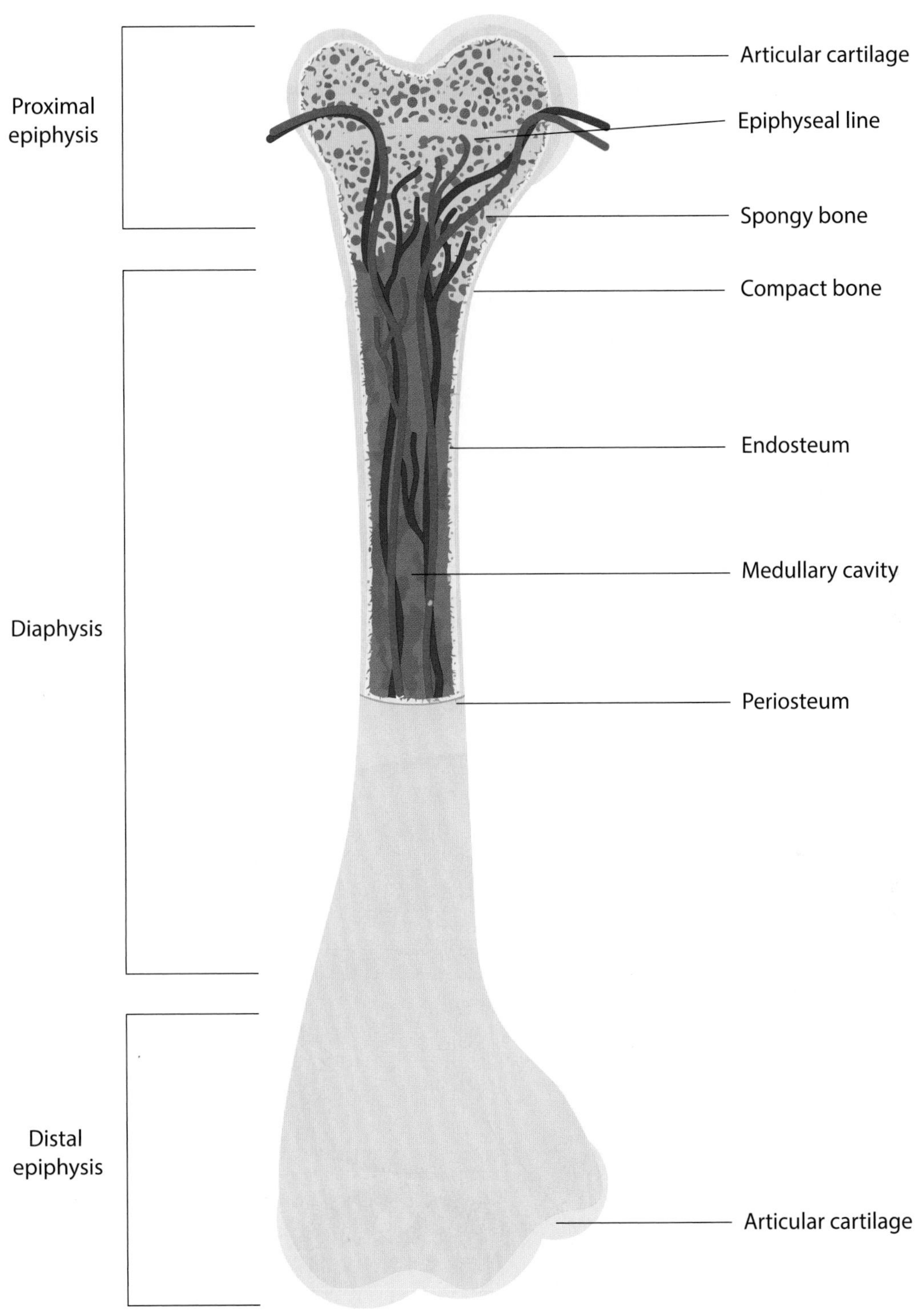
Proximal epiphysis
Diaphysis
Distal epiphysis
Articular cartilage
Epiphyseal line
Spongy bone
Compact bone
Endosteum
Medullary cavity
Periosteum
Articular cartilage

Skeletal System — Skull

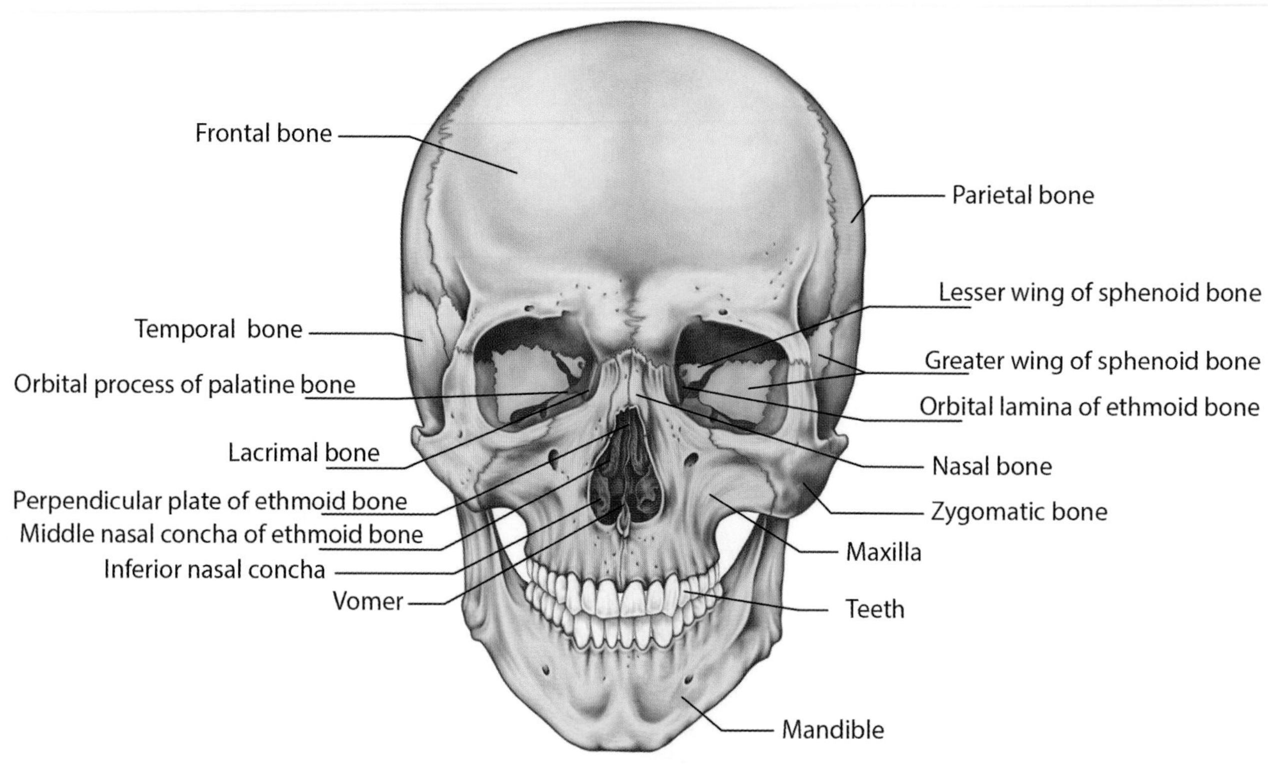
Frontal bone
Parietal bone
Lesser wing of sphenoid bone
Temporal bone
Greater wing of sphenoid bone
Orbital process of palatine bone
Orbital lamina of ethmoid bone
Lacrimal bone
Nasal bone
Perpendicular plate of ethmoid bone
Zygomatic bone
Middle nasal concha of ethmoid bone
Maxilla
Inferior nasal concha
Vomer
Teeth
Mandible

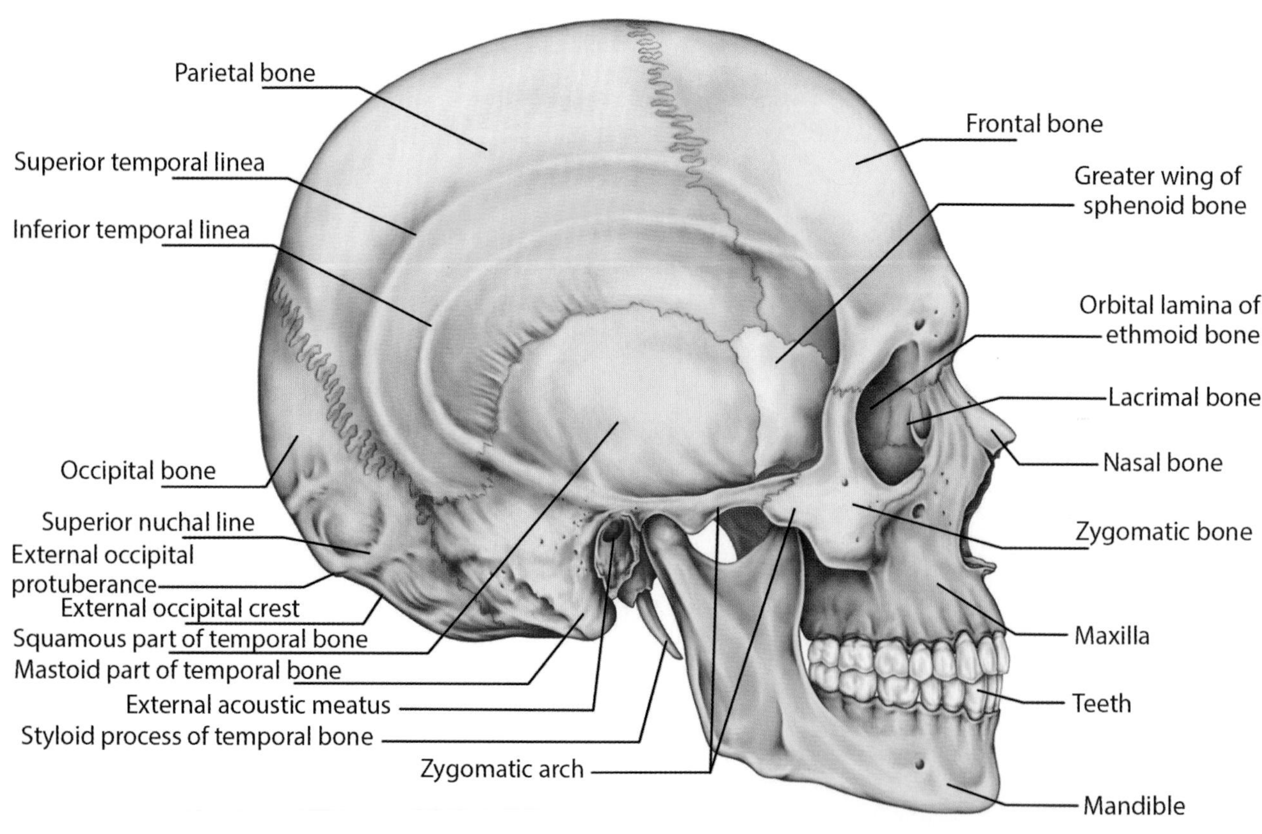
Parietal bone
Frontal bone
Superior temporal linea
Greater wing of sphenoid bone
Inferior temporal linea
Orbital lamina of ethmoid bone
Lacrimal bone
Occipital bone
Nasal bone
Superior nuchal line
Zygomatic bone
External occipital protuberance
External occipital crest
Squamous part of temporal bone
Maxilla
Mastoid part of temporal bone
Teeth
External acoustic meatus
Styloid process of temporal bone
Zygomatic arch
Mandible

Skeletal System — Cervical, Thoracic, and Lumbar Spine

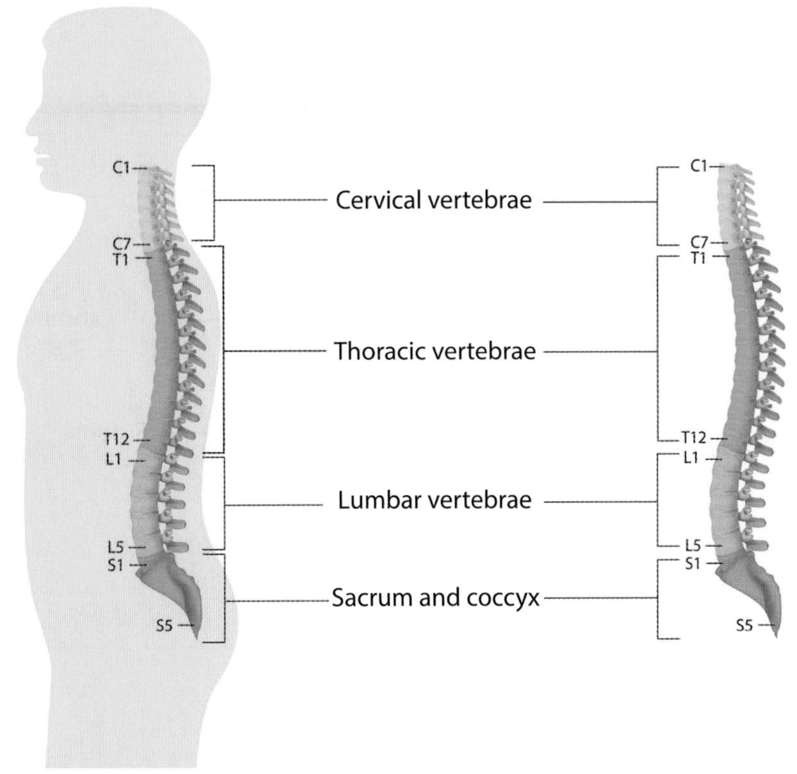
C1
C7
T1
T12
L1
L5
S1
S5
Cervical vertebrae
Thoracic vertebrae
Lumbar vertebrae
Sacrum and coccyx
C1
C7
T1
T12
L1
L5
S1
S5

Skeletal System — Pelvic Girdle

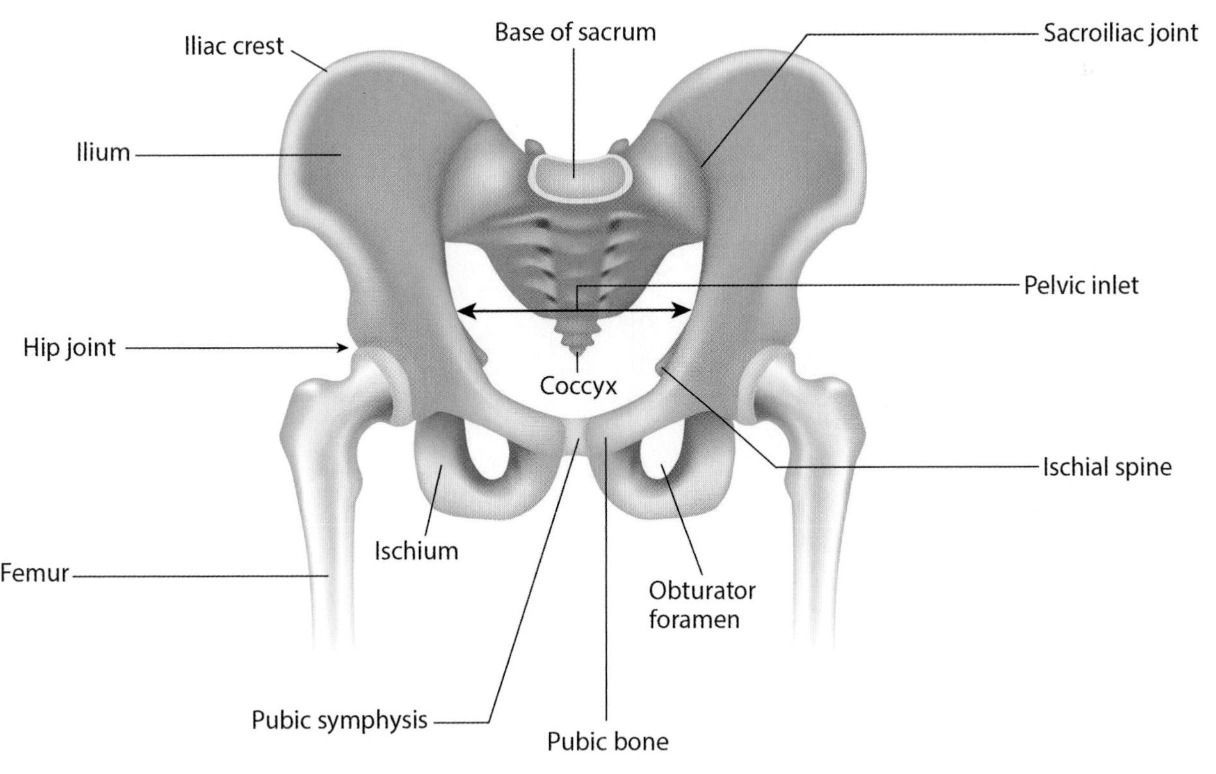
Iliac crest
Base of sacrum
Sacroiliac joint
Ilium
Pelvic inlet
Hip joint
Coccyx
Ischial spine
Ischium
Femur
Obturator foramen
Pubic symphysis
Pubic bone

Muscular System — Shoulder Joint Structure

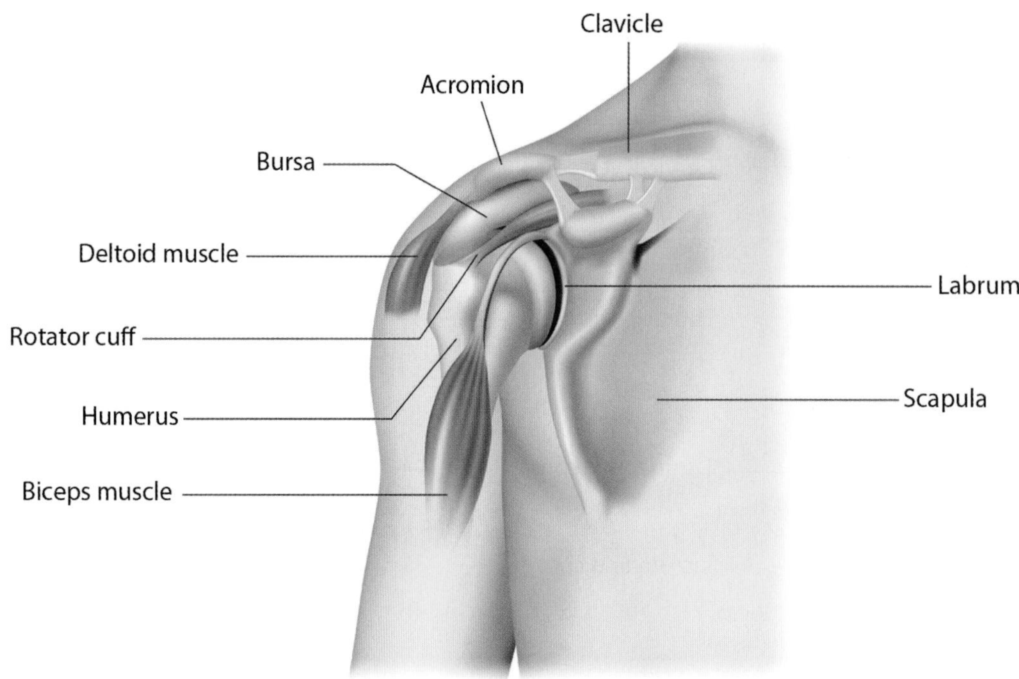
Clavicle
Acromion
Bursa
Deltoid muscle
Labrum
Rotator cuff
Humerus
Scapula
Biceps muscle

Muscular System — Elbow Joint Structure

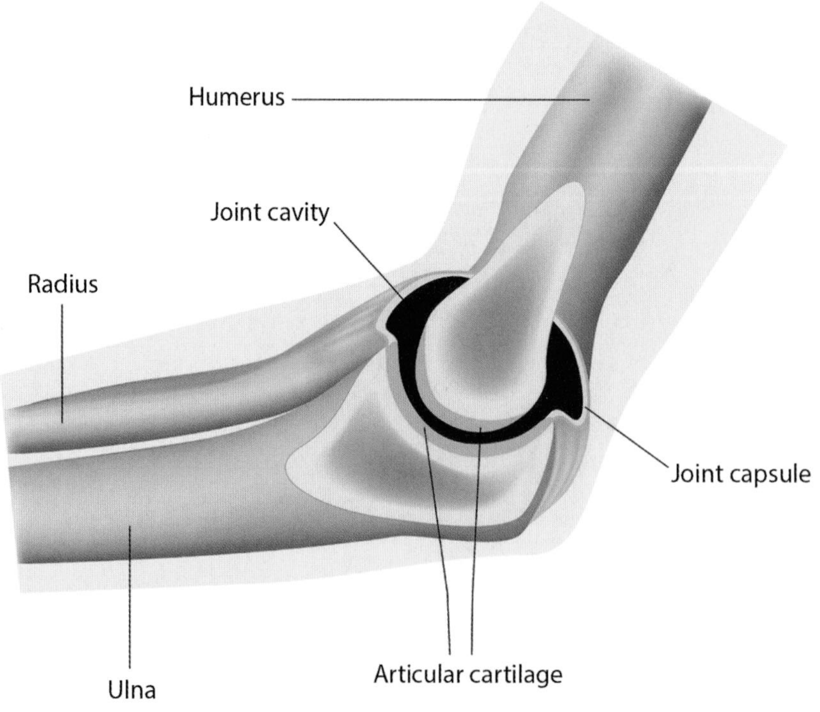
Humerus
Joint cavity
Radius
Joint capsule
Ulna
Articular cartilage

Muscular System — Hand Bones

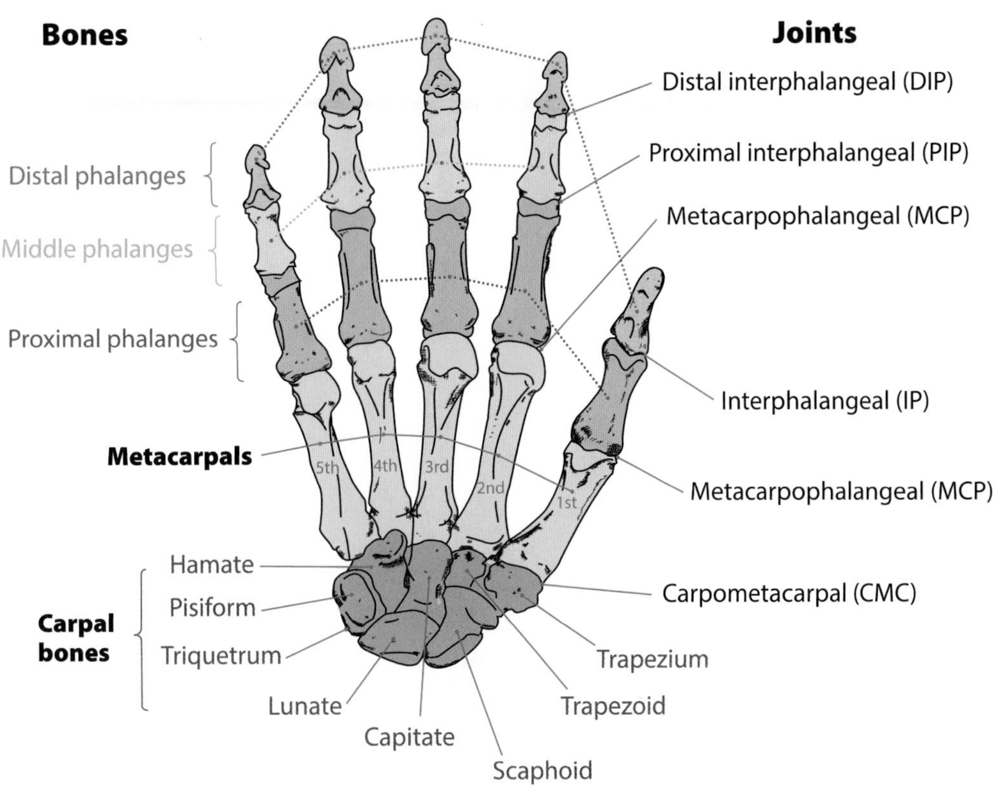
Bones
Joints
Distal interphalangeal (DIP)
Proximal interphalangeal (PIP)
Metacarpophalangeal (MCP)
Distal phalanges
Middle phalanges
Proximal phalanges
Interphalangeal (IP)
Metacarpals
5th
4th
3rd
2nd
1st
Metacarpophalangeal (MCP)
Hamate
Pisiform
Carpal bones
Triquetrum
Lunate
Capitate
Scaphoid
Trapezoid
Trapezium
Carpometacarpal (CMC)

Skeletal System — Foot Bones (Right Foot, Lateral View)

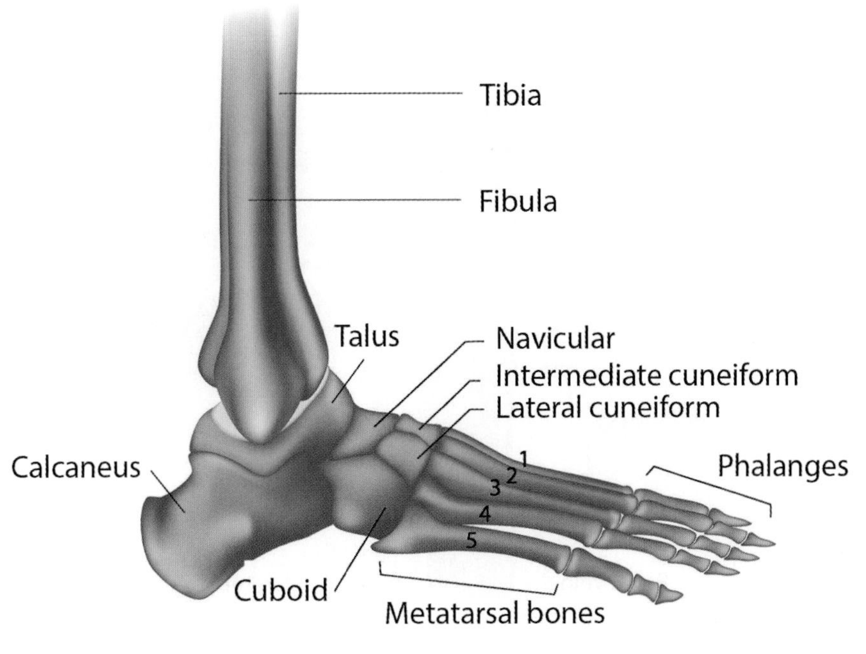
Tibia
Fibula
Talus
Navicular
Intermediate cuneiform
Lateral cuneiform
Calcaneus
1
2
3
4
5
Phalanges
Cuboid
Metatarsal bones

Urinary System Anatomy

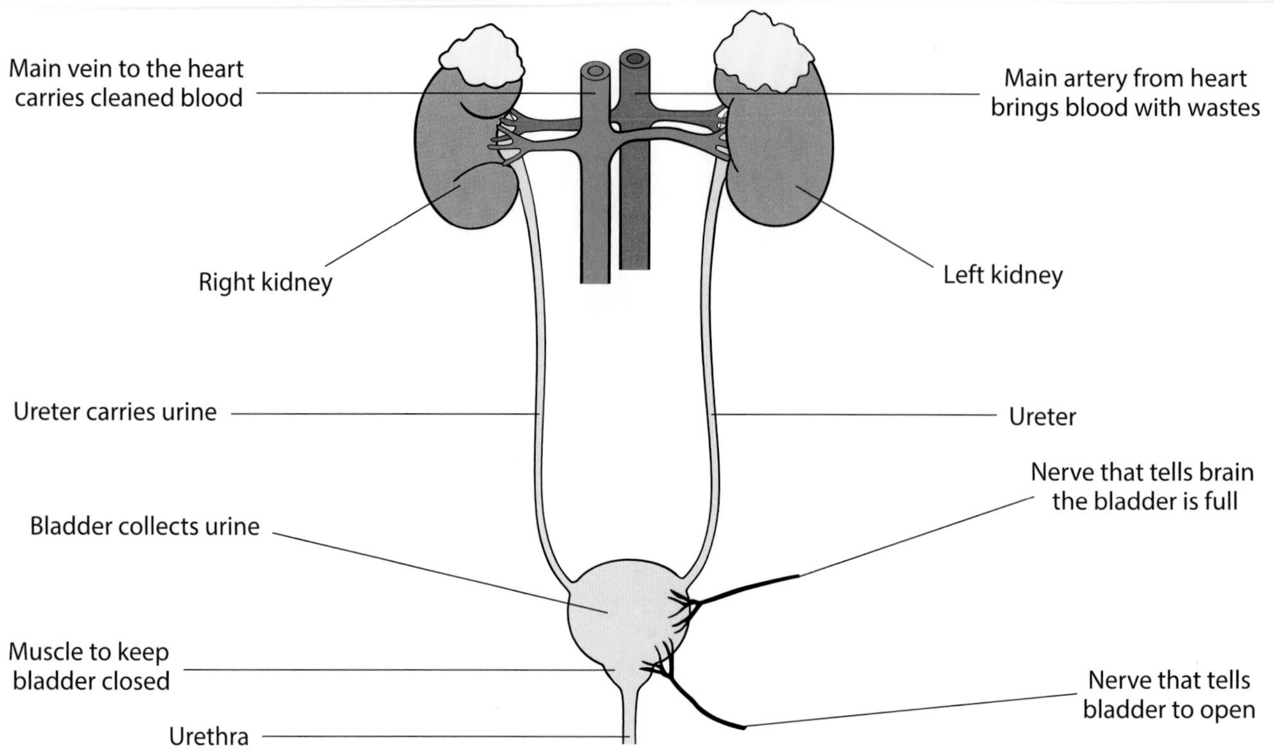
Main vein to the heart carries cleaned blood
Main artery from heart brings blood with wastes
Right kidney
Left kidney
Ureter carries urine
Ureter
Nerve that tells brain the bladder is full
Bladder collects urine
Muscle to keep bladder closed
Nerve that tells bladder to open
Urethra

Urinary System — Kidney Anatomy

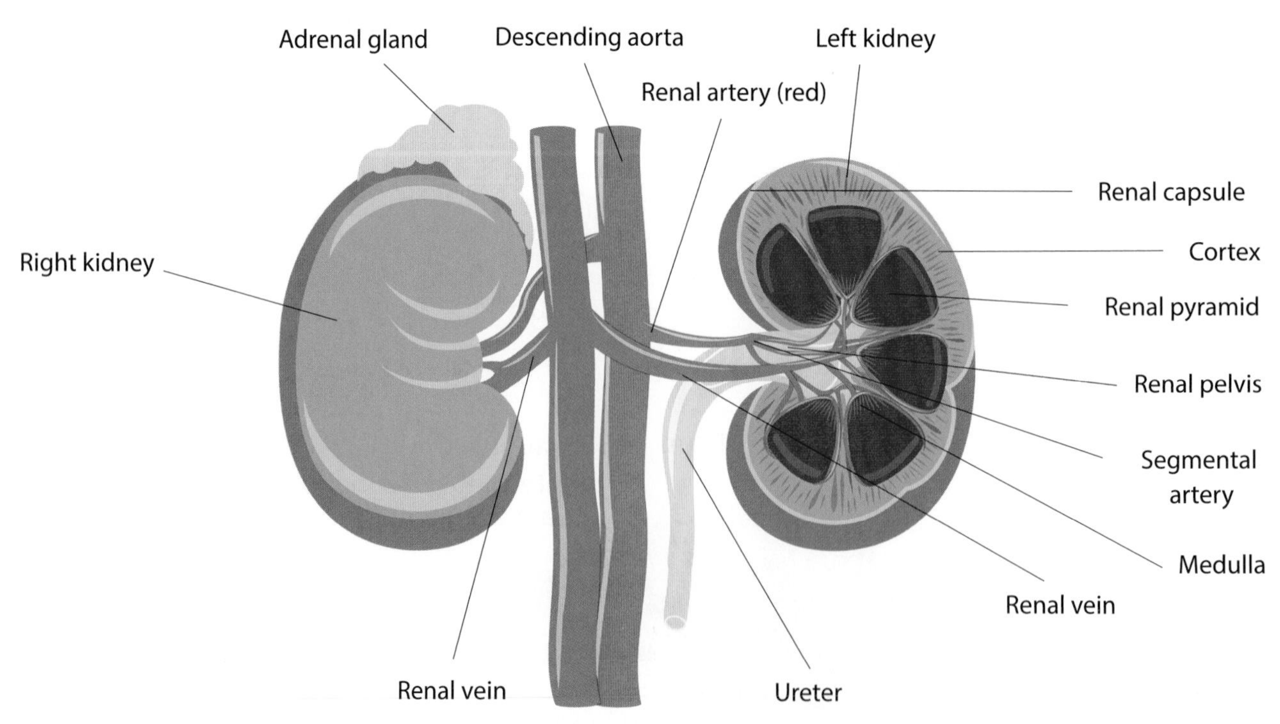
Adrenal gland
Descending aorta
Left kidney
Renal artery (red)
Renal capsule
Right kidney
Cortex
Renal pyramid
Renal pelvis
Segmental artery
Medulla
Renal vein
Renal vein
Ureter

Approach Table

Section 0 - Medical and Surgical
Character 5 - Approach

Approach	5th Character	Definition	Examples
External	X	Procedures performed directly on the skin or mucous membrane and procedures performed indirectly by the application of external force through the skin or mucous membrane	• Cauterization of epistaxis • Reduction of a dislocated shoulder • Destruction of renal calculi with lithotripsy
Open	0	Cutting through the skin or mucous membrane and any other body layers necessary to expose the site of the procedure	• Open reduction and internal fixation of a fracture • Abdominal appendectomy • Open coronary artery bypass graft
Percutaneous	3	Entry, by puncture or minor incision, of instrumentation through the skin or mucous membrane and/or any other body layers necessary to reach the site of the procedure	• Percutaneous paracentesis • Tracheostomy formation with tracheostomy tube placement • Needle biopsy of breast mass
Percutaneous, Endoscopic	4	Entry, by puncture or minor incision, of instrumentation through the skin or mucous membrane and/or any other body layers necessary to reach and visualize the site of the procedure	• Shoulder arthroscopy • Autograft nerve graft to right median nerve • Mapping of left cerebral hemisphere
Via Natural or Artificial Opening	7	Entry of instrumentation through a natural or artificial external opening to reach the site of the procedure	• Placement of a Foley catheter • Endotracheal intubation • Transvaginal cervical cerclage
Via Natural or Artificial Opening, Endoscopic	8	Entry of instrumentation through a natural or artificial external opening to reach and visualize the site of the procedure	• Colonoscopy • Bronchoscopy • Esophagogastroduodenoscopy (EGD)
Via Natural or Artificial Opening, with Percutaneous Endoscopic Assistance	F	Entry of instrumentation through a natural or artificial external opening to reach and visualize the site of the procedure, and entry, by puncture or minor incision, of instrumentation through the skin or mucous membrane and any other body layers necessary to aid in the performance of the procedure	• Resections of the female reproductive system • Laparoscopic-assisted vaginal salpingo-oophorectomy and hysterectomy

This page intentionally left blank

ICD-10-PCS Index

3

3f® (Aortic) Bioprosthesis valve
use Zooplastic Tissue in Heart and Great Vessels

A

Abdominal aortic plexus
use Abdominal Sympathetic Nerve
Abdominal esophagus
use Esophagus, Lower
Abdominohysterectomy
see Resection, Uterus 0UT9
Abdominoplasty
see Alteration, Abdominal Wall 0W0F
see Repair, Abdominal Wall 0WQF
see Supplement, Abdominal Wall 0WUF
Abductor hallucis muscle
use Foot Muscle, Right
use Foot Muscle, Left
AbioCor® Total Replacement Heart
use Synthetic Substitute
Ablation
see Destruction
Abortion
Products of Conception 10A0
Abortifacient 10A07ZX
Laminaria 10A07ZW
Vacuum 10A07Z6
Abrasion
see Extraction
Absolute Pro® Vascular (OTW) Self-Expanding Stent System
use Intraluminal Device
Accessory cephalic vein
use Cephalic Vein, Right
use Cephalic Vein, Left
Accessory obturator nerve
use Lumbar Plexus
Accessory phrenic nerve
use Phrenic Nerve
Accessory spleen
use Spleen
Acculink™ (RX) Carotid Stent System
use Intraluminal Device
Acellular hydrated dermis
use Nonautologous Tissue Substitute
Acetabular cup
use Liner in Lower Joints
Acetabulectomy
see Excision, Lower Bones 0QB
see Resection, Lower Bones 0QT
Acetabulofemoral joint
use Hip Joint, Right
use Hip Joint, Left
Acetabuloplasty
see Repair, Lower Bones 0QQ
see Replacement, Lower Bones 0QR
see Supplement, Lower Bones 0QU
Achilles tendon
use Lower Leg Tendon, Right
use Lower Leg Tendon, Left
Achillorrhaphy
see Repair, Tendons 0LQ
Achillotenotomy, achillotomy
see Division, Tendons 0L8
see Drainage, Tendons 0L9
Acromioclavicular ligament
use Shoulder Bursa and Ligament, Right
use Shoulder Bursa and Ligament, Left
Acromion (process)
use Scapula, Right
use Scapula, Left
Acromionectomy
see Excision, Upper Joints 0RB
see Resection, Upper Joints 0RT
Acromioplasty
see Repair, Upper Joints 0RQ
see Replacement, Upper Joints 0RR
see Supplement, Upper Joints 0RU
Activa PC® neurostimulator
use Stimulator Generator, Multiple Array in 0JH
Activa RC® neurostimulator
use Stimulator Generator, Multiple Array Rechargeable in 0JH
Activa SC® neurostimulator
use Stimulator Generator, Single Array in 0JH
Activities of daily living assessment F02
Activities of daily living treatment F08
ACUITY™ Steerable Lead
use Cardiac Lead, Pacemaker in 02H
use Cardiac Lead, Defibrillator in 02H
Acupuncture
Breast
Anesthesia 8E0H300
No Qualifier 8E0H30Z
Integumentary System
Anesthesia 8E0H300
No Qualifier 8E0H30Z
Adductor brevis muscle
use Upper Leg Muscle, Right
use Upper Leg Muscle, Left
Adductor hallucis muscle
use Foot Muscle, Right
use Foot Muscle, Left
Adductor longus muscle
use Upper Leg Muscle, Right
use Upper Leg Muscle, Left
Adductor magnus muscle
use Upper Leg Muscle, Right
use Upper Leg Muscle, Left
Adenohypophysis
use Pituitary Gland
Adenoidectomy
see Excision, Adenoids 0CBQ
see Resection, Adenoids 0CTQ
Adenoidotomy
see Drainage, Adenoids 0C9Q
Adhesiolysis
see Release
Administration
Blood products *see* Transfusion
Other substance *see* Introduction of substance in or on
Adrenalectomy
see Excision, Endocrine System 0GB
see Resection, Endocrine System 0GT
Adrenalorrhaphy
see Repair, Endocrine System 0GQ
Adrenalotomy
see Drainage, Endocrine System 0G9
Advancement
see Reposition
see Transfer
Advisa (MRI)™
use Pacemaker, Dual Chamber in 0JH
AFX® Endovascular AAA System
use Intraluminal Device
AIGISRx® Antibacterial Envelope
use Anti-Infective Envelope
Alar ligament of axis
use Head and Neck Bursa and Ligament
Alfieri stitch valvuloplasty
see Restriction, Valve, Mitral 02VG
Alimentation
see Introduction of substance in or on
Alteration
Abdominal Wall 0W0F
Ankle Region
Left 0Y0L
Right 0Y0K
Arm
Lower
Left 0X0F
Right 0X0D
Upper
Left 0X09
Right 0X08
Axilla
Left 0X05
Right 0X04
Back
Lower 0W0L
Upper 0W0K
Breast
Bilateral 0H0V
Left 0H0U
Right 0H0T
Buttock
Left 0Y01
Right 0Y00
Chest Wall 0W08
Ear
Bilateral 0902
Left 0901
Right 0900
Elbow Region
Left 0X0C
Right 0X0B
Extremity
Lower
Left 0Y0B
Right 0Y09
Upper
Left 0X07
Right 0X06
Eyelid
Lower
Left 080R
Right 080Q
Upper
Left 080P
Right 080N
Face 0W02
Head 0W00
Jaw
Lower 0W05
Upper 0W04
Knee Region
Left 0Y0G
Right 0Y0F
Leg
Lower
Left 0Y0J
Right 0Y0H
Upper
Left 0Y0D
Right 0Y0C
Lip
Lower 0C01X
Upper 0C00X
Nasal Mucosa and Soft Tissue 090K
Neck 0W06

Alteration — *continued*
Perineum
Female 0W0N
Male 0W0M
Shoulder Region
Left 0X03
Right 0X02
Subcutaneous Tissue and Fascia
Abdomen 0J08
Back 0J07
Buttock 0J09
Chest 0J06
Face 0J01
Lower Arm
Left 0J0H
Right 0J0G
Lower Leg
Left 0J0P
Right 0J0N
Neck
Left 0J05
Right 0J04
Upper Arm
Left 0J0F
Right 0J0D
Upper Leg
Left 0J0M
Right 0J0L
Wrist Region
Left 0X0H
Right 0X0G
Alveolar process of mandible
use Mandible, Right
use Mandible, Left
Alveolar process of maxilla
use Maxilla
Alveolectomy
see Excision, Head and Facial Bones 0NB
see Resection, Head and Facial Bones 0NT
Alveoloplasty
see Repair, Head and Facial Bones 0NQ
see Replacement, Head and Facial Bones 0NR
see Supplement, Head and Facial Bones 0NU
Alveolotomy
see Division, Head and Facial Bones 0N8
see Drainage, Head and Facial Bones 0N9
Ambulatory cardiac monitoring 4A12X45
Amniocentesis
see Drainage, Products of Conception 1090
Amnioinfusion
see Introduction of substance in or on, Products of Conception 3E0E
Amnioscopy 10J08ZZ
Amniotomy
see Drainage, Products of Conception 1090
AMPLATZER® Muscular VSD Occluder
use Synthetic Substitute
Amputation
see Detachment
AMS 800® Urinary Control System
use Artificial Sphincter in Urinary System
Anal orifice
use Anus
Analog radiography
see Plain Radiography
Analog radiology
see Plain Radiography
Anastomosis
see Bypass
Anatomical snuffbox
use Lower Arm and Wrist Muscle, Right
use Lower Arm and Wrist Muscle, Left
Andexanet Alfa, Factor Xa Inhibitor Reversal Agent XW0
AneuRx® AAA Advantage®
use Intraluminal Device
Angiectomy
see Excision, Heart and Great Vessels 02B
see Excision, Upper Arteries 03B
see Excision, Lower Arteries 04B
see Excision, Upper Veins 05B
see Excision, Lower Veins 06B
Angiocardiography
Combined right and left heart *see* Fluoroscopy, Heart, Right and Left B216
Left Heart *see* Fluoroscopy, Heart, Left B215
Right Heart *see* Fluoroscopy, Heart, Right B214
SPY system intravascular fluorescence *see* Monitoring, Physiological Systems 4A1
Angiography
see Plain Radiography, Heart B20
see Fluoroscopy, Heart B21
Angioplasty
see Dilation, Heart and Great Vessels 027
see Repair, Heart and Great Vessels 02Q
see Replacement, Heart and Great Vessels 02R
see Supplement, Heart and Great Vessels 02U
see Dilation, Upper Arteries 037
see Repair, Upper Arteries 03Q
see Replacement, Upper Arteries 03R
see Supplement, Upper Arteries 03U
see Dilation, Lower Arteries 047
see Repair, Lower Arteries 04Q
see Replacement, Lower Arteries 04R
see Supplement, Lower Arteries 04U
Angiorrhaphy
see Repair, Heart and Great Vessels 02Q
see Repair, Upper Arteries 03Q
see Repair, Lower Arteries 04Q
Angioscopy
02JY4ZZ
03JY4ZZ
04JY4ZZ
Angiotensin II
use Synthetic Human Angiotensin II
Angiotripsy
see Occlusion, Upper Arteries 03L
see Occlusion, Lower Arteries 04L
Angular artery
use Face Artery
Angular vein
use Face Vein, Right
use Face Vein, Left
Annular ligament
use Elbow Bursa and Ligament, Right
use Elbow Bursa and Ligament, Left
Annuloplasty
see Repair, Heart and Great Vessels 02Q
see Supplement, Heart and Great Vessels 02U
Annuloplasty ring
use Synthetic Substitute
Anoplasty
see Repair, Anus 0DQQ
see Supplement, Anus 0DUQ
Anorectal junction
use Rectum
Anoscopy 0DJD8ZZ
Ansa cervicalis
use Cervical Plexus
Antabuse therapy HZ93ZZZ
Antebrachial fascia
use Subcutaneous Tissue and Fascia, Right Lower Arm
use Subcutaneous Tissue and Fascia, Left Lower Arm
Anterior (pectoral) lymph node
use Lymphatic, Right Axillary
use Lymphatic, Left Axillary
Anterior cerebral artery
use Intracranial Artery
Anterior cerebral vein
use Intracranial Vein
Anterior choroidal artery
use Intracranial Artery
Anterior circumflex humeral artery
use Axillary Artery, Right
use Axillary Artery, Left
Anterior communicating artery
use Intracranial Artery
Anterior cruciate ligament (ACL)
use Knee Bursa and Ligament, Right
use Knee Bursa and Ligament, Left
Anterior crural nerve
use Femoral Nerve
Anterior facial vein
use Face Vein, Right
use Face Vein, Left
Anterior intercostal artery
use Internal Mammary Artery, Right
use Internal Mammary Artery, Left
Anterior interosseous nerve
use Median Nerve
Anterior lateral malleolar artery
use Anterior Tibial Artery, Right
use Anterior Tibial Artery, Left
Anterior lingual gland
use Minor Salivary Gland
Anterior medial malleolar artery
use Anterior Tibial Artery, Right
use Anterior Tibial Artery, Left
Anterior spinal artery
use Vertebral Artery, Right
use Vertebral Artery, Left
Anterior tibial recurrent artery
use Anterior Tibial Artery, Right
use Anterior Tibial Artery, Left
Anterior ulnar recurrent artery
use Ulnar Artery, Right
use Ulnar Artery, Left
Anterior vagal trunk
use Vagus Nerve
Anterior vertebral muscle
use Neck Muscle, Right
use Neck Muscle, Left
Antigen-free air conditioning
see Atmospheric Control, Physiological Systems 6A0
Antihelix
use External Ear, Right
use External Ear, Left
use External Ear, Bilateral
Antimicrobial envelope
use Anti-Infective Envelope
Antitragus
use External Ear, Right
use External Ear, Left
use External Ear, Bilateral
Antrostomy
see Drainage, Ear, Nose, Sinus 099
Antrotomy
see Drainage, Ear, Nose, Sinus 099
Antrum of highmore
use Maxillary Sinus, Right
use Maxillary Sinus, Left
Aortic annulus
use Aortic Valve
Aortic arch
use Thoracic Aorta, Ascending/Arch
Aortic intercostal artery
use Upper Artery
Aortography
see Plain Radiography, Upper Arteries B30
see Fluoroscopy, Upper Arteries B31
see Plain Radiography, Lower Arteries B40
see Fluoroscopy, Lower Arteries B41

Aortoplasty
see Repair, Aorta, Thoracic, Descending 02QW
see Repair, Aorta, Thoracic, Ascending/Arch 02QX
see Replacement, Aorta, Thoracic, Descending 02RW
see Replacement, Aorta, Thoracic, Ascending/Arch 02RX
see Supplement, Aorta, Thoracic, Descending 02UW
see Supplement, Aorta, Thoracic, Ascending/Arch 02UX
see Repair, Aorta, Abdominal 04Q0
see Replacement, Aorta, Abdominal 04R0
see Supplement, Aorta, Abdominal 04U0
Apical (subclavicular) lymph node
use Lymphatic, Right Axillary
use Lymphatic, Left Axillary
Apneustic center
use Pons
Appendectomy
see Excision, Appendix 0DBJ
see Resection, Appendix 0DTJ
Appendicolysis
see Release, Appendix 0DNJ
Appendicotomy
see Drainage, Appendix 0D9J
Application
see Introduction of substance in or on
Aquablation therapy, prostate XV508A4
Aquapheresis 6A550Z3
Aqueduct of sylvius
use Cerebral Ventricle
Aqueous humour
use Anterior Chamber, Right
use Anterior Chamber, Left
Arachnoid mater, intracranial
use Cerebral Meninges
Arachnoid mater, spinal
use Spinal Meninges
Arcuate artery
use Foot Artery, Right
use Foot Artery, Left
Areola
use Nipple, Right
use Nipple, Left
AROM (artificial rupture of membranes) 10907ZC
Arterial canal (duct)
use Pulmonary Artery, Left
Arterial pulse tracing
see Measurement, Arterial 4A03
Arteriectomy
see Excision, Heart and Great Vessels 02B
see Excision, Upper Arteries 03B
see Excision, Lower Arteries 04B
Arteriography
see Plain Radiography, Heart B20
see Fluoroscopy, Heart B21
see Plain Radiography, Upper Arteries B30
see Fluoroscopy, Upper Arteries B31
see Plain Radiography, Lower Arteries B40
see Fluoroscopy, Lower Arteries B41
Arterioplasty
see Repair, Heart and Great Vessels 02Q
see Replacement, Heart and Great Vessels 02R
see Supplement, Heart and Great Vessels 02U
see Repair, Upper Arteries 03Q
see Replacement, Upper Arteries 03R
see Supplement, Upper Arteries 03U
see Repair, Lower Arteries 04Q
see Replacement, Lower Arteries 04R
see Supplement, Lower Arteries 04U
Arteriorrhaphy
see Repair, Heart and Great Vessels 02Q
see Repair, Upper Arteries 03Q
see Repair, Lower Arteries 04Q
Arterioscopy
see Inspection, Great Vessel 02JY
see Inspection, Artery, Upper 03JY
see Inspection, Artery, Lower 04JY
Arthrectomy
see Excision, Upper Joints 0RB
see Resection, Upper Joints 0RT
see Excision, Lower Joints 0SB
see Resection, Lower Joints 0ST
Arthrocentesis
see Drainage, Upper Joints 0R9
see Drainage, Lower Joints 0S9
Arthrodesis
see Fusion, Upper Joints 0RG
see Fusion, Lower Joints 0SG
Arthrography
see Plain Radiography, Skull and Facial Bones BN0
see Plain Radiography, Non-Axial Upper Bones BP0
see Plain Radiography, Non-Axial Lower Bones BQ0
Arthrolysis
see Release, Upper Joints 0RN
see Release, Lower Joints 0SN
Arthropexy
see Repair, Upper Joints 0RQ
see Reposition, Upper Joints 0RS
see Repair, Lower Joints 0SQ
see Reposition, Lower Joints 0SS
Arthroplasty
see Repair, Upper Joints 0RQ
see Replacement, Upper Joints 0RR
see Supplement, Upper Joints 0RU
see Repair, Lower Joints 0SQ
see Replacement, Lower Joints 0SR
see Supplement, Lower Joints 0SU
Arthroplasty, radial head
see Replacement, Radius, Right 0PRH
see Replacement, Radius, Left 0PRJ
Arthroscopy
see Inspection, Upper Joints 0RJ
see Inspection, Lower Joints 0SJ
Arthrotomy
see Drainage, Upper Joints 0R9
see Drainage, Lower Joints 0S9
Articulating spacer (antibiotic)
use Articulating Spacer in Lower Joints
Artificial anal sphincter (AAS)
use Artificial Sphincter in Gastrointestinal System
Artificial bowel sphincter (neosphincter)
use Artificial Sphincter in Gastrointestinal System
Artificial sphincter
Insertion of device in
Anus 0DHQ
Bladder 0THB
Bladder Neck 0THC
Urethra 0THD
Removal of device from
Anus 0DPQ
Bladder 0TPB
Urethra 0TPD
Revision of device in
Anus 0DWQ
Bladder 0TWB
Urethra 0TWD
Artificial urinary sphincter (AUS)
use Artificial Sphincter in Urinary System
Aryepiglottic fold
use Larynx
Arytenoid cartilage
use Larynx
Arytenoid muscle
use Neck Muscle, Right
use Neck Muscle, Left
Arytenoidectomy
see Excision, Larynx 0CBS
Arytenoidopexy
see Repair, Larynx 0CQS
Ascenda intrathecal catheter
use Infusion Device
Ascending aorta
use Thoracic Aorta, Ascending/Arch
Ascending palatine artery
use Face Artery
Ascending pharyngeal artery
use External Carotid Artery, Right
use External Carotid Artery, Left
Aspiration, fine needle
Fluid or gas *see* Drainage
Tissue biopsy
see Extraction
see Excision
Assessment
Activities of daily living *see* Activities of Daily Living Assessment, Rehabilitation F02
Hearing *see* Hearing Assessment, Diagnostic Audiology F13
Hearing aid *see* Hearing Aid Assessment, Diagnostic Audiology F14
Intravascular perfusion, using indocyanine green (ICG) dye *see* Monitoring, Physiological Systems 4A1
Motor function *see* Motor Function Assessment, Rehabilitation F01
Nerve function *see* Motor Function Assessment, Rehabilitation F01
Speech *see* Speech Assessment, Rehabilitation F00
Vestibular *see* Vestibular Assessment, Diagnostic Audiology F15
Vocational *see* Activities of Daily Living Treatment, Rehabilitation F08
Assistance
Cardiac
Continuous
Balloon Pump 5A02210
Impeller Pump 5A0221D
Other Pump 5A02216
Pulsatile Compression 5A02215
Intermittent
Balloon Pump 5A02110
Impeller Pump 5A0211D
Other Pump 5A02116
Pulsatile Compression 5A02115
Circulatory
Continuous
Hyperbaric 5A05221
Supersaturated 5A0522C
Intermittent
Hyperbaric 5A05121
Supersaturated 5A0512C
Respiratory
24-96 Consecutive Hours
Continuous Negative Airway Pressure 5A09459
Continuous Positive Airway Pressure 5A09457
Intermittent Negative Airway Pressure 5A0945B
Intermittent Positive Airway Pressure 5A09458
No Qualifier 5A0945Z
Continuous, Filtration 5A0920Z

Assistance — *continued*
Respiratory — *continued*
Greater than 96 Consecutive Hours
Continuous Negative Airway Pressure 5A09559
Continuous Positive Airway Pressure 5A09557
Intermittent Negative Airway Pressure 5A0955B
Intermittent Positive Airway Pressure 5A09558
No Qualifier 5A0955Z
Less than 24 Consecutive Hours
Continuous Negative Airway Pressure 5A09359
Continuous Positive Airway Pressure 5A09357
Intermittent Negative Airway Pressure 5A0935B
Intermittent Positive Airway Pressure 5A09358
No Qualifier 5A0935Z
Assurant (cobalt)® stent
use Intraluminal Device
Atherectomy
see Extirpation, Heart and Great Vessels 02C
see Extirpation, Upper Arteries 03C
see Extirpation, Lower Arteries 04C
Atlantoaxial joint
use Cervical Vertebral Joint
Atmospheric control 6A0Z
AtriClip® LAA Exclusion System
use Extraluminal Device
Atrioseptoplasty
see Repair, Heart and Great Vessels 02Q
see Replacement, Heart and Great Vessels 02R
see Supplement, Heart and Great Vessels 02U
Atrioventricular node
use Conduction Mechanism
Atrium dextrum cordis
use Atrium, Right
Atrium pulmonale
use Atrium, Left
Attain Ability® lead
use Cardiac Lead, Pacemaker in 02H
use Cardiac Lead, Defibrillator in 02H
Attain StarFix® (OTW) lead
use Cardiac Lead, Pacemaker in 02H
use Cardiac Lead, Defibrillator in 02H
Audiology, diagnostic
see Hearing Assessment, Diagnostic Audiology F13
see Hearing Aid Assessment, Diagnostic Audiology F14
see Vestibular Assessment, Diagnostic Audiology F15
Audiometry
see Hearing Assessment, Diagnostic Audiology F13
Auditory tube
use Eustachian Tube, Right
use Eustachian Tube, Left
Auerbach's (myenteric) plexus
use Abdominal Sympathetic Nerve
Auricle
use External Ear, Right
use External Ear, Left
use External Ear, Bilateral
Auricularis muscle
use Head Muscle
Autograft
use Autologous Tissue Substitute
Autologous artery graft
use Autologous Arterial Tissue in Heart and Great Vessels
use Autologous Arterial Tissue in Upper Arteries
use Autologous Arterial Tissue in Lower Arteries
use Autologous Arterial Tissue in Upper Veins
use Autologous Arterial Tissue in Lower Veins
Autologous vein graft
use Autologous Venous Tissue in Heart and Great Vessels
use Autologous Venous Tissue in Upper Arteries
use Autologous Venous Tissue in Lower Arteries
use Autologous Venous Tissue in Upper Veins
use Autologous Venous Tissue in Lower Veins
Autotransfusion
see Transfusion
Autotransplant
Adrenal tissue *see* Reposition, Endocrine System 0GS
Kidney *see* Reposition, Urinary System 0TS
Pancreatic tissue *see* Reposition, Pancreas 0FSG
Parathyroid tissue *see* Reposition, Endocrine System 0GS
Thyroid tissue *see* Reposition, Endocrine System 0GS
Tooth *see* Reattachment, Mouth and Throat 0CM
Avulsion
see Extraction
Axial lumbar interbody fusion system
use Interbody Fusion Device in Lower Joints
AxiaLIF® System
use Interbody Fusion Device in Lower Joints
Axicabtagene Ciloeucel
use Engineered Autologous Chimeric Antigen Receptor T-cell Immunotherapy
Axillary fascia
use Subcutaneous Tissue and Fascia, Right Upper Arm
use Subcutaneous Tissue and Fascia, Left Upper Arm
Axillary nerve
use Brachial Plexus

B

BAK/C® Interbody Cervical Fusion System
use Interbody Fusion Device in Upper Joints
BAL (bronchial alveolar lavage), diagnostic
see Drainage, Respiratory System 0B9
Balanoplasty
see Repair, Penis 0VQS
see Supplement, Penis 0VUS
Balloon atrial septostomy (BAS) 02163Z7
Balloon pump
Continuous, Output 5A02210
Intermittent, Output 5A02110
Bandage, elastic
see Compression
Banding
see Occlusion
see Restriction
Banding, esophageal varices
see Occlusion, Vein, Esophageal 06L3
Banding, laparoscopic (adjustable) gastric
Initial procedure 0DV64CZ
Surgical correction *see* Revision of device in, Stomach 0DW6
Bard® Composix® (E/X)(LP) mesh
use Synthetic Substitute
Bard® Composix® Kugel® patch
use Synthetic Substitute
Bard® Dulex™ mesh
use Synthetic Substitute
Bard® Ventralex™ hernia patch
use Synthetic Substitute
Barium swallow
see Fluoroscopy, Gastrointestinal System BD1
Baroreflex Activation Therapy® (BAT®)
use Stimulator Lead in Upper Arteries
use Stimulator Generator in Subcutaneous Tissue and Fascia
Bartholin's (greater vestibular) gland
use Vestibular Gland
Basal (internal) cerebral vein
use Intracranial Vein
Basal metabolic rate (BMR)
see Measurement, Physiological Systems 4A0Z
Basal nuclei
use Basal Ganglia
Base of tongue
use Pharynx
Basilar artery
use Intracranial Artery
Basis pontis
use Pons
Beam radiation
Abdomen DW03
Intraoperative DW033Z0
Adrenal Gland DG02
Intraoperative DG023Z0
Bile Ducts DF02
Intraoperative DF023Z0
Bladder DT02
Intraoperative DT023Z0
Bone
Other DP0C
Intraoperative DP0C3Z0
Bone Marrow D700
Intraoperative D7003Z0
Brain D000
Intraoperative D0003Z0
Brain Stem D001
Intraoperative D0013Z0
Breast
Left DM00
Intraoperative DM003Z0
Right DM01
Intraoperative DM013Z0
Bronchus DB01
Intraoperative DB013Z0
Cervix DU01
Intraoperative DU013Z0
Chest DW02
Intraoperative DW023Z0
Chest Wall DB07
Intraoperative DB073Z0
Colon DD05
Intraoperative DD053Z0
Diaphragm DB08
Intraoperative DB083Z0
Duodenum DD02
Intraoperative DD023Z0
Ear D900
Intraoperative D9003Z0
Esophagus DD00
Intraoperative DD003Z0
Eye D800
Intraoperative D8003Z0
Femur DP09
Intraoperative DP093Z0
Fibula DP0B
Intraoperative DP0B3Z0

Beam radiation — *continued*
Gallbladder DF01
Intraoperative DF013Z0
Gland
Adrenal DG02
Intraoperative DG023Z0
Parathyroid DG04
Intraoperative DG043Z0
Pituitary DG00
Intraoperative DG003Z0
Thyroid DG05
Intraoperative DG053Z0
Glands
Salivary D906
Intraoperative D9063Z0
Head and Neck DW01
Intraoperative DW013Z0
Hemibody DW04
Intraoperative DW043Z0
Humerus DP06
Intraoperative DP063Z0
Hypopharynx D903
Intraoperative D9033Z0
Ileum DD04
Intraoperative DD043Z0
Jejunum DD03
Intraoperative DD033Z0
Kidney DT00
Intraoperative DT003Z0
Larynx D90B
Intraoperative D90B3Z0
Liver DF00
Intraoperative DF003Z0
Lung DB02
Intraoperative DB023Z0
Lymphatics
Abdomen D706
Intraoperative D7063Z0
Axillary D704
Intraoperative D7043Z0
Inguinal D708
Intraoperative D7083Z0
Neck D703
Intraoperative D7033Z0
Pelvis D707
Intraoperative D7073Z0
Thorax D705
Intraoperative D7053Z0
Mandible DP03
Intraoperative DP033Z0
Maxilla DP02
Intraoperative DP023Z0
Mediastinum DB06
Intraoperative DB063Z0
Mouth D904
Intraoperative D9043Z0
Nasopharynx D90D
Intraoperative D90D3Z0
Neck and Head DW01
Intraoperative DW013Z0
Nerve
Peripheral D007
Intraoperative D0073Z0
Nose D901
Intraoperative D9013Z0
Oropharynx D90F
Intraoperative D90F3Z0
Ovary DU00
Intraoperative DU003Z0
Palate
Hard D908
Intraoperative D9083Z0
Soft D909
Intraoperative D9093Z0
Pancreas DF03
Intraoperative DF033Z0

Beam radiation — *continued*
Parathyroid Gland DG04
Intraoperative DG043Z0
Pelvic Bones DP08
Intraoperative DP083Z0
Pelvic Region DW06
Intraoperative DW063Z0
Pineal Body DG01
Intraoperative DG013Z0
Pituitary Gland DG00
Intraoperative DG003Z0
Pleura DB05
Intraoperative DB053Z0
Prostate DV00
Intraoperative DV003Z0
Radius DP07
Intraoperative DP073Z0
Rectum DD07
Intraoperative DD073Z0
Rib DP05
Intraoperative DP053Z0
Sinuses D907
Intraoperative D9073Z0
Skin
Abdomen DH08
Intraoperative DH083Z0
Arm DH04
Intraoperative DH043Z0
Back DH07
Intraoperative DH073Z0
Buttock DH09
Intraoperative DH093Z0
Chest DH06
Intraoperative DH063Z0
Face DH02
Intraoperative DH023Z0
Leg DH0B
Intraoperative DH0B3Z0
Neck DH03
Intraoperative DH033Z0
Skull DP00
Intraoperative DP003Z0
Spinal Cord D006
Intraoperative D0063Z0
Spleen D702
Intraoperative D7023Z0
Sternum DP04
Intraoperative DP043Z0
Stomach DD01
Intraoperative DD013Z0
Testis DV01
Intraoperative DV013Z0
Thymus D701
Intraoperative D7013Z0
Thyroid Gland DG05
Intraoperative DG053Z0
Tibia DP0B
Intraoperative DP0B3Z0
Tongue D905
Intraoperative D9053Z0
Trachea DB00
Intraoperative DB003Z0
Ulna DP07
Intraoperative DP073Z0
Ureter DT01
Intraoperative DT013Z0
Urethra DT03
Intraoperative DT033Z0
Uterus DU02
Intraoperative DU023Z0
Whole Body DW05
Intraoperative DW053Z0
Bedside swallow F00ZJWZ
Berlin Heart ventricular assist device
use Implantable Heart Assist System in Heart and Great Vessels
Bezlotoxumab monoclonal antibody XW0

Biceps brachii muscle
use Upper Arm Muscle, Right
use Upper Arm Muscle, Left
Biceps femoris muscle
use Upper Leg Muscle, Right
use Upper Leg Muscle, Left
Bicipital aponeurosis
use Subcutaneous Tissue and Fascia, Right Lower Arm
use Subcutaneous Tissue and Fascia, Left Lower Arm
Bicuspid valve
use Mitral Valve
Bili light therapy
see Phototherapy, Skin 6A60
Bioactive embolization coil(s)
use Intraluminal Device, Bioactive in Upper Arteries
Biofeedback GZC9ZZZ
Biopsy
see Drainage with qualifier Diagnostic
see Excision with qualifier Diagnostic
see Extraction with qualifier Diagnostic
BiPAP
see Assistance, Respiratory 5A09
Bisection
see Division
Biventricular external heart assist system
use Short-term External Heart Assist System in Heart and Great Vessels
Blepharectomy
see Excision, Eye 08B
see Resection, Eye 08T
Blepharoplasty
see Repair, Eye 08Q
see Replacement, Eye 08R
see Reposition, Eye 08S
see Supplement, Eye 08U
Blepharorrhaphy
see Repair, Eye 08Q
Blepharotomy
see Drainage, Eye 089
Blinatumomab antineoplastic immunotherapy XW0
Block, nerve, anesthetic injection 3E0T3CZ
Blood glucose monitoring system
use Monitoring Device
Blood pressure
see Measurement, Arterial 4A03
BMR (basal metabolic rate)
see Measurement, Physiological Systems 4A0Z
Body of femur
use Femoral Shaft, Right
use Femoral Shaft, Left
Body of fibula
use Fibula, Right
use Fibula, Left
Bone anchored hearing device
use Hearing Device, Bone Conduction in 09H
use Hearing Device in Head and Facial Bones
Bone bank bone graft
use Nonautologous Tissue Substitute
Bone growth stimulator
Insertion of device in
Bone
Facial 0NHW
Lower 0QHY
Nasal 0NHB
Upper 0PHY
Skull 0NH0
Removal of device from
Bone
Facial 0NPW
Lower 0QPY
Nasal 0NPB

Bone growth stimulator — *continued*
Removal of device from — *continued*
Upper 0PPY
Skull 0NP0
Revision of device in
Bone
Facial 0NWW
Lower 0QWY
Nasal 0NWB
Upper 0PWY
Skull 0NW0
Bone marrow transplant
see Transfusion, Circulatory 302
Bone morphogenetic protein 2 (BMP 2)
use Recombinant Bone Morphogenetic Protein
Bone screw (interlocking)(lag)(pedicle)(recessed)
use Internal Fixation Device in Head and Facial Bones
use Internal Fixation Device in Upper Bones
use Internal Fixation Device in Lower Bones
Bony labyrinth
use Inner Ear, Right
use Inner Ear, Left
Bony orbit
use Orbit, Right
use Orbit, Left
Bony vestibule
use Inner Ear, Right
use Inner Ear, Left
Botallo's duct
use Pulmonary Artery, Left
Bovine pericardial valve
use Zooplastic Tissue in Heart and Great Vessels
Bovine pericardium graft
use Zooplastic Tissue in Heart and Great Vessels
BP (blood pressure)
see Measurement, Arterial 4A03
Brachial (lateral) lymph node
use Lymphatic, Right Axillary
use Lymphatic, Left Axillary
Brachialis muscle
use Upper Arm Muscle, Right
use Upper Arm Muscle, Left
Brachiocephalic artery
use Innominate Artery
Brachiocephalic trunk
use Innominate Artery
Brachiocephalic vein
use Innominate Vein, Right
use Innominate Vein, Left
Brachioradialis muscle
use Lower Arm and Wrist Muscle, Right
use Lower Arm and Wrist Muscle, Left
Brachytherapy
Abdomen DW13
Adrenal Gland DG12
Bile Ducts DF12
Bladder DT12
Bone Marrow D710
Brain D010
Brain Stem D011
Breast
Left DM10
Right DM11
Bronchus DB11
Cervix DU11
Chest DW12
Chest Wall DB17
Colon DD15
Diaphragm DB18
Duodenum DD12
Ear D910
Esophagus DD10
Brachytherapy — *continued*
Eye D810
Gallbladder DF11
Gland
Adrenal DG12
Parathyroid DG14
Pituitary DG10
Thyroid DG15
Glands, Salivary D916
Head and Neck DW11
Hypopharynx D913
Ileum DD14
Jejunum DD13
Kidney DT10
Larynx D91B
Liver DF10
Lung DB12
Lymphatics
Abdomen D716
Axillary D714
Inguinal D718
Neck D713
Pelvis D717
Thorax D715
Mediastinum DB16
Mouth D914
Nasopharynx D91D
Neck and Head DW11
Nerve, Peripheral D017
Nose D911
Oropharynx D91F
Ovary DU10
Palate
Hard D918
Soft D919
Pancreas DF13
Parathyroid Gland DG14
Pelvic Region DW16
Pineal Body DG11
Pituitary Gland DG10
Pleura DB15
Prostate DV10
Rectum DD17
Sinuses D917
Spinal Cord D016
Spleen D712
Stomach DD11
Testis DV11
Thymus D711
Thyroid Gland DG15
Tongue D915
Trachea DB10
Ureter DT11
Urethra DT13
Uterus DU12
Brachytherapy seeds
use Radioactive Element
Broad ligament
use Uterine Supporting Structure
Bronchial artery
use Upper Artery
Bronchography
see Plain Radiography, Respiratory System BB0
see Fluoroscopy, Respiratory System BB1
Bronchoplasty
see Repair, Respiratory System 0BQ
see Supplement, Respiratory System 0BU
Bronchorrhaphy
see Repair, Respiratory System 0BQ
Bronchoscopy 0BJ08ZZ
Bronchotomy
see Drainage, Respiratory System 0B9
Bronchus intermedius
use Main Bronchus, Right
BRYAN® Cervical Disc System
use Synthetic Substitute
Buccal gland
use Buccal Mucosa
Buccinator lymph node
use Lymphatic, Head
Buccinator muscle
use Facial Muscle
Buckling, scleral with implant
see Supplement, Eye 08U
Bulbospongiosus muscle
use Perineum Muscle
Bulbourethral (Cowper's) gland
use Urethra
Bundle of His
use Conduction Mechanism
Bundle of Kent
use Conduction Mechanism
Bunionectomy
see Excision, Lower Bones 0QB
Bursectomy
see Excision, Bursae and Ligaments 0MB
see Resection, Bursae and Ligaments 0MT
Bursocentesis
see Drainage, Bursae and Ligaments 0M9
Bursography
see Plain Radiography, Non-Axial Upper Bones BP0
see Plain Radiography, Non-Axial Lower Bones BQ0
Bursotomy
see Division, Bursae and Ligaments 0M8
see Drainage, Bursae and Ligaments 0M9
BVS 5000 Ventricular Assist Device
use Short-term External Heart Assist System in Heart and Great Vessels
Bypass
Anterior Chamber
Left 08133
Right 08123
Aorta
Abdominal 0410
Thoracic
Ascending/Arch 021X
Descending 021W
Artery
Anterior Tibial
Left 041Q
Right 041P
Axillary
Left 03160
Right 03150
Brachial
Left 03180
Right 03170
Common Carotid
Left 031J0
Right 031H0
Common Iliac
Left 041D
Right 041C
Coronary
Four or More Arteries 0213
One Artery 0210
Three Arteries 0212
Two Arteries 0211
External Carotid
Left 031N0
Right 031M0
External Iliac
Left 041J
Right 041H
Femoral
Left 041L
Right 041K
Foot
Left 041W
Right 041V
Hepatic 0413

Bypass — *continued*
Artery — *continued*
Innominate 03120
Internal Carotid
Left 031L0
Right 031K0
Internal Iliac
Left 041F
Right 041E
Intracranial 031G0
Peroneal
Left 041U
Right 041T
Popliteal
Left 041N
Right 041M
Posterior Tibial
Left 041S
Right 041R
Pulmonary
Left 021R
Right 021Q
Pulmonary Trunk 021P
Radial
Left 031C0
Right 031B0
Splenic 0414
Subclavian
Left 03140
Right 03130
Temporal
Left 031T0
Right 031S0
Ulnar
Left 031A0
Right 03190
Atrium
Left 0217
Right 0216
Bladder 0T1B
Cavity, Cranial 0W110J
Cecum 0D1H
Cerebral Ventricle 0016
Colon
Ascending 0D1K
Descending 0D1M
Sigmoid 0D1N
Transverse 0D1L
Duct
Common Bile 0F19
Cystic 0F18
Hepatic
Common 0F17
Left 0F16
Right 0F15
Lacrimal
Left 081Y
Right 081X
Pancreatic 0F1D
Accessory 0F1F
Duodenum 0D19
Ear
Left 091E0
Right 091D0
Esophagus 0D15
Lower 0D13
Middle 0D12
Upper 0D11
Fallopian Tube
Left 0U16
Right 0U15
Gallbladder 0F14
Ileum 0D1B
Jejunum 0D1A
Kidney Pelvis
Left 0T14
Right 0T13

Bypass — *continued*
Pancreas 0F1G
Pelvic Cavity 0W1J
Peritoneal Cavity 0W1G
Pleural Cavity
Left 0W1B
Right 0W19
Spinal Canal 001U
Stomach 0D16
Trachea 0B11
Ureter
Left 0T17
Right 0T16
Ureters, Bilateral 0T18
Vas Deferens
Bilateral 0V1Q
Left 0V1P
Right 0V1N
Vein
Axillary
Left 0518
Right 0517
Azygos 0510
Basilic
Left 051C
Right 051B
Brachial
Left 051A
Right 0519
Cephalic
Left 051F
Right 051D
Colic 0617
Common Iliac
Left 061D
Right 061C
Esophageal 0613
External Iliac
Left 061G
Right 061F
External Jugular
Left 051Q
Right 051P
Face
Left 051V
Right 051T
Femoral
Left 061N
Right 061M
Foot
Left 061V
Right 061T
Gastric 0612
Hand
Left 051H
Right 051G
Hemiazygos 0511
Hepatic 0614
Hypogastric
Left 061J
Right 061H
Inferior Mesenteric 0616
Innominate
Left 0514
Right 0513
Internal Jugular
Left 051N
Right 051M
Intracranial 051L
Portal 0618
Renal
Left 061B
Right 0619
Saphenous
Left 061Q
Right 061P
Splenic 0611

Bypass — *continued*
Vein — *continued*
Subclavian
Left 0516
Right 0515
Superior Mesenteric 0615
Vertebral
Left 051S
Right 051R
Vena Cava
Inferior 0610
Superior 021V
Ventricle
Left 021L
Right 021K
Bypass, cardiopulmonary 5A1221Z

C

Caesarean section
see Extraction, Products of Conception 10D0
Calcaneocuboid joint
use Tarsal Joint, Right
use Tarsal Joint, Left
Calcaneocuboid ligament
use Foot Bursa and Ligament, Right
use Foot Bursa and Ligament, Left
Calcaneofibular ligament
use Ankle Bursa and Ligament, Right
use Ankle Bursa and Ligament, Left
Calcaneus
use Tarsal, Right
use Tarsal, Left
Cannulation
see Bypass
see Dilation
see Drainage
see Irrigation
Canthorrhaphy
see Repair, Eye 08Q
Canthotomy
see Release, Eye 08N
Capitate bone
use Carpal, Right
use Carpal, Left
Capsulectomy, lens
see Excision, Eye 08B
Capsulorrhaphy, joint
see Repair, Upper Joints 0RQ
see Repair, Lower Joints 0SQ
Cardia
use Esophagogastric Junction
Cardiac contractility modulation lead
use Cardiac Lead in Heart and Great Vessels
Cardiac event recorder
use Monitoring Device
Cardiac lead
Defibrillator
Atrium
Left 02H7
Right 02H6
Pericardium 02HN
Vein, Coronary 02H4
Ventricle
Left 02HL
Right 02HK
Insertion of device in
Atrium
Left 02H7
Right 02H6
Pericardium 02HN
Vein, Coronary 02H4
Ventricle
Left 02HL
Right 02HK

Cardiac lead — *continued*
Pacemaker
Atrium
Left 02H7
Right 02H6
Pericardium 02HN
Vein, Coronary 02H4
Ventricle
Left 02HL
Right 02HK
Removal of device from, Heart 02PA
Revision of device in, Heart 02WA
Cardiac plexus
use Thoracic Sympathetic Nerve
Cardiac resynchronization defibrillator pulse generator
Abdomen 0JH8
Chest 0JH6
Cardiac resynchronization pacemaker pulse generator
Abdomen 0JH8
Chest 0JH6
Cardiac resynchronization therapy (CRT) lead
use Cardiac Lead, Pacemaker in 02H
use Cardiac Lead, Defibrillator in 02H
Cardiac rhythm related device
Insertion of device in
Abdomen 0JH8
Chest 0JH6
Removal of device from, Subcutaneous Tissue and Fascia, Trunk 0JPT
Revision of device in, Subcutaneous Tissue and Fascia, Trunk 0JWT
Cardiocentesis
see Drainage, Pericardial Cavity 0W9D
Cardioesophageal junction
use Esophagogastric Junction
Cardiolysis
see Release, Heart and Great Vessels 02N
CardioMEMS® pressure sensor
use Monitoring Device, Pressure Sensor in 02H
Cardiomyotomy
see Division, Esophagogastric Junction 0D84
Cardioplegia
see Introduction of substance in or on, Heart 3E08
Cardiorrhaphy
see Repair, Heart and Great Vessels 02Q
Cardioversion 5A2204Z
Caregiver training F0FZ
Caroticotympanic artery
use Internal Carotid Artery, Right
use Internal Carotid Artery, Left
Carotid (artery) sinus (baroreceptor) lead
use Stimulator Lead in Upper Arteries
Carotid glomus
use Carotid Body, Left
use Carotid Body, Right
use Carotid Bodies, Bilateral
Carotid sinus
use Internal Carotid Artery, Right
use Internal Carotid Artery, Left
Carotid sinus nerve
use Glossopharyngeal Nerve
Carotid WALLSTENT® Monorail® Endoprosthesis
use Intraluminal Device
Carpectomy
see Excision, Upper Bones 0PB
see Resection, Upper Bones 0PT
Carpometacarpal ligament
use Hand Bursa and Ligament, Right
use Hand Bursa and Ligament, Left
Casting
see Immobilization
CAT scan
see Computerized Tomography (CT Scan)
Catheterization
see Dilation
see Drainage
see Insertion of device in
see Irrigation
Heart *see* Measurement, Cardiac 4A02
Umbilical vein, for infusion 06H033T
Cauda equina
use Lumbar Spinal Cord
Cauterization
see Destruction
see Repair
Cavernous plexus
use Head and Neck Sympathetic Nerve
CBMA (concentrated bone marrow aspirate)
use Concentrated Bone Marrow Aspirate
CBMA (concentrated bone marrow aspirate) injection, intramuscular XK02303
Cecectomy
see Excision, Cecum 0DBH
see Resection, Cecum 0DTH
Cecocolostomy
see Bypass, Gastrointestinal System 0D1
see Drainage, Gastrointestinal System 0D9
Cecopexy
see Repair, Cecum 0DQH
see Reposition, Cecum 0DSH
Cecoplication
see Restriction, Cecum 0DVH
Cecorrhaphy
see Repair, Cecum 0DQH
Cecostomy
see Bypass, Cecum 0D1H
see Drainage, Cecum 0D9H
Cecotomy
see Drainage, Cecum 0D9H
Ceftazidime-Avibactam anti-infective XW0
Celiac (solar) plexus
use Abdominal Sympathetic Nerve
Celiac ganglion
use Abdominal Sympathetic Nerve
Celiac lymph node
use Lymphatic, Aortic
Celiac trunk
use Celiac Artery
Central axillary lymph node
use Lymphatic, Right Axillary
use Lymphatic, Left Axillary
Central venous pressure
see Measurement, Venous 4A04
Centrimag® Blood Pump
use Short-term External Heart Assist System in Heart and Great Vessels
Cephalogram BN00ZZZ
Ceramic on ceramic bearing surface
use Synthetic Substitute, Ceramic in 0SR
Cerclage
see Restriction
Cerebral aqueduct (sylvius)
use Cerebral Ventricle
Cerebral embolic filtration, dual filter X2A5312
Cerebrum
use Brain
Cervical esophagus
use Esophagus, Upper
Cervical facet joint
use Cervical Vertebral Joint
use Cervical Vertebral Joints, 2 or more
Cervical ganglion
use Head and Neck Sympathetic Nerve
Cervical interspinous ligament
use Head and Neck Bursa and Ligament
Cervical intertransverse ligament
use Head and Neck Bursa and Ligament
Cervical ligamentum flavum
use Head and Neck Bursa and Ligament
Cervical lymph node
use Lymphatic, Right Neck
use Lymphatic, Left Neck
Cervicectomy
see Excision, Cervix 0UBC
see Resection, Cervix 0UTC
Cervicothoracic facet joint
use Cervicothoracic Vertebral Joint
Cesarean section
see Extraction, Products of Conception 10D0
Cesium-131 collagen implant
use Radioactive Element, Cesium-131 Collagen Implant in 00H
Change device in
Abdominal Wall 0W2FX
Back
Lower 0W2LX
Upper 0W2KX
Bladder 0T2BX
Bone
Facial 0N2WX
Lower 0Q2YX
Nasal 0N2BX
Upper 0P2YX
Bone Marrow 072TX
Brain 0020X
Breast
Left 0H2UX
Right 0H2TX
Bursa and Ligament
Lower 0M2YX
Upper 0M2XX
Cavity, Cranial 0W21X
Chest Wall 0W28X
Cisterna Chyli 072LX
Diaphragm 0B2TX
Duct
Hepatobiliary 0F2BX
Pancreatic 0F2DX
Ear
Left 092JX
Right 092HX
Epididymis and Spermatic Cord 0V2MX
Extremity
Lower
Left 0Y2BX
Right 0Y29X
Upper
Left 0X27X
Right 0X26X
Eye
Left 0821X
Right 0820X
Face 0W22X
Fallopian Tube 0U28X
Gallbladder 0F24X
Gland
Adrenal 0G25X
Endocrine 0G2SX
Pituitary 0G20X
Salivary 0C2AX
Head 0W20X
Intestinal Tract
Lower 0D2DXUZ
Upper 0D20XUZ
Jaw
Lower 0W25X
Upper 0W24X
Joint
Lower 0S2YX
Upper 0R2YX

Change device in — *continued*
Kidney 0T25X
Larynx 0C2SX
Liver 0F20X
Lung
Left 0B2LX
Right 0B2KX
Lymphatic 072NX
Thoracic Duct 072KX
Mediastinum 0W2CX
Mesentery 0D2VX
Mouth and Throat 0C2YX
Muscle
Lower 0K2YX
Upper 0K2XX
Nasal Mucosa and Soft Tissue 092KX
Neck 0W26X
Nerve
Cranial 002EX
Peripheral 012YX
Omentum 0D2UX
Ovary 0U23X
Pancreas 0F2GX
Parathyroid Gland 0G2RX
Pelvic Cavity 0W2JX
Penis 0V2SX
Pericardial Cavity 0W2DX
Perineum
Female 0W2NX
Male 0W2MX
Peritoneal Cavity 0W2GX
Peritoneum 0D2WX
Pineal Body 0G21X
Pleura 0B2QX
Pleural Cavity
Left 0W2BX
Right 0W29X
Products of Conception 10207
Prostate and Seminal Vesicles 0V24X
Retroperitoneum 0W2HX
Scrotum and Tunica Vaginalis 0V28X
Sinus 092YX
Skin 0H2PX
Skull 0N20X
Spinal Canal 002UX
Spleen 072PX
Subcutaneous Tissue and Fascia
Head and Neck 0J2SX
Lower Extremity 0J2WX
Trunk 0J2TX
Upper Extremity 0J2VX
Tendon
Lower 0L2YX
Upper 0L2XX
Testis 0V2DX
Thymus 072MX
Thyroid Gland 0G2KX
Trachea 0B21
Tracheobronchial Tree 0B20X
Ureter 0T29X
Urethra 0T2DX
Uterus and Cervix 0U2DXHZ
Vagina and Cul-de-sac 0U2HXGZ
Vas Deferens 0V2RX
Vulva 0U2MX
Change device in or on
Abdominal Wall 2W03X
Anorectal 2Y03X5Z
Arm
Lower
Left 2W0DX
Right 2W0CX
Upper
Left 2W0BX
Right 2W0AX
Back 2W05X
Chest Wall 2W04X
Change device in or on — *continued*
Ear 2Y02X5Z
Extremity
Lower
Left 2W0MX
Right 2W0LX
Upper
Left 2W09X
Right 2W08X
Face 2W01X
Finger
Left 2W0KX
Right 2W0JX
Foot
Left 2W0TX
Right 2W0SX
Genital Tract, Female 2Y04X5Z
Hand
Left 2W0FX
Right 2W0EX
Head 2W00X
Inguinal Region
Left 2W07X
Right 2W06X
Leg
Lower
Left 2W0RX
Right 2W0QX
Upper
Left 2W0PX
Right 2W0NX
Mouth and Pharynx 2Y00X5Z
Nasal 2Y01X5Z
Neck 2W02X
Thumb
Left 2W0HX
Right 2W0GX
Toe
Left 2W0VX
Right 2W0UX
Urethra 2Y05X5Z
Chemoembolization
see Introduction of substance in or on
Chemosurgery, skin 3E00XTZ
Chemothalamectomy
see Destruction, Thalamus 0059
Chemotherapy, infusion for cancer
see Introduction of substance in or on
Chest X-ray
see Plain Radiography, Chest BW03
Chiropractic manipulation
Abdomen 9WB9X
Cervical 9WB1X
Extremities
Lower 9WB6X
Upper 9WB7X
Head 9WB0X
Lumbar 9WB3X
Pelvis 9WB5X
Rib Cage 9WB8X
Sacrum 9WB4X
Thoracic 9WB2X
Choana
use Nasopharynx
Cholangiogram
see Plain Radiography, Hepatobiliary System and Pancreas BF0
see Fluoroscopy, Hepatobiliary System and Pancreas BF1
Cholecystectomy
see Excision, Gallbladder 0FB4
see Resection, Gallbladder 0FT4
Cholecystojejunostomy
see Bypass, Hepatobiliary System and Pancreas 0F1
see Drainage, Hepatobiliary System and Pancreas 0F9
Cholecystopexy
see Repair, Gallbladder 0FQ4
see Reposition, Gallbladder 0FS4
Cholecystoscopy 0FJ44ZZ
Cholecystostomy
see Bypass, Gallbladder 0F14
see Drainage, Gallbladder 0F94
Cholecystotomy
see Drainage, Gallbladder 0F94
Choledochectomy
see Excision, Hepatobiliary System and Pancreas 0FB
see Resection, Hepatobiliary System and Pancreas 0FT
Choledocholithotomy
see Extirpation, Duct, Common Bile 0FC9
Choledochoplasty
see Repair, Hepatobiliary System and Pancreas 0FQ
see Replacement, Hepatobiliary System and Pancreas 0FR
see Supplement, Hepatobiliary System and Pancreas 0FU
Choledochoscopy 0FJB8ZZ
Choledochotomy
see Drainage, Hepatobiliary System and Pancreas 0F9
Cholelithotomy
see Extirpation, Hepatobiliary System and Pancreas 0FC
Chondrectomy
see Excision, Upper Joints 0RB
see Excision, Lower Joints 0SB
Knee *see* Excision, Lower Joints 0SB
Semilunar cartilage *see* Excision, Lower Joints 0SB
Chondroglossus muscle
use Tongue, Palate, Pharynx Muscle
Chorda tympani
use Facial Nerve
Chordotomy
see Division, Central Nervous System and Cranial Nerves 008
Choroid plexus
use Cerebral Ventricle
Choroidectomy
see Excision, Eye 08B
see Resection, Eye 08T
Ciliary body
use Eye, Right
use Eye, Left
Ciliary ganglion
use Head and Neck Sympathetic Nerve
Circle of Willis
use Intracranial Artery
Circumcision 0VTTXZZ
Circumflex iliac artery
use Femoral Artery, Right
use Femoral Artery, Left
Clamp and rod internal fixation system (CRIF)
use Internal Fixation Device in Upper Bones
use Internal Fixation Device in Lower Bones
Clamping
see Occlusion
Claustrum
use Basal Ganglia
Claviculectomy
see Excision, Upper Bones 0PB
see Resection, Upper Bones 0PT
Claviculotomy
see Division, Upper Bones 0P8
see Drainage, Upper Bones 0P9
Clipping, aneurysm
see Occlusion using Extraluminal Device
see Restriction using Extraluminal Device

Clitorectomy, clitoridectomy
see Excision, Clitoris 0UBJ
see Resection, Clitoris 0UTJ
Clolar®
use Clofarabine
Closure
see Occlusion
see Repair
Clysis
see Introduction of substance in or on
Coagulation
see Destruction
COALESCE® radiolucent interbody fusion device
use Interbody Fusion Device, Radiolucent Porous in New Technology
CoAxia NeuroFlo catheter
use Intraluminal Device
Cobalt/chromium head and polyethylene socket
use Synthetic Substitute, Metal on Polyethylene in 0SR
Cobalt/chromium head and socket
use Synthetic Substitute, Metal in 0SR
Coccygeal body
use Coccygeal Glomus
Coccygeus muscle
use Trunk Muscle, Right
use Trunk Muscle, Left
Cochlea
use Inner Ear, Right
use Inner Ear, Left
Cochlear implant (CI), multiple channel (electrode)
use Hearing Device, Multiple Channel Cochlear Prosthesis in 09H
Cochlear implant (CI), single channel (electrode)
use Hearing Device, Single Channel Cochlear Prosthesis in 09H
Cochlear implant treatment F0BZ0
Cochlear nerve
use Acoustic Nerve
COGNIS® CRT-D
use Cardiac Resynchronization Defibrillator Pulse Generator in 0JH
COHERE® radiolucent interbody fusion device
use Interbody Fusion Device, Radiolucent Porous in New Technology
Colectomy
see Excision, Gastrointestinal System 0DB
see Resection, Gastrointestinal System 0DT
Collapse
see Occlusion
Collection from
Breast, Breast Milk 8E0HX62
Indwelling Device
Circulatory System
Blood 8C02X6K
Other Fluid 8C02X6L
Nervous System
Cerebrospinal Fluid 8C01X6J
Other Fluid 8C01X6L
Integumentary System, Breast Milk 8E0HX62
Reproductive System, Male, Sperm 8E0VX63
Colocentesis
see Drainage, Gastrointestinal System 0D9
Colofixation
see Repair, Gastrointestinal System 0DQ
see Reposition, Gastrointestinal System 0DS
Cololysis
see Release, Gastrointestinal System 0DN
Colonic Z-Stent®
use Intraluminal Device
Colonoscopy 0DJD8ZZ
Colopexy
see Repair, Gastrointestinal System 0DQ
see Reposition, Gastrointestinal System 0DS
Coloplication
see Restriction, Gastrointestinal System 0DV
Coloproctectomy
see Excision, Gastrointestinal System 0DB
see Resection, Gastrointestinal System 0DT
Coloproctostomy
see Bypass, Gastrointestinal System 0D1
see Drainage, Gastrointestinal System 0D9
Colopuncture
see Drainage, Gastrointestinal System 0D9
Colorrhaphy
see Repair, Gastrointestinal System 0DQ
Colostomy
see Bypass, Gastrointestinal System 0D1
see Drainage, Gastrointestinal System 0D9
Colpectomy
see Excision, Vagina 0UBG
see Resection, Vagina 0UTG
Colpocentesis
see Drainage, Vagina 0U9G
Colpopexy
see Repair, Vagina 0UQG
see Reposition, Vagina 0USG
Colpoplasty
see Repair, Vagina 0UQG
see Supplement, Vagina 0UUG
Colporrhaphy
see Repair, Vagina 0UQG
Colposcopy 0UJH8ZZ
Columella
use Nasal Mucosa and Soft Tissue
Common digital vein
use Foot Vein, Right
use Foot Vein, Left
Common facial vein
use Face Vein, Right
use Face Vein, Left
Common fibular nerve
use Peroneal Nerve
Common hepatic artery
use Hepatic Artery
Common iliac (subaortic) lymph node
use Lymphatic, Pelvis
Common interosseous artery
use Ulnar Artery, Right
use Ulnar Artery, Left
Common peroneal nerve
use Peroneal Nerve
Complete® (SE) stent
use Intraluminal Device
Compression
see Restriction
Abdominal Wall 2W13X
Arm
Lower
Left 2W1DX
Right 2W1CX
Upper
Left 2W1BX
Right 2W1AX
Back 2W15X
Chest Wall 2W14X
Extremity
Lower
Left 2W1MX
Right 2W1LX
Upper
Left 2W19X
Right 2W18X
Face 2W11X
Finger
Left 2W1KX
Compression — *continued*
Finger — *continued*
Right 2W1JX
Foot
Left 2W1TX
Right 2W1SX
Hand
Left 2W1FX
Right 2W1EX
Head 2W10X
Inguinal Region
Left 2W17X
Right 2W16X
Leg
Lower
Left 2W1RX
Right 2W1QX
Upper
Left 2W1PX
Right 2W1NX
Neck 2W12X
Thumb
Left 2W1HX
Right 2W1GX
Toe
Left 2W1VX
Right 2W1UX
Computer assisted procedure
Extremity
Lower
No Qualifier 8E0YXBZ
With Computerized Tomography 8E0YXBG
With Fluoroscopy 8E0YXBF
With Magnetic Resonance Imaging 8E0YXBH
Upper
No Qualifier 8E0XXBZ
With Computerized Tomography 8E0XXBG
With Fluoroscopy 8E0XXBF
With Magnetic Resonance Imaging 8E0XXBH
Head and Neck Region
No Qualifier 8E09XBZ
With Computerized Tomography 8E09XBG
With Fluoroscopy 8E09XBF
With Magnetic Resonance Imaging 8E09XBH
Trunk Region
No Qualifier 8E0WXBZ
With Computerized Tomography 8E0WXBG
With Fluoroscopy 8E0WXBF
With Magnetic Resonance Imaging 8E0WXBH
Computerized Tomography (CT Scan)
Abdomen BW20
Chest and Pelvis BW25
Abdomen and Chest BW24
Abdomen and Pelvis BW21
Airway, Trachea BB2F
Ankle
Left BQ2H
Right BQ2G
Aorta
Abdominal B420
Intravascular Optical Coherence B420Z2Z
Thoracic B320
Intravascular Optical Coherence B320Z2Z
Arm
Left BP2F
Right BP2E

Computerized Tomography (CT Scan) — *continued*
Artery
Celiac B421
Intravascular Optical Coherence B421Z2Z
Common Carotid
Bilateral B325
Intravascular Optical Coherence B325Z2Z
Coronary
Bypass Graft
Multiple B223
Intravascular Optical Coherence B223Z2Z
Multiple B221
Intravascular Optical Coherence B221Z2Z
Internal Carotid
Bilateral B328
Intravascular Optical Coherence B328Z2Z
Intracranial B32R
Intravascular Optical Coherence B32RZ2Z
Lower Extremity
Bilateral B42H
Intravascular Optical Coherence B42HZ2Z
Left B42G
Intravascular Optical Coherence B42GZ2Z
Right B42F
Intravascular Optical Coherence B42FZ2Z
Pelvic B42C
Intravascular Optical Coherence B42CZ2Z
Pulmonary
Left B32T
Intravascular Optical Coherence B32TZ2Z
Right B32S
Intravascular Optical Coherence B32SZ2Z
Renal
Bilateral B428
Intravascular Optical Coherence B428Z2Z
Transplant B42M
Intravascular Optical Coherence B42MZ2Z
Superior Mesenteric B424
Intravascular Optical Coherence B424Z2Z
Vertebral
Bilateral B32G
Intravascular Optical Coherence B32GZ2Z
Bladder BT20
Bone
Facial BN25
Temporal BN2F
Brain B020
Calcaneus
Left BQ2K
Right BQ2J
Cerebral Ventricle B028
Chest, Abdomen and Pelvis BW25
Chest and Abdomen BW24
Cisterna B027
Clavicle
Left BP25
Right BP24
Coccyx BR2F
Colon BD24
Ear B920

Computerized Tomography (CT Scan) — *continued*
Elbow
Left BP2H
Right BP2G
Extremity
Lower
Left BQ2S
Right BQ2R
Upper
Bilateral BP2V
Left BP2U
Right BP2T
Eye
Bilateral B827
Left B826
Right B825
Femur
Left BQ24
Right BQ23
Fibula
Left BQ2C
Right BQ2B
Finger
Left BP2S
Right BP2R
Foot
Left BQ2M
Right BQ2L
Forearm
Left BP2K
Right BP2J
Gland
Adrenal, Bilateral BG22
Parathyroid BG23
Parotid, Bilateral B926
Salivary, Bilateral B92D
Submandibular, Bilateral B929
Thyroid BG24
Hand
Left BP2P
Right BP2N
Hands and Wrists, Bilateral BP2Q
Head BW28
Head and Neck BW29
Heart
Right and Left B226
Intravascular Optical Coherence B226Z2Z
Hepatobiliary System, All BF2C
Hip
Left BQ21
Right BQ20
Humerus
Left BP2B
Right BP2A
Intracranial Sinus B522
Intravascular Optical Coherence B522Z2Z
Joint
Acromioclavicular, Bilateral BP23
Finger
Left BP2DZZZ
Right BP2CZZZ
Foot
Left BQ2Y
Right BQ2X
Hand
Left BP2DZZZ
Right BP2CZZZ
Sacroiliac BR2D
Sternoclavicular
Bilateral BP22
Left BP21
Right BP20
Temporomandibular, Bilateral BN29

Computerized Tomography (CT Scan) — *continued*
Joint — *continued*
Toe
Left BQ2Y
Right BQ2X
Kidney
Bilateral BT23
Left BT22
Right BT21
Transplant BT29
Knee
Left BQ28
Right BQ27
Larynx B92J
Leg
Left BQ2F
Right BQ2D
Liver BF25
Liver and Spleen BF26
Lung, Bilateral BB24
Mandible BN26
Nasopharynx B92F
Neck BW2F
Neck and Head BW29
Orbit, Bilateral BN23
Oropharynx B92F
Pancreas BF27
Patella
Left BQ2W
Right BQ2V
Pelvic Region BW2G
Pelvis BR2C
Chest and Abdomen BW25
Pelvis and Abdomen BW21
Pituitary Gland B029
Prostate BV23
Ribs
Left BP2Y
Right BP2X
Sacrum BR2F
Scapula
Left BP27
Right BP26
Sella Turcica B029
Shoulder
Left BP29
Right BP28
Sinus
Intracranial B522
Intravascular Optical Coherence B522Z2Z
Paranasal B922
Skull BN20
Spinal Cord B02B
Spine
Cervical BR20
Lumbar BR29
Thoracic BR27
Spleen and Liver BF26
Thorax BP2W
Tibia
Left BQ2C
Right BQ2B
Toe
Left BQ2Q
Right BQ2P
Trachea BB2F
Tracheobronchial Tree
Bilateral BB29
Left BB28
Right BB27
Vein
Pelvic (Iliac)
Left B52G
Intravascular Optical Coherence B52GZ2Z
Right B52F

Computerized Tomography (CT Scan) — *continued*
Vein — *continued*
Intravascular Optical Coherence B52FZ2Z
Pelvic (Iliac) Bilateral B52H
Intravascular Optical Coherence B52HZ2Z
Portal B52T
Intravascular Optical Coherence B52TZ2Z
Pulmonary
Bilateral B52S
Intravascular Optical Coherence B52SZ2Z
Left B52R
Intravascular Optical Coherence B52RZ2Z
Right B52Q
Intravascular Optical Coherence B52QZ2Z
Renal
Bilateral B52L
Intravascular Optical Coherence B52LZ2Z
Left B52K
Intravascular Optical Coherence B52KZ2Z
Right B52J
Intravascular Optical Coherence B52JZ2Z
Splanchnic B52T
Intravascular Optical Coherence B52TZ2Z
Vena Cava
Inferior B529
Intravascular Optical Coherence B529Z2Z
Superior B528
Intravascular Optical Coherence B528Z2Z
Ventricle, Cerebral B028
Wrist
Left BP2M
Right BP2L
Concentrated bone marrow aspirate (CBMA) injection, intramuscular XK02303
Concerto® II CRT-D
use Cardiac Resynchronization Defibrillator Pulse Generator in 0JH
Condylectomy
see Excision, Head and Facial Bones 0NB
see Excision, Upper Bones 0PB
see Excision, Lower Bones 0QB
Condyloid process
use Mandible, Right
use Mandible, Left
Condylotomy
see Division, Head and Facial Bones 0N8
see Drainage, Head and Facial Bones 0N9
see Division, Upper Bones 0P8
see Drainage, Upper Bones 0P9
see Division, Lower Bones 0Q8
see Drainage, Lower Bones 0Q9
Condylysis
see Release, Head and Facial Bones 0NN
see Release, Upper Bones 0PN
see Release, Lower Bones 0QN
Conization, cervix
see Excision, Cervix 0UBC
Conjunctivoplasty
see Repair, Eye 08Q
see Replacement, Eye 08R
CONSERVE® PLUS Total Resurfacing Hip System
use Resurfacing Device in Lower Joints
Construction
Auricle, ear *see* Replacement, Ear, Nose, Sinus 09R
Ileal conduit *see* Bypass, Urinary System 0T1
Consulta® CRT-D
use Cardiac Resynchronization Defibrillator Pulse Generator in 0JH
Consulta CRT-P
use Cardiac Resynchronization Pacemaker Pulse Generator in 0JH
Contact radiation
Abdomen DWY37ZZ
Adrenal Gland DGY27ZZ
Bile Ducts DFY27ZZ
Bladder DTY27ZZ
Bone, Other DPYC7ZZ
Brain D0Y07ZZ
Brain Stem D0Y17ZZ
Breast
Left DMY07ZZ
Right DMY17ZZ
Bronchus DBY17ZZ
Cervix DUY17ZZ
Chest DWY27ZZ
Chest Wall DBY77ZZ
Colon DDY57ZZ
Diaphragm DBY87ZZ
Duodenum DDY27ZZ
Ear D9Y07ZZ
Esophagus DDY07ZZ
Eye D8Y07ZZ
Femur DPY97ZZ
Fibula DPYB7ZZ
Gallbladder DFY17ZZ
Gland
Adrenal DGY27ZZ
Parathyroid DGY47ZZ
Pituitary DGY07ZZ
Thyroid DGY57ZZ
Glands, Salivary D9Y67ZZ
Head and Neck DWY17ZZ
Hemibody DWY47ZZ
Humerus DPY67ZZ
Hypopharynx D9Y37ZZ
Ileum DDY47ZZ
Jejunum DDY37ZZ
Kidney DTY07ZZ
Larynx D9YB7ZZ
Liver DFY07ZZ
Lung DBY27ZZ
Mandible DPY37ZZ
Maxilla DPY27ZZ
Mediastinum DBY67ZZ
Mouth D9Y47ZZ
Nasopharynx D9YD7ZZ
Neck and Head DWY17ZZ
Nerve, Peripheral D0Y77ZZ
Nose D9Y17ZZ
Oropharynx D9YF7ZZ
Ovary DUY07ZZ
Palate
Hard D9Y87ZZ
Soft D9Y97ZZ
Pancreas DFY37ZZ
Parathyroid Gland DGY47ZZ
Pelvic Bones DPY87ZZ
Pelvic Region DWY67ZZ
Pineal Body DGY17ZZ
Pituitary Gland DGY07ZZ
Pleura DBY57ZZ
Prostate DVY07ZZ
Radius DPY77ZZ
Rectum DDY77ZZ
Rib DPY57ZZ
Sinuses D9Y77ZZ
Contact radiation — *continued*
Skin
Abdomen DHY87ZZ
Arm DHY47ZZ
Back DHY77ZZ
Buttock DHY97ZZ
Chest DHY67ZZ
Face DHY27ZZ
Leg DHYB7ZZ
Neck DHY37ZZ
Skull DPY07ZZ
Spinal Cord D0Y67ZZ
Sternum DPY47ZZ
Stomach DDY17ZZ
Testis DVY17ZZ
Thyroid Gland DGY57ZZ
Tibia DPYB7ZZ
Tongue D9Y57ZZ
Trachea DBY07ZZ
Ulna DPY77ZZ
Ureter DTY17ZZ
Urethra DTY37ZZ
Uterus DUY27ZZ
Whole Body DWY57ZZ
CONTAK RENEWAL® 3 RF (HE) CRT-D
use Cardiac Resynchronization Defibrillator Pulse Generator in 0JH
Contegra® Pulmonary Valved Conduit
use Zooplastic Tissue in Heart and Great Vessels
Continuous glucose monitoring (CGM) device
use Monitoring Device
Continuous negative airway pressure
24-96 Consecutive Hours, Ventilation 5A09459
Greater than 96 Consecutive Hours, Ventilation 5A09559
Less than 24 Consecutive Hours, Ventilation 5A09359
Continuous positive airway pressure
24-96 Consecutive Hours, Ventilation 5A09457
Greater than 96 Consecutive Hours, Ventilation 5A09557
Less than 24 Consecutive Hours, Ventilation 5A09357
Continuous renal replacement therapy (CRRT) 5A1D90Z
Contraceptive device
Change device in, Uterus and Cervix 0U2DXHZ
Insertion of device in
Cervix 0UHC
Subcutaneous Tissue and Fascia
Abdomen 0JH8
Chest 0JH6
Lower Arm
Left 0JHH
Right 0JHG
Lower Leg
Left 0JHP
Right 0JHN
Upper Arm
Left 0JHF
Right 0JHD
Upper Leg
Left 0JHM
Right 0JHL
Uterus 0UH9
Removal of device from
Subcutaneous Tissue and Fascia
Lower Extremity 0JPW
Trunk 0JPT
Upper Extremity 0JPV
Uterus and Cervix 0UPD

Contraceptive device — *continued*
Revision of device in
Subcutaneous Tissue and Fascia
Lower Extremity 0JWW
Trunk 0JWT
Upper Extremity 0JWV
Uterus and Cervix 0UWD
Contractility modulation device
Abdomen 0JH8
Chest 0JH6
Control, epistaxis
see Control bleeding in, Nasal Mucosa and Soft Tissue 093K
Control bleeding in
Abdominal Wall 0W3F
Ankle Region
Left 0Y3L
Right 0Y3K
Arm
Lower
Left 0X3F
Right 0X3D
Upper
Left 0X39
Right 0X38
Axilla
Left 0X35
Right 0X34
Back
Lower 0W3L
Upper 0W3K
Buttock
Left 0Y31
Right 0Y30
Cavity, Cranial 0W31
Chest Wall 0W38
Elbow Region
Left 0X3C
Right 0X3B
Extremity
Lower
Left 0Y3B
Right 0Y39
Upper
Left 0X37
Right 0X36
Face 0W32
Femoral Region
Left 0Y38
Right 0Y37
Foot
Left 0Y3N
Right 0Y3M
Gastrointestinal Tract 0W3P
Genitourinary Tract 0W3R
Hand
Left 0X3K
Right 0X3J
Head 0W30
Inguinal Region
Left 0Y36
Right 0Y35
Jaw
Lower 0W35
Upper 0W34
Knee Region
Left 0Y3G
Right 0Y3F
Leg
Lower
Left 0Y3J
Right 0Y3H
Upper
Left 0Y3D
Right 0Y3C
Mediastinum 0W3C
Nasal Mucosa and Soft Tissue 093K

Control bleeding in — *continued*
Neck 0W36
Oral Cavity and Throat 0W33
Pelvic Cavity 0W3J
Pericardial Cavity 0W3D
Perineum
Female 0W3N
Male 0W3M
Peritoneal Cavity 0W3G
Pleural Cavity
Left 0W3B
Right 0W39
Respiratory Tract 0W3Q
Retroperitoneum 0W3H
Shoulder Region
Left 0X33
Right 0X32
Wrist Region
Left 0X3H
Right 0X3G
Conus arteriosus
use Ventricle, Right
Conus medullaris
use Lumbar Spinal Cord
Conversion
Cardiac rhythm 5A2204Z
Gastrostomy to jejunostomy feeding device *see* Insertion of device in, Jejunum 0DHA
Cook Biodesign® Fistula Plug(s)
use Nonautologous Tissue Substitute
Cook Biodesign® Hernia Graft(s)
use Nonautologous Tissue Substitute
Cook Biodesign® Layered Graft(s)
use Nonautologous Tissue Substitute
Cook Zenapro™ Layered Graft(s)
use Nonautologous Tissue Substitute
Cook Zenith AAA endovascular graft
use Intraluminal Device, Branched or Fenestrated, One or Two Arteries in 04V
use Intraluminal Device, Branched or Fenestrated, Three or More Arteries in 04V
use Intraluminal Device
Coracoacromial ligament
use Shoulder Bursa and Ligament, Right
use Shoulder Bursa and Ligament, Left
Coracobrachialis muscle
use Upper Arm Muscle, Right
use Upper Arm Muscle, Left
Coracoclavicular ligament
use Shoulder Bursa and Ligament, Right
use Shoulder Bursa and Ligament, Left
Coracohumeral ligament
use Shoulder Bursa and Ligament, Right
use Shoulder Bursa and Ligament, Left
Coracoid process
use Scapula, Right
use Scapula, Left
Cordotomy
see Division, Central Nervous System and Cranial Nerves 008
Core needle biopsy
see Excision with qualifier Diagnostic
CoreValve™ transcatheter aortic valve
use Zooplastic Tissue in Heart and Great Vessels
Cormet™ Hip Resurfacing System
use Resurfacing Device in Lower Joints
Corniculate cartilage
use Larynx
CoRoent® XL
use Interbody Fusion Device in Lower Joints
Coronary arteriography
see Plain Radiography, Heart B20
see Fluoroscopy, Heart B21

Corox® (OTW) Bipolar Lead
use Cardiac Lead, Pacemaker in 02H
use Cardiac Lead, Defibrillator in 02H
Corpus callosum
use Brain
Corpus cavernosum
use Penis
Corpus spongiosum
use Penis
Corpus striatum
use Basal Ganglia
Corrugator supercilii muscle
use Facial Muscle
Cortical strip neurostimulator lead
use Neurostimulator Lead in Central Nervous System and Cranial Nerves
Costatectomy
see Excision, Upper Bones 0PB
see Resection, Upper Bones 0PT
Costectomy
see Excision, Upper Bones 0PB
see Resection, Upper Bones 0PT
Costocervical trunk
use Subclavian Artery, Right
use Subclavian Artery, Left
Costochondrectomy
see Excision, Upper Bones 0PB
see Resection, Upper Bones 0PT
Costoclavicular ligament
use Shoulder Bursa and Ligament, Right
use Shoulder Bursa and Ligament, Left
Costosternoplasty
see Repair, Upper Bones 0PQ
see Replacement, Upper Bones 0PR
see Supplement, Upper Bones 0PU
Costotomy
see Division, Upper Bones 0P8
see Drainage, Upper Bones 0P9
Costotransverse joint
use Thoracic Vertebral Joint
Costotransverse ligament
use Rib(s) Bursa and Ligament
Costovertebral joint
use Thoracic Vertebral Joint
Costoxiphoid ligament
use Sternum Bursa and Ligament
Counseling
Family, for substance abuse, Other Family Counseling HZ63ZZZ
Group
12-Step HZ43ZZZ
Behavioral HZ41ZZZ
Cognitive HZ40ZZZ
Cognitive-Behavioral HZ42ZZZ
Confrontational HZ48ZZZ
Continuing Care HZ49ZZZ
Infectious Disease
Post-Test HZ4CZZZ
Pre-Test HZ4CZZZ
Interpersonal HZ44ZZZ
Motivational Enhancement HZ47ZZZ
Psychoeducation HZ46ZZZ
Spiritual HZ4BZZZ
Vocational HZ45ZZZ
Individual
12-Step HZ33ZZZ
Behavioral HZ31ZZZ
Cognitive HZ30ZZZ
Cognitive-Behavioral HZ32ZZZ
Confrontational HZ38ZZZ
Continuing Care HZ39ZZZ
Infectious Disease
Post-Test HZ3CZZZ
Pre-Test HZ3CZZZ
Interpersonal HZ34ZZZ
Motivational Enhancement HZ37ZZZ
Psychoeducation HZ36ZZZ

Counseling — *continued*
- Individual — *continued*
  - Spiritual HZ3BZZZ
  - Vocational HZ35ZZZ
- Mental Health Services
  - Educational GZ60ZZZ
  - Other Counseling GZ63ZZZ
  - Vocational GZ61ZZZ

Countershock, cardiac 5A2204Z

Cowper's (bulbourethral) gland
- *use* Urethra

CPAP (continuous positive airway pressure)
- *see* Assistance, Respiratory 5A09

Craniectomy
- *see* Excision, Head and Facial Bones 0NB
- *see* Resection, Head and Facial Bones 0NT

Cranioplasty
- *see* Repair, Head and Facial Bones 0NQ
- *see* Replacement, Head and Facial Bones 0NR
- *see* Supplement, Head and Facial Bones 0NU

Craniotomy
- *see* Drainage, Central Nervous System and Cranial Nerves 009
- *see* Division, Head and Facial Bones 0N8
- *see* Drainage, Head and Facial Bones 0N9

Creation
- Perineum
  - Female 0W4N0
  - Male 0W4M0
- Valve
  - Aortic 024F0
  - Mitral 024G0
  - Tricuspid 024J0

Cremaster muscle
- *use* Perineum Muscle

Cribriform plate
- *use* Ethmoid Bone, Right
- *use* Ethmoid Bone, Left

Cricoid cartilage
- *use* Trachea

Cricoidectomy
- *see* Excision, Larynx 0CBS

Cricothyroid artery
- *use* Thyroid Artery, Right
- *use* Thyroid Artery, Left

Cricothyroid muscle
- *use* Neck Muscle, Right
- *use* Neck Muscle, Left

Crisis intervention GZ2ZZZZ

CRRT (continuous renal replacement therapy) 5A1D90Z

Crural fascia
- *use* Subcutaneous Tissue and Fascia, Right Upper Leg
- *use* Subcutaneous Tissue and Fascia, Left Upper Leg

Crushing, nerve
- Cranial *see* Destruction, Central Nervous System and Cranial Nerves 005
- Peripheral *see* Destruction, Peripheral Nervous System 015

Cryoablation
- *see* Destruction

Cryotherapy
- *see* Destruction

Cryptorchidectomy
- *see* Excision, Male Reproductive System 0VB
- *see* Resection, Male Reproductive System 0VT

Cryptorchiectomy
- *see* Excision, Male Reproductive System 0VB
- *see* Resection, Male Reproductive System 0VT

Cryptotomy
- *see* Division, Gastrointestinal System 0D8
- *see* Drainage, Gastrointestinal System 0D9

CT scan
- *see* Computerized Tomography (CT Scan)

CT sialogram
- *see* Computerized Tomography (CT Scan), Ear, Nose, Mouth and Throat B92

Cubital lymph node
- *use* Lymphatic, Right Upper Extremity
- *use* Lymphatic, Left Upper Extremity

Cubital nerve
- *use* Ulnar Nerve

Cuboid bone
- *use* Tarsal, Right
- *use* Tarsal, Left

Cuboideonavicular joint
- *use* Tarsal Joint, Right
- *use* Tarsal Joint, Left

Culdocentesis
- *see* Drainage, Cul-de-sac 0U9F

Culdoplasty
- *see* Repair, Cul-de-sac 0UQF
- *see* Supplement, Cul-de-sac 0UUF

Culdoscopy 0UJH8ZZ

Culdotomy
- *see* Drainage, Cul-de-sac 0U9F

Culmen
- *use* Cerebellum

Cultured epidermal cell autograft
- *use* Autologous Tissue Substitute

Cuneiform cartilage
- *use* Larynx

Cuneonavicular joint
- *use* Tarsal Joint, Right
- *use* Tarsal Joint, Left

Cuneonavicular ligament
- *use* Foot Bursa and Ligament, Right
- *use* Foot Bursa and Ligament, Left

Curettage
- *see* Excision
- *see* Extraction

Cutaneous (transverse) cervical nerve
- *use* Cervical Plexus

CVP (central venous pressure)
- *see* Measurement, Venous 4A04

Cyclodiathermy
- *see* Destruction, Eye 085

Cyclophotocoagulation
- *see* Destruction, Eye 085

CYPHER® Stent
- *use* Intraluminal Device, Drug-eluting in Heart and Great Vessels

Cystectomy
- *see* Excision, Bladder 0TBB
- *see* Resection, Bladder 0TTB

Cystocele repair
- *see* Repair, Subcutaneous Tissue and Fascia, Pelvic Region 0JQC

Cystography
- *see* Plain Radiography, Urinary System BT0
- *see* Fluoroscopy, Urinary System BT1

Cystolithotomy
- *see* Extirpation, Bladder 0TCB

Cystopexy
- *see* Repair, Bladder 0TQB
- *see* Reposition, Bladder 0TSB

Cystoplasty
- *see* Repair, Bladder 0TQB
- *see* Replacement, Bladder 0TRB
- *see* Supplement, Bladder 0TUB

Cystorrhaphy
- *see* Repair, Bladder 0TQB

Cystoscopy 0TJB8ZZ

Cystostomy
- *see* Bypass, Bladder 0T1B

Cystostomy tube
- *use* Drainage Device

Cystotomy
- *see* Drainage, Bladder 0T9B

Cystourethrography
- *see* Plain Radiography, Urinary System BT0
- *see* Fluoroscopy, Urinary System BT1

Cystourethroplasty
- *see* Repair, Urinary System 0TQ
- *see* Replacement, Urinary System 0TR
- *see* Supplement, Urinary System 0TU

Cytarabine and Daunorubicin Liposome Antineoplastic XW0

DBS lead
- *use* Neurostimulator Lead in Central Nervous System and Cranial Nerves

DeBakey Left Ventricular Assist Device
- *use* Implantable Heart Assist System in Heart and Great Vessels

Debridement
- Excisional *see* Excision
- Non-excisional *see* Extraction

Decompression, circulatory 6A15

Decortication, lung
- *see* Extirpation, Respiratory System 0BC
- *see* Release, Respiratory System 0BN

Deep brain neurostimulator lead
- *use* Neurostimulator Lead in Central Nervous System and Cranial Nerves

Deep cervical fascia
- *use* Subcutaneous Tissue and Fascia, Right Neck
- *use* Subcutaneous Tissue and Fascia, Left Neck

Deep cervical vein
- *use* Vertebral Vein, Right
- *use* Vertebral Vein, Left

Deep circumflex iliac artery
- *use* External Iliac Artery, Right
- *use* External Iliac Artery, Left

Deep facial vein
- *use* Face Vein, Right
- *use* Face Vein, Left

Deep femoral (profunda femoris) vein
- *use* Femoral Vein, Right
- *use* Femoral Vein, Left

Deep femoral artery
- *use* Femoral Artery, Right
- *use* Femoral Artery, Left

Deep inferior epigastric artery perforator flap
- Replacement
  - Bilateral 0HRV077
  - Left 0HRU077
  - Right 0HRT077
- Transfer
  - Left 0KXG
  - Right 0KXF

Deep palmar arch
- *use* Hand Artery, Right
- *use* Hand Artery, Left

Deep transverse perineal muscle
- *use* Perineum Muscle

Deferential artery
- *use* Internal Iliac Artery, Right
- *use* Internal Iliac Artery, Left

Defibrillator generator
- Abdomen 0JH8
- Chest 0JH6

Defibrotide Sodium anticoagulant XW0

Defitelio®
- *use* Defibrotide Sodium Anticoagulant

Delivery
Cesarean *see* Extraction, Products of Conception 10D0
Forceps *see* Extraction, Products of Conception 10D0
Manually assisted 10E0XZZ
Products of Conception 10E0XZZ
Vacuum assisted *see* Extraction, Products of Conception 10D0
Delta frame external fixator
use External Fixation Device, Hybrid in 0PH
use External Fixation Device, Hybrid in 0PS
use External Fixation Device, Hybrid in 0QH
use External Fixation Device, Hybrid in 0QS
Delta III™ reverse shoulder prosthesis
use Synthetic Substitute, Reverse Ball and Socket in 0RR
Deltoid fascia
use Subcutaneous Tissue and Fascia, Right Upper Arm
use Subcutaneous Tissue and Fascia, Left Upper Arm
Deltoid ligament
use Ankle Bursa and Ligament, Right
use Ankle Bursa and Ligament, Left
Deltoid muscle
use Shoulder Muscle, Right
use Shoulder Muscle, Left
Deltopectoral (infraclavicular) lymph node
use Lymphatic, Right Upper Extremity
use Lymphatic, Left Upper Extremity
Denervation
Cranial nerve *see* Destruction, Central Nervous System and Cranial Nerves 005
Peripheral nerve *see* Destruction, Peripheral Nervous System 015
Dens
use Cervical Vertebra
Densitometry
Plain Radiography
Femur
Left BQ04ZZ1
Right BQ03ZZ1
Hip
Left BQ01ZZ1
Right BQ00ZZ1
Spine
Cervical BR00ZZ1
Lumbar BR09ZZ1
Thoracic BR07ZZ1
Whole BR0GZZ1
Ultrasonography
Elbow
Left BP4HZZ1
Right BP4GZZ1
Hand
Left BP4PZZ1
Right BP4NZZ1
Shoulder
Left BP49ZZ1
Right BP48ZZ1
Wrist
Left BP4MZZ1
Right BP4LZZ1
Denticulate (dentate) ligament
use Spinal Meninges
Depressor anguli oris muscle
use Facial Muscle
Depressor labii inferioris muscle
use Facial Muscle
Depressor septi nasi muscle
use Facial Muscle
Depressor supercilii muscle
use Facial Muscle
Dermabrasion
see Extraction, Skin and Breast 0HD
Dermis
use Skin
Descending genicular artery
use Femoral Artery, Right
use Femoral Artery, Left
Destruction
Acetabulum
Left 0Q55
Right 0Q54
Adenoids 0C5Q
Ampulla of Vater 0F5C
Anal Sphincter 0D5R
Anterior Chamber
Left 08533ZZ
Right 08523ZZ
Anus 0D5Q
Aorta
Abdominal 0450
Thoracic
Ascending/Arch 025X
Descending 025W
Aortic Body 0G5D
Appendix 0D5J
Artery
Anterior Tibial
Left 045Q
Right 045P
Axillary
Left 0356
Right 0355
Brachial
Left 0358
Right 0357
Celiac 0451
Colic
Left 0457
Middle 0458
Right 0456
Common Carotid
Left 035J
Right 035H
Common Iliac
Left 045D
Right 045C
External Carotid
Left 035N
Right 035M
External Iliac
Left 045J
Right 045H
Face 035R
Femoral
Left 045L
Right 045K
Foot
Left 045W
Right 045V
Gastric 0452
Hand
Left 035F
Right 035D
Hepatic 0453
Inferior Mesenteric 045B
Innominate 0352
Internal Carotid
Left 035L
Right 035K
Internal Iliac
Left 045F
Right 045E
Internal Mammary
Left 0351
Right 0350
Intracranial 035G
Lower 045Y
Peroneal
Left 045U
Destruction — *continued*
Artery — *continued*
Right 045T
Popliteal
Left 045N
Right 045M
Posterior Tibial
Left 045S
Right 045R
Pulmonary
Left 025R
Right 025Q
Pulmonary Trunk 025P
Radial
Left 035C
Right 035B
Renal
Left 045A
Right 0459
Splenic 0454
Subclavian
Left 0354
Right 0353
Superior Mesenteric 0455
Temporal
Left 035T
Right 035S
Thyroid
Left 035V
Right 035U
Ulnar
Left 035A
Right 0359
Upper 035Y
Vertebral
Left 035Q
Right 035P
Atrium
Left 0257
Right 0256
Auditory Ossicle
Left 095A
Right 0959
Basal Ganglia 0058
Bladder 0T5B
Bladder Neck 0T5C
Bone
Ethmoid
Left 0N5G
Right 0N5F
Frontal 0N51
Hyoid 0N5X
Lacrimal
Left 0N5J
Right 0N5H
Nasal 0N5B
Occipital 0N57
Palatine
Left 0N5L
Right 0N5K
Parietal
Left 0N54
Right 0N53
Pelvic
Left 0Q53
Right 0Q52
Sphenoid 0N5C
Temporal
Left 0N56
Right 0N55
Zygomatic
Left 0N5N
Right 0N5M
Brain 0050
Breast
Bilateral 0H5V
Left 0H5U

Destruction — *continued*
Breast — *continued*
Right 0H5T
Bronchus
Lingula 0B59
Lower Lobe
Left 0B5B
Right 0B56
Main
Left 0B57
Right 0B53
Middle Lobe, Right 0B55
Upper Lobe
Left 0B58
Right 0B54
Buccal Mucosa 0C54
Bursa and Ligament
Abdomen
Left 0M5J
Right 0M5H
Ankle
Left 0M5R
Right 0M5Q
Elbow
Left 0M54
Right 0M53
Foot
Left 0M5T
Right 0M5S
Hand
Left 0M58
Right 0M57
Head and Neck 0M50
Hip
Left 0M5M
Right 0M5L
Knee
Left 0M5P
Right 0M5N
Lower Extremity
Left 0M5W
Right 0M5V
Perineum 0M5K
Rib(s) 0M5G
Shoulder
Left 0M52
Right 0M51
Spine
Lower 0M5D
Upper 0M5C
Sternum 0M5F
Upper Extremity
Left 0M5B
Right 0M59
Wrist
Left 0M56
Right 0M55
Carina 0B52
Carotid Bodies, Bilateral 0G58
Carotid Body
Left 0G56
Right 0G57
Carpal
Left 0P5N
Right 0P5M
Cecum 0D5H
Cerebellum 005C
Cerebral Hemisphere 0057
Cerebral Meninges 0051
Cerebral Ventricle 0056
Cervix 0U5C
Chordae Tendineae 0259
Choroid
Left 085B
Right 085A
Cisterna Chyli 075L

Destruction — *continued*
Clavicle
Left 0P5B
Right 0P59
Clitoris 0U5J
Coccygeal Glomus 0G5B
Coccyx 0Q5S
Colon
Ascending 0D5K
Descending 0D5M
Sigmoid 0D5N
Transverse 0D5L
Conduction Mechanism 0258
Conjunctiva
Left 085TXZZ
Right 085SXZZ
Cord
Bilateral 0V5H
Left 0V5G
Right 0V5F
Cornea
Left 0859XZZ
Right 0858XZZ
Cul-de-sac 0U5F
Diaphragm 0B5T
Disc
Cervical Vertebral 0R53
Cervicothoracic Vertebral 0R55
Lumbar Vertebral 0S52
Lumbosacral 0S54
Thoracic Vertebral 0R59
Thoracolumbar Vertebral 0R5B
Duct
Common Bile 0F59
Cystic 0F58
Hepatic
Common 0F57
Left 0F56
Right 0F55
Lacrimal
Left 085Y
Right 085X
Pancreatic 0F5D
Accessory 0F5F
Parotid
Left 0C5C
Right 0C5B
Duodenum 0D59
Dura Mater 0052
Ear
External
Left 0951
Right 0950
External Auditory Canal
Left 0954
Right 0953
Inner
Left 095E
Right 095D
Middle
Left 0956
Right 0955
Endometrium 0U5B
Epididymis
Bilateral 0V5L
Left 0V5K
Right 0V5J
Epiglottis 0C5R
Esophagogastric Junction 0D54
Esophagus 0D55
Lower 0D53
Middle 0D52
Upper 0D51
Eustachian Tube
Left 095G
Right 095F

Destruction — *continued*
Eye
Left 0851XZZ
Right 0850XZZ
Eyelid
Lower
Left 085R
Right 085Q
Upper
Left 085P
Right 085N
Fallopian Tube
Left 0U56
Right 0U55
Fallopian Tubes, Bilateral 0U57
Femoral Shaft
Left 0Q59
Right 0Q58
Femur
Lower
Left 0Q5C
Right 0Q5B
Upper
Left 0Q57
Right 0Q56
Fibula
Left 0Q5K
Right 0Q5J
Finger Nail 0H5QXZZ
Gallbladder 0F54
Gingiva
Lower 0C56
Upper 0C55
Gland
Adrenal
Bilateral 0G54
Left 0G52
Right 0G53
Lacrimal
Left 085W
Right 085V
Minor Salivary 0C5J
Parotid
Left 0C59
Right 0C58
Pituitary 0G50
Sublingual
Left 0C5F
Right 0C5D
Submaxillary
Left 0C5H
Right 0C5G
Vestibular 0U5L
Glenoid Cavity
Left 0P58
Right 0P57
Glomus Jugulare 0G5C
Humeral Head
Left 0P5D
Right 0P5C
Humeral Shaft
Left 0P5G
Right 0P5F
Hymen 0U5K
Hypothalamus 005A
Ileocecal Valve 0D5C
Ileum 0D5B
Intestine
Large 0D5E
Left 0D5G
Right 0D5F
Small 0D58
Iris
Left 085D3ZZ
Right 085C3ZZ
Jejunum 0D5A

Destruction — *continued*
Joint
Acromioclavicular
Left 0R5H
Right 0R5G
Ankle
Left 0S5G
Right 0S5F
Carpal
Left 0R5R
Right 0R5Q
Carpometacarpal
Left 0R5T
Right 0R5S
Cervical Vertebral 0R51
Cervicothoracic Vertebral 0R54
Coccygeal 0S56
Elbow
Left 0R5M
Right 0R5L
Finger Phalangeal
Left 0R5X
Right 0R5W
Hip
Left 0S5B
Right 0S59
Knee
Left 0S5D
Right 0S5C
Lumbar Vertebral 0S50
Lumbosacral 0S53
Metacarpophalangeal
Left 0R5V
Right 0R5U
Metatarsal-Phalangeal
Left 0S5N
Right 0S5M
Occipital-cervical 0R50
Sacrococcygeal 0S55
Sacroiliac
Left 0S58
Right 0S57
Shoulder
Left 0R5K
Right 0R5J
Sternoclavicular
Left 0R5F
Right 0R5E
Tarsal
Left 0S5J
Right 0S5H
Tarsometatarsal
Left 0S5L
Right 0S5K
Temporomandibular
Left 0R5D
Right 0R5C
Thoracic Vertebral 0R56
Thoracolumbar Vertebral 0R5A
Toe Phalangeal
Left 0S5Q
Right 0S5P
Wrist
Left 0R5P
Right 0R5N
Kidney
Left 0T51
Right 0T50
Kidney Pelvis
Left 0T54
Right 0T53
Larynx 0C5S
Lens
Left 085K3ZZ
Right 085J3ZZ
Lip
Lower 0C51

Destruction — *continued*
Lip — *continued*
Upper 0C50
Liver 0F50
Left Lobe 0F52
Right Lobe 0F51
Lung
Bilateral 0B5M
Left 0B5L
Lower Lobe
Left 0B5J
Right 0B5F
Middle Lobe, Right 0B5D
Right 0B5K
Upper Lobe
Left 0B5G
Right 0B5C
Lung Lingula 0B5H
Lymphatic
Aortic 075D
Axillary
Left 0756
Right 0755
Head 0750
Inguinal
Left 075J
Right 075H
Internal Mammary
Left 0759
Right 0758
Lower Extremity
Left 075G
Right 075F
Mesenteric 075B
Neck
Left 0752
Right 0751
Pelvis 075C
Thoracic Duct 075K
Thorax 0757
Upper Extremity
Left 0754
Right 0753
Mandible
Left 0N5V
Right 0N5T
Maxilla 0N5R
Medulla Oblongata 005D
Mesentery 0D5V
Metacarpal
Left 0P5Q
Right 0P5P
Metatarsal
Left 0Q5P
Right 0Q5N
Muscle
Abdomen
Left 0K5L
Right 0K5K
Extraocular
Left 085M
Right 085L
Facial 0K51
Foot
Left 0K5W
Right 0K5V
Hand
Left 0K5D
Right 0K5C
Head 0K50
Hip
Left 0K5P
Right 0K5N
Lower Arm and Wrist
Left 0K5B
Right 0K59
Lower Leg

Destruction — *continued*
Muscle — *continued*
Left 0K5T
Right 0K5S
Neck
Left 0K53
Right 0K52
Papillary 025D
Perineum 0K5M
Shoulder
Left 0K56
Right 0K55
Thorax
Left 0K5J
Right 0K5H
Tongue, Palate, Pharynx 0K54
Trunk
Left 0K5G
Right 0K5F
Upper Arm
Left 0K58
Right 0K57
Upper Leg
Left 0K5R
Right 0K5Q
Nasal Mucosa and Soft Tissue 095K
Nasopharynx 095N
Nerve
Abdominal Sympathetic 015M
Abducens 005L
Accessory 005R
Acoustic 005N
Brachial Plexus 0153
Cervical 0151
Cervical Plexus 0150
Facial 005M
Femoral 015D
Glossopharyngeal 005P
Head and Neck Sympathetic 015K
Hypoglossal 005S
Lumbar 015B
Lumbar Plexus 0159
Lumbar Sympathetic 015N
Lumbosacral Plexus 015A
Median 0155
Oculomotor 005H
Olfactory 005F
Optic 005G
Peroneal 015H
Phrenic 0152
Pudendal 015C
Radial 0156
Sacral 015R
Sacral Plexus 015Q
Sacral Sympathetic 015P
Sciatic 015F
Thoracic 0158
Thoracic Sympathetic 015L
Tibial 015G
Trigeminal 005K
Trochlear 005J
Ulnar 0154
Vagus 005Q
Nipple
Left 0H5X
Right 0H5W
Omentum 0D5U
Orbit
Left 0N5Q
Right 0N5P
Ovary
Bilateral 0U52
Left 0U51
Right 0U50
Palate
Hard 0C52
Soft 0C53

Destruction — *continued*
- Pancreas 0F5G
- Para-aortic Body 0G59
- Paraganglion Extremity 0G5F
- Parathyroid Gland 0G5R
  - Inferior
    - Left 0G5P
    - Right 0G5N
  - Multiple 0G5Q
  - Superior
    - Left 0G5M
    - Right 0G5L
- Patella
  - Left 0Q5F
  - Right 0Q5D
- Penis 0V5S
- Pericardium 025N
- Peritoneum 0D5W
- Phalanx
  - Finger
    - Left 0P5V
    - Right 0P5T
  - Thumb
    - Left 0P5S
    - Right 0P5R
  - Toe
    - Left 0Q5R
    - Right 0Q5Q
- Pharynx 0C5M
- Pineal Body 0G51
- Pleura
  - Left 0B5P
  - Right 0B5N
- Pons 005B
- Prepuce 0V5T
- Prostate 0V50
  - Robotic Waterjet Ablation XV508A4
- Radius
  - Left 0P5J
  - Right 0P5H
- Rectum 0D5P
- Retina
  - Left 085F3ZZ
  - Right 085E3ZZ
- Retinal Vessel
  - Left 085H3ZZ
  - Right 085G3ZZ
- Ribs
  - 1 to 2 0P51
  - 3 or More 0P52
- Sacrum 0Q51
- Scapula
  - Left 0P56
  - Right 0P55
- Sclera
  - Left 0857XZZ
  - Right 0856XZZ
- Scrotum 0V55
- Septum
  - Atrial 0255
  - Nasal 095M
  - Ventricular 025M
- Sinus
  - Accessory 095P
  - Ethmoid
    - Left 095V
    - Right 095U
  - Frontal
    - Left 095T
    - Right 095S
  - Mastoid
    - Left 095C
    - Right 095B
  - Maxillary
    - Left 095R
    - Right 095Q

Destruction — *continued*
- Sinus — *continued*
  - Sphenoid
    - Left 095X
    - Right 095W
- Skin
  - Abdomen 0H57XZ
  - Back 0H56XZ
  - Buttock 0H58XZ
  - Chest 0H55XZ
  - Ear
    - Left 0H53XZ
    - Right 0H52XZ
  - Face 0H51XZ
  - Foot
    - Left 0H5NXZ
    - Right 0H5MXZ
  - Hand
    - Left 0H5GXZ
    - Right 0H5FXZ
  - Inguinal 0H5AXZ
  - Lower Arm
    - Left 0H5EXZ
    - Right 0H5DXZ
  - Lower Leg
    - Left 0H5LXZ
    - Right 0H5KXZ
  - Neck 0H54XZ
  - Perineum 0H59XZ
  - Scalp 0H50XZ
  - Upper Arm
    - Left 0H5CXZ
    - Right 0H5BXZ
  - Upper Leg
    - Left 0H5JXZ
    - Right 0H5HXZ
- Skull 0N50
- Spinal Cord
  - Cervical 005W
  - Lumbar 005Y
  - Thoracic 005X
- Spinal Meninges 005T
- Spleen 075P
- Sternum 0P50
- Stomach 0D56
  - Pylorus 0D57
- Subcutaneous Tissue and Fascia
  - Abdomen 0J58
  - Back 0J57
  - Buttock 0J59
  - Chest 0J56
  - Face 0J51
  - Foot
    - Left 0J5R
    - Right 0J5Q
  - Hand
    - Left 0J5K
    - Right 0J5J
  - Lower Arm
    - Left 0J5H
    - Right 0J5G
  - Lower Leg
    - Left 0J5P
    - Right 0J5N
  - Neck
    - Left 0J55
    - Right 0J54
  - Pelvic Region 0J5C
  - Perineum 0J5B
  - Scalp 0J50
  - Upper Arm
    - Left 0J5F
    - Right 0J5D
  - Upper Leg
    - Left 0J5M
    - Right 0J5L
- Tarsal
  - Left 0Q5M

Destruction — *continued*
- Tarsal— *continued*
  - Right 0Q5L
- Tendon
  - Abdomen
    - Left 0L5G
    - Right 0L5F
  - Ankle
    - Left 0L5T
    - Right 0L5S
  - Foot
    - Left 0L5W
    - Right 0L5V
  - Hand
    - Left 0L58
    - Right 0L57
  - Head and Neck 0L50
  - Hip
    - Left 0L5K
    - Right 0L5J
  - Knee
    - Left 0L5R
    - Right 0L5Q
  - Lower Arm and Wrist
    - Left 0L56
    - Right 0L55
  - Lower Leg
    - Left 0L5P
    - Right 0L5N
  - Perineum 0L5H
  - Shoulder
    - Left 0L52
    - Right 0L51
  - Thorax
    - Left 0L5D
    - Right 0L5C
  - Trunk
    - Left 0L5B
    - Right 0L59
  - Upper Arm
    - Left 0L54
    - Right 0L53
  - Upper Leg
    - Left 0L5M
    - Right 0L5L
- Testis
  - Bilateral 0V5C
  - Left 0V5B
  - Right 0V59
- Thalamus 0059
- Thymus 075M
- Thyroid Gland 0G5K
  - Left Lobe 0G5G
  - Right Lobe 0G5H
- Tibia
  - Left 0Q5H
  - Right 0Q5G
- Toe Nail 0H5RXZZ
- Tongue 0C57
- Tonsils 0C5P
- Tooth
  - Lower 0C5X
  - Upper 0C5W
- Trachea 0B51
- Tunica Vaginalis
  - Left 0V57
  - Right 0V56
- Turbinate, Nasal 095L
- Tympanic Membrane
  - Left 0958
  - Right 0957
- Ulna
  - Left 0P5L
  - Right 0P5K
- Ureter
  - Left 0T57
  - Right 0T56

Destruction — *continued*
Urethra 0T5D
Uterine Supporting Structure 0U54
Uterus 0U59
Uvula 0C5N
Vagina 0U5G
Valve
Aortic 025F
Mitral 025G
Pulmonary 025H
Tricuspid 025J
Vas Deferens
Bilateral 0V5Q
Left 0V5P
Right 0V5N
Vein
Axillary
Left 0558
Right 0557
Azygos 0550
Basilic
Left 055C
Right 055B
Brachial
Left 055A
Right 0559
Cephalic
Left 055F
Right 055D
Colic 0657
Common Iliac
Left 065D
Right 065C
Coronary 0254
Esophageal 0653
External Iliac
Left 065G
Right 065F
External Jugular
Left 055Q
Right 055P
Face
Left 055V
Right 055T
Femoral
Left 065N
Right 065M
Foot
Left 065V
Right 065T
Gastric 0652
Hand
Left 055H
Right 055G
Hemiazygos 0551
Hepatic 0654
Hypogastric
Left 065J
Right 065H
Inferior Mesenteric 0656
Innominate
Left 0554
Right 0553
Internal Jugular
Left 055N
Right 055M
Intracranial 055L
Lower 065Y
Portal 0658
Pulmonary
Left 025T
Right 025S
Renal
Left 065B
Right 0659
Saphenous
Left 065Q

Destruction — *continued*
Vein— *continued*
Right 065P
Splenic 0651
Subclavian
Left 0556
Right 0555
Superior Mesenteric 0655
Upper 055Y
Vertebral
Left 055S
Right 055R
Vena Cava
Inferior 0650
Superior 025V
Ventricle
Left 025L
Right 025K
Vertebra
Cervical 0P53
Lumbar 0Q50
Thoracic 0P54
Vesicle
Bilateral 0V53
Left 0V52
Right 0V51
Vitreous
Left 08553ZZ
Right 08543ZZ
Vocal Cord
Left 0C5V
Right 0C5T
Vulva 0U5M
Detachment
Arm
Lower
Left 0X6F0Z
Right 0X6D0Z
Upper
Left 0X690Z
Right 0X680Z
Elbow Region
Left 0X6C0ZZ
Right 0X6B0ZZ
Femoral Region
Left 0Y680ZZ
Right 0Y670ZZ
Finger
Index
Left 0X6P0Z
Right 0X6N0Z
Little
Left 0X6W0Z
Right 0X6V0Z
Middle
Left 0X6R0Z
Right 0X6Q0Z
Ring
Left 0X6T0Z
Right 0X6S0Z
Foot
Left 0Y6N0Z
Right 0Y6M0Z
Forequarter
Left 0X610ZZ
Right 0X600ZZ
Hand
Left 0X6K0Z
Right 0X6J0Z
Hindquarter
Bilateral 0Y640ZZ
Left 0Y630ZZ
Right 0Y620ZZ
Knee Region
Left 0Y6G0ZZ
Right 0Y6F0ZZ

Detachment — *continued*
Leg
Lower
Left 0Y6J0Z
Right 0Y6H0Z
Upper
Left 0Y6D0Z
Right 0Y6C0Z
Shoulder Region
Left 0X630ZZ
Right 0X620ZZ
Thumb
Left 0X6M0Z
Right 0X6L0Z
Toe
1st
Left 0Y6Q0Z
Right 0Y6P0Z
2nd
Left 0Y6S0Z
Right 0Y6R0Z
3rd
Left 0Y6U0Z
Right 0Y6T0Z
4th
Left 0Y6W0Z
Right 0Y6V0Z
5th
Left 0Y6Y0Z
Right 0Y6X0Z
Determination, mental status GZ14ZZZ
Detorsion
see Release
see Reposition
Detoxification services, for substance abuse HZ2ZZZZ
Device fitting F0DZ
Diagnostic audiology
see Audiology, Diagnostic
Diagnostic imaging
see Imaging, Diagnostic
Diagnostic radiology
see Imaging, Diagnostic
Dialysis
Hemodialysis *see* Performance, Urinary 5A1D
Peritoneal 3E1M39Z
Diaphragma sellae
use Dura Mater
Diaphragmatic pacemaker generator
use Stimulator Generator in Subcutaneous Tissue and Fascia
Diaphragmatic pacemaker lead
Insertion of device in, Diaphragm 0BHT
Removal of device from, Diaphragm 0BPT
Revision of device in, Diaphragm 0BWT
Digital radiography, plain
see Plain Radiography
Dilation
Ampulla of Vater 0F7C
Anus 0D7Q
Aorta
Abdominal 0470
Thoracic
Ascending/Arch 027X
Descending 027W
Artery
Anterior Tibial
Left 047Q
Right 047P
Axillary
Left 0376
Right 0375
Brachial
Left 0378
Right 0377
Celiac 0471

Dilation — *continued*
Artery — *continued*
Colic
Left 0477
Middle 0478
Right 0476
Common Carotid
Left 037J
Right 037H
Common Iliac
Left 047D
Right 047C
Coronary
Four or More Arteries 0273
One Artery 0270
Three Arteries 0272
Two Arteries 0271
External Carotid
Left 037N
Right 037M
External Iliac
Left 047J
Right 047H
Face 037R
Femoral
Left 047L
Right 047K
Foot
Left 047W
Right 047V
Gastric 0472
Hand
Left 037F
Right 037D
Hepatic 0473
Inferior Mesenteric 047B
Innominate 0372
Internal Carotid
Left 037L
Right 037K
Internal Iliac
Left 047F
Right 047E
Internal Mammary
Left 0371
Right 0370
Intracranial 037G
Lower 047Y
Peroneal
Left 047U
Right 047T
Popliteal
Left 047N
Right 047M
Posterior Tibial
Left 047S
Right 047R
Pulmonary
Left 027R
Right 027Q
Pulmonary Trunk 027P
Radial
Left 037C
Right 037B
Renal
Left 047A
Right 0479
Splenic 0474
Subclavian
Left 0374
Right 0373
Superior Mesenteric 0475
Temporal
Left 037T
Right 037S
Thyroid
Left 037V

Dilation — *continued*
Artery — *continued*
Right 037U
Ulnar
Left 037A
Right 0379
Upper 037Y
Vertebral
Left 037Q
Right 037P
Bladder 0T7B
Bladder Neck 0T7C
Bronchus
Lingula 0B79
Lower Lobe
Left 0B7B
Right 0B76
Main
Left 0B77
Right 0B73
Middle Lobe, Right 0B75
Upper Lobe
Left 0B78
Right 0B74
Carina 0B72
Cecum 0D7H
Cerebral Ventricle 0076
Cervix 0U7C
Colon
Ascending 0D7K
Descending 0D7M
Sigmoid 0D7N
Transverse 0D7L
Duct
Common Bile 0F79
Cystic 0F78
Hepatic
Common 0F77
Left 0F76
Right 0F75
Lacrimal
Left 087Y
Right 087X
Pancreatic 0F7D
Accessory 0F7F
Parotid
Left 0C7C
Right 0C7B
Duodenum 0D79
Esophagogastric Junction 0D74
Esophagus 0D75
Lower 0D73
Middle 0D72
Upper 0D71
Eustachian Tube
Left 097G
Right 097F
Fallopian Tube
Left 0U76
Right 0U75
Fallopian Tubes, Bilateral 0U77
Hymen 0U7K
Ileocecal Valve 0D7C
Ileum 0D7B
Intestine
Large 0D7E
Left 0D7G
Right 0D7F
Small 0D78
Jejunum 0D7A
Kidney Pelvis
Left 0T74
Right 0T73
Larynx 0C7S
Pharynx 0C7M
Rectum 0D7P

Dilation — *continued*
Stomach 0D76
Pylorus 0D77
Trachea 0B71
Ureter
Left 0T77
Right 0T76
Ureters, Bilateral 0T78
Urethra 0T7D
Uterus 0U79
Vagina 0U7G
Valve
Aortic 027F
Mitral 027G
Pulmonary 027H
Tricuspid 027J
Vas Deferens
Bilateral 0V7Q
Left 0V7P
Right 0V7N
Vein
Axillary
Left 0578
Right 0577
Azygos 0570
Basilic
Left 057C
Right 057B
Brachial
Left 057A
Right 0579
Cephalic
Left 057F
Right 057D
Colic 0677
Common Iliac
Left 067D
Right 067C
Esophageal 0673
External Iliac
Left 067G
Right 067F
External Jugular
Left 057Q
Right 057P
Face
Left 057V
Right 057T
Femoral
Left 067N
Right 067M
Foot
Left 067V
Right 067T
Gastric 0672
Hand
Left 057H
Right 057G
Hemiazygos 0571
Hepatic 0674
Hypogastric
Left 067J
Right 067H
Inferior Mesenteric 0676
Innominate
Left 0574
Right 0573
Internal Jugular
Left 057N
Right 057M
Intracranial 057L
Lower 067Y
Portal 0678
Pulmonary
Left 027T
Right 027S

Dilation — *continued*
Vein — *continued*
Renal
Left 067B
Right 0679
Saphenous
Left 067Q
Right 067P
Splenic 0671
Subclavian
Left 0576
Right 0575
Superior Mesenteric 0675
Upper 057Y
Vertebral
Left 057S
Right 057R
Vena Cava
Inferior 0670
Superior 027V
Ventricle
Left 027L
Right 027K
Direct Lateral Interbody Fusion (DLIF) device
use Interbody Fusion Device in Lower Joints
Disarticulation
see Detachment
Discectomy, diskectomy
see Excision, Upper Joints 0RB
see Resection, Upper Joints 0RT
see Excision, Lower Joints 0SB
see Resection, Lower Joints 0ST
Discography
see Plain Radiography, Axial Skeleton, Except Skull and Facial Bones BR0
see Fluoroscopy, Axial Skeleton, Except Skull and Facial Bones BR1
Distal humerus
use Humeral Shaft, Right
use Humeral Shaft, Left
Distal humerus, involving joint
use Elbow Joint, Right
use Elbow Joint, Left
Distal radioulnar joint
use Wrist Joint, Right
use Wrist Joint, Left
Diversion
see Bypass
Diverticulectomy
see Excision, Gastrointestinal System 0DB
Division
Acetabulum
Left 0Q85
Right 0Q84
Anal Sphincter 0D8R
Basal Ganglia 0088
Bladder Neck 0T8C
Bone
Ethmoid
Left 0N8G
Right 0N8F
Frontal 0N81
Hyoid 0N8X
Lacrimal
Left 0N8J
Right 0N8H
Nasal 0N8B
Occipital 0N87
Palatine
Left 0N8L
Right 0N8K
Parietal
Left 0N84
Right 0N83
Pelvic
Left 0Q83

Division — *continued*
Bone — *continued*
Right 0Q82
Sphenoid 0N8C
Temporal
Left 0N86
Right 0N85
Zygomatic
Left 0N8N
Right 0N8M
Brain 0080
Bursa and Ligament
Abdomen
Left 0M8J
Right 0M8H
Ankle
Left 0M8R
Right 0M8Q
Elbow
Left 0M84
Right 0M83
Foot
Left 0M8T
Right 0M8S
Hand
Left 0M88
Right 0M87
Head and Neck 0M80
Hip
Left 0M8M
Right 0M8L
Knee
Left 0M8P
Right 0M8N
Lower Extremity
Left 0M8W
Right 0M8V
Perineum 0M8K
Rib(s) 0M8G
Shoulder
Left 0M82
Right 0M81
Spine
Lower 0M8D
Upper 0M8C
Sternum 0M8F
Upper Extremity
Left 0M8B
Right 0M89
Wrist
Left 0M86
Right 0M85
Carpal
Left 0P8N
Right 0P8M
Cerebral Hemisphere 0087
Chordae Tendineae 0289
Clavicle
Left 0P8B
Right 0P89
Coccyx 0Q8S
Conduction Mechanism 0288
Esophagogastric Junction 0D84
Femoral Shaft
Left 0Q89
Right 0Q88
Femur
Lower
Left 0Q8C
Right 0Q8B
Upper
Left 0Q87
Right 0Q86
Fibula
Left 0Q8K
Right 0Q8J
Gland, Pituitary 0G80

Division — *continued*
Glenoid Cavity
Left 0P88
Right 0P87
Humeral Head
Left 0P8D
Right 0P8C
Humeral Shaft
Left 0P8G
Right 0P8F
Hymen 0U8K
Kidneys, Bilateral 0T82
Mandible
Left 0N8V
Right 0N8T
Maxilla 0N8R
Metacarpal
Left 0P8Q
Right 0P8P
Metatarsal
Left 0Q8P
Right 0Q8N
Muscle
Abdomen
Left 0K8L
Right 0K8K
Facial 0K81
Foot
Left 0K8W
Right 0K8V
Hand
Left 0K8D
Right 0K8C
Head 0K80
Hip
Left 0K8P
Right 0K8N
Lower Arm and Wrist
Left 0K8B
Right 0K89
Lower Leg
Left 0K8T
Right 0K8S
Neck
Left 0K83
Right 0K82
Papillary 028D
Perineum 0K8M
Shoulder
Left 0K86
Right 0K85
Thorax
Left 0K8J
Right 0K8H
Tongue, Palate, Pharynx 0K84
Trunk
Left 0K8G
Right 0K8F
Upper Arm
Left 0K88
Right 0K87
Upper Leg
Left 0K8R
Right 0K8Q
Nerve
Abdominal Sympathetic 018M
Abducens 008L
Accessory 008R
Acoustic 008N
Brachial Plexus 0183
Cervical 0181
Cervical Plexus 0180
Facial 008M
Femoral 018D
Glossopharyngeal 008P
Head and Neck Sympathetic 018K
Hypoglossal 008S

Division — *continued*
Nerve — *continued*
Lumbar 018B
Lumbar Plexus 0189
Lumbar Sympathetic 018N
Lumbosacral Plexus 018A
Median 0185
Oculomotor 008H
Olfactory 008F
Optic 008G
Peroneal 018H
Phrenic 0182
Pudendal 018C
Radial 0186
Sacral 018R
Sacral Plexus 018Q
Sacral Sympathetic 018P
Sciatic 018F
Thoracic 0188
Thoracic Sympathetic 018L
Tibial 018G
Trigeminal 008K
Trochlear 008J
Ulnar 0184
Vagus 008Q
Orbit
Left 0N8Q
Right 0N8P
Ovary
Bilateral 0U82
Left 0U81
Right 0U80
Pancreas 0F8G
Patella
Left 0Q8F
Right 0Q8D
Perineum, Female 0W8NXZZ
Phalanx
Finger
Left 0P8V
Right 0P8T
Thumb
Left 0P8S
Right 0P8R
Toe
Left 0Q8R
Right 0Q8Q
Radius
Left 0P8J
Right 0P8H
Ribs
1 to 2 0P81
3 or More 0P82
Sacrum 0Q81
Scapula
Left 0P86
Right 0P85
Skin
Abdomen 0H87XZZ
Back 0H86XZZ
Buttock 0H88XZZ
Chest 0H85XZZ
Ear
Left 0H83XZZ
Right 0H82XZZ
Face 0H81XZZ
Foot
Left 0H8NXZZ
Right 0H8MXZZ
Hand
Left 0H8GXZZ
Right 0H8FXZZ
Inguinal 0H8AXZZ
Lower Arm
Left 0H8EXZZ
Right 0H8DXZZ

Division — *continued*
Skin — *continued*
Lower Leg
Left 0H8LXZZ
Right 0H8KXZZ
Neck 0H84XZZ
Perineum 0H89XZZ
Scalp 0H80XZZ
Upper Arm
Left 0H8CXZZ
Right 0H8BXZZ
Upper Leg
Left 0H8JXZZ
Right 0H8HXZZ
Skull 0N80
Spinal Cord
Cervical 008W
Lumbar 008Y
Thoracic 008X
Sternum 0P80
Stomach, Pylorus 0D87
Subcutaneous Tissue and Fascia
Abdomen 0J88
Back 0J87
Buttock 0J89
Chest 0J86
Face 0J81
Foot
Left 0J8R
Right 0J8Q
Hand
Left 0J8K
Right 0J8J
Head and Neck 0J8S
Lower Arm
Left 0J8H
Right 0J8G
Lower Extremity 0J8W
Lower Leg
Left 0J8P
Right 0J8N
Neck
Left 0J85
Right 0J84
Pelvic Region 0J8C
Perineum 0J8B
Scalp 0J80
Trunk 0J8T
Upper Arm
Left 0J8F
Right 0J8D
Upper Extremity 0J8V
Upper Leg
Left 0J8M
Right 0J8L
Tarsal
Left 0Q8M
Right 0Q8L
Tendon
Abdomen
Left 0L8G
Right 0L8F
Ankle
Left 0L8T
Right 0L8S
Foot
Left 0L8W
Right 0L8V
Hand
Left 0L88
Right 0L87
Head and Neck 0L80
Hip
Left 0L8K
Right 0L8J
Knee
Left 0L8R
Right 0L8Q

Division — *continued*
Tendon — *continued*
Lower Arm and Wrist
Left 0L86
Right 0L85
Lower Leg
Left 0L8P
Right 0L8N
Perineum 0L8H
Shoulder
Left 0L82
Right 0L81
Thorax
Left 0L8D
Right 0L8C
Trunk
Left 0L8B
Right 0L89
Upper Arm
Left 0L84
Right 0L83
Upper Leg
Left 0L8M
Right 0L8L
Thyroid Gland Isthmus 0G8J
Tibia
Left 0Q8H
Right 0Q8G
Turbinate, Nasal 098L
Ulna
Left 0P8L
Right 0P8K
Uterine Supporting Structure 0U84
Vertebra
Cervical 0P83
Lumbar 0Q80
Thoracic 0P84
Doppler study
see Ultrasonography
Dorsal digital nerve
use Radial Nerve
Dorsal metacarpal vein
use Hand Vein, Right
use Hand Vein, Left
Dorsal metatarsal artery
use Foot Artery, Right
use Foot Artery, Left
Dorsal metatarsal vein
use Foot Vein, Right
use Foot Vein, Left
Dorsal scapular artery
use Subclavian Artery, Right
use Subclavian Artery, Left
Dorsal scapular nerve
use Brachial Plexus
Dorsal venous arch
use Foot Vein, Right
use Foot Vein, Left
Dorsalis pedis artery
use Anterior Tibial Artery, Right
use Anterior Tibial Artery, Left
DownStream® System
5A0512C
5A0522C
Drainage
Abdominal Wall 0W9F
Acetabulum
Left 0Q95
Right 0Q94
Adenoids 0C9Q
Ampulla of Vater 0F9C
Anal Sphincter 0D9R
Ankle Region
Left 0Y9L
Right 0Y9K
Anterior Chamber
Left 0893

Drainage — *continued*
Anterior Chamber — *continued*
Right 0892
Anus 0D9Q
Aorta, Abdominal 0490
Aortic Body 0G9D
Appendix 0D9J
Arm
Lower
Left 0X9F
Right 0X9D
Upper
Left 0X99
Right 0X98
Artery
Anterior Tibial
Left 049Q
Right 049P
Axillary
Left 0396
Right 0395
Brachial
Left 0398
Right 0397
Celiac 0491
Colic
Left 0497
Middle 0498
Right 0496
Common Carotid
Left 039J
Right 039H
Common Iliac
Left 049D
Right 049C
External Carotid
Left 039N
Right 039M
External Iliac
Left 049J
Right 049H
Face 039R
Femoral
Left 049L
Right 049K
Foot
Left 049W
Right 049V
Gastric 0492
Hand
Left 039F
Right 039D
Hepatic 0493
Inferior Mesenteric 049B
Innominate 0392
Internal Carotid
Left 039L
Right 039K
Internal Iliac
Left 049F
Right 049E
Internal Mammary
Left 0391
Right 0390
Intracranial 039G
Lower 049Y
Peroneal
Left 049U
Right 049T
Popliteal
Left 049N
Right 049M
Posterior Tibial
Left 049S
Right 049R
Radial
Left 039C

Drainage — *continued*
Artery — *continued*
Right 039B
Renal
Left 049A
Right 0499
Splenic 0494
Subclavian
Left 0394
Right 0393
Superior Mesenteric 0495
Temporal
Left 039T
Right 039S
Thyroid
Left 039V
Right 039U
Ulnar
Left 039A
Right 0399
Upper 039Y
Vertebral
Left 039Q
Right 039P
Auditory Ossicle
Left 099A
Right 0999
Axilla
Left 0X95
Right 0X94
Back
Lower 0W9L
Upper 0W9K
Basal Ganglia 0098
Bladder 0T9B
Bladder Neck 0T9C
Bone
Ethmoid
Left 0N9G
Right 0N9F
Frontal 0N91
Hyoid 0N9X
Lacrimal
Left 0N9J
Right 0N9H
Nasal 0N9B
Occipital 0N97
Palatine
Left 0N9L
Right 0N9K
Parietal
Left 0N94
Right 0N93
Pelvic
Left 0Q93
Right 0Q92
Sphenoid 0N9C
Temporal
Left 0N96
Right 0N95
Zygomatic
Left 0N9N
Right 0N9M
Bone Marrow 079T
Brain 0090
Breast
Bilateral 0H9V
Left 0H9U
Right 0H9T
Bronchus
Lingula 0B99
Lower Lobe
Left 0B9B
Right 0B96
Main
Left 0B97
Right 0B93

Drainage — *continued*
Bronchus — *continued*
Middle Lobe, Right 0B95
Upper Lobe
Left 0B98
Right 0B94
Buccal Mucosa 0C94
Bursa and Ligament
Abdomen
Left 0M9J
Right 0M9H
Ankle
Left 0M9R
Right 0M9Q
Elbow
Left 0M94
Right 0M93
Foot
Left 0M9T
Right 0M9S
Hand
Left 0M98
Right 0M97
Head and Neck 0M90
Hip
Left 0M9M
Right 0M9L
Knee
Left 0M9P
Right 0M9N
Lower Extremity
Left 0M9W
Right 0M9V
Perineum 0M9K
Rib(s) 0M9G
Shoulder
Left 0M92
Right 0M91
Spine
Lower 0M9D
Upper 0M9C
Sternum 0M9F
Upper Extremity
Left 0M9B
Right 0M99
Wrist
Left 0M96
Right 0M95
Buttock
Left 0Y91
Right 0Y90
Carina 0B92
Carotid Bodies, Bilateral 0G98
Carotid Body
Left 0G96
Right 0G97
Carpal
Left 0P9N
Right 0P9M
Cavity, Cranial 0W91
Cecum 0D9H
Cerebellum 009C
Cerebral Hemisphere 0097
Cerebral Meninges 0091
Cerebral Ventricle 0096
Cervix 0U9C
Chest Wall 0W98
Choroid
Left 089B
Right 089A
Cisterna Chyli 079L
Clavicle
Left 0P9B
Right 0P99
Clitoris 0U9J
Coccygeal Glomus 0G9B
Coccyx 0Q9S

Drainage — *continued*
Colon
Ascending 0D9K
Descending 0D9M
Sigmoid 0D9N
Transverse 0D9L
Conjunctiva
Left 089T
Right 089S
Cord
Bilateral 0V9H
Left 0V9G
Right 0V9F
Cornea
Left 0899
Right 0898
Cul-de-sac 0U9F
Diaphragm 0B9T
Disc
Cervical Vertebral 0R93
Cervicothoracic Vertebral 0R95
Lumbar Vertebral 0S92
Lumbosacral 0S94
Thoracic Vertebral 0R99
Thoracolumbar Vertebral 0R9B
Duct
Common Bile 0F99
Cystic 0F98
Hepatic
Common 0F97
Left 0F96
Right 0F95
Lacrimal
Left 089Y
Right 089X
Pancreatic 0F9D
Accessory 0F9F
Parotid
Left 0C9C
Right 0C9B
Duodenum 0D99
Dura Mater 0092
Ear
External
Left 0991
Right 0990
External Auditory Canal
Left 0994
Right 0993
Inner
Left 099E
Right 099D
Middle
Left 0996
Right 0995
Elbow Region
Left 0X9C
Right 0X9B
Epididymis
Bilateral 0V9L
Left 0V9K
Right 0V9J
Epidural Space, Intracranial 0093
Epiglottis 0C9R
Esophagogastric Junction 0D94
Esophagus 0D95
Lower 0D93
Middle 0D92
Upper 0D91
Eustachian Tube
Left 099G
Right 099F
Extremity
Lower
Left 0Y9B
Right 0Y99

Drainage — *continued*
Extremity — *continued*
Upper
Left 0X97
Right 0X96
Eye
Left 0891
Right 0890
Eyelid
Lower
Left 089R
Right 089Q
Upper
Left 089P
Right 089N
Face 0W92
Fallopian Tube
Left 0U96
Right 0U95
Fallopian Tubes, Bilateral 0U97
Femoral Region
Left 0Y98
Right 0Y97
Femoral Shaft
Left 0Q99
Right 0Q98
Femur
Lower
Left 0Q9C
Right 0Q9B
Upper
Left 0Q97
Right 0Q96
Fibula
Left 0Q9K
Right 0Q9J
Finger Nail 0H9Q
Foot
Left 0Y9N
Right 0Y9M
Gallbladder 0F94
Gingiva
Lower 0C96
Upper 0C95
Gland
Adrenal
Bilateral 0G94
Left 0G92
Right 0G93
Lacrimal
Left 089W
Right 089V
Minor Salivary 0C9J
Parotid
Left 0C99
Right 0C98
Pituitary 0G90
Sublingual
Left 0C9F
Right 0C9D
Submaxillary
Left 0C9H
Right 0C9G
Vestibular 0U9L
Glenoid Cavity
Left 0P98
Right 0P97
Glomus Jugulare 0G9C
Hand
Left 0X9K
Right 0X9J
Head 0W90
Humeral Head
Left 0P9D
Right 0P9C
Humeral Shaft
Left 0P9G
Right 0P9F

Drainage — *continued*
Hymen 0U9K
Hypothalamus 009A
Ileocecal Valve 0D9C
Ileum 0D9B
Inguinal Region
Left 0Y96
Right 0Y95
Intestine
Large 0D9E
Left 0D9G
Right 0D9F
Small 0D98
Iris
Left 089D
Right 089C
Jaw
Lower 0W95
Upper 0W94
Jejunum 0D9A
Joint
Acromioclavicular
Left 0R9H
Right 0R9G
Ankle
Left 0S9G
Right 0S9F
Carpal
Left 0R9R
Right 0R9Q
Carpometacarpal
Left 0R9T
Right 0R9S
Cervical Vertebral 0R91
Cervicothoracic Vertebral 0R94
Coccygeal 0S96
Elbow
Left 0R9M
Right 0R9L
Finger Phalangeal
Left 0R9X
Right 0R9W
Hip
Left 0S9B
Right 0S99
Knee
Left 0S9D
Right 0S9C
Lumbar Vertebral 0S90
Lumbosacral 0S93
Metacarpophalangeal
Left 0R9V
Right 0R9U
Metatarsal-Phalangeal
Left 0S9N
Right 0S9M
Occipital-cervical 0R90
Sacrococcygeal 0S95
Sacroiliac
Left 0S98
Right 0S97
Shoulder
Left 0R9K
Right 0R9J
Sternoclavicular
Left 0R9F
Right 0R9E
Tarsal
Left 0S9J
Right 0S9H
Tarsometatarsal
Left 0S9L
Right 0S9K
Temporomandibular
Left 0R9D
Right 0R9C
Thoracic Vertebral 0R96

Drainage — *continued*
Joint — *continued*
Thoracolumbar Vertebral 0R9A
Toe Phalangeal
Left 0S9Q
Right 0S9P
Wrist
Left 0R9P
Right 0R9N
Kidney
Left 0T91
Right 0T90
Kidney Pelvis
Left 0T94
Right 0T93
Knee Region
Left 0Y9G
Right 0Y9F
Larynx 0C9S
Leg
Lower
Left 0Y9J
Right 0Y9H
Upper
Left 0Y9D
Right 0Y9C
Lens
Left 089K
Right 089J
Lip
Lower 0C91
Upper 0C90
Liver 0F90
Left Lobe 0F92
Right Lobe 0F91
Lung
Bilateral 0B9M
Left 0B9L
Lower Lobe
Left 0B9J
Right 0B9F
Middle Lobe, Right 0B9D
Right 0B9K
Upper Lobe
Left 0B9G
Right 0B9C
Lung Lingula 0B9H
Lymphatic
Aortic 079D
Axillary
Left 0796
Right 0795
Head 0790
Inguinal
Left 079J
Right 079H
Internal Mammary
Left 0799
Right 0798
Lower Extremity
Left 079G
Right 079F
Mesenteric 079B
Neck
Left 0792
Right 0791
Pelvis 079C
Thoracic Duct 079K
Thorax 0797
Upper Extremity
Left 0794
Right 0793
Mandible
Left 0N9V
Right 0N9T
Maxilla 0N9R
Mediastinum 0W9C

Drainage — *continued*
Medulla Oblongata 009D
Mesentery 0D9V
Metacarpal
Left 0P9Q
Right 0P9P
Metatarsal
Left 0Q9P
Right 0Q9N
Muscle
Abdomen
Left 0K9L
Right 0K9K
Extraocular
Left 089M
Right 089L
Facial 0K91
Foot
Left 0K9W
Right 0K9V
Hand
Left 0K9D
Right 0K9C
Head 0K90
Hip
Left 0K9P
Right 0K9N
Lower Arm and Wrist
Left 0K9B
Right 0K99
Lower Leg
Left 0K9T
Right 0K9S
Neck
Left 0K93
Right 0K92
Perineum 0K9M
Shoulder
Left 0K96
Right 0K95
Thorax
Left 0K9J
Right 0K9H
Tongue, Palate, Pharynx 0K94
Trunk
Left 0K9G
Right 0K9F
Upper Arm
Left 0K98
Right 0K97
Upper Leg
Left 0K9R
Right 0K9Q
Nasal Mucosa and Soft Tissue 099K
Nasopharynx 099N
Neck 0W96
Nerve
Abdominal Sympathetic 019M
Abducens 009L
Accessory 009R
Acoustic 009N
Brachial Plexus 0193
Cervical 0191
Cervical Plexus 0190
Facial 009M
Femoral 019D
Glossopharyngeal 009P
Head and Neck Sympathetic 019K
Hypoglossal 009S
Lumbar 019B
Lumbar Plexus 0199
Lumbar Sympathetic 019N
Lumbosacral Plexus 019A
Median 0195
Oculomotor 009H
Olfactory 009F
Optic 009G

Drainage — *continued*
Nerve — *continued*
Peroneal 019H
Phrenic 0192
Pudendal 019C
Radial 0196
Sacral 019R
Sacral Plexus 019Q
Sacral Sympathetic 019P
Sciatic 019F
Thoracic 0198
Thoracic Sympathetic 019L
Tibial 019G
Trigeminal 009K
Trochlear 009J
Ulnar 0194
Vagus 009Q
Nipple
Left 0H9X
Right 0H9W
Omentum 0D9U
Oral Cavity and Throat 0W93
Orbit
Left 0N9Q
Right 0N9P
Ovary
Bilateral 0U92
Left 0U91
Right 0U90
Palate
Hard 0C92
Soft 0C93
Pancreas 0F9G
Para-aortic Body 0G99
Paraganglion Extremity 0G9F
Parathyroid Gland 0G9R
Inferior
Left 0G9P
Right 0G9N
Multiple 0G9Q
Superior
Left 0G9M
Right 0G9L
Patella
Left 0Q9F
Right 0Q9D
Pelvic Cavity 0W9J
Penis 0V9S
Pericardial Cavity 0W9D
Perineum
Female 0W9N
Male 0W9M
Peritoneal Cavity 0W9G
Peritoneum 0D9W
Phalanx
Finger
Left 0P9V
Right 0P9T
Thumb
Left 0P9S
Right 0P9R
Toe
Left 0Q9R
Right 0Q9Q
Pharynx 0C9M
Pineal Body 0G91
Pleura
Left 0B9P
Right 0B9N
Pleural Cavity
Left 0W9B
Right 0W99
Pons 009B
Prepuce 0V9T

- **Drainage** — *continued*
  - Products of Conception
    - Amniotic Fluid
      - Diagnostic 1090
      - Therapeutic 1090
    - Fetal Blood 1090
    - Fetal Cerebrospinal Fluid 1090
    - Fetal Fluid, Other 1090
    - Fluid, Other 1090
  - Prostate 0V90
  - Radius
    - Left 0P9J
    - Right 0P9H
  - Rectum 0D9P
  - Retina
    - Left 089F
    - Right 089E
  - Retinal Vessel
    - Left 089H
    - Right 089G
  - Retroperitoneum 0W9H
  - Ribs
    - 1 to 2 0P91
    - 3 or More 0P92
  - Sacrum 0Q91
  - Scapula
    - Left 0P96
    - Right 0P95
  - Sclera
    - Left 0897
    - Right 0896
  - Scrotum 0V95
  - Septum, Nasal 099M
  - Shoulder Region
    - Left 0X93
    - Right 0X92
  - Sinus
    - Accessory 099P
    - Ethmoid
      - Left 099V
      - Right 099U
    - Frontal
      - Left 099T
      - Right 099S
    - Mastoid
      - Left 099C
      - Right 099B
    - Maxillary
      - Left 099R
      - Right 099Q
    - Sphenoid
      - Left 099X
      - Right 099W
  - Skin
    - Abdomen 0H97
    - Back 0H96
    - Buttock 0H98
    - Chest 0H95
    - Ear
      - Left 0H93
      - Right 0H92
    - Face 0H91
    - Foot
      - Left 0H9N
      - Right 0H9M
    - Hand
      - Left 0H9G
      - Right 0H9F
    - Inguinal 0H9A
    - Lower Arm
      - Left 0H9E
      - Right 0H9D
    - Lower Leg
      - Left 0H9L
      - Right 0H9K
    - Neck 0H94
    - Perineum 0H99
    - Scalp 0H90

- **Drainage** — *continued*
  - Skin — *continued*
    - Upper Arm
      - Left 0H9C
      - Right 0H9B
    - Upper Leg
      - Left 0H9J
      - Right 0H9H
  - Skull 0N90
  - Spinal Canal 009U
  - Spinal Cord
    - Cervical 009W
    - Lumbar 009Y
    - Thoracic 009X
  - Spinal Meninges 009T
  - Spleen 079P
  - Sternum 0P90
  - Stomach 0D96
    - Pylorus 0D97
  - Subarachnoid Space, Intracranial 0095
  - Subcutaneous Tissue and Fascia
    - Abdomen 0J98
    - Back 0J97
    - Buttock 0J99
    - Chest 0J96
    - Face 0J91
    - Foot
      - Left 0J9R
      - Right 0J9Q
    - Hand
      - Left 0J9K
      - Right 0J9J
    - Lower Arm
      - Left 0J9H
      - Right 0J9G
    - Lower Leg
      - Left 0J9P
      - Right 0J9N
    - Neck
      - Left 0J95
      - Right 0J94
    - Pelvic Region 0J9C
    - Perineum 0J9B
    - Scalp 0J90
    - Upper Arm
      - Left 0J9F
      - Right 0J9D
    - Upper Leg
      - Left 0J9M
      - Right 0J9L
  - Subdural Space, Intracranial 0094
  - Tarsal
    - Left 0Q9M
    - Right 0Q9L
  - Tendon
    - Abdomen
      - Left 0L9G
      - Right 0L9F
    - Ankle
      - Left 0L9T
      - Right 0L9S
    - Foot
      - Left 0L9W
      - Right 0L9V
    - Hand
      - Left 0L98
      - Right 0L97
    - Head and Neck 0L90
    - Hip
      - Left 0L9K
      - Right 0L9J
    - Knee
      - Left 0L9R
      - Right 0L9Q
    - Lower Arm and Wrist
      - Left 0L96
      - Right 0L95

- **Drainage** — *continued*
  - Tendon — *continued*
    - Lower Leg
      - Left 0L9P
      - Right 0L9N
    - Perineum 0L9H
    - Shoulder
      - Left 0L92
      - Right 0L91
    - Thorax
      - Left 0L9D
      - Right 0L9C
    - Trunk
      - Left 0L9B
      - Right 0L99
    - Upper Arm
      - Left 0L94
      - Right 0L93
    - Upper Leg
      - Left 0L9M
      - Right 0L9L
  - Testis
    - Bilateral 0V9C
    - Left 0V9B
    - Right 0V99
  - Thalamus 0099
  - Thymus 079M
  - Thyroid Gland 0G9K
    - Left Lobe 0G9G
    - Right Lobe 0G9H
  - Tibia
    - Left 0Q9H
    - Right 0Q9G
  - Toe Nail 0H9R
  - Tongue 0C97
  - Tonsils 0C9P
  - Tooth
    - Lower 0C9X
    - Upper 0C9W
  - Trachea 0B91
  - Tunica Vaginalis
    - Left 0V97
    - Right 0V96
  - Turbinate, Nasal 099L
  - Tympanic Membrane
    - Left 0998
    - Right 0997
  - Ulna
    - Left 0P9L
    - Right 0P9K
  - Ureter
    - Left 0T97
    - Right 0T96
  - Ureters, Bilateral 0T98
  - Urethra 0T9D
  - Uterine Supporting Structure 0U94
  - Uterus 0U99
  - Uvula 0C9N
  - Vagina 0U9G
  - Vas Deferens
    - Bilateral 0V9Q
    - Left 0V9P
    - Right 0V9N
  - Vein
    - Axillary
      - Left 0598
      - Right 0597
    - Azygos 0590
    - Basilic
      - Left 059C
      - Right 059B
    - Brachial
      - Left 059A
      - Right 0599
    - Cephalic
      - Left 059F
      - Right 059D
    - Colic 0697

Drainage — *continued*
Vein — *continued*
Common Iliac
Left 069D
Right 069C
Esophageal 0693
External Iliac
Left 069G
Right 069F
External Jugular
Left 059Q
Right 059P
Face
Left 059V
Right 059T
Femoral
Left 069N
Right 069M
Foot
Left 069V
Right 069T
Gastric 0692
Hand
Left 059H
Right 059G
Hemiazygos 0591
Hepatic 0694
Hypogastric
Left 069J
Right 069H
Inferior Mesenteric 0696
Innominate
Left 0594
Right 0593
Internal Jugular
Left 059N
Right 059M
Intracranial 059L
Lower 069Y
Portal 0698
Renal
Left 069B
Right 0699
Saphenous
Left 069Q
Right 069P
Splenic 0691
Subclavian
Left 0596
Right 0595
Superior Mesenteric 0695
Upper 059Y
Vertebral
Left 059S
Right 059R
Vena Cava, Inferior 0690
Vertebra
Cervical 0P93
Lumbar 0Q90
Thoracic 0P94
Vesicle
Bilateral 0V93
Left 0V92
Right 0V91
Vitreous
Left 0895
Right 0894
Vocal Cord
Left 0C9V
Right 0C9T
Vulva 0U9M
Wrist Region
Left 0X9H
Right 0X9G
Dressing
Abdominal Wall 2W23X4Z
Dressing — *continued*
Arm
Lower
Left 2W2DX4Z
Right 2W2CX4Z
Upper
Left 2W2BX4Z
Right 2W2AX4Z
Back 2W25X4Z
Chest Wall 2W24X4Z
Extremity
Lower
Left 2W2MX4Z
Right 2W2LX4Z
Upper
Left 2W29X4Z
Right 2W28X4Z
Face 2W21X4Z
Finger
Left 2W2KX4Z
Right 2W2JX4Z
Foot
Left 2W2TX4Z
Right 2W2SX4Z
Hand
Left 2W2FX4Z
Right 2W2EX4Z
Head 2W20X4Z
Inguinal Region
Left 2W27X4Z
Right 2W26X4Z
Leg
Lower
Left 2W2RX4Z
Right 2W2QX4Z
Upper
Left 2W2PX4Z
Right 2W2NX4Z
Neck 2W22X4Z
Thumb
Left 2W2HX4Z
Right 2W2GX4Z
Toe
Left 2W2VX4Z
Right 2W2UX4Z
Driver® stent (RX) (OTW)
use Intraluminal Device
Drotrecogin alfa, infusion
see Introduction of Recombinant Human-activated Protein C
Duct of Santorini
use Pancreatic Duct, Accessory
Duct of Wirsung
use Pancreatic Duct
Ductogram, mammary
see Plain Radiography, Skin, Subcutaneous Tissue and Breast BH0
Ductography, mammary
see Plain Radiography, Skin, Subcutaneous Tissue and Breast BH0
Ductus deferens
use Vas Deferens, Right
use Vas Deferens, Left
use Vas Deferens, Bilateral
use Vas Deferens
Duodenal ampulla
use Ampulla of Vater
Duodenectomy
see Excision, Duodenum 0DB9
see Resection, Duodenum 0DT9
Duodenocholedochotomy
see Drainage, Gallbladder 0F94
Duodenocystostomy
see Bypass, Gallbladder 0F14
see Drainage, Gallbladder 0F94
Duodenoenterostomy
see Bypass, Gastrointestinal System 0D1
Duodenoenterostomy — *continued*
see Drainage, Gastrointestinal System 0D9
Duodenojejunal flexure
use Jejunum
Duodenolysis
see Release, Duodenum 0DN9
Duodenorrhaphy
see Repair, Duodenum 0DQ9
Duodenostomy
see Bypass, Duodenum 0D19
see Drainage, Duodenum 0D99
Duodenotomy
see Drainage, Duodenum 0D99
Dura mater, intracranial
use Dura Mater
Dura mater, spinal
use Spinal Meninges
DuraGraft® Endothelial Damage Inhibitor
use Endothelial Damage Inhibitor
DuraHeart™ Left Ventricular Assist System
use Implantable Heart Assist System in Heart and Great Vessels
Dural venous sinus
use Intracranial Vein
Durata® Defibrillation Lead
use Cardiac Lead, Defibrillator in 02H
Dynesys® Dynamic Stabilization System
use Spinal Stabilization Device, Pedicle-Based in 0RH
use Spinal Stabilization Device, Pedicle-Based in 0SH

E

E-Luminexx™ (Biliary)(Vascular) Stent
use Intraluminal Device
Earlobe
use External Ear, Right
use External Ear, Left
use External Ear, Bilateral
ECCO2R (extracorporeal carbon dioxide removal) 5A0920Z
Echocardiogram
see Ultrasonography, Heart B24
Echography
see Ultrasonography
ECMO
see Performance, Circulatory 5A15
EDWARDS INTUITY Elite™ valve system
use Zooplastic Tissue, Rapid Deployment Technique in New Technology
EEG (electroencephalogram)
see Measurement, Central Nervous 4A00
EGD (esophagogastroduodenoscopy) 0DJ08ZZ
Eighth cranial nerve
use Acoustic Nerve
Ejaculatory duct
use Vas Deferens, Right
use Vas Deferens, Left
use Vas Deferens, Bilateral
use Vas Deferens
EKG (electrocardiogram)
see Measurement, Cardiac 4A02
Electrical bone growth stimulator (EBGS)
use Bone Growth Stimulator in Head and Facial Bones
use Bone Growth Stimulator in Upper Bones
use Bone Growth Stimulator in Lower Bones
Electrical muscle stimulation (EMS) lead
use Stimulator Lead in Muscles
Electrocautery
Destruction *see* Destruction
Repair *see* Repair

Electroconvulsive therapy
Bilateral-Multiple Seizure GZB3ZZZ
Bilateral-Single Seizure GZB2ZZZ
Electroconvulsive Therapy, Other GZB4ZZZ
Unilateral-Multiple Seizure GZB1ZZZ
Unilateral-Single Seizure GZB0ZZZ
Electroencephalogram (EEG)
see Measurement, Central Nervous 4A00
Electromagnetic therapy
Central Nervous 6A22
Urinary 6A21
Electronic muscle stimulator lead
use Stimulator Lead in Muscles
Electrophysiologic stimulation (EPS)
see Measurement, Cardiac 4A02
Electroshock therapy
see Electroconvulsive Therapy
Elevation, bone fragments, skull
see Reposition, Head and Facial Bones 0NS
Eleventh cranial nerve
use Accessory Nerve
Embolectomy
see Extirpation
Embolization
see Occlusion
see Restriction
Embolization coil(s)
use Intraluminal Device
EMG (electromyogram)
see Measurement, Musculoskeletal 4A0F
Encephalon
use Brain
Endarterectomy
see Extirpation, Upper Arteries 03C
see Extirpation, Lower Arteries 04C
Endeavor® (III)(IV) (Sprint) Zotarolimus-eluting Coronary Stent System
use Intraluminal Device, Drug-eluting in Heart and Great Vessels
Endologix AFX® Endovascular AAA System
use Intraluminal Device
EndoSure® sensor
use Monitoring Device, Pressure Sensor in 02H
ENDOTAK RELIANCE® (G) Defibrillation Lead
use Cardiac Lead, Defibrillator in 02H
Endothelial damage inhibitor, applied to vein graft XY0VX83
Endotracheal tube (cuffed)(double-lumen)
use Intraluminal Device, Endotracheal Airway in Respiratory System
Endurant® Endovascular Stent Graft
use Intraluminal Device
Endurant® II AAA stent graft system
use Intraluminal Device
Engineered Autologous Chimeric Antigen Receptor T-cell Immunotherapy XW0
Enlargement
see Dilation
see Repair
EnRhythm®
use Pacemaker, Dual Chamber in 0JH
Enterorrhaphy
see Repair, Gastrointestinal System 0DQ
Enterra® gastric neurostimulator
use Stimulator Generator, Multiple Array in 0JH
Enucleation
Eyeball *see* Resection, Eye 08T
Eyeball with prosthetic implant *see* Replacement, Eye 08R
Ependyma
use Cerebral Ventricle
Epic™ Stented Tissue Valve (aortic)
use Zooplastic Tissue in Heart and Great Vessels
Epicel® cultured epidermal autograft
use Autologous Tissue Substitute
Epidermis
use Skin
Epididymectomy
see Excision, Male Reproductive System 0VB
see Resection, Male Reproductive System 0VT
Epididymoplasty
see Repair, Male Reproductive System 0VQ
see Supplement, Male Reproductive System 0VU
Epididymorrhaphy
see Repair, Male Reproductive System 0VQ
Epididymotomy
see Drainage, Male Reproductive System 0V9
Epidural space, spinal
use Spinal Canal
Epiphysiodesis
see Insertion of device in, Upper Bones 0PH
see Repair, Upper Bones 0PQ
see Insertion of device in, Lower Bones 0QH
see Repair, Lower Bones 0QQ
Epiploic foramen
use Peritoneum
Epiretinal visual prosthesis
Left 08H105Z
Right 08H005Z
Episiorrhaphy
see Repair, Perineum, Female 0WQN
Episiotomy
see Division, Perineum, Female 0W8N
Epithalamus
use Thalamus
Epitrochlear lymph node
use Lymphatic, Right Upper Extremity
use Lymphatic, Left Upper Extremity
EPS (electrophysiologic stimulation)
see Measurement, Cardiac 4A02
Eptifibatide, infusion
see Introduction of Platelet Inhibitor
ERCP (endoscopic retrograde cholangiopancreatography)
see Fluoroscopy, Hepatobiliary System and Pancreas BF1
Erector spinae muscle
use Trunk Muscle, Right
use Trunk Muscle, Left
Esophageal artery
use Upper Artery
Esophageal obturator airway (EOA)
use Intraluminal Device, Airway in Gastrointestinal System
Esophageal plexus
use Thoracic Sympathetic Nerve
Esophagectomy
see Excision, Gastrointestinal System 0DB
see Resection, Gastrointestinal System 0DT
Esophagocoloplasty
see Repair, Gastrointestinal System 0DQ
see Supplement, Gastrointestinal System 0DU
Esophagoenterostomy
see Bypass, Gastrointestinal System 0D1
see Drainage, Gastrointestinal System 0D9
Esophagoesophagostomy
see Bypass, Gastrointestinal System 0D1
see Drainage, Gastrointestinal System 0D9
Esophagogastrectomy
see Excision, Gastrointestinal System 0DB
see Resection, Gastrointestinal System 0DT
Esophagogastroduodenoscopy (EGD) 0DJ08ZZ
Esophagogastroplasty
see Repair, Gastrointestinal System 0DQ
Esophagogastroplasty — *continued*
see Supplement, Gastrointestinal System 0DU
Esophagogastroscopy 0DJ68ZZ
Esophagogastrostomy
see Bypass, Gastrointestinal System 0D1
see Drainage, Gastrointestinal System 0D9
Esophagojejunoplasty
see Supplement, Gastrointestinal System 0DU
Esophagojejunostomy
see Bypass, Gastrointestinal System 0D1
see Drainage, Gastrointestinal System 0D9
Esophagomyotomy
see Division, Esophagogastric Junction 0D84
Esophagoplasty
see Repair, Gastrointestinal System 0DQ
see Replacement, Esophagus 0DR5
see Supplement, Gastrointestinal System 0DU
Esophagoplication
see Restriction, Gastrointestinal System 0DV
Esophagorrhaphy
see Repair, Gastrointestinal System 0DQ
Esophagoscopy 0DJ08ZZ
Esophagotomy
see Drainage, Gastrointestinal System 0D9
Esteem® implantable hearing system
use Hearing Device in Ear, Nose, Sinus
ESWL (extracorporeal shock wave lithotripsy)
see Fragmentation
Ethmoidal air cell
use Ethmoid Sinus, Right
use Ethmoid Sinus, Left
Ethmoidectomy
see Excision, Ear, Nose, Sinus 09B
see Resection, Ear, Nose, Sinus 09T
see Excision, Head and Facial Bones 0NB
see Resection, Head and Facial Bones 0NT
Ethmoidotomy
see Drainage, Ear, Nose, Sinus 099
Evacuation
Hematoma *see* Extirpation
Other Fluid *see* Drainage
Evera™ (XT)(S)(DR/VR)
use Defibrillator Generator in 0JH
Everolimus-eluting coronary stent
use Intraluminal Device, Drug-eluting in Heart and Great Vessels
Evisceration
Eyeball *see* Resection, Eye 08T
Eyeball with prosthetic implant *see* Replacement, Eye 08R
Ex-PRESS™ mini glaucoma shunt
use Synthetic Substitute
Examination
see Inspection
Exchange
see Change device in
Excision
Abdominal Wall 0WBF
Acetabulum
Left 0QB5
Right 0QB4
Adenoids 0CBQ
Ampulla of Vater 0FBC
Anal Sphincter 0DBR
Ankle Region
Left 0YBL
Right 0YBK
Anus 0DBQ
Aorta
Abdominal 04B0

Excision — *continued*
Aorta — *continued*
Thoracic
Ascending/Arch 02BX
Descending 02BW
Aortic Body 0GBD
Appendix 0DBJ
Arm
Lower
Left 0XBF
Right 0XBD
Upper
Left 0XB9
Right 0XB8
Artery
Anterior Tibial
Left 04BQ
Right 04BP
Axillary
Left 03B6
Right 03B5
Brachial
Left 03B8
Right 03B7
Celiac 04B1
Colic
Left 04B7
Middle 04B8
Right 04B6
Common Carotid
Left 03BJ
Right 03BH
Common Iliac
Left 04BD
Right 04BC
External Carotid
Left 03BN
Right 03BM
External Iliac
Left 04BJ
Right 04BH
Face 03BR
Femoral
Left 04BL
Right 04BK
Foot
Left 04BW
Right 04BV
Gastric 04B2
Hand
Left 03BF
Right 03BD
Hepatic 04B3
Inferior Mesenteric 04BB
Innominate 03B2
Internal Carotid
Left 03BL
Right 03BK
Internal Iliac
Left 04BF
Right 04BE
Internal Mammary
Left 03B1
Right 03B0
Intracranial 03BG
Lower 04BY
Peroneal
Left 04BU
Right 04BT
Popliteal
Left 04BN
Right 04BM
Posterior Tibial
Left 04BS
Right 04BR
Pulmonary
Left 02BR
Right 02BQ

Excision — *continued*
Artery — *continued*
Pulmonary Trunk 02BP
Radial
Left 03BC
Right 03BB
Renal
Left 04BA
Right 04B9
Splenic 04B4
Subclavian
Left 03B4
Right 03B3
Superior Mesenteric 04B5
Temporal
Left 03BT
Right 03BS
Thyroid
Left 03BV
Right 03BU
Ulnar
Left 03BA
Right 03B9
Upper 03BY
Vertebral
Left 03BQ
Right 03BP
Atrium
Left 02B7
Right 02B6
Auditory Ossicle
Left 09BA
Right 09B9
Axilla
Left 0XB5
Right 0XB4
Back
Lower 0WBL
Upper 0WBK
Basal Ganglia 00B8
Bladder 0TBB
Bladder Neck 0TBC
Bone
Ethmoid
Left 0NBG
Right 0NBF
Frontal 0NB1
Hyoid 0NBX
Lacrimal
Left 0NBJ
Right 0NBH
Nasal 0NBB
Occipital 0NB7
Palatine
Left 0NBL
Right 0NBK
Parietal
Left 0NB4
Right 0NB3
Pelvic
Left 0QB3
Right 0QB2
Sphenoid 0NBC
Temporal
Left 0NB6
Right 0NB5
Zygomatic
Left 0NBN
Right 0NBM
Brain 00B0
Breast
Bilateral 0HBV
Left 0HBU
Right 0HBT
Supernumerary 0HBY
Bronchus
Lingula 0BB9

Excision — *continued*
Bronchus — *continued*
Lower Lobe
Left 0BBB
Right 0BB6
Main
Left 0BB7
Right 0BB3
Middle Lobe, Right 0BB5
Upper Lobe
Left 0BB8
Right 0BB4
Buccal Mucosa 0CB4
Bursa and Ligament
Abdomen
Left 0MBJ
Right 0MBH
Ankle
Left 0MBR
Right 0MBQ
Elbow
Left 0MB4
Right 0MB3
Foot
Left 0MBT
Right 0MBS
Hand
Left 0MB8
Right 0MB7
Head and Neck 0MB0
Hip
Left 0MBM
Right 0MBL
Knee
Left 0MBP
Right 0MBN
Lower Extremity
Left 0MBW
Right 0MBV
Perineum 0MBK
Rib(s) 0MBG
Shoulder
Left 0MB2
Right 0MB1
Spine
Lower 0MBD
Upper 0MBC
Sternum 0MBF
Upper Extremity
Left 0MBB
Right 0MB9
Wrist
Left 0MB6
Right 0MB5
Buttock
Left 0YB1
Right 0YB0
Carina 0BB2
Carotid Bodies, Bilateral 0GB8
Carotid Body
Left 0GB6
Right 0GB7
Carpal
Left 0PBN
Right 0PBM
Cecum 0DBH
Cerebellum 00BC
Cerebral Hemisphere 00B7
Cerebral Meninges 00B1
Cerebral Ventricle 00B6
Cervix 0UBC
Chest Wall 0WB8
Chordae Tendineae 02B9
Choroid
Left 08BB
Right 08BA
Cisterna Chyli 07BL

Excision — *continued*
- Clavicle
  - Left 0PBB
  - Right 0PB9
- Clitoris 0UBJ
- Coccygeal Glomus 0GBB
- Coccyx 0QBS
- Colon
  - Ascending 0DBK
  - Descending 0DBM
  - Sigmoid 0DBN
  - Transverse 0DBL
- Conduction Mechanism 02B8
- Conjunctiva
  - Left 08BTXZ
  - Right 08BSXZ
- Cord
  - Bilateral 0VBH
  - Left 0VBG
  - Right 0VBF
- Cornea
  - Left 08B9XZ
  - Right 08B8XZ
- Cul-de-sac 0UBF
- Diaphragm 0BBT
- Disc
  - Cervical Vertebral 0RB3
  - Cervicothoracic Vertebral 0RB5
  - Lumbar Vertebral 0SB2
  - Lumbosacral 0SB4
  - Thoracic Vertebral 0RB9
  - Thoracolumbar Vertebral 0RBB
- Duct
  - Common Bile 0FB9
  - Cystic 0FB8
  - Hepatic
    - Common 0FB7
    - Left 0FB6
    - Right 0FB5
  - Lacrimal
    - Left 08BY
    - Right 08BX
  - Pancreatic 0FBD
    - Accessory 0FBF
  - Parotid
    - Left 0CBC
    - Right 0CBB
- Duodenum 0DB9
- Dura Mater 00B2
- Ear
  - External
    - Left 09B1
    - Right 09B0
  - External Auditory Canal
    - Left 09B4
    - Right 09B3
  - Inner
    - Left 09BE
    - Right 09BD
  - Middle
    - Left 09B6
    - Right 09B5
- Elbow Region
  - Left 0XBC
  - Right 0XBB
- Epididymis
  - Bilateral 0VBL
  - Left 0VBK
  - Right 0VBJ
- Epiglottis 0CBR
- Esophagogastric Junction 0DB4
- Esophagus 0DB5
  - Lower 0DB3
  - Middle 0DB2
  - Upper 0DB1
- Eustachian Tube
  - Left 09BG

Excision — *continued*
- Eustachian Tube — *continued*
  - Right 09BF
- Extremity
  - Lower
    - Left 0YBB
    - Right 0YB9
  - Upper
    - Left 0XB7
    - Right 0XB6
- Eye
  - Left 08B1
  - Right 08B0
- Eyelid
  - Lower
    - Left 08BR
    - Right 08BQ
  - Upper
    - Left 08BP
    - Right 08BN
- Face 0WB2
- Fallopian Tube
  - Left 0UB6
  - Right 0UB5
- Fallopian Tubes, Bilateral 0UB7
- Femoral Region
  - Left 0YB8
  - Right 0YB7
- Femoral Shaft
  - Left 0QB9
  - Right 0QB8
- Femur
  - Lower
    - Left 0QBC
    - Right 0QBB
  - Upper
    - Left 0QB7
    - Right 0QB6
- Fibula
  - Left 0QBK
  - Right 0QBJ
- Finger Nail 0HBQXZ
- Floor of mouth *see* Excision, Oral Cavity and Throat 0WB3
- Foot
  - Left 0YBN
  - Right 0YBM
- Gallbladder 0FB4
- Gingiva
  - Lower 0CB6
  - Upper 0CB5
- Gland
  - Adrenal
    - Bilateral 0GB4
    - Left 0GB2
    - Right 0GB3
  - Lacrimal
    - Left 08BW
    - Right 08BV
  - Minor Salivary 0CBJ
  - Parotid
    - Left 0CB9
    - Right 0CB8
  - Pituitary 0GB0
  - Sublingual
    - Left 0CBF
    - Right 0CBD
  - Submaxillary
    - Left 0CBH
    - Right 0CBG
  - Vestibular 0UBL
- Glenoid Cavity
  - Left 0PB8
  - Right 0PB7
- Glomus Jugulare 0GBC
- Hand
  - Left 0XBK

Excision — *continued*
- Hand — *continued*
  - Right 0XBJ
- Head 0WB0
- Humeral Head
  - Left 0PBD
  - Right 0PBC
- Humeral Shaft
  - Left 0PBG
  - Right 0PBF
- Hymen 0UBK
- Hypothalamus 00BA
- Ileocecal Valve 0DBC
- Ileum 0DBB
- Inguinal Region
  - Left 0YB6
  - Right 0YB5
- Intestine
  - Large 0DBE
    - Left 0DBG
    - Right 0DBF
  - Small 0DB8
- Iris
  - Left 08BD3Z
  - Right 08BC3Z
- Jaw
  - Lower 0WB5
  - Upper 0WB4
- Jejunum 0DBA
- Joint
  - Acromioclavicular
    - Left 0RBH
    - Right 0RBG
  - Ankle
    - Left 0SBG
    - Right 0SBF
  - Carpal
    - Left 0RBR
    - Right 0RBQ
  - Carpometacarpal
    - Left 0RBT
    - Right 0RBS
  - Cervical Vertebral 0RB1
  - Cervicothoracic Vertebral 0RB4
  - Coccygeal 0SB6
  - Elbow
    - Left 0RBM
    - Right 0RBL
  - Finger Phalangeal
    - Left 0RBX
    - Right 0RBW
  - Hip
    - Left 0SBB
    - Right 0SB9
  - Knee
    - Left 0SBD
    - Right 0SBC
  - Lumbar Vertebral 0SB0
  - Lumbosacral 0SB3
  - Metacarpophalangeal
    - Left 0RBV
    - Right 0RBU
  - Metatarsal-Phalangeal
    - Left 0SBN
    - Right 0SBM
  - Occipital-cervical 0RB0
  - Sacrococcygeal 0SB5
  - Sacroiliac
    - Left 0SB8
    - Right 0SB7
  - Shoulder
    - Left 0RBK
    - Right 0RBJ
  - Sternoclavicular
    - Left 0RBF
    - Right 0RBE

Excision — *continued*
Joint — *continued*
Tarsal
Left 0SBJ
Right 0SBH
Tarsometatarsal
Left 0SBL
Right 0SBK
Temporomandibular
Left 0RBD
Right 0RBC
Thoracic Vertebral 0RB6
Thoracolumbar Vertebral 0RBA
Toe Phalangeal
Left 0SBQ
Right 0SBP
Wrist
Left 0RBP
Right 0RBN
Kidney
Left 0TB1
Right 0TB0
Kidney Pelvis
Left 0TB4
Right 0TB3
Knee Region
Left 0YBG
Right 0YBF
Larynx 0CBS
Leg
Lower
Left 0YBJ
Right 0YBH
Upper
Left 0YBD
Right 0YBC
Lens
Left 08BK3Z
Right 08BJ3Z
Lip
Lower 0CB1
Upper 0CB0
Liver 0FB0
Left Lobe 0FB2
Right Lobe 0FB1
Lung
Bilateral 0BBM
Left 0BBL
Lower Lobe
Left 0BBJ
Right 0BBF
Middle Lobe, Right 0BBD
Right 0BBK
Upper Lobe
Left 0BBG
Right 0BBC
Lung Lingula 0BBH
Lymphatic
Aortic 07BD
Axillary
Left 07B6
Right 07B5
Head 07B0
Inguinal
Left 07BJ
Right 07BH
Internal Mammary
Left 07B9
Right 07B8
Lower Extremity
Left 07BG
Right 07BF
Mesenteric 07BB
Neck
Left 07B2
Right 07B1
Pelvis 07BC
Thoracic Duct 07BK

Excision — *continued*
Lymphatic — *continued*
Thorax 07B7
Upper Extremity
Left 07B4
Right 07B3
Mandible
Left 0NBV
Right 0NBT
Maxilla 0NBR
Mediastinum 0WBC
Medulla Oblongata 00BD
Mesentery 0DBV
Metacarpal
Left 0PBQ
Right 0PBP
Metatarsal
Left 0QBP
Right 0QBN
Muscle
Abdomen
Left 0KBL
Right 0KBK
Extraocular
Left 08BM
Right 08BL
Facial 0KB1
Foot
Left 0KBW
Right 0KBV
Hand
Left 0KBD
Right 0KBC
Head 0KB0
Hip
Left 0KBP
Right 0KBN
Lower Arm and Wrist
Left 0KBB
Right 0KB9
Lower Leg
Left 0KBT
Right 0KBS
Neck
Left 0KB3
Right 0KB2
Papillary 02BD
Perineum 0KBM
Shoulder
Left 0KB6
Right 0KB5
Thorax
Left 0KBJ
Right 0KBH
Tongue, Palate, Pharynx 0KB4
Trunk
Left 0KBG
Right 0KBF
Upper Arm
Left 0KB8
Right 0KB7
Upper Leg
Left 0KBR
Right 0KBQ
Nasal Mucosa and Soft Tissue 09BK
Nasopharynx 09BN
Neck 0WB6
Nerve
Abdominal Sympathetic 01BM
Abducens 00BL
Accessory 00BR
Acoustic 00BN
Brachial Plexus 01B3
Cervical 01B1
Cervical Plexus 01B0
Facial 00BM
Femoral 01BD

Excision — *continued*
Nerve — *continued*
Glossopharyngeal 00BP
Head and Neck Sympathetic 01BK
Hypoglossal 00BS
Lumbar 01BB
Lumbar Plexus 01B9
Lumbar Sympathetic 01BN
Lumbosacral Plexus 01BA
Median 01B5
Oculomotor 00BH
Olfactory 00BF
Optic 00BG
Peroneal 01BH
Phrenic 01B2
Pudendal 01BC
Radial 01B6
Sacral 01BR
Sacral Plexus 01BQ
Sacral Sympathetic 01BP
Sciatic 01BF
Thoracic 01B8
Thoracic Sympathetic 01BL
Tibial 01BG
Trigeminal 00BK
Trochlear 00BJ
Ulnar 01B4
Vagus 00BQ
Nipple
Left 0HBX
Right 0HBW
Omentum 0DBU
Oral Cavity and Throat 0WB3
Orbit
Left 0NBQ
Right 0NBP
Ovary
Bilateral 0UB2
Left 0UB1
Right 0UB0
Palate
Hard 0CB2
Soft 0CB3
Pancreas 0FBG
Para-aortic Body 0GB9
Paraganglion Extremity 0GBF
Parathyroid Gland 0GBR
Inferior
Left 0GBP
Right 0GBN
Multiple 0GBQ
Superior
Left 0GBM
Right 0GBL
Patella
Left 0QBF
Right 0QBD
Penis 0VBS
Pericardium 02BN
Perineum
Female 0WBN
Male 0WBM
Peritoneum 0DBW
Phalanx
Finger
Left 0PBV
Right 0PBT
Thumb
Left 0PBS
Right 0PBR
Toe
Left 0QBR
Right 0QBQ
Pharynx 0CBM
Pineal Body 0GB1
Pleura
Left 0BBP

Excision — *continued*
Pleura — *continued*
Right 0BBN
Pons 00BB
Prepuce 0VBT
Prostate 0VB0
Radius
Left 0PBJ
Right 0PBH
Rectum 0DBP
Retina
Left 08BF3Z
Right 08BE3Z
Retroperitoneum 0WBH
Ribs
1 to 2 0PB1
3 or More 0PB2
Sacrum 0QB1
Scapula
Left 0PB6
Right 0PB5
Sclera
Left 08B7XZ
Right 08B6XZ
Scrotum 0VB5
Septum
Atrial 02B5
Nasal 09BM
Ventricular 02BM
Shoulder Region
Left 0XB3
Right 0XB2
Sinus
Accessory 09BP
Ethmoid
Left 09BV
Right 09BU
Frontal
Left 09BT
Right 09BS
Mastoid
Left 09BC
Right 09BB
Maxillary
Left 09BR
Right 09BQ
Sphenoid
Left 09BX
Right 09BW
Skin
Abdomen 0HB7XZ
Back 0HB6XZ
Buttock 0HB8XZ
Chest 0HB5XZ
Ear
Left 0HB3XZ
Right 0HB2XZ
Face 0HB1XZ
Foot
Left 0HBNXZ
Right 0HBMXZ
Hand
Left 0HBGXZ
Right 0HBFXZ
Inguinal 0HBAXZ
Lower Arm
Left 0HBEXZ
Right 0HBDXZ
Lower Leg
Left 0HBLXZ
Right 0HBKXZ
Neck 0HB4XZ
Perineum 0HB9XZ
Scalp 0HB0XZ
Upper Arm
Left 0HBCXZ
Right 0HBBXZ

Excision — *continued*
Skin — *continued*
Upper Leg
Left 0HBJXZ
Right 0HBHXZ
Skull 0NB0
Spinal Cord
Cervical 00BW
Lumbar 00BY
Thoracic 00BX
Spinal Meninges 00BT
Spleen 07BP
Sternum 0PB0
Stomach 0DB6
Pylorus 0DB7
Subcutaneous Tissue and Fascia
Abdomen 0JB8
Back 0JB7
Buttock 0JB9
Chest 0JB6
Face 0JB1
Foot
Left 0JBR
Right 0JBQ
Hand
Left 0JBK
Right 0JBJ
Lower Arm
Left 0JBH
Right 0JBG
Lower Leg
Left 0JBP
Right 0JBN
Neck
Left 0JB5
Right 0JB4
Pelvic Region 0JBC
Perineum 0JBB
Scalp 0JB0
Upper Arm
Left 0JBF
Right 0JBD
Upper Leg
Left 0JBM
Right 0JBL
Tarsal
Left 0QBM
Right 0QBL
Tendon
Abdomen
Left 0LBG
Right 0LBF
Ankle
Left 0LBT
Right 0LBS
Foot
Left 0LBW
Right 0LBV
Hand
Left 0LB8
Right 0LB7
Head and Neck 0LB0
Hip
Left 0LBK
Right 0LBJ
Knee
Left 0LBR
Right 0LBQ
Lower Arm and Wrist
Left 0LB6
Right 0LB5
Lower Leg
Left 0LBP
Right 0LBN
Perineum 0LBH
Shoulder
Left 0LB2

Excision — *continued*
Tendon — *continued*
Right 0LB1
Thorax
Left 0LBD
Right 0LBC
Trunk
Left 0LBB
Right 0LB9
Upper Arm
Left 0LB4
Right 0LB3
Upper Leg
Left 0LBM
Right 0LBL
Testis
Bilateral 0VBC
Left 0VBB
Right 0VB9
Thalamus 00B9
Thymus 07BM
Thyroid Gland
Left Lobe 0GBG
Right Lobe 0GBH
Thyroid Gland Isthmus 0GBJ
Tibia
Left 0QBH
Right 0QBG
Toe Nail 0HBRXZ
Tongue 0CB7
Tonsils 0CBP
Tooth
Lower 0CBX
Upper 0CBW
Trachea 0BB1
Tunica Vaginalis
Left 0VB7
Right 0VB6
Turbinate, Nasal 09BL
Tympanic Membrane
Left 09B8
Right 09B7
Ulna
Left 0PBL
Right 0PBK
Ureter
Left 0TB7
Right 0TB6
Urethra 0TBD
Uterine Supporting Structure 0UB4
Uterus 0UB9
Uvula 0CBN
Vagina 0UBG
Valve
Aortic 02BF
Mitral 02BG
Pulmonary 02BH
Tricuspid 02BJ
Vas Deferens
Bilateral 0VBQ
Left 0VBP
Right 0VBN
Vein
Axillary
Left 05B8
Right 05B7
Azygos 05B0
Basilic
Left 05BC
Right 05BB
Brachial
Left 05BA
Right 05B9
Cephalic
Left 05BF
Right 05BD
Colic 06B7

Excision — *continued*
Vein — *continued*
Common Iliac
Left 06BD
Right 06BC
Coronary 02B4
Esophageal 06B3
External Iliac
Left 06BG
Right 06BF
External Jugular
Left 05BQ
Right 05BP
Face
Left 05BV
Right 05BT
Femoral
Left 06BN
Right 06BM
Foot
Left 06BV
Right 06BT
Gastric 06B2
Hand
Left 05BH
Right 05BG
Hemiazygos 05B1
Hepatic 06B4
Hypogastric
Left 06BJ
Right 06BH
Inferior Mesenteric 06B6
Innominate
Left 05B4
Right 05B3
Internal Jugular
Left 05BN
Right 05BM
Intracranial 05BL
Lower 06BY
Portal 06B8
Pulmonary
Left 02BT
Right 02BS
Renal
Left 06BB
Right 06B9
Saphenous
Left 06BQ
Right 06BP
Splenic 06B1
Subclavian
Left 05B6
Right 05B5
Superior Mesenteric 06B5
Upper 05BY
Vertebral
Left 05BS
Right 05BR
Vena Cava
Inferior 06B0
Superior 02BV
Ventricle
Left 02BL
Right 02BK
Vertebra
Cervical 0PB3
Lumbar 0QB0
Thoracic 0PB4
Vesicle
Bilateral 0VB3
Left 0VB2
Right 0VB1
Vitreous
Left 08B53Z
Right 08B43Z

Excision — *continued*
Vocal Cord
Left 0CBV
Right 0CBT
Vulva 0UBM
Wrist Region
Left 0XBH
Right 0XBG
EXCLUDER® AAA Endoprosthesis
use Intraluminal Device, Branched or Fenestrated, One or Two Arteries in 04V
use Intraluminal Device, Branched or Fenestrated, Three or More Arteries in 04V
use Intraluminal Device
EXCLUDER® IBE Endoprosthesis
use Intraluminal Device, Branched or Fenestrated, One or Two Arteries in 04V
Exclusion, left atrial appendage (LAA)
see Occlusion, Atrium, Left 02L7
Exercise, rehabilitation
see Motor Treatment, Rehabilitation F07
Exploration
see Inspection
Express® (LD) Premounted Stent System
use Intraluminal Device
Express® Biliary SD Monorail® Premounted Stent System
use Intraluminal Device
Express® SD Renal Monorail® Premounted Stent System
use Intraluminal Device
Extensor carpi radialis muscle
use Lower Arm and Wrist Muscle, Right
use Lower Arm and Wrist Muscle, Left
Extensor carpi ulnaris muscle
use Lower Arm and Wrist Muscle, Right
use Lower Arm and Wrist Muscle, Left
Extensor digitorum brevis muscle
use Foot Muscle, Right
use Foot Muscle, Left
Extensor digitorum longus muscle
use Lower Leg Muscle, Right
use Lower Leg Muscle, Left
Extensor hallucis brevis muscle
use Foot Muscle, Right
use Foot Muscle, Left
Extensor hallucis longus muscle
use Lower Leg Muscle, Right
use Lower Leg Muscle, Left
External anal sphincter
use Anal Sphincter
External auditory meatus
use External Auditory Canal, Right
use External Auditory Canal, Left
External fixator
use External Fixation Device in Head and Facial Bones
use External Fixation Device in Upper Bones
use External Fixation Device in Lower Bones
use External Fixation Device in Upper Joints
use External Fixation Device in Lower Joints
External maxillary artery
use Face Artery
External naris
use Nasal Mucosa and Soft Tissue
External oblique aponeurosis
use Subcutaneous Tissue and Fascia, Trunk
External oblique muscle
use Abdomen Muscle, Right
use Abdomen Muscle, Left
External popliteal nerve
use Peroneal Nerve
External pudendal artery
use Femoral Artery, Right
use Femoral Artery, Left

External pudendal vein
use Saphenous Vein, Right
use Saphenous Vein, Left
External urethral sphincter
use Urethra
Extirpation
Acetabulum
Left 0QC5
Right 0QC4
Adenoids 0CCQ
Ampulla of Vater 0FCC
Anal Sphincter 0DCR
Anterior Chamber
Left 08C3
Right 08C2
Anus 0DCQ
Aorta
Abdominal 04C0
Thoracic
Ascending/Arch 02CX
Descending 02CW
Aortic Body 0GCD
Appendix 0DCJ
Artery
Anterior Tibial
Left 04CQ
Right 04CP
Axillary
Left 03C6
Right 03C5
Brachial
Left 03C8
Right 03C7
Celiac 04C1
Colic
Left 04C7
Middle 04C8
Right 04C6
Common Carotid
Left 03CJ
Right 03CH
Common Iliac
Left 04CD
Right 04CC
Coronary
Four or More Arteries 02C3
One Artery 02C0
Three Arteries 02C2
Two Arteries 02C1
External Carotid
Left 03CN
Right 03CM
External Iliac
Left 04CJ
Right 04CH
Face 03CR
Femoral
Left 04CL
Right 04CK
Foot
Left 04CW
Right 04CV
Gastric 04C2
Hand
Left 03CF
Right 03CD
Hepatic 04C3
Inferior Mesenteric 04CB
Innominate 03C2
Internal Carotid
Left 03CL
Right 03CK
Internal Iliac
Left 04CF
Right 04CE

Extirpation — *continued*
Artery — *continued*
Internal Mammary
Left 03C1
Right 03C0
Intracranial 03CG
Lower 04CY
Peroneal
Left 04CU
Right 04CT
Popliteal
Left 04CN
Right 04CM
Posterior Tibial
Left 04CS
Right 04CR
Pulmonary
Left 02CR
Right 02CQ
Pulmonary Trunk 02CP
Radial
Left 03CC
Right 03CB
Renal
Left 04CA
Right 04C9
Splenic 04C4
Subclavian
Left 03C4
Right 03C3
Superior Mesenteric 04C5
Temporal
Left 03CT
Right 03CS
Thyroid
Left 03CV
Right 03CU
Ulnar
Left 03CA
Right 03C9
Upper 03CY
Vertebral
Left 03CQ
Right 03CP
Atrium
Left 02C7
Right 02C6
Auditory Ossicle
Left 09CA
Right 09C9
Basal Ganglia 00C8
Bladder 0TCB
Bladder Neck 0TCC
Bone
Ethmoid
Left 0NCG
Right 0NCF
Frontal 0NC1
Hyoid 0NCX
Lacrimal
Left 0NCJ
Right 0NCH
Nasal 0NCB
Occipital 0NC7
Palatine
Left 0NCL
Right 0NCK
Parietal
Left 0NC4
Right 0NC3
Pelvic
Left 0QC3
Right 0QC2
Sphenoid 0NCC
Temporal
Left 0NC6
Right 0NC5

Extirpation — *continued*
Zygomatic
Left 0NCN
Right 0NCM
Brain 00C0
Breast
Bilateral 0HCV
Left 0HCU
Right 0HCT
Bronchus
Lingula 0BC9
Lower Lobe
Left 0BCB
Right 0BC6
Main
Left 0BC7
Right 0BC3
Middle Lobe, Right 0BC5
Upper Lobe
Left 0BC8
Right 0BC4
Buccal Mucosa 0CC4
Bursa and Ligament
Abdomen
Left 0MCJ
Right 0MCH
Ankle
Left 0MCR
Right 0MCQ
Elbow
Left 0MC4
Right 0MC3
Foot
Left 0MCT
Right 0MCS
Hand
Left 0MC8
Right 0MC7
Head and Neck 0MC0
Hip
Left 0MCM
Right 0MCL
Knee
Left 0MCP
Right 0MCN
Lower Extremity
Left 0MCW
Right 0MCV
Perineum 0MCK
Rib(s) 0MCG
Shoulder
Left 0MC2
Right 0MC1
Spine
Lower 0MCD
Upper 0MCC
Sternum 0MCF
Upper Extremity
Left 0MCB
Right 0MC9
Wrist
Left 0MC6
Right 0MC5
Carina 0BC2
Carotid Bodies, Bilateral 0GC8
Carotid Body
Left 0GC6
Right 0GC7
Carpal
Left 0PCN
Right 0PCM
Cavity, Cranial 0WC1
Cecum 0DCH
Cerebellum 00CC
Cerebral Hemisphere 00C7
Cerebral Meninges 00C1
Cerebral Ventricle 00C6
Cervix 0UCC

Extirpation — *continued*
Chordae Tendineae 02C9
Choroid
Left 08CB
Right 08CA
Cisterna Chyli 07CL
Clavicle
Left 0PCB
Right 0PC9
Clitoris 0UCJ
Coccygeal Glomus 0GCB
Coccyx 0QCS
Colon
Ascending 0DCK
Descending 0DCM
Sigmoid 0DCN
Transverse 0DCL
Conduction Mechanism 02C8
Conjunctiva
Left 08CTXZZ
Right 08CSXZZ
Cord
Bilateral 0VCH
Left 0VCG
Right 0VCF
Cornea
Left 08C9XZZ
Right 08C8XZZ
Cul-de-sac 0UCF
Diaphragm 0BCT
Disc
Cervical Vertebral 0RC3
Cervicothoracic Vertebral 0RC5
Lumbar Vertebral 0SC2
Lumbosacral 0SC4
Thoracic Vertebral 0RC9
Thoracolumbar Vertebral 0RCB
Duct
Common Bile 0FC9
Cystic 0FC8
Hepatic
Common 0FC7
Left 0FC6
Right 0FC5
Lacrimal
Left 08CY
Right 08CX
Pancreatic 0FCD
Accessory 0FCF
Parotid
Left 0CCC
Right 0CCB
Duodenum 0DC9
Dura Mater 00C2
Ear
External
Left 09C1
Right 09C0
External Auditory Canal
Left 09C4
Right 09C3
Inner
Left 09CE
Right 09CD
Middle
Left 09C6
Right 09C5
Endometrium 0UCB
Epididymis
Bilateral 0VCL
Left 0VCK
Right 0VCJ
Epidural Space, Intracranial 00C3
Epiglottis 0CCR
Esophagogastric Junction 0DC4
Esophagus 0DC5
Lower 0DC3

Extirpation — *continued*
- Esophagus — *continued*
  - Middle 0DC2
  - Upper 0DC1
- Eustachian Tube
  - Left 09CG
  - Right 09CF
- Eye
  - Left 08C1XZZ
  - Right 08C0XZZ
- Eyelid
  - Lower
    - Left 08CR
    - Right 08CQ
  - Upper
    - Left 08CP
    - Right 08CN
- Fallopian Tube
  - Left 0UC6
  - Right 0UC5
- Fallopian Tubes, Bilateral 0UC7
- Femoral Shaft
  - Left 0QC9
  - Right 0QC8
- Femur
  - Lower
    - Left 0QCC
    - Right 0QCB
  - Upper
    - Left 0QC7
    - Right 0QC6
- Fibula
  - Left 0QCK
  - Right 0QCJ
- Finger Nail 0HCQXZZ
- Gallbladder 0FC4
- Gastrointestinal Tract 0WCP
- Genitourinary Tract 0WCR
- Gingiva
  - Lower 0CC6
  - Upper 0CC5
- Gland
  - Adrenal
    - Bilateral 0GC4
    - Left 0GC2
    - Right 0GC3
  - Lacrimal
    - Left 08CW
    - Right 08CV
  - Minor Salivary 0CCJ
  - Parotid
    - Left 0CC9
    - Right 0CC8
  - Pituitary 0GC0
  - Sublingual
    - Left 0CCF
    - Right 0CCD
  - Submaxillary
    - Left 0CCH
    - Right 0CCG
  - Vestibular 0UCL
- Glenoid Cavity
  - Left 0PC8
  - Right 0PC7
- Glomus Jugulare 0GCC
- Humeral Head
  - Left 0PCD
  - Right 0PCC
- Humeral Shaft
  - Left 0PCG
  - Right 0PCF
- Hymen 0UCK
- Hypothalamus 00CA
- Ileocecal Valve 0DCC
- Ileum 0DCB
- Intestine
  - Large 0DCE

Extirpation — *continued*
- Intestine — *continued*
    - Left 0DCG
    - Right 0DCF
  - Small 0DC8
- Iris
  - Left 08CD
  - Right 08CC
- Jejunum 0DCA
- Joint
  - Acromioclavicular
    - Left 0RCH
    - Right 0RCG
  - Ankle
    - Left 0SCG
    - Right 0SCF
  - Carpal
    - Left 0RCR
    - Right 0RCQ
  - Carpometacarpal
    - Left 0RCT
    - Right 0RCS
  - Cervical Vertebral 0RC1
  - Cervicothoracic Vertebral 0RC4
  - Coccygeal 0SC6
  - Elbow
    - Left 0RCM
    - Right 0RCL
  - Finger Phalangeal
    - Left 0RCX
    - Right 0RCW
  - Hip
    - Left 0SCB
    - Right 0SC9
  - Knee
    - Left 0SCD
    - Right 0SCC
  - Lumbar Vertebral 0SC0
  - Lumbosacral 0SC3
  - Metacarpophalangeal
    - Left 0RCV
    - Right 0RCU
  - Metatarsal-Phalangeal
    - Left 0SCN
    - Right 0SCM
  - Occipital-cervical 0RC0
  - Sacrococcygeal 0SC5
  - Sacroiliac
    - Left 0SC8
    - Right 0SC7
  - Shoulder
    - Left 0RCK
    - Right 0RCJ
  - Sternoclavicular
    - Left 0RCF
    - Right 0RCE
  - Tarsal
    - Left 0SCJ
    - Right 0SCH
  - Tarsometatarsal
    - Left 0SCL
    - Right 0SCK
  - Temporomandibular
    - Left 0RCD
    - Right 0RCC
  - Thoracic Vertebral 0RC6
  - Thoracolumbar Vertebral 0RCA
  - Toe Phalangeal
    - Left 0SCQ
    - Right 0SCP
  - Wrist
    - Left 0RCP
    - Right 0RCN
- Kidney
  - Left 0TC1
  - Right 0TC0

Extirpation — *continued*
- Kidney Pelvis
  - Left 0TC4
  - Right 0TC3
- Larynx 0CCS
- Lens
  - Left 08CK
  - Right 08CJ
- Lip
  - Lower 0CC1
  - Upper 0CC0
- Liver 0FC0
  - Left Lobe 0FC2
  - Right Lobe 0FC1
- Lung
  - Bilateral 0BCM
  - Left 0BCL
  - Lower Lobe
    - Left 0BCJ
    - Right 0BCF
  - Middle Lobe, Right 0BCD
  - Right 0BCK
  - Upper Lobe
    - Left 0BCG
    - Right 0BCC
- Lung Lingula 0BCH
- Lymphatic
  - Aortic 07CD
  - Axillary
    - Left 07C6
    - Right 07C5
  - Head 07C0
  - Inguinal
    - Left 07CJ
    - Right 07CH
  - Internal Mammary
    - Left 07C9
    - Right 07C8
  - Lower Extremity
    - Left 07CG
    - Right 07CF
  - Mesenteric 07CB
  - Neck
    - Left 07C2
    - Right 07C1
  - Pelvis 07CC
  - Thoracic Duct 07CK
  - Thorax 07C7
  - Upper Extremity
    - Left 07C4
    - Right 07C3
- Mandible
  - Left 0NCV
  - Right 0NCT
- Maxilla 0NCR
- Mediastinum 0WCC
- Medulla Oblongata 00CD
- Mesentery 0DCV
- Metacarpal
  - Left 0PCQ
  - Right 0PCP
- Metatarsal
  - Left 0QCP
  - Right 0QCN
- Muscle
  - Abdomen
    - Left 0KCL
    - Right 0KCK
  - Extraocular
    - Left 08CM
    - Right 08CL
  - Facial 0KC1
  - Foot
    - Left 0KCW
    - Right 0KCV
  - Hand
    - Left 0KCD

Extirpation — *continued*
- Muscle — *continued*
    - Right 0KCC
  - Head 0KC0
  - Hip
    - Left 0KCP
    - Right 0KCN
  - Lower Arm and Wrist
    - Left 0KCB
    - Right 0KC9
  - Lower Leg
    - Left 0KCT
    - Right 0KCS
  - Neck
    - Left 0KC3
    - Right 0KC2
  - Papillary 02CD
  - Perineum 0KCM
  - Shoulder
    - Left 0KC6
    - Right 0KC5
  - Thorax
    - Left 0KCJ
    - Right 0KCH
  - Tongue, Palate, Pharynx 0KC4
  - Trunk
    - Left 0KCG
    - Right 0KCF
  - Upper Arm
    - Left 0KC8
    - Right 0KC7
  - Upper Leg
    - Left 0KCR
    - Right 0KCQ
- Nasal Mucosa and Soft Tissue 09CK
- Nasopharynx 09CN
- Nerve
  - Abdominal Sympathetic 01CM
  - Abducens 00CL
  - Accessory 00CR
  - Acoustic 00CN
  - Brachial Plexus 01C3
  - Cervical 01C1
  - Cervical Plexus 01C0
  - Facial 00CM
  - Femoral 01CD
  - Glossopharyngeal 00CP
  - Head and Neck Sympathetic 01CK
  - Hypoglossal 00CS
  - Lumbar 01CB
  - Lumbar Plexus 01C9
  - Lumbar Sympathetic 01CN
  - Lumbosacral Plexus 01CA
  - Median 01C5
  - Oculomotor 00CH
  - Olfactory 00CF
  - Optic 00CG
  - Peroneal 01CH
  - Phrenic 01C2
  - Pudendal 01CC
  - Radial 01C6
  - Sacral 01CR
  - Sacral Plexus 01CQ
  - Sacral Sympathetic 01CP
  - Sciatic 01CF
  - Thoracic 01C8
  - Thoracic Sympathetic 01CL
  - Tibial 01CG
  - Trigeminal 00CK
  - Trochlear 00CJ
  - Ulnar 01C4
  - Vagus 00CQ
- Nipple
  - Left 0HCX
  - Right 0HCW
- Omentum 0DCU
- Oral Cavity and Throat 0WC3

Extirpation — *continued*
- Orbit
  - Left 0NCQ
  - Right 0NCP
- Orbital Atherectomy Technology X2C
- Ovary
  - Bilateral 0UC2
  - Left 0UC1
  - Right 0UC0
- Palate
  - Hard 0CC2
  - Soft 0CC3
- Pancreas 0FCG
- Para-aortic Body 0GC9
- Paraganglion Extremity 0GCF
- Parathyroid Gland 0GCR
  - Inferior
    - Left 0GCP
    - Right 0GCN
  - Multiple 0GCQ
  - Superior
    - Left 0GCM
    - Right 0GCL
- Patella
  - Left 0QCF
  - Right 0QCD
- Pelvic Cavity 0WCJ
- Penis 0VCS
- Pericardial Cavity 0WCD
- Pericardium 02CN
- Peritoneal Cavity 0WCG
- Peritoneum 0DCW
- Phalanx
  - Finger
    - Left 0PCV
    - Right 0PCT
  - Thumb
    - Left 0PCS
    - Right 0PCR
  - Toe
    - Left 0QCR
    - Right 0QCQ
- Pharynx 0CCM
- Pineal Body 0GC1
- Pleura
  - Left 0BCP
  - Right 0BCN
- Pleural Cavity
  - Left 0WCB
  - Right 0WC9
- Pons 00CB
- Prepuce 0VCT
- Prostate 0VC0
- Radius
  - Left 0PCJ
  - Right 0PCH
- Rectum 0DCP
- Respiratory Tract 0WCQ
- Retina
  - Left 08CF
  - Right 08CE
- Retinal Vessel
  - Left 08CH
  - Right 08CG
- Retroperitoneum 0WCH
- Ribs
  - 1 to 2 0PC1
  - 3 or More 0PC2
- Sacrum 0QC1
- Scapula
  - Left 0PC6
  - Right 0PC5
- Sclera
  - Left 08C7XZZ
  - Right 08C6XZZ
- Scrotum 0VC5

Extirpation — *continued*
- Septum
  - Atrial 02C5
  - Nasal 09CM
  - Ventricular 02CM
- Sinus
  - Accessory 09CP
  - Ethmoid
    - Left 09CV
    - Right 09CU
  - Frontal
    - Left 09CT
    - Right 09CS
  - Mastoid
    - Left 09CC
    - Right 09CB
  - Maxillary
    - Left 09CR
    - Right 09CQ
  - Sphenoid
    - Left 09CX
    - Right 09CW
- Skin
  - Abdomen 0HC7XZZ
  - Back 0HC6XZZ
  - Buttock 0HC8XZZ
  - Chest 0HC5XZZ
  - Ear
    - Left 0HC3XZZ
    - Right 0HC2XZZ
  - Face 0HC1XZZ
  - Foot
    - Left 0HCNXZZ
    - Right 0HCMXZZ
  - Hand
    - Left 0HCGXZZ
    - Right 0HCFXZZ
  - Inguinal 0HCAXZZ
  - Lower Arm
    - Left 0HCEXZZ
    - Right 0HCDXZZ
  - Lower Leg
    - Left 0HCLXZZ
    - Right 0HCKXZZ
  - Neck 0HC4XZZ
  - Perineum 0HC9XZZ
  - Scalp 0HC0XZZ
  - Upper Arm
    - Left 0HCCXZZ
    - Right 0HCBXZZ
  - Upper Leg
    - Left 0HCJXZZ
    - Right 0HCHXZZ
- Spinal Canal 00CU
- Spinal Cord
  - Cervical 00CW
  - Lumbar 00CY
  - Thoracic 00CX
- Spinal Meninges 00CT
- Spleen 07CP
- Sternum 0PC0
- Stomach 0DC6
  - Pylorus 0DC7
- Subarachnoid Space, Intracranial 00C5
- Subcutaneous Tissue and Fascia
  - Abdomen 0JC8
  - Back 0JC7
  - Buttock 0JC9
  - Chest 0JC6
  - Face 0JC1
  - Foot
    - Left 0JCR
    - Right 0JCQ
  - Hand
    - Left 0JCK
    - Right 0JCJ

Extirpation — *continued*
Subcutaneous Tissue and Fascia — *continued*
Lower Arm
Left 0JCH
Right 0JCG
Lower Leg
Left 0JCP
Right 0JCN
Neck
Left 0JC5
Right 0JC4
Pelvic Region 0JCC
Perineum 0JCB
Scalp 0JC0
Upper Arm
Left 0JCF
Right 0JCD
Upper Leg
Left 0JCM
Right 0JCL
Subdural Space, Intracranial 00C4
Tarsal
Left 0QCM
Right 0QCL
Tendon
Abdomen
Left 0LCG
Right 0LCF
Ankle
Left 0LCT
Right 0LCS
Foot
Left 0LCW
Right 0LCV
Hand
Left 0LC8
Right 0LC7
Head and Neck 0LC0
Hip
Left 0LCK
Right 0LCJ
Knee
Left 0LCR
Right 0LCQ
Lower Arm and Wrist
Left 0LC6
Right 0LC5
Lower Leg
Left 0LCP
Right 0LCN
Perineum 0LCH
Shoulder
Left 0LC2
Right 0LC1
Thorax
Left 0LCD
Right 0LCC
Trunk
Left 0LCB
Right 0LC9
Upper Arm
Left 0LC4
Right 0LC3
Upper Leg
Left 0LCM
Right 0LCL
Testis
Bilateral 0VCC
Left 0VCB
Right 0VC9
Thalamus 00C9
Thymus 07CM
Thyroid Gland 0GCK
Left Lobe 0GCG
Right Lobe 0GCH
Tibia
Left 0QCH
Right 0QCG

Extirpation — *continued*
Toe Nail 0HCRXZZ
Tongue 0CC7
Tonsils 0CCP
Tooth
Lower 0CCX
Upper 0CCW
Trachea 0BC1
Tunica Vaginalis
Left 0VC7
Right 0VC6
Turbinate, Nasal 09CL
Tympanic Membrane
Left 09C8
Right 09C7
Ulna
Left 0PCL
Right 0PCK
Ureter
Left 0TC7
Right 0TC6
Urethra 0TCD
Uterine Supporting Structure 0UC4
Uterus 0UC9
Uvula 0CCN
Vagina 0UCG
Valve
Aortic 02CF
Mitral 02CG
Pulmonary 02CH
Tricuspid 02CJ
Vas Deferens
Bilateral 0VCQ
Left 0VCP
Right 0VCN
Vein
Axillary
Left 05C8
Right 05C7
Azygos 05C0
Basilic
Left 05CC
Right 05CB
Brachial
Left 05CA
Right 05C9
Cephalic
Left 05CF
Right 05CD
Colic 06C7
Common Iliac
Left 06CD
Right 06CC
Coronary 02C4
Esophageal 06C3
External Iliac
Left 06CG
Right 06CF
External Jugular
Left 05CQ
Right 05CP
Face
Left 05CV
Right 05CT
Femoral
Left 06CN
Right 06CM
Foot
Left 06CV
Right 06CT
Gastric 06C2
Hand
Left 05CH
Right 05CG
Hemiazygos 05C1
Hepatic 06C4

Extirpation — *continued*
Vein — *continued*
Hypogastric
Left 06CJ
Right 06CH
Inferior Mesenteric 06C6
Innominate
Left 05C4
Right 05C3
Internal Jugular
Left 05CN
Right 05CM
Intracranial 05CL
Lower 06CY
Portal 06C8
Pulmonary
Left 02CT
Right 02CS
Renal
Left 06CB
Right 06C9
Saphenous
Left 06CQ
Right 06CP
Splenic 06C1
Subclavian
Left 05C6
Right 05C5
Superior Mesenteric 06C5
Upper 05CY
Vertebral
Left 05CS
Right 05CR
Vena Cava
Inferior 06C0
Superior 02CV
Ventricle
Left 02CL
Right 02CK
Vertebra
Cervical 0PC3
Lumbar 0QC0
Thoracic 0PC4
Vesicle
Bilateral 0VC3
Left 0VC2
Right 0VC1
Vitreous
Left 08C5
Right 08C4
Vocal Cord
Left 0CCV
Right 0CCT
Vulva 0UCM
Extracorporeal carbon dioxide removal (ECCO2R) 5A0920Z
Extracorporeal shock wave lithotripsy
see Fragmentation
Extracranial-intracranial bypass (EC-IC)
see Bypass, Upper Arteries 031
Extraction
Acetabulum
Left 0QD50ZZ
Right 0QD40ZZ
Ampulla of Vater 0FDC
Anus 0DDQ
Appendix 0DDJ
Auditory Ossicle
Left 09DA0ZZ
Right 09D90ZZ
Bone
Ethmoid
Left 0NDG0ZZ
Right 0NDF0ZZ
Frontal 0ND10ZZ
Hyoid 0NDX0ZZ
Lacrimal
Left 0NDJ0ZZ

- **Extraction** — *continued*
  - Bone — *continued*
    - Right 0NDH0ZZ
    - Nasal 0NDB0ZZ
    - Occipital 0ND70ZZ
    - Palatine
      - Left 0NDL0ZZ
      - Right 0NDK0ZZ
    - Parietal
      - Left 0ND40ZZ
      - Right 0ND30ZZ
    - Pelvic
      - Left 0QD30ZZ
      - Right 0QD20ZZ
    - Sphenoid 0NDC0ZZ
    - Temporal
      - Left 0ND60ZZ
      - Right 0ND50ZZ
    - Zygomatic
      - Left 0NDN0ZZ
      - Right 0NDM0ZZ
  - Bone Marrow
    - Iliac 07DR
    - Sternum 07DQ
    - Vertebral 07DS
  - Bronchus
    - Lingula 0BD9
    - Lower Lobe
      - Left 0BDB
      - Right 0BD6
    - Main
      - Left 0BD7
      - Right 0BD3
    - Middle Lobe, Right 0BD5
    - Upper Lobe
      - Left 0BD8
      - Right 0BD4
  - Bursa and Ligament
    - Abdomen
      - Left 0MDJ
      - Right 0MDH
    - Ankle
      - Left 0MDR
      - Right 0MDQ
    - Elbow
      - Left 0MD4
      - Right 0MD3
    - Foot
      - Left 0MDT
      - Right 0MDS
    - Hand
      - Left 0MD8
      - Right 0MD7
    - Head and Neck 0MD0
    - Hip
      - Left 0MDM
      - Right 0MDL
    - Knee
      - Left 0MDP
      - Right 0MDN
    - Lower Extremity
      - Left 0MDW
      - Right 0MDV
    - Perineum 0MDK
    - Rib(s) 0MDG
    - Shoulder
      - Left 0MD2
      - Right 0MD1
    - Spine
      - Lower 0MDD
      - Upper 0MDC
    - Sternum 0MDF
    - Upper Extremity
      - Left 0MDB
      - Right 0MD9
    - Wrist
      - Left 0MD6

- **Extraction** — *continued*
  - Bursa and Ligament — *continued*
    - Right 0MD5
  - Carina 0BD2
  - Carpal
    - Left 0PDN0ZZ
    - Right 0PDM0ZZ
  - Cecum 0DDH
  - Cerebral Meninges 00D1
  - Cisterna Chyli 07DL
  - Clavicle
    - Left 0PDB0ZZ
    - Right 0PD90ZZ
  - Coccyx 0QDS0ZZ
  - Colon
    - Ascending 0DDK
    - Descending 0DDM
    - Sigmoid 0DDN
    - Transverse 0DDL
  - Cornea
    - Left 08D9XZ
    - Right 08D8XZ
  - Duct
    - Common Bile 0FD9
    - Cystic 0FD8
    - Hepatic
      - Common 0FD7
      - Left 0FD6
      - Right 0FD5
    - Pancreatic 0FDD
      - Accessory 0FDF
  - Duodenum 0DD9
  - Dura Mater 00D2
  - Endometrium 0UDB
  - Esophagogastric Junction 0DD4
  - Esophagus 0DD5
    - Lower 0DD3
    - Middle 0DD2
    - Upper 0DD1
  - Femoral Shaft
    - Left 0QD90ZZ
    - Right 0QD80ZZ
  - Femur
    - Lower
      - Left 0QDC0ZZ
      - Right 0QDB0ZZ
    - Upper
      - Left 0QD70ZZ
      - Right 0QD60ZZ
  - Fibula
    - Left 0QDK0ZZ
    - Right 0QDJ0ZZ
  - Finger Nail 0HDQXZZ
  - Gallbladder 0FD4
  - Glenoid Cavity
    - Left 0PD80ZZ
    - Right 0PD70ZZ
  - Hair 0HDSXZZ
  - Humeral Head
    - Left 0PDD0ZZ
    - Right 0PDC0ZZ
  - Humeral Shaft
    - Left 0PDG0ZZ
    - Right 0PDF0ZZ
  - Ileocecal Valve 0DDC
  - Ileum 0DDB
  - Intestine
    - Large 0DDE
      - Left 0DDG
      - Right 0DDF
    - Small 0DD8
  - Jejunum 0DDA
  - Kidney
    - Left 0TD1
    - Right 0TD0
  - Lens
    - Left 08DK3ZZ

- **Extraction** — *continued*
  - Lens — *continued*
    - Right 08DJ3ZZ
  - Liver 0FD0
    - Left Lobe 0FD2
    - Right Lobe 0FD1
  - Lung
    - Bilateral 0BDM
    - Left 0BDL
    - Lower Lobe
      - Left 0BDJ
      - Right 0BDF
    - Middle Lobe, Right 0BDD
    - Right 0BDK
    - Upper Lobe
      - Left 0BDG
      - Right 0BDC
  - Lung Lingula 0BDH
  - Lymphatic
    - Aortic 07DD
    - Axillary
      - Left 07D6
      - Right 07D5
    - Head 07D0
    - Inguinal
      - Left 07DJ
      - Right 07DH
    - Internal Mammary
      - Left 07D9
      - Right 07D8
    - Lower Extremity
      - Left 07DG
      - Right 07DF
    - Mesenteric 07DB
    - Neck
      - Left 07D2
      - Right 07D1
    - Pelvis 07DC
    - Thoracic Duct 07DK
    - Thorax 07D7
    - Upper Extremity
      - Left 07D4
      - Right 07D3
  - Mandible
    - Left 0NDV0ZZ
    - Right 0NDT0ZZ
  - Maxilla 0NDR0ZZ
  - Metacarpal
    - Left 0PDQ0ZZ
    - Right 0PDP0ZZ
  - Metatarsal
    - Left 0QDP0ZZ
    - Right 0QDN0ZZ
  - Muscle
    - Abdomen
      - Left 0KDL0ZZ
      - Right 0KDK0ZZ
    - Facial 0KD10ZZ
    - Foot
      - Left 0KDW0ZZ
      - Right 0KDV0ZZ
    - Hand
      - Left 0KDD0ZZ
      - Right 0KDC0ZZ
    - Head 0KD00ZZ
    - Hip
      - Left 0KDP0ZZ
      - Right 0KDN0ZZ
    - Lower Arm and Wrist
      - Left 0KDB0ZZ
      - Right 0KD90ZZ
    - Lower Leg
      - Left 0KDT0ZZ
      - Right 0KDS0ZZ
    - Neck
      - Left 0KD30ZZ
      - Right 0KD20ZZ

Extraction — *continued*
- Muscle — *continued*
  - Perineum 0KDM0ZZ
  - Shoulder
    - Left 0KD60ZZ
    - Right 0KD50ZZ
  - Thorax
    - Left 0KDJ0ZZ
    - Right 0KDH0ZZ
  - Tongue, Palate, Pharynx 0KD40ZZ
  - Trunk
    - Left 0KDG0ZZ
    - Right 0KDF0ZZ
  - Upper Arm
    - Left 0KD80ZZ
    - Right 0KD70ZZ
  - Upper Leg
    - Left 0KDR0ZZ
    - Right 0KDQ0ZZ
- Nerve
  - Abdominal Sympathetic 01DM
  - Abducens 00DL
  - Accessory 00DR
  - Acoustic 00DN
  - Brachial Plexus 01D3
  - Cervical 01D1
  - Cervical Plexus 01D0
  - Facial 00DM
  - Femoral 01DD
  - Glossopharyngeal 00DP
  - Head and Neck Sympathetic 01DK
  - Hypoglossal 00DS
  - Lumbar 01DB
  - Lumbar Plexus 01D9
  - Lumbar Sympathetic 01DN
  - Lumbosacral Plexus 01DA
  - Median 01D5
  - Oculomotor 00DH
  - Olfactory 00DF
  - Optic 00DG
  - Peroneal 01DH
  - Phrenic 01D2
  - Pudendal 01DC
  - Radial 01D6
  - Sacral 01DR
  - Sacral Plexus 01DQ
  - Sacral Sympathetic 01DP
  - Sciatic 01DF
  - Thoracic 01D8
  - Thoracic Sympathetic 01DL
  - Tibial 01DG
  - Trigeminal 00DK
  - Trochlear 00DJ
  - Ulnar 01D4
  - Vagus 00DQ
- Orbit
  - Left 0NDQ0ZZ
  - Right 0NDP0ZZ
- Ova 0UDN
- Pancreas 0FDG
- Patella
  - Left 0QDF0ZZ
  - Right 0QDD0ZZ
- Phalanx
  - Finger
    - Left 0PDV0ZZ
    - Right 0PDT0ZZ
  - Thumb
    - Left 0PDS0ZZ
    - Right 0PDR0ZZ
  - Toe
    - Left 0QDR0ZZ
    - Right 0QDQ0ZZ
- Pleura
  - Left 0BDP
  - Right 0BDN

Extraction — *continued*
- Products of Conception
  - Ectopic 10D2
  - Extraperitoneal 10D00Z2
  - High 10D00Z0
  - High Forceps 10D07Z5
  - Internal Version 10D07Z7
  - Low 10D00Z1
  - Low Forceps 10D07Z3
  - Mid Forceps 10D07Z4
  - Other 10D07Z8
  - Retained 10D1
  - Vacuum 10D07Z6
- Radius
  - Left 0PDJ0ZZ
  - Right 0PDH0ZZ
- Rectum 0DDP
- Ribs
  - 1 to 2 0PD10ZZ
  - 3 or More 0PD20ZZ
- Sacrum 0QD10ZZ
- Scapula
  - Left 0PD60ZZ
  - Right 0PD50ZZ
- Septum, Nasal 09DM
- Sinus
  - Accessory 09DP
  - Ethmoid
    - Left 09DV
    - Right 09DU
  - Frontal
    - Left 09DT
    - Right 09DS
  - Mastoid
    - Left 09DC
    - Right 09DB
  - Maxillary
    - Left 09DR
    - Right 09DQ
  - Sphenoid
    - Left 09DX
    - Right 09DW
- Skin
  - Abdomen 0HD7XZZ
  - Back 0HD6XZZ
  - Buttock 0HD8XZZ
  - Chest 0HD5XZZ
  - Ear
    - Left 0HD3XZZ
    - Right 0HD2XZZ
  - Face 0HD1XZZ
  - Foot
    - Left 0HDNXZZ
    - Right 0HDMXZZ
  - Hand
    - Left 0HDGXZZ
    - Right 0HDFXZZ
  - Inguinal 0HDAXZZ
  - Lower Arm
    - Left 0HDEXZZ
    - Right 0HDDXZZ
  - Lower Leg
    - Left 0HDLXZZ
    - Right 0HDKXZZ
  - Neck 0HD4XZZ
  - Perineum 0HD9XZZ
  - Scalp 0HD0XZZ
  - Upper Arm
    - Left 0HDCXZZ
    - Right 0HDBXZZ
  - Upper Leg
    - Left 0HDJXZZ
    - Right 0HDHXZZ
- Skull 0ND00ZZ
- Spinal Meninges 00DT
- Spleen 07DP
- Sternum 0PD00ZZ

Extraction — *continued*
- Stomach 0DD6
  - Pylorus 0DD7
- Subcutaneous Tissue and Fascia
  - Abdomen 0JD8
  - Back 0JD7
  - Buttock 0JD9
  - Chest 0JD6
  - Face 0JD1
  - Foot
    - Left 0JDR
    - Right 0JDQ
  - Hand
    - Left 0JDK
    - Right 0JDJ
  - Lower Arm
    - Left 0JDH
    - Right 0JDG
  - Lower Leg
    - Left 0JDP
    - Right 0JDN
  - Neck
    - Left 0JD5
    - Right 0JD4
  - Pelvic Region 0JDC
  - Perineum 0JDB
  - Scalp 0JD0
  - Upper Arm
    - Left 0JDF
    - Right 0JDD
  - Upper Leg
    - Left 0JDM
    - Right 0JDL
- Tarsal
  - Left 0QDM0ZZ
  - Right 0QDL0ZZ
- Tendon
  - Abdomen
    - Left 0LDG0ZZ
    - Right 0LDF0ZZ
  - Ankle
    - Left 0LDT0ZZ
    - Right 0LDS0ZZ
  - Foot
    - Left 0LDW0ZZ
    - Right 0LDV0ZZ
  - Hand
    - Left 0LD80ZZ
    - Right 0LD70ZZ
  - Head and Neck 0LD00ZZ
  - Hip
    - Left 0LDK0ZZ
    - Right 0LDJ0ZZ
  - Knee
    - Left 0LDR0ZZ
    - Right 0LDQ0ZZ
  - Lower Arm and Wrist
    - Left 0LD60ZZ
    - Right 0LD50ZZ
  - Lower Leg
    - Left 0LDP0ZZ
    - Right 0LDN0ZZ
  - Perineum 0LDH0ZZ
  - Shoulder
    - Left 0LD20ZZ
    - Right 0LD10ZZ
  - Thorax
    - Left 0LDD0ZZ
    - Right 0LDC0ZZ
  - Trunk
    - Left 0LDB0ZZ
    - Right 0LD90ZZ
  - Upper Arm
    - Left 0LD40ZZ
    - Right 0LD30ZZ
  - Upper Leg
    - Left 0LDM0ZZ

Extraction — *continued*
Tendon — *continued*
Right 0LDL0ZZ
Thymus 07DM
Tibia
Left 0QDH0ZZ
Right 0QDG0ZZ
Toe Nail 0HDRXZZ
Tooth
Lower 0CDXXZ
Upper 0CDWXZ
Trachea 0BD1
Turbinate, Nasal 09DL
Tympanic Membrane
Left 09D8
Right 09D7
Ulna
Left 0PDL0ZZ
Right 0PDK0ZZ
Vein
Basilic
Left 05DC
Right 05DB
Brachial
Left 05DA
Right 05D9
Cephalic
Left 05DF
Right 05DD
Femoral
Left 06DN
Right 06DM
Foot
Left 06DV
Right 06DT
Hand
Left 05DH
Right 05DG
Lower 06DY
Saphenous
Left 06DQ
Right 06DP
Upper 05DY
Vertebra
Cervical 0PD30ZZ
Lumbar 0QD00ZZ
Thoracic 0PD40ZZ
Vocal Cord
Left 0CDV
Right 0CDT
Extradural space, intracranial
use Epidural Space, Intracranial
Extradural space, spinal
use Spinal Canal
EXtreme Lateral Interbody Fusion (XLIF®) device
use Interbody Fusion Device in Lower Joints

F

Face lift
see Alteration, Face 0W02
Facet replacement spinal stabilization device
use Spinal Stabilization Device, Facet Replacement in 0RH
use Spinal Stabilization Device, Facet Replacement in 0SH
Facial artery
use Face Artery
Factor Xa Inhibitor Reversal Agent, Andexanet Alfa
use Andexanet Alfa, Factor Xa Inhibitor Reversal Agent
False vocal cord
use Larynx
Falx cerebri
use Dura Mater
Fascia lata
use Subcutaneous Tissue and Fascia, Right Upper Leg
use Subcutaneous Tissue and Fascia, Left Upper Leg
Fasciaplasty, fascioplasty
see Repair, Subcutaneous Tissue and Fascia 0JQ
see Replacement, Subcutaneous Tissue and Fascia 0JR
Fasciectomy
see Excision, Subcutaneous Tissue and Fascia 0JB
Fasciorrhaphy
see Repair, Subcutaneous Tissue and Fascia 0JQ
Fasciotomy
see Division, Subcutaneous Tissue and Fascia 0J8
see Drainage, Subcutaneous Tissue and Fascia 0J9
see Release
Feeding device
Change device in
Lower 0D2DXUZ
Upper 0D20XUZ
Insertion of device in
Duodenum 0DH9
Esophagus 0DH5
Ileum 0DHB
Intestine, Small 0DH8
Jejunum 0DHA
Stomach 0DH6
Removal of device from
Esophagus 0DP5
Intestinal Tract
Lower 0DPD
Upper 0DP0
Stomach 0DP6
Revision of device in
Intestinal Tract
Lower 0DWD
Upper 0DW0
Stomach 0DW6
Femoral head
use Upper Femur, Right
use Upper Femur, Left
Femoral lymph node
use Lymphatic, Right Lower Extremity
use Lymphatic, Left Lower Extremity
Femoropatellar joint
use Knee Joint, Right
use Knee Joint, Left
use Knee Joint, Femoral Surface, Right
use Knee Joint, Femoral Surface, Left
Femorotibial joint
use Knee Joint, Right
use Knee Joint, Left
use Knee Joint, Tibial Surface, Right
use Knee Joint, Tibial Surface, Left
Fibular artery
use Peroneal Artery, Right
use Peroneal Artery, Left
Fibularis brevis muscle
use Lower Leg Muscle, Right
use Lower Leg Muscle, Left
Fibularis longus muscle
use Lower Leg Muscle, Right
use Lower Leg Muscle, Left
Fifth cranial nerve
use Trigeminal Nerve
Filum terminale
use Spinal Meninges
Fimbriectomy
see Excision, Female Reproductive System 0UB
see Resection, Female Reproductive System 0UT
Fine needle aspiration
Fluid or gas *see* Drainage
Tissue biopsy
see Extraction
see Excision
First cranial nerve
use Olfactory Nerve
First intercostal nerve
use Brachial Plexus
Fistulization
see Bypass
see Drainage
see Repair
Fitting
Arch bars, for fracture reduction *see* Reposition, Mouth and Throat 0CS
Arch bars, for immobilization *see* Immobilization, Face 2W31
Artificial limb *see* Device Fitting, Rehabilitation F0D
Hearing aid *see* Device Fitting, Rehabilitation F0D
Ocular prosthesis F0DZ8UZ
Prosthesis, limb *see* Device Fitting, Rehabilitation F0D
Prosthesis, ocular F0DZ8UZ
Fixation, bone
External, with fracture reduction *see* Reposition
External, without fracture reduction *see* Insertion
Internal, with fracture reduction *see* Reposition
Internal, without fracture reduction *see* Insertion
FLAIR® Endovascular Stent Graft
use Intraluminal Device
Flexible composite mesh
use Synthetic Substitute
Flexor carpi radialis muscle
use Lower Arm and Wrist Muscle, Right
use Lower Arm and Wrist Muscle, Left
Flexor carpi ulnaris muscle
use Lower Arm and Wrist Muscle, Right
use Lower Arm and Wrist Muscle, Left
Flexor digitorum brevis muscle
use Foot Muscle, Right
use Foot Muscle, Left
Flexor digitorum longus muscle
use Lower Leg Muscle, Right
use Lower Leg Muscle, Left
Flexor hallucis brevis muscle
use Foot Muscle, Right
use Foot Muscle, Left
Flexor hallucis longus muscle
use Lower Leg Muscle, Right
use Lower Leg Muscle, Left
Flexor pollicis longus muscle
use Lower Arm and Wrist Muscle, Right
use Lower Arm and Wrist Muscle, Left
Fluoroscopy
Abdomen and Pelvis BW11
Airway, Upper BB1DZZZ
Ankle
Left BQ1H
Right BQ1G
Aorta
Abdominal B410
Laser, Intraoperative B410
Thoracic B310
Laser, Intraoperative B310
Thoraco-Abdominal B31P

Fluoroscopy — *continued*
Aorta — *continued*
Laser, Intraoperative B31P
Aorta and Bilateral Lower Extremity Arteries B41D
Laser, Intraoperative B41D
Arm
Left BP1FZZZ
Right BP1EZZZ
Artery
Brachiocephalic-Subclavian
Right B311
Laser, Intraoperative B311
Bronchial B31L
Laser, Intraoperative B31L
Bypass Graft, Other B21F
Cervico-Cerebral Arch B31Q
Laser, Intraoperative B31Q
Common Carotid
Bilateral B315
Laser, Intraoperative B315
Left B314
Laser, Intraoperative B314
Right B313
Laser, Intraoperative B313
Coronary
Bypass Graft
Multiple B213
Laser, Intraoperative B213
Single B212
Laser, Intraoperative B212
Multiple B211
Laser, Intraoperative B211
Single B210
Laser, Intraoperative B210
External Carotid
Bilateral B31C
Laser, Intraoperative B31C
Left B31B
Laser, Intraoperative B31B
Right B319
Laser, Intraoperative B319
Hepatic B412
Laser, Intraoperative B412
Inferior Mesenteric B415
Laser, Intraoperative B415
Intercostal B31L
Laser, Intraoperative B31L
Internal Carotid
Bilateral B318
Laser, Intraoperative B318
Left B317
Laser, Intraoperative B317
Right B316
Laser, Intraoperative B316
Internal Mammary Bypass Graft
Left B218
Right B217
Intra-Abdominal
Other B41B
Laser, Intraoperative B41B
Intracranial B31R
Laser, Intraoperative B31R
Lower
Other B41J
Laser, Intraoperative B41J
Lower Extremity
Bilateral and Aorta B41D
Laser, Intraoperative B41D
Left B41G
Laser, Intraoperative B41G
Right B41F
Laser, Intraoperative B41F
Lumbar B419
Laser, Intraoperative B419
Pelvic B41C
Laser, Intraoperative B41C

Fluoroscopy — *continued*
Artery — *continued*
Pulmonary
Left B31T
Laser, Intraoperative B31T
Right B31S
Laser, Intraoperative B31S
Pulmonary Trunk B31U
Laser, Intraoperative B31U
Renal
Bilateral B418
Laser, Intraoperative B418
Left B417
Laser, Intraoperative B417
Right B416
Laser, Intraoperative B416
Spinal B31M
Laser, Intraoperative B31M
Splenic B413
Laser, Intraoperative B413
Subclavian
Left B312
Laser, Intraoperative B312
Superior Mesenteric B414
Laser, Intraoperative B414
Upper
Other B31N
Laser, Intraoperative B31N
Upper Extremity
Bilateral B31K
Laser, Intraoperative B31K
Left B31J
Laser, Intraoperative B31J
Right B31H
Laser, Intraoperative B31H
Vertebral
Bilateral B31G
Laser, Intraoperative B31G
Left B31F
Laser, Intraoperative B31F
Right B31D
Laser, Intraoperative B31D
Bile Duct BF10
Pancreatic Duct and Gallbladder BF14
Bile Duct and Gallbladder BF13
Biliary Duct BF11
Bladder BT10
Kidney and Ureter BT14
Left BT1F
Right BT1D
Bladder and Urethra BT1B
Bowel, Small BD1
Calcaneus
Left BQ1KZZZ
Right BQ1JZZZ
Clavicle
Left BP15ZZZ
Right BP14ZZZ
Coccyx BR1F
Colon BD14
Corpora Cavernosa BV10
Dialysis Fistula B51W
Dialysis Shunt B51W
Diaphragm BB16ZZZ
Disc
Cervical BR11
Lumbar BR13
Thoracic BR12
Duodenum BD19
Elbow
Left BP1H
Right BP1G
Epiglottis B91G
Esophagus BD11
Extremity
Lower BW1C
Upper BW1J

Fluoroscopy — *continued*
Facet Joint
Cervical BR14
Lumbar BR16
Thoracic BR15
Fallopian Tube
Bilateral BU12
Left BU11
Right BU10
Fallopian Tube and Uterus BU18
Femur
Left BQ14ZZZ
Right BQ13ZZZ
Finger
Left BP1SZZZ
Right BP1RZZZ
Foot
Left BQ1MZZZ
Right BQ1LZZZ
Forearm
Left BP1KZZZ
Right BP1JZZZ
Gallbladder BF12
Bile Duct and Pancreatic Duct BF14
Gallbladder and Bile Duct BF13
Gastrointestinal, Upper BD1
Hand
Left BP1PZZZ
Right BP1NZZZ
Head and Neck BW19
Heart
Left B215
Right B214
Right and Left B216
Hip
Left BQ11
Right BQ10
Humerus
Left BP1BZZZ
Right BP1AZZZ
Ileal Diversion Loop BT1C
Ileal Loop, Ureters and Kidney BT1G
Intracranial Sinus B512
Joint
Acromioclavicular, Bilateral BP13ZZZ
Finger
Left BP1D
Right BP1C
Foot
Left BQ1Y
Right BQ1X
Hand
Left BP1D
Right BP1C
Lumbosacral BR1B
Sacroiliac BR1D
Sternoclavicular
Bilateral BP12ZZZ
Left BP11ZZZ
Right BP10ZZZ
Temporomandibular
Bilateral BN19
Left BN18
Right BN17
Thoracolumbar BR18
Toe
Left BQ1Y
Right BQ1X
Kidney
Bilateral BT13
Ileal Loop and Ureter BT1G
Left BT12
Right BT11
Ureter and Bladder BT14
Left BT1F
Right BT1D

Fluoroscopy — *continued*
Knee
Left BQ18
Right BQ17
Larynx B91J
Leg
Left BQ1FZZZ
Right BQ1DZZZ
Lung
Bilateral BB14ZZZ
Left BB13ZZZ
Right BB12ZZZ
Mediastinum BB1CZZZ
Mouth BD1B
Neck and Head BW19
Oropharynx BD1B
Pancreatic Duct BF1
Gallbladder and Bile Buct BF14
Patella
Left BQ1WZZZ
Right BQ1VZZZ
Pelvis BR1C
Pelvis and Abdomen BW11
Pharynx B91G
Ribs
Left BP1YZZZ
Right BP1XZZZ
Sacrum BR1F
Scapula
Left BP17ZZZ
Right BP16ZZZ
Shoulder
Left BP19
Right BP18
Sinus, Intracranial B512
Spinal Cord B01B
Spine
Cervical BR10
Lumbar BR19
Thoracic BR17
Whole BR1G
Sternum BR1H
Stomach BD12
Toe
Left BQ1QZZZ
Right BQ1PZZZ
Tracheobronchial Tree
Bilateral BB19YZZ
Left BB18YZZ
Right BB17YZZ
Ureter
Ileal Loop and Kidney BT1G
Kidney and Bladder BT14
Left BT1F
Right BT1D
Left BT17
Right BT16
Urethra BT15
Urethra and Bladder BT1B
Uterus BU16
Uterus and Fallopian Tube BU18
Vagina BU19
Vasa Vasorum BV18
Vein
Cerebellar B511
Cerebral B511
Epidural B510
Jugular
Bilateral B515
Left B514
Right B513
Lower Extremity
Bilateral B51D
Left B51C
Right B51B
Other B51V

Fluoroscopy — *continued*
Vein — *continued*
Pelvic (Iliac)
Left B51G
Right B51F
Pelvic (Iliac) Bilateral B51H
Portal B51T
Pulmonary
Bilateral B51S
Left B51R
Right B51Q
Renal
Bilateral B51L
Left B51K
Right B51J
Splanchnic B51T
Subclavian
Left B517
Right B516
Upper Extremity
Bilateral B51P
Left B51N
Right B51M
Vena Cava
Inferior B519
Superior B518
Wrist
Left BP1M
Right BP1L
Fluoroscopy, laser intraoperative
see Fluoroscopy, Heart B21
see Fluoroscopy, Upper Arteries B31
see Fluoroscopy, Lower Arteries B41
Flushing
see Irrigation
Foley catheter
use Drainage Device
Fontan completion procedure Stage II
see Bypass, Vena Cava, Inferior 0610
Foramen magnum
use Occipital Bone
Foramen of Monro (intraventricular)
use Cerebral Ventricle
Foreskin
use Prepuce
Formula™ Balloon-Expandable Renal Stent System
use Intraluminal Device
Fossa of Rosenmuller
use Nasopharynx
Fourth cranial nerve
use Trochlear Nerve
Fourth ventricle
use Cerebral Ventricle
Fovea
use Retina, Right
use Retina, Left
Fragmentation
Ampulla of Vater 0FFC
Anus 0DFQ
Appendix 0DFJ
Bladder 0TFB
Bladder Neck 0TFC
Bronchus
Lingula 0BF9
Lower Lobe
Left 0BFB
Right 0BF6
Main
Left 0BF7
Right 0BF3
Middle Lobe, Right 0BF5
Upper Lobe
Left 0BF8
Right 0BF4
Carina 0BF2
Cavity, Cranial 0WF1
Cecum 0DFH

Fragmentation — *continued*
Cerebral Ventricle 00F6
Colon
Ascending 0DFK
Descending 0DFM
Sigmoid 0DFN
Transverse 0DFL
Duct
Common Bile 0FF9
Cystic 0FF8
Hepatic
Common 0FF7
Left 0FF6
Right 0FF5
Pancreatic 0FFD
Accessory 0FFF
Parotid
Left 0CFC
Right 0CFB
Duodenum 0DF9
Epidural Space, Intracranial 00F3
Esophagus 0DF5
Fallopian Tube
Left 0UF6
Right 0UF5
Fallopian Tubes, Bilateral 0UF7
Gallbladder 0FF4
Gastrointestinal Tract 0WFP
Genitourinary Tract 0WFR
Ileum 0DFB
Intestine
Large 0DFE
Left 0DFG
Right 0DFF
Small 0DF8
Jejunum 0DFA
Kidney Pelvis
Left 0TF4
Right 0TF3
Mediastinum 0WFC
Oral Cavity and Throat 0WF3
Pelvic Cavity 0WFJ
Pericardial Cavity 0WFD
Pericardium 02FN
Peritoneal Cavity 0WFG
Pleural Cavity
Left 0WFB
Right 0WF9
Rectum 0DFP
Respiratory Tract 0WFQ
Spinal Canal 00FU
Stomach 0DF6
Subarachnoid Space, Intracranial 00F5
Subdural Space, Intracranial 00F4
Trachea 0BF1
Ureter
Left 0TF7
Right 0TF6
Urethra 0TFD
Uterus 0UF9
Vitreous
Left 08F5
Right 08F4
Freestyle (stentless) aortic root bioprosthesis
use Zooplastic Tissue in Heart and Great Vessels
Frenectomy
see Excision, Mouth and Throat 0CB
see Resection, Mouth and Throat 0CT
Frenoplasty, frenuloplasty
see Repair, Mouth and Throat 0CQ
see Replacement, Mouth and Throat 0CR
see Supplement, Mouth and Throat 0CU
Frenotomy
see Drainage, Mouth and Throat 0C9
see Release, Mouth and Throat 0CN

Frenulotomy
see Drainage, Mouth and Throat 0C9
see Release, Mouth and Throat 0CN
Frenulum labii inferioris
use Lower Lip
Frenulum labii superioris
use Upper Lip
Frenulum linguae
use Tongue
Frenulumectomy
see Excision, Mouth and Throat 0CB
see Resection, Mouth and Throat 0CT
Frontal lobe
use Cerebral Hemisphere
Frontal vein
use Face Vein, Right
use Face Vein, Left
Fulguration
see Destruction
Fundoplication, gastroesophageal
see Restriction, Esophagogastric Junction 0DV4
Fundus uteri
use Uterus
Fusion
Acromioclavicular
Left 0RGH
Right 0RGG
Ankle
Left 0SGG
Right 0SGF
Carpal
Left 0RGR
Right 0RGQ
Carpometacarpal
Left 0RGT
Right 0RGS
Cervical Vertebral 0RG1
2 or more 0RG2
Interbody Fusion Device
Nanotextured Surface XRG2092
Radiolucent Porous XRG20F3
Interbody Fusion Device
Nanotextured Surface XRG1092
Radiolucent Porous XRG10F3
Cervicothoracic Vertebral 0RG4
Interbody Fusion Device
Nanotextured Surface XRG4092
Radiolucent Porous XRG40F3
Coccygeal 0SG6
Elbow
Left 0RGM
Right 0RGL
Finger Phalangeal
Left 0RGX
Right 0RGW
Hip
Left 0SGB
Right 0SG9
Knee
Left 0SGD
Right 0SGC
Lumbar Vertebral 0SG0
2 or more 0SG1
Interbody Fusion Device
Nanotextured Surface XRGC092
Radiolucent Porous XRGC0F3
Interbody Fusion Device
Nanotextured Surface XRGB092
Radiolucent Porous XRGB0F3
Lumbosacral 0SG3
Interbody Fusion Device
Nanotextured Surface XRGD092
Radiolucent Porous XRGD0F3
Metacarpophalangeal
Left 0RGV
Right 0RGU

Fusion — *continued*
Metatarsal-Phalangeal
Left 0SGN
Right 0SGM
Occipital-cervical 0RG0
Interbody Fusion Device
Nanotextured Surface XRG0092
Radiolucent Porous XRG00F3
Sacrococcygeal 0SG5
Sacroiliac
Left 0SG8
Right 0SG7
Shoulder
Left 0RGK
Right 0RGJ
Sternoclavicular
Left 0RGF
Right 0RGE
Tarsal
Left 0SGJ
Right 0SGH
Tarsometatarsal
Left 0SGL
Right 0SGK
Temporomandibular
Left 0RGD
Right 0RGC
Thoracic Vertebral 0RG6
2 to 7 0RG7
Interbody Fusion Device
Nanotextured Surface XRG7092
Radiolucent Porous XRG70F3
8 or more 0RG8
Interbody Fusion Device
Nanotextured Surface XRG8092
Radiolucent Porous XRG80F3
Interbody Fusion Device
Nanotextured Surface XRG6092
Radiolucent Porous XRG60F3
Thoracolumbar Vertebral 0RGA
Interbody Fusion Device
Nanotextured Surface XRGA092
Radiolucent Porous XRGA0F3
Toe Phalangeal
Left 0SGQ
Right 0SGP
Wrist
Left 0RGP
Right 0RGN
Fusion screw (compression)(lag)(locking)
use Internal Fixation Device in Upper Joints
use Internal Fixation Device in Lower Joints

G

Gait training
see Motor Treatment, Rehabilitation F07
Galea aponeurotica
use Subcutaneous Tissue and Fascia, Scalp
GammaTile™

use Radioactive Element, Cesium-131 Collagen Implant in 00H
Ganglion impar (ganglion of Walther)
use Sacral Sympathetic Nerve
Ganglionectomy
Destruction of lesion *see* Destruction
Excision of lesion *see* Excision
Gasserian ganglion
use Trigeminal Nerve
Gastrectomy
Partial *see* Excision, Stomach 0DB6
Total *see* Resection, Stomach 0DT6
Vertical (sleeve) *see* Excision, Stomach 0DB6
Gastric electrical stimulation (GES) lead
use Stimulator Lead in Gastrointestinal System
Gastric lymph node
use Lymphatic, Aortic
Gastric pacemaker lead
use Stimulator Lead in Gastrointestinal System
Gastric plexus
use Abdominal Sympathetic Nerve
Gastrocnemius muscle
use Lower Leg Muscle, Right
use Lower Leg Muscle, Left
Gastrocolic ligament
use Omentum
Gastrocolic omentum
use Omentum
Gastrocolostomy
see Bypass, Gastrointestinal System 0D1
see Drainage, Gastrointestinal System 0D9
Gastroduodenal artery
use Hepatic Artery
Gastroduodenectomy
see Excision, Gastrointestinal System 0DB
see Resection, Gastrointestinal System 0DT
Gastroduodenoscopy 0DJ08ZZ
Gastroenteroplasty
see Repair, Gastrointestinal System 0DQ
see Supplement, Gastrointestinal System 0DU
Gastroenterostomy
see Bypass, Gastrointestinal System 0D1
see Drainage, Gastrointestinal System 0D9
Gastroesophageal (GE) junction
use Esophagogastric Junction
Gastrogastrostomy
see Bypass, Stomach 0D16
see Drainage, Stomach 0D96
Gastrohepatic omentum
use Omentum
Gastrojejunostomy
see Bypass, Stomach 0D16
see Drainage, Stomach 0D96
Gastrolysis
see Release, Stomach 0DN6
Gastropexy
see Repair, Stomach 0DQ6
see Reposition, Stomach 0DS6
Gastrophrenic ligament
use Omentum
Gastroplasty
see Repair, Stomach 0DQ6
see Supplement, Stomach 0DU6
Gastroplication
see Restriction, Stomach 0DV6
Gastropylorectomy
see Excision, Gastrointestinal System 0DB
Gastrorrhaphy
see Repair, Stomach 0DQ6
Gastroscopy 0DJ68ZZ
Gastrosplenic ligament
use Omentum
Gastrostomy
see Bypass, Stomach 0D16
see Drainage, Stomach 0D96
Gastrotomy
see Drainage, Stomach 0D96
Gemellus muscle
use Hip Muscle, Right
use Hip Muscle, Left
Geniculate ganglion
use Facial Nerve
Geniculate nucleus
use Thalamus
Genioglossus muscle
use Tongue, Palate, Pharynx Muscle

Genioplasty
see Alteration, Jaw, Lower 0W05
Genitofemoral nerve
use Lumbar Plexus
GIAPREZA™
use Synthetic Human Angiotensin II
Gingivectomy
see Excision, Mouth and Throat 0CB
Gingivoplasty
see Repair, Mouth and Throat 0CQ
see Replacement, Mouth and Throat 0CR
see Supplement, Mouth and Throat 0CU
Glans penis
use Prepuce
Glenohumeral joint
use Shoulder Joint, Right
use Shoulder Joint, Left
Glenohumeral ligament
use Shoulder Bursa and Ligament, Right
use Shoulder Bursa and Ligament, Left
Glenoid fossa (of scapula)
use Glenoid Cavity, Right
use Glenoid Cavity, Left
Glenoid ligament (labrum)
use Shoulder Joint, Right
use Shoulder Joint, Left
Globus pallidus
use Basal Ganglia
Glomectomy
see Excision, Endocrine System 0GB
see Resection, Endocrine System 0GT
Glossectomy
see Excision, Tongue 0CB7
see Resection, Tongue 0CT7
Glossoepiglottic fold
use Epiglottis
Glossopexy
see Repair, Tongue 0CQ7
see Reposition, Tongue 0CS7
Glossoplasty
see Repair, Tongue 0CQ7
see Replacement, Tongue 0CR7
see Supplement, Tongue 0CU7
Glossorrhaphy
see Repair, Tongue 0CQ7
Glossotomy
see Drainage, Tongue 0C97
Glottis
use Larynx
Gluteal artery perforator flap
Replacement
Bilateral 0HRV079
Left 0HRU079
Right 0HRT079
Transfer
Left 0KXG
Right 0KXF
Gluteal lymph node
use Lymphatic, Pelvis
Gluteal vein
use Hypogastric Vein, Right
use Hypogastric Vein, Left
Gluteus maximus muscle
use Hip Muscle, Right
use Hip Muscle, Left
Gluteus medius muscle
use Hip Muscle, Right
use Hip Muscle, Left
Gluteus minimus muscle
use Hip Muscle, Right
use Hip Muscle, Left
GORE EXCLUDER® AAA Endoprosthesis
use Intraluminal Device, Branched or Fenestrated, One or Two Arteries in 04V
use Intraluminal Device, Branched or Fenestrated, Three or More Arteries in 04V
use Intraluminal Device
GORE EXCLUDER® IBE Endoprosthesis
use Intraluminal Device, Branched or Fenestrated, One or Two Arteries in 04V
GORE TAG® Thoracic Endoprosthesis
use Intraluminal Device
GORE® DUALMESH®
use Synthetic Substitute
Gracilis muscle
use Upper Leg Muscle, Right
use Upper Leg Muscle, Left
Graft
see Replacement
see Supplement
Great auricular nerve
use Cervical Plexus
Great cerebral vein
use Intracranial Vein
Great(er) saphenous vein
use Saphenous Vein, Right
use Saphenous Vein, Left
Greater alar cartilage
use Nasal Mucosa and Soft Tissue
Greater occipital nerve
use Cervical Nerve
Greater omentum
use Omentum
Greater splanchnic nerve
use Thoracic Sympathetic Nerve
Greater superficial petrosal nerve
use Facial Nerve
Greater trochanter
use Upper Femur, Right
use Upper Femur, Left
Greater tuberosity
use Humeral Head, Right
use Humeral Head, Left
Greater vestibular (Bartholin's) gland
use Vestibular Gland
Greater wing
use Sphenoid Bone
Guedel airway
use Intraluminal Device, Airway in Mouth and Throat
Guidance, catheter placement
EKG *see* Measurement, Physiological Systems 4A0
Fluoroscopy *see* Fluoroscopy, Veins B51
Ultrasound *see* Ultrasonography, Veins B54

Hallux
use 1st Toe, Right
use 1st Toe, Left
Hamate bone
use Carpal, Right
use Carpal, Left
Hancock® Bioprosthesis (aortic) (mitral) valve
use Zooplastic Tissue in Heart and Great Vessels
Hancock® Bioprosthetic Valved Conduit
use Zooplastic Tissue in Heart and Great Vessels
Harvesting, stem cells
see Pheresis, Circulatory 6A55
Head of fibula
use Fibula, Right
use Fibula, Left
Hearing aid assessment F14Z
Hearing assessment F13Z
Hearing device
Bone Conduction
Left 09HE
Right 09HD
Hearing device — *continued*
Insertion of device in
Left 0NH6
Right 0NH5
Multiple Channel Cochlear Prosthesis
Left 09HE
Right 09HD
Removal of device from, Skull 0NP0
Revision of device in, Skull 0NW0
Single Channel Cochlear Prosthesis
Left 09HE
Right 09HD
Hearing treatment F09Z
Heart assist system
Implantable
Insertion of device in, Heart 02HA
Removal of device from, Heart 02PA
Revision of device in, Heart 02WA
Short-term External
Insertion of device in, Heart 02HA
Removal of device from, Heart 02PA
Revision of device in, Heart 02WA
HeartMate 3™ LVAS
use Implantable Heart Assist System in Heart and Great Vessels
HeartMate II® Left Ventricular Assist Device (LVAD)
use Implantable Heart Assist System in Heart and Great Vessels
HeartMate XVE® Left Ventricular Assist Device (LVAD)
use Implantable Heart Assist System in Heart and Great Vessels
HeartMate® implantable heart assist system
see Insertion of device in, Heart 02HA
Helix
use External Ear, Right
use External Ear, Left
use External Ear, Bilateral
Hematopoietic cell transplant (HCT)
see Transfusion, Circulatory 302
Hemicolectomy
see Resection, Gastrointestinal System 0DT
Hemicystectomy
see Excision, Urinary System 0TB
Hemigastrectomy
see Excision, Gastrointestinal System 0DB
Hemiglossectomy
see Excision, Mouth and Throat 0CB
Hemilaminectomy
see Excision, Upper Bones 0PB
see Excision, Lower Bones 0QB
Hemilaminotomy
see Release, Central Nervous System and Cranial Nerves 00N
see Release, Peripheral Nervous System 01N
see Drainage, Upper Bones 0P9
see Excision, Upper Bones 0PB
see Release, Upper Bones 0PN
see Drainage, Lower Bones 0Q9
see Excision, Lower Bones 0QB
see Release, Lower Bones 0QN
Hemilaryngectomy
see Excision, Larynx 0CBS
Hemimandibulectomy
see Excision, Head and Facial Bones 0NB
Hemimaxillectomy
see Excision, Head and Facial Bones 0NB
Hemipylorectomy
see Excision, Gastrointestinal System 0DB
Hemispherectomy
see Excision, Central Nervous System and Cranial Nerves 00B
see Resection, Central Nervous System and Cranial Nerves 00T

Hemithyroidectomy
see Excision, Endocrine System 0GB
see Resection, Endocrine System 0GT
Hemodialysis
see Performance, Urinary 5A1D
Hemolung® Respiratory Assist System (RAS) 5A0920Z
Hepatectomy
see Excision, Hepatobiliary System and Pancreas 0FB
see Resection, Hepatobiliary System and Pancreas 0FT
Hepatic artery proper
use Hepatic Artery
Hepatic flexure
use Transverse Colon
Hepatic lymph node
use Lymphatic, Aortic
Hepatic plexus
use Abdominal Sympathetic Nerve
Hepatic portal vein
use Portal Vein
Hepaticoduodenostomy
see Bypass, Hepatobiliary System and Pancreas 0F1
see Drainage, Hepatobiliary System and Pancreas 0F9
Hepaticotomy
see Drainage, Hepatobiliary System and Pancreas 0F9
Hepatocholedochostomy
see Drainage, Duct, Common Bile 0F99
Hepatogastric ligament
use Omentum
Hepatopancreatic ampulla
use Ampulla of Vater
Hepatopexy
see Repair, Hepatobiliary System and Pancreas 0FQ
see Reposition, Hepatobiliary System and Pancreas 0FS
Hepatorrhaphy
see Repair, Hepatobiliary System and Pancreas 0FQ
Hepatotomy
see Drainage, Hepatobiliary System and Pancreas 0F9
Herculink® (RX) Elite® Renal Stent System
use Intraluminal Device
Herniorrhaphy
see Repair, Anatomical Regions, General 0WQ
see Repair, Anatomical Regions, Lower Extremities 0YQ
With synthetic substitute
see Supplement, Anatomical Regions, General 0WU
see Supplement, Anatomical Regions, Lower Extremities 0YU
Hip (joint) liner
use Liner in Lower Joints
Holter monitoring 4A12X45
Holter valve ventricular shunt
use Synthetic Substitute
Human angiotensin II, synthetic
use Synthetic Human Angiotensin II
Humeroradial joint
use Elbow Joint, Right
use Elbow Joint, Left
Humeroulnar joint
use Elbow Joint, Right
use Elbow Joint, Left
Humerus, distal
use Humeral Shaft, Right
use Humeral Shaft, Left
Hydrocelectomy
see Excision, Male Reproductive System 0VB
Hydrotherapy
Assisted exercise in pool *see* Motor Treatment, Rehabilitation F07
Whirlpool *see* Activities of Daily Living Treatment, Rehabilitation F08
Hymenectomy
see Excision, Hymen 0UBK
see Resection, Hymen 0UTK
Hymenoplasty
see Repair, Hymen 0UQK
see Supplement, Hymen 0UUK
Hymenorrhaphy
see Repair, Hymen 0UQK
Hymenotomy
see Division, Hymen 0U8K
see Drainage, Hymen 0U9K
Hyoglossus muscle
use Tongue, Palate, Pharynx Muscle
Hyoid artery
use Thyroid Artery, Right
use Thyroid Artery, Left
Hyperalimentation
see Introduction of substance in or on
Hyperbaric oxygenation
Decompression sickness treatment *see* Decompression, Circulatory 6A15
Wound treatment *see* Assistance, Circulatory 5A05
Hyperthermia
Radiation Therapy
Abdomen DWY38ZZ
Adrenal Gland DGY28ZZ
Bile Ducts DFY28ZZ
Bladder DTY28ZZ
Bone, Other DPYC8ZZ
Bone Marrow D7Y08ZZ
Brain D0Y08ZZ
Brain Stem D0Y18ZZ
Breast
Left DMY08ZZ
Right DMY18ZZ
Bronchus DBY18ZZ
Cervix DUY18ZZ
Chest DWY28ZZ
Chest Wall DBY78ZZ
Colon DDY58ZZ
Diaphragm DBY88ZZ
Duodenum DDY28ZZ
Ear D9Y08ZZ
Esophagus DDY08ZZ
Eye D8Y08ZZ
Femur DPY98ZZ
Fibula DPYB8ZZ
Gallbladder DFY18ZZ
Gland
Adrenal DGY28ZZ
Parathyroid DGY48ZZ
Pituitary DGY08ZZ
Thyroid DGY58ZZ
Glands, Salivary D9Y68ZZ
Head and Neck DWY18ZZ
Hemibody DWY48ZZ
Humerus DPY68ZZ
Hypopharynx D9Y38ZZ
Ileum DDY48ZZ
Jejunum DDY38ZZ
Kidney DTY08ZZ
Larynx D9YB8ZZ
Liver DFY08ZZ
Lung DBY28ZZ
Lymphatics
Abdomen D7Y68ZZ
Axillary D7Y48ZZ
Hyperthermia — *continued*
Radiation Therapy — *continued*
Inguinal D7Y88ZZ
Neck D7Y38ZZ
Pelvis D7Y78ZZ
Thorax D7Y58ZZ
Mandible DPY38ZZ
Maxilla DPY28ZZ
Mediastinum DBY68ZZ
Mouth D9Y48ZZ
Nasopharynx D9YD8ZZ
Neck and Head DWY18ZZ
Nerve, Peripheral D0Y78ZZ
Nose D9Y18ZZ
Oropharynx D9YF8ZZ
Ovary DUY08ZZ
Palate
Hard D9Y88ZZ
Soft D9Y98ZZ
Pancreas DFY38ZZ
Parathyroid Gland DGY48ZZ
Pelvic Bones DPY88ZZ
Pelvic Region DWY68ZZ
Pineal Body DGY18ZZ
Pituitary Gland DGY08ZZ
Pleura DBY58ZZ
Prostate DVY08ZZ
Radius DPY78ZZ
Rectum DDY78ZZ
Rib DPY58ZZ
Sinuses D9Y78ZZ
Skin
Abdomen DHY88ZZ
Arm DHY48ZZ
Back DHY78ZZ
Buttock DHY98ZZ
Chest DHY68ZZ
Face DHY28ZZ
Leg DHYB8ZZ
Neck DHY38ZZ
Skull DPY08ZZ
Spinal Cord D0Y68ZZ
Spleen D7Y28ZZ
Sternum DPY48ZZ
Stomach DDY18ZZ
Testis DVY18ZZ
Thymus D7Y18ZZ
Thyroid Gland DGY58ZZ
Tibia DPYB8ZZ
Tongue D9Y58ZZ
Trachea DBY08ZZ
Ulna DPY78ZZ
Ureter DTY18ZZ
Urethra DTY38ZZ
Uterus DUY28ZZ
Whole Body DWY58ZZ
Whole Body 6A3Z
Hypnosis GZFZZZZ
Hypogastric artery
use Internal Iliac Artery, Right
use Internal Iliac Artery, Left
Hypopharynx
use Pharynx
Hypophysectomy
see Excision, Gland, Pituitary 0GB0
see Resection, Gland, Pituitary 0GT0
Hypophysis
use Pituitary Gland
Hypothalamotomy
see Destruction, Thalamus 0059
Hypothenar muscle
use Hand Muscle, Right
use Hand Muscle, Left
Hypothermia, whole body 6A4Z
Hysterectomy
Supracervical *see* Resection, Uterus 0UT9
Total *see* Resection, Uterus 0UT9

Hysterolysis
see Release, Uterus 0UN9
Hysteropexy
see Repair, Uterus 0UQ9
see Reposition, Uterus 0US9
Hysteroplasty
see Repair, Uterus 0UQ9
Hysterorrhaphy
see Repair, Uterus 0UQ9
Hysteroscopy 0UJD8ZZ
Hysterotomy
see Drainage, Uterus 0U99
Hysterotrachelectomy
see Resection, Uterus 0UT9
see Resection, Cervix 0UTC
Hysterotracheloplasty
see Repair, Uterus 0UQ9
Hysterotrachelorrhaphy
see Repair, Uterus 0UQ9

I

IABP (Intra-aortic balloon pump)
see Assistance, Cardiac 5A02
IAEMT (Intraoperative anesthetic effect monitoring and titration)
see Monitoring, Central Nervous 4A10
Idarucizumab, Dabigatran Reversal Agent XW0
IHD (Intermittent hemodialysis) 5A1D70Z
Ileal artery
use Superior Mesenteric Artery
Ileectomy
see Excision, Ileum 0DBB
see Resection, Ileum 0DTB
Ileocolic artery
use Superior Mesenteric Artery
Ileocolic vein
use Colic Vein
Ileopexy
see Repair, Ileum 0DQB
see Reposition, Ileum 0DSB
Ileorrhaphy
see Repair, Ileum 0DQB
Ileoscopy 0DJD8ZZ
Ileostomy
see Bypass, Ileum 0D1B
see Drainage, Ileum 0D9B
Ileotomy
see Drainage, Ileum 0D9B
Ileoureterostomy
see Bypass, Urinary System 0T1
Iliac crest
use Pelvic Bone, Right
use Pelvic Bone, Left
Iliac fascia
use Subcutaneous Tissue and Fascia, Right Upper Leg
use Subcutaneous Tissue and Fascia, Left Upper Leg
Iliac lymph node
use Lymphatic, Pelvis
Iliacus muscle
use Hip Muscle, Right
use Hip Muscle, Left
Iliofemoral ligament
use Hip Bursa and Ligament, Right
use Hip Bursa and Ligament, Left
Iliohypogastric nerve
use Lumbar Plexus
Ilioinguinal nerve
use Lumbar Plexus
Iliolumbar artery
use Internal Iliac Artery, Right
use Internal Iliac Artery, Left
Iliolumbar ligament
use Lower Spine Bursa and Ligament
Iliotibial tract (band)
use Subcutaneous Tissue and Fascia, Right Upper Leg
use Subcutaneous Tissue and Fascia, Left Upper Leg
Ilium
use Pelvic Bone, Right
use Pelvic Bone, Left
Ilizarov external fixator
use External Fixation Device, Ring in 0PH
use External Fixation Device, Ring in 0PS
use External Fixation Device, Ring in 0QH
use External Fixation Device, Ring in 0QS
Ilizarov-Vecklich device
use External Fixation Device, Limb Lengthening in 0PH
use External Fixation Device, Limb Lengthening in 0QH
Imaging, diagnostic
see Plain Radiography
see Fluoroscopy
see Computerized Tomography (CT Scan)
see Magnetic Resonance Imaging (MRI)
see Ultrasonography
Immobilization
Abdominal Wall 2W33X
Arm
Lower
Left 2W3DX
Right 2W3CX
Upper
Left 2W3BX
Right 2W3AX
Back 2W35X
Chest Wall 2W34X
Extremity
Lower
Left 2W3MX
Right 2W3LX
Upper
Left 2W39X
Right 2W38X
Face 2W31X
Finger
Left 2W3KX
Right 2W3JX
Foot
Left 2W3TX
Right 2W3SX
Hand
Left 2W3FX
Right 2W3EX
Head 2W30X
Inguinal Region
Left 2W37X
Right 2W36X
Leg
Lower
Left 2W3RX
Right 2W3QX
Upper
Left 2W3PX
Right 2W3NX
Neck 2W32X
Thumb
Left 2W3HX
Right 2W3GX
Toe
Left 2W3VX
Right 2W3UX
Immunization
see Introduction of Serum, Toxoid, and Vaccine
Immunotherapy
see Introduction of Immunotherapeutic Substance
Immunotherapy, antineoplastic
Interferon *see* Introduction of Low-dose Interleukin-2
Interleukin-2, high-dose *see* Introduction of High-dose Interleukin-2
Interleukin-2, low-dose *see* Introduction of Low dose Interleukin-2
Monoclonal antibody *see* Introduction of Monoclonal Antibody
Proleukin, high-dose *see* Introduction of High-dose Interleukin-2
Proleukin, low-dose *see* Introduction of Low-dose Interleukin-2
Impella® heart pump
use Short-term External Heart Assist System in Heart and Great Vessels
Impeller pump
Continuous, Output 5A0221D
Intermittent, Output 5A0211D
Implantable cardioverter-defibrillator (ICD)
use Defibrillator Generator in 0JH
Implantable drug infusion pump (anti-spasmodic)(chemotherapy)(pain)
use Infusion Device, Pump in Subcutaneous Tissue and Fascia
Implantable glucose monitoring device
use Monitoring Device
Implantable hemodynamic monitor (IHM)
use Monitoring Device, Hemodynamic in 0JH
Implantable hemodynamic monitoring system (IHMS)
use Monitoring Device, Hemodynamic in 0JH
Implantable Miniature Telescope™ (IMT)
use Synthetic Substitute, Intraocular Telescope in 08R
Implantation
see Replacement
see Insertion
Implanted (venous)(access) port
use Vascular Access Device, Totally Implantable in Subcutaneous Tissue and Fascia
IMV (intermittent mandatory ventilation)
see Assistance, Respiratory 5A09
In Vitro fertilization 8E0ZXY1
Incision, abscess
see Drainage
Incudectomy
see Excision, Ear, Nose, Sinus 09B
see Resection, Ear, Nose, Sinus 09T
Incudopexy
see Repair, Ear, Nose, Sinus 09Q
see Reposition, Ear, Nose, Sinus 09S
Incus
use Auditory Ossicle, Right
use Auditory Ossicle, Left
Induction of labor
Artificial rupture of membranes *see* Drainage, Pregnancy 109
Oxytocin *see* Introduction of Hormone
InDura®, intrathecal catheter (1P) (spinal)
use Infusion Device
Inferior cardiac nerve
use Thoracic Sympathetic Nerve
Inferior cerebellar vein
use Intracranial Vein
Inferior cerebral vein
use Intracranial Vein
Inferior epigastric artery
use External Iliac Artery, Right
use External Iliac Artery, Left

Inferior epigastric lymph node
use Lymphatic, Pelvis
Inferior genicular artery
use Popliteal Artery, Right
use Popliteal Artery, Left
Inferior gluteal artery
use Internal Iliac Artery, Right
use Internal Iliac Artery, Left
Inferior gluteal nerve
use Sacral Plexus
Inferior hypogastric plexus
use Abdominal Sympathetic Nerve
Inferior labial artery
use Face Artery
Inferior longitudinal muscle
use Tongue, Palate, Pharynx Muscle
Inferior mesenteric ganglion
use Abdominal Sympathetic Nerve
Inferior mesenteric lymph node
use Lymphatic, Mesenteric
Inferior mesenteric plexus
use Abdominal Sympathetic Nerve
Inferior oblique muscle
use Extraocular Muscle, Right
use Extraocular Muscle, Left
Inferior pancreaticoduodenal artery
use Superior Mesenteric Artery
Inferior phrenic artery
use Abdominal Aorta
Inferior rectus muscle
use Extraocular Muscle, Right
use Extraocular Muscle, Left
Inferior suprarenal artery
use Renal Artery, Right
use Renal Artery, Left
Inferior tarsal plate
use Lower Eyelid, Right
use Lower Eyelid, Left
Inferior thyroid vein
use Innominate Vein, Right
use Innominate Vein, Left
Inferior tibiofibular joint
use Ankle Joint, Right
use Ankle Joint, Left
Inferior turbinate
use Nasal Turbinate
Inferior ulnar collateral artery
use Brachial Artery, Right
use Brachial Artery, Left
Inferior vesical artery
use Internal Iliac Artery, Right
use Internal Iliac Artery, Left
Infraauricular lymph node
use Lymphatic, Head
Infraclavicular (deltopectoral) lymph node
use Lymphatic, Right Upper Extremity
use Lymphatic, Left Upper Extremity
Infrahyoid muscle
use Neck Muscle, Right
use Neck Muscle, Left
Infraparotid lymph node
use Lymphatic, Head
Infraspinatus fascia
use Subcutaneous Tissue and Fascia, Right Upper Arm
use Subcutaneous Tissue and Fascia, Left Upper Arm
Infraspinatus muscle
use Shoulder Muscle, Right
use Shoulder Muscle, Left
Infundibulopelvic ligament
use Uterine Supporting Structure
Infusion
see Introduction of substance in or on
Infusion device, pump
Insertion of device in
Abdomen 0JH8
Infusion device, pump — *continued*
Insertion of device in — *continued*
Back 0JH7
Chest 0JH6
Lower Arm
Left 0JHH
Right 0JHG
Lower Leg
Left 0JHP
Right 0JHN
Trunk 0JHT
Upper Arm
Left 0JHF
Right 0JHD
Upper Leg
Left 0JHM
Right 0JHL
Removal of device from
Lower Extremity 0JPW
Trunk 0JPT
Upper Extremity 0JPV
Revision of device in
Lower Extremity 0JWW
Trunk 0JWT
Upper Extremity 0JWV
Infusion, glucarpidase
Central vein 3E043GQ
Peripheral vein 3E033GQ
Inguinal canal
use Inguinal Region, Right
use Inguinal Region, Left
use Inguinal Region, Bilateral
Inguinal triangle
use Inguinal Region, Right
use Inguinal Region, Left
use Inguinal Region, Bilateral
Injection
see Introduction of substance in or on
Injection reservoir, port
use Vascular Access Device, Totally Implantable in Subcutaneous Tissue and Fascia
Injection reservoir, pump
use Infusion Device, Pump in Subcutaneous Tissue and Fascia
Injection, concentrated bone marrow aspirate (CBMA), intramuscular XK02303
Insemination, artificial 3E0P7LZ
Insertion
Antimicrobial envelope *see* Introduction of Anti-infective
Aqueous drainage shunt
see Bypass, Eye 081
see Drainage, Eye 089
Products of Conception 10H0
Spinal Stabilization Device
see Insertion of device in, Upper Joints 0RH
see Insertion of device in, Lower Joints 0SH
Insertion of device in
Abdominal Wall 0WHF
Acetabulum
Left 0QH5
Right 0QH4
Anal Sphincter 0DHR
Ankle Region
Left 0YHL
Right 0YHK
Anus 0DHQ
Aorta
Abdominal 04H0
Thoracic
Ascending/Arch 02HX
Descending 02HW
Insertion of device in — *continued*
Arm
Lower
Left 0XHF
Right 0XHD
Upper
Left 0XH9
Right 0XH8
Artery
Anterior Tibial
Left 04HQ
Right 04HP
Axillary
Left 03H6
Right 03H5
Brachial
Left 03H8
Right 03H7
Celiac 04H1
Colic
Left 04H7
Middle 04H8
Right 04H6
Common Carotid
Left 03HJ
Right 03HH
Common Iliac
Left 04HD
Right 04HC
External Carotid
Left 03HN
Right 03HM
External Iliac
Left 04HJ
Right 04HH
Face 03HR
Femoral
Left 04HL
Right 04HK
Foot
Left 04HW
Right 04HV
Gastric 04H2
Hand
Left 03HF
Right 03HD
Hepatic 04H3
Inferior Mesenteric 04HB
Innominate 03H2
Internal Carotid
Left 03HL
Right 03HK
Internal Iliac
Left 04HF
Right 04HE
Internal Mammary
Left 03H1
Right 03H0
Intracranial 03HG
Lower 04HY
Peroneal
Left 04HU
Right 04HT
Popliteal
Left 04HN
Right 04HM
Posterior Tibial
Left 04HS
Right 04HR
Pulmonary
Left 02HR
Right 02HQ
Pulmonary Trunk 02HP
Radial
Left 03HC
Right 03HB
Renal
Left 04HA

Insertion of device in — *continued*
- Artery — *continued*
  - Right 04H9
  - Splenic 04H4
  - Subclavian
    - Left 03H4
    - Right 03H3
  - Superior Mesenteric 04H5
  - Temporal
    - Left 03HT
    - Right 03HS
  - Thyroid
    - Left 03HV
    - Right 03HU
  - Ulnar
    - Left 03HA
    - Right 03H9
  - Upper 03HY
  - Vertebral
    - Left 03HQ
    - Right 03HP
- Atrium
  - Left 02H7
  - Right 02H6
- Axilla
  - Left 0XH5
  - Right 0XH4
- Back
  - Lower 0WHL
  - Upper 0WHK
- Bladder 0THB
- Bladder Neck 0THC
- Bone
  - Ethmoid
    - Left 0NHG
    - Right 0NHF
  - Facial 0NHW
  - Frontal 0NH1
  - Hyoid 0NHX
  - Lacrimal
    - Left 0NHJ
    - Right 0NHH
  - Lower 0QHY
  - Nasal 0NHB
  - Occipital 0NH7
  - Palatine
    - Left 0NHL
    - Right 0NHK
  - Parietal
    - Left 0NH4
    - Right 0NH3
  - Pelvic
    - Left 0QH3
    - Right 0QH2
  - Sphenoid 0NHC
  - Temporal
    - Left 0NH6
    - Right 0NH5
  - Upper 0PHY
  - Zygomatic
    - Left 0NHN
    - Right 0NHM
- Brain 00H0
- Breast
  - Bilateral 0HHV
  - Left 0HHU
  - Right 0HHT
- Bronchus
  - Lingula 0BH9
  - Lower Lobe
    - Left 0BHB
    - Right 0BH6
  - Main
    - Left 0BH7
    - Right 0BH3
  - Middle Lobe, Right 0BH5

Insertion of device in — *continued*
- Bronchus — *continued*
  - Upper Lobe
    - Left 0BH8
    - Right 0BH4
- Bursa and Ligament
  - Lower 0MHY
  - Upper 0MHX
- Buttock
  - Left 0YH1
  - Right 0YH0
- Carpal
  - Left 0PHN
  - Right 0PHM
- Cavity, Cranial 0WH1
- Cerebral Ventricle 00H6
- Cervix 0UHC
- Chest Wall 0WH8
- Cisterna Chyli 07HL
- Clavicle
  - Left 0PHB
  - Right 0PH9
- Coccyx 0QHS
- Cul-de-sac 0UHF
- Diaphragm 0BHT
- Disc
  - Cervical Vertebral 0RH3
  - Cervicothoracic Vertebral 0RH5
  - Lumbar Vertebral 0SH2
  - Lumbosacral 0SH4
  - Thoracic Vertebral 0RH9
  - Thoracolumbar Vertebral 0RHB
- Duct
  - Hepatobiliary 0FHB
  - Pancreatic 0FHD
- Duodenum 0DH9
- Ear
  - Inner
    - Left 09HE
    - Right 09HD
  - Left 09HJ
  - Right 09HH
- Elbow Region
  - Left 0XHC
  - Right 0XHB
- Epididymis and Spermatic Cord 0VHM
- Esophagus 0DH5
- Extremity
  - Lower
    - Left 0YHB
    - Right 0YH9
  - Upper
    - Left 0XH7
    - Right 0XH6
- Eye
  - Left 08H1
  - Right 08H0
- Face 0WH2
- Fallopian Tube 0UH8
- Femoral Region
  - Left 0YH8
  - Right 0YH7
- Femoral Shaft
  - Left 0QH9
  - Right 0QH8
- Femur
  - Lower
    - Left 0QHC
    - Right 0QHB
  - Upper
    - Left 0QH7
    - Right 0QH6
- Fibula
  - Left 0QHK
  - Right 0QHJ
- Foot
  - Left 0YHN
  - Right 0YHM

Insertion of device in — *continued*
- Gallbladder 0FH4
- Gastrointestinal Tract 0WHP
- Genitourinary Tract 0WHR
- Gland
  - Endocrine 0GHS
  - Salivary 0CHA
- Glenoid Cavity
  - Left 0PH8
  - Right 0PH7
- Hand
  - Left 0XHK
  - Right 0XHJ
- Head 0WH0
- Heart 02HA
- Humeral Head
  - Left 0PHD
  - Right 0PHC
- Humeral Shaft
  - Left 0PHG
  - Right 0PHF
- Ileum 0DHB
- Inguinal Region
  - Left 0YH6
  - Right 0YH5
- Intestinal Tract
  - Lower 0DHD
  - Upper 0DH0
- Intestine
  - Large 0DHE
  - Small 0DH8
- Jaw
  - Lower 0WH5
  - Upper 0WH4
- Jejunum 0DHA
- Joint
  - Acromioclavicular
    - Left 0RHH
    - Right 0RHG
  - Ankle
    - Left 0SHG
    - Right 0SHF
  - Carpal
    - Left 0RHR
    - Right 0RHQ
  - Carpometacarpal
    - Left 0RHT
    - Right 0RHS
  - Cervical Vertebral 0RH1
  - Cervicothoracic Vertebral 0RH4
  - Coccygeal 0SH6
  - Elbow
    - Left 0RHM
    - Right 0RHL
  - Finger Phalangeal
    - Left 0RHX
    - Right 0RHW
  - Hip
    - Left 0SHB
    - Right 0SH9
  - Knee
    - Left 0SHD
    - Right 0SHC
  - Lumbar Vertebral 0SH0
  - Lumbosacral 0SH3
  - Metacarpophalangeal
    - Left 0RHV
    - Right 0RHU
  - Metatarsal-Phalangeal
    - Left 0SHN
    - Right 0SHM
  - Occipital-cervical 0RH0
  - Sacrococcygeal 0SH5
  - Sacroiliac
    - Left 0SH8
    - Right 0SH7

Insertion of device in — *continued*
Joint — *continued*
Shoulder
Left 0RHK
Right 0RHJ
Sternoclavicular
Left 0RHF
Right 0RHE
Tarsal
Left 0SHJ
Right 0SHH
Tarsometatarsal
Left 0SHL
Right 0SHK
Temporomandibular
Left 0RHD
Right 0RHC
Thoracic Vertebral 0RH6
Thoracolumbar Vertebral 0RHA
Toe Phalangeal
Left 0SHQ
Right 0SHP
Wrist
Left 0RHP
Right 0RHN
Kidney 0TH5
Knee Region
Left 0YHG
Right 0YHF
Larynx 0CHS
Leg
Lower
Left 0YHJ
Right 0YHH
Upper
Left 0YHD
Right 0YHC
Liver 0FH0
Left Lobe 0FH2
Right Lobe 0FH1
Lung
Left 0BHL
Right 0BHK
Lymphatic 07HN
Thoracic Duct 07HK
Mandible
Left 0NHV
Right 0NHT
Maxilla 0NHR
Mediastinum 0WHC
Metacarpal
Left 0PHQ
Right 0PHP
Metatarsal
Left 0QHP
Right 0QHN
Mouth and Throat 0CHY
Muscle
Lower 0KHY
Upper 0KHX
Nasal Mucosa and Soft Tissue 09HK
Nasopharynx 09HN
Neck 0WH6
Nerve
Cranial 00HE
Peripheral 01HY
Nipple
Left 0HHX
Right 0HHW
Oral Cavity and Throat 0WH3
Orbit
Left 0NHQ
Right 0NHP
Ovary 0UH3
Pancreas 0FHG
Patella
Left 0QHF

Insertion of device in — *continued*
Patella — *continued*
Right 0QHD
Pelvic Cavity 0WHJ
Penis 0VHS
Pericardial Cavity 0WHD
Pericardium 02HN
Perineum
Female 0WHN
Male 0WHM
Peritoneal Cavity 0WHG
Phalanx
Finger
Left 0PHV
Right 0PHT
Thumb
Left 0PHS
Right 0PHR
Toe
Left 0QHR
Right 0QHQ
Pleura 0BHQ
Pleural Cavity
Left 0WHB
Right 0WH9
Prostate 0VH0
Prostate and Seminal Vesicles 0VH4
Radius
Left 0PHJ
Right 0PHH
Rectum 0DHP
Respiratory Tract 0WHQ
Retroperitoneum 0WHH
Ribs
1 to 2 0PH1
3 or More 0PH2
Sacrum 0QH1
Scapula
Left 0PH6
Right 0PH5
Scrotum and Tunica Vaginalis 0VH8
Shoulder Region
Left 0XH3
Right 0XH2
Sinus 09HY
Skin 0HHPXYZ
Skull 0NH0
Spinal Canal 00HU
Spinal Cord 00HV
Spleen 07HP
Sternum 0PH0
Stomach 0DH6
Subcutaneous Tissue and Fascia
Abdomen 0JH8
Back 0JH7
Buttock 0JH9
Chest 0JH6
Face 0JH1
Foot
Left 0JHR
Right 0JHQ
Hand
Left 0JHK
Right 0JHJ
Head and Neck 0JHS
Lower Arm
Left 0JHH
Right 0JHG
Lower Extremity 0JHW
Lower Leg
Left 0JHP
Right 0JHN
Neck
Left 0JH5
Right 0JH4
Pelvic Region 0JHC
Perineum 0JHB

Insertion of device in — *continued*
Subcutaneous Tissue and Fascia — *continued*
Scalp 0JH0
Trunk 0JHT
Upper Arm
Left 0JHF
Right 0JHD
Upper Extremity 0JHV
Upper Leg
Left 0JHM
Right 0JHL
Tarsal
Left 0QHM
Right 0QHL
Tendon
Lower 0LHY
Upper 0LHX
Testis 0VHD
Thymus 07HM
Tibia
Left 0QHH
Right 0QHG
Tongue 0CH7
Trachea 0BH1
Tracheobronchial Tree 0BH0
Ulna
Left 0PHL
Right 0PHK
Ureter 0TH9
Urethra 0THD
Uterus 0UH9
Uterus and Cervix 0UHD
Vagina 0UHG
Vagina and Cul-de-sac 0UHH
Vas Deferens 0VHR
Vein
Axillary
Left 05H8
Right 05H7
Azygos 05H0
Basilic
Left 05HC
Right 05HB
Brachial
Left 05HA
Right 05H9
Cephalic
Left 05HF
Right 05HD
Colic 06H7
Common Iliac
Left 06HD
Right 06HC
Coronary 02H4
Esophageal 06H3
External Iliac
Left 06HG
Right 06HF
External Jugular
Left 05HQ
Right 05HP
Face
Left 05HV
Right 05HT
Femoral
Left 06HN
Right 06HM
Foot
Left 06HV
Right 06HT
Gastric 06H2
Hand
Left 05HH
Right 05HG
Hemiazygos 05H1
Hepatic 06H4

Insertion of device in — *continued*
Vein — *continued*
Hypogastric
Left 06HJ
Right 06HH
Inferior Mesenteric 06H6
Innominate
Left 05H4
Right 05H3
Internal Jugular
Left 05HN
Right 05HM
Intracranial 05HL
Lower 06HY
Portal 06H8
Pulmonary
Left 02HT
Right 02HS
Renal
Left 06HB
Right 06H9
Saphenous
Left 06HQ
Right 06HP
Splenic 06H1
Subclavian
Left 05H6
Right 05H5
Superior Mesenteric 06H5
Upper 05HY
Vertebral
Left 05HS
Right 05HR
Vena Cava
Inferior 06H0
Superior 02HV
Ventricle
Left 02HL
Right 02HK
Vertebra
Cervical 0PH3
Lumbar 0QH0
Thoracic 0PH4
Wrist Region
Left 0XHH
Right 0XHG

Inspection
Abdominal Wall 0WJF
Ankle Region
Left 0YJL
Right 0YJK
Arm
Lower
Left 0XJF
Right 0XJD
Upper
Left 0XJ9
Right 0XJ8
Artery
Lower 04JY
Upper 03JY
Axilla
Left 0XJ5
Right 0XJ4
Back
Lower 0WJL
Upper 0WJK
Bladder 0TJB
Bone
Facial 0NJW
Lower 0QJY
Nasal 0NJB
Upper 0PJY
Bone Marrow 07JT
Brain 00J0
Breast
Left 0HJU
Right 0HJT

Inspection — *continued*
Bursa and Ligament
Lower 0MJY
Upper 0MJX
Buttock
Left 0YJ1
Right 0YJ0
Cavity, Cranial 0WJ1
Chest Wall 0WJ8
Cisterna Chyli 07JL
Diaphragm 0BJT
Disc
Cervical Vertebral 0RJ3
Cervicothoracic Vertebral 0RJ5
Lumbar Vertebral 0SJ2
Lumbosacral 0SJ4
Thoracic Vertebral 0RJ9
Thoracolumbar Vertebral 0RJB
Duct
Hepatobiliary 0FJB
Pancreatic 0FJD
Ear
Inner
Left 09JE
Right 09JD
Left 09JJ
Right 09JH
Elbow Region
Left 0XJC
Right 0XJB
Epididymis and Spermatic Cord 0VJM
Extremity
Lower
Left 0YJB
Right 0YJ9
Upper
Left 0XJ7
Right 0XJ6
Eye
Left 08J1XZZ
Right 08J0XZZ
Face 0WJ2
Fallopian Tube 0UJ8
Femoral Region
Bilateral 0YJE
Left 0YJ8
Right 0YJ7
Finger Nail 0HJQXZZ
Foot
Left 0YJN
Right 0YJM
Gallbladder 0FJ4
Gastrointestinal Tract 0WJP
Genitourinary Tract 0WJR
Gland
Adrenal 0GJ5
Endocrine 0GJS
Pituitary 0GJ0
Salivary 0CJA
Great Vessel 02JY
Hand
Left 0XJK
Right 0XJJ
Head 0WJ0
Heart 02JA
Inguinal Region
Bilateral 0YJA
Left 0YJ6
Right 0YJ5
Intestinal Tract
Lower 0DJD
Upper 0DJ0
Jaw
Lower 0WJ5
Upper 0WJ4

Inspection — *continued*
Joint
Acromioclavicular
Left 0RJH
Right 0RJG
Ankle
Left 0SJG
Right 0SJF
Carpal
Left 0RJR
Right 0RJQ
Carpometacarpal
Left 0RJT
Right 0RJS
Cervical Vertebral 0RJ1
Cervicothoracic Vertebral 0RJ4
Coccygeal 0SJ6
Elbow
Left 0RJM
Right 0RJL
Finger Phalangeal
Left 0RJX
Right 0RJW
Hip
Left 0SJB
Right 0SJ9
Knee
Left 0SJD
Right 0SJC
Lumbar Vertebral 0SJ0
Lumbosacral 0SJ3
Metacarpophalangeal
Left 0RJV
Right 0RJU
Metatarsal-Phalangeal
Left 0SJN
Right 0SJM
Occipital-cervical 0RJ0
Sacrococcygeal 0SJ5
Sacroiliac
Left 0SJ8
Right 0SJ7
Shoulder
Left 0RJK
Right 0RJJ
Sternoclavicular
Left 0RJF
Right 0RJE
Tarsal
Left 0SJJ
Right 0SJH
Tarsometatarsal
Left 0SJL
Right 0SJK
Temporomandibular
Left 0RJD
Right 0RJC
Thoracic Vertebral 0RJ6
Thoracolumbar Vertebral 0RJA
Toe Phalangeal
Left 0SJQ
Right 0SJP
Wrist
Left 0RJP
Right 0RJN
Kidney 0TJ5
Knee Region
Left 0YJG
Right 0YJF
Larynx 0CJS
Leg
Lower
Left 0YJJ
Right 0YJH
Upper
Left 0YJD
Right 0YJC

Inspection — *continued*
- Lens
  - Left 08JKXZZ
  - Right 08JJXZZ
- Liver 0FJ0
- Lung
  - Left 0BJL
  - Right 0BJK
- Lymphatic 07JN
  - Thoracic Duct 07JK
- Mediastinum 0WJC
- Mesentery 0DJV
- Mouth and Throat 0CJY
- Muscle
  - Extraocular
    - Left 08JM
    - Right 08JL
  - Lower 0KJY
  - Upper 0KJX
- Nasal Mucosa and Soft Tissue 09JK
- Neck 0WJ6
- Nerve
  - Cranial 00JE
  - Peripheral 01JY
- Omentum 0DJU
- Oral Cavity and Throat 0WJ3
- Ovary 0UJ3
- Pancreas 0FJG
- Parathyroid Gland 0GJR
- Pelvic Cavity 0WJJ
- Penis 0VJS
- Pericardial Cavity 0WJD
- Perineum
  - Female 0WJN
  - Male 0WJM
- Peritoneal Cavity 0WJG
- Peritoneum 0DJW
- Pineal Body 0GJ1
- Pleura 0BJQ
- Pleural Cavity
  - Left 0WJB
  - Right 0WJ9
- Products of Conception 10J0
  - Ectopic 10J2
  - Retained 10J1
- Prostate and Seminal Vesicles 0VJ4
- Respiratory Tract 0WJQ
- Retroperitoneum 0WJH
- Scrotum and Tunica Vaginalis 0VJ8
- Shoulder Region
  - Left 0XJ3
  - Right 0XJ2
- Sinus 09JY
- Skin 0HJPXZZ
- Skull 0NJ0
- Spinal Canal 00JU
- Spinal Cord 00JV
- Spleen 07JP
- Stomach 0DJ6
- Subcutaneous Tissue and Fascia
  - Head and Neck 0JJS
  - Lower Extremity 0JJW
  - Trunk 0JJT
  - Upper Extremity 0JJV
- Tendon
  - Lower 0LJY
  - Upper 0LJX
- Testis 0VJD
- Thymus 07JM
- Thyroid Gland 0GJK
- Toe Nail 0HJRXZZ
- Trachea 0BJ1
- Tracheobronchial Tree 0BJ0
- Tympanic Membrane
  - Left 09J8
  - Right 09J7
- Ureter 0TJ9

Inspection — *continued*
- Urethra 0TJD
- Uterus and Cervix 0UJD
- Vagina and Cul-de-sac 0UJH
- Vas Deferens 0VJR
- Vein
  - Lower 06JY
  - Upper 05JY
- Vulva 0UJM
- Wrist Region
  - Left 0XJH
  - Right 0XJG

Instillation
- *see* Introduction of substance in or on

Insufflation
- *see* Introduction of substance in or on

Interatrial septum
- *use* Atrial Septum

Interbody fusion (spine) cage
- *use* Interbody Fusion Device in Upper Joints
- *use* Interbody Fusion Device in Lower Joints

Interbody fusion device
- Nanotextured Surface
  - Cervical Vertebral XRG1092
    - 2 or more XRG2092
  - Cervicothoracic Vertebral XRG4092
  - Lumbar Vertebral XRGB092
    - 2 or more XRGC092
  - Lumbosacral XRGD092
  - Occipital-cervical XRG0092
  - Thoracic Vertebral XRG6092
    - 2 to 7 XRG7092
    - 8 or more XRG8092
  - Thoracolumbar Vertebral XRGA092
- Radiolucent Porous
  - Cervical Vertebral XRG10F3
    - 2 or more XRG20F3
  - Cervicothoracic Vertebral XRG40F3
  - Lumbar Vertebral XRGB0F3
    - 2 or more XRGC0F3
  - Lumbosacral XRGD0F3
  - Occipital-cervical XRG00F3
  - Thoracic Vertebral XRG60F3
    - 2 to 7 XRG70F3
    - 8 or more XRG80F3
  - Thoracolumbar Vertebral XRGA0F3

Intercarpal joint
- *use* Carpal Joint, Right
- *use* Carpal Joint, Left

Intercarpal ligament
- *use* Hand Bursa and Ligament, Right
- *use* Hand Bursa and Ligament, Left

Interclavicular ligament
- *use* Shoulder Bursa and Ligament, Right
- *use* Shoulder Bursa and Ligament, Left

Intercostal lymph node
- *use* Lymphatic, Thorax

Intercostal muscle
- *use* Thorax Muscle, Right
- *use* Thorax Muscle, Left

Intercostal nerve
- *use* Thoracic Nerve

Intercostobrachial nerve
- *use* Thoracic Nerve

Intercuneiform joint
- *use* Tarsal Joint, Right
- *use* Tarsal Joint, Left

Intercuneiform ligament
- *use* Foot Bursa and Ligament, Right
- *use* Foot Bursa and Ligament, Left

Intermediate bronchus
- *use* Main Bronchus, Right

Intermediate cuneiform bone
- *use* Tarsal, Right
- *use* Tarsal, Left

Intermittent hemodialysis (IHD) 5A1D70Z

Intermittent mandatory ventilation
- *see* Assistance, Respiratory 5A09

Intermittent negative airway pressure
- 24-96 Consecutive Hours, Ventilation 5A0945B
- Greater than 96 Consecutive Hours, Ventilation 5A0955B
- Less than 24 Consecutive Hours, Ventilation 5A0935B

Intermittent positive airway pressure
- 24-96 Consecutive Hours, Ventilation 5A09458
- Greater than 96 Consecutive Hours, Ventilation 5A09558
- Less than 24 Consecutive Hours, Ventilation 5A09358

Intermittent positive pressure breathing
- *see* Assistance, Respiratory 5A09

Internal (basal) cerebral vein
- *use* Intracranial Vein

Internal anal sphincter
- *use* Anal Sphincter

Internal carotid artery, intracranial portion
- *use* Intracranial Artery

Internal carotid plexus
- *use* Head and Neck Sympathetic Nerve

Internal iliac vein
- *use* Hypogastric Vein, Right
- *use* Hypogastric Vein, Left

Internal maxillary artery
- *use* External Carotid Artery, Right
- *use* External Carotid Artery, Left

Internal naris
- *use* Nasal Mucosa and Soft Tissue

Internal oblique muscle
- *use* Abdomen Muscle, Right
- *use* Abdomen Muscle, Left

Internal pudendal artery
- *use* Internal Iliac Artery, Right
- *use* Internal Iliac Artery, Left

Internal pudendal vein
- *use* Hypogastric Vein, Right
- *use* Hypogastric Vein, Left

Internal thoracic artery
- *use* Internal Mammary Artery, Right
- *use* Internal Mammary Artery, Left
- *use* Subclavian Artery, Right
- *use* Subclavian Artery, Left

Internal urethral sphincter
- *use* Urethra

Interphalangeal (IP) joint
- *use* Finger Phalangeal Joint, Right
- *use* Finger Phalangeal Joint, Left
- *use* Toe Phalangeal Joint, Right
- *use* Toe Phalangeal Joint, Left

Interphalangeal ligament
- *use* Hand Bursa and Ligament, Right
- *use* Hand Bursa and Ligament, Left
- *use* Foot Bursa and Ligament, Right
- *use* Foot Bursa and Ligament, Left

Interrogation, cardiac rhythm related device
- Interrogation only *see* Measurement, Cardiac 4B02
- With cardiac function testing *see* Measurement, Cardiac 4A02

Interruption
- *see* Occlusion

Interspinalis muscle
- *use* Trunk Muscle, Right
- *use* Trunk Muscle, Left

Interspinous ligament, cervical
- *use* Head and Neck Bursa and Ligament

Interspinous ligament, lumbar
- *use* Lower Spine Bursa and Ligament

Interspinous ligament, thoracic
- *use* Upper Spine Bursa and Ligament

Interspinous process spinal stabilization device
- *use* Spinal Stabilization Device, Interspinous Process in 0RH
- *use* Spinal Stabilization Device, Interspinous Process in 0SH

InterStim® Therapy lead
- *use* Neurostimulator Lead in Peripheral Nervous System

InterStim® Therapy neurostimulator
- *use* Stimulator Generator, Single Array in 0JH

Intertransversarius muscle
- *use* Trunk Muscle, Right
- *use* Trunk Muscle, Left

Intertransverse ligament, cervical
- *use* Head and Neck Bursa and Ligament

Intertransverse ligament, lumbar
- *use* Lower Spine Bursa and Ligament

Intertransverse ligament, thoracic
- *use* Upper Spine Bursa and Ligament

Interventricular foramen (Monro)
- *use* Cerebral Ventricle

Interventricular septum
- *use* Ventricular Septum

Intestinal lymphatic trunk
- *use* Cisterna Chyli

Intraluminal device
- Airway
  - Esophagus 0DH5
  - Mouth and Throat 0CHY
  - Nasopharynx 09HN
- Bioactive
  - Occlusion
    - Common Carotid
      - Left 03LJ
      - Right 03LH
    - External Carotid
      - Left 03LN
      - Right 03LM
    - Internal Carotid
      - Left 03LL
      - Right 03LK
    - Intracranial 03LG
    - Vertebral
      - Left 03LQ
      - Right 03LP
  - Restriction
    - Common Carotid
      - Left 03VJ
      - Right 03VH
    - External Carotid
      - Left 03VN
      - Right 03VM
    - Internal Carotid
      - Left 03VL
      - Right 03VK
    - Intracranial 03VG
    - Vertebral
      - Left 03VQ
      - Right 03VP
- Endobronchial Valve
  - Lingula 0BH9
  - Lower Lobe
    - Left 0BHB
    - Right 0BH6
  - Main
    - Left 0BH7
    - Right 0BH3
  - Middle Lobe, Right 0BH5
  - Upper Lobe
    - Left 0BH8
    - Right 0BH4
- Endotracheal Airway
  - Change device in, Trachea 0B21XEZ

Intraluminal device — *continued*
- Endotracheal Airway — *continued*
  - Insertion of device in, Trachea 0BH1
- Pessary
  - Change device in, Vagina and Cul-de-sac 0U2HXGZ
  - Insertion of device in
    - Cul-de-sac 0UHF
    - Vagina 0UHG

Intramedullary (IM) rod (nail)
- *use* Internal Fixation Device, Intramedullary in Upper Bones
- *use* Internal Fixation Device, Intramedullary in Lower Bones

Intramedullary skeletal kinetic distractor (ISKD)
- *use* Internal Fixation Device, Intramedullary in Upper Bones
- *use* Internal Fixation Device, Intramedullary in Lower Bones

Intraocular telescope
- Left 08RK30Z
- Right 08RJ30Z

Intraoperative knee replacement sensor XR2

Intraoperative radiation therapy (IORT)
- Anus DDY8CZZ
- Bile Ducts DFY2CZZ
- Bladder DTY2CZZ
- Cervix DUY1CZZ
- Colon DDY5CZZ
- Duodenum DDY2CZZ
- Gallbladder DFY1CZZ
- Ileum DDY4CZZ
- Jejunum DDY3CZZ
- Kidney DTY0CZZ
- Larynx D9YBCZZ
- Liver DFY0CZZ
- Mouth D9Y4CZZ
- Nasopharynx D9YDCZZ
- Ovary DUY0CZZ
- Pancreas DFY3CZZ
- Pharynx D9YCCZZ
- Prostate DVY0CZZ
- Rectum DDY7CZZ
- Stomach DDY1CZZ
- Ureter DTY1CZZ
- Urethra DTY3CZZ
- Uterus DUY2CZZ

Intrauterine device (IUD)
- *use* Contraceptive Device in Female Reproductive System

Intravascular fluorescence angiography (IFA)
- *see* Monitoring, Physiological Systems 4A1

Introduction of substance in or on
- Artery
  - Central 3E06
    - Analgesics 3E06
    - Anesthetic, Intracirculatory 3E06
    - Anti-infective 3E06
    - Anti-inflammatory 3E06
    - Antiarrhythmic 3E06
    - Antineoplastic 3E06
    - Destructive Agent 3E06
    - Diagnostic Substance, Other 3E06
    - Electrolytic Substance 3E06
    - Hormone 3E06
    - Hypnotics 3E06
    - Immunotherapeutic 3E06
    - Nutritional Substance 3E06
    - Platelet Inhibitor 3E06
    - Radioactive Substance 3E06
    - Sedatives 3E06
    - Serum 3E06
    - Thrombolytic 3E06
    - Toxoid 3E06

Introduction of substance in or on — *continued*
- Artery — *continued*
    - Vaccine 3E06
    - Vasopressor 3E06
    - Water Balance Substance 3E06
  - Coronary 3E07
    - Diagnostic Substance, Other 3E07
    - Platelet Inhibitor 3E07
    - Thrombolytic 3E07
  - Peripheral 3E05
    - Analgesics 3E05
    - Anesthetic, Intracirculatory 3E05
    - Anti-infective 3E05
    - Anti-inflammatory 3E05
    - Antiarrhythmic 3E05
    - Antineoplastic 3E05
    - Destructive Agent 3E05
    - Diagnostic Substance, Other 3E05
    - Electrolytic Substance 3E05
    - Hormone 3E05
    - Hypnotics 3E05
    - Immunotherapeutic 3E05
    - Nutritional Substance 3E05
    - Platelet Inhibitor 3E05
    - Radioactive Substance 3E05
    - Sedatives 3E05
    - Serum 3E05
    - Thrombolytic 3E05
    - Toxoid 3E05
    - Vaccine 3E05
    - Vasopressor 3E05
    - Water Balance Substance 3E05
- Biliary Tract 3E0J
  - Analgesics 3E0J
  - Anesthetic Agent 3E0J
  - Anti-infective 3E0J
  - Anti-inflammatory 3E0J
  - Antineoplastic 3E0J
  - Destructive Agent 3E0J
  - Diagnostic Substance, Other 3E0J
  - Electrolytic Substance 3E0J
  - Gas 3E0J
  - Hypnotics 3E0J
  - Islet Cells, Pancreatic 3E0J
  - Nutritional Substance 3E0J
  - Radioactive Substance 3E0J
  - Sedatives 3E0J
  - Water Balance Substance 3E0J
- Bone 3E0V
  - Analgesics 3E0V3NZ
  - Anesthetic Agent 3E0V3BZ
  - Anti-infective 3E0V32
  - Anti-inflammatory 3E0V33Z
  - Antineoplastic 3E0V30
  - Destructive Agent 3E0V3TZ
  - Diagnostic Substance, Other 3E0V3KZ
  - Electrolytic Substance 3E0V37Z
  - Hypnotics 3E0V3NZ
  - Nutritional Substance 3E0V36Z
  - Radioactive Substance 3E0V3HZ
  - Sedatives 3E0V3NZ
  - Water Balance Substance 3E0V37Z
- Bone Marrow 3E0A3GC
  - Antineoplastic 3E0A30
- Brain 3E0Q
  - Analgesics 3E0Q
  - Anesthetic Agent 3E0Q
  - Anti-infective 3E0Q
  - Anti-inflammatory 3E0Q
  - Antineoplastic 3E0Q
  - Destructive Agent 3E0Q
  - Diagnostic Substance, Other 3E0Q
  - Electrolytic Substance 3E0Q
  - Gas 3E0Q
  - Hypnotics 3E0Q
  - Nutritional Substance 3E0Q
  - Radioactive Substance 3E0Q

Introduction of substance in or on — *continued*
Brain — *continued*
Sedatives 3E0Q
Stem Cells
Embryonic 3E0Q
Somatic 3E0Q
Water Balance Substance 3E0Q
Cranial Cavity 3E0Q
Analgesics 3E0Q
Anesthetic Agent 3E0Q
Anti-infective 3E0Q
Anti-inflammatory 3E0Q
Antineoplastic 3E0Q
Destructive Agent 3E0Q
Diagnostic Substance, Other 3E0Q
Electrolytic Substance 3E0Q
Gas 3E0Q
Hypnotics 3E0Q
Nutritional Substance 3E0Q
Radioactive Substance 3E0Q
Sedatives 3E0Q
Stem Cells
Embryonic 3E0Q
Somatic 3E0Q
Water Balance Substance 3E0Q
Ear 3E0B
Analgesics 3E0B
Anesthetic Agent 3E0B
Anti-infective 3E0B
Anti-inflammatory 3E0B
Antineoplastic 3E0B
Destructive Agent 3E0B
Diagnostic Substance, Other 3E0B
Hypnotics 3E0B
Radioactive Substance 3E0B
Sedatives 3E0B
Epidural Space 3E0S3GC
Analgesics 3E0S3NZ
Anesthetic Agent 3E0S3BZ
Anti-infective 3E0S32
Anti-inflammatory 3E0S33Z
Antineoplastic 3E0S30
Destructive Agent 3E0S3TZ
Diagnostic Substance, Other 3E0S3KZ
Electrolytic Substance 3E0S37Z
Gas 3E0S
Hypnotics 3E0S3NZ
Nutritional Substance 3E0S36Z
Radioactive Substance 3E0S3HZ
Sedatives 3E0S3NZ
Water Balance Substance 3E0S37Z
Eye 3E0C
Analgesics 3E0C
Anesthetic Agent 3E0C
Anti-infective 3E0C
Anti-inflammatory 3E0C
Antineoplastic 3E0C
Destructive Agent 3E0C
Diagnostic Substance, Other 3E0C
Gas 3E0C
Hypnotics 3E0C
Pigment 3E0C
Radioactive Substance 3E0C
Sedatives 3E0C
Gastrointestinal Tract
Lower 3E0H
Analgesics 3E0H
Anesthetic Agent 3E0H
Anti-infective 3E0H
Anti-inflammatory 3E0H
Antineoplastic 3E0H
Destructive Agent 3E0H
Diagnostic Substance, Other 3E0H
Electrolytic Substance 3E0H
Gas 3E0H
Hypnotics 3E0H
Nutritional Substance 3E0H

Introduction of substance in or on — *continued*
Gastrointestinal Tract — *continued*
Radioactive Substance 3E0H
Sedatives 3E0H
Water Balance Substance 3E0H
Upper 3E0G
Analgesics 3E0G
Anesthetic Agent 3E0G
Anti-infective 3E0G
Anti-inflammatory 3E0G
Antineoplastic 3E0G
Destructive Agent 3E0G
Diagnostic Substance, Other 3E0G
Electrolytic Substance 3E0G
Gas 3E0G
Hypnotics 3E0G
Nutritional Substance 3E0G
Radioactive Substance 3E0G
Sedatives 3E0G
Water Balance Substance 3E0G
Genitourinary Tract 3E0K
Analgesics 3E0K
Anesthetic Agent 3E0K
Anti-infective 3E0K
Anti-inflammatory 3E0K
Antineoplastic 3E0K
Destructive Agent 3E0K
Diagnostic Substance, Other 3E0K
Electrolytic Substance 3E0K
Gas 3E0K
Hypnotics 3E0K
Nutritional Substance 3E0K
Radioactive Substance 3E0K
Sedatives 3E0K
Water Balance Substance 3E0K
Heart 3E08
Diagnostic Substance, Other 3E08
Platelet Inhibitor 3E08
Thrombolytic 3E08
Joint 3E0U
Analgesics 3E0U3NZ
Anesthetic Agent 3E0U3BZ
Anti-infective 3E0U
Anti-inflammatory 3E0U33Z
Antineoplastic 3E0U30
Destructive Agent 3E0U3TZ
Diagnostic Substance, Other 3E0U3KZ
Electrolytic Substance 3E0U37Z
Gas 3E0U3SF
Hypnotics 3E0U3NZ
Nutritional Substance 3E0U36Z
Radioactive Substance 3E0U3HZ
Sedatives 3E0U3NZ
Water Balance Substance 3E0U37Z
Lymphatic 3E0W3GC
Analgesics 3E0W3NZ
Anesthetic Agent 3E0W3BZ
Anti-infective 3E0W32
Anti-inflammatory 3E0W33Z
Antineoplastic 3E0W30
Destructive Agent 3E0W3TZ
Diagnostic Substance, Other 3E0W3KZ
Electrolytic Substance 3E0W37Z
Hypnotics 3E0W3NZ
Nutritional Substance 3E0W36Z
Radioactive Substance 3E0W3HZ
Sedatives 3E0W3NZ
Water Balance Substance 3E0W37Z
Mouth 3E0D
Analgesics 3E0D
Anesthetic Agent 3E0D
Anti-infective 3E0D
Anti-inflammatory 3E0D
Antiarrhythmic 3E0D
Antineoplastic 3E0D
Destructive Agent 3E0D
Diagnostic Substance, Other 3E0D

Introduction of substance in or on — *continued*
Mouth — *continued*
Electrolytic Substance 3E0D
Hypnotics 3E0D
Nutritional Substance 3E0D
Radioactive Substance 3E0D
Sedatives 3E0D
Serum 3E0D
Toxoid 3E0D
Vaccine 3E0D
Water Balance Substance 3E0D
Mucous Membrane 3E00XGC
Analgesics 3E00XNZ
Anesthetic Agent 3E00XBZ
Anti-infective 3E00X2
Anti-inflammatory 3E00X3Z
Antineoplastic 3E00X0
Destructive Agent 3E00XTZ
Diagnostic Substance, Other 3E00XKZ
Hypnotics 3E00XNZ
Pigment 3E00XMZ
Sedatives 3E00XNZ
Serum 3E00X4Z
Toxoid 3E00X4Z
Vaccine 3E00X4Z
Muscle 3E023GC
Analgesics 3E023NZ
Anesthetic Agent 3E023BZ
Anti-infective 3E0232
Anti-inflammatory 3E0233Z
Antineoplastic 3E0230
Destructive Agent 3E023TZ
Diagnostic Substance, Other 3E023KZ
Electrolytic Substance 3E0237Z
Hypnotics 3E023NZ
Nutritional Substance 3E0236Z
Radioactive Substance 3E023HZ
Sedatives 3E023NZ
Serum 3E0234Z
Toxoid 3E0234Z
Vaccine 3E0234Z
Water Balance Substance 3E0237Z
Nerve
Cranial 3E0X3GC
Anesthetic Agent 3E0X3BZ
Anti-inflammatory 3E0X33Z
Destructive Agent 3E0X3TZ
Peripheral 3E0T3GC
Anesthetic Agent 3E0T3BZ
Anti-inflammatory 3E0T33Z
Destructive Agent 3E0T3TZ
Plexus 3E0T3GC
Anesthetic Agent 3E0T3BZ
Anti-inflammatory 3E0T33Z
Destructive Agent 3E0T3TZ
Nose 3E09
Analgesics 3E09
Anesthetic Agent 3E09
Anti-infective 3E09
Anti-inflammatory 3E09
Antineoplastic 3E09
Destructive Agent 3E09
Diagnostic Substance, Other 3E09
Hypnotics 3E09
Radioactive Substance 3E09
Sedatives 3E09
Serum 3E09
Toxoid 3E09
Vaccine 3E09
Pancreatic Tract 3E0J
Analgesics 3E0J
Anesthetic Agent 3E0J
Anti-infective 3E0J
Anti-inflammatory 3E0J
Antineoplastic 3E0J
Destructive Agent 3E0J
Diagnostic Substance, Other 3E0J

Introduction of substance in or on — *continued*
Pancreatic Tract — *continued*
Electrolytic Substance 3E0J
Gas 3E0J
Hypnotics 3E0J
Islet Cells, Pancreatic 3E0J
Nutritional Substance 3E0J
Radioactive Substance 3E0J
Sedatives 3E0J
Water Balance Substance 3E0J
Pericardial Cavity 3E0Y
Analgesics 3E0Y3NZ
Anesthetic Agent 3E0Y3BZ
Anti-infective 3E0Y32
Anti-inflammatory 3E0Y33Z
Antineoplastic 3E0Y
Destructive Agent 3E0Y3TZ
Diagnostic Substance, Other 3E0Y3KZ
Electrolytic Substance 3E0Y37Z
Gas 3E0Y
Hypnotics 3E0Y3NZ
Nutritional Substance 3E0Y36Z
Radioactive Substance 3E0Y3HZ
Sedatives 3E0Y3NZ
Water Balance Substance 3E0Y37Z
Peritoneal Cavity 3E0M
Adhesion Barrier 3E0M
Analgesics 3E0M3NZ
Anesthetic Agent 3E0M3BZ
Anti-infective 3E0M32
Anti-inflammatory 3E0M33Z
Antineoplastic 3E0M
Destructive Agent 3E0M3TZ
Diagnostic Substance, Other 3E0M3KZ
Electrolytic Substance 3E0M37Z
Gas 3E0M
Hypnotics 3E0M3NZ
Nutritional Substance 3E0M36Z
Radioactive Substance 3E0M3HZ
Sedatives 3E0M3NZ
Water Balance Substance 3E0M37Z
Pharynx 3E0D
Analgesics 3E0D
Anesthetic Agent 3E0D
Anti-infective 3E0D
Anti-inflammatory 3E0D
Antiarrhythmic 3E0D
Antineoplastic 3E0D
Destructive Agent 3E0D
Diagnostic Substance, Other 3E0D
Electrolytic Substance 3E0D
Hypnotics 3E0D
Nutritional Substance 3E0D
Radioactive Substance 3E0D
Sedatives 3E0D
Serum 3E0D
Toxoid 3E0D
Vaccine 3E0D
Water Balance Substance 3E0D
Pleural Cavity 3E0L
Adhesion Barrier 3E0L
Analgesics 3E0L3NZ
Anesthetic Agent 3E0L3BZ
Anti-infective 3E0L32
Anti-inflammatory 3E0L33Z
Antineoplastic 3E0L
Destructive Agent 3E0L3TZ
Diagnostic Substance, Other 3E0L3KZ
Electrolytic Substance 3E0L37Z
Gas 3E0L
Hypnotics 3E0L3NZ
Nutritional Substance 3E0L36Z
Radioactive Substance 3E0L3HZ
Sedatives 3E0L3NZ
Water Balance Substance 3E0L37Z
Products of Conception 3E0E
Analgesics 3E0E

Introduction of substance in or on — *continued*
Products of Conception — *continued*
Anesthetic Agent 3E0E
Anti-infective 3E0E
Anti-inflammatory 3E0E
Antineoplastic 3E0E
Destructive Agent 3E0E
Diagnostic Substance, Other 3E0E
Electrolytic Substance 3E0E
Gas 3E0E
Hypnotics 3E0E
Nutritional Substance 3E0E
Radioactive Substance 3E0E
Sedatives 3E0E
Water Balance Substance 3E0E
Reproductive
Female 3E0P
Adhesion Barrier 3E0P
Analgesics 3E0P
Anesthetic Agent 3E0P
Anti-infective 3E0P
Anti-inflammatory 3E0P
Antineoplastic 3E0P
Destructive Agent 3E0P
Diagnostic Substance, Other 3E0P
Electrolytic Substance 3E0P
Gas 3E0P
Hormone 3E0P
Hypnotics 3E0P
Nutritional Substance 3E0P
Ovum, Fertilized 3E0P
Radioactive Substance 3E0P
Sedatives 3E0P
Sperm 3E0P
Water Balance Substance 3E0P
Male 3E0N
Analgesics 3E0N
Anesthetic Agent 3E0N
Anti-infective 3E0N
Anti-inflammatory 3E0N
Antineoplastic 3E0N
Destructive Agent 3E0N
Diagnostic Substance, Other 3E0N
Electrolytic Substance 3E0N
Gas 3E0N
Hypnotics 3E0N
Nutritional Substance 3E0N
Radioactive Substance 3E0N
Sedatives 3E0N
Water Balance Substance 3E0N
Respiratory Tract 3E0F
Analgesics 3E0F
Anesthetic Agent 3E0F
Anti-infective 3E0F
Anti-inflammatory 3E0F
Antineoplastic 3E0F
Destructive Agent 3E0F
Diagnostic Substance, Other 3E0F
Electrolytic Substance 3E0F
Gas 3E0F
Hypnotics 3E0F
Nutritional Substance 3E0F
Radioactive Substance 3E0F
Sedatives 3E0F
Water Balance Substance 3E0F
Skin 3E00XGC
Analgesics 3E00XNZ
Anesthetic Agent 3E00XBZ
Anti-infective 3E00X2
Anti-inflammatory 3E00X3Z
Antineoplastic 3E00X0
Destructive Agent 3E00XTZ
Diagnostic Substance, Other 3E00XKZ
Hypnotics 3E00XNZ
Pigment 3E00XMZ
Sedatives 3E00XNZ
Serum 3E00X4Z

Introduction of substance in or on — *continued*
Skin — *continued*
Toxoid 3E00X4Z
Vaccine 3E00X4Z
Spinal Canal 3E0R3GC
Analgesics 3E0R3NZ
Anesthetic Agent 3E0R3BZ
Anti-infective 3E0R32
Anti-inflammatory 3E0R33Z
Antineoplastic 3E0R30
Destructive Agent 3E0R3TZ
Diagnostic Substance, Other 3E0R3KZ
Electrolytic Substance 3E0R37Z
Gas 3E0R
Hypnotics 3E0R3NZ
Nutritional Substance 3E0R36Z
Radioactive Substance 3E0R3HZ
Sedatives 3E0R3NZ
Stem Cells
Embryonic 3E0R
Somatic 3E0R
Water Balance Substance 3E0R37Z
Subcutaneous Tissue 3E013GC
Analgesics 3E013NZ
Anesthetic Agent 3E013BZ
Anti-infective 3E01
Anti-inflammatory 3E0133Z
Antineoplastic 3E0130
Destructive Agent 3E013TZ
Diagnostic Substance, Other 3E013KZ
Electrolytic Substance 3E0137Z
Hormone 3E013V
Hypnotics 3E013NZ
Nutritional Substance 3E0136Z
Radioactive Substance 3E013HZ
Sedatives 3E013NZ
Serum 3E0134Z
Toxoid 3E0134Z
Vaccine 3E0134Z
Water Balance Substance 3E0137Z
Vein
Central 3E04
Analgesics 3E04
Anesthetic, Intracirculatory 3E04
Anti-infective 3E04
Anti-inflammatory 3E04
Antiarrhythmic 3E04
Antineoplastic 3E04
Destructive Agent 3E04
Diagnostic Substance, Other 3E04
Electrolytic Substance 3E04
Hormone 3E04
Hypnotics 3E04
Immunotherapeutic 3E04
Nutritional Substance 3E04
Platelet Inhibitor 3E04
Radioactive Substance 3E04
Sedatives 3E04
Serum 3E04
Thrombolytic 3E04
Toxoid 3E04
Vaccine 3E04
Vasopressor 3E04
Water Balance Substance 3E04
Peripheral 3E03
Analgesics 3E03
Anesthetic, Intracirculatory 3E03
Anti-infective 3E03
Anti-inflammatory 3E03
Antiarrhythmic 3E03
Antineoplastic 3E03
Destructive Agent 3E03
Diagnostic Substance, Other 3E03
Electrolytic Substance 3E03
Hormone 3E03
Hypnotics 3E03
Immunotherapeutic 3E03

Introduction of substance in or on — *continued*
Vein — *continued*
Islet Cells, Pancreatic 3E03
Nutritional Substance 3E03
Platelet Inhibitor 3E03
Radioactive Substance 3E03
Sedatives 3E03
Serum 3E03
Thrombolytic 3E03
Toxoid 3E03
Vaccine 3E03
Vasopressor 3E03
Water Balance Substance 3E03
Intubation
Airway
see Insertion of device in, Trachea 0BH1
see Insertion of device in, Mouth and Throat 0CHY
see Insertion of device in, Esophagus 0DH5
Drainage device *see* Drainage
Feeding Device *see* Insertion of device in, Gastrointestinal System 0DH
INTUITY Elite® valve system, EDWARDS
use Zooplastic Tissue, Rapid Deployment Technique in New Technology
IPPB (intermittent positive pressure breathing)
see Assistance, Respiratory 5A09
IRE (irreversible electroporation)
see Destruction, Hepatobiliary System and Pancreas 0F5
Iridectomy
see Excision, Eye 08B
see Resection, Eye 08T
Iridoplasty
see Repair, Eye 08Q
see Replacement, Eye 08R
see Supplement, Eye 08U
Iridotomy
see Drainage, Eye 089
Irreversible electroporation (IRE)
see Destruction, Hepatobiliary System and Pancreas 0F5
Irrigation
Biliary Tract, Irrigating Substance 3E1J
Brain, Irrigating Substance 3E1Q38Z
Cranial Cavity, Irrigating Substance 3E1Q38Z
Ear, Irrigating Substance 3E1B
Epidural Space, Irrigating Substance 3E1S38Z
Eye, Irrigating Substance 3E1C
Gastrointestinal Tract
Lower, Irrigating Substance 3E1H
Upper, Irrigating Substance 3E1G
Genitourinary Tract, Irrigating Substance 3E1K
Irrigating Substance 3C1ZX8Z
Joint, Irrigating Substance 3E1U38Z
Mucous Membrane, Irrigating Substance 3E10
Nose, Irrigating Substance 3E19
Pancreatic Tract, Irrigating Substance 3E1J
Pericardial Cavity, Irrigating Substance 3E1Y38Z
Peritoneal Cavity
Dialysate 3E1M39Z
Irrigating Substance 3E1M38Z
Pleural Cavity, Irrigating Substance 3E1L38Z
Reproductive
Female, Irrigating Substance 3E1P
Male, Irrigating Substance 3E1N
Respiratory Tract, Irrigating Substance 3E1F
Skin, Irrigating Substance 3E10
Spinal Canal, Irrigating Substance 3E1R38Z
Isavuconazole anti-infective XW0
Ischiatic nerve
use Sciatic Nerve
Ischiocavernosus muscle
use Perineum Muscle
Ischiofemoral ligament
use Hip Bursa and Ligament, Right
use Hip Bursa and Ligament, Left
Ischium
use Pelvic Bone, Right
use Pelvic Bone, Left
Isolation 8E0ZXY6
Isotope administration, whole body DWY5G
Itrel (3)(4) neurostimulator
use Stimulator Generator, Single Array in 0JH

J

Jejunal artery
use Superior Mesenteric Artery
Jejunectomy
see Excision, Jejunum 0DBA
see Resection, Jejunum 0DTA
Jejunocolostomy
see Bypass, Gastrointestinal System 0D1
see Drainage, Gastrointestinal System 0D9
Jejunopexy
see Repair, Jejunum 0DQA
see Reposition, Jejunum 0DSA
Jejunostomy
see Bypass, Jejunum 0D1A
see Drainage, Jejunum 0D9A
Jejunotomy
see Drainage, Jejunum 0D9A
Joint fixation plate
use Internal Fixation Device in Upper Joints
use Internal Fixation Device in Lower Joints
Joint liner (insert)
use Liner in Lower Joints
Joint spacer (antibiotic)
use Spacer in Upper Joints
use Spacer in Lower Joints
Jugular body
use Glomus Jugulare
Jugular lymph node
use Lymphatic, Right Neck
use Lymphatic, Left Neck

K

Kappa®
use Pacemaker, Dual Chamber in 0JH
Kcentra®
use 4-Factor Prothrombin Complex Concentrate
Keratectomy, kerectomy
see Excision, Eye 08B
see Resection, Eye 08T
Keratocentesis
see Drainage, Eye 089
Keratoplasty
see Repair, Eye 08Q
see Replacement, Eye 08R
see Supplement, Eye 08U
Keratotomy
see Drainage, Eye 089
see Repair, Eye 08Q
Kirschner wire (K-wire)
use Internal Fixation Device in Head and Facial Bones
use Internal Fixation Device in Upper Bones
use Internal Fixation Device in Lower Bones
use Internal Fixation Device in Upper Joints
use Internal Fixation Device in Lower Joints
Knee (implant) insert
use Liner in Lower Joints
KUB X-ray
see Plain Radiography, Kidney, Ureter and Bladder BT04
Kuntscher nail
use Internal Fixation Device, Intramedullary in Upper Bones
use Internal Fixation Device, Intramedullary in Lower Bones
KYMRIAH™
use Engineered Autologous Chimeric Antigen Receptor T-cell Immunotherapy

L

Labia majora
use Vulva
Labia minora
use Vulva
Labial gland
use Upper Lip
use Lower Lip
Labiectomy
see Excision, Female Reproductive System 0UB
see Resection, Female Reproductive System 0UT
Lacrimal canaliculus
use Lacrimal Duct, Right
use Lacrimal Duct, Left
Lacrimal punctum
use Lacrimal Duct, Right
use Lacrimal Duct, Left
Lacrimal sac
use Lacrimal Duct, Right
use Lacrimal Duct, Left
LAGB (laparoscopic adjustable gastric banding)
Initial procedure 0DV64CZ
Surgical correction *see* Revision of device in, Stomach 0DW6
Laminectomy
see Release, Central Nervous System and Cranial Nerves 00N
see Release, Peripheral Nervous System 01N
see Excision, Upper Bones 0PB
see Excision, Lower Bones 0QB
Laminotomy
see Release, Central Nervous System and Cranial Nerves 00N
see Release, Peripheral Nervous System 01N
see Drainage, Upper Bones 0P9
see Excision, Upper Bones 0PB
see Release, Upper Bones 0PN
see Drainage, Lower Bones 0Q9
see Excision, Lower Bones 0QB
see Release, Lower Bones 0QN
LAP-BAND® adjustable gastric banding system
use Extraluminal Device
Laparoscopic-assisted transanal pull-through
see Excision, Gastrointestinal System 0DB
see Resection, Gastrointestinal System 0DT
Laparoscopy
see Inspection
Laparotomy
Drainage *see* Drainage, Peritoneal Cavity 0W9G
Exploratory *see* Inspection, Peritoneal Cavity 0WJG
Laryngectomy
see Excision, Larynx 0CBS
see Resection, Larynx 0CTS

Laryngocentesis
see Drainage, Larynx 0C9S
Laryngogram
see Fluoroscopy, Larynx B91J
Laryngopexy
see Repair, Larynx 0CQS
Laryngopharynx
use Pharynx
Laryngoplasty
see Repair, Larynx 0CQS
see Replacement, Larynx 0CRS
see Supplement, Larynx 0CUS
Laryngorrhaphy
see Repair, Larynx 0CQS
Laryngoscopy 0CJS8ZZ
Laryngotomy
see Drainage, Larynx 0C9S
Laser interstitial thermal therapy
Adrenal Gland DGY2KZZ
Anus DDY8KZZ
Bile Ducts DFY2KZZ
Brain D0Y0KZZ
Brain Stem D0Y1KZZ
Breast
Left DMY0KZZ
Right DMY1KZZ
Bronchus DBY1KZZ
Chest Wall DBY7KZZ
Colon DDY5KZZ
Diaphragm DBY8KZZ
Duodenum DDY2KZZ
Esophagus DDY0KZZ
Gallbladder DFY1KZZ
Gland
Adrenal DGY2KZZ
Parathyroid DGY4KZZ
Pituitary DGY0KZZ
Thyroid DGY5KZZ
Ileum DDY4KZZ
Jejunum DDY3KZZ
Liver DFY0KZZ
Lung DBY2KZZ
Mediastinum DBY6KZZ
Nerve, Peripheral D0Y7KZZ
Pancreas DFY3KZZ
Parathyroid Gland DGY4KZZ
Pineal Body DGY1KZZ
Pituitary Gland DGY0KZZ
Pleura DBY5KZZ
Prostate DVY0KZZ
Rectum DDY7KZZ
Spinal Cord D0Y6KZZ
Stomach DDY1KZZ
Thyroid Gland DGY5KZZ
Trachea DBY0KZZ
Lateral (brachial) lymph node
use Lymphatic, Right Axillary
use Lymphatic, Left Axillary
Lateral canthus
use Upper Eyelid, Right
use Upper Eyelid, Left
Lateral collateral ligament (LCL)
use Knee Bursa and Ligament, Right
use Knee Bursa and Ligament, Left
Lateral condyle of femur
use Lower Femur, Right
use Lower Femur, Left
Lateral condyle of tibia
use Tibia, Right
use Tibia, Left
Lateral cuneiform bone
use Tarsal, Right
use Tarsal, Left
Lateral epicondyle of femur
use Lower Femur, Right
use Lower Femur, Left
Lateral epicondyle of humerus
use Humeral Shaft, Right
use Humeral Shaft, Left
Lateral femoral cutaneous nerve
use Lumbar Plexus
Lateral malleolus
use Fibula, Right
use Fibula, Left
Lateral meniscus
use Knee Joint, Right
use Knee Joint, Left
Lateral nasal cartilage
use Nasal Mucosa and Soft Tissue
Lateral plantar artery
use Foot Artery, Right
use Foot Artery, Left
Lateral plantar nerve
use Tibial Nerve
Lateral rectus muscle
use Extraocular Muscle, Right
use Extraocular Muscle, Left
Lateral sacral artery
use Internal Iliac Artery, Right
use Internal Iliac Artery, Left
Lateral sacral vein
use Hypogastric Vein, Right
use Hypogastric Vein, Left
Lateral sural cutaneous nerve
use Peroneal Nerve
Lateral tarsal artery
use Foot Artery, Right
use Foot Artery, Left
Lateral temporomandibular ligament
use Head and Neck Bursa and Ligament
Lateral thoracic artery
use Axillary Artery, Right
use Axillary Artery, Left
Latissimus dorsi muscle
use Trunk Muscle, Right
use Trunk Muscle, Left
Latissimus dorsi myocutaneous flap
Replacement
Bilateral 0HRV075
Left 0HRU075
Right 0HRT075
Transfer
Left 0KXG
Right 0KXF
Lavage
see Irrigation
Bronchial alveolar, diagnostic *see* Drainage, Respiratory System 0B9
Least splanchnic nerve
use Thoracic Sympathetic Nerve
Left ascending lumbar vein
use Hemiazygos Vein
Left atrioventricular valve
use Mitral Valve
Left auricular appendix
use Atrium, Left
Left colic vein
use Colic Vein
Left coronary sulcus
use Heart, Left
Left gastric artery
use Gastric Artery
Left gastroepiploic artery
use Splenic Artery
Left gastroepiploic vein
use Splenic Vein
Left inferior phrenic vein
use Renal Vein, Left
Left inferior pulmonary vein
use Pulmonary Vein, Left
Left jugular trunk
use Thoracic Duct
Left lateral ventricle
use Cerebral Ventricle
Left ovarian vein
use Renal Vein, Left
Left second lumbar vein
use Renal Vein, Left
Left subclavian trunk
use Thoracic Duct
Left subcostal vein
use Hemiazygos Vein
Left superior pulmonary vein
use Pulmonary Vein, Left
Left suprarenal vein
use Renal Vein, Left
Left testicular vein
use Renal Vein, Left
Lengthening
Bone, with device *see* Insertion of Limb Lengthening Device
Muscle, by incision *see* Division, Muscles 0K8
Tendon, by incision *see* Division, Tendons 0L8
Leptomeninges, intracranial
use Cerebral Meninges
Leptomeninges, spinal
use Spinal Meninges
Lesser alar cartilage
use Nasal Mucosa and Soft Tissue
Lesser occipital nerve
use Cervical Plexus
Lesser omentum
use Omentum
Lesser saphenous vein
use Saphenous Vein, Right
use Saphenous Vein, Left
Lesser splanchnic nerve
use Thoracic Sympathetic Nerve
Lesser trochanter
use Upper Femur, Right
use Upper Femur, Left
Lesser tuberosity
use Humeral Head, Right
use Humeral Head, Left
Lesser wing
use Sphenoid Bone
Leukopheresis, therapeutic
see Pheresis, Circulatory 6A55
Levator anguli oris muscle
use Facial Muscle
Levator ani muscle
use Perineum Muscle
Levator labii superioris alaeque nasi muscle
use Facial Muscle
Levator labii superioris muscle
use Facial Muscle
Levator palpebrae superioris muscle
use Upper Eyelid, Right
use Upper Eyelid, Left
Levator scapulae muscle
use Neck Muscle, Right
use Neck Muscle, Left
Levator veli palatini muscle
use Tongue, Palate, Pharynx Muscle
Levatores costarum muscle
use Thorax Muscle, Right
use Thorax Muscle, Left
LifeStent® (Flexstar)(XL) Vascular Stent System
use Intraluminal Device
Ligament of head of fibula
use Knee Bursa and Ligament, Right
use Knee Bursa and Ligament, Left
Ligament of the lateral malleolus
use Ankle Bursa and Ligament, Right
use Ankle Bursa and Ligament, Left

Ligamentum flavum, cervical
use Head and Neck Bursa and Ligament
Ligamentum flavum, lumbar
use Lower Spine Bursa and Ligament
Ligamentum flavum, thoracic
use Upper Spine Bursa and Ligament
Ligation
see Occlusion
Ligation, hemorrhoid
see Occlusion, Lower Veins, Hemorrhoidal Plexus
Light therapy GZJZZZZ
Liner
Removal of device from
Hip
Left 0SPB09Z
Right 0SP909Z
Knee
Left 0SPD09Z
Right 0SPC09Z
Revision of device in
Hip
Left 0SWB09Z
Right 0SW909Z
Knee
Left 0SWD09Z
Right 0SWC09Z
Supplement
Hip
Left 0SUB09Z
Acetabular Surface 0SUE09Z
Femoral Surface 0SUS09Z
Right 0SU909Z
Acetabular Surface 0SUA09Z
Femoral Surface 0SUR09Z
Knee
Left 0SUD09
Femoral Surface 0SUU09Z
Tibial Surface 0SUW09Z
Right 0SUC09
Femoral Surface 0SUT09Z
Tibial Surface 0SUV09Z
Lingual artery
use External Carotid Artery, Right
use External Carotid Artery, Left
Lingual tonsil
use Pharynx
Lingulectomy, lung
see Excision, Lung Lingula 0BBH
see Resection, Lung Lingula 0BTH
Lithotripsy
see Fragmentation
With removal of fragments *see* Extirpation
LITT (laser interstitial thermal therapy)
see Laser Interstitial Thermal Therapy
LIVIAN™ CRT-D
use Cardiac Resynchronization Defibrillator Pulse Generator in 0JH
Lobectomy
see Excision, Central Nervous System and Cranial Nerves 00B
see Excision, Respiratory System 0BB
see Resection, Respiratory System 0BT
see Excision, Hepatobiliary System and Pancreas 0FB
see Resection, Hepatobiliary System and Pancreas 0FT
see Excision, Endocrine System 0GB
see Resection, Endocrine System 0GT
Lobotomy
see Division, Brain 0080
Localization
see Map
see Imaging
Locus ceruleus
use Pons
Long thoracic nerve
use Brachial Plexus
Loop ileostomy
see Bypass, Ileum 0D1B
Loop recorder, implantable
use Monitoring Device
Lower GI series
see Fluoroscopy, Colon BD14
Lumbar artery
use Abdominal Aorta
Lumbar facet joint
use Lumbar Vertebral Joint
Lumbar ganglion
use Lumbar Sympathetic Nerve
Lumbar lymph node
use Lymphatic, Aortic
Lumbar lymphatic trunk
use Cisterna Chyli
Lumbar splanchnic nerve
use Lumbar Sympathetic Nerve
Lumbosacral facet joint
use Lumbosacral Joint
Lumbosacral trunk
use Lumbar Nerve
Lumpectomy
see Excision
Lunate bone
use Carpal, Right
use Carpal, Left
Lunotriquetral ligament
use Hand Bursa and Ligament, Right
use Hand Bursa and Ligament, Left
Lymphadenectomy
see Excision, Lymphatic and Hemic Systems 07B
see Resection, Lymphatic and Hemic Systems 07T
Lymphadenotomy
see Drainage, Lymphatic and Hemic Systems 079
Lymphangiectomy
see Excision, Lymphatic and Hemic Systems 07B
see Resection, Lymphatic and Hemic Systems 07T
Lymphangiogram
see Plain Radiography, Lymphatic System B70
Lymphangioplasty
see Repair, Lymphatic and Hemic Systems 07Q
see Supplement, Lymphatic and Hemic Systems 07U
Lymphangiorrhaphy
see Repair, Lymphatic and Hemic Systems 07Q
Lymphangiotomy
see Drainage, Lymphatic and Hemic Systems 079
Lysis
see Release

M

Macula
use Retina, Right
use Retina, Left
MAGEC® Spinal Bracing and Distraction System
use Magnetically Controlled Growth Rod(s) in New Technology
Magnet extraction, ocular foreign body
see Extirpation, Eye 08C
Magnetic resonance imaging (MRI)
Abdomen BW30
Magnetic resonance imaging (MRI) *— continued*
Ankle
Left BQ3H
Right BQ3G
Aorta
Abdominal B430
Thoracic B330
Arm
Left BP3F
Right BP3E
Artery
Celiac B431
Cervico-Cerebral Arch B33Q
Common Carotid, Bilateral B335
Coronary
Bypass Graft, Multiple B233
Multiple B231
Internal Carotid, Bilateral B338
Intracranial B33R
Lower Extremity
Bilateral B43H
Left B43G
Right B43F
Pelvic B43C
Renal, Bilateral B438
Spinal B33M
Superior Mesenteric B434
Upper Extremity
Bilateral B33K
Left B33J
Right B33H
Vertebral, Bilateral B33G
Bladder BT30
Brachial Plexus BW3P
Brain B030
Breast
Bilateral BH32
Left BH31
Right BH30
Calcaneus
Left BQ3K
Right BQ3J
Chest BW33Y
Coccyx BR3F
Connective Tissue
Lower Extremity BL31
Upper Extremity BL30
Corpora Cavernosa BV30
Disc
Cervical BR31
Lumbar BR33
Thoracic BR32
Ear B930
Elbow
Left BP3H
Right BP3G
Eye
Bilateral B837
Left B836
Right B835
Femur
Left BQ34
Right BQ33
Fetal Abdomen BY33
Fetal Extremity BY35
Fetal Head BY30
Fetal Heart BY31
Fetal Spine BY34
Fetal Thorax BY32
Fetus, Whole BY36
Foot
Left BQ3M
Right BQ3L
Forearm
Left BP3K
Right BP3J

Magnetic resonance imaging (MRI) *— continued*
Gland
Adrenal, Bilateral BG32
Parathyroid BG33
Parotid, Bilateral B936
Salivary, Bilateral B93D
Submandibular, Bilateral B939
Thyroid BG34
Head BW38
Heart, Right and Left B236
Hip
Left BQ31
Right BQ30
Intracranial Sinus B532
Joint
Finger
Left BP3D
Right BP3C
Hand
Left BP3D
Right BP3C
Temporomandibular, Bilateral BN39
Kidney
Bilateral BT33
Left BT32
Right BT31
Transplant BT39
Knee
Left BQ38
Right BQ37
Larynx B93J
Leg
Left BQ3F
Right BQ3D
Liver BF35
Liver and Spleen BF36
Lung Apices BB3G
Nasopharynx B93F
Neck BW3F
Nerve
Acoustic B03C
Brachial Plexus BW3P
Oropharynx B93F
Ovary
Bilateral BU35
Left BU34
Right BU33
Ovary and Uterus BU3C
Pancreas BF37
Patella
Left BQ3W
Right BQ3V
Pelvic Region BW3G
Pelvis BR3C
Pituitary Gland B039
Plexus, Brachial BW3P
Prostate BV33
Retroperitoneum BW3H
Sacrum BR3F
Scrotum BV34
Sella Turcica B039
Shoulder
Left BP39
Right BP38
Sinus
Intracranial B532
Paranasal B932
Spinal Cord B03B
Spine
Cervical BR30
Lumbar BR39
Thoracic BR37
Spleen and Liver BF36
Subcutaneous Tissue
Abdomen BH3H
Extremity

Magnetic resonance imaging (MRI) *— continued*
Subcutaneous Tissue *— continued*
Lower BH3J
Upper BH3F
Head BH3D
Neck BH3D
Pelvis BH3H
Thorax BH3G
Tendon
Lower Extremity BL33
Upper Extremity BL32
Testicle
Bilateral BV37
Left BV36
Right BV35
Toe
Left BQ3Q
Right BQ3P
Uterus BU36
Pregnant BU3B
Uterus and Ovary BU3C
Vagina BU39
Vein
Cerebellar B531
Cerebral B531
Jugular, Bilateral B535
Lower Extremity
Bilateral B53D
Left B53C
Right B53B
Other B53V
Pelvic (Iliac) Bilateral B53H
Portal B53T
Pulmonary, Bilateral B53S
Renal, Bilateral B53L
Splanchnic B53T
Upper Extremity
Bilateral B53P
Left B53N
Right B53M
Vena Cava
Inferior B539
Superior B538
Wrist
Left BP3M
Right BP3L
Magnetically controlled growth rod(s)
Cervical XNS3
Lumbar XNS0
Thoracic XNS4
Malleotomy
see Drainage, Ear, Nose, Sinus 099
Malleus
use Auditory Ossicle, Right
use Auditory Ossicle, Left
Mammaplasty, mammoplasty
see Alteration, Skin and Breast 0H0
see Repair, Skin and Breast 0HQ
see Replacement, Skin and Breast 0HR
see Supplement, Skin and Breast 0HU
Mammary duct
use Breast, Right
use Breast, Left
use Breast, Bilateral
Mammary gland
use Breast, Right
use Breast, Left
use Breast, Bilateral
Mammectomy
see Excision, Skin and Breast 0HB
see Resection, Skin and Breast 0HT
Mammillary body
use Hypothalamus
Mammography
see Plain Radiography, Skin, Subcutaneous Tissue and Breast BH0

Mammotomy
see Drainage, Skin and Breast 0H9
Mandibular nerve
use Trigeminal Nerve
Mandibular notch
use Mandible, Right
use Mandible, Left
Mandibulectomy
see Excision, Head and Facial Bones 0NB
see Resection, Head and Facial Bones 0NT
Manipulation
Adhesions *see* Release
Chiropractic *see* Chiropractic Manipulation
Manual removal, retained placenta
see Extraction, Products of Conception, Retained 10D1
Manubrium
use Sternum
Map
Basal Ganglia 00K8
Brain 00K0
Cerebellum 00KC
Cerebral Hemisphere 00K7
Conduction Mechanism 02K8
Hypothalamus 00KA
Medulla Oblongata 00KD
Pons 00KB
Thalamus 00K9
Mapping
Doppler ultrasound *see* Ultrasonography
Electrocardiogram only *see* Measurement, Cardiac 4A02
Mark IV™ Breathing Pacemaker System
use Stimulator Generator in Subcutaneous Tissue and Fascia
Marsupialization
see Drainage
see Excision
Massage, cardiac
External 5A12012
Open 02QA0ZZ
Masseter muscle
use Head Muscle
Masseteric fascia
use Subcutaneous Tissue and Fascia, Face
Mastectomy
see Excision, Skin and Breast 0HB
see Resection, Skin and Breast 0HT
Mastoid (postauricular) lymph node
use Lymphatic, Right Neck
use Lymphatic, Left Neck
Mastoid air cells
use Mastoid Sinus, Right
use Mastoid Sinus, Left
Mastoid process
use Temporal Bone, Right
use Temporal Bone, Left
Mastoidectomy
see Excision, Ear, Nose, Sinus 09B
see Resection, Ear, Nose, Sinus 09T
Mastoidotomy
see Drainage, Ear, Nose, Sinus 099
Mastopexy
see Repair, Skin and Breast 0HQ
see Reposition, Skin and Breast 0HS
Mastorrhaphy
see Repair, Skin and Breast 0HQ
Mastotomy
see Drainage, Skin and Breast 0H9
Maxillary artery
use External Carotid Artery, Right
use External Carotid Artery, Left
Maxillary nerve
use Trigeminal Nerve
Maximo® II DR (VR)
use Defibrillator Generator in 0JH

Maximo® II DR CRT-D
use Cardiac Resynchronization Defibrillator Pulse Generator in 0JH
Measurement
Arterial
Flow
Coronary 4A03
Peripheral 4A03
Pulmonary 4A03
Pressure
Coronary 4A03
Peripheral 4A03
Pulmonary 4A03
Thoracic, Other 4A03
Pulse
Coronary 4A03
Peripheral 4A03
Pulmonary 4A03
Saturation, Peripheral 4A03
Sound, Peripheral 4A03
Biliary
Flow 4A0C
Pressure 4A0C
Cardiac
Action Currents 4A02
Defibrillator 4B02XTZ
Electrical Activity 4A02
Guidance 4A02X4A
No Qualifier 4A02X4Z
Output 4A02
Pacemaker 4B02XSZ
Rate 4A02
Rhythm 4A02
Sampling and Pressure
Bilateral 4A02
Left Heart 4A02
Right Heart 4A02
Sound 4A02
Total Activity, Stress 4A02XM4
Central Nervous
Conductivity 4A00
Electrical Activity 4A00
Pressure 4A000BZ
Intracranial 4A00
Saturation, Intracranial 4A00
Stimulator 4B00XVZ
Temperature, Intracranial 4A00
Circulatory, Volume 4A05XLZ
Gastrointestinal
Motility 4A0B
Pressure 4A0B
Secretion 4A0B
Lymphatic
Flow 4A06
Pressure 4A06
Metabolism 4A0Z
Musculoskeletal
Contractility 4A0F
Stimulator 4B0FXVZ
Olfactory, Acuity 4A08X0Z
Peripheral Nervous
Conductivity
Motor 4A01
Sensory 4A01
Electrical Activity 4A01
Stimulator 4B01XVZ
Products of Conception
Cardiac
Electrical Activity 4A0H
Rate 4A0H
Rhythm 4A0H
Sound 4A0H
Nervous
Conductivity 4A0J
Electrical Activity 4A0J
Pressure 4A0J

Measurement — *continued*
Respiratory
Capacity 4A09
Flow 4A09
Pacemaker 4B09XSZ
Rate 4A09
Resistance 4A09
Total Activity 4A09
Volume 4A09
Sleep 4A0ZXQZ
Temperature 4A0Z
Urinary
Contractility 4A0D
Flow 4A0D
Pressure 4A0D
Resistance 4A0D
Volume 4A0D
Venous
Flow
Central 4A04
Peripheral 4A04
Portal 4A04
Pulmonary 4A04
Pressure
Central 4A04
Peripheral 4A04
Portal 4A04
Pulmonary 4A04
Pulse
Central 4A04
Peripheral 4A04
Portal 4A04
Pulmonary 4A04
Saturation, Peripheral 4A04
Visual
Acuity 4A07X0Z
Mobility 4A07X7Z
Pressure 4A07XBZ
Meatoplasty, urethra
see Repair, Urethra 0TQD
Meatotomy
see Drainage, Urinary System 0T9
Mechanical ventilation
see Performance, Respiratory 5A19
Medial canthus
use Lower Eyelid, Right
use Lower Eyelid, Left
Medial collateral ligament (MCL)
use Knee Bursa and Ligament, Right
use Knee Bursa and Ligament, Left
Medial condyle of femur
use Lower Femur, Right
use Lower Femur, Left
Medial condyle of tibia
use Tibia, Right
use Tibia, Left
Medial cuneiform bone
use Tarsal, Right
use Tarsal, Left
Medial epicondyle of femur
use Lower Femur, Right
use Lower Femur, Left
Medial epicondyle of humerus
use Humeral Shaft, Right
use Humeral Shaft, Left
Medial malleolus
use Tibia, Right
use Tibia, Left
Medial meniscus
use Knee Joint, Right
use Knee Joint, Left
Medial plantar artery
use Foot Artery, Right
use Foot Artery, Left
Medial plantar nerve
use Tibial Nerve

Medial popliteal nerve
use Tibial Nerve
Medial rectus muscle
use Extraocular Muscle, Right
use Extraocular Muscle, Left
Medial sural cutaneous nerve
use Tibial Nerve
Median antebrachial vein
use Basilic Vein, Right
use Basilic Vein, Left
Median cubital vein
use Basilic Vein, Right
use Basilic Vein, Left
Median sacral artery
use Abdominal Aorta
Mediastinal cavity
use Mediastinum
Mediastinal lymph node
use Lymphatic, Thorax
Mediastinal space
use Mediastinum
Mediastinoscopy 0WJC4ZZ
Medication management GZ3ZZZZ
for substance abuse
Antabuse HZ83ZZZ
Bupropion HZ87ZZZ
Clonidine HZ86ZZZ
Levo-alpha-acetyl-methadol (LAAM) HZ82ZZZ
Methadone Maintenance HZ81ZZZ
Naloxone HZ85ZZZ
Naltrexone HZ84ZZZ
Nicotine Replacement HZ80ZZZ
Other Replacement Medication HZ89ZZZ
Psychiatric Medication HZ88ZZZ
Meditation 8E0ZXY5
Medtronic Endurant® II AAA stent graft system
use Intraluminal Device
Meissner's (submucous) plexus
use Abdominal Sympathetic Nerve
Melody® transcatheter pulmonary valve
use Zooplastic Tissue in Heart and Great Vessels
Membranous urethra
use Urethra
Meningeorrhaphy
see Repair, Cerebral Meninges 00Q1
see Repair, Spinal Meninges 00QT
Meniscectomy, knee
see Excision, Joint, Knee, Right 0SBC
see Excision, Joint, Knee, Left 0SBD
Mental foramen
use Mandible, Right
use Mandible, Left
Mentalis muscle
use Facial Muscle
Mentoplasty
see Alteration, Jaw, Lower 0W05
Mesenterectomy
see Excision, Mesentery 0DBV
Mesenteriorrhaphy, mesenterorrhaphy
see Repair, Mesentery 0DQV
Mesenteriplication
see Repair, Mesentery 0DQV
Mesoappendix
use Mesentery
Mesocolon
use Mesentery
Metacarpal ligament
use Hand Bursa and Ligament, Right
use Hand Bursa and Ligament, Left
Metacarpophalangeal ligament
use Hand Bursa and Ligament, Right
use Hand Bursa and Ligament, Left

Metal on metal bearing surface
  use Synthetic Substitute, Metal in 0SR
Metatarsal ligament
  use Foot Bursa and Ligament, Right
  use Foot Bursa and Ligament, Left
Metatarsectomy
  see Excision, Lower Bones 0QB
  see Resection, Lower Bones 0QT
Metatarsophalangeal (MTP) joint
  use Metatarsal-Phalangeal Joint, Right
  use Metatarsal-Phalangeal Joint, Left
Metatarsophalangeal ligament
  use Foot Bursa and Ligament, Right
  use Foot Bursa and Ligament, Left
Metathalamus
  use Thalamus
Micro-Driver® stent (RX) (OTW)
  use Intraluminal Device
MicroMed HeartAssist™
  use Implantable Heart Assist System in Heart and Great Vessels
Micrus CERECYTE® microcoil
  use Intraluminal Device, Bioactive in Upper Arteries
Midcarpal joint
  use Carpal Joint, Right
  use Carpal Joint, Left
Middle cardiac nerve
  use Thoracic Sympathetic Nerve
Middle cerebral artery
  use Intracranial Artery
Middle cerebral vein
  use Intracranial Vein
Middle colic vein
  use Colic Vein
Middle genicular artery
  use Popliteal Artery, Right
  use Popliteal Artery, Left
Middle hemorrhoidal vein
  use Hypogastric Vein, Right
  use Hypogastric Vein, Left
Middle rectal artery
  use Internal Iliac Artery, Right
  use Internal Iliac Artery, Left
Middle suprarenal artery
  use Abdominal Aorta
Middle temporal artery
  use Temporal Artery, Right
  use Temporal Artery, Left
Middle turbinate
  use Nasal Turbinate
MIRODERM™ Biologic Wound Matrix
  use Skin Substitute, Porcine Liver Derived in New Technology
MitraClip® valve repair system
  use Synthetic Substitute
Mitral annulus
  use Mitral Valve
Mitroflow® Aortic Pericardial Heart Valve
  use Zooplastic Tissue in Heart and Great Vessels
Mobilization, adhesions
  see Release
Molar gland
  use Buccal Mucosa
Monitoring
  Arterial
    Flow
      Coronary 4A13
      Peripheral 4A13
      Pulmonary 4A13
    Pressure
      Coronary 4A13
      Peripheral 4A13
      Pulmonary 4A13
    Pulse
      Coronary 4A13
      Peripheral 4A13
      Pulmonary 4A13
    Saturation, Peripheral 4A13
    Sound, Peripheral 4A13
  Cardiac
    Electrical Activity 4A12
      Ambulatory 4A12X45
      No Qualifier 4A12X4Z
    Output 4A12
    Rate 4A12
    Rhythm 4A12
    Sound 4A12
    Total Activity, Stress 4A12XM4
    Vascular Perfusion, Indocyanine Green Dye 4A12XSH
  Central Nervous
    Conductivity 4A10
    Electrical Activity
      Intraoperative 4A10
      No Qualifier 4A10
    Pressure 4A100BZ
      Intracranial 4A10
    Saturation, Intracranial 4A10
    Temperature, Intracranial 4A10
  Gastrointestinal
    Motility 4A1B
    Pressure 4A1B
    Secretion 4A1B
    Vascular Perfusion, Indocyanine Green Dye 4A1BXSH
  Intraoperative Knee Replacement Sensor XR2
  Lymphatic
    Flow 4A16
    Pressure 4A16
  Peripheral Nervous
    Conductivity
      Motor 4A11
      Sensory 4A11
    Electrical Activity
      Intraoperative 4A11
      No Qualifier 4A11
  Products of Conception
    Cardiac
      Electrical Activity 4A1H
      Rate 4A1H
      Rhythm 4A1H
      Sound 4A1H
    Nervous
      Conductivity 4A1J
      Electrical Activity 4A1J
      Pressure 4A1J
  Respiratory
    Capacity 4A19
    Flow 4A19
    Rate 4A19
    Resistance 4A19
    Volume 4A19
  Skin and Breast, Vascular Perfusion, Indocyanine Green Dye 4A1GXSH
  Sleep 4A1ZXQZ
  Temperature 4A1Z
  Urinary
    Contractility 4A1D
    Flow 4A1D
    Pressure 4A1D
    Resistance 4A1D
    Volume 4A1D
  Venous
    Flow
      Central 4A14
      Peripheral 4A14
      Portal 4A14
      Pulmonary 4A14
    Pressure
      Central 4A14
      Peripheral 4A14
      Portal 4A14
      Pulmonary 4A14
    Pulse
      Central 4A14
      Peripheral 4A14
      Portal 4A14
      Pulmonary 4A14
    Saturation
      Central 4A14
      Portal 4A14
      Pulmonary 4A14
Monitoring device, hemodynamic
  Abdomen 0JH8
  Chest 0JH6
Mosaic® Bioprosthesis (aortic) (mitral) valve
  use Zooplastic Tissue in Heart and Great Vessels
Motor function assessment F01
Motor Treatment F07
MR angiography
  see Magnetic Resonance Imaging (MRI), Heart B23
  see Magnetic Resonance Imaging (MRI), Upper Arteries B33
  see Magnetic Resonance Imaging (MRI), Lower Arteries B43
MULTI-LINK (VISION®)(MINI-VISION®) (ULTRA™) Coronary Stent System
  use Intraluminal Device
Multiple sleep latency test 4A0ZXQZ
Musculocutaneous nerve
  use Brachial Plexus
Musculopexy
  see Repair, Muscles 0KQ
  see Reposition, Muscles 0KS
Musculophrenic artery
  use Internal Mammary Artery, Right
  use Internal Mammary Artery, Left
Musculoplasty
  see Repair, Muscles 0KQ
  see Supplement, Muscles 0KU
Musculorrhaphy
  see Repair, Muscles 0KQ
Musculospiral nerve
  use Radial Nerve
Myectomy
  see Excision, Muscles 0KB
  see Resection, Muscles 0KT
Myelencephalon
  use Medulla Oblongata
Myelogram
  CT *see* Computerized Tomography (CT Scan), Central Nervous System B02
  MRI *see* Magnetic Resonance Imaging (MRI), Central Nervous System B03
Myenteric (Auerbach's) plexus
  use Abdominal Sympathetic Nerve
Myocardial bridge release
  see Release, Artery, Coronary
Myomectomy
  see Excision, Female Reproductive System 0UB
Myometrium
  use Uterus
Myopexy
  see Repair, Muscles 0KQ
  see Reposition, Muscles 0KS
Myoplasty
  see Repair, Muscles 0KQ
  see Supplement, Muscles 0KU
Myorrhaphy
  see Repair, Muscles 0KQ

Myoscopy
see Inspection, Muscles 0KJ
Myotomy
see Division, Muscles 0K8
see Drainage, Muscles 0K9
Myringectomy
see Excision, Ear, Nose, Sinus 09B
see Resection, Ear, Nose, Sinus 09T
Myringoplasty
see Repair, Ear, Nose, Sinus 09Q
see Replacement, Ear, Nose, Sinus 09R
see Supplement, Ear, Nose, Sinus 09U
Myringostomy
see Drainage, Ear, Nose, Sinus 099
Myringotomy
see Drainage, Ear, Nose, Sinus 099

N

Nail bed
use Finger Nail
use Toe Nail
Nail plate
use Finger Nail
use Toe Nail
nanoLOCK™ interbody fusion device
use Interbody Fusion Device, Nanotextured Surface in New Technology
Narcosynthesis GZGZZZZ
Nasal cavity
use Nasal Mucosa and Soft Tissue
Nasal concha
use Nasal Turbinate
Nasalis muscle
use Facial Muscle
Nasolacrimal duct
use Lacrimal Duct, Right
use Lacrimal Duct, Left
Nasopharyngeal airway (NPA)
use Intraluminal Device, Airway in Ear, Nose, Sinus
Navicular bone
use Tarsal, Right
use Tarsal, Left
Near infrared spectroscopy, circulatory system 8E023DZ
Neck of femur
use Upper Femur, Right
use Upper Femur, Left
Neck of humerus (anatomical)(surgical)
use Humeral Head, Right
use Humeral Head, Left
Nephrectomy
see Excision, Urinary System 0TB
see Resection, Urinary System 0TT
Nephrolithotomy
see Extirpation, Urinary System 0TC
Nephrolysis
see Release, Urinary System 0TN
Nephropexy
see Repair, Urinary System 0TQ
see Reposition, Urinary System 0TS
Nephroplasty
see Repair, Urinary System 0TQ
see Supplement, Urinary System 0TU
Nephropyeloureterostomy
see Bypass, Urinary System 0T1
see Drainage, Urinary System 0T9
Nephrorrhaphy
see Repair, Urinary System 0TQ
Nephroscopy, transurethral 0TJ58ZZ
Nephrostomy
see Bypass, Urinary System 0T1
see Drainage, Urinary System 0T9
Nephrotomography
see Plain Radiography, Urinary System BT0
Nephrotomography — *continued*
see Fluoroscopy, Urinary System BT1
Nephrotomy
see Division, Urinary System 0T8
see Drainage, Urinary System 0T9
Nerve conduction study
see Measurement, Central Nervous 4A00
see Measurement, Peripheral Nervous 4A01
Nerve function assessment F01
Nerve to the stapedius
use Facial Nerve
Nesiritide
use Human B-type Natriuretic Peptide
Neurectomy
see Excision, Central Nervous System and Cranial Nerves 00B
see Excision, Peripheral Nervous System 01B
Neurexeresis
see Extraction, Central Nervous System and Cranial Nerves 00D
see Extraction, Peripheral Nervous System 01D
Neurohypophysis
use Pituitary Gland
Neurolysis
see Release, Central Nervous System and Cranial Nerves 00N
see Release, Peripheral Nervous System 01N
Neuromuscular electrical stimulation (NEMS) lead
use Stimulator Lead in Muscles
Neurophysiologic monitoring
see Monitoring, Central Nervous 4A10
Neuroplasty
see Repair, Central Nervous System and Cranial Nerves 00Q
see Supplement, Central Nervous System and Cranial Nerves 00U
see Repair, Peripheral Nervous System 01Q
see Supplement, Peripheral Nervous System 01U
Neurorrhaphy
see Repair, Central Nervous System and Cranial Nerves 00Q
see Repair, Peripheral Nervous System 01Q
Neurostimulator generator
Insertion of device in, Skull 0NH00NZ
Removal of device from, Skull 0NP00NZ
Revision of device in, Skull 0NW00NZ
Neurostimulator generator, multiple channel
use Stimulator Generator, Multiple Array in 0JH
Neurostimulator generator, multiple channel rechargeable
use Stimulator Generator, Multiple Array Rechargeable in 0JH
Neurostimulator generator, single channel
use Stimulator Generator, Single Array in 0JH
Neurostimulator generator, single channel rechargeable
use Stimulator Generator, Single Array Rechargeable in 0JH
Neurostimulator lead
Insertion of device in
Brain 00H0
Cerebral Ventricle 00H6
Nerve
Cranial 00HE
Peripheral 01HY
Spinal Canal 00HU
Spinal Cord 00HV
Vein
Azygos 05H0
Neurostimulator lead — *continued*
Insertion of device in — *continued*
Innominate
Left 05H4
Right 05H3
Removal of device from
Brain 00P0
Cerebral Ventricle 00P6
Nerve
Cranial 00PE
Peripheral 01PY
Spinal Canal 00PU
Spinal Cord 00PV
Vein
Azygos 05P0
Innominate
Left 05P4
Right 05P3
Revision of device in
Brain 00W0
Cerebral Ventricle 00W6
Nerve
Cranial 00WE
Peripheral 01WY
Spinal Canal 00WU
Spinal Cord 00WV
Vein
Azygos 05W0
Innominate
Left 05W4
Right 05W3
Neurotomy
see Division, Central Nervous System and Cranial Nerves 008
see Division, Peripheral Nervous System 018
Neurotripsy
see Destruction, Central Nervous System and Cranial Nerves 005
see Destruction, Peripheral Nervous System 015
Neutralization plate
use Internal Fixation Device in Head and Facial Bones
use Internal Fixation Device in Upper Bones
use Internal Fixation Device in Lower Bones
New technology
Andexanet Alfa, Factor Xa Inhibitor Reversal Agent XW0
Bezlotoxumab Monoclonal Antibody XW0
Blinatumomab Antineoplastic Immunotherapy XW0
Ceftazidime-Avibactam Anti-infective XW0
Cerebral Embolic Filtration, Dual Filter X2A5312
Concentrated Bone Marrow Aspirate XK02303
Cytarabine and Daunorubicin Liposome Antineoplastic XW0
Defibrotide Sodium Anticoagulant XW0
Destruction, Prostate, Robotic Waterjet Ablation XV508A4
Endothelial Damage Inhibitor XY0VX83
Engineered Autologous Chimeric Antigen Receptor T-cell Immunotherapy XW0
Fusion
Cervical Vertebral
2 or more
Nanotextured Surface XRG2092
Radiolucent Porous XRG20F3
Interbody Fusion Device
Nanotextured Surface XRG1092
Radiolucent Porous XRG10F3
Cervicothoracic Vertebral
Nanotextured Surface XRG4092
Radiolucent Porous XRG40F3

New technology — *continued*
Fusion — *continued*
Lumbar Vertebral
2 or more
Nanotextured Surface XRGC092
Radiolucent Porous XRGC0F3
Interbody Fusion Device
Nanotextured Surface XRGB092
Radiolucent Porous XRGB0F3
Lumbosacral
Nanotextured Surface XRGD092
Radiolucent Porous XRGD0F3
Occipital-cervical
Nanotextured Surface XRG0092
Radiolucent Porous XRG00F3
Thoracic Vertebral
2 to 7
Nanotextured Surface XRG7092
Radiolucent Porous XRG70F3
8 or more
Nanotextured Surface XRG8092
Radiolucent Porous XRG80F3
Interbody Fusion Device
Nanotextured Surface XRG6092
Radiolucent Porous XRG60F3
Thoracolumbar Vertebral
Nanotextured Surface XRGA092
Radiolucent Porous XRGA0F3
Idarucizumab, Dabigatran Reversal Agent XW0
Intraoperative Knee Replacement Sensor XR2
Isavuconazole Anti-infective XW0
Orbital Atherectomy Technology X2C
Other New Technology Therapeutic Substance XW0
Plazomicin Anti-infective XW0
Replacement
Skin Substitute, Porcine Liver Derived XHRPXL2
Zooplastic Tissue, Rapid Deployment Technique X2RF
Reposition
Cervical, Magnetically Controlled Growth Rod(s) XNS3
Lumbar, Magnetically Controlled Growth Rod(s) XNS0
Thoracic, Magnetically Controlled Growth Rod(s) XNS4
Synthetic Human Angiotensin II XW0
Uridine Triacetate XW0DX82
Ninth cranial nerve
use Glossopharyngeal Nerve
Nitinol framed polymer mesh
use Synthetic Substitute
Non-tunneled central venous catheter
use Infusion Device
Nonimaging nuclear medicine assay
Bladder, Kidneys and Ureters CT63
Blood C763
Kidneys, Ureters and Bladder CT63
Lymphatics and Hematologic System C76YYZZ
Ureters, Kidneys and Bladder CT63
Urinary System CT6YYZZ
Nonimaging nuclear medicine probe
Abdomen CW50
Abdomen and Chest CW54
Abdomen and Pelvis CW51
Brain C050
Central Nervous System C05YYZZ
Chest CW53
Chest and Abdomen CW54
Chest and Neck CW56
Extremity
Lower CP5PZZZ
Upper CP5NZZZ
Head and Neck CW5B
Nonimaging nuclear medicine probe — *continued*
Heart C25YYZZ
Right and Left C256
Lymphatics
Head C75J
Head and Neck C755
Lower Extremity C75P
Neck C75K
Pelvic C75D
Trunk C75M
Upper Chest C75L
Upper Extremity C75N
Lymphatics and Hematologic System C75YYZZ
Musculoskeletal System, Other CP5YYZZ
Neck and Chest CW56
Neck and Head CW5B
Pelvic Region CW5J
Pelvis and Abdomen CW51
Spine CP55ZZZ
Nonimaging nuclear medicine uptake
Endocrine System CG4YYZZ
Gland, Thyroid CG42
Nostril
use Nasal Mucosa and Soft Tissue
Novacor® Left Ventricular Assist Device
use Implantable Heart Assist System in Heart and Great Vessels
Novation® Ceramic AHS® (Articulation Hip System)
use Synthetic Substitute, Ceramic in 0SR
Nuclear medicine
see Planar Nuclear Medicine Imaging
see Tomographic (Tomo) Nuclear Medicine Imaging
see Positron Emission Tomographic (PET) Imaging
see Nonimaging Nuclear Medicine Uptake
see Nonimaging Nuclear Medicine Probe
see Nonimaging Nuclear Medicine Assay
see Systemic Nuclear Medicine Therapy
Nuclear scintigraphy
see Nuclear Medicine
Nutrition, concentrated substances
Enteral infusion 3E0G36Z
Parenteral (peripheral) infusion *see* Introduction of Nutritional Substance

O

Obliteration
see Destruction
Obturator artery
use Internal Iliac Artery, Right
use Internal Iliac Artery, Left
Obturator lymph node
use Lymphatic, Pelvis
Obturator muscle
use Hip Muscle, Right
use Hip Muscle, Left
Obturator nerve
use Lumbar Plexus
Obturator vein
use Hypogastric Vein, Right
use Hypogastric Vein, Left
Obtuse margin
use Heart, Left
Occipital artery
use External Carotid Artery, Right
use External Carotid Artery, Left
Occipital lobe
use Cerebral Hemisphere
Occipital lymph node
use Lymphatic, Right Neck
use Lymphatic, Left Neck
Occipitofrontalis muscle
use Facial Muscle
Occlusion
Ampulla of Vater 0FLC
Anus 0DLQ
Aorta
Abdominal 04L0
Thoracic, Descending 02LW3DJ
Artery
Anterior Tibial
Left 04LQ
Right 04LP
Axillary
Left 03L6
Right 03L5
Brachial
Left 03L8
Right 03L7
Celiac 04L1
Colic
Left 04L7
Middle 04L8
Right 04L6
Common Carotid
Left 03LJ
Right 03LH
Common Iliac
Left 04LD
Right 04LC
External Carotid
Left 03LN
Right 03LM
External Iliac
Left 04LJ
Right 04LH
Face 03LR
Femoral
Left 04LL
Right 04LK
Foot
Left 04LW
Right 04LV
Gastric 04L2
Hand
Left 03LF
Right 03LD
Hepatic 04L3
Inferior Mesenteric 04LB
Innominate 03L2
Internal Carotid
Left 03LL
Right 03LK
Internal Iliac
Left 04LF
Right 04LE
Internal Mammary
Left 03L1
Right 03L0
Intracranial 03LG
Lower 04LY
Peroneal
Left 04LU
Right 04LT
Popliteal
Left 04LN
Right 04LM
Posterior Tibial
Left 04LS
Right 04LR
Pulmonary
Left 02LR
Right 02LQ
Pulmonary Trunk 02LP
Radial
Left 03LC
Right 03LB

Occlusion — *continued*
Artery — *continued*
Renal
Left 04LA
Right 04L9
Splenic 04L4
Subclavian
Left 03L4
Right 03L3
Superior Mesenteric 04L5
Temporal
Left 03LT
Right 03LS
Thyroid
Left 03LV
Right 03LU
Ulnar
Left 03LA
Right 03L9
Upper 03LY
Vertebral
Left 03LQ
Right 03LP
Atrium, Left 02L7
Bladder 0TLB
Bladder Neck 0TLC
Bronchus
Lingula 0BL9
Lower Lobe
Left 0BLB
Right 0BL6
Main
Left 0BL7
Right 0BL3
Middle Lobe, Right 0BL5
Upper Lobe
Left 0BL8
Right 0BL4
Carina 0BL2
Cecum 0DLH
Cisterna Chyli 07LL
Colon
Ascending 0DLK
Descending 0DLM
Sigmoid 0DLN
Transverse 0DLL
Cord
Bilateral 0VLH
Left 0VLG
Right 0VLF
Cul-de-sac 0ULF
Duct
Common Bile 0FL9
Cystic 0FL8
Hepatic
Common 0FL7
Left 0FL6
Right 0FL5
Lacrimal
Left 08LY
Right 08LX
Pancreatic 0FLD
Accessory 0FLF
Parotid
Left 0CLC
Right 0CLB
Duodenum 0DL9
Esophagogastric Junction 0DL4
Esophagus 0DL5
Lower 0DL3
Middle 0DL2
Upper 0DL1
Fallopian Tube
Left 0UL6
Right 0UL5
Fallopian Tubes, Bilateral 0UL7
Ileocecal Valve 0DLC

Occlusion — *continued*
Ileum 0DLB
Intestine
Large 0DLE
Left 0DLG
Right 0DLF
Small 0DL8
Jejunum 0DLA
Kidney Pelvis
Left 0TL4
Right 0TL3
Left atrial appendage (LAA) *see* Occlusion, Atrium, Left 02L7
Lymphatic
Aortic 07LD
Axillary
Left 07L6
Right 07L5
Head 07L0
Inguinal
Left 07LJ
Right 07LH
Internal Mammary
Left 07L9
Right 07L8
Lower Extremity
Left 07LG
Right 07LF
Mesenteric 07LB
Neck
Left 07L2
Right 07L1
Pelvis 07LC
Thoracic Duct 07LK
Thorax 07L7
Upper Extremity
Left 07L4
Right 07L3
Rectum 0DLP
Stomach 0DL6
Pylorus 0DL7
Trachea 0BL1
Ureter
Left 0TL7
Right 0TL6
Urethra 0TLD
Vagina 0ULG
Valve, Pulmonary 02LH
Vas Deferens
Bilateral 0VLQ
Left 0VLP
Right 0VLN
Vein
Axillary
Left 05L8
Right 05L7
Azygos 05L0
Basilic
Left 05LC
Right 05LB
Brachial
Left 05LA
Right 05L9
Cephalic
Left 05LF
Right 05LD
Colic 06L7
Common Iliac
Left 06LD
Right 06LC
Esophageal 06L3
External Iliac
Left 06LG
Right 06LF
External Jugular
Left 05LQ
Right 05LP

Occlusion — *continued*
Vein — *continued*
Face
Left 05LV
Right 05LT
Femoral
Left 06LN
Right 06LM
Foot
Left 06LV
Right 06LT
Gastric 06L2
Hand
Left 05LH
Right 05LG
Hemiazygos 05L1
Hepatic 06L4
Hypogastric
Left 06LJ
Right 06LH
Inferior Mesenteric 06L6
Innominate
Left 05L4
Right 05L3
Internal Jugular
Left 05LN
Right 05LM
Intracranial 05LL
Lower 06LY
Portal 06L8
Pulmonary
Left 02LT
Right 02LS
Renal
Left 06LB
Right 06L9
Saphenous
Left 06LQ
Right 06LP
Splenic 06L1
Subclavian
Left 05L6
Right 05L5
Superior Mesenteric 06L5
Upper 05LY
Vertebral
Left 05LS
Right 05LR
Vena Cava
Inferior 06L0
Superior 02LV
Occlusion, REBOA (resuscitative endovascular balloon occlusion of the aorta)
02LW3DJ
04L03DJ
Occupational therapy
see Activities of Daily Living Treatment, Rehabilitation F08
Odentectomy
see Excision, Mouth and Throat 0CB
see Resection, Mouth and Throat 0CT
Odontoid process
use Cervical Vertebra
Olecranon bursa
use Elbow Bursa and Ligament, Right
use Elbow Bursa and Ligament, Left
Olecranon process
use Ulna, Right
use Ulna, Left
Olfactory bulb
use Olfactory Nerve
Omentectomy, omentumectomy
see Excision, Gastrointestinal System 0DB
see Resection, Gastrointestinal System 0DT
Omentofixation
see Repair, Gastrointestinal System 0DQ

Omentoplasty
see Repair, Gastrointestinal System 0DQ
see Replacement, Gastrointestinal System 0DR
see Supplement, Gastrointestinal System 0DU
Omentorrhaphy
see Repair, Gastrointestinal System 0DQ
Omentotomy
see Drainage, Gastrointestinal System 0D9
Omnilink Elite® Vascular Balloon Expandable Stent System
use Intraluminal Device
Onychectomy
see Excision, Skin and Breast 0HB
see Resection, Skin and Breast 0HT
Onychoplasty
see Repair, Skin and Breast 0HQ
see Replacement, Skin and Breast 0HR
Onychotomy
see Drainage, Skin and Breast 0H9
Oophorectomy
see Excision, Female Reproductive System 0UB
see Resection, Female Reproductive System 0UT
Oophoropexy
see Repair, Female Reproductive System 0UQ
see Reposition, Female Reproductive System 0US
Oophoroplasty
see Repair, Female Reproductive System 0UQ
see Supplement, Female Reproductive System 0UU
Oophororrhaphy
see Repair, Female Reproductive System 0UQ
Oophorostomy
see Drainage, Female Reproductive System 0U9
Oophorotomy
see Division, Female Reproductive System 0U8
see Drainage, Female Reproductive System 0U9
Oophorrhaphy
see Repair, Female Reproductive System 0UQ
Open Pivot™ (mechanical) valve
use Synthetic Substitute
Open Pivot™ Aortic Valve Graft (AVG)
use Synthetic Substitute
Ophthalmic artery
use Intracranial Artery
Ophthalmic nerve
use Trigeminal Nerve
Ophthalmic vein
use Intracranial Vein
Opponensplasty
Tendon replacement *see* Replacement, Tendons 0LR
Tendon transfer *see* Transfer, Tendons 0LX
Optic chiasma
use Optic Nerve
Optic disc
use Retina, Right
use Retina, Left
Optic foramen
use Sphenoid Bone
Optical coherence tomography, intravascular
see Computerized Tomography (CT Scan)
Optimizer™ III implantable pulse generator
use Contractility Modulation Device in 0JH
Orbicularis oculi muscle
use Upper Eyelid, Right
use Upper Eyelid, Left
Orbicularis oris muscle
use Facial Muscle
Orbital atherectomy technology X2C
Orbital fascia
use Subcutaneous Tissue and Fascia, Face
Orbital portion of ethmoid bone
use Orbit, Right
use Orbit, Left
Orbital portion of frontal bone
use Orbit, Right
use Orbit, Left
Orbital portion of lacrimal bone
use Orbit, Right
use Orbit, Left
Orbital portion of maxilla
use Orbit, Right
use Orbit, Left
Orbital portion of palatine bone
use Orbit, Right
use Orbit, Left
Orbital portion of sphenoid bone
use Orbit, Right
use Orbit, Left
Orbital portion of zygomatic bone
use Orbit, Right
use Orbit, Left
Orchectomy, orchidectomy, orchiectomy
see Excision, Male Reproductive System 0VB
see Resection, Male Reproductive System 0VT
Orchidoplasty, orchioplasty
see Repair, Male Reproductive System 0VQ
see Replacement, Male Reproductive System 0VR
see Supplement, Male Reproductive System 0VU
Orchidorrhaphy, orchiorrhaphy
see Repair, Male Reproductive System 0VQ
Orchidotomy, orchiotomy, orchotomy
see Drainage, Male Reproductive System 0V9
Orchiopexy
see Repair, Male Reproductive System 0VQ
see Reposition, Male Reproductive System 0VS
Oropharyngeal airway (OPA)
use Intraluminal Device, Airway in Mouth and Throat
Oropharynx
use Pharynx
Ossiculectomy
see Excision, Ear, Nose, Sinus 09B
see Resection, Ear, Nose, Sinus 09T
Ossiculotomy
see Drainage, Ear, Nose, Sinus 099
Ostectomy
see Excision, Head and Facial Bones 0NB
see Resection, Head and Facial Bones 0NT
see Excision, Upper Bones 0PB
see Resection, Upper Bones 0PT
see Excision, Lower Bones 0QB
see Resection, Lower Bones 0QT
Osteoclasis
see Division, Head and Facial Bones 0N8
see Division, Upper Bones 0P8
see Division, Lower Bones 0Q8
Osteolysis
see Release, Head and Facial Bones 0NN
see Release, Upper Bones 0PN
see Release, Lower Bones 0QN
Osteopathic treatment
Abdomen 7W09X
Cervical 7W01X
Osteopathic treatment — *continued*
Extremity
Lower 7W06X
Upper 7W07X
Head 7W00X
Lumbar 7W03X
Pelvis 7W05X
Rib Cage 7W08X
Sacrum 7W04X
Thoracic 7W02X
Osteopexy
see Repair, Head and Facial Bones 0NQ
see Reposition, Head and Facial Bones 0NS
see Repair, Upper Bones 0PQ
see Reposition, Upper Bones 0PS
see Repair, Lower Bones 0QQ
see Reposition, Lower Bones 0QS
Osteoplasty
see Repair, Head and Facial Bones 0NQ
see Replacement, Head and Facial Bones 0NR
see Supplement, Head and Facial Bones 0NU
see Repair, Upper Bones 0PQ
see Replacement, Upper Bones 0PR
see Supplement, Upper Bones 0PU
see Repair, Lower Bones 0QQ
see Replacement, Lower Bones 0QR
see Supplement, Lower Bones 0QU
Osteorrhaphy
see Repair, Head and Facial Bones 0NQ
see Repair, Upper Bones 0PQ
see Repair, Lower Bones 0QQ
Osteotomy, ostotomy
see Division, Head and Facial Bones 0N8
see Drainage, Head and Facial Bones 0N9
see Division, Upper Bones 0P8
see Drainage, Upper Bones 0P9
see Division, Lower Bones 0Q8
see Drainage, Lower Bones 0Q9
Otic ganglion
use Head and Neck Sympathetic Nerve
Otoplasty
see Repair, Ear, Nose, Sinus 09Q
see Replacement, Ear, Nose, Sinus 09R
see Supplement, Ear, Nose, Sinus 09U
Otoscopy
see Inspection, Ear, Nose, Sinus 09J
Oval window
use Middle Ear, Right
use Middle Ear, Left
Ovarian artery
use Abdominal Aorta
Ovarian ligament
use Uterine Supporting Structure
Ovariectomy
see Excision, Female Reproductive System 0UB
see Resection, Female Reproductive System 0UT
Ovariocentesis
see Drainage, Female Reproductive System 0U9
Ovariopexy
see Repair, Female Reproductive System 0UQ
see Reposition, Female Reproductive System 0US
Ovariotomy
see Division, Female Reproductive System 0U8
see Drainage, Female Reproductive System 0U9
Ovatio™ CRT-D
use Cardiac Resynchronization Defibrillator Pulse Generator in 0JH

Oversewing
Gastrointestinal ulcer *see* Repair, Gastrointestinal System 0DQ
Pleural bleb *see* Repair, Respiratory System 0BQ
Oviduct
use Fallopian Tube, Right
use Fallopian Tube, Left
Oximetry, fetal pulse 10H073Z
OXINIUM™
use Synthetic Substitute, Oxidized Zirconium on Polyethylene in 0SR
Oxygenation
Extracorporeal membrane (ECMO) *see* Performance, Circulatory 5A15
Hyperbaric *see* Assistance, Circulatory 5A05
Supersaturated *see* Assistance, Circulatory 5A05

P

Pacemaker
Dual Chamber
Abdomen 0JH8
Chest 0JH6
Intracardiac
Insertion of device in
Atrium
Left 02H7
Right 02H6
Vein, Coronary 02H4
Ventricle
Left 02HL
Right 02HK
Removal of device from, Heart 02PA
Revision of device in, Heart 02WA
Single Chamber
Abdomen 0JH8
Chest 0JH6
Single Chamber Rate Responsive
Abdomen 0JH8
Chest 0JH6
Packing
Abdominal Wall 2W43X5Z
Anorectal 2Y43X5Z
Arm
Lower
Left 2W4DX5Z
Right 2W4CX5Z
Upper
Left 2W4BX5Z
Right 2W4AX5Z
Back 2W45X5Z
Chest Wall 2W44X5Z
Ear 2Y42X5Z
Extremity
Lower
Left 2W4MX5Z
Right 2W4LX5Z
Upper
Left 2W49X5Z
Right 2W48X5Z
Face 2W41X5Z
Finger
Left 2W4KX5Z
Right 2W4JX5Z
Foot
Left 2W4TX5Z
Right 2W4SX5Z
Genital Tract, Female 2Y44X5Z
Hand
Left 2W4FX5Z
Right 2W4EX5Z
Head 2W40X5Z
Inguinal Region
Left 2W47X5Z
Packing — *continued*
Inguinal Region — *continued*
Right 2W46X5Z
Leg
Lower
Left 2W4RX5Z
Right 2W4QX5Z
Upper
Left 2W4PX5Z
Right 2W4NX5Z
Mouth and Pharynx 2Y40X5Z
Nasal 2Y41X5Z
Neck 2W42X5Z
Thumb
Left 2W4HX5Z
Right 2W4GX5Z
Toe
Left 2W4VX5Z
Right 2W4UX5Z
Urethra 2Y45X5Z
Paclitaxel-eluting coronary stent
use Intraluminal Device, Drug-eluting in Heart and Great Vessels
Paclitaxel-eluting peripheral stent
use Intraluminal Device, Drug-eluting in Upper Arteries
use Intraluminal Device, Drug-eluting in Lower Arteries
Palatine gland
use Buccal Mucosa
Palatine tonsil
use Tonsils
Palatine uvula
use Uvula
Palatoglossal muscle
use Tongue, Palate, Pharynx Muscle
Palatopharyngeal muscle
use Tongue, Palate, Pharynx Muscle
Palatoplasty
see Repair, Mouth and Throat 0CQ
see Replacement, Mouth and Throat 0CR
see Supplement, Mouth and Throat 0CU
Palatorrhaphy
see Repair, Mouth and Throat 0CQ
Palmar (volar) digital vein
use Hand Vein, Right
use Hand Vein, Left
Palmar (volar) metacarpal vein
use Hand Vein, Right
use Hand Vein, Left
Palmar cutaneous nerve
use Median Nerve
use Radial Nerve
Palmar fascia (aponeurosis)
use Subcutaneous Tissue and Fascia, Right Hand
use Subcutaneous Tissue and Fascia, Left Hand
Palmar interosseous muscle
use Hand Muscle, Right
use Hand Muscle, Left
Palmar ulnocarpal ligament
use Wrist Bursa and Ligament, Right
use Wrist Bursa and Ligament, Left
Palmaris longus muscle
use Lower Arm and Wrist Muscle, Right
use Lower Arm and Wrist Muscle, Left
Pancreatectomy
see Excision, Pancreas 0FBG
see Resection, Pancreas 0FTG
Pancreatic artery
use Splenic Artery
Pancreatic plexus
use Abdominal Sympathetic Nerve
Pancreatic vein
use Splenic Vein
Pancreaticoduodenostomy
see Bypass, Hepatobiliary System and Pancreas 0F1
Pancreaticosplenic lymph node
use Lymphatic, Aortic
Pancreatogram, endoscopic retrograde
see Fluoroscopy, Pancreatic Duct BF18
Pancreatolithotomy
see Extirpation, Pancreas 0FCG
Pancreatotomy
see Division, Pancreas 0F8G
see Drainage, Pancreas 0F9G
Panniculectomy
see Excision, Skin, Abdomen 0HB7
see Excision, Abdominal Wall 0WBF
Paraaortic lymph node
use Lymphatic, Aortic
Paracentesis
Eye *see* Drainage, Eye 089
Peritoneal Cavity *see* Drainage, Peritoneal Cavity 0W9G
Tympanum *see* Drainage, Ear, Nose, Sinus 099
Pararectal lymph node
use Lymphatic, Mesenteric
Parasternal lymph node
use Lymphatic, Thorax
Parathyroidectomy
see Excision, Endocrine System 0GB
see Resection, Endocrine System 0GT
Paratracheal lymph node
use Lymphatic, Thorax
Paraurethral (Skene's) gland
use Vestibular Gland
Parenteral nutrition, total
see Introduction of Nutritional Substance
Parietal lobe
use Cerebral Hemisphere
Parotid lymph node
use Lymphatic, Head
Parotid plexus
use Facial Nerve
Parotidectomy
see Excision, Mouth and Throat 0CB
see Resection, Mouth and Throat 0CT
Pars flaccida
use Tympanic Membrane, Right
use Tympanic Membrane, Left
Partial joint replacement
Hip *see* Replacement, Lower Joints 0SR
Knee *see* Replacement, Lower Joints 0SR
Shoulder *see* Replacement, Upper Joints 0RR
Partially absorbable mesh
use Synthetic Substitute
Patch, blood, spinal 3E0R3GC
Patellapexy
see Repair, Lower Bones 0QQ
see Reposition, Lower Bones 0QS
Patellaplasty
see Repair, Lower Bones 0QQ
see Replacement, Lower Bones 0QR
see Supplement, Lower Bones 0QU
Patellar ligament
use Knee Bursa and Ligament, Right
use Knee Bursa and Ligament, Left
Patellar tendon
use Knee Tendon, Right
use Knee Tendon, Left
Patellectomy
see Excision, Lower Bones 0QB
see Resection, Lower Bones 0QT
Patellofemoral joint
use Knee Joint, Right
use Knee Joint, Left
use Knee Joint, Femoral Surface, Right
use Knee Joint, Femoral Surface, Left

Pectineus muscle
use Upper Leg Muscle, Right
use Upper Leg Muscle, Left
Pectoral (anterior) lymph node
use Lymphatic, Right Axillary
use Lymphatic, Left Axillary
Pectoral fascia
use Subcutaneous Tissue and Fascia, Chest
Pectoralis major muscle
use Thorax Muscle, Right
use Thorax Muscle, Left
Pectoralis minor muscle
use Thorax Muscle, Right
use Thorax Muscle, Left
Pedicle-based dynamic stabilization device
use Spinal Stabilization Device, Pedicle-Based in 0RH
use Spinal Stabilization Device, Pedicle-Based in 0SH
PEEP (positive end expiratory pressure)
see Assistance, Respiratory 5A09
PEG (percutaneous endoscopic gastrostomy) 0DH63UZ
PEJ (percutaneous endoscopic jejunostomy) 0DHA3UZ
Pelvic splanchnic nerve
use Abdominal Sympathetic Nerve
use Sacral Sympathetic Nerve
Penectomy
see Excision, Male Reproductive System 0VB
see Resection, Male Reproductive System 0VT
Penile urethra
use Urethra
Perceval sutureless valve
use Zooplastic Tissue, Rapid Deployment Technique in New Technology
Percutaneous endoscopic gastrojejunostomy (PEG/J) tube
use Feeding Device in Gastrointestinal System
Percutaneous endoscopic gastrostomy (PEG) tube
use Feeding Device in Gastrointestinal System
Percutaneous nephrostomy catheter
use Drainage Device
Percutaneous transluminal coronary angioplasty (PTCA)
see Dilation, Heart and Great Vessels 027
Performance
Biliary
Multiple, Filtration 5A1C60Z
Single, Filtration 5A1C00Z
Cardiac
Continuous
Output 5A1221Z
Pacing 5A1223Z
Intermittent, Pacing 5A1213Z
Single, Output, Manual 5A12012
Circulatory
Central Membrane 5A1522F
Peripheral Veno-arterial Membrane 5A1522G
Peripheral Veno-venous Membrane 5A1522H
Respiratory
24-96 Consecutive Hours, Ventilation 5A1945Z
Greater than 96 Consecutive Hours, Ventilation 5A1955Z
Less than 24 Consecutive Hours, Ventilation 5A1935Z
Single, Ventilation, Nonmechanical 5A19054
Performance — *continued*
Urinary
Continuous, Greater than 18 hours per day, Filtration 5A1D90Z
Intermittent, Less than 6 Hours Per Day, Filtration 5A1D70Z
Prolonged Intermittent, 6-18 hours per day, Filtration 5A1D80Z
Perfusion
see Introduction of substance in or on
Perfusion, donor organ
Heart 6AB50BZ
Kidney(s) 6ABT0BZ
Liver 6ABF0BZ
Lung(s) 6ABB0BZ
Pericardiectomy
see Excision, Pericardium 02BN
see Resection, Pericardium 02TN
Pericardiocentesis
see Drainage, Pericardial Cavity 0W9D
Pericardiolysis
see Release, Pericardium 02NN
Pericardiophrenic artery
use Internal Mammary Artery, Right
use Internal Mammary Artery, Left
Pericardioplasty
see Repair, Pericardium 02QN
see Replacement, Pericardium 02RN
see Supplement, Pericardium 02UN
Pericardiorrhaphy
see Repair, Pericardium 02QN
Pericardiostomy
see Drainage, Pericardial Cavity 0W9D
Pericardiotomy
see Drainage, Pericardial Cavity 0W9D
Perimetrium
use Uterus
Peripheral parenteral nutrition
see Introduction of Nutritional Substance
Peripherally inserted central catheter (PICC)
use Infusion Device
Peritoneal dialysis 3E1M39Z
Peritoneocentesis
see Drainage, Peritoneum 0D9W
see Drainage, Peritoneal Cavity 0W9G
Peritoneoplasty
see Repair, Peritoneum 0DQW
see Replacement, Peritoneum 0DRW
see Supplement, Peritoneum 0DUW
Peritoneoscopy 0DJW4ZZ
Peritoneotomy
see Drainage, Peritoneum 0D9W
Peritoneumectomy
see Excision, Peritoneum 0DBW
Peroneus brevis muscle
use Lower Leg Muscle, Right
use Lower Leg Muscle, Left
Peroneus longus muscle
use Lower Leg Muscle, Right
use Lower Leg Muscle, Left
Pessary ring
use Intraluminal Device, Pessary in Female Reproductive System
PET scan
see Positron Emission Tomographic (PET) Imaging
Petrous part of temporal bone
use Temporal Bone, Right
use Temporal Bone, Left
Phacoemulsification, lens
With IOL implant *see* Replacement, Eye 08R
Without IOL implant *see* Extraction, Eye 08D
Phalangectomy
see Excision, Upper Bones 0PB
see Resection, Upper Bones 0PT
Phalangectomy — *continued*
see Excision, Lower Bones 0QB
see Resection, Lower Bones 0QT
Phallectomy
see Excision, Penis 0VBS
see Resection, Penis 0VTS
Phalloplasty
see Repair, Penis 0VQS
see Supplement, Penis 0VUS
Phallotomy
see Drainage, Penis 0V9S
Pharmacotherapy, for substance abuse
Antabuse HZ93ZZZ
Bupropion HZ97ZZZ
Clonidine HZ96ZZZ
Levo-alpha-acetyl-methadol (LAAM) HZ92ZZZ
Methadone Maintenance HZ91ZZZ
Naloxone HZ95ZZZ
Naltrexone HZ94ZZZ
Nicotine Replacement HZ90ZZZ
Psychiatric Medication HZ98ZZZ
Replacement Medication, Other HZ99ZZZ
Pharyngeal constrictor muscle
use Tongue, Palate, Pharynx Muscle
Pharyngeal plexus
use Vagus Nerve
Pharyngeal recess
use Nasopharynx
Pharyngeal tonsil
use Adenoids
Pharyngogram
see Fluoroscopy, Pharynx B91G
Pharyngoplasty
see Repair, Mouth and Throat 0CQ
see Replacement, Mouth and Throat 0CR
see Supplement, Mouth and Throat 0CU
Pharyngorrhaphy
see Repair, Mouth and Throat 0CQ
Pharyngotomy
see Drainage, Mouth and Throat 0C9
Pharyngotympanic tube
use Eustachian Tube, Right
use Eustachian Tube, Left
Pheresis
Erythrocytes 6A55
Leukocytes 6A55
Plasma 6A55
Platelets 6A55
Stem Cells
Cord Blood 6A55
Hematopoietic 6A55
Phlebectomy
see Excision, Upper Veins 05B
see Extraction, Upper Veins 05D
see Excision, Lower Veins 06B
see Extraction, Lower Veins 06D
Phlebography
see Plain Radiography, Veins B50
Impedance 4A04X51
Phleborrhaphy
see Repair, Upper Veins 05Q
see Repair, Lower Veins 06Q
Phlebotomy
see Drainage, Upper Veins 059
see Drainage, Lower Veins 069
Photocoagulation
For Destruction *see* Destruction
For Repair *see* Repair
Photopheresis, therapeutic
see Phototherapy, Circulatory 6A65
Phototherapy
Circulatory 6A65
Skin 6A60
Ultraviolet light *see* Ultraviolet Light Therapy, Physiological Systems 6A8

- **Phrenectomy, phrenoneurectomy**
  - *see* Excision, Nerve, Phrenic 01B2
- **Phrenemphraxis**
  - *see* Destruction, Nerve, Phrenic 0152
- **Phrenic nerve stimulator generator**
  - *use* Stimulator Generator in Subcutaneous Tissue and Fascia
- **Phrenic nerve stimulator lead**
  - *use* Diaphragmatic Pacemaker Lead in Respiratory System
- **Phreniclasis**
  - *see* Destruction, Nerve, Phrenic 0152
- **Phrenicoexeresis**
  - *see* Extraction, Nerve, Phrenic 01D2
- **Phrenicotomy**
  - *see* Division, Nerve, Phrenic 0182
- **Phrenicotripsy**
  - *see* Destruction, Nerve, Phrenic 0152
- **Phrenoplasty**
  - *see* Repair, Respiratory System 0BQ
  - *see* Supplement, Respiratory System 0BU
- **Phrenotomy**
  - *see* Drainage, Respiratory System 0B9
- **Physiatry**
  - *see* Motor Treatment, Rehabilitation F07
- **Physical medicine**
  - *see* Motor Treatment, Rehabilitation F07
- **Physical therapy**
  - *see* Motor Treatment, Rehabilitation F07
- **PHYSIOMESH™ Flexible Composite Mesh**
  - *use* Synthetic Substitute
- **Pia mater, intracranial**
  - *use* Cerebral Meninges
- **Pia mater, spinal**
  - *use* Spinal Meninges
- **Pinealectomy**
  - *see* Excision, Pineal Body 0GB1
  - *see* Resection, Pineal Body 0GT1
- **Pinealoscopy** 0GJ14ZZ
- **Pinealotomy**
  - *see* Drainage, Pineal Body 0G91
- **Pinna**
  - *use* External Ear, Right
  - *use* External Ear, Left
  - *use* External Ear, Bilateral
- **Pipeline™ Embolization device (PED)**
  - *use* Intraluminal Device
- **Piriform recess (sinus)**
  - *use* Pharynx
- **Piriformis muscle**
  - *use* Hip Muscle, Right
  - *use* Hip Muscle, Left
- **PIRRT (Prolonged intermittent renal replacement therapy)** 5A1D80Z
- **Pisiform bone**
  - *use* Carpal, Right
  - *use* Carpal, Left
- **Pisohamate ligament**
  - *use* Hand Bursa and Ligament, Right
  - *use* Hand Bursa and Ligament, Left
- **Pisometacarpal ligament**
  - *use* Hand Bursa and Ligament, Right
  - *use* Hand Bursa and Ligament, Left
- **Pituitectomy**
  - *see* Excision, Gland, Pituitary 0GB0
  - *see* Resection, Gland, Pituitary 0GT0
- **Plain film radiology**
  - *see* Plain Radiography
- **Plain radiography**
  - Abdomen BW00ZZZ
  - Abdomen and Pelvis BW01ZZZ
  - Abdominal Lymphatic
    - Bilateral B701
    - Unilateral B700
  - Airway, Upper BB0DZZZ
  - Ankle
    - Left BQ0H

Plain radiography — *continued*
  - Ankle — *continued*
    - Right BQ0G
  - Aorta
    - Abdominal B400
    - Thoracic B300
    - Thoraco-Abdominal B30P
  - Aorta and Bilateral Lower Extremity Arteries B40D
  - Arch
    - Bilateral BN0DZZZ
    - Left BN0CZZZ
    - Right BN0BZZZ
  - Arm
    - Left BP0FZZZ
    - Right BP0EZZZ
  - Artery
    - Brachiocephalic-Subclavian, Right B301
    - Bronchial B30L
    - Bypass Graft, Other B20F
    - Cervico-Cerebral Arch B30Q
    - Common Carotid
      - Bilateral B305
      - Left B304
      - Right B303
    - Coronary
      - Bypass Graft
        - Multiple B203
        - Single B202
      - Multiple B201
      - Single B200
    - External Carotid
      - Bilateral B30C
      - Left B30B
      - Right B309
    - Hepatic B402
    - Inferior Mesenteric B405
    - Intercostal B30L
    - Internal Carotid
      - Bilateral B308
      - Left B307
      - Right B306
    - Internal Mammary Bypass Graft
      - Left B208
      - Right B207
    - Intra-Abdominal, Other B40B
    - Intracranial B30R
    - Lower, Other B40J
    - Lower Extremity
      - Bilateral and Aorta B40D
      - Left B40G
      - Right B40F
    - Lumbar B409
    - Pelvic B40C
    - Pulmonary
      - Left B30T
      - Right B30S
    - Renal
      - Bilateral B408
      - Left B407
      - Right B406
      - Transplant B40M
    - Spinal B30M
    - Splenic B403
    - Subclavian, Left B302
    - Superior Mesenteric B404
    - Upper, Other B30N
    - Upper Extremity
      - Bilateral B30K
      - Left B30J
      - Right B30H
    - Vertebral
      - Bilateral B30G
      - Left B30F
      - Right B30D
  - Bile Duct BF00
  - Bile Duct and Gallbladder BF03

Plain radiography — *continued*
  - Bladder BT00
    - Kidney and Ureter BT04
  - Bladder and Urethra BT0B
  - Bone
    - Facial BN05ZZZ
    - Nasal BN04ZZZ
  - Bones, Long, All BW0BZZZ
  - Breast
    - Bilateral BH02ZZZ
    - Left BH01ZZZ
    - Right BH00ZZZ
  - Calcaneus
    - Left BQ0KZZZ
    - Right BQ0JZZZ
  - Chest BW03ZZZ
  - Clavicle
    - Left BP05ZZZ
    - Right BP04ZZZ
  - Coccyx BR0FZZZ
  - Corpora Cavernosa BV00
  - Dialysis Fistula B50W
  - Dialysis Shunt B50W
  - Disc
    - Cervical BR01
    - Lumbar BR03
    - Thoracic BR02
  - Duct
    - Lacrimal
      - Bilateral B802
      - Left B801
      - Right B800
    - Mammary
      - Multiple
        - Left BH06
        - Right BH05
      - Single
        - Left BH04
        - Right BH03
  - Elbow
    - Left BP0H
    - Right BP0G
  - Epididymis
    - Left BV02
    - Right BV01
  - Extremity
    - Lower BW0CZZZ
    - Upper BW0JZZZ
  - Eye
    - Bilateral B807ZZZ
    - Left B806ZZZ
    - Right B805ZZZ
  - Facet Joint
    - Cervical BR04
    - Lumbar BR06
    - Thoracic BR05
  - Fallopian Tube
    - Bilateral BU02
    - Left BU01
    - Right BU00
  - Fallopian Tube and Uterus BU08
  - Femur
    - Left, Densitometry BQ04ZZ1
    - Right, Densitometry BQ03ZZ1
  - Finger
    - Left BP0SZZZ
    - Right BP0RZZZ
  - Foot
    - Left BQ0MZZZ
    - Right BQ0LZZZ
  - Forearm
    - Left BP0KZZZ
    - Right BP0JZZZ
  - Gallbladder and Bile Duct BF03
  - Gland
    - Parotid
      - Bilateral B906

- **Plain radiography** — *continued*
  - Gland — *continued*
      - Left B905
      - Right B904
    - Salivary
      - Bilateral B90D
      - Left B90C
      - Right B90B
    - Submandibular
      - Bilateral B909
      - Left B908
      - Right B907
  - Hand
    - Left BP0PZZZ
    - Right BP0NZZZ
  - Heart
    - Left B205
    - Right B204
    - Right and Left B206
  - Hepatobiliary System, All BF0C
  - Hip
    - Left BQ01
      - Densitometry BQ01ZZ1
    - Right BQ00
      - Densitometry BQ00ZZ1
  - Humerus
    - Left BP0BZZZ
    - Right BP0AZZZ
  - Ileal Diversion Loop BT0C
  - Intracranial Sinus B502
  - Joint
    - Acromioclavicular, Bilateral BP03ZZZ
    - Finger
      - Left BP0D
      - Right BP0C
    - Foot
      - Left BQ0Y
      - Right BQ0X
    - Hand
      - Left BP0D
      - Right BP0C
    - Lumbosacral BR0BZZZ
    - Sacroiliac BR0D
    - Sternoclavicular
      - Bilateral BP02ZZZ
      - Left BP01ZZZ
      - Right BP00ZZZ
    - Temporomandibular
      - Bilateral BN09
      - Left BN08
      - Right BN07
    - Thoracolumbar BR08ZZZ
    - Toe
      - Left BQ0Y
      - Right BQ0X
  - Kidney
    - Bilateral BT03
    - Left BT02
    - Right BT01
    - Ureter and Bladder BT04
  - Knee
    - Left BQ08
    - Right BQ07
  - Leg
    - Left BQ0FZZZ
    - Right BQ0DZZZ
  - Lymphatic
    - Head B704
    - Lower Extremity
      - Bilateral B70B
      - Left B709
      - Right B708
    - Neck B704
    - Pelvic B70C
    - Upper Extremity
      - Bilateral B707
      - Left B706

- **Plain radiography** — *continued*
  - Lymphatic — *continued*
      - Right B705
  - Mandible BN06ZZZ
  - Mastoid B90HZZZ
  - Nasopharynx B90FZZZ
  - Optic Foramina
    - Left B804ZZZ
    - Right B803ZZZ
  - Orbit
    - Bilateral BN03ZZZ
    - Left BN02ZZZ
    - Right BN01ZZZ
  - Oropharynx B90FZZZ
  - Patella
    - Left BQ0WZZZ
    - Right BQ0VZZZ
  - Pelvis BR0CZZZ
  - Pelvis and Abdomen BW01ZZZ
  - Prostate BV03
  - Retroperitoneal Lymphatic
    - Bilateral B701
    - Unilateral B700
  - Ribs
    - Left BP0YZZZ
    - Right BP0XZZZ
  - Sacrum BR0FZZZ
  - Scapula
    - Left BP07ZZZ
    - Right BP06ZZZ
  - Shoulder
    - Left BP09
    - Right BP08
  - Sinus
    - Intracranial B502
    - Paranasal B902ZZZ
  - Skull BN00ZZZ
  - Spinal Cord B00B
  - Spine
    - Cervical, Densitometry BR00ZZ1
    - Lumbar, Densitometry BR09ZZ1
    - Thoracic, Densitometry BR07ZZ1
    - Whole, Densitometry BR0GZZ1
  - Sternum BR0HZZZ
  - Teeth
    - All BN0JZZZ
    - Multiple BN0HZZZ
  - Testicle
    - Left BV06
    - Right BV05
  - Toe
    - Left BQ0QZZZ
    - Right BQ0PZZZ
  - Tooth, Single BN0GZZZ
  - Tracheobronchial Tree
    - Bilateral BB09YZZ
    - Left BB08YZZ
    - Right BB07YZZ
  - Ureter
    - Bilateral BT08
    - Kidney and Bladder BT04
    - Left BT07
    - Right BT06
  - Urethra BT05
  - Urethra and Bladder BT0B
  - Uterus BU06
  - Uterus and Fallopian Tube BU08
  - Vagina BU09
  - Vasa Vasorum BV08
  - Vein
    - Cerebellar B501
    - Cerebral B501
    - Epidural B500
    - Jugular
      - Bilateral B505
      - Left B504
      - Right B503

- **Plain radiography** — *continued*
  - Vein — *continued*
    - Lower Extremity
      - Bilateral B50D
      - Left B50C
      - Right B50B
    - Other B50V
    - Pelvic (Iliac)
      - Left B50G
      - Right B50F
    - Pelvic (Iliac) Bilateral B50H
    - Portal B50T
    - Pulmonary
      - Bilateral B50S
      - Left B50R
      - Right B50Q
    - Renal
      - Bilateral B50L
      - Left B50K
      - Right B50J
    - Splanchnic B50T
    - Subclavian
      - Left B507
      - Right B506
    - Upper Extremity
      - Bilateral B50P
      - Left B50N
      - Right B50M
  - Vena Cava
    - Inferior B509
    - Superior B508
  - Whole Body BW0KZZZ
    - Infant BW0MZZZ
  - Whole Skeleton BW0LZZZ
  - Wrist
    - Left BP0M
    - Right BP0L
- **Planar nuclear medicine imaging**
  - Abdomen CW10
  - Abdomen and Chest CW14
  - Abdomen and Pelvis CW11
  - Anatomical Region, Other CW1ZZZZ
  - Anatomical Regions, Multiple CW1YYZZ
  - Bladder, Kidneys and Ureters CT13
  - Bladder and Ureters CT1H
  - Blood C713
  - Bone Marrow C710
  - Brain C010
  - Breast CH1YYZZ
    - Bilateral CH12
    - Left CH11
    - Right CH10
  - Bronchi and Lungs CB12
  - Central Nervous System C01YYZZ
  - Cerebrospinal Fluid C015
  - Chest CW13
  - Chest and Abdomen CW14
  - Chest and Neck CW16
  - Digestive System CD1YYZZ
  - Ducts, Lacrimal, Bilateral C819
  - Ear, Nose, Mouth and Throat C91YYZZ
  - Endocrine System CG1YYZZ
  - Extremity
    - Lower CW1D
      - Bilateral CP1F
      - Left CP1D
      - Right CP1C
    - Upper CW1M
      - Bilateral CP1B
      - Left CP19
      - Right CP18
  - Eye C81YYZZ
  - Gallbladder CF14
  - Gastrointestinal Tract CD17
    - Upper CD15
  - Gland
    - Adrenal, Bilateral CG14

Planar nuclear medicine imaging — *continued*
Gland — *continued*
Parathyroid CG11
Thyroid CG12
Glands, Salivary, Bilateral C91B
Head and Neck CW1B
Heart C21YYZZ
Right and Left C216
Hepatobiliary System, All CF1C
Hepatobiliary System and Pancreas CF1YYZZ
Kidneys, Ureters and Bladder CT13
Liver CF15
Liver and Spleen CF16
Lungs and Bronchi CB12
Lymphatics
Head C71J
Head and Neck C715
Lower Extremity C71P
Neck C71K
Pelvic C71D
Trunk C71M
Upper Chest C71L
Upper Extremity C71N
Lymphatics and Hematologic System C71YYZZ
Musculoskeletal System
All CP1Z
Other CP1YYZZ
Myocardium C21G
Neck and Chest CW16
Neck and Head CW1B
Pancreas and Hepatobiliary System CF1YYZZ
Pelvic Region CW1J
Pelvis CP16
Pelvis and Abdomen CW11
Pelvis and Spine CP17
Reproductive System, Male CV1YYZZ
Respiratory System CB1YYZZ
Skin CH1YYZZ
Skull CP11
Spine CP15
Spine and Pelvis CP17
Spleen C712
Spleen and Liver CF16
Subcutaneous Tissue CH1YYZZ
Testicles, Bilateral CV19
Thorax CP14
Ureters, Kidneys and Bladder CT13
Ureters and Bladder CT1H
Urinary System CT1YYZZ
Veins C51YYZZ
Central C51R
Lower Extremity
Bilateral C51D
Left C51C
Right C51B
Upper Extremity
Bilateral C51Q
Left C51P
Right C51N
Whole Body CW1N
Plantar digital vein
use Foot Vein, Right
use Foot Vein, Left
Plantar fascia (aponeurosis)
use Subcutaneous Tissue and Fascia, Right Foot
use Subcutaneous Tissue and Fascia, Left Foot
Plantar metatarsal vein
use Foot Vein, Right
use Foot Vein, Left
Plantar venous arch
use Foot Vein, Right
use Foot Vein, Left
Plaque radiation
Abdomen DWY3FZZ
Adrenal Gland DGY2FZZ
Anus DDY8FZZ
Bile Ducts DFY2FZZ
Bladder DTY2FZZ
Bone, Other DPYCFZZ
Bone Marrow D7Y0FZZ
Brain D0Y0FZZ
Brain Stem D0Y1FZZ
Breast
Left DMY0FZZ
Right DMY1FZZ
Bronchus DBY1FZZ
Cervix DUY1FZZ
Chest DWY2FZZ
Chest Wall DBY7FZZ
Colon DDY5FZZ
Diaphragm DBY8FZZ
Duodenum DDY2FZZ
Ear D9Y0FZZ
Esophagus DDY0FZZ
Eye D8Y0FZZ
Femur DPY9FZZ
Fibula DPYBFZZ
Gallbladder DFY1FZZ
Gland
Adrenal DGY2FZZ
Parathyroid DGY4FZZ
Pituitary DGY0FZZ
Thyroid DGY5FZZ
Glands, Salivary D9Y6FZZ
Head and Neck DWY1FZZ
Hemibody DWY4FZZ
Humerus DPY6FZZ
Ileum DDY4FZZ
Jejunum DDY3FZZ
Kidney DTY0FZZ
Larynx D9YBFZZ
Liver DFY0FZZ
Lung DBY2FZZ
Lymphatics
Abdomen D7Y6FZZ
Axillary D7Y4FZZ
Inguinal D7Y8FZZ
Neck D7Y3FZZ
Pelvis D7Y7FZZ
Thorax D7Y5FZZ
Mandible DPY3FZZ
Maxilla DPY2FZZ
Mediastinum DBY6FZZ
Mouth D9Y4FZZ
Nasopharynx D9YDFZZ
Neck and Head DWY1FZZ
Nerve, Peripheral D0Y7FZZ
Nose D9Y1FZZ
Ovary DUY0FZZ
Palate
Hard D9Y8FZZ
Soft D9Y9FZZ
Pancreas DFY3FZZ
Parathyroid Gland DGY4FZZ
Pelvic Bones DPY8FZZ
Pelvic Region DWY6FZZ
Pharynx D9YCFZZ
Pineal Body DGY1FZZ
Pituitary Gland DGY0FZZ
Pleura DBY5FZZ
Prostate DVY0FZZ
Radius DPY7FZZ
Rectum DDY7FZZ
Rib DPY5FZZ
Sinuses D9Y7FZZ
Skin
Abdomen DHY8FZZ
Arm DHY4FZZ
Back DHY7FZZ
Plaque radiation — *continued*
Skin — *continued*
Buttock DHY9FZZ
Chest DHY6FZZ
Face DHY2FZZ
Foot DHYCFZZ
Hand DHY5FZZ
Leg DHYBFZZ
Neck DHY3FZZ
Skull DPY0FZZ
Spinal Cord D0Y6FZZ
Spleen D7Y2FZZ
Sternum DPY4FZZ
Stomach DDY1FZZ
Testis DVY1FZZ
Thymus D7Y1FZZ
Thyroid Gland DGY5FZZ
Tibia DPYBFZZ
Tongue D9Y5FZZ
Trachea DBY0FZZ
Ulna DPY7FZZ
Ureter DTY1FZZ
Urethra DTY3FZZ
Uterus DUY2FZZ
Whole Body DWY5FZZ
Plasmapheresis, therapeutic
see Pheresis, Physiological Systems 6A5
Plateletpheresis, therapeutic
see Pheresis, Physiological Systems 6A5
Platysma muscle
use Neck Muscle, Right
use Neck Muscle, Left
Plazomicin anti-infective XW0
Pleurectomy
see Excision, Respiratory System 0BB
see Resection, Respiratory System 0BT
Pleurocentesis
see Drainage, Anatomical Regions, General 0W9
Pleurodesis, pleurosclerosis
Chemical injection *see* Introduction of substance in or on, Pleural Cavity 3E0L
Surgical *see* Destruction, Respiratory System 0B5
Pleurolysis
see Release, Respiratory System 0BN
Pleuroscopy 0BJQ4ZZ
Pleurotomy
see Drainage, Respiratory System 0B9
Plica semilunaris
use Conjunctiva, Right
use Conjunctiva, Left
Plication
see Restriction
Pneumectomy
see Excision, Respiratory System 0BB
see Resection, Respiratory System 0BT
Pneumocentesis
see Drainage, Respiratory System 0B9
Pneumogastric nerve
use Vagus Nerve
Pneumolysis
see Release, Respiratory System 0BN
Pneumonectomy
see Resection, Respiratory System 0BT
Pneumonolysis
see Release, Respiratory System 0BN
Pneumonopexy
see Repair, Respiratory System 0BQ
see Reposition, Respiratory System 0BS
Pneumonorrhaphy
see Repair, Respiratory System 0BQ
Pneumonotomy
see Drainage, Respiratory System 0B9
Pneumotaxic center
use Pons

Pneumotomy
see Drainage, Respiratory System 0B9
Pollicization
see Transfer, Anatomical Regions, Upper Extremities 0XX
Polyethylene socket
use Synthetic Substitute, Polyethylene in 0SR
Polymethylmethacrylate (PMMA)
use Synthetic Substitute
Polypectomy, gastrointestinal
see Excision, Gastrointestinal System 0DB
Polypropylene mesh
use Synthetic Substitute
Polysomnogram 4A1ZXQZ
Pontine tegmentum
use Pons
Popliteal ligament
use Knee Bursa and Ligament, Right
use Knee Bursa and Ligament, Left
Popliteal lymph node
use Lymphatic, Right Lower Extremity
use Lymphatic, Left Lower Extremity
Popliteal vein
use Femoral Vein, Right
use Femoral Vein, Left
Popliteus muscle
use Lower Leg Muscle, Right
use Lower Leg Muscle, Left
Porcine (bioprosthetic) valve
use Zooplastic Tissue in Heart and Great Vessels
Positive end expiratory pressure
see Performance, Respiratory 5A19
Positron Emission Tomographic (PET) Imaging
Brain C030
Bronchi and Lungs CB32
Central Nervous System C03YYZZ
Heart C23YYZZ
Lungs and Bronchi CB32
Myocardium C23G
Respiratory System CB3YYZZ
Whole Body CW3NYZZ
Positron emission tomography
see Positron Emission Tomographic (PET) Imaging
Postauricular (mastoid) lymph node
use Lymphatic, Right Neck
use Lymphatic, Left Neck
Postcava
use Inferior Vena Cava
Posterior (subscapular) lymph node
use Lymphatic, Right Axillary
use Lymphatic, Left Axillary
Posterior auricular artery
use External Carotid Artery, Right
use External Carotid Artery, Left
Posterior auricular nerve
use Facial Nerve
Posterior auricular vein
use External Jugular Vein, Right
use External Jugular Vein, Left
Posterior cerebral artery
use Intracranial Artery
Posterior chamber
use Eye, Right
use Eye, Left
Posterior circumflex humeral artery
use Axillary Artery, Right
use Axillary Artery, Left
Posterior communicating artery
use Intracranial Artery
Posterior cruciate ligament (PCL)
use Knee Bursa and Ligament, Right
use Knee Bursa and Ligament, Left
Posterior facial (retromandibular) vein
use Face Vein, Right
use Face Vein, Left
Posterior femoral cutaneous nerve
use Sacral Plexus
Posterior inferior cerebellar artery (PICA)
use Intracranial Artery
Posterior interosseous nerve
use Radial Nerve
Posterior labial nerve
use Pudendal Nerve
Posterior scrotal nerve
use Pudendal Nerve
Posterior spinal artery
use Vertebral Artery, Right
use Vertebral Artery, Left
Posterior tibial recurrent artery
use Anterior Tibial Artery, Right
use Anterior Tibial Artery, Left
Posterior ulnar recurrent artery
use Ulnar Artery, Right
use Ulnar Artery, Left
Posterior vagal trunk
use Vagus Nerve
PPN (peripheral parenteral nutrition)
see Introduction of Nutritional Substance
Preauricular lymph node
use Lymphatic, Head
Precava
use Superior Vena Cava
Prepatellar bursa
use Knee Bursa and Ligament, Right
use Knee Bursa and Ligament, Left
Preputiotomy
see Drainage, Male Reproductive System 0V9
Pressure support ventilation
see Performance, Respiratory 5A19
PRESTIGE® Cervical Disc
use Synthetic Substitute
Pretracheal fascia
use Subcutaneous Tissue and Fascia, Right Neck
use Subcutaneous Tissue and Fascia, Left Neck
Prevertebral fascia
use Subcutaneous Tissue and Fascia, Right Neck
use Subcutaneous Tissue and Fascia, Left Neck
PrimeAdvanced™ neurostimulator (SureScan™)(MRI Safe)
use Stimulator Generator, Multiple Array in 0JH
Princeps pollicis artery
use Hand Artery, Right
use Hand Artery, Left
Probing, duct
Diagnostic *see* Inspection
Dilation *see* Dilation
PROCEED™ Ventral Patch
use Synthetic Substitute
Procerus muscle
use Facial Muscle
Proctectomy
see Excision, Rectum 0DBP
see Resection, Rectum 0DTP
Proctoclysis
see Introduction of substance in or on, Gastrointestinal Tract, Lower 3E0H
Proctocolectomy
see Excision, Gastrointestinal System 0DB
see Resection, Gastrointestinal System 0DT
Proctocolpoplasty
see Repair, Gastrointestinal System 0DQ
see Supplement, Gastrointestinal System 0DU
Proctoperineoplasty
see Repair, Gastrointestinal System 0DQ
see Supplement, Gastrointestinal System 0DU
Proctoperineorrhaphy
see Repair, Gastrointestinal System 0DQ
Proctopexy
see Repair, Rectum 0DQP
see Reposition, Rectum 0DSP
Proctoplasty
see Repair, Rectum 0DQP
see Supplement, Rectum 0DUP
Proctorrhaphy
see Repair, Rectum 0DQP
Proctoscopy 0DJD8ZZ
Proctosigmoidectomy
see Excision, Gastrointestinal System 0DB
see Resection, Gastrointestinal System 0DT
Proctosigmoidoscopy 0DJD8ZZ
Proctostomy
see Drainage, Rectum 0D9P
Proctotomy
see Drainage, Rectum 0D9P
Prodisc-C®
use Synthetic Substitute
Prodisc-L®
use Synthetic Substitute
Production, atrial septal defect
see Excision, Septum, Atrial 02B5
Profunda brachii
use Brachial Artery, Right
use Brachial Artery, Left
Profunda femoris (deep femoral) vein
use Femoral Vein, Right
use Femoral Vein, Left
PROLENE® Polypropylene Hernia System (PHS)
use Synthetic Substitute
Prolonged intermittent renal replacement therapy (PIRRT) 5A1D80Z
Pronator quadratus muscle
use Lower Arm and Wrist Muscle, Right
use Lower Arm and Wrist Muscle, Left
Pronator teres muscle
use Lower Arm and Wrist Muscle, Right
use Lower Arm and Wrist Muscle, Left
Prostatectomy
see Excision, Prostate 0VB0
see Resection, Prostate 0VT0
Prostatic urethra
use Urethra
Prostatomy, prostatotomy
see Drainage, Prostate 0V90
Protecta™ XT CRT-D
use Cardiac Resynchronization Defibrillator Pulse Generator in 0JH
Protecta XT™ DR (XT VR)
use Defibrillator Generator in 0JH
Protege® RX Carotid Stent System
use Intraluminal Device
Proximal radioulnar joint
use Elbow Joint, Right
use Elbow Joint, Left
Psoas muscle
use Hip Muscle, Right
use Hip Muscle, Left
PSV (pressure support ventilation)
see Performance, Respiratory 5A19
Psychoanalysis GZ54ZZZ
Psychological tests
Cognitive Status GZ14ZZZ
Developmental GZ10ZZZ
Intellectual and Psychoeducational GZ12ZZZ
Neurobehavioral Status GZ14ZZZ
Neuropsychological GZ13ZZZ
Personality and Behavioral GZ11ZZZ

Psychotherapy
- Family, Mental Health Services GZ72ZZZ
- Group
  - GZHZZZZ
  - Mental Health Services GZHZZZZ
- Individual
  - *see* Psychotherapy, Individual, Mental Health Services
  - for substance abuse
    - 12-Step HZ53ZZZ
    - Behavioral HZ51ZZZ
    - Cognitive HZ50ZZZ
    - Cognitive-Behavioral HZ52ZZZ
    - Confrontational HZ58ZZZ
    - Interactive HZ55ZZZ
    - Interpersonal HZ54ZZZ
    - Motivational Enhancement HZ57ZZZ
    - Psychoanalysis HZ5BZZZ
    - Psychodynamic HZ5CZZZ
    - Psychoeducation HZ56ZZZ
    - Psychophysiological HZ5DZZZ
    - Supportive HZ59ZZZ
  - Mental Health Services
    - Behavioral GZ51ZZZ
    - Cognitive GZ52ZZZ
    - Cognitive-Behavioral GZ58ZZZ
    - Interactive GZ50ZZZ
    - Interpersonal GZ53ZZZ
    - Psychoanalysis GZ54ZZZ
    - Psychodynamic GZ55ZZZ
    - Psychophysiological GZ59ZZZ
    - Supportive GZ56ZZZ

PTCA (percutaneous transluminal coronary angioplasty)
- *see* Dilation, Heart and Great Vessels 027

Pterygoid muscle
- *use* Head Muscle

Pterygoid process
- *use* Sphenoid Bone

Pterygopalatine (sphenopalatine) ganglion
- *use* Head and Neck Sympathetic Nerve

Pubis
- *use* Pelvic Bone, Right
- *use* Pelvic Bone, Left

Pubofemoral ligament
- *use* Hip Bursa and Ligament, Right
- *use* Hip Bursa and Ligament, Left

Pudendal nerve
- *use* Sacral Plexus

Pull-through, laparoscopic-assisted transanal
- *see* Excision, Gastrointestinal System 0DB
- *see* Resection, Gastrointestinal System 0DT

Pull-through, rectal
- *see* Resection, Rectum 0DTP

Pulmoaortic canal
- *use* Pulmonary Artery, Left

Pulmonary annulus
- *use* Pulmonary Valve

Pulmonary artery wedge monitoring
- *see* Monitoring, Arterial 4A13

Pulmonary plexus
- *use* Vagus Nerve
- *use* Thoracic Sympathetic Nerve

Pulmonic valve
- *use* Pulmonary Valve

Pulpectomy
- *see* Excision, Mouth and Throat 0CB

Pulverization
- *see* Fragmentation

Pulvinar
- *use* Thalamus

Pump reservoir
- *use* Infusion Device, Pump in Subcutaneous Tissue and Fascia

Punch biopsy
- *see* Excision with qualifier Diagnostic

Puncture
- *see* Drainage

Puncture, lumbar
- *see* Drainage, Spinal Canal 009U

Pyelography
- *see* Plain Radiography, Urinary System BT0
- *see* Fluoroscopy, Urinary System BT1

Pyeloileostomy, urinary diversion
- *see* Bypass, Urinary System 0T1

Pyeloplasty
- *see* Repair, Urinary System 0TQ
- *see* Replacement, Urinary System 0TR
- *see* Supplement, Urinary System 0TU

Pyelorrhaphy
- *see* Repair, Urinary System 0TQ

Pyeloscopy 0TJ58ZZ

Pyelostomy
- *see* Bypass, Urinary System 0T1
- *see* Drainage, Urinary System 0T9

Pyelotomy
- *see* Drainage, Urinary System 0T9

Pylorectomy
- *see* Excision, Stomach, Pylorus 0DB7
- *see* Resection, Stomach, Pylorus 0DT7

Pyloric antrum
- *use* Stomach, Pylorus

Pyloric canal
- *use* Stomach, Pylorus

Pyloric sphincter
- *use* Stomach, Pylorus

Pylorodiosis
- *see* Dilation, Stomach, Pylorus 0D77

Pylorogastrectomy
- *see* Excision, Gastrointestinal System 0DB
- *see* Resection, Gastrointestinal System 0DT

Pyloroplasty
- *see* Repair, Stomach, Pylorus 0DQ7
- *see* Supplement, Stomach, Pylorus 0DU7

Pyloroscopy 0DJ68ZZ

Pylorotomy
- *see* Drainage, Stomach, Pylorus 0D97

Pyramidalis muscle
- *use* Abdomen Muscle, Right
- *use* Abdomen Muscle, Left

Q

Quadrangular cartilage
- *use* Nasal Septum

Quadrant resection of breast
- *see* Excision, Skin and Breast 0HB

Quadrate lobe
- *use* Liver

Quadratus femoris muscle
- *use* Hip Muscle, Right
- *use* Hip Muscle, Left

Quadratus lumborum muscle
- *use* Trunk Muscle, Right
- *use* Trunk Muscle, Left

Quadratus plantae muscle
- *use* Foot Muscle, Right
- *use* Foot Muscle, Left

Quadriceps (femoris)
- *use* Upper Leg Muscle, Right
- *use* Upper Leg Muscle, Left

Quarantine 8E0ZXY6

R

Radial collateral carpal ligament
- *use* Wrist Bursa and Ligament, Right
- *use* Wrist Bursa and Ligament, Left

Radial collateral ligament
- *use* Elbow Bursa and Ligament, Right

Radial collateral ligament — *continued*
- *use* Elbow Bursa and Ligament, Left

Radial notch
- *use* Ulna, Right
- *use* Ulna, Left

Radial recurrent artery
- *use* Radial Artery, Right
- *use* Radial Artery, Left

Radial vein
- *use* Brachial Vein, Right
- *use* Brachial Vein, Left

Radialis indicis
- *use* Hand Artery, Right
- *use* Hand Artery, Left

Radiation therapy
- *see* Beam Radiation
- *see* Brachytherapy
- *see* Stereotactic Radiosurgery

Radiation treatment
- *see* Radiation Therapy

Radiocarpal joint
- *use* Wrist Joint, Right
- *use* Wrist Joint, Left

Radiocarpal ligament
- *use* Wrist Bursa and Ligament, Right
- *use* Wrist Bursa and Ligament, Left

Radiography
- *see* Plain Radiography

Radiology, analog
- *see* Plain Radiography

Radiology, diagnostic
- *see* Imaging, Diagnostic

Radioulnar ligament
- *use* Wrist Bursa and Ligament, Right
- *use* Wrist Bursa and Ligament, Left

Range of motion testing
- *see* Motor Function Assessment, Rehabilitation F01

REALIZE® Adjustable Gastric Band
- *use* Extraluminal Device

Reattachment
- Abdominal Wall 0WMF0ZZ
- Ampulla of Vater 0FMC
- Ankle Region
  - Left 0YML0ZZ
  - Right 0YMK0ZZ
- Arm
  - Lower
    - Left 0XMF0ZZ
    - Right 0XMD0ZZ
  - Upper
    - Left 0XM90ZZ
    - Right 0XM80ZZ
- Axilla
  - Left 0XM50ZZ
  - Right 0XM40ZZ
- Back
  - Lower 0WML0ZZ
  - Upper 0WMK0ZZ
- Bladder 0TMB
- Bladder Neck 0TMC
- Breast
  - Bilateral 0HMVXZZ
  - Left 0HMUXZZ
  - Right 0HMTXZZ
- Bronchus
  - Lingula 0BM90ZZ
  - Lower Lobe
    - Left 0BMB0ZZ
    - Right 0BM60ZZ
  - Main
    - Left 0BM70ZZ
    - Right 0BM30ZZ
  - Middle Lobe, Right 0BM50ZZ
  - Upper Lobe
    - Left 0BM80ZZ
    - Right 0BM40ZZ

Reattachment — *continued*
Bursa and Ligament
Abdomen
Left 0MMJ
Right 0MMH
Ankle
Left 0MMR
Right 0MMQ
Elbow
Left 0MM4
Right 0MM3
Foot
Left 0MMT
Right 0MMS
Hand
Left 0MM8
Right 0MM7
Head and Neck 0MM0
Hip
Left 0MMM
Right 0MML
Knee
Left 0MMP
Right 0MMN
Lower Extremity
Left 0MMW
Right 0MMV
Perineum 0MMK
Rib(s) 0MMG
Shoulder
Left 0MM2
Right 0MM1
Spine
Lower 0MMD
Upper 0MMC
Sternum 0MMF
Upper Extremity
Left 0MMB
Right 0MM9
Wrist
Left 0MM6
Right 0MM5
Buttock
Left 0YM10ZZ
Right 0YM00ZZ
Carina 0BM20ZZ
Cecum 0DMH
Cervix 0UMC
Chest Wall 0WM80ZZ
Clitoris 0UMJXZZ
Colon
Ascending 0DMK
Descending 0DMM
Sigmoid 0DMN
Transverse 0DML
Cord
Bilateral 0VMH
Left 0VMG
Right 0VMF
Cul-de-sac 0UMF
Diaphragm 0BMT0ZZ
Duct
Common Bile 0FM9
Cystic 0FM8
Hepatic
Common 0FM7
Left 0FM6
Right 0FM5
Pancreatic 0FMD
Accessory 0FMF
Duodenum 0DM9
Ear
Left 09M1XZZ
Right 09M0XZZ
Elbow Region
Left 0XMC0ZZ
Right 0XMB0ZZ

Reattachment — *continued*
Esophagus 0DM5
Extremity
Lower
Left 0YMB0ZZ
Right 0YM90ZZ
Upper
Left 0XM70ZZ
Right 0XM60ZZ
Eyelid
Lower
Left 08MRXZZ
Right 08MQXZZ
Upper
Left 08MPXZZ
Right 08MNXZZ
Face 0WM20ZZ
Fallopian Tube
Left 0UM6
Right 0UM5
Fallopian Tubes, Bilateral 0UM7
Femoral Region
Left 0YM80ZZ
Right 0YM70ZZ
Finger
Index
Left 0XMP0ZZ
Right 0XMN0ZZ
Little
Left 0XMW0ZZ
Right 0XMV0ZZ
Middle
Left 0XMR0ZZ
Right 0XMQ0ZZ
Ring
Left 0XMT0ZZ
Right 0XMS0ZZ
Foot
Left 0YMN0ZZ
Right 0YMM0ZZ
Forequarter
Left 0XM10ZZ
Right 0XM00ZZ
Gallbladder 0FM4
Gland
Left 0GM2
Right 0GM3
Hand
Left 0XMK0ZZ
Right 0XMJ0ZZ
Hindquarter
Bilateral 0YM40ZZ
Left 0YM30ZZ
Right 0YM20ZZ
Hymen 0UMK
Ileum 0DMB
Inguinal Region
Left 0YM60ZZ
Right 0YM50ZZ
Intestine
Large 0DME
Left 0DMG
Right 0DMF
Small 0DM8
Jaw
Lower 0WM50ZZ
Upper 0WM40ZZ
Jejunum 0DMA
Kidney
Left 0TM1
Right 0TM0
Kidney Pelvis
Left 0TM4
Right 0TM3
Kidneys, Bilateral 0TM2
Knee Region
Left 0YMG0ZZ

Reattachment — *continued*
Knee Region — *continued*
Right 0YMF0ZZ
Leg
Lower
Left 0YMJ0ZZ
Right 0YMH0ZZ
Upper
Left 0YMD0ZZ
Right 0YMC0ZZ
Lip
Lower 0CM10ZZ
Upper 0CM00ZZ
Liver 0FM0
Left Lobe 0FM2
Right Lobe 0FM1
Lung
Left 0BML0ZZ
Lower Lobe
Left 0BMJ0ZZ
Right 0BMF0ZZ
Middle Lobe, Right 0BMD0ZZ
Right 0BMK0ZZ
Upper Lobe
Left 0BMG0ZZ
Right 0BMC0ZZ
Lung Lingula 0BMH0ZZ
Muscle
Abdomen
Left 0KML
Right 0KMK
Facial 0KM1
Foot
Left 0KMW
Right 0KMV
Hand
Left 0KMD
Right 0KMC
Head 0KM0
Hip
Left 0KMP
Right 0KMN
Lower Arm and Wrist
Left 0KMB
Right 0KM9
Lower Leg
Left 0KMT
Right 0KMS
Neck
Left 0KM3
Right 0KM2
Perineum 0KMM
Shoulder
Left 0KM6
Right 0KM5
Thorax
Left 0KMJ
Right 0KMH
Tongue, Palate, Pharynx 0KM4
Trunk
Left 0KMG
Right 0KMF
Upper Arm
Left 0KM8
Right 0KM7
Upper Leg
Left 0KMR
Right 0KMQ
Nasal Mucosa and Soft Tissue 09MKXZZ
Neck 0WM60ZZ
Nipple
Left 0HMXXZZ
Right 0HMWXZZ
Ovary
Bilateral 0UM2
Left 0UM1
Right 0UM0

Reattachment — *continued*
Palate, Soft 0CM30ZZ
Pancreas 0FMG
Parathyroid Gland 0GMR
Inferior
Left 0GMP
Right 0GMN
Multiple 0GMQ
Superior
Left 0GMM
Right 0GML
Penis 0VMSXZZ
Perineum
Female 0WMN0ZZ
Male 0WMM0ZZ
Rectum 0DMP
Scrotum 0VM5XZZ
Shoulder Region
Left 0XM30ZZ
Right 0XM20ZZ
Skin
Abdomen 0HM7XZZ
Back 0HM6XZZ
Buttock 0HM8XZZ
Chest 0HM5XZZ
Ear
Left 0HM3XZZ
Right 0HM2XZZ
Face 0HM1XZZ
Foot
Left 0HMNXZZ
Right 0HMMXZZ
Hand
Left 0HMGXZZ
Right 0HMFXZZ
Inguinal 0HMAXZZ
Lower Arm
Left 0HMEXZZ
Right 0HMDXZZ
Lower Leg
Left 0HMLXZZ
Right 0HMKXZZ
Neck 0HM4XZZ
Perineum 0HM9XZZ
Scalp 0HM0XZZ
Upper Arm
Left 0HMCXZZ
Right 0HMBXZZ
Upper Leg
Left 0HMJXZZ
Right 0HMHXZZ
Stomach 0DM6
Tendon
Abdomen
Left 0LMG
Right 0LMF
Ankle
Left 0LMT
Right 0LMS
Foot
Left 0LMW
Right 0LMV
Hand
Left 0LM8
Right 0LM7
Head and Neck 0LM0
Hip
Left 0LMK
Right 0LMJ
Knee
Left 0LMR
Right 0LMQ
Lower Arm and Wrist
Left 0LM6
Right 0LM5
Lower Leg
Left 0LMP

Reattachment — *continued*
Tendon — *continued*
Right 0LMN
Perineum 0LMH
Shoulder
Left 0LM2
Right 0LM1
Thorax
Left 0LMD
Right 0LMC
Trunk
Left 0LMB
Right 0LM9
Upper Arm
Left 0LM4
Right 0LM3
Upper Leg
Left 0LMM
Right 0LML
Testis
Bilateral 0VMC
Left 0VMB
Right 0VM9
Thumb
Left 0XMM0ZZ
Right 0XML0ZZ
Thyroid Gland
Left Lobe 0GMG
Right Lobe 0GMH
Toe
1st
Left 0YMQ0ZZ
Right 0YMP0ZZ
2nd
Left 0YMS0ZZ
Right 0YMR0ZZ
3rd
Left 0YMU0ZZ
Right 0YMT0ZZ
4th
Left 0YMW0ZZ
Right 0YMV0ZZ
5th
Left 0YMY0ZZ
Right 0YMX0ZZ
Tongue 0CM70ZZ
Tooth
Lower 0CMX
Upper 0CMW
Trachea 0BM10ZZ
Tunica Vaginalis
Left 0VM7
Right 0VM6
Ureter
Left 0TM7
Right 0TM6
Ureters, Bilateral 0TM8
Urethra 0TMD
Uterine Supporting Structure 0UM4
Uterus 0UM9
Uvula 0CMN0ZZ
Vagina 0UMG
Vulva 0UMMXZZ
Wrist Region
Left 0XMH0ZZ
Right 0XMG0ZZ
REBOA (resuscitative endovascular balloon occlusion of the aorta)
02LW3DJ
04L03DJ
Rebound HRD® (Hernia Repair Device)
use Synthetic Substitute
Recession
see Repair
see Reposition
Reclosure, disrupted abdominal wall
0WQFXZZ

Reconstruction
see Repair
see Replacement
see Supplement
Rectectomy
see Excision, Rectum 0DBP
see Resection, Rectum 0DTP
Rectocele repair
see Repair, Subcutaneous Tissue and Fascia, Pelvic Region 0JQC
Rectopexy
see Repair, Gastrointestinal System 0DQ
see Reposition, Gastrointestinal System 0DS
Rectoplasty
see Repair, Gastrointestinal System 0DQ
see Supplement, Gastrointestinal System 0DU
Rectorrhaphy
see Repair, Gastrointestinal System 0DQ
Rectoscopy 0DJD8ZZ
Rectosigmoid junction
use Sigmoid Colon
Rectosigmoidectomy
see Excision, Gastrointestinal System 0DB
see Resection, Gastrointestinal System 0DT
Rectostomy
see Drainage, Rectum 0D9P
Rectotomy
see Drainage, Rectum 0D9P
Rectus abdominis muscle
use Abdomen Muscle, Right
use Abdomen Muscle, Left
Rectus femoris muscle
use Upper Leg Muscle, Right
use Upper Leg Muscle, Left
Recurrent laryngeal nerve
use Vagus Nerve
Reduction
Dislocation *see* Reposition
Fracture *see* Reposition
Intussusception, intestinal *see* Reposition, Gastrointestinal System 0DS
Mammoplasty *see* Excision, Skin and Breast 0HB
Prolapse *see* Reposition
Torsion *see* Reposition
Volvulus, gastrointestinal *see* Reposition, Gastrointestinal System 0DS
Refusion
see Fusion
Rehabilitation
see Speech Assessment, Rehabilitation F00
see Motor Function Assessment, Rehabilitation F01
see Activities of Daily Living Assessment, Rehabilitation F02
see Speech Treatment, Rehabilitation F06
see Motor Treatment, Rehabilitation F07
see Activities of Daily Living Treatment, Rehabilitation F08
see Hearing Treatment, Rehabilitation F09
see Cochlear Implant Treatment, Rehabilitation F0B
see Vestibular Treatment, Rehabilitation F0C
see Device Fitting, Rehabilitation F0D
see Caregiver Training, Rehabilitation F0F
Reimplantation
see Reattachment
see Reposition
see Transfer
Reinforcement
see Repair
see Supplement
Relaxation, scar tissue
see Release

Release
- Acetabulum
  - Left 0QN5
  - Right 0QN4
- Adenoids 0CNQ
- Ampulla of Vater 0FNC
- Anal Sphincter 0DNR
- Anterior Chamber
  - Left 08N33ZZ
  - Right 08N23ZZ
- Anus 0DNQ
- Aorta
  - Abdominal 04N0
  - Thoracic
    - Ascending/Arch 02NX
    - Descending 02NW
- Aortic Body 0GND
- Appendix 0DNJ
- Artery
  - Anterior Tibial
    - Left 04NQ
    - Right 04NP
  - Axillary
    - Left 03N6
    - Right 03N5
  - Brachial
    - Left 03N8
    - Right 03N7
  - Celiac 04N1
  - Colic
    - Left 04N7
    - Middle 04N8
    - Right 04N6
  - Common Carotid
    - Left 03NJ
    - Right 03NH
  - Common Iliac
    - Left 04ND
    - Right 04NC
  - Coronary
    - Four or More Arteries 02N3
    - One Artery 02N0
    - Three Arteries 02N2
    - Two Arteries 02N1
  - External Carotid
    - Left 03NN
    - Right 03NM
  - External Iliac
    - Left 04NJ
    - Right 04NH
  - Face 03NR
  - Femoral
    - Left 04NL
    - Right 04NK
  - Foot
    - Left 04NW
    - Right 04NV
  - Gastric 04N2
  - Hand
    - Left 03NF
    - Right 03ND
  - Hepatic 04N3
  - Inferior Mesenteric 04NB
  - Innominate 03N2
  - Internal Carotid
    - Left 03NL
    - Right 03NK
  - Internal Iliac
    - Left 04NF
    - Right 04NE
  - Internal Mammary
    - Left 03N1
    - Right 03N0
  - Intracranial 03NG
  - Lower 04NY
  - Peroneal

Release — *continued*
- Artery — *continued*
    - Left 04NU
    - Right 04NT
  - Popliteal
    - Left 04NN
    - Right 04NM
  - Posterior Tibial
    - Left 04NS
    - Right 04NR
  - Pulmonary
    - Left 02NR
    - Right 02NQ
  - Pulmonary Trunk 02NP
  - Radial
    - Left 03NC
    - Right 03NB
  - Renal
    - Left 04NA
    - Right 04N9
  - Splenic 04N4
  - Subclavian
    - Left 03N4
    - Right 03N3
  - Superior Mesenteric 04N5
  - Temporal
    - Left 03NT
    - Right 03NS
  - Thyroid
    - Left 03NV
    - Right 03NU
  - Ulnar
    - Left 03NA
    - Right 03N9
  - Upper 03NY
  - Vertebral
    - Left 03NQ
    - Right 03NP
- Atrium
  - Left 02N7
  - Right 02N6
- Auditory Ossicle
  - Left 09NA
  - Right 09N9
- Basal Ganglia 00N8
- Bladder 0TNB
- Bladder Neck 0TNC
- Bone
  - Ethmoid
    - Left 0NNG
    - Right 0NNF
  - Frontal 0NN1
  - Hyoid 0NNX
  - Lacrimal
    - Left 0NNJ
    - Right 0NNH
  - Nasal 0NNB
  - Occipital 0NN7
  - Palatine
    - Left 0NNL
    - Right 0NNK
  - Parietal
    - Left 0NN4
    - Right 0NN3
  - Pelvic
    - Left 0QN3
    - Right 0QN2
  - Sphenoid 0NNC
  - Temporal
    - Left 0NN6
    - Right 0NN5
  - Zygomatic
    - Left 0NNN
    - Right 0NNM
- Brain 00N0
- Breast
  - Bilateral 0HNV

Release — *continued*
- Breast — *continued*
  - Left 0HNU
  - Right 0HNT
- Bronchus
  - Lingula 0BN9
  - Lower Lobe
    - Left 0BNB
    - Right 0BN6
  - Main
    - Left 0BN7
    - Right 0BN3
  - Middle Lobe, Right 0BN5
  - Upper Lobe
    - Left 0BN8
    - Right 0BN4
- Buccal Mucosa 0CN4
- Bursa and Ligament
  - Abdomen
    - Left 0MNJ
    - Right 0MNH
  - Ankle
    - Left 0MNR
    - Right 0MNQ
  - Elbow
    - Left 0MN4
    - Right 0MN3
  - Foot
    - Left 0MNT
    - Right 0MNS
  - Hand
    - Left 0MN8
    - Right 0MN7
  - Head and Neck 0MN0
  - Hip
    - Left 0MNM
    - Right 0MNL
  - Knee
    - Left 0MNP
    - Right 0MNN
  - Lower Extremity
    - Left 0MNW
    - Right 0MNV
  - Perineum 0MNK
  - Rib(s) 0MNG
  - Shoulder
    - Left 0MN2
    - Right 0MN1
  - Spine
    - Lower 0MND
    - Upper 0MNC
  - Sternum 0MNF
  - Upper Extremity
    - Left 0MNB
    - Right 0MN9
  - Wrist
    - Left 0MN6
    - Right 0MN5
- Carina 0BN2
- Carotid Bodies, Bilateral 0GN8
- Carotid Body
  - Left 0GN6
  - Right 0GN7
- Carpal
  - Left 0PNN
  - Right 0PNM
- Cecum 0DNH
- Cerebellum 00NC
- Cerebral Hemisphere 00N7
- Cerebral Meninges 00N1
- Cerebral Ventricle 00N6
- Cervix 0UNC
- Chordae Tendineae 02N9
- Choroid
  - Left 08NB
  - Right 08NA
- Cisterna Chyli 07NL

Release — *continued*
Clavicle
Left 0PNB
Right 0PN9
Clitoris 0UNJ
Coccygeal Glomus 0GNB
Coccyx 0QNS
Colon
Ascending 0DNK
Descending 0DNM
Sigmoid 0DNN
Transverse 0DNL
Conduction Mechanism 02N8
Conjunctiva
Left 08NTXZZ
Right 08NSXZZ
Cord
Bilateral 0VNH
Left 0VNG
Right 0VNF
Cornea
Left 08N9XZZ
Right 08N8XZZ
Cul-de-sac 0UNF
Diaphragm 0BNT
Disc
Cervical Vertebral 0RN3
Cervicothoracic Vertebral 0RN5
Lumbar Vertebral 0SN2
Lumbosacral 0SN4
Thoracic Vertebral 0RN9
Thoracolumbar Vertebral 0RNB
Duct
Common Bile 0FN9
Cystic 0FN8
Hepatic
Common 0FN7
Left 0FN6
Right 0FN5
Lacrimal
Left 08NY
Right 08NX
Pancreatic 0FND
Accessory 0FNF
Parotid
Left 0CNC
Right 0CNB
Duodenum 0DN9
Dura Mater 00N2
Ear
External
Left 09N1
Right 09N0
External Auditory Canal
Left 09N4
Right 09N3
Inner
Left 09NE
Right 09ND
Middle
Left 09N6
Right 09N5
Epididymis
Bilateral 0VNL
Left 0VNK
Right 0VNJ
Epiglottis 0CNR
Esophagogastric Junction 0DN4
Esophagus 0DN5
Lower 0DN3
Middle 0DN2
Upper 0DN1
Eustachian Tube
Left 09NG
Right 09NF
Eye
Left 08N1XZZ

Release — *continued*
Eye — *continued*
Right 08N0XZZ
Eyelid
Lower
Left 08NR
Right 08NQ
Upper
Left 08NP
Right 08NN
Fallopian Tube
Left 0UN6
Right 0UN5
Fallopian Tubes, Bilateral 0UN7
Femoral Shaft
Left 0QN9
Right 0QN8
Femur
Lower
Left 0QNC
Right 0QNB
Upper
Left 0QN7
Right 0QN6
Fibula
Left 0QNK
Right 0QNJ
Finger Nail 0HNQXZZ
Gallbladder 0FN4
Gingiva
Lower 0CN6
Upper 0CN5
Gland
Adrenal
Bilateral 0GN4
Left 0GN2
Right 0GN3
Lacrimal
Left 08NW
Right 08NV
Minor Salivary 0CNJ
Parotid
Left 0CN9
Right 0CN8
Pituitary 0GN0
Sublingual
Left 0CNF
Right 0CND
Submaxillary
Left 0CNH
Right 0CNG
Vestibular 0UNL
Glenoid Cavity
Left 0PN8
Right 0PN7
Glomus Jugulare 0GNC
Humeral Head
Left 0PND
Right 0PNC
Humeral Shaft
Left 0PNG
Right 0PNF
Hymen 0UNK
Hypothalamus 00NA
Ileocecal Valve 0DNC
Ileum 0DNB
Intestine
Large 0DNE
Left 0DNG
Right 0DNF
Small 0DN8
Iris
Left 08ND3ZZ
Right 08NC3ZZ
Jejunum 0DNA
Joint
Acromioclavicular

Release — *continued*
Joint — *continued*
Left 0RNH
Right 0RNG
Ankle
Left 0SNG
Right 0SNF
Carpal
Left 0RNR
Right 0RNQ
Carpometacarpal
Left 0RNT
Right 0RNS
Cervical Vertebral 0RN1
Cervicothoracic Vertebral 0RN4
Coccygeal 0SN6
Elbow
Left 0RNM
Right 0RNL
Finger Phalangeal
Left 0RNX
Right 0RNW
Hip
Left 0SNB
Right 0SN9
Knee
Left 0SND
Right 0SNC
Lumbar Vertebral 0SN0
Lumbosacral 0SN3
Metacarpophalangeal
Left 0RNV
Right 0RNU
Metatarsal-Phalangeal
Left 0SNN
Right 0SNM
Occipital-cervical 0RN0
Sacrococcygeal 0SN5
Sacroiliac
Left 0SN8
Right 0SN7
Shoulder
Left 0RNK
Right 0RNJ
Sternoclavicular
Left 0RNF
Right 0RNE
Tarsal
Left 0SNJ
Right 0SNH
Tarsometatarsal
Left 0SNL
Right 0SNK
Temporomandibular
Left 0RND
Right 0RNC
Thoracic Vertebral 0RN6
Thoracolumbar Vertebral 0RNA
Toe Phalangeal
Left 0SNQ
Right 0SNP
Wrist
Left 0RNP
Right 0RNN
Kidney
Left 0TN1
Right 0TN0
Kidney Pelvis
Left 0TN4
Right 0TN3
Larynx 0CNS
Lens
Left 08NK3ZZ
Right 08NJ3ZZ
Lip
Lower 0CN1
Upper 0CN0

Release — *continued*
Liver 0FN0
Left Lobe 0FN2
Right Lobe 0FN1
Lung
Bilateral 0BNM
Left 0BNL
Lower Lobe
Left 0BNJ
Right 0BNF
Middle Lobe, Right 0BND
Right 0BNK
Upper Lobe
Left 0BNG
Right 0BNC
Lung Lingula 0BNH
Lymphatic
Aortic 07ND
Axillary
Left 07N6
Right 07N5
Head 07N0
Inguinal
Left 07NJ
Right 07NH
Internal Mammary
Left 07N9
Right 07N8
Lower Extremity
Left 07NG
Right 07NF
Mesenteric 07NB
Neck
Left 07N2
Right 07N1
Pelvis 07NC
Thoracic Duct 07NK
Thorax 07N7
Upper Extremity
Left 07N4
Right 07N3
Mandible
Left 0NNV
Right 0NNT
Maxilla 0NNR
Medulla Oblongata 00ND
Mesentery 0DNV
Metacarpal
Left 0PNQ
Right 0PNP
Metatarsal
Left 0QNP
Right 0QNN
Muscle
Abdomen
Left 0KNL
Right 0KNK
Extraocular
Left 08NM
Right 08NL
Facial 0KN1
Foot
Left 0KNW
Right 0KNV
Hand
Left 0KND
Right 0KNC
Head 0KN0
Hip
Left 0KNP
Right 0KNN
Lower Arm and Wrist
Left 0KNB
Right 0KN9
Lower Leg
Left 0KNT
Right 0KNS

Release — *continued*
Muscle — *continued*
Neck
Left 0KN3
Right 0KN2
Papillary 02ND
Perineum 0KNM
Shoulder
Left 0KN6
Right 0KN5
Thorax
Left 0KNJ
Right 0KNH
Tongue, Palate, Pharynx 0KN4
Trunk
Left 0KNG
Right 0KNF
Upper Arm
Left 0KN8
Right 0KN7
Upper Leg
Left 0KNR
Right 0KNQ
Myocardial Bridge *see* Release, Artery, Coronary
Nasal Mucosa and Soft Tissue 09NK
Nasopharynx 09NN
Nerve
Abdominal Sympathetic 01NM
Abducens 00NL
Accessory 00NR
Acoustic 00NN
Brachial Plexus 01N3
Cervical 01N1
Cervical Plexus 01N0
Facial 00NM
Femoral 01ND
Glossopharyngeal 00NP
Head and Neck Sympathetic 01NK
Hypoglossal 00NS
Lumbar 01NB
Lumbar Plexus 01N9
Lumbar Sympathetic 01NN
Lumbosacral Plexus 01NA
Median 01N5
Oculomotor 00NH
Olfactory 00NF
Optic 00NG
Peroneal 01NH
Phrenic 01N2
Pudendal 01NC
Radial 01N6
Sacral 01NR
Sacral Plexus 01NQ
Sacral Sympathetic 01NP
Sciatic 01NF
Thoracic 01N8
Thoracic Sympathetic 01NL
Tibial 01NG
Trigeminal 00NK
Trochlear 00NJ
Ulnar 01N4
Vagus 00NQ
Nipple
Left 0HNX
Right 0HNW
Omentum 0DNU
Orbit
Left 0NNQ
Right 0NNP
Ovary
Bilateral 0UN2
Left 0UN1
Right 0UN0
Palate
Hard 0CN2
Soft 0CN3

Release — *continued*
Pancreas 0FNG
Para-aortic Body 0GN9
Paraganglion Extremity 0GNF
Parathyroid Gland 0GNR
Inferior
Left 0GNP
Right 0GNN
Multiple 0GNQ
Superior
Left 0GNM
Right 0GNL
Patella
Left 0QNF
Right 0QND
Penis 0VNS
Pericardium 02NN
Peritoneum 0DNW
Phalanx
Finger
Left 0PNV
Right 0PNT
Thumb
Left 0PNS
Right 0PNR
Toe
Left 0QNR
Right 0QNQ
Pharynx 0CNM
Pineal Body 0GN1
Pleura
Left 0BNP
Right 0BNN
Pons 00NB
Prepuce 0VNT
Prostate 0VN0
Radius
Left 0PNJ
Right 0PNH
Rectum 0DNP
Retina
Left 08NF3ZZ
Right 08NE3ZZ
Retinal Vessel
Left 08NH3ZZ
Right 08NG3ZZ
Ribs
1 to 2 0PN1
3 or More 0PN2
Sacrum 0QN1
Scapula
Left 0PN6
Right 0PN5
Sclera
Left 08N7XZZ
Right 08N6XZZ
Scrotum 0VN5
Septum
Atrial 02N5
Nasal 09NM
Ventricular 02NM
Sinus
Accessory 09NP
Ethmoid
Left 09NV
Right 09NU
Frontal
Left 09NT
Right 09NS
Mastoid
Left 09NC
Right 09NB
Maxillary
Left 09NR
Right 09NQ
Sphenoid
Left 09NX

Release — *continued*
Sinus — *continued*
Right 09NW
Skin
Abdomen 0HN7XZZ
Back 0HN6XZZ
Buttock 0HN8XZZ
Chest 0HN5XZZ
Ear
Left 0HN3XZZ
Right 0HN2XZZ
Face 0HN1XZZ
Foot
Left 0HNNXZZ
Right 0HNMXZZ
Hand
Left 0HNGXZZ
Right 0HNFXZZ
Inguinal 0HNAXZZ
Lower Arm
Left 0HNEXZZ
Right 0HNDXZZ
Lower Leg
Left 0HNLXZZ
Right 0HNKXZZ
Neck 0HN4XZZ
Perineum 0HN9XZZ
Scalp 0HN0XZZ
Upper Arm
Left 0HNCXZZ
Right 0HNBXZZ
Upper Leg
Left 0HNJXZZ
Right 0HNHXZZ
Spinal Cord
Cervical 00NW
Lumbar 00NY
Thoracic 00NX
Spinal Meninges 00NT
Spleen 07NP
Sternum 0PN0
Stomach 0DN6
Pylorus 0DN7
Subcutaneous Tissue and Fascia
Abdomen 0JN8
Back 0JN7
Buttock 0JN9
Chest 0JN6
Face 0JN1
Foot
Left 0JNR
Right 0JNQ
Hand
Left 0JNK
Right 0JNJ
Lower Arm
Left 0JNH
Right 0JNG
Lower Leg
Left 0JNP
Right 0JNN
Neck
Left 0JN5
Right 0JN4
Pelvic Region 0JNC
Perineum 0JNB
Scalp 0JN0
Upper Arm
Left 0JNF
Right 0JND
Upper Leg
Left 0JNM
Right 0JNL
Tarsal
Left 0QNM
Right 0QNL

Release — *continued*
Tendon
Abdomen
Left 0LNG
Right 0LNF
Ankle
Left 0LNT
Right 0LNS
Foot
Left 0LNW
Right 0LNV
Hand
Left 0LN8
Right 0LN7
Head and Neck 0LN0
Hip
Left 0LNK
Right 0LNJ
Knee
Left 0LNR
Right 0LNQ
Lower Arm and Wrist
Left 0LN6
Right 0LN5
Lower Leg
Left 0LNP
Right 0LNN
Perineum 0LNH
Shoulder
Left 0LN2
Right 0LN1
Thorax
Left 0LND
Right 0LNC
Trunk
Left 0LNB
Right 0LN9
Upper Arm
Left 0LN4
Right 0LN3
Upper Leg
Left 0LNM
Right 0LNL
Testis
Bilateral 0VNC
Left 0VNB
Right 0VN9
Thalamus 00N9
Thymus 07NM
Thyroid Gland 0GNK
Left Lobe 0GNG
Right Lobe 0GNH
Tibia
Left 0QNH
Right 0QNG
Toe Nail 0HNRXZZ
Tongue 0CN7
Tonsils 0CNP
Tooth
Lower 0CNX
Upper 0CNW
Trachea 0BN1
Tunica Vaginalis
Left 0VN7
Right 0VN6
Turbinate, Nasal 09NL
Tympanic Membrane
Left 09N8
Right 09N7
Ulna
Left 0PNL
Right 0PNK
Ureter
Left 0TN7
Right 0TN6
Urethra 0TND
Uterine Supporting Structure 0UN4

Release — *continued*
Uterus 0UN9
Uvula 0CNN
Vagina 0UNG
Valve
Aortic 02NF
Mitral 02NG
Pulmonary 02NH
Tricuspid 02NJ
Vas Deferens
Bilateral 0VNQ
Left 0VNP
Right 0VNN
Vein
Axillary
Left 05N8
Right 05N7
Azygos 05N0
Basilic
Left 05NC
Right 05NB
Brachial
Left 05NA
Right 05N9
Cephalic
Left 05NF
Right 05ND
Colic 06N7
Common Iliac
Left 06ND
Right 06NC
Coronary 02N4
Esophageal 06N3
External Iliac
Left 06NG
Right 06NF
External Jugular
Left 05NQ
Right 05NP
Face
Left 05NV
Right 05NT
Femoral
Left 06NN
Right 06NM
Foot
Left 06NV
Right 06NT
Gastric 06N2
Hand
Left 05NH
Right 05NG
Hemiazygos 05N1
Hepatic 06N4
Hypogastric
Left 06NJ
Right 06NH
Inferior Mesenteric 06N6
Innominate
Left 05N4
Right 05N3
Internal Jugular
Left 05NN
Right 05NM
Intracranial 05NL
Lower 06NY
Portal 06N8
Pulmonary
Left 02NT
Right 02NS
Renal
Left 06NB
Right 06N9
Saphenous
Left 06NQ
Right 06NP
Splenic 06N1

Release — *continued*
- Vein — *continued*
  - Subclavian
    - Left 05N6
    - Right 05N5
  - Superior Mesenteric 06N5
  - Upper 05NY
  - Vertebral
    - Left 05NS
    - Right 05NR
- Vena Cava
  - Inferior 06N0
  - Superior 02NV
- Ventricle
  - Left 02NL
  - Right 02NK
- Vertebra
  - Cervical 0PN3
  - Lumbar 0QN0
  - Thoracic 0PN4
- Vesicle
  - Bilateral 0VN3
  - Left 0VN2
  - Right 0VN1
- Vitreous
  - Left 08N53ZZ
  - Right 08N43ZZ
- Vocal Cord
  - Left 0CNV
  - Right 0CNT
- Vulva 0UNM

Relocation
- *see* Reposition

Removal
- Abdominal Wall 2W53X
- Anorectal 2Y53X5Z
- Arm
  - Lower
    - Left 2W5DX
    - Right 2W5CX
  - Upper
    - Left 2W5BX
    - Right 2W5AX
- Back 2W55X
- Chest Wall 2W54X
- Ear 2Y52X5Z
- Extremity
  - Lower
    - Left 2W5MX
    - Right 2W5LX
  - Upper
    - Left 2W59X
    - Right 2W58X
- Face 2W51X
- Finger
  - Left 2W5KX
  - Right 2W5JX
- Foot
  - Left 2W5TX
  - Right 2W5SX
- Genital Tract, Female 2Y54X5Z
- Hand
  - Left 2W5FX
  - Right 2W5EX
- Head 2W50X
- Inguinal Region
  - Left 2W57X
  - Right 2W56X
- Leg
  - Lower
    - Left 2W5RX
    - Right 2W5QX
  - Upper
    - Left 2W5PX
    - Right 2W5NX
- Mouth and Pharynx 2Y50X5Z
- Nasal 2Y51X5Z

Removal — *continued*
- Neck 2W52X
- Thumb
  - Left 2W5HX
  - Right 2W5GX
- Toe
  - Left 2W5VX
  - Right 2W5UX
- Urethra 2Y55X5Z

Removal of device from
- Abdominal Wall 0WPF
- Acetabulum
  - Left 0QP5
  - Right 0QP4
- Anal Sphincter 0DPR
- Anus 0DPQ
- Artery
  - Lower 04PY
  - Upper 03PY
- Back
  - Lower 0WPL
  - Upper 0WPK
- Bladder 0TPB
- Bone
  - Facial 0NPW
  - Lower 0QPY
  - Nasal 0NPB
  - Pelvic
    - Left 0QP3
    - Right 0QP2
  - Upper 0PPY
- Bone Marrow 07PT
- Brain 00P0
- Breast
  - Left 0HPU
  - Right 0HPT
- Bursa and Ligament
  - Lower 0MPY
  - Upper 0MPX
- Carpal
  - Left 0PPN
  - Right 0PPM
- Cavity, Cranial 0WP1
- Cerebral Ventricle 00P6
- Chest Wall 0WP8
- Cisterna Chyli 07PL
- Clavicle
  - Left 0PPB
  - Right 0PP9
- Coccyx 0QPS
- Diaphragm 0BPT
- Disc
  - Cervical Vertebral 0RP3
  - Cervicothoracic Vertebral 0RP5
  - Lumbar Vertebral 0SP2
  - Lumbosacral 0SP4
  - Thoracic Vertebral 0RP9
  - Thoracolumbar Vertebral 0RPB
- Duct
  - Hepatobiliary 0FPB
  - Pancreatic 0FPD
- Ear
  - Inner
    - Left 09PE
    - Right 09PD
  - Left 09PJ
  - Right 09PH
- Epididymis and Spermatic Cord 0VPM
- Esophagus 0DP5
- Extremity
  - Lower
    - Left 0YPB
    - Right 0YP9
  - Upper
    - Left 0XP7
    - Right 0XP6

Removal of device from — *continued*
- Eye
  - Left 08P1
  - Right 08P0
- Face 0WP2
- Fallopian Tube 0UP8
- Femoral Shaft
  - Left 0QP9
  - Right 0QP8
- Femur
  - Lower
    - Left 0QPC
    - Right 0QPB
  - Upper
    - Left 0QP7
    - Right 0QP6
- Fibula
  - Left 0QPK
  - Right 0QPJ
- Finger Nail 0HPQX
- Gallbladder 0FP4
- Gastrointestinal Tract 0WPP
- Genitourinary Tract 0WPR
- Gland
  - Adrenal 0GP5
  - Endocrine 0GPS
  - Pituitary 0GP0
  - Salivary 0CPA
- Glenoid Cavity
  - Left 0PP8
  - Right 0PP7
- Great Vessel 02PY
- Hair 0HPSX
- Head 0WP0
- Heart 02PA
- Humeral Head
  - Left 0PPD
  - Right 0PPC
- Humeral Shaft
  - Left 0PPG
  - Right 0PPF
- Intestinal Tract
  - Lower 0DPD
  - Upper 0DP0
- Jaw
  - Lower 0WP5
  - Upper 0WP4
- Joint
  - Acromioclavicular
    - Left 0RPH
    - Right 0RPG
  - Ankle
    - Left 0SPG
    - Right 0SPF
  - Carpal
    - Left 0RPR
    - Right 0RPQ
  - Carpometacarpal
    - Left 0RPT
    - Right 0RPS
  - Cervical Vertebral 0RP1
  - Cervicothoracic Vertebral 0RP4
  - Coccygeal 0SP6
  - Elbow
    - Left 0RPM
    - Right 0RPL
  - Finger Phalangeal
    - Left 0RPX
    - Right 0RPW
  - Hip
    - Left 0SPB
      - Acetabular Surface 0SPE
      - Femoral Surface 0SPS
    - Right 0SP9
      - Acetabular Surface 0SPA
      - Femoral Surface 0SPR

Removal of device from — *continued*
Joint — *continued*
Knee
Left 0SPD
Femoral Surface 0SPU
Tibial Surface 0SPW
Right 0SPC
Femoral Surface 0SPT
Tibial Surface 0SPV
Lumbar Vertebral 0SP0
Lumbosacral 0SP3
Metacarpophalangeal
Left 0RPV
Right 0RPU
Metatarsal-Phalangeal
Left 0SPN
Right 0SPM
Occipital-cervical 0RP0
Sacrococcygeal 0SP5
Sacroiliac
Left 0SP8
Right 0SP7
Shoulder
Left 0RPK
Right 0RPJ
Sternoclavicular
Left 0RPF
Right 0RPE
Tarsal
Left 0SPJ
Right 0SPH
Tarsometatarsal
Left 0SPL
Right 0SPK
Temporomandibular
Left 0RPD
Right 0RPC
Thoracic Vertebral 0RP6
Thoracolumbar Vertebral 0RPA
Toe Phalangeal
Left 0SPQ
Right 0SPP
Wrist
Left 0RPP
Right 0RPN
Kidney 0TP5
Larynx 0CPS
Lens
Left 08PK3
Right 08PJ3
Liver 0FP0
Lung
Left 0BPL
Right 0BPK
Lymphatic 07PN
Thoracic Duct 07PK
Mediastinum 0WPC
Mesentery 0DPV
Metacarpal
Left 0PPQ
Right 0PPP
Metatarsal
Left 0QPP
Right 0QPN
Mouth and Throat 0CPY
Muscle
Extraocular
Left 08PM
Right 08PL
Lower 0KPY
Upper 0KPX
Nasal Mucosa and Soft Tissue 09PK
Neck 0WP6
Nerve
Cranial 00PE
Peripheral 01PY
Omentum 0DPU
Ovary 0UP3

Removal of device from — *continued*
Pancreas 0FPG
Parathyroid Gland 0GPR
Patella
Left 0QPF
Right 0QPD
Pelvic Cavity 0WPJ
Penis 0VPS
Pericardial Cavity 0WPD
Perineum
Female 0WPN
Male 0WPM
Peritoneal Cavity 0WPG
Peritoneum 0DPW
Phalanx
Finger
Left 0PPV
Right 0PPT
Thumb
Left 0PPS
Right 0PPR
Toe
Left 0QPR
Right 0QPQ
Pineal Body 0GP1
Pleura 0BPQ
Pleural Cavity
Left 0WPB
Right 0WP9
Products of Conception 10P0
Prostate and Seminal Vesicles 0VP4
Radius
Left 0PPJ
Right 0PPH
Rectum 0DPP
Respiratory Tract 0WPQ
Retroperitoneum 0WPH
Ribs
1 to 2 0PP1
3 or More 0PP2
Sacrum 0QP1
Scapula
Left 0PP6
Right 0PP5
Scrotum and Tunica Vaginalis 0VP8
Sinus 09PY
Skin 0HPPX
Skull 0NP0
Spinal Canal 00PU
Spinal Cord 00PV
Spleen 07PP
Sternum 0PP0
Stomach 0DP6
Subcutaneous Tissue and Fascia
Head and Neck 0JPS
Lower Extremity 0JPW
Trunk 0JPT
Upper Extremity 0JPV
Tarsal
Left 0QPM
Right 0QPL
Tendon
Lower 0LPY
Upper 0LPX
Testis 0VPD
Thymus 07PM
Thyroid Gland 0GPK
Tibia
Left 0QPH
Right 0QPG
Toe Nail 0HPRX
Trachea 0BP1
Tracheobronchial Tree 0BP0
Tympanic Membrane
Left 09P8
Right 09P7

Removal of device from — *continued*
Ulna
Left 0PPL
Right 0PPK
Ureter 0TP9
Urethra 0TPD
Uterus and Cervix 0UPD
Vagina and Cul-de-sac 0UPH
Vas Deferens 0VPR
Vein
Azygos 05P0
Innominate
Left 05P4
Right 05P3
Lower 06PY
Upper 05PY
Vertebra
Cervical 0PP3
Lumbar 0QP0
Thoracic 0PP4
Vulva 0UPM
Renal calyx
use Kidney, Right
use Kidney, Left
use Kidneys, Bilateral
use Kidney
Renal capsule
use Kidney, Right
use Kidney, Left
use Kidneys, Bilateral
use Kidney
Renal cortex
use Kidney, Right
use Kidney, Left
use Kidneys, Bilateral
use Kidney
Renal dialysis
see Performance, Urinary 5A1D
Renal plexus
use Abdominal Sympathetic Nerve
Renal segment
use Kidney, Right
use Kidney, Left
use Kidneys, Bilateral
use Kidney
Renal segmental artery
use Renal Artery, Right
use Renal Artery, Left
Reopening, operative site
Control of bleeding *see* Control bleeding in
Inspection only *see* Inspection
Repair
Abdominal Wall 0WQF
Acetabulum
Left 0QQ5
Right 0QQ4
Adenoids 0CQQ
Ampulla of Vater 0FQC
Anal Sphincter 0DQR
Ankle Region
Left 0YQL
Right 0YQK
Anterior Chamber
Left 08Q33ZZ
Right 08Q23ZZ
Anus 0DQQ
Aorta
Abdominal 04Q0
Thoracic
Ascending/Arch 02QX
Descending 02QW
Aortic Body 0GQD
Appendix 0DQJ
Arm
Lower
Left 0XQF
Right 0XQD

Repair — *continued*
- Arm — *continued*
  - Upper
    - Left 0XQ9
    - Right 0XQ8
- Artery
  - Anterior Tibial
    - Left 04QQ
    - Right 04QP
  - Axillary
    - Left 03Q6
    - Right 03Q5
  - Brachial
    - Left 03Q8
    - Right 03Q7
  - Celiac 04Q1
  - Colic
    - Left 04Q7
    - Middle 04Q8
    - Right 04Q6
  - Common Carotid
    - Left 03QJ
    - Right 03QH
  - Common Iliac
    - Left 04QD
    - Right 04QC
  - Coronary
    - Four or More Arteries 02Q3
    - One Artery 02Q0
    - Three Arteries 02Q2
    - Two Arteries 02Q1
  - External Carotid
    - Left 03QN
    - Right 03QM
  - External Iliac
    - Left 04QJ
    - Right 04QH
  - Face 03QR
  - Femoral
    - Left 04QL
    - Right 04QK
  - Foot
    - Left 04QW
    - Right 04QV
  - Gastric 04Q2
  - Hand
    - Left 03QF
    - Right 03QD
  - Hepatic 04Q3
  - Inferior Mesenteric 04QB
  - Innominate 03Q2
  - Internal Carotid
    - Left 03QL
    - Right 03QK
  - Internal Iliac
    - Left 04QF
    - Right 04QE
  - Internal Mammary
    - Left 03Q1
    - Right 03Q0
  - Intracranial 03QG
  - Lower 04QY
  - Peroneal
    - Left 04QU
    - Right 04QT
  - Popliteal
    - Left 04QN
    - Right 04QM
  - Posterior Tibial
    - Left 04QS
    - Right 04QR
  - Pulmonary
    - Left 02QR
    - Right 02QQ
  - Pulmonary Trunk 02QP
  - Radial
    - Left 03QC

Repair — *continued*
- Artery — *continued*
    - Right 03QB
  - Renal
    - Left 04QA
    - Right 04Q9
  - Splenic 04Q4
  - Subclavian
    - Left 03Q4
    - Right 03Q3
  - Superior Mesenteric 04Q5
  - Temporal
    - Left 03QT
    - Right 03QS
  - Thyroid
    - Left 03QV
    - Right 03QU
  - Ulnar
    - Left 03QA
    - Right 03Q9
  - Upper 03QY
  - Vertebral
    - Left 03QQ
    - Right 03QP
- Atrium
  - Left 02Q7
  - Right 02Q6
- Auditory Ossicle
  - Left 09QA
  - Right 09Q9
- Axilla
  - Left 0XQ5
  - Right 0XQ4
- Back
  - Lower 0WQL
  - Upper 0WQK
- Basal Ganglia 00Q8
- Bladder 0TQB
- Bladder Neck 0TQC
- Bone
  - Ethmoid
    - Left 0NQG
    - Right 0NQF
  - Frontal 0NQ1
  - Hyoid 0NQX
  - Lacrimal
    - Left 0NQJ
    - Right 0NQH
  - Nasal 0NQB
  - Occipital 0NQ7
  - Palatine
    - Left 0NQL
    - Right 0NQK
  - Parietal
    - Left 0NQ4
    - Right 0NQ3
  - Pelvic
    - Left 0QQ3
    - Right 0QQ2
  - Sphenoid 0NQC
  - Temporal
    - Left 0NQ6
    - Right 0NQ5
  - Zygomatic
    - Left 0NQN
    - Right 0NQM
- Brain 00Q0
- Breast
  - Bilateral 0HQV
  - Left 0HQU
  - Right 0HQT
  - Supernumerary 0HQY
- Bronchus
  - Lingula 0BQ9
  - Lower Lobe
    - Left 0BQB
    - Right 0BQ6

Repair — *continued*
- Bronchus — *continued*
  - Main
    - Left 0BQ7
    - Right 0BQ3
  - Middle Lobe, Right 0BQ5
  - Upper Lobe
    - Left 0BQ8
    - Right 0BQ4
- Buccal Mucosa 0CQ4
- Bursa and Ligament
  - Abdomen
    - Left 0MQJ
    - Right 0MQH
  - Ankle
    - Left 0MQR
    - Right 0MQQ
  - Elbow
    - Left 0MQ4
    - Right 0MQ3
  - Foot
    - Left 0MQT
    - Right 0MQS
  - Hand
    - Left 0MQ8
    - Right 0MQ7
  - Head and Neck 0MQ0
  - Hip
    - Left 0MQM
    - Right 0MQL
  - Knee
    - Left 0MQP
    - Right 0MQN
  - Lower Extremity
    - Left 0MQW
    - Right 0MQV
  - Perineum 0MQK
  - Rib(s) 0MQG
  - Shoulder
    - Left 0MQ2
    - Right 0MQ1
  - Spine
    - Lower 0MQD
    - Upper 0MQC
  - Sternum 0MQF
  - Upper Extremity
    - Left 0MQB
    - Right 0MQ9
  - Wrist
    - Left 0MQ6
    - Right 0MQ5
- Buttock
  - Left 0YQ1
  - Right 0YQ0
- Carina 0BQ2
- Carotid Bodies, Bilateral 0GQ8
- Carotid Body
  - Left 0GQ6
  - Right 0GQ7
- Carpal
  - Left 0PQN
  - Right 0PQM
- Cecum 0DQH
- Cerebellum 00QC
- Cerebral Hemisphere 00Q7
- Cerebral Meninges 00Q1
- Cerebral Ventricle 00Q6
- Cervix 0UQC
- Chest Wall 0WQ8
- Chordae Tendineae 02Q9
- Choroid
  - Left 08QB
  - Right 08QA
- Cisterna Chyli 07QL
- Clavicle
  - Left 0PQB
  - Right 0PQ9

Repair — *continued*
- Clitoris 0UQJ
- Coccygeal Glomus 0GQB
- Coccyx 0QQS
- Colon
  - Ascending 0DQK
  - Descending 0DQM
  - Sigmoid 0DQN
  - Transverse 0DQL
- Conduction Mechanism 02Q8
- Conjunctiva
  - Left 08QTXZZ
  - Right 08QSXZZ
- Cord
  - Bilateral 0VQH
  - Left 0VQG
  - Right 0VQF
- Cornea
  - Left 08Q9XZZ
  - Right 08Q8XZZ
- Cul-de-sac 0UQF
- Diaphragm 0BQT
- Disc
  - Cervical Vertebral 0RQ3
  - Cervicothoracic Vertebral 0RQ5
  - Lumbar Vertebral 0SQ2
  - Lumbosacral 0SQ4
  - Thoracic Vertebral 0RQ9
  - Thoracolumbar Vertebral 0RQB
- Duct
  - Common Bile 0FQ9
  - Cystic 0FQ8
  - Hepatic
    - Common 0FQ7
    - Left 0FQ6
    - Right 0FQ5
  - Lacrimal
    - Left 08QY
    - Right 08QX
  - Pancreatic 0FQD
    - Accessory 0FQF
  - Parotid
    - Left 0CQC
    - Right 0CQB
- Duodenum 0DQ9
- Dura Mater 00Q2
- Ear
  - External
    - Bilateral 09Q2
    - Left 09Q1
    - Right 09Q0
  - External Auditory Canal
    - Left 09Q4
    - Right 09Q3
  - Inner
    - Left 09QE
    - Right 09QD
  - Middle
    - Left 09Q6
    - Right 09Q5
- Elbow Region
  - Left 0XQC
  - Right 0XQB
- Epididymis
  - Bilateral 0VQL
  - Left 0VQK
  - Right 0VQJ
- Epiglottis 0CQR
- Esophagogastric Junction 0DQ4
- Esophagus 0DQ5
  - Lower 0DQ3
  - Middle 0DQ2
  - Upper 0DQ1
- Eustachian Tube
  - Left 09QG
  - Right 09QF

Repair — *continued*
- Extremity
  - Lower
    - Left 0YQB
    - Right 0YQ9
  - Upper
    - Left 0XQ7
    - Right 0XQ6
- Eye
  - Left 08Q1XZZ
  - Right 08Q0XZZ
- Eyelid
  - Lower
    - Left 08QR
    - Right 08QQ
  - Upper
    - Left 08QP
    - Right 08QN
- Face 0WQ2
- Fallopian Tube
  - Left 0UQ6
  - Right 0UQ5
- Fallopian Tubes, Bilateral 0UQ7
- Femoral Region
  - Bilateral 0YQE
  - Left 0YQ8
  - Right 0YQ7
- Femoral Shaft
  - Left 0QQ9
  - Right 0QQ8
- Femur
  - Lower
    - Left 0QQC
    - Right 0QQB
  - Upper
    - Left 0QQ7
    - Right 0QQ6
- Fibula
  - Left 0QQK
  - Right 0QQJ
- Finger
  - Index
    - Left 0XQP
    - Right 0XQN
  - Little
    - Left 0XQW
    - Right 0XQV
  - Middle
    - Left 0XQR
    - Right 0XQQ
  - Ring
    - Left 0XQT
    - Right 0XQS
- Finger Nail 0HQQXZZ
- Floor of mouth *see* Repair, Oral Cavity and Throat 0WQ3
- Foot
  - Left 0YQN
  - Right 0YQM
- Gallbladder 0FQ4
- Gingiva
  - Lower 0CQ6
  - Upper 0CQ5
- Gland
  - Adrenal
    - Bilateral 0GQ4
    - Left 0GQ2
    - Right 0GQ3
  - Lacrimal
    - Left 08QW
    - Right 08QV
  - Minor Salivary 0CQJ
  - Parotid
    - Left 0CQ9
    - Right 0CQ8
  - Pituitary 0GQ0
  - Sublingual

Repair — *continued*
- Gland — *continued*
    - Left 0CQF
    - Right 0CQD
  - Submaxillary
    - Left 0CQH
    - Right 0CQG
  - Vestibular 0UQL
- Glenoid Cavity
  - Left 0PQ8
  - Right 0PQ7
- Glomus Jugulare 0GQC
- Hand
  - Left 0XQK
  - Right 0XQJ
- Head 0WQ0
- Heart 02QA
  - Left 02QC
  - Right 02QB
- Humeral Head
  - Left 0PQD
  - Right 0PQC
- Humeral Shaft
  - Left 0PQG
  - Right 0PQF
- Hymen 0UQK
- Hypothalamus 00QA
- Ileocecal Valve 0DQC
- Ileum 0DQB
- Inguinal Region
  - Bilateral 0YQA
  - Left 0YQ6
  - Right 0YQ5
- Intestine
  - Large 0DQE
    - Left 0DQG
    - Right 0DQF
  - Small 0DQ8
- Iris
  - Left 08QD3ZZ
  - Right 08QC3ZZ
- Jaw
  - Lower 0WQ5
  - Upper 0WQ4
- Jejunum 0DQA
- Joint
  - Acromioclavicular
    - Left 0RQH
    - Right 0RQG
  - Ankle
    - Left 0SQG
    - Right 0SQF
  - Carpal
    - Left 0RQR
    - Right 0RQQ
  - Carpometacarpal
    - Left 0RQT
    - Right 0RQS
  - Cervical Vertebral 0RQ1
  - Cervicothoracic Vertebral 0RQ4
  - Coccygeal 0SQ6
  - Elbow
    - Left 0RQM
    - Right 0RQL
  - Finger Phalangeal
    - Left 0RQX
    - Right 0RQW
  - Hip
    - Left 0SQB
    - Right 0SQ9
  - Knee
    - Left 0SQD
    - Right 0SQC
  - Lumbar Vertebral 0SQ0
  - Lumbosacral 0SQ3
  - Metacarpophalangeal
    - Left 0RQV

Repair — *continued*
Joint — *continued*
Right 0RQU
Metatarsal-Phalangeal
Left 0SQN
Right 0SQM
Occipital-cervical 0RQ0
Sacrococcygeal 0SQ5
Sacroiliac
Left 0SQ8
Right 0SQ7
Shoulder
Left 0RQK
Right 0RQJ
Sternoclavicular
Left 0RQF
Right 0RQE
Tarsal
Left 0SQJ
Right 0SQH
Tarsometatarsal
Left 0SQL
Right 0SQK
Temporomandibular
Left 0RQD
Right 0RQC
Thoracic Vertebral 0RQ6
Thoracolumbar Vertebral 0RQA
Toe Phalangeal
Left 0SQQ
Right 0SQP
Wrist
Left 0RQP
Right 0RQN
Kidney
Left 0TQ1
Right 0TQ0
Kidney Pelvis
Left 0TQ4
Right 0TQ3
Knee Region
Left 0YQG
Right 0YQF
Larynx 0CQS
Leg
Lower
Left 0YQJ
Right 0YQH
Upper
Left 0YQD
Right 0YQC
Lens
Left 08QK3ZZ
Right 08QJ3ZZ
Lip
Lower 0CQ1
Upper 0CQ0
Liver 0FQ0
Left Lobe 0FQ2
Right Lobe 0FQ1
Lung
Bilateral 0BQM
Left 0BQL
Lower Lobe
Left 0BQJ
Right 0BQF
Middle Lobe, Right 0BQD
Right 0BQK
Upper Lobe
Left 0BQG
Right 0BQC
Lung Lingula 0BQH
Lymphatic
Aortic 07QD
Axillary
Left 07Q6
Right 07Q5

Repair — *continued*
Lymphatic — *continued*
Head 07Q0
Inguinal
Left 07QJ
Right 07QH
Internal Mammary
Left 07Q9
Right 07Q8
Lower Extremity
Left 07QG
Right 07QF
Mesenteric 07QB
Neck
Left 07Q2
Right 07Q1
Pelvis 07QC
Thoracic Duct 07QK
Thorax 07Q7
Upper Extremity
Left 07Q4
Right 07Q3
Mandible
Left 0NQV
Right 0NQT
Maxilla 0NQR
Mediastinum 0WQC
Medulla Oblongata 00QD
Mesentery 0DQV
Metacarpal
Left 0PQQ
Right 0PQP
Metatarsal
Left 0QQP
Right 0QQN
Muscle
Abdomen
Left 0KQL
Right 0KQK
Extraocular
Left 08QM
Right 08QL
Facial 0KQ1
Foot
Left 0KQW
Right 0KQV
Hand
Left 0KQD
Right 0KQC
Head 0KQ0
Hip
Left 0KQP
Right 0KQN
Lower Arm and Wrist
Left 0KQB
Right 0KQ9
Lower Leg
Left 0KQT
Right 0KQS
Neck
Left 0KQ3
Right 0KQ2
Papillary 02QD
Perineum 0KQM
Shoulder
Left 0KQ6
Right 0KQ5
Thorax
Left 0KQJ
Right 0KQH
Tongue, Palate, Pharynx 0KQ4
Trunk
Left 0KQG
Right 0KQF
Upper Arm
Left 0KQ8
Right 0KQ7

Repair — *continued*
Muscle — *continued*
Upper Leg
Left 0KQR
Right 0KQQ
Nasal Mucosa and Soft Tissue 09QK
Nasopharynx 09QN
Neck 0WQ6
Nerve
Abdominal Sympathetic 01QM
Abducens 00QL
Accessory 00QR
Acoustic 00QN
Brachial Plexus 01Q3
Cervical 01Q1
Cervical Plexus 01Q0
Facial 00QM
Femoral 01QD
Glossopharyngeal 00QP
Head and Neck Sympathetic 01QK
Hypoglossal 00QS
Lumbar 01QB
Lumbar Plexus 01Q9
Lumbar Sympathetic 01QN
Lumbosacral Plexus 01QA
Median 01Q5
Oculomotor 00QH
Olfactory 00QF
Optic 00QG
Peroneal 01QH
Phrenic 01Q2
Pudendal 01QC
Radial 01Q6
Sacral 01QR
Sacral Plexus 01QQ
Sacral Sympathetic 01QP
Sciatic 01QF
Thoracic 01Q8
Thoracic Sympathetic 01QL
Tibial 01QG
Trigeminal 00QK
Trochlear 00QJ
Ulnar 01Q4
Vagus 00QQ
Nipple
Left 0HQX
Right 0HQW
Omentum 0DQU
Oral Cavity and Throat 0WQ3
Orbit
Left 0NQQ
Right 0NQP
Ovary
Bilateral 0UQ2
Left 0UQ1
Right 0UQ0
Palate
Hard 0CQ2
Soft 0CQ3
Pancreas 0FQG
Para-aortic Body 0GQ9
Paraganglion Extremity 0GQF
Parathyroid Gland 0GQR
Inferior
Left 0GQP
Right 0GQN
Multiple 0GQQ
Superior
Left 0GQM
Right 0GQL
Patella
Left 0QQF
Right 0QQD
Penis 0VQS
Pericardium 02QN
Perineum
Female 0WQN

Repair — *continued*
- Perineum — *continued*
  - Male 0WQM
- Peritoneum 0DQW
- Phalanx
  - Finger
    - Left 0PQV
    - Right 0PQT
  - Thumb
    - Left 0PQS
    - Right 0PQR
  - Toe
    - Left 0QQR
    - Right 0QQQ
- Pharynx 0CQM
- Pineal Body 0GQ1
- Pleura
  - Left 0BQP
  - Right 0BQN
- Pons 00QB
- Prepuce 0VQT
- Products of Conception 10Q0
- Prostate 0VQ0
- Radius
  - Left 0PQJ
  - Right 0PQH
- Rectum 0DQP
- Retina
  - Left 08QF3ZZ
  - Right 08QE3ZZ
- Retinal Vessel
  - Left 08QH3ZZ
  - Right 08QG3ZZ
- Ribs
  - 1 to 2 0PQ1
  - 3 or More 0PQ2
- Sacrum 0QQ1
- Scapula
  - Left 0PQ6
  - Right 0PQ5
- Sclera
  - Left 08Q7XZZ
  - Right 08Q6XZZ
- Scrotum 0VQ5
- Septum
  - Atrial 02Q5
  - Nasal 09QM
  - Ventricular 02QM
- Shoulder Region
  - Left 0XQ3
  - Right 0XQ2
- Sinus
  - Accessory 09QP
  - Ethmoid
    - Left 09QV
    - Right 09QU
  - Frontal
    - Left 09QT
    - Right 09QS
  - Mastoid
    - Left 09QC
    - Right 09QB
  - Maxillary
    - Left 09QR
    - Right 09QQ
  - Sphenoid
    - Left 09QX
    - Right 09QW
- Skin
  - Abdomen 0HQ7XZZ
  - Back 0HQ6XZZ
  - Buttock 0HQ8XZZ
  - Chest 0HQ5XZZ
  - Ear
    - Left 0HQ3XZZ
    - Right 0HQ2XZZ
  - Face 0HQ1XZZ

Repair — *continued*
- Skin — *continued*
  - Foot
    - Left 0HQNXZZ
    - Right 0HQMXZZ
  - Hand
    - Left 0HQGXZZ
    - Right 0HQFXZZ
  - Inguinal 0HQAXZZ
  - Lower Arm
    - Left 0HQEXZZ
    - Right 0HQDXZZ
  - Lower Leg
    - Left 0HQLXZZ
    - Right 0HQKXZZ
  - Neck 0HQ4XZZ
  - Perineum 0HQ9XZZ
  - Scalp 0HQ0XZZ
  - Upper Arm
    - Left 0HQCXZZ
    - Right 0HQBXZZ
  - Upper Leg
    - Left 0HQJXZZ
    - Right 0HQHXZZ
- Skull 0NQ0
- Spinal Cord
  - Cervical 00QW
  - Lumbar 00QY
  - Thoracic 00QX
- Spinal Meninges 00QT
- Spleen 07QP
- Sternum 0PQ0
- Stomach 0DQ6
  - Pylorus 0DQ7
- Subcutaneous Tissue and Fascia
  - Abdomen 0JQ8
  - Back 0JQ7
  - Buttock 0JQ9
  - Chest 0JQ6
  - Face 0JQ1
  - Foot
    - Left 0JQR
    - Right 0JQQ
  - Hand
    - Left 0JQK
    - Right 0JQJ
  - Lower Arm
    - Left 0JQH
    - Right 0JQG
  - Lower Leg
    - Left 0JQP
    - Right 0JQN
  - Neck
    - Left 0JQ5
    - Right 0JQ4
  - Pelvic Region 0JQC
  - Perineum 0JQB
  - Scalp 0JQ0
  - Upper Arm
    - Left 0JQF
    - Right 0JQD
  - Upper Leg
    - Left 0JQM
    - Right 0JQL
- Tarsal
  - Left 0QQM
  - Right 0QQL
- Tendon
  - Abdomen
    - Left 0LQG
    - Right 0LQF
  - Ankle
    - Left 0LQT
    - Right 0LQS
  - Foot
    - Left 0LQW
    - Right 0LQV

Repair — *continued*
- Tendon — *continued*
  - Hand
    - Left 0LQ8
    - Right 0LQ7
  - Head and Neck 0LQ0
  - Hip
    - Left 0LQK
    - Right 0LQJ
  - Knee
    - Left 0LQR
    - Right 0LQQ
  - Lower Arm and Wrist
    - Left 0LQ6
    - Right 0LQ5
  - Lower Leg
    - Left 0LQP
    - Right 0LQN
  - Perineum 0LQH
  - Shoulder
    - Left 0LQ2
    - Right 0LQ1
  - Thorax
    - Left 0LQD
    - Right 0LQC
  - Trunk
    - Left 0LQB
    - Right 0LQ9
  - Upper Arm
    - Left 0LQ4
    - Right 0LQ3
  - Upper Leg
    - Left 0LQM
    - Right 0LQL
- Testis
  - Bilateral 0VQC
  - Left 0VQB
  - Right 0VQ9
- Thalamus 00Q9
- Thumb
  - Left 0XQM
  - Right 0XQL
- Thymus 07QM
- Thyroid Gland 0GQK
  - Left Lobe 0GQG
  - Right Lobe 0GQH
- Thyroid Gland Isthmus 0GQJ
- Tibia
  - Left 0QQH
  - Right 0QQG
- Toe
  - 1st
    - Left 0YQQ
    - Right 0YQP
  - 2nd
    - Left 0YQS
    - Right 0YQR
  - 3rd
    - Left 0YQU
    - Right 0YQT
  - 4th
    - Left 0YQW
    - Right 0YQV
  - 5th
    - Left 0YQY
    - Right 0YQX
- Toe Nail 0HQRXZZ
- Tongue 0CQ7
- Tonsils 0CQP
- Tooth
  - Lower 0CQX
  - Upper 0CQW
- Trachea 0BQ1
- Tunica Vaginalis
  - Left 0VQ7
  - Right 0VQ6
- Turbinate, Nasal 09QL

Repair — *continued*
Tympanic Membrane
Left 09Q8
Right 09Q7
Ulna
Left 0PQL
Right 0PQK
Ureter
Left 0TQ7
Right 0TQ6
Urethra 0TQD
Uterine Supporting Structure 0UQ4
Uterus 0UQ9
Uvula 0CQN
Vagina 0UQG
Valve
Aortic 02QF
Mitral 02QG
Pulmonary 02QH
Tricuspid 02QJ
Vas Deferens
Bilateral 0VQQ
Left 0VQP
Right 0VQN
Vein
Axillary
Left 05Q8
Right 05Q7
Azygos 05Q0
Basilic
Left 05QC
Right 05QB
Brachial
Left 05QA
Right 05Q9
Cephalic
Left 05QF
Right 05QD
Colic 06Q7
Common Iliac
Left 06QD
Right 06QC
Coronary 02Q4
Esophageal 06Q3
External Iliac
Left 06QG
Right 06QF
External Jugular
Left 05QQ
Right 05QP
Face
Left 05QV
Right 05QT
Femoral
Left 06QN
Right 06QM
Foot
Left 06QV
Right 06QT
Gastric 06Q2
Hand
Left 05QH
Right 05QG
Hemiazygos 05Q1
Hepatic 06Q4
Hypogastric
Left 06QJ
Right 06QH
Inferior Mesenteric 06Q6
Innominate
Left 05Q4
Right 05Q3
Internal Jugular
Left 05QN
Right 05QM
Intracranial 05QL
Lower 06QY

Repair — *continued*
Vein — *continued*
Portal 06Q8
Pulmonary
Left 02QT
Right 02QS
Renal
Left 06QB
Right 06Q9
Saphenous
Left 06QQ
Right 06QP
Splenic 06Q1
Subclavian
Left 05Q6
Right 05Q5
Superior Mesenteric 06Q5
Upper 05QY
Vertebral
Left 05QS
Right 05QR
Vena Cava
Inferior 06Q0
Superior 02QV
Ventricle
Left 02QL
Right 02QK
Vertebra
Cervical 0PQ3
Lumbar 0QQ0
Thoracic 0PQ4
Vesicle
Bilateral 0VQ3
Left 0VQ2
Right 0VQ1
Vitreous
Left 08Q53ZZ
Right 08Q43ZZ
Vocal Cord
Left 0CQV
Right 0CQT
Vulva 0UQM
Wrist Region
Left 0XQH
Right 0XQG
Repair, obstetric laceration, periurethral 0UQMXZZ
Replacement
Acetabulum
Left 0QR5
Right 0QR4
Ampulla of Vater 0FRC
Anal Sphincter 0DRR
Aorta
Abdominal 04R0
Thoracic
Ascending/Arch 02RX
Descending 02RW
Artery
Anterior Tibial
Left 04RQ
Right 04RP
Axillary
Left 03R6
Right 03R5
Brachial
Left 03R8
Right 03R7
Celiac 04R1
Colic
Left 04R7
Middle 04R8
Right 04R6
Common Carotid
Left 03RJ
Right 03RH

Replacement — *continued*
Artery — *continued*
Common Iliac
Left 04RD
Right 04RC
External Carotid
Left 03RN
Right 03RM
External Iliac
Left 04RJ
Right 04RH
Face 03RR
Femoral
Left 04RL
Right 04RK
Foot
Left 04RW
Right 04RV
Gastric 04R2
Hand
Left 03RF
Right 03RD
Hepatic 04R3
Inferior Mesenteric 04RB
Innominate 03R2
Internal Carotid
Left 03RL
Right 03RK
Internal Iliac
Left 04RF
Right 04RE
Internal Mammary
Left 03R1
Right 03R0
Intracranial 03RG
Lower 04RY
Peroneal
Left 04RU
Right 04RT
Popliteal
Left 04RN
Right 04RM
Posterior Tibial
Left 04RS
Right 04RR
Pulmonary
Left 02RR
Right 02RQ
Pulmonary Trunk 02RP
Radial
Left 03RC
Right 03RB
Renal
Left 04RA
Right 04R9
Splenic 04R4
Subclavian
Left 03R4
Right 03R3
Superior Mesenteric 04R5
Temporal
Left 03RT
Right 03RS
Thyroid
Left 03RV
Right 03RU
Ulnar
Left 03RA
Right 03R9
Upper 03RY
Vertebral
Left 03RQ
Right 03RP
Atrium
Left 02R7
Right 02R6
Auditory Ossicle
Left 09RA0

Replacement — *continued*
Auditory Ossicle — *continued*
Right 09R90
Bladder 0TRB
Bladder Neck 0TRC
Bone
Ethmoid
Left 0NRG
Right 0NRF
Frontal 0NR1
Hyoid 0NRX
Lacrimal
Left 0NRJ
Right 0NRH
Nasal 0NRB
Occipital 0NR7
Palatine
Left 0NRL
Right 0NRK
Parietal
Left 0NR4
Right 0NR3
Pelvic
Left 0QR3
Right 0QR2
Sphenoid 0NRC
Temporal
Left 0NR6
Right 0NR5
Zygomatic
Left 0NRN
Right 0NRM
Breast
Bilateral 0HRV
Left 0HRU
Right 0HRT
Bronchus
Lingula 0BR9
Lower Lobe
Left 0BRB
Right 0BR6
Main
Left 0BR7
Right 0BR3
Middle Lobe, Right 0BR5
Upper Lobe
Left 0BR8
Right 0BR4
Buccal Mucosa 0CR4
Bursa and Ligament
Abdomen
Left 0MRJ
Right 0MRH
Ankle
Left 0MRR
Right 0MRQ
Elbow
Left 0MR4
Right 0MR3
Foot
Left 0MRT
Right 0MRS
Hand
Left 0MR8
Right 0MR7
Head and Neck 0MR0
Hip
Left 0MRM
Right 0MRL
Knee
Left 0MRP
Right 0MRN
Lower Extremity
Left 0MRW
Right 0MRV
Perineum 0MRK
Rib(s) 0MRG

Replacement — *continued*
Bursa and Ligament — *continued*
Shoulder
Left 0MR2
Right 0MR1
Spine
Lower 0MRD
Upper 0MRC
Sternum 0MRF
Upper Extremity
Left 0MRB
Right 0MR9
Wrist
Left 0MR6
Right 0MR5
Carina 0BR2
Carpal
Left 0PRN
Right 0PRM
Cerebral Meninges 00R1
Cerebral Ventricle 00R6
Chordae Tendineae 02R9
Choroid
Left 08RB
Right 08RA
Clavicle
Left 0PRB
Right 0PR9
Coccyx 0QRS
Conjunctiva
Left 08RTX
Right 08RSX
Cornea
Left 08R9
Right 08R8
Diaphragm 0BRT
Disc
Cervical Vertebral 0RR30
Cervicothoracic Vertebral 0RR50
Lumbar Vertebral 0SR20
Lumbosacral 0SR40
Thoracic Vertebral 0RR90
Thoracolumbar Vertebral 0RRB0
Duct
Common Bile 0FR9
Cystic 0FR8
Hepatic
Common 0FR7
Left 0FR6
Right 0FR5
Lacrimal
Left 08RY
Right 08RX
Pancreatic 0FRD
Accessory 0FRF
Parotid
Left 0CRC
Right 0CRB
Dura Mater 00R2
Ear
External
Bilateral 09R2
Left 09R1
Right 09R0
Inner
Left 09RE0
Right 09RD0
Middle
Left 09R60
Right 09R50
Epiglottis 0CRR
Esophagus 0DR5
Eye
Left 08R1
Right 08R0

Replacement — *continued*
Eyelid
Lower
Left 08RR
Right 08RQ
Upper
Left 08RP
Right 08RN
Femoral Shaft
Left 0QR9
Right 0QR8
Femur
Lower
Left 0QRC
Right 0QRB
Upper
Left 0QR7
Right 0QR6
Fibula
Left 0QRK
Right 0QRJ
Finger Nail 0HRQX
Gingiva
Lower 0CR6
Upper 0CR5
Glenoid Cavity
Left 0PR8
Right 0PR7
Hair 0HRSX
Humeral Head
Left 0PRD
Right 0PRC
Humeral Shaft
Left 0PRG
Right 0PRF
Iris
Left 08RD3
Right 08RC3
Joint
Acromioclavicular
Left 0RRH0
Right 0RRG0
Ankle
Left 0SRG
Right 0SRF
Carpal
Left 0RRR0
Right 0RRQ0
Carpometacarpal
Left 0RRT0
Right 0RRS0
Cervical Vertebral 0RR10
Cervicothoracic Vertebral 0RR40
Coccygeal 0SR60
Elbow
Left 0RRM0
Right 0RRL0
Finger Phalangeal
Left 0RRX0
Right 0RRW0
Hip
Left 0SRB
Acetabular Surface 0SRE
Femoral Surface 0SRS
Right 0SR9
Acetabular Surface 0SRA
Femoral Surface 0SRR
Knee
Left 0SRD
Femoral Surface 0SRU
Tibial Surface 0SRW
Right 0SRC
Femoral Surface 0SRT
Tibial Surface 0SRV
Lumbar Vertebral 0SR00
Lumbosacral 0SR30
Metacarpophalangeal
Left 0RRV0

Replacement — *continued*
Joint — *continued*
Right 0RRU0
Metatarsal-Phalangeal
Left 0SRN0
Right 0SRM0
Occipital-cervical 0RR00
Sacrococcygeal 0SR50
Sacroiliac
Left 0SR80
Right 0SR70
Shoulder
Left 0RRK
Right 0RRJ
Sternoclavicular
Left 0RRF0
Right 0RRE0
Tarsal
Left 0SRJ0
Right 0SRH0
Tarsometatarsal
Left 0SRL0
Right 0SRK0
Temporomandibular
Left 0RRD0
Right 0RRC0
Thoracic Vertebral 0RR60
Thoracolumbar Vertebral 0RRA0
Toe Phalangeal
Left 0SRQ0
Right 0SRP0
Wrist
Left 0RRP0
Right 0RRN0
Kidney Pelvis
Left 0TR4
Right 0TR3
Larynx 0CRS
Lens
Left 08RK30Z
Right 08RJ30Z
Lip
Lower 0CR1
Upper 0CR0
Mandible
Left 0NRV
Right 0NRT
Maxilla 0NRR
Mesentery 0DRV
Metacarpal
Left 0PRQ
Right 0PRP
Metatarsal
Left 0QRP
Right 0QRN
Muscle
Abdomen
Left 0KRL
Right 0KRK
Facial 0KR1
Foot
Left 0KRW
Right 0KRV
Hand
Left 0KRD
Right 0KRC
Head 0KR0
Hip
Left 0KRP
Right 0KRN
Lower Arm and Wrist
Left 0KRB
Right 0KR9
Lower Leg
Left 0KRT
Right 0KRS

Replacement — *continued*
Muscle — *continued*
Neck
Left 0KR3
Right 0KR2
Papillary 02RD
Perineum 0KRM
Shoulder
Left 0KR6
Right 0KR5
Thorax
Left 0KRJ
Right 0KRH
Tongue, Palate, Pharynx 0KR4
Trunk
Left 0KRG
Right 0KRF
Upper Arm
Left 0KR8
Right 0KR7
Upper Leg
Left 0KRR
Right 0KRQ
Nasal Mucosa and Soft Tissue 09RK
Nasopharynx 09RN
Nerve
Abducens 00RL
Accessory 00RR
Acoustic 00RN
Cervical 01R1
Facial 00RM
Femoral 01RD
Glossopharyngeal 00RP
Hypoglossal 00RS
Lumbar 01RB
Median 01R5
Oculomotor 00RH
Olfactory 00RF
Optic 00RG
Peroneal 01RH
Phrenic 01R2
Pudendal 01RC
Radial 01R6
Sacral 01RR
Sciatic 01RF
Thoracic 01R8
Tibial 01RG
Trigeminal 00RK
Trochlear 00RJ
Ulnar 01R4
Vagus 00RQ
Nipple
Left 0HRX
Right 0HRW
Omentum 0DRU
Orbit
Left 0NRQ
Right 0NRP
Palate
Hard 0CR2
Soft 0CR3
Patella
Left 0QRF
Right 0QRD
Pericardium 02RN
Peritoneum 0DRW
Phalanx
Finger
Left 0PRV
Right 0PRT
Thumb
Left 0PRS
Right 0PRR
Toe
Left 0QRR
Right 0QRQ
Pharynx 0CRM

Replacement — *continued*
Radius
Left 0PRJ
Right 0PRH
Retinal Vessel
Left 08RH3
Right 08RG3
Ribs
1 to 2 0PR1
3 or More 0PR2
Sacrum 0QR1
Scapula
Left 0PR6
Right 0PR5
Sclera
Left 08R7X
Right 08R6X
Septum
Atrial 02R5
Nasal 09RM
Ventricular 02RM
Skin
Abdomen 0HR7
Back 0HR6
Buttock 0HR8
Chest 0HR5
Ear
Left 0HR3
Right 0HR2
Face 0HR1
Foot
Left 0HRN
Right 0HRM
Hand
Left 0HRG
Right 0HRF
Inguinal 0HRA
Lower Arm
Left 0HRE
Right 0HRD
Lower Leg
Left 0HRL
Right 0HRK
Neck 0HR4
Perineum 0HR9
Scalp 0HR0
Upper Arm
Left 0HRC
Right 0HRB
Upper Leg
Left 0HRJ
Right 0HRH
Skin Substitute, Porcine Liver Derived XHRPXL2
Skull 0NR0
Spinal Meninges 00RT
Sternum 0PR0
Subcutaneous Tissue and Fascia
Abdomen 0JR8
Back 0JR7
Buttock 0JR9
Chest 0JR6
Face 0JR1
Foot
Left 0JRR
Right 0JRQ
Hand
Left 0JRK
Right 0JRJ
Lower Arm
Left 0JRH
Right 0JRG
Lower Leg
Left 0JRP
Right 0JRN
Neck
Left 0JR5

Replacement — *continued*
Subcutaneous Tissue and Fascia — *continued*
Right 0JR4
Pelvic Region 0JRC
Perineum 0JRB
Scalp 0JR0
Upper Arm
Left 0JRF
Right 0JRD
Upper Leg
Left 0JRM
Right 0JRL
Tarsal
Left 0QRM
Right 0QRL
Tendon
Abdomen
Left 0LRG
Right 0LRF
Ankle
Left 0LRT
Right 0LRS
Foot
Left 0LRW
Right 0LRV
Hand
Left 0LR8
Right 0LR7
Head and Neck 0LR0
Hip
Left 0LRK
Right 0LRJ
Knee
Left 0LRR
Right 0LRQ
Lower Arm and Wrist
Left 0LR6
Right 0LR5
Lower Leg
Left 0LRP
Right 0LRN
Perineum 0LRH
Shoulder
Left 0LR2
Right 0LR1
Thorax
Left 0LRD
Right 0LRC
Trunk
Left 0LRB
Right 0LR9
Upper Arm
Left 0LR4
Right 0LR3
Upper Leg
Left 0LRM
Right 0LRL
Testis
Bilateral 0VRC0JZ
Left 0VRB0JZ
Right 0VR90JZ
Thumb
Left 0XRM
Right 0XRL
Tibia
Left 0QRH
Right 0QRG
Toe Nail 0HRRX
Tongue 0CR7
Tooth
Lower 0CRX
Upper 0CRW
Trachea 0BR1
Turbinate, Nasal 09RL
Tympanic Membrane
Left 09R8
Right 09R7

Replacement — *continued*
Ulna
Left 0PRL
Right 0PRK
Ureter
Left 0TR7
Right 0TR6
Urethra 0TRD
Uvula 0CRN
Valve
Aortic 02RF
Mitral 02RG
Pulmonary 02RH
Tricuspid 02RJ
Vein
Axillary
Left 05R8
Right 05R7
Azygos 05R0
Basilic
Left 05RC
Right 05RB
Brachial
Left 05RA
Right 05R9
Cephalic
Left 05RF
Right 05RD
Colic 06R7
Common Iliac
Left 06RD
Right 06RC
Esophageal 06R3
External Iliac
Left 06RG
Right 06RF
External Jugular
Left 05RQ
Right 05RP
Face
Left 05RV
Right 05RT
Femoral
Left 06RN
Right 06RM
Foot
Left 06RV
Right 06RT
Gastric 06R2
Hand
Left 05RH
Right 05RG
Hemiazygos 05R1
Hepatic 06R4
Hypogastric
Left 06RJ
Right 06RH
Inferior Mesenteric 06R6
Innominate
Left 05R4
Right 05R3
Internal Jugular
Left 05RN
Right 05RM
Intracranial 05RL
Lower 06RY
Portal 06R8
Pulmonary
Left 02RT
Right 02RS
Renal
Left 06RB
Right 06R9
Saphenous
Left 06RQ
Right 06RP
Splenic 06R1

Replacement — *continued*
Vein — *continued*
Subclavian
Left 05R6
Right 05R5
Superior Mesenteric 06R5
Upper 05RY
Vertebral
Left 05RS
Right 05RR
Vena Cava
Inferior 06R0
Superior 02RV
Ventricle
Left 02RL
Right 02RK
Vertebra
Cervical 0PR3
Lumbar 0QR0
Thoracic 0PR4
Vitreous
Left 08R53
Right 08R43
Vocal Cord
Left 0CRV
Right 0CRT
Zooplastic Tissue, Rapid Deployment Technique X2RF
Replacement, hip
Partial or total *see* Replacement, Lower Joints 0SR
Resurfacing only *see* Supplement, Lower Joints 0SU
Replantation
see Reposition
Replantation, scalp
see Reattachment, Skin, Scalp 0HM0
Reposition
Acetabulum
Left 0QS5
Right 0QS4
Ampulla of Vater 0FSC
Anus 0DSQ
Aorta
Abdominal 04S0
Thoracic
Ascending/Arch 02SX0ZZ
Descending 02SW0ZZ
Artery
Anterior Tibial
Left 04SQ
Right 04SP
Axillary
Left 03S6
Right 03S5
Brachial
Left 03S8
Right 03S7
Celiac 04S1
Colic
Left 04S7
Middle 04S8
Right 04S6
Common Carotid
Left 03SJ
Right 03SH
Common Iliac
Left 04SD
Right 04SC
Coronary
One Artery 02S00ZZ
Two Arteries 02S10ZZ
External Carotid
Left 03SN
Right 03SM
External Iliac
Left 04SJ

Reposition — *continued*
Artery — *continued*
Right 04SH
Face 03SR
Femoral
Left 04SL
Right 04SK
Foot
Left 04SW
Right 04SV
Gastric 04S2
Hand
Left 03SF
Right 03SD
Hepatic 04S3
Inferior Mesenteric 04SB
Innominate 03S2
Internal Carotid
Left 03SL
Right 03SK
Internal Iliac
Left 04SF
Right 04SE
Internal Mammary
Left 03S1
Right 03S0
Intracranial 03SG
Lower 04SY
Peroneal
Left 04SU
Right 04ST
Popliteal
Left 04SN
Right 04SM
Posterior Tibial
Left 04SS
Right 04SR
Pulmonary
Left 02SR0ZZ
Right 02SQ0ZZ
Pulmonary Trunk 02SP0ZZ
Radial
Left 03SC
Right 03SB
Renal
Left 04SA
Right 04S9
Splenic 04S4
Subclavian
Left 03S4
Right 03S3
Superior Mesenteric 04S5
Temporal
Left 03ST
Right 03SS
Thyroid
Left 03SV
Right 03SU
Ulnar
Left 03SA
Right 03S9
Upper 03SY
Vertebral
Left 03SQ
Right 03SP
Auditory Ossicle
Left 09SA
Right 09S9
Bladder 0TSB
Bladder Neck 0TSC
Bone
Ethmoid
Left 0NSG
Right 0NSF
Frontal 0NS1
Hyoid 0NSX
Lacrimal

Reposition — *continued*
Bone — *continued*
Left 0NSJ
Right 0NSH
Nasal 0NSB
Occipital 0NS7
Palatine
Left 0NSL
Right 0NSK
Parietal
Left 0NS4
Right 0NS3
Pelvic
Left 0QS3
Right 0QS2
Sphenoid 0NSC
Temporal
Left 0NS6
Right 0NS5
Zygomatic
Left 0NSN
Right 0NSM
Breast
Bilateral 0HSV0ZZ
Left 0HSU0ZZ
Right 0HST0ZZ
Bronchus
Lingula 0BS90ZZ
Lower Lobe
Left 0BSB0ZZ
Right 0BS60ZZ
Main
Left 0BS70ZZ
Right 0BS30ZZ
Middle Lobe, Right 0BS50ZZ
Upper Lobe
Left 0BS80ZZ
Right 0BS40ZZ
Bursa and Ligament
Abdomen
Left 0MSJ
Right 0MSH
Ankle
Left 0MSR
Right 0MSQ
Elbow
Left 0MS4
Right 0MS3
Foot
Left 0MST
Right 0MSS
Hand
Left 0MS8
Right 0MS7
Head and Neck 0MS0
Hip
Left 0MSM
Right 0MSL
Knee
Left 0MSP
Right 0MSN
Lower Extremity
Left 0MSW
Right 0MSV
Perineum 0MSK
Rib(s) 0MSG
Shoulder
Left 0MS2
Right 0MS1
Spine
Lower 0MSD
Upper 0MSC
Sternum 0MSF
Upper Extremity
Left 0MSB
Right 0MS9

Reposition — *continued*
Bursa and Ligament — *continued*
Wrist
Left 0MS6
Right 0MS5
Carina 0BS20ZZ
Carpal
Left 0PSN
Right 0PSM
Cecum 0DSH
Cervix 0USC
Clavicle
Left 0PSB
Right 0PS9
Coccyx 0QSS
Colon
Ascending 0DSK
Descending 0DSM
Sigmoid 0DSN
Transverse 0DSL
Cord
Bilateral 0VSH
Left 0VSG
Right 0VSF
Cul-de-sac 0USF
Diaphragm 0BST0ZZ
Duct
Common Bile 0FS9
Cystic 0FS8
Hepatic
Common 0FS7
Left 0FS6
Right 0FS5
Lacrimal
Left 08SY
Right 08SX
Pancreatic 0FSD
Accessory 0FSF
Parotid
Left 0CSC
Right 0CSB
Duodenum 0DS9
Ear
Bilateral 09S2
Left 09S1
Right 09S0
Epiglottis 0CSR
Esophagus 0DS5
Eustachian Tube
Left 09SG
Right 09SF
Eyelid
Lower
Left 08SR
Right 08SQ
Upper
Left 08SP
Right 08SN
Fallopian Tube
Left 0US6
Right 0US5
Fallopian Tubes, Bilateral 0US7
Femoral Shaft
Left 0QS9
Right 0QS8
Femur
Lower
Left 0QSC
Right 0QSB
Upper
Left 0QS7
Right 0QS6
Fibula
Left 0QSK
Right 0QSJ
Gallbladder 0FS4
Gland
Adrenal

Reposition — *continued*
Gland — *continued*
Left 0GS2
Right 0GS3
Lacrimal
Left 08SW
Right 08SV
Glenoid Cavity
Left 0PS8
Right 0PS7
Hair 0HSSXZZ
Humeral Head
Left 0PSD
Right 0PSC
Humeral Shaft
Left 0PSG
Right 0PSF
Ileum 0DSB
Intestine
Large 0DSE
Small 0DS8
Iris
Left 08SD3ZZ
Right 08SC3ZZ
Jejunum 0DSA
Joint
Acromioclavicular
Left 0RSH
Right 0RSG
Ankle
Left 0SSG
Right 0SSF
Carpal
Left 0RSR
Right 0RSQ
Carpometacarpal
Left 0RST
Right 0RSS
Cervical Vertebral 0RS1
Cervicothoracic Vertebral 0RS4
Coccygeal 0SS6
Elbow
Left 0RSM
Right 0RSL
Finger Phalangeal
Left 0RSX
Right 0RSW
Hip
Left 0SSB
Right 0SS9
Knee
Left 0SSD
Right 0SSC
Lumbar Vertebral 0SS0
Lumbosacral 0SS3
Metacarpophalangeal
Left 0RSV
Right 0RSU
Metatarsal-Phalangeal
Left 0SSN
Right 0SSM
Occipital-cervical 0RS0
Sacrococcygeal 0SS5
Sacroiliac
Left 0SS8
Right 0SS7
Shoulder
Left 0RSK
Right 0RSJ
Sternoclavicular
Left 0RSF
Right 0RSE
Tarsal
Left 0SSJ
Right 0SSH
Tarsometatarsal
Left 0SSL

Reposition — *continued*
Joint — *continued*
Right 0SSK
Temporomandibular
Left 0RSD
Right 0RSC
Thoracic Vertebral 0RS6
Thoracolumbar Vertebral 0RSA
Toe Phalangeal
Left 0SSQ
Right 0SSP
Wrist
Left 0RSP
Right 0RSN
Kidney
Left 0TS1
Right 0TS0
Kidney Pelvis
Left 0TS4
Right 0TS3
Kidneys, Bilateral 0TS2
Lens
Left 08SK3ZZ
Right 08SJ3ZZ
Lip
Lower 0CS1
Upper 0CS0
Liver 0FS0
Lung
Left 0BSL0ZZ
Lower Lobe
Left 0BSJ0ZZ
Right 0BSF0ZZ
Middle Lobe, Right 0BSD0ZZ
Right 0BSK0ZZ
Upper Lobe
Left 0BSG0ZZ
Right 0BSC0ZZ
Lung Lingula 0BSH0ZZ
Mandible
Left 0NSV
Right 0NST
Maxilla 0NSR
Metacarpal
Left 0PSQ
Right 0PSP
Metatarsal
Left 0QSP
Right 0QSN
Muscle
Abdomen
Left 0KSL
Right 0KSK
Extraocular
Left 08SM
Right 08SL
Facial 0KS1
Foot
Left 0KSW
Right 0KSV
Hand
Left 0KSD
Right 0KSC
Head 0KS0
Hip
Left 0KSP
Right 0KSN
Lower Arm and Wrist
Left 0KSB
Right 0KS9
Lower Leg
Left 0KST
Right 0KSS
Neck
Left 0KS3
Right 0KS2
Perineum 0KSM

Reposition — *continued*
Muscle — *continued*
Shoulder
Left 0KS6
Right 0KS5
Thorax
Left 0KSJ
Right 0KSH
Tongue, Palate, Pharynx 0KS4
Trunk
Left 0KSG
Right 0KSF
Upper Arm
Left 0KS8
Right 0KS7
Upper Leg
Left 0KSR
Right 0KSQ
Nasal Mucosa and Soft Tissue 09SK
Nerve
Abducens 00SL
Accessory 00SR
Acoustic 00SN
Brachial Plexus 01S3
Cervical 01S1
Cervical Plexus 01S0
Facial 00SM
Femoral 01SD
Glossopharyngeal 00SP
Hypoglossal 00SS
Lumbar 01SB
Lumbar Plexus 01S9
Lumbosacral Plexus 01SA
Median 01S5
Oculomotor 00SH
Olfactory 00SF
Optic 00SG
Peroneal 01SH
Phrenic 01S2
Pudendal 01SC
Radial 01S6
Sacral 01SR
Sacral Plexus 01SQ
Sciatic 01SF
Thoracic 01S8
Tibial 01SG
Trigeminal 00SK
Trochlear 00SJ
Ulnar 01S4
Vagus 00SQ
Nipple
Left 0HSXXZZ
Right 0HSWXZZ
Orbit
Left 0NSQ
Right 0NSP
Ovary
Bilateral 0US2
Left 0US1
Right 0US0
Palate
Hard 0CS2
Soft 0CS3
Pancreas 0FSG
Parathyroid Gland 0GSR
Inferior
Left 0GSP
Right 0GSN
Multiple 0GSQ
Superior
Left 0GSM
Right 0GSL
Patella
Left 0QSF
Right 0QSD

Reposition — *continued*
Phalanx
Finger
Left 0PSV
Right 0PST
Thumb
Left 0PSS
Right 0PSR
Toe
Left 0QSR
Right 0QSQ
Products of Conception 10S0
Ectopic 10S2
Radius
Left 0PSJ
Right 0PSH
Rectum 0DSP
Retinal Vessel
Left 08SH3ZZ
Right 08SG3ZZ
Ribs
1 to 2 0PS1
3 or More 0PS2
Sacrum 0QS1
Scapula
Left 0PS6
Right 0PS5
Septum, Nasal 09SM
Sesamoid Bone(s) 1st Toe
see Reposition, Metatarsal, Right 0QSN
see Reposition, Metatarsal, Left 0QSP
Skull 0NS0
Spinal Cord
Cervical 00SW
Lumbar 00SY
Thoracic 00SX
Spleen 07SP0ZZ
Sternum 0PS0
Stomach 0DS6
Tarsal
Left 0QSM
Right 0QSL
Tendon
Abdomen
Left 0LSG
Right 0LSF
Ankle
Left 0LST
Right 0LSS
Foot
Left 0LSW
Right 0LSV
Hand
Left 0LS8
Right 0LS7
Head and Neck 0LS0
Hip
Left 0LSK
Right 0LSJ
Knee
Left 0LSR
Right 0LSQ
Lower Arm and Wrist
Left 0LS6
Right 0LS5
Lower Leg
Left 0LSP
Right 0LSN
Perineum 0LSH
Shoulder
Left 0LS2
Right 0LS1
Thorax
Left 0LSD
Right 0LSC
Trunk
Left 0LSB
Right 0LS9

Reposition — *continued*
Tendon — *continued*
Upper Arm
Left 0LS4
Right 0LS3
Upper Leg
Left 0LSM
Right 0LSL
Testis
Bilateral 0VSC
Left 0VSB
Right 0VS9
Thymus 07SM0ZZ
Thyroid Gland
Left Lobe 0GSG
Right Lobe 0GSH
Tibia
Left 0QSH
Right 0QSG
Tongue 0CS7
Tooth
Lower 0CSX
Upper 0CSW
Trachea 0BS10ZZ
Turbinate, Nasal 09SL
Tympanic Membrane
Left 09S8
Right 09S7
Ulna
Left 0PSL
Right 0PSK
Ureter
Left 0TS7
Right 0TS6
Ureters, Bilateral 0TS8
Urethra 0TSD
Uterine Supporting Structure 0US4
Uterus 0US9
Uvula 0CSN
Vagina 0USG
Vein
Axillary
Left 05S8
Right 05S7
Azygos 05S0
Basilic
Left 05SC
Right 05SB
Brachial
Left 05SA
Right 05S9
Cephalic
Left 05SF
Right 05SD
Colic 06S7
Common Iliac
Left 06SD
Right 06SC
Esophageal 06S3
External Iliac
Left 06SG
Right 06SF
External Jugular
Left 05SQ
Right 05SP
Face
Left 05SV
Right 05ST
Femoral
Left 06SN
Right 06SM
Foot
Left 06SV
Right 06ST
Gastric 06S2
Hand
Left 05SH

Reposition — *continued*
Vein — *continued*
Right 05SG
Hemiazygos 05S1
Hepatic 06S4
Hypogastric
Left 06SJ
Right 06SH
Inferior Mesenteric 06S6
Innominate
Left 05S4
Right 05S3
Internal Jugular
Left 05SN
Right 05SM
Intracranial 05SL
Lower 06SY
Portal 06S8
Pulmonary
Left 02ST0ZZ
Right 02SS0ZZ
Renal
Left 06SB
Right 06S9
Saphenous
Left 06SQ
Right 06SP
Splenic 06S1
Subclavian
Left 05S6
Right 05S5
Superior Mesenteric 06S5
Upper 05SY
Vertebral
Left 05SS
Right 05SR
Vena Cava
Inferior 06S0
Superior 02SV0ZZ
Vertebra
Cervical 0PS3
Magnetically Controlled Growth Rod(s) XNS3
Lumbar 0QS0
Magnetically Controlled Growth Rod(s) XNS0
Thoracic 0PS4
Magnetically Controlled Growth Rod(s) XNS4
Vocal Cord
Left 0CSV
Right 0CST
Resection
Acetabulum
Left 0QT50ZZ
Right 0QT40ZZ
Adenoids 0CTQ
Ampulla of Vater 0FTC
Anal Sphincter 0DTR
Anus 0DTQ
Aortic Body 0GTD
Appendix 0DTJ
Auditory Ossicle
Left 09TA
Right 09T9
Bladder 0TTB
Bladder Neck 0TTC
Bone
Ethmoid
Left 0NTG0ZZ
Right 0NTF0ZZ
Frontal 0NT10ZZ
Hyoid 0NTX0ZZ
Lacrimal
Left 0NTJ0ZZ
Right 0NTH0ZZ
Nasal 0NTB0ZZ

Resection — *continued*
Bone — *continued*
Occipital 0NT70ZZ
Palatine
Left 0NTL0ZZ
Right 0NTK0ZZ
Parietal
Left 0NT40ZZ
Right 0NT30ZZ
Pelvic
Left 0QT30ZZ
Right 0QT20ZZ
Sphenoid 0NTC0ZZ
Temporal
Left 0NT60ZZ
Right 0NT50ZZ
Zygomatic
Left 0NTN0ZZ
Right 0NTM0ZZ
Breast
Bilateral 0HTV0ZZ
Left 0HTU0ZZ
Right 0HTT0ZZ
Supernumerary 0HTY0ZZ
Bronchus
Lingula 0BT9
Lower Lobe
Left 0BTB
Right 0BT6
Main
Left 0BT7
Right 0BT3
Middle Lobe, Right 0BT5
Upper Lobe
Left 0BT8
Right 0BT4
Bursa and Ligament
Abdomen
Left 0MTJ
Right 0MTH
Ankle
Left 0MTR
Right 0MTQ
Elbow
Left 0MT4
Right 0MT3
Foot
Left 0MTT
Right 0MTS
Hand
Left 0MT8
Right 0MT7
Head and Neck 0MT0
Hip
Left 0MTM
Right 0MTL
Knee
Left 0MTP
Right 0MTN
Lower Extremity
Left 0MTW
Right 0MTV
Perineum 0MTK
Rib(s) 0MTG
Shoulder
Left 0MT2
Right 0MT1
Spine
Lower 0MTD
Upper 0MTC
Sternum 0MTF
Upper Extremity
Left 0MTB
Right 0MT9
Wrist
Left 0MT6
Right 0MT5

Resection — *continued*
Carina 0BT2
Carotid Bodies, Bilateral 0GT8
Carotid Body
Left 0GT6
Right 0GT7
Carpal
Left 0PTN0ZZ
Right 0PTM0ZZ
Cecum 0DTH
Cerebral Hemisphere 00T7
Cervix 0UTC
Chordae Tendineae 02T9
Cisterna Chyli 07TL
Clavicle
Left 0PTB0ZZ
Right 0PT90ZZ
Clitoris 0UTJ
Coccygeal Glomus 0GTB
Coccyx 0QTS0ZZ
Colon
Ascending 0DTK
Descending 0DTM
Sigmoid 0DTN
Transverse 0DTL
Conduction Mechanism 02T8
Cord
Bilateral 0VTH
Left 0VTG
Right 0VTF
Cornea
Left 08T9XZZ
Right 08T8XZZ
Cul-de-sac 0UTF
Diaphragm 0BTT
Disc
Cervical Vertebral 0RT30ZZ
Cervicothoracic Vertebral 0RT50ZZ
Lumbar Vertebral 0ST20ZZ
Lumbosacral 0ST40ZZ
Thoracic Vertebral 0RT90ZZ
Thoracolumbar Vertebral 0RTB0ZZ
Duct
Common Bile 0FT9
Cystic 0FT8
Hepatic
Common 0FT7
Left 0FT6
Right 0FT5
Lacrimal
Left 08TY
Right 08TX
Pancreatic 0FTD
Accessory 0FTF
Parotid
Left 0CTC0ZZ
Right 0CTB0ZZ
Duodenum 0DT9
Ear
External
Left 09T1
Right 09T0
Inner
Left 09TE
Right 09TD
Middle
Left 09T6
Right 09T5
Epididymis
Bilateral 0VTL
Left 0VTK
Right 0VTJ
Epiglottis 0CTR
Esophagogastric Junction 0DT4
Esophagus 0DT5
Lower 0DT3
Middle 0DT2

Resection — *continued*
Esophagus — *continued*
Upper 0DT1
Eustachian Tube
Left 09TG
Right 09TF
Eye
Left 08T1XZZ
Right 08T0XZZ
Eyelid
Lower
Left 08TR
Right 08TQ
Upper
Left 08TP
Right 08TN
Fallopian Tube
Left 0UT6
Right 0UT5
Fallopian Tubes, Bilateral 0UT7
Femoral Shaft
Left 0QT90ZZ
Right 0QT80ZZ
Femur
Lower
Left 0QTC0ZZ
Right 0QTB0ZZ
Upper
Left 0QT70ZZ
Right 0QT60ZZ
Fibula
Left 0QTK0ZZ
Right 0QTJ0ZZ
Finger Nail 0HTQXZZ
Gallbladder 0FT4
Gland
Adrenal
Bilateral 0GT4
Left 0GT2
Right 0GT3
Lacrimal
Left 08TW
Right 08TV
Minor Salivary 0CTJ0ZZ
Parotid
Left 0CT90ZZ
Right 0CT80ZZ
Pituitary 0GT0
Sublingual
Left 0CTF0ZZ
Right 0CTD0ZZ
Submaxillary
Left 0CTH0ZZ
Right 0CTG0ZZ
Vestibular 0UTL
Glenoid Cavity
Left 0PT80ZZ
Right 0PT70ZZ
Glomus Jugulare 0GTC
Humeral Head
Left 0PTD0ZZ
Right 0PTC0ZZ
Humeral Shaft
Left 0PTG0ZZ
Right 0PTF0ZZ
Hymen 0UTK
Ileocecal Valve 0DTC
Ileum 0DTB
Intestine
Large 0DTE
Left 0DTG
Right 0DTF
Small 0DT8
Iris
Left 08TD3ZZ
Right 08TC3ZZ
Jejunum 0DTA

- **Resection** — *continued*
  - Joint
    - Acromioclavicular
      - Left 0RTH0ZZ
      - Right 0RTG0ZZ
    - Ankle
      - Left 0STG0ZZ
      - Right 0STF0ZZ
    - Carpal
      - Left 0RTR0ZZ
      - Right 0RTQ0ZZ
    - Carpometacarpal
      - Left 0RTT0ZZ
      - Right 0RTS0ZZ
    - Cervicothoracic Vertebral 0RT40ZZ
    - Coccygeal 0ST60ZZ
    - Elbow
      - Left 0RTM0ZZ
      - Right 0RTL0ZZ
    - Finger Phalangeal
      - Left 0RTX0ZZ
      - Right 0RTW0ZZ
    - Hip
      - Left 0STB0ZZ
      - Right 0ST90ZZ
    - Knee
      - Left 0STD0ZZ
      - Right 0STC0ZZ
    - Metacarpophalangeal
      - Left 0RTV0ZZ
      - Right 0RTU0ZZ
    - Metatarsal-Phalangeal
      - Left 0STN0ZZ
      - Right 0STM0ZZ
    - Sacrococcygeal 0ST50ZZ
    - Sacroiliac
      - Left 0ST80ZZ
      - Right 0ST70ZZ
    - Shoulder
      - Left 0RTK0ZZ
      - Right 0RTJ0ZZ
    - Sternoclavicular
      - Left 0RTF0ZZ
      - Right 0RTE0ZZ
    - Tarsal
      - Left 0STJ0ZZ
      - Right 0STH0ZZ
    - Tarsometatarsal
      - Left 0STL0ZZ
      - Right 0STK0ZZ
    - Temporomandibular
      - Left 0RTD0ZZ
      - Right 0RTC0ZZ
    - Toe Phalangeal
      - Left 0STQ0ZZ
      - Right 0STP0ZZ
    - Wrist
      - Left 0RTP0ZZ
      - Right 0RTN0ZZ
  - Kidney
    - Left 0TT1
    - Right 0TT0
  - Kidney Pelvis
    - Left 0TT4
    - Right 0TT3
  - Kidneys, Bilateral 0TT2
  - Larynx 0CTS
  - Lens
    - Left 08TK3ZZ
    - Right 08TJ3ZZ
  - Lip
    - Lower 0CT1
    - Upper 0CT0
  - Liver 0FT0
    - Left Lobe 0FT2
    - Right Lobe 0FT1

- **Resection** — *continued*
  - Lung
    - Bilateral 0BTM
    - Left 0BTL
    - Lower Lobe
      - Left 0BTJ
      - Right 0BTF
    - Middle Lobe, Right 0BTD
    - Right 0BTK
    - Upper Lobe
      - Left 0BTG
      - Right 0BTC
  - Lung Lingula 0BTH
  - Lymphatic
    - Aortic 07TD
    - Axillary
      - Left 07T6
      - Right 07T5
    - Head 07T0
    - Inguinal
      - Left 07TJ
      - Right 07TH
    - Internal Mammary
      - Left 07T9
      - Right 07T8
    - Lower Extremity
      - Left 07TG
      - Right 07TF
    - Mesenteric 07TB
    - Neck
      - Left 07T2
      - Right 07T1
    - Pelvis 07TC
    - Thoracic Duct 07TK
    - Thorax 07T7
    - Upper Extremity
      - Left 07T4
      - Right 07T3
  - Mandible
    - Left 0NTV0ZZ
    - Right 0NTT0ZZ
  - Maxilla 0NTR0ZZ
  - Metacarpal
    - Left 0PTQ0ZZ
    - Right 0PTP0ZZ
  - Metatarsal
    - Left 0QTP0ZZ
    - Right 0QTN0ZZ
  - Muscle
    - Abdomen
      - Left 0KTL
      - Right 0KTK
    - Extraocular
      - Left 08TM
      - Right 08TL
    - Facial 0KT1
    - Foot
      - Left 0KTW
      - Right 0KTV
    - Hand
      - Left 0KTD
      - Right 0KTC
    - Head 0KT0
    - Hip
      - Left 0KTP
      - Right 0KTN
    - Lower Arm and Wrist
      - Left 0KTB
      - Right 0KT9
    - Lower Leg
      - Left 0KTT
      - Right 0KTS
    - Neck
      - Left 0KT3
      - Right 0KT2
    - Papillary 02TD
    - Perineum 0KTM

- **Resection** — *continued*
  - Muscle — *continued*
    - Shoulder
      - Left 0KT6
      - Right 0KT5
    - Thorax
      - Left 0KTJ
      - Right 0KTH
    - Tongue, Palate, Pharynx 0KT4
    - Trunk
      - Left 0KTG
      - Right 0KTF
    - Upper Arm
      - Left 0KT8
      - Right 0KT7
    - Upper Leg
      - Left 0KTR
      - Right 0KTQ
  - Nasal Mucosa and Soft Tissue 09TK
  - Nasopharynx 09TN
  - Nipple
    - Left 0HTXXZZ
    - Right 0HTWXZZ
  - Omentum 0DTU
  - Orbit
    - Left 0NTQ0ZZ
    - Right 0NTP0ZZ
  - Ovary
    - Bilateral 0UT2
    - Left 0UT1
    - Right 0UT0
  - Palate
    - Hard 0CT2
    - Soft 0CT3
  - Pancreas 0FTG
  - Para-aortic Body 0GT9
  - Paraganglion Extremity 0GTF
  - Parathyroid Gland 0GTR
    - Inferior
      - Left 0GTP
      - Right 0GTN
    - Multiple 0GTQ
    - Superior
      - Left 0GTM
      - Right 0GTL
  - Patella
    - Left 0QTF0ZZ
    - Right 0QTD0ZZ
  - Penis 0VTS
  - Pericardium 02TN
  - Phalanx
    - Finger
      - Left 0PTV0ZZ
      - Right 0PTT0ZZ
    - Thumb
      - Left 0PTS0ZZ
      - Right 0PTR0ZZ
    - Toe
      - Left 0QTR0ZZ
      - Right 0QTQ0ZZ
  - Pharynx 0CTM
  - Pineal Body 0GT1
  - Prepuce 0VTT
  - Products of Conception, Ectopic 10T2
  - Prostate 0VT0
  - Radius
    - Left 0PTJ0ZZ
    - Right 0PTH0ZZ
  - Rectum 0DTP
  - Ribs
    - 1 to 2 0PT10ZZ
    - 3 or More 0PT20ZZ
  - Scapula
    - Left 0PT60ZZ
    - Right 0PT50ZZ
  - Scrotum 0VT5

Resection — *continued*
Septum
Atrial 02T5
Nasal 09TM
Ventricular 02TM
Sinus
Accessory 09TP
Ethmoid
Left 09TV
Right 09TU
Frontal
Left 09TT
Right 09TS
Mastoid
Left 09TC
Right 09TB
Maxillary
Left 09TR
Right 09TQ
Sphenoid
Left 09TX
Right 09TW
Spleen 07TP
Sternum 0PT00ZZ
Stomach 0DT6
Pylorus 0DT7
Tarsal
Left 0QTM0ZZ
Right 0QTL0ZZ
Tendon
Abdomen
Left 0LTG
Right 0LTF
Ankle
Left 0LTT
Right 0LTS
Foot
Left 0LTW
Right 0LTV
Hand
Left 0LT8
Right 0LT7
Head and Neck 0LT0
Hip
Left 0LTK
Right 0LTJ
Knee
Left 0LTR
Right 0LTQ
Lower Arm and Wrist
Left 0LT6
Right 0LT5
Lower Leg
Left 0LTP
Right 0LTN
Perineum 0LTH
Shoulder
Left 0LT2
Right 0LT1
Thorax
Left 0LTD
Right 0LTC
Trunk
Left 0LTB
Right 0LT9
Upper Arm
Left 0LT4
Right 0LT3
Upper Leg
Left 0LTM
Right 0LTL
Testis
Bilateral 0VTC
Left 0VTB
Right 0VT9
Thymus 07TM

Resection — *continued*
Thyroid Gland 0GTK
Left Lobe 0GTG
Right Lobe 0GTH
Thyroid Gland Isthmus 0GTJ
Tibia
Left 0QTH0ZZ
Right 0QTG0ZZ
Toe Nail 0HTRXZZ
Tongue 0CT7
Tonsils 0CTP
Tooth
Lower 0CTX0Z
Upper 0CTW0Z
Trachea 0BT1
Tunica Vaginalis
Left 0VT7
Right 0VT6
Turbinate, Nasal 09TL
Tympanic Membrane
Left 09T8
Right 09T7
Ulna
Left 0PTL0ZZ
Right 0PTK0ZZ
Ureter
Left 0TT7
Right 0TT6
Urethra 0TTD
Uterine Supporting Structure 0UT4
Uterus 0UT9
Uvula 0CTN
Vagina 0UTG
Valve, Pulmonary 02TH
Vas Deferens
Bilateral 0VTQ
Left 0VTP
Right 0VTN
Vesicle
Bilateral 0VT3
Left 0VT2
Right 0VT1
Vitreous
Left 08T53ZZ
Right 08T43ZZ
Vocal Cord
Left 0CTV
Right 0CTT
Vulva 0UTM

Resection, left ventricular outflow tract obstruction (LVOT)
see Dilation, Ventricle, Left 027L

Resection, subaortic membrane (Left ventricular outflow tract obstruction)
see Dilation, Ventricle, Left 027L

Restoration, cardiac, single, rhythm 5A2204Z

RestoreAdvanced® neurostimulator (SureScan®)(MRI Safe)
use Stimulator Generator, Multiple Array Rechargeable in 0JH

RestoreSensor® neurostimulator (SureScan®)(MRI Safe)
use Stimulator Generator, Multiple Array Rechargeable in 0JH

RestoreUltra® neurostimulator (SureScan®) (MRI Safe)
use Stimulator Generator, Multiple Array Rechargeable in 0JH

Restriction
Ampulla of Vater 0FVC
Anus 0DVQ
Aorta
Abdominal 04V0
Intraluminal Device, Branched or Fenestrated 04V0

Restriction — *continued*
Aorta — *continued*
Thoracic
Ascending/Arch, Intraluminal Device, Branched or Fenestrated 02VX
Descending, Intraluminal Device, Branched or Fenestrated 02VW
Artery
Anterior Tibial
Left 04VQ
Right 04VP
Axillary
Left 03V6
Right 03V5
Brachial
Left 03V8
Right 03V7
Celiac 04V1
Colic
Left 04V7
Middle 04V8
Right 04V6
Common Carotid
Left 03VJ
Right 03VH
Common Iliac
Left 04VD
Right 04VC
External Carotid
Left 03VN
Right 03VM
External Iliac
Left 04VJ
Right 04VH
Face 03VR
Femoral
Left 04VL
Right 04VK
Foot
Left 04VW
Right 04VV
Gastric 04V2
Hand
Left 03VF
Right 03VD
Hepatic 04V3
Inferior Mesenteric 04VB
Innominate 03V2
Internal Carotid
Left 03VL
Right 03VK
Internal Iliac
Left 04VF
Right 04VE
Internal Mammary
Left 03V1
Right 03V0
Intracranial 03VG
Lower 04VY
Peroneal
Left 04VU
Right 04VT
Popliteal
Left 04VN
Right 04VM
Posterior Tibial
Left 04VS
Right 04VR
Pulmonary
Left 02VR
Right 02VQ
Pulmonary Trunk 02VP
Radial
Left 03VC
Right 03VB
Renal
Left 04VA
Right 04V9

Restriction — *continued*
Artery — *continued*
Splenic 04V4
Subclavian
Left 03V4
Right 03V3
Superior Mesenteric 04V5
Temporal
Left 03VT
Right 03VS
Thyroid
Left 03VV
Right 03VU
Ulnar
Left 03VA
Right 03V9
Upper 03VY
Vertebral
Left 03VQ
Right 03VP
Bladder 0TVB
Bladder Neck 0TVC
Bronchus
Lingula 0BV9
Lower Lobe
Left 0BVB
Right 0BV6
Main
Left 0BV7
Right 0BV3
Middle Lobe, Right 0BV5
Upper Lobe
Left 0BV8
Right 0BV4
Carina 0BV2
Cecum 0DVH
Cervix 0UVC
Cisterna Chyli 07VL
Colon
Ascending 0DVK
Descending 0DVM
Sigmoid 0DVN
Transverse 0DVL
Duct
Common Bile 0FV9
Cystic 0FV8
Hepatic
Common 0FV7
Left 0FV6
Right 0FV5
Lacrimal
Left 08VY
Right 08VX
Pancreatic 0FVD
Accessory 0FVF
Parotid
Left 0CVC
Right 0CVB
Duodenum 0DV9
Esophagogastric Junction 0DV4
Esophagus 0DV5
Lower 0DV3
Middle 0DV2
Upper 0DV1
Heart 02VA
Ileocecal Valve 0DVC
Ileum 0DVB
Intestine
Large 0DVE
Left 0DVG
Right 0DVF
Small 0DV8
Jejunum 0DVA
Kidney Pelvis
Left 0TV4
Right 0TV3

Restriction — *continued*
Lymphatic
Aortic 07VD
Axillary
Left 07V6
Right 07V5
Head 07V0
Inguinal
Left 07VJ
Right 07VH
Internal Mammary
Left 07V9
Right 07V8
Lower Extremity
Left 07VG
Right 07VF
Mesenteric 07VB
Neck
Left 07V2
Right 07V1
Pelvis 07VC
Thoracic Duct 07VK
Thorax 07V7
Upper Extremity
Left 07V4
Right 07V3
Rectum 0DVP
Stomach 0DV6
Pylorus 0DV7
Trachea 0BV1
Ureter
Left 0TV7
Right 0TV6
Urethra 0TVD
Valve, Mitral 02VG
Vein
Axillary
Left 05V8
Right 05V7
Azygos 05V0
Basilic
Left 05VC
Right 05VB
Brachial
Left 05VA
Right 05V9
Cephalic
Left 05VF
Right 05VD
Colic 06V7
Common Iliac
Left 06VD
Right 06VC
Esophageal 06V3
External Iliac
Left 06VG
Right 06VF
External Jugular
Left 05VQ
Right 05VP
Face
Left 05VV
Right 05VT
Femoral
Left 06VN
Right 06VM
Foot
Left 06VV
Right 06VT
Gastric 06V2
Hand
Left 05VH
Right 05VG
Hemiazygos 05V1
Hepatic 06V4

Restriction — *continued*
Vein — *continued*
Hypogastric
Left 06VJ
Right 06VH
Inferior Mesenteric 06V6
Innominate
Left 05V4
Right 05V3
Internal Jugular
Left 05VN
Right 05VM
Intracranial 05VL
Lower 06VY
Portal 06V8
Pulmonary
Left 02VT
Right 02VS
Renal
Left 06VB
Right 06V9
Saphenous
Left 06VQ
Right 06VP
Splenic 06V1
Subclavian
Left 05V6
Right 05V5
Superior Mesenteric 06V5
Upper 05VY
Vertebral
Left 05VS
Right 05VR
Vena Cava
Inferior 06V0
Superior 02VV
Resurfacing device
Removal of device from
Left 0SPB0BZ
Right 0SP90BZ
Revision of device in
Left 0SWB0BZ
Right 0SW90BZ
Supplement
Left 0SUB0BZ
Acetabular Surface 0SUE0BZ
Femoral Surface 0SUS0BZ
Right 0SU90BZ
Acetabular Surface 0SUA0BZ
Femoral Surface 0SUR0BZ
Resuscitation
Cardiopulmonary *see* Assistance, Cardiac 5A02
Cardioversion 5A2204Z
Defibrillation 5A2204Z
Endotracheal intubation *see* Insertion of device in, Trachea 0BH1
External chest compression 5A12012
Pulmonary 5A19054
Resuscitative endovascular balloon occlusion of the aorta (REBOA)
02LW3DJ
04L03DJ
Resuture, heart valve prosthesis
see Revision of device in, Heart and Great Vessels 02W
Retained placenta, manual removal
see Extraction, Products of Conception, Retained 10D1
Retraining
Cardiac *see* Motor Treatment, Rehabilitation F07
Vocational *see* Activities of Daily Living Treatment, Rehabilitation F08
Retrogasserian rhizotomy
see Division, Nerve, Trigeminal 008K
Retroperitoneal cavity
use Retroperitoneum

Retroperitoneal lymph node
use Lymphatic, Aortic
Retroperitoneal space
use Retroperitoneum
Retropharyngeal lymph node
use Lymphatic, Right Neck
use Lymphatic, Left Neck
Retropubic space
use Pelvic Cavity
Reveal® (DX)(XT)
use Monitoring Device
Reverse® total shoulder replacement
see Replacement, Upper Joints 0RR
Reverse® Shoulder Prosthesis
use Synthetic Substitute, Reverse Ball and Socket in 0RR
Revision
Correcting a portion of existing device *see* Revision of device in
Removal of device without replacement *see* Removal of device from
Replacement of existing device
see Removal of device from
see Root operation to place new device, e.g., Insertion, Replacement, Supplement
Revision of device in
Abdominal Wall 0WWF
Acetabulum
Left 0QW5
Right 0QW4
Anal Sphincter 0DWR
Anus 0DWQ
Artery
Lower 04WY
Upper 03WY
Auditory Ossicle
Left 09WA
Right 09W9
Back
Lower 0WWL
Upper 0WWK
Bladder 0TWB
Bone
Facial 0NWW
Lower 0QWY
Nasal 0NWB
Pelvic
Left 0QW3
Right 0QW2
Upper 0PWY
Bone Marrow 07WT
Brain 00W0
Breast
Left 0HWU
Right 0HWT
Bursa and Ligament
Lower 0MWY
Upper 0MWX
Carpal
Left 0PWN
Right 0PWM
Cavity, Cranial 0WW1
Cerebral Ventricle 00W6
Chest Wall 0WW8
Cisterna Chyli 07WL
Clavicle
Left 0PWB
Right 0PW9
Coccyx 0QWS
Diaphragm 0BWT
Disc
Cervical Vertebral 0RW3
Cervicothoracic Vertebral 0RW5
Lumbar Vertebral 0SW2
Lumbosacral 0SW4
Thoracic Vertebral 0RW9
Thoracolumbar Vertebral 0RWB

Revision of device in — *continued*
Duct
Hepatobiliary 0FWB
Pancreatic 0FWD
Ear
Inner
Left 09WE
Right 09WD
Left 09WJ
Right 09WH
Epididymis and Spermatic Cord 0VWM
Esophagus 0DW5
Extremity
Lower
Left 0YWB
Right 0YW9
Upper
Left 0XW7
Right 0XW6
Eye
Left 08W1
Right 08W0
Face 0WW2
Fallopian Tube 0UW8
Femoral Shaft
Left 0QW9
Right 0QW8
Femur
Lower
Left 0QWC
Right 0QWB
Upper
Left 0QW7
Right 0QW6
Fibula
Left 0QWK
Right 0QWJ
Finger Nail 0HWQX
Gallbladder 0FW4
Gastrointestinal Tract 0WWP
Genitourinary Tract 0WWR
Gland
Adrenal 0GW5
Endocrine 0GWS
Pituitary 0GW0
Salivary 0CWA
Glenoid Cavity
Left 0PW8
Right 0PW7
Great Vessel 02WY
Hair 0HWSX
Head 0WW0
Heart 02WA
Humeral Head
Left 0PWD
Right 0PWC
Humeral Shaft
Left 0PWG
Right 0PWF
Intestinal Tract
Lower 0DWD
Upper 0DW0
Intestine
Large 0DWE
Small 0DW8
Jaw
Lower 0WW5
Upper 0WW4
Joint
Acromioclavicular
Left 0RWH
Right 0RWG
Ankle
Left 0SWG
Right 0SWF
Carpal
Left 0RWR

Revision of device in — *continued*
Joint — *continued*
Right 0RWQ
Carpometacarpal
Left 0RWT
Right 0RWS
Cervical Vertebral 0RW1
Cervicothoracic Vertebral 0RW4
Coccygeal 0SW6
Elbow
Left 0RWM
Right 0RWL
Finger Phalangeal
Left 0RWX
Right 0RWW
Hip
Left 0SWB
Acetabular Surface 0SWE
Femoral Surface 0SWS
Right 0SW9
Acetabular Surface 0SWA
Femoral Surface 0SWR
Knee
Left 0SWD
Femoral Surface 0SWU
Tibial Surface 0SWW
Right 0SWC
Femoral Surface 0SWT
Tibial Surface 0SWV
Lumbar Vertebral 0SW0
Lumbosacral 0SW3
Metacarpophalangeal
Left 0RWV
Right 0RWU
Metatarsal-Phalangeal
Left 0SWN
Right 0SWM
Occipital-cervical 0RW0
Sacrococcygeal 0SW5
Sacroiliac
Left 0SW8
Right 0SW7
Shoulder
Left 0RWK
Right 0RWJ
Sternoclavicular
Left 0RWF
Right 0RWE
Tarsal
Left 0SWJ
Right 0SWH
Tarsometatarsal
Left 0SWL
Right 0SWK
Temporomandibular
Left 0RWD
Right 0RWC
Thoracic Vertebral 0RW6
Thoracolumbar Vertebral 0RWA
Toe Phalangeal
Left 0SWQ
Right 0SWP
Wrist
Left 0RWP
Right 0RWN
Kidney 0TW5
Larynx 0CWS
Lens
Left 08WK
Right 08WJ
Liver 0FW0
Lung
Left 0BWL
Right 0BWK
Lymphatic 07WN
Thoracic Duct 07WK
Mediastinum 0WWC

Revision of device in — *continued*
Mesentery 0DWV
Metacarpal
Left 0PWQ
Right 0PWP
Metatarsal
Left 0QWP
Right 0QWN
Mouth and Throat 0CWY
Muscle
Extraocular
Left 08WM
Right 08WL
Lower 0KWY
Upper 0KWX
Nasal Mucosa and Soft Tissue 09WK
Neck 0WW6
Nerve
Cranial 00WE
Peripheral 01WY
Omentum 0DWU
Ovary 0UW3
Pancreas 0FWG
Parathyroid Gland 0GWR
Patella
Left 0QWF
Right 0QWD
Pelvic Cavity 0WWJ
Penis 0VWS
Pericardial Cavity 0WWD
Perineum
Female 0WWN
Male 0WWM
Peritoneal Cavity 0WWG
Peritoneum 0DWW
Phalanx
Finger
Left 0PWV
Right 0PWT
Thumb
Left 0PWS
Right 0PWR
Toe
Left 0QWR
Right 0QWQ
Pineal Body 0GW1
Pleura 0BWQ
Pleural Cavity
Left 0WWB
Right 0WW9
Prostate and Seminal Vesicles 0VW4
Radius
Left 0PWJ
Right 0PWH
Respiratory Tract 0WWQ
Retroperitoneum 0WWH
Ribs
1 to 2 0PW1
3 or More 0PW2
Sacrum 0QW1
Scapula
Left 0PW6
Right 0PW5
Scrotum and Tunica Vaginalis 0VW8
Septum
Atrial 02W5
Ventricular 02WM
Sinus 09WY
Skin 0HWPX
Skull 0NW0
Spinal Canal 00WU
Spinal Cord 00WV
Spleen 07WP
Sternum 0PW0
Stomach 0DW6
Subcutaneous Tissue and Fascia
Head and Neck 0JWS

Revision of device in — *continued*
Subcutaneous Tissue and Fascia — *continued*
Lower Extremity 0JWW
Trunk 0JWT
Upper Extremity 0JWV
Tarsal
Left 0QWM
Right 0QWL
Tendon
Lower 0LWY
Upper 0LWX
Testis 0VWD
Thymus 07WM
Thyroid Gland 0GWK
Tibia
Left 0QWH
Right 0QWG
Toe Nail 0HWRX
Trachea 0BW1
Tracheobronchial Tree 0BW0
Tympanic Membrane
Left 09W8
Right 09W7
Ulna
Left 0PWL
Right 0PWK
Ureter 0TW9
Urethra 0TWD
Uterus and Cervix 0UWD
Vagina and Cul-de-sac 0UWH
Valve
Aortic 02WF
Mitral 02WG
Pulmonary 02WH
Tricuspid 02WJ
Vas Deferens 0VWR
Vein
Azygos 05W0
Innominate
Left 05W4
Right 05W3
Lower 06WY
Upper 05WY
Vertebra
Cervical 0PW3
Lumbar 0QW0
Thoracic 0PW4
Vulva 0UWM
Revo MRI™ SureScan® pacemaker
use Pacemaker, Dual Chamber in 0JH
rhBMP-2
use Recombinant Bone Morphogenetic Protein
Rheos® System device
use Stimulator Generator in Subcutaneous Tissue and Fascia
Rheos® System lead
use Stimulator Lead in Upper Arteries
Rhinopharynx
use Nasopharynx
Rhinoplasty
see Alteration, Nasal Mucosa and Soft Tissue 090K
see Repair, Nasal Mucosa and Soft Tissue 09QK
see Replacement, Nasal Mucosa and Soft Tissue 09RK
see Supplement, Nasal Mucosa and Soft Tissue 09UK
Rhinorrhaphy
see Repair, Nasal Mucosa and Soft Tissue 09QK
Rhinoscopy 09JKXZZ
Rhizotomy
see Division, Central Nervous System and Cranial Nerves 008
see Division, Peripheral Nervous System 018

Rhomboid major muscle
use Trunk Muscle, Right
use Trunk Muscle, Left
Rhomboid minor muscle
use Trunk Muscle, Right
use Trunk Muscle, Left
Rhythm electrocardiogram
see Measurement, Cardiac 4A02
Rhytidectomy
see Alteration, Face 0W02
Right ascending lumbar vein
use Azygos Vein
Right atrioventricular valve
use Tricuspid Valve
Right auricular appendix
use Atrium, Right
Right colic vein
use Colic Vein
Right coronary sulcus
use Heart, Right
Right gastric artery
use Gastric Artery
Right gastroepiploic vein
use Superior Mesenteric Vein
Right inferior phrenic vein
use Inferior Vena Cava
Right inferior pulmonary vein
use Pulmonary Vein, Right
Right jugular trunk
use Lymphatic, Right Neck
Right lateral ventricle
use Cerebral Ventricle
Right lymphatic duct
use Lymphatic, Right Neck
Right ovarian vein
use Inferior Vena Cava
Right second lumbar vein
use Inferior Vena Cava
Right subclavian trunk
use Lymphatic, Right Neck
Right subcostal vein
use Azygos Vein
Right superior pulmonary vein
use Pulmonary Vein, Right
Right suprarenal vein
use Inferior Vena Cava
Right testicular vein
use Inferior Vena Cava
Rima glottidis
use Larynx
Risorius muscle
use Facial Muscle
RNS® System lead
use Neurostimulator Lead in Central Nervous System and Cranial Nerves
RNS® system neurostimulator generator
use Neurostimulator Generator in Head and Facial Bones
Robotic assisted procedure
Extremity
Lower 8E0Y
Upper 8E0X
Head and Neck Region 8E09
Trunk Region 8E0W
Robotic waterjet ablation, destruction, prostate XV508A4
Rotation of fetal head
Forceps 10S07ZZ
Manual 10S0XZZ
Round ligament of uterus
use Uterine Supporting Structure
Round window
use Inner Ear, Right
use Inner Ear, Left
Roux-en-Y operation
see Bypass, Gastrointestinal System 0D1

Roux-en-Y operation — *continued*
see Bypass, Hepatobiliary System and Pancreas 0F1
Rupture
Adhesions *see* Release
Fluid collection *see* Drainage

S

Sacral ganglion
use Sacral Sympathetic Nerve
Sacral lymph node
use Lymphatic, Pelvis
Sacral nerve modulation (SNM) lead
use Stimulator Lead in Urinary System
Sacral neuromodulation lead
use Stimulator Lead in Urinary System
Sacral splanchnic nerve
use Sacral Sympathetic Nerve
Sacrectomy
see Excision, Lower Bones 0QB
Sacrococcygeal ligament
use Lower Spine Bursa and Ligament
Sacrococcygeal symphysis
use Sacrococcygeal Joint
Sacroiliac ligament
use Lower Spine Bursa and Ligament
Sacrospinous ligament
use Lower Spine Bursa and Ligament
Sacrotuberous ligament
use Lower Spine Bursa and Ligament
Salpingectomy
see Excision, Female Reproductive System 0UB
see Resection, Female Reproductive System 0UT
Salpingolysis
see Release, Female Reproductive System 0UN
Salpingopexy
see Repair, Female Reproductive System 0UQ
see Reposition, Female Reproductive System 0US
Salpingopharyngeus muscle
use Tongue, Palate, Pharynx Muscle
Salpingoplasty
see Repair, Female Reproductive System 0UQ
see Supplement, Female Reproductive System 0UU
Salpingorrhaphy
see Repair, Female Reproductive System 0UQ
Salpingoscopy 0UJ88ZZ
Salpingostomy
see Drainage, Female Reproductive System 0U9
Salpingotomy
see Drainage, Female Reproductive System 0U9
Salpinx
use Fallopian Tube, Right
use Fallopian Tube, Left
Saphenous nerve
use Femoral Nerve
SAPIEN® transcatheter aortic valve
use Zooplastic Tissue in Heart and Great Vessels
Sartorius muscle
use Upper Leg Muscle, Right
use Upper Leg Muscle, Left
Scalene muscle
use Neck Muscle, Right
use Neck Muscle, Left
Scan
Computerized Tomography (CT) *see* Computerized Tomography (CT Scan)
Radioisotope *see* Planar Nuclear Medicine Imaging
Scaphoid bone
use Carpal, Right
use Carpal, Left
Scapholunate ligament
use Hand Bursa and Ligament, Right
use Hand Bursa and Ligament, Left
Scaphotrapezium ligament
use Hand Bursa and Ligament, Right
use Hand Bursa and Ligament, Left
Scapulectomy
see Excision, Upper Bones 0PB
see Resection, Upper Bones 0PT
Scapulopexy
see Repair, Upper Bones 0PQ
see Reposition, Upper Bones 0PS
Scarpa's (vestibular) ganglion
use Acoustic Nerve
Sclerectomy
see Excision, Eye 08B
Sclerotherapy, mechanical
see Destruction
Sclerotherapy, via injection of sclerosing agent
see Introduction, Destructive Agent
Sclerotomy
see Drainage, Eye 089
Scrotectomy
see Excision, Male Reproductive System 0VB
see Resection, Male Reproductive System 0VT
Scrotoplasty
see Repair, Male Reproductive System 0VQ
see Supplement, Male Reproductive System 0VU
Scrotorrhaphy
see Repair, Male Reproductive System 0VQ
Scrototomy
see Drainage, Male Reproductive System 0V9
Sebaceous gland
use Skin
Second cranial nerve
use Optic Nerve
Section, cesarean
see Extraction, Pregnancy 10D
Secura™ (DR) (VR)
use Defibrillator Generator in 0JH
Sella turcica
use Sphenoid Bone
Semicircular canal
use Inner Ear, Right
use Inner Ear, Left
Semimembranosus muscle
use Upper Leg Muscle, Right
use Upper Leg Muscle, Left
Semitendinosus muscle
use Upper Leg Muscle, Right
use Upper Leg Muscle, Left
Seprafilm®
use Adhesion Barrier
Septal cartilage
use Nasal Septum
Septectomy
see Excision, Heart and Great Vessels 02B
see Resection, Heart and Great Vessels 02T
see Excision, Ear, Nose, Sinus 09B
see Resection, Ear, Nose, Sinus 09T
Septoplasty
see Repair, Heart and Great Vessels 02Q
see Replacement, Heart and Great Vessels 02R
Septoplasty — *continued*
see Supplement, Heart and Great Vessels 02U
see Repair, Ear, Nose, Sinus 09Q
see Replacement, Ear, Nose, Sinus 09R
see Reposition, Ear, Nose, Sinus 09S
see Supplement, Ear, Nose, Sinus 09U
Septostomy, balloon atrial 02163Z7
Septotomy
see Drainage, Ear, Nose, Sinus 099
Sequestrectomy, bone
see Extirpation
Serratus anterior muscle
use Thorax Muscle, Right
use Thorax Muscle, Left
Serratus posterior muscle
use Trunk Muscle, Right
use Trunk Muscle, Left
Seventh cranial nerve
use Facial Nerve
Sheffield hybrid external fixator
use External Fixation Device, Hybrid in 0PH
use External Fixation Device, Hybrid in 0PS
use External Fixation Device, Hybrid in 0QH
use External Fixation Device, Hybrid in 0QS
Sheffield ring external fixator
use External Fixation Device, Ring in 0PH
use External Fixation Device, Ring in 0PS
use External Fixation Device, Ring in 0QH
use External Fixation Device, Ring in 0QS
Shirodkar cervical cerclage 0UVC7ZZ
Shock wave therapy, musculoskeletal 6A93
Short gastric artery
use Splenic Artery
Shortening
see Excision
see Repair
see Reposition
Shunt creation
see Bypass
Sialoadenectomy
Complete *see* Resection, Mouth and Throat 0CT
Partial *see* Excision, Mouth and Throat 0CB
Sialodochoplasty
see Repair, Mouth and Throat 0CQ
see Replacement, Mouth and Throat 0CR
see Supplement, Mouth and Throat 0CU
Sialectomy
see Excision, Mouth and Throat 0CB
see Resection, Mouth and Throat 0CT
Sialography
see Plain Radiography, Ear, Nose, Mouth and Throat B90
Sialolithotomy
see Extirpation, Mouth and Throat 0CC
Sigmoid artery
use Inferior Mesenteric Artery
Sigmoid flexure
use Sigmoid Colon
Sigmoid vein
use Inferior Mesenteric Vein
Sigmoidectomy
see Excision, Gastrointestinal System 0DB
see Resection, Gastrointestinal System 0DT
Sigmoidorrhaphy
see Repair, Gastrointestinal System 0DQ
Sigmoidoscopy 0DJD8ZZ
Sigmoidotomy
see Drainage, Gastrointestinal System 0D9
Single lead pacemaker (atrium)(ventricle)
use Pacemaker, Single Chamber in 0JH
Single lead rate responsive pacemaker (atrium)(ventricle)
use Pacemaker, Single Chamber Rate Responsive in 0JH

Sinoatrial node
use Conduction Mechanism
Sinogram
Abdominal Wall *see* Fluoroscopy, Abdomen and Pelvis BW11
Chest Wall *see* Plain Radiography, Chest BW03
Retroperitoneum *see* Fluoroscopy, Abdomen and Pelvis BW11
Sinus venosus
use Atrium, Right
Sinusectomy
see Excision, Ear, Nose, Sinus 09B
see Resection, Ear, Nose, Sinus 09T
Sinusoscopy 09JY4ZZ
Sinusotomy
see Drainage, Ear, Nose, Sinus 099
Sirolimus-eluting coronary stent
use Intraluminal Device, Drug-eluting in Heart and Great Vessels
Sixth cranial nerve
use Abducens Nerve
Size reduction, breast
see Excision, Skin and Breast 0HB
SJM Biocor® Stented Valve System
use Zooplastic Tissue in Heart and Great Vessels
Skene's (paraurethral) gland
use Vestibular Gland
Skin substitute, porcine liver derived, replacement XHRPXL2
Sling
Fascial, orbicularis muscle (mouth) *see* Supplement, Muscle, Facial 0KU1
Levator muscle, for urethral suspension *see* Reposition, Bladder Neck 0TSC
Pubococcygeal, for urethral suspension *see* Reposition, Bladder Neck 0TSC
Rectum *see* Reposition, Rectum 0DSP
Small bowel series
see Fluoroscopy, Bowel, Small BD13
Small saphenous vein
use Saphenous Vein, Right
use Saphenous Vein, Left
Snaring, polyp, colon
see Excision, Gastrointestinal System 0DB
Solar (celiac) plexus
use Abdominal Sympathetic Nerve
Soleus muscle
use Lower Leg Muscle, Right
use Lower Leg Muscle, Left
Spacer
Insertion of device in
Disc
Lumbar Vertebral 0SH2
Lumbosacral 0SH4
Joint
Acromioclavicular
Left 0RHH
Right 0RHG
Ankle
Left 0SHG
Right 0SHF
Carpal
Left 0RHR
Right 0RHQ
Carpometacarpal
Left 0RHT
Right 0RHS
Cervical Vertebral 0RH1
Cervicothoracic Vertebral 0RH4
Coccygeal 0SH6
Elbow
Left 0RHM
Right 0RHL
Finger Phalangeal
Left 0RHX
Spacer — *continued*
Insertion of device in — *continued*
Right 0RHW
Hip
Left 0SHB
Right 0SH9
Knee
Left 0SHD
Right 0SHC
Lumbar Vertebral 0SH0
Lumbosacral 0SH3
Metacarpophalangeal
Left 0RHV
Right 0RHU
Metatarsal-Phalangeal
Left 0SHN
Right 0SHM
Occipital-cervical 0RH0
Sacrococcygeal 0SH5
Sacroiliac
Left 0SH8
Right 0SH7
Shoulder
Left 0RHK
Right 0RHJ
Sternoclavicular
Left 0RHF
Right 0RHE
Tarsal
Left 0SHJ
Right 0SHH
Tarsometatarsal
Left 0SHL
Right 0SHK
Temporomandibular
Left 0RHD
Right 0RHC
Thoracic Vertebral 0RH6
Thoracolumbar Vertebral 0RHA
Toe Phalangeal
Left 0SHQ
Right 0SHP
Wrist
Left 0RHP
Right 0RHN
Removal of device from
Acromioclavicular
Left 0RPH
Right 0RPG
Ankle
Left 0SPG
Right 0SPF
Carpal
Left 0RPR
Right 0RPQ
Carpometacarpal
Left 0RPT
Right 0RPS
Cervical Vertebral 0RP1
Cervicothoracic Vertebral 0RP4
Coccygeal 0SP6
Elbow
Left 0RPM
Right 0RPL
Finger Phalangeal
Left 0RPX
Right 0RPW
Hip
Left 0SPB
Right 0SP9
Knee
Left 0SPD
Right 0SPC
Lumbar Vertebral 0SP0
Lumbosacral 0SP3
Metacarpophalangeal
Left 0RPV
Spacer — *continued*
Removal of device from — *continued*
Right 0RPU
Metatarsal-Phalangeal
Left 0SPN
Right 0SPM
Occipital-cervical 0RP0
Sacrococcygeal 0SP5
Sacroiliac
Left 0SP8
Right 0SP7
Shoulder
Left 0RPK
Right 0RPJ
Sternoclavicular
Left 0RPF
Right 0RPE
Tarsal
Left 0SPJ
Right 0SPH
Tarsometatarsal
Left 0SPL
Right 0SPK
Temporomandibular
Left 0RPD
Right 0RPC
Thoracic Vertebral 0RP6
Thoracolumbar Vertebral 0RPA
Toe Phalangeal
Left 0SPQ
Right 0SPP
Wrist
Left 0RPP
Right 0RPN
Revision of device in
Acromioclavicular
Left 0RWH
Right 0RWG
Ankle
Left 0SWG
Right 0SWF
Carpal
Left 0RWR
Right 0RWQ
Carpometacarpal
Left 0RWT
Right 0RWS
Cervical Vertebral 0RW1
Cervicothoracic Vertebral 0RW4
Coccygeal 0SW6
Elbow
Left 0RWM
Right 0RWL
Finger Phalangeal
Left 0RWX
Right 0RWW
Hip
Left 0SWB
Right 0SW9
Knee
Left 0SWD
Right 0SWC
Lumbar Vertebral 0SW0
Lumbosacral 0SW3
Metacarpophalangeal
Left 0RWV
Right 0RWU
Metatarsal-Phalangeal
Left 0SWN
Right 0SWM
Occipital-cervical 0RW0
Sacrococcygeal 0SW5
Sacroiliac
Left 0SW8
Right 0SW7
Shoulder
Left 0RWK

Spacer — *continued*
Revision of device in — *continued*
Right 0RWJ
Sternoclavicular
Left 0RWF
Right 0RWE
Tarsal
Left 0SWJ
Right 0SWH
Tarsometatarsal
Left 0SWL
Right 0SWK
Temporomandibular
Left 0RWD
Right 0RWC
Thoracic Vertebral 0RW6
Thoracolumbar Vertebral 0RWA
Toe Phalangeal
Left 0SWQ
Right 0SWP
Wrist
Left 0RWP
Right 0RWN
Spacer, articulating (antibiotic)
use Articulating Spacer in Lower Joints
Spacer, static (antibiotic)
use Spacer in Lower Joints
Spectroscopy
Intravascular 8E023DZ
Near infrared 8E023DZ
Speech assessment F00
Speech therapy
see Speech Treatment, Rehabilitation F06
Speech treatment F06
Sphenoidectomy
see Excision, Ear, Nose, Sinus 09B
see Resection, Ear, Nose, Sinus 09T
see Excision, Head and Facial Bones 0NB
see Resection, Head and Facial Bones 0NT
Sphenoidotomy
see Drainage, Ear, Nose, Sinus 099
Sphenomandibular ligament
use Head and Neck Bursa and Ligament
Sphenopalatine (pterygopalatine) ganglion
use Head and Neck Sympathetic Nerve
Sphincterorrhaphy, anal
see Repair, Anal Sphincter 0DQR
Sphincterotomy, anal
see Division, Anal Sphincter 0D8R
see Drainage, Anal Sphincter 0D9R
Spinal cord neurostimulator lead
use Neurostimulator Lead in Central Nervous System and Cranial Nerves
Spinal growth rods, magnetically controlled
use Magnetically Controlled Growth Rod(s) in New Technology
Spinal nerve, cervical
use Cervical Nerve
Spinal nerve, lumbar
use Lumbar Nerve
Spinal nerve, sacral
use Sacral Nerve
Spinal nerve, thoracic
use Thoracic Nerve
Spinal stabilization device
Facet Replacement
Cervical Vertebral 0RH1
Cervicothoracic Vertebral 0RH4
Lumbar Vertebral 0SH0
Lumbosacral 0SH3
Occipital-cervical 0RH0
Thoracic Vertebral 0RH6
Thoracolumbar Vertebral 0RHA
Interspinous Process
Cervical Vertebral 0RH1
Spinal stabilization device — *continued*
Interspinous Process — *continued*
Cervicothoracic Vertebral 0RH4
Lumbar Vertebral 0SH0
Lumbosacral 0SH3
Occipital-cervical 0RH0
Thoracic Vertebral 0RH6
Thoracolumbar Vertebral 0RHA
Pedicle-Based
Cervical Vertebral 0RH1
Cervicothoracic Vertebral 0RH4
Lumbar Vertebral 0SH0
Lumbosacral 0SH3
Occipital-cervical 0RH0
Thoracic Vertebral 0RH6
Thoracolumbar Vertebral 0RHA
Spinous process
use Cervical Vertebra
use Thoracic Vertebra
use Lumbar Vertebra
Spiral ganglion
use Acoustic Nerve
Spiration IBV™ Valve System
use Intraluminal Device, Endobronchial Valve in Respiratory System
Splenectomy
see Excision, Lymphatic and Hemic Systems 07B
see Resection, Lymphatic and Hemic Systems 07T
Splenic flexure
use Transverse Colon
Splenic plexus
use Abdominal Sympathetic Nerve
Splenius capitis muscle
use Head Muscle
Splenius cervicis muscle
use Neck Muscle, Right
use Neck Muscle, Left
Splenolysis
see Release, Lymphatic and Hemic Systems 07N
Splenopexy
see Repair, Lymphatic and Hemic Systems 07Q
see Reposition, Lymphatic and Hemic Systems 07S
Splenoplasty
see Repair, Lymphatic and Hemic Systems 07Q
Splenorrhaphy
see Repair, Lymphatic and Hemic Systems 07Q
Splenotomy
see Drainage, Lymphatic and Hemic Systems 079
Splinting, musculoskeletal
see Immobilization, Anatomical Regions 2W3
SPY system intravascular fluorescence angiography
see Monitoring, Physiological Systems 4A1
Stapedectomy
see Excision, Ear, Nose, Sinus 09B
see Resection, Ear, Nose, Sinus 09T
Stapediolysis
see Release, Ear, Nose, Sinus 09N
Stapedioplasty
see Repair, Ear, Nose, Sinus 09Q
see Replacement, Ear, Nose, Sinus 09R
see Supplement, Ear, Nose, Sinus 09U
Stapedotomy
see Drainage, Ear, Nose, Sinus 099
Stapes
use Auditory Ossicle, Right
use Auditory Ossicle, Left
Static spacer (antibiotic)
use Spacer in Lower Joints
STELARA®
use Other New Technology Therapeutic Substance
Stellate ganglion
use Head and Neck Sympathetic Nerve
Stem cell transplant
see Transfusion, Circulatory 302
Stensen's duct
use Parotid Duct, Right
use Parotid Duct, Left
Stent retriever thrombectomy
see Extirpation, Upper Arteries 03C
Stent, intraluminal (cardiovascular)(gastrointestinal)(hepatobiliary)(urinary)
use Intraluminal Device
Stented tissue valve
use Zooplastic Tissue in Heart and Great Vessels
Stereotactic radiosurgery
Abdomen DW23
Adrenal Gland DG22
Bile Ducts DF22
Bladder DT22
Bone Marrow D720
Brain D020
Brain Stem D021
Breast
Left DM20
Right DM21
Bronchus DB21
Cervix DU21
Chest DW22
Chest Wall DB27
Colon DD25
Diaphragm DB28
Duodenum DD22
Ear D920
Esophagus DD20
Eye D820
Gallbladder DF21
Gamma Beam
Abdomen DW23JZZ
Adrenal Gland DG22JZZ
Bile Ducts DF22JZZ
Bladder DT22JZZ
Bone Marrow D720JZZ
Brain D020JZZ
Brain Stem D021JZZ
Breast
Left DM20JZZ
Right DM21JZZ
Bronchus DB21JZZ
Cervix DU21JZZ
Chest DW22JZZ
Chest Wall DB27JZZ
Colon DD25JZZ
Diaphragm DB28JZZ
Duodenum DD22JZZ
Ear D920JZZ
Esophagus DD20JZZ
Eye D820JZZ
Gallbladder DF21JZZ
Gland
Adrenal DG22JZZ
Parathyroid DG24JZZ
Pituitary DG20JZZ
Thyroid DG25JZZ
Glands, Salivary D926JZZ
Head and Neck DW21JZZ
Ileum DD24JZZ
Jejunum DD23JZZ
Kidney DT20JZZ
Larynx D92BJZZ
Liver DF20JZZ
Lung DB22JZZ

Stereotactic radiosurgery — *continued*
Gamma Beam — *continued*
Lymphatics
Abdomen D726JZZ
Axillary D724JZZ
Inguinal D728JZZ
Neck D723JZZ
Pelvis D727JZZ
Thorax D725JZZ
Mediastinum DB26JZZ
Mouth D924JZZ
Nasopharynx D92DJZZ
Neck and Head DW21JZZ
Nerve, Peripheral D027JZZ
Nose D921JZZ
Ovary DU20JZZ
Palate
Hard D928JZZ
Soft D929JZZ
Pancreas DF23JZZ
Parathyroid Gland DG24JZZ
Pelvic Region DW26JZZ
Pharynx D92CJZZ
Pineal Body DG21JZZ
Pituitary Gland DG20JZZ
Pleura DB25JZZ
Prostate DV20JZZ
Rectum DD27JZZ
Sinuses D927JZZ
Spinal Cord D026JZZ
Spleen D722JZZ
Stomach DD21JZZ
Testis DV21JZZ
Thymus D721JZZ
Thyroid Gland DG25JZZ
Tongue D925JZZ
Trachea DB20JZZ
Ureter DT21JZZ
Urethra DT23JZZ
Uterus DU22JZZ
Gland
Adrenal DG22
Parathyroid DG24
Pituitary DG20
Thyroid DG25
Glands, Salivary D926
Head and Neck DW21
Ileum DD24
Jejunum DD23
Kidney DT20
Larynx D92B
Liver DF20
Lung DB22
Lymphatics
Abdomen D726
Axillary D724
Inguinal D728
Neck D723
Pelvis D727
Thorax D725
Mediastinum DB26
Mouth D924
Nasopharynx D92D
Neck and Head DW21
Nerve, Peripheral D027
Nose D921
Other Photon
Abdomen DW23DZZ
Adrenal Gland DG22DZZ
Bile Ducts DF22DZZ
Bladder DT22DZZ
Bone Marrow D720DZZ
Brain D020DZZ
Brain Stem D021DZZ
Breast
Left DM20DZZ
Right DM21DZZ

Stereotactic radiosurgery — *continued*
Other Photon — *continued*
Bronchus DB21DZZ
Cervix DU21DZZ
Chest DW22DZZ
Chest Wall DB27DZZ
Colon DD25DZZ
Diaphragm DB28DZZ
Duodenum DD22DZZ
Ear D920DZZ
Esophagus DD20DZZ
Eye D820DZZ
Gallbladder DF21DZZ
Gland
Adrenal DG22DZZ
Parathyroid DG24DZZ
Pituitary DG20DZZ
Thyroid DG25DZZ
Glands, Salivary D926DZZ
Head and Neck DW21DZZ
Ileum DD24DZZ
Jejunum DD23DZZ
Kidney DT20DZZ
Larynx D92BDZZ
Liver DF20DZZ
Lung DB22DZZ
Lymphatics
Abdomen D726DZZ
Axillary D724DZZ
Inguinal D728DZZ
Neck D723DZZ
Pelvis D727DZZ
Thorax D725DZZ
Mediastinum DB26DZZ
Mouth D924DZZ
Nasopharynx D92DDZZ
Neck and Head DW21DZZ
Nerve, Peripheral D027DZZ
Nose D921DZZ
Ovary DU20DZZ
Palate
Hard D928DZZ
Soft D929DZZ
Pancreas DF23DZZ
Parathyroid Gland DG24DZZ
Pelvic Region DW26DZZ
Pharynx D92CDZZ
Pineal Body DG21DZZ
Pituitary Gland DG20DZZ
Pleura DB25DZZ
Prostate DV20DZZ
Rectum DD27DZZ
Sinuses D927DZZ
Spinal Cord D026DZZ
Spleen D722DZZ
Stomach DD21DZZ
Testis DV21DZZ
Thymus D721DZZ
Thyroid Gland DG25DZZ
Tongue D925DZZ
Trachea DB20DZZ
Ureter DT21DZZ
Urethra DT23DZZ
Uterus DU22DZZ
Ovary DU20
Palate
Hard D928
Soft D929
Pancreas DF23
Parathyroid Gland DG24
Particulate
Abdomen DW23HZZ
Adrenal Gland DG22HZZ
Bile Ducts DF22HZZ
Bladder DT22HZZ
Bone Marrow D720HZZ
Brain D020HZZ

Stereotactic radiosurgery — *continued*
Particulate — *continued*
Brain Stem D021HZZ
Breast
Left DM20HZZ
Right DM21HZZ
Bronchus DB21HZZ
Cervix DU21HZZ
Chest DW22HZZ
Chest Wall DB27HZZ
Colon DD25HZZ
Diaphragm DB28HZZ
Duodenum DD22HZZ
Ear D920HZZ
Esophagus DD20HZZ
Eye D820HZZ
Gallbladder DF21HZZ
Gland
Adrenal DG22HZZ
Parathyroid DG24HZZ
Pituitary DG20HZZ
Thyroid DG25HZZ
Glands, Salivary D926HZZ
Head and Neck DW21HZZ
Ileum DD24HZZ
Jejunum DD23HZZ
Kidney DT20HZZ
Larynx D92BHZZ
Liver DF20HZZ
Lung DB22HZZ
Lymphatics
Abdomen D726HZZ
Axillary D724HZZ
Inguinal D728HZZ
Neck D723HZZ
Pelvis D727HZZ
Thorax D725HZZ
Mediastinum DB26HZZ
Mouth D924HZZ
Nasopharynx D92DHZZ
Neck and Head DW21HZZ
Nerve, Peripheral D027HZZ
Nose D921HZZ
Ovary DU20HZZ
Palate
Hard D928HZZ
Soft D929HZZ
Pancreas DF23HZZ
Parathyroid Gland DG24HZZ
Pelvic Region DW26HZZ
Pharynx D92CHZZ
Pineal Body DG21HZZ
Pituitary Gland DG20HZZ
Pleura DB25HZZ
Prostate DV20HZZ
Rectum DD27HZZ
Sinuses D927HZZ
Spinal Cord D026HZZ
Spleen D722HZZ
Stomach DD21HZZ
Testis DV21HZZ
Thymus D721HZZ
Thyroid Gland DG25HZZ
Tongue D925HZZ
Trachea DB20HZZ
Ureter DT21HZZ
Urethra DT23HZZ
Uterus DU22HZZ
Pelvic Region DW26
Pharynx D92C
Pineal Body DG21
Pituitary Gland DG20
Pleura DB25
Prostate DV20
Rectum DD27
Sinuses D927
Spinal Cord D026

Stereotactic radiosurgery — *continued*
Spleen D722
Stomach DD21
Testis DV21
Thymus D721
Thyroid Gland DG25
Tongue D925
Trachea DB20
Ureter DT21
Urethra DT23
Uterus DU22
Sternoclavicular ligament
use Shoulder Bursa and Ligament, Right
use Shoulder Bursa and Ligament, Left
Sternocleidomastoid artery
use Thyroid Artery, Right
use Thyroid Artery, Left
Sternocleidomastoid muscle
use Neck Muscle, Right
use Neck Muscle, Left
Sternocostal ligament
use Sternum Bursa and Ligament
Sternotomy
see Division, Sternum 0P80
see Drainage, Sternum 0P90
Stimulation, cardiac
Cardioversion 5A2204Z
Electrophysiologic testing *see* Measurement, Cardiac 4A02
Stimulator generator
Insertion of device in
Abdomen 0JH8
Back 0JH7
Chest 0JH6
Multiple Array
Abdomen 0JH8
Back 0JH7
Chest 0JH6
Multiple Array Rechargeable
Abdomen 0JH8
Back 0JH7
Chest 0JH6
Removal of device from, Subcutaneous Tissue and Fascia, Trunk 0JPT
Revision of device in, Subcutaneous Tissue and Fascia, Trunk 0JWT
Single Array
Abdomen 0JH8
Back 0JH7
Chest 0JH6
Single Array Rechargeable
Abdomen 0JH8
Back 0JH7
Chest 0JH6
Stimulator lead
Insertion of device in
Anal Sphincter 0DHR
Artery
Left 03HL
Right 03HK
Bladder 0THB
Muscle
Lower 0KHY
Upper 0KHX
Stomach 0DH6
Ureter 0TH9
Removal of device from
Anal Sphincter 0DPR
Artery, Upper 03PY
Bladder 0TPB
Muscle
Lower 0KPY
Upper 0KPX
Stomach 0DP6
Ureter 0TP9
Revision of device in
Anal Sphincter 0DWR
Stimulator lead — *continued*
Revision of device in — *continued*
Artery, Upper 03WY
Bladder 0TWB
Muscle
Lower 0KWY
Upper 0KWX
Stomach 0DW6
Ureter 0TW9
Stoma
Excision
Abdominal Wall 0WBFXZ2
Neck 0WB6XZ2
Repair
Abdominal Wall 0WQFXZ2
Neck 0WQ6XZ2
Stomatoplasty
see Repair, Mouth and Throat 0CQ
see Replacement, Mouth and Throat 0CR
see Supplement, Mouth and Throat 0CU
Stomatorrhaphy
see Repair, Mouth and Throat 0CQ
Stratos LV®
use Cardiac Resynchronization Pacemaker Pulse Generator in 0JH
Stress test
4A02XM4
4A12XM4
Stripping
see Extraction
Study
Electrophysiologic stimulation, cardiac *see* Measurement, Cardiac 4A02
Ocular motility 4A07X7Z
Pulmonary airway flow measurement *see* Measurement, Respiratory 4A09
Visual acuity 4A07X0Z
Styloglossus muscle
use Tongue, Palate, Pharynx Muscle
Stylomandibular ligament
use Head and Neck Bursa and Ligament
Stylopharyngeus muscle
use Tongue, Palate, Pharynx Muscle
Subacromial bursa
use Shoulder Bursa and Ligament, Right
use Shoulder Bursa and Ligament, Left
Subaortic (common iliac) lymph node
use Lymphatic, Pelvis
Subarachnoid space, spinal
use Spinal Canal
Subclavicular (apical) lymph node
use Lymphatic, Right Axillary
use Lymphatic, Left Axillary
Subclavius muscle
use Thorax Muscle, Right
use Thorax Muscle, Left
Subclavius nerve
use Brachial Plexus
Subcostal artery
use Upper Artery
Subcostal muscle
use Thorax Muscle, Right
use Thorax Muscle, Left
Subcostal nerve
use Thoracic Nerve
Subcutaneous injection reservoir, port
use Vascular Access Device, Totally Implantable in Subcutaneous Tissue and Fascia
Subcutaneous injection reservoir, pump
use Infusion Device, Pump in Subcutaneous Tissue and Fascia
Subdermal progesterone implant
use Contraceptive Device in Subcutaneous Tissue and Fascia
Subdural space, spinal
use Spinal Canal
Submandibular ganglion
use Facial Nerve
use Head and Neck Sympathetic Nerve
Submandibular gland
use Submaxillary Gland, Right
use Submaxillary Gland, Left
Submandibular lymph node
use Lymphatic, Head
Submaxillary ganglion
use Head and Neck Sympathetic Nerve
Submaxillary lymph node
use Lymphatic, Head
Submental artery
use Face Artery
Submental lymph node
use Lymphatic, Head
Submucous (Meissner's) plexus
use Abdominal Sympathetic Nerve
Suboccipital nerve
use Cervical Nerve
Suboccipital venous plexus
use Vertebral Vein, Right
use Vertebral Vein, Left
Subparotid lymph node
use Lymphatic, Head
Subscapular (posterior) lymph node
use Lymphatic, Right Axillary
use Lymphatic, Left Axillary
Subscapular aponeurosis
use Subcutaneous Tissue and Fascia, Right Upper Arm
use Subcutaneous Tissue and Fascia, Left Upper Arm
Subscapular artery
use Axillary Artery, Right
use Axillary Artery, Left
Subscapularis muscle
use Shoulder Muscle, Right
use Shoulder Muscle, Left
Substance abuse treatment
Counseling
Family, for substance abuse, Other Family Counseling HZ63ZZZ
Group
12-Step HZ43ZZZ
Behavioral HZ41ZZZ
Cognitive HZ40ZZZ
Cognitive-Behavioral HZ42ZZZ
Confrontational HZ48ZZZ
Continuing Care HZ49ZZZ
Infectious Disease
Post-Test HZ4CZZZ
Pre-Test HZ4CZZZ
Interpersonal HZ44ZZZ
Motivational Enhancement HZ47ZZZ
Psychoeducation HZ46ZZZ
Spiritual HZ4BZZZ
Vocational HZ45ZZZ
Individual
12-Step HZ33ZZZ
Behavioral HZ31ZZZ
Cognitive HZ30ZZZ
Cognitive-Behavioral HZ32ZZZ
Confrontational HZ38ZZZ
Continuing Care HZ39ZZZ
Infectious Disease
Post-Test HZ3CZZZ
Pre-Test HZ3CZZZ
Interpersonal HZ34ZZZ
Motivational Enhancement HZ37ZZZ
Psychoeducation HZ36ZZZ
Spiritual HZ3BZZZ
Vocational HZ35ZZZ
Detoxification Services, for substance abuse HZ2ZZZZ

Substance abuse treatment — *continued*
Medication Management
Antabuse HZ83ZZZ
Bupropion HZ87ZZZ
Clonidine HZ86ZZZ
Levo-alpha-acetyl-methadol (LAAM) HZ82ZZZ
Methadone Maintenance HZ81ZZZ
Naloxone HZ85ZZZ
Naltrexone HZ84ZZZ
Nicotine Replacement HZ80ZZZ
Other Replacement Medication HZ89ZZZ
Psychiatric Medication HZ88ZZZ
Pharmacotherapy
Antabuse HZ93ZZZ
Bupropion HZ97ZZZ
Clonidine HZ96ZZZ
Levo-alpha-acetyl-methadol (LAAM) HZ92ZZZ
Methadone Maintenance HZ91ZZZ
Naloxone HZ95ZZZ
Naltrexone HZ94ZZZ
Nicotine Replacement HZ90ZZZ
Psychiatric Medication HZ98ZZZ
Replacement Medication, Other HZ99ZZZ
Psychotherapy
12-Step HZ53ZZZ
Behavioral HZ51ZZZ
Cognitive HZ50ZZZ
Cognitive-Behavioral HZ52ZZZ
Confrontational HZ58ZZZ
Interactive HZ55ZZZ
Interpersonal HZ54ZZZ
Motivational Enhancement HZ57ZZZ
Psychoanalysis HZ5BZZZ
Psychodynamic HZ5CZZZ
Psychoeducation HZ56ZZZ
Psychophysiological HZ5DZZZ
Supportive HZ59ZZZ
Substantia nigra
use Basal Ganglia
Subtalar (talocalcaneal) joint
use Tarsal Joint, Right
use Tarsal Joint, Left
Subtalar ligament
use Foot Bursa and Ligament, Right
use Foot Bursa and Ligament, Left
Subthalamic nucleus
use Basal Ganglia
Suction curettage (D&C), nonobstetric
see Extraction, Endometrium 0UDB
Suction curettage, obstetric post-delivery
see Extraction, Products of Conception, Retained 10D1
Superficial circumflex iliac vein
use Saphenous Vein, Right
use Saphenous Vein, Left
Superficial epigastric artery
use Femoral Artery, Right
use Femoral Artery, Left
Superficial epigastric vein
use Saphenous Vein, Right
use Saphenous Vein, Left
Superficial inferior epigastric artery flap
Replacement
Bilateral 0HRV078
Left 0HRU078
Right 0HRT078
Transfer
Left 0KXG
Right 0KXF
Superficial palmar arch
use Hand Artery, Right
use Hand Artery, Left
Superficial palmar venous arch
use Hand Vein, Right
use Hand Vein, Left
Superficial temporal artery
use Temporal Artery, Right
use Temporal Artery, Left
Superficial transverse perineal muscle
use Perineum Muscle
Superior cardiac nerve
use Thoracic Sympathetic Nerve
Superior cerebellar vein
use Intracranial Vein
Superior cerebral vein
use Intracranial Vein
Superior clunic (cluneal) nerve
use Lumbar Nerve
Superior epigastric artery
use Internal Mammary Artery, Right
use Internal Mammary Artery, Left
Superior genicular artery
use Popliteal Artery, Right
use Popliteal Artery, Left
Superior gluteal artery
use Internal Iliac Artery, Right
use Internal Iliac Artery, Left
Superior gluteal nerve
use Lumbar Plexus
Superior hypogastric plexus
use Abdominal Sympathetic Nerve
Superior labial artery
use Face Artery
Superior laryngeal artery
use Thyroid Artery, Right
use Thyroid Artery, Left
Superior laryngeal nerve
use Vagus Nerve
Superior longitudinal muscle
use Tongue, Palate, Pharynx Muscle
Superior mesenteric ganglion
use Abdominal Sympathetic Nerve
Superior mesenteric lymph node
use Lymphatic, Mesenteric
Superior mesenteric plexus
use Abdominal Sympathetic Nerve
Superior oblique muscle
use Extraocular Muscle, Right
use Extraocular Muscle, Left
Superior olivary nucleus
use Pons
Superior rectal artery
use Inferior Mesenteric Artery
Superior rectal vein
use Inferior Mesenteric Vein
Superior rectus muscle
use Extraocular Muscle, Right
use Extraocular Muscle, Left
Superior tarsal plate
use Upper Eyelid, Right
use Upper Eyelid, Left
Superior thoracic artery
use Axillary Artery, Right
use Axillary Artery, Left
Superior thyroid artery
use External Carotid Artery, Right
use External Carotid Artery, Left
use Thyroid Artery, Right
use Thyroid Artery, Left
Superior turbinate
use Nasal Turbinate
Superior ulnar collateral artery
use Brachial Artery, Right
use Brachial Artery, Left
Supersaturated oxygen therapy
5A0512C
5A0522C
Supplement
Abdominal Wall 0WUF
Supplement — *continued*
Acetabulum
Left 0QU5
Right 0QU4
Ampulla of Vater 0FUC
Anal Sphincter 0DUR
Ankle Region
Left 0YUL
Right 0YUK
Anus 0DUQ
Aorta
Abdominal 04U0
Thoracic
Ascending/Arch 02UX
Descending 02UW
Arm
Lower
Left 0XUF
Right 0XUD
Upper
Left 0XU9
Right 0XU8
Artery
Anterior Tibial
Left 04UQ
Right 04UP
Axillary
Left 03U6
Right 03U5
Brachial
Left 03U8
Right 03U7
Celiac 04U1
Colic
Left 04U7
Middle 04U8
Right 04U6
Common Carotid
Left 03UJ
Right 03UH
Common Iliac
Left 04UD
Right 04UC
External Carotid
Left 03UN
Right 03UM
External Iliac
Left 04UJ
Right 04UH
Face 03UR
Femoral
Left 04UL
Right 04UK
Foot
Left 04UW
Right 04UV
Gastric 04U2
Hand
Left 03UF
Right 03UD
Hepatic 04U3
Inferior Mesenteric 04UB
Innominate 03U2
Internal Carotid
Left 03UL
Right 03UK
Internal Iliac
Left 04UF
Right 04UE
Internal Mammary
Left 03U1
Right 03U0
Intracranial 03UG
Lower 04UY
Peroneal
Left 04UU
Right 04UT

Supplement — *continued*
Artery — *continued*
Popliteal
Left 04UN
Right 04UM
Posterior Tibial
Left 04US
Right 04UR
Pulmonary
Left 02UR
Right 02UQ
Pulmonary Trunk 02UP
Radial
Left 03UC
Right 03UB
Renal
Left 04UA
Right 04U9
Splenic 04U4
Subclavian
Left 03U4
Right 03U3
Superior Mesenteric 04U5
Temporal
Left 03UT
Right 03US
Thyroid
Left 03UV
Right 03UU
Ulnar
Left 03UA
Right 03U9
Upper 03UY
Vertebral
Left 03UQ
Right 03UP
Atrium
Left 02U7
Right 02U6
Auditory Ossicle
Left 09UA
Right 09U9
Axilla
Left 0XU5
Right 0XU4
Back
Lower 0WUL
Upper 0WUK
Bladder 0TUB
Bladder Neck 0TUC
Bone
Ethmoid
Left 0NUG
Right 0NUF
Frontal 0NU1
Hyoid 0NUX
Lacrimal
Left 0NUJ
Right 0NUH
Nasal 0NUB
Occipital 0NU7
Palatine
Left 0NUL
Right 0NUK
Parietal
Left 0NU4
Right 0NU3
Pelvic
Left 0QU3
Right 0QU2
Sphenoid 0NUC
Temporal
Left 0NU6
Right 0NU5
Zygomatic
Left 0NUN
Right 0NUM

Supplement — *continued*
Breast
Bilateral 0HUV
Left 0HUU
Right 0HUT
Bronchus
Lingula 0BU9
Lower Lobe
Left 0BUB
Right 0BU6
Main
Left 0BU7
Right 0BU3
Middle Lobe, Right 0BU5
Upper Lobe
Left 0BU8
Right 0BU4
Buccal Mucosa 0CU4
Bursa and Ligament
Abdomen
Left 0MUJ
Right 0MUH
Ankle
Left 0MUR
Right 0MUQ
Elbow
Left 0MU4
Right 0MU3
Foot
Left 0MUT
Right 0MUS
Hand
Left 0MU8
Right 0MU7
Head and Neck 0MU0
Hip
Left 0MUM
Right 0MUL
Knee
Left 0MUP
Right 0MUN
Lower Extremity
Left 0MUW
Right 0MUV
Perineum 0MUK
Rib(s) 0MUG
Shoulder
Left 0MU2
Right 0MU1
Spine
Lower 0MUD
Upper 0MUC
Sternum 0MUF
Upper Extremity
Left 0MUB
Right 0MU9
Wrist
Left 0MU6
Right 0MU5
Buttock
Left 0YU1
Right 0YU0
Carina 0BU2
Carpal
Left 0PUN
Right 0PUM
Cecum 0DUH
Cerebral Meninges 00U1
Cerebral Ventricle 00U6
Chest Wall 0WU8
Chordae Tendineae 02U9
Cisterna Chyli 07UL
Clavicle
Left 0PUB
Right 0PU9
Clitoris 0UUJ
Coccyx 0QUS

Supplement — *continued*
Colon
Ascending 0DUK
Descending 0DUM
Sigmoid 0DUN
Transverse 0DUL
Cord
Bilateral 0VUH
Left 0VUG
Right 0VUF
Cornea
Left 08U9
Right 08U8
Cul-de-sac 0UUF
Diaphragm 0BUT
Disc
Cervical Vertebral 0RU3
Cervicothoracic Vertebral 0RU5
Lumbar Vertebral 0SU2
Lumbosacral 0SU4
Thoracic Vertebral 0RU9
Thoracolumbar Vertebral 0RUB
Duct
Common Bile 0FU9
Cystic 0FU8
Hepatic
Common 0FU7
Left 0FU6
Right 0FU5
Lacrimal
Left 08UY
Right 08UX
Pancreatic 0FUD
Accessory 0FUF
Duodenum 0DU9
Dura Mater 00U2
Ear
External
Bilateral 09U2
Left 09U1
Right 09U0
Inner
Left 09UE
Right 09UD
Middle
Left 09U6
Right 09U5
Elbow Region
Left 0XUC
Right 0XUB
Epididymis
Bilateral 0VUL
Left 0VUK
Right 0VUJ
Epiglottis 0CUR
Esophagogastric Junction 0DU4
Esophagus 0DU5
Lower 0DU3
Middle 0DU2
Upper 0DU1
Extremity
Lower
Left 0YUB
Right 0YU9
Upper
Left 0XU7
Right 0XU6
Eye
Left 08U1
Right 08U0
Eyelid
Lower
Left 08UR
Right 08UQ
Upper
Left 08UP
Right 08UN

Supplement — *continued*
Face 0WU2
Fallopian Tube
Left 0UU6
Right 0UU5
Fallopian Tubes, Bilateral 0UU7
Femoral Region
Bilateral 0YUE
Left 0YU8
Right 0YU7
Femoral Shaft
Left 0QU9
Right 0QU8
Femur
Lower
Left 0QUC
Right 0QUB
Upper
Left 0QU7
Right 0QU6
Fibula
Left 0QUK
Right 0QUJ
Finger
Index
Left 0XUP
Right 0XUN
Little
Left 0XUW
Right 0XUV
Middle
Left 0XUR
Right 0XUQ
Ring
Left 0XUT
Right 0XUS
Foot
Left 0YUN
Right 0YUM
Gingiva
Lower 0CU6
Upper 0CU5
Glenoid Cavity
Left 0PU8
Right 0PU7
Hand
Left 0XUK
Right 0XUJ
Head 0WU0
Heart 02UA
Humeral Head
Left 0PUD
Right 0PUC
Humeral Shaft
Left 0PUG
Right 0PUF
Hymen 0UUK
Ileocecal Valve 0DUC
Ileum 0DUB
Inguinal Region
Bilateral 0YUA
Left 0YU6
Right 0YU5
Intestine
Large 0DUE
Left 0DUG
Right 0DUF
Small 0DU8
Iris
Left 08UD
Right 08UC
Jaw
Lower 0WU5
Upper 0WU4
Jejunum 0DUA

Supplement — *continued*
Joint
Acromioclavicular
Left 0RUH
Right 0RUG
Ankle
Left 0SUG
Right 0SUF
Carpal
Left 0RUR
Right 0RUQ
Carpometacarpal
Left 0RUT
Right 0RUS
Cervical Vertebral 0RU1
Cervicothoracic Vertebral 0RU4
Coccygeal 0SU6
Elbow
Left 0RUM
Right 0RUL
Finger Phalangeal
Left 0RUX
Right 0RUW
Hip
Left 0SUB
Acetabular Surface 0SUE
Femoral Surface 0SUS
Right 0SU9
Acetabular Surface 0SUA
Femoral Surface 0SUR
Knee
Left 0SUD
Femoral Surface 0SUU09Z
Tibial Surface 0SUW09Z
Right 0SUC
Femoral Surface 0SUT09Z
Tibial Surface 0SUV09Z
Lumbar Vertebral 0SU0
Lumbosacral 0SU3
Metacarpophalangeal
Left 0RUV
Right 0RUU
Metatarsal-Phalangeal
Left 0SUN
Right 0SUM
Occipital-cervical 0RU0
Sacrococcygeal 0SU5
Sacroiliac
Left 0SU8
Right 0SU7
Shoulder
Left 0RUK
Right 0RUJ
Sternoclavicular
Left 0RUF
Right 0RUE
Tarsal
Left 0SUJ
Right 0SUH
Tarsometatarsal
Left 0SUL
Right 0SUK
Temporomandibular
Left 0RUD
Right 0RUC
Thoracic Vertebral 0RU6
Thoracolumbar Vertebral 0RUA
Toe Phalangeal
Left 0SUQ
Right 0SUP
Wrist
Left 0RUP
Right 0RUN
Kidney Pelvis
Left 0TU4
Right 0TU3
Knee Region
Left 0YUG

Supplement — *continued*
Knee Region — *continued*
Right 0YUF
Larynx 0CUS
Leg
Lower
Left 0YUJ
Right 0YUH
Upper
Left 0YUD
Right 0YUC
Lip
Lower 0CU1
Upper 0CU0
Lymphatic
Aortic 07UD
Axillary
Left 07U6
Right 07U5
Head 07U0
Inguinal
Left 07UJ
Right 07UH
Internal Mammary
Left 07U9
Right 07U8
Lower Extremity
Left 07UG
Right 07UF
Mesenteric 07UB
Neck
Left 07U2
Right 07U1
Pelvis 07UC
Thoracic Duct 07UK
Thorax 07U7
Upper Extremity
Left 07U4
Right 07U3
Mandible
Left 0NUV
Right 0NUT
Maxilla 0NUR
Mediastinum 0WUC
Mesentery 0DUV
Metacarpal
Left 0PUQ
Right 0PUP
Metatarsal
Left 0QUP
Right 0QUN
Muscle
Abdomen
Left 0KUL
Right 0KUK
Extraocular
Left 08UM
Right 08UL
Facial 0KU1
Foot
Left 0KUW
Right 0KUV
Hand
Left 0KUD
Right 0KUC
Head 0KU0
Hip
Left 0KUP
Right 0KUN
Lower Arm and Wrist
Left 0KUB
Right 0KU9
Lower Leg
Left 0KUT
Right 0KUS
Neck
Left 0KU3

Supplement — *continued*
Muscle — *continued*
Right 0KU2
Papillary 02UD
Perineum 0KUM
Shoulder
Left 0KU6
Right 0KU5
Thorax
Left 0KUJ
Right 0KUH
Tongue, Palate, Pharynx 0KU4
Trunk
Left 0KUG
Right 0KUF
Upper Arm
Left 0KU8
Right 0KU7
Upper Leg
Left 0KUR
Right 0KUQ
Nasal Mucosa and Soft Tissue 09UK
Nasopharynx 09UN
Neck 0WU6
Nerve
Abducens 00UL
Accessory 00UR
Acoustic 00UN
Cervical 01U1
Facial 00UM
Femoral 01UD
Glossopharyngeal 00UP
Hypoglossal 00US
Lumbar 01UB
Median 01U5
Oculomotor 00UH
Olfactory 00UF
Optic 00UG
Peroneal 01UH
Phrenic 01U2
Pudendal 01UC
Radial 01U6
Sacral 01UR
Sciatic 01UF
Thoracic 01U8
Tibial 01UG
Trigeminal 00UK
Trochlear 00UJ
Ulnar 01U4
Vagus 00UQ
Nipple
Left 0HUX
Right 0HUW
Omentum 0DUU
Orbit
Left 0NUQ
Right 0NUP
Palate
Hard 0CU2
Soft 0CU3
Patella
Left 0QUF
Right 0QUD
Penis 0VUS
Pericardium 02UN
Perineum
Female 0WUN
Male 0WUM
Peritoneum 0DUW
Phalanx
Finger
Left 0PUV
Right 0PUT
Thumb
Left 0PUS
Right 0PUR

Supplement — *continued*
Phalanx — *continued*
Toe
Left 0QUR
Right 0QUQ
Pharynx 0CUM
Prepuce 0VUT
Radius
Left 0PUJ
Right 0PUH
Rectum 0DUP
Retina
Left 08UF
Right 08UE
Retinal Vessel
Left 08UH
Right 08UG
Ribs
1 to 2 0PU1
3 or More 0PU2
Sacrum 0QU1
Scapula
Left 0PU6
Right 0PU5
Scrotum 0VU5
Septum
Atrial 02U5
Nasal 09UM
Ventricular 02UM
Shoulder Region
Left 0XU3
Right 0XU2
Skull 0NU0
Spinal Meninges 00UT
Sternum 0PU0
Stomach 0DU6
Pylorus 0DU7
Subcutaneous Tissue and Fascia
Abdomen 0JU8
Back 0JU7
Buttock 0JU9
Chest 0JU6
Face 0JU1
Foot
Left 0JUR
Right 0JUQ
Hand
Left 0JUK
Right 0JUJ
Lower Arm
Left 0JUH
Right 0JUG
Lower Leg
Left 0JUP
Right 0JUN
Neck
Left 0JU5
Right 0JU4
Pelvic Region 0JUC
Perineum 0JUB
Scalp 0JU0
Upper Arm
Left 0JUF
Right 0JUD
Upper Leg
Left 0JUM
Right 0JUL
Tarsal
Left 0QUM
Right 0QUL
Tendon
Abdomen
Left 0LUG
Right 0LUF
Ankle
Left 0LUT
Right 0LUS

Supplement — *continued*
Tendon — *continued*
Foot
Left 0LUW
Right 0LUV
Hand
Left 0LU8
Right 0LU7
Head and Neck 0LU0
Hip
Left 0LUK
Right 0LUJ
Knee
Left 0LUR
Right 0LUQ
Lower Arm and Wrist
Left 0LU6
Right 0LU5
Lower Leg
Left 0LUP
Right 0LUN
Perineum 0LUH
Shoulder
Left 0LU2
Right 0LU1
Thorax
Left 0LUD
Right 0LUC
Trunk
Left 0LUB
Right 0LU9
Upper Arm
Left 0LU4
Right 0LU3
Upper Leg
Left 0LUM
Right 0LUL
Testis
Bilateral 0VUC0
Left 0VUB0
Right 0VU90
Thumb
Left 0XUM
Right 0XUL
Tibia
Left 0QUH
Right 0QUG
Toe
1st
Left 0YUQ
Right 0YUP
2nd
Left 0YUS
Right 0YUR
3rd
Left 0YUU
Right 0YUT
4th
Left 0YUW
Right 0YUV
5th
Left 0YUY
Right 0YUX
Tongue 0CU7
Trachea 0BU1
Tunica Vaginalis
Left 0VU7
Right 0VU6
Turbinate, Nasal 09UL
Tympanic Membrane
Left 09U8
Right 09U7
Ulna
Left 0PUL
Right 0PUK
Ureter
Left 0TU7
Right 0TU6

Supplement — *continued*
Urethra 0TUD
Uterine Supporting Structure 0UU4
Uvula 0CUN
Vagina 0UUG
Valve
Aortic 02UF
Mitral 02UG
Pulmonary 02UH
Tricuspid 02UJ
Vas Deferens
Bilateral 0VUQ
Left 0VUP
Right 0VUN
Vein
Axillary
Left 05U8
Right 05U7
Azygos 05U0
Basilic
Left 05UC
Right 05UB
Brachial
Left 05UA
Right 05U9
Cephalic
Left 05UF
Right 05UD
Colic 06U7
Common Iliac
Left 06UD
Right 06UC
Esophageal 06U3
External Iliac
Left 06UG
Right 06UF
External Jugular
Left 05UQ
Right 05UP
Face
Left 05UV
Right 05UT
Femoral
Left 06UN
Right 06UM
Foot
Left 06UV
Right 06UT
Gastric 06U2
Hand
Left 05UH
Right 05UG
Hemiazygos 05U1
Hepatic 06U4
Hypogastric
Left 06UJ
Right 06UH
Inferior Mesenteric 06U6
Innominate
Left 05U4
Right 05U3
Internal Jugular
Left 05UN
Right 05UM
Intracranial 05UL
Lower 06UY
Portal 06U8
Pulmonary
Left 02UT
Right 02US
Renal
Left 06UB
Right 06U9
Saphenous
Left 06UQ
Right 06UP
Splenic 06U1

Supplement — *continued*
Vein — *continued*
Subclavian
Left 05U6
Right 05U5
Superior Mesenteric 06U5
Upper 05UY
Vertebral
Left 05US
Right 05UR
Vena Cava
Inferior 06U0
Superior 02UV
Ventricle
Left 02UL
Right 02UK
Vertebra
Cervical 0PU3
Lumbar 0QU0
Thoracic 0PU4
Vesicle
Bilateral 0VU3
Left 0VU2
Right 0VU1
Vocal Cord
Left 0CUV
Right 0CUT
Vulva 0UUM
Wrist Region
Left 0XUH
Right 0XUG

Supraclavicular (Virchow's) lymph node
use Lymphatic, Right Neck
use Lymphatic, Left Neck

Supraclavicular nerve
use Cervical Plexus

Suprahyoid lymph node
use Lymphatic, Head

Suprahyoid muscle
use Neck Muscle, Right
use Neck Muscle, Left

Suprainguinal lymph node
use Lymphatic, Pelvis

Supraorbital vein
use Face Vein, Right
use Face Vein, Left

Suprarenal gland
use Adrenal Gland, Left
use Adrenal Gland, Right
use Adrenal Glands, Bilateral
use Adrenal Gland

Suprarenal plexus
use Abdominal Sympathetic Nerve

Suprascapular nerve
use Brachial Plexus

Supraspinatus fascia
use Subcutaneous Tissue and Fascia, Right Upper Arm
use Subcutaneous Tissue and Fascia, Left Upper Arm

Supraspinatus muscle
use Shoulder Muscle, Right
use Shoulder Muscle, Left

Supraspinous ligament
use Upper Spine Bursa and Ligament
use Lower Spine Bursa and Ligament

Suprasternal notch
use Sternum

Supratrochlear lymph node
use Lymphatic, Right Upper Extremity
use Lymphatic, Left Upper Extremity

Sural artery
use Popliteal Artery, Right
use Popliteal Artery, Left

Suspension
Bladder Neck *see* Reposition, Bladder Neck 0TSC

Suspension — *continued*
Kidney *see* Reposition, Urinary System 0TS
Urethra *see* Reposition, Urinary System 0TS
Urethrovesical *see* Reposition, Bladder Neck 0TSC
Uterus *see* Reposition, Uterus 0US9
Vagina *see* Reposition, Vagina 0USG

Suture
Laceration repair *see* Repair
Ligation *see* Occlusion

Suture removal
Extremity
Lower 8E0YXY8
Upper 8E0XXY8
Head and Neck Region 8E09XY8
Trunk Region 8E0WXY8

Sutureless valve, Perceval
use Zooplastic Tissue, Rapid Deployment Technique in New Technology

Sweat gland
use Skin

Sympathectomy
see Excision, Peripheral Nervous System 01B

SynCardia™ Total Artificial Heart
use Synthetic Substitute

Synchra™ CRT-P
use Cardiac Resynchronization Pacemaker Pulse Generator in 0JH

SynchroMed® pump
use Infusion Device, Pump in Subcutaneous Tissue and Fascia

Synechiotomy, iris
see Release, Eye 08N

Synovectomy
Lower joint *see* Excision, Lower Joints 0SB
Upper joint *see* Excision, Upper Joints 0RB

Synthetic Human Angiotensin II XW0

Systemic nuclear medicine therapy
Abdomen CW70
Anatomical Regions, Multiple CW7YYZZ
Chest CW73
Thyroid CW7G
Whole Body CW7N

T

Takedown
Arteriovenous shunt *see* Removal of device from, Upper Arteries 03P
Arteriovenous shunt, with creation of new shunt *see* Bypass, Upper Arteries 031
Stoma
see Excision
see Reposition

Talent® Converter
use Intraluminal Device

Talent® Occluder
use Intraluminal Device

Talent® Stent Graft (abdominal)(thoracic)
use Intraluminal Device

Talocalcaneal (subtalar) joint
use Tarsal Joint, Right
use Tarsal Joint, Left

Talocalcaneal ligament
use Foot Bursa and Ligament, Right
use Foot Bursa and Ligament, Left

Talocalcaneonavicular joint
use Tarsal Joint, Right
use Tarsal Joint, Left

Talocalcaneonavicular ligament
use Foot Bursa and Ligament, Right
use Foot Bursa and Ligament, Left

Talocrural joint
use Ankle Joint, Right
use Ankle Joint, Left

Talofibular ligament
use Ankle Bursa and Ligament, Right
use Ankle Bursa and Ligament, Left
Talus bone
use Tarsal, Right
use Tarsal, Left
TandemHeart® System
use Short-term External Heart Assist System in Heart and Great Vessels
Tarsectomy
see Excision, Lower Bones 0QB
see Resection, Lower Bones 0QT
Tarsometatarsal ligament
use Foot Bursa and Ligament, Right
use Foot Bursa and Ligament, Left
Tarsorrhaphy
see Repair, Eye 08Q
Tattooing
Cornea 3E0CXMZ
Skin *see* Introduction of substance in or on, Skin 3E00
TAXUS® Liberte® Paclitaxel-eluting Coronary Stent System
use Intraluminal Device, Drug-eluting in Heart and Great Vessels
TBNA (transbronchial needle aspiration)
Fluid or gas *see* Drainage, Respiratory System 0B9
Tissue biopsy *see* Extraction, Respiratory System 0BD
Telemetry
4A12X4Z
Ambulatory 4A12X45
Temperature gradient study 4A0ZXKZ
Temporal lobe
use Cerebral Hemisphere
Temporalis muscle
use Head Muscle
Temporoparietalis muscle
use Head Muscle
Tendolysis
see Release, Tendons 0LN
Tendonectomy
see Excision, Tendons 0LB
see Resection, Tendons 0LT
Tendonoplasty, tenoplasty
see Repair, Tendons 0LQ
see Replacement, Tendons 0LR
see Supplement, Tendons 0LU
Tendorrhaphy
see Repair, Tendons 0LQ
Tendototomy
see Division, Tendons 0L8
see Drainage, Tendons 0L9
Tenectomy, tenonectomy
see Excision, Tendons 0LB
see Resection, Tendons 0LT
Tenolysis
see Release, Tendons 0LN
Tenontorrhaphy
see Repair, Tendons 0LQ
Tenontotomy
see Division, Tendons 0L8
see Drainage, Tendons 0L9
Tenorrhaphy
see Repair, Tendons 0LQ
Tenosynovectomy
see Excision, Tendons 0LB
see Resection, Tendons 0LT
Tenotomy
see Division, Tendons 0L8
see Drainage, Tendons 0L9
Tensor fasciae latae muscle
use Hip Muscle, Right
use Hip Muscle, Left
Tensor veli palatini muscle
use Tongue, Palate, Pharynx Muscle
Tenth cranial nerve
use Vagus Nerve
Tentorium cerebelli
use Dura Mater
Teres major muscle
use Shoulder Muscle, Right
use Shoulder Muscle, Left
Teres minor muscle
use Shoulder Muscle, Right
use Shoulder Muscle, Left
Termination of pregnancy
Aspiration curettage 10A07ZZ
Dilation and curettage 10A07ZZ
Hysterotomy 10A00ZZ
Intra-amniotic injection 10A03ZZ
Laminaria 10A07ZW
Vacuum 10A07Z6
Testectomy
see Excision, Male Reproductive System 0VB
see Resection, Male Reproductive System 0VT
Testicular artery
use Abdominal Aorta
Testing
Glaucoma 4A07XBZ
Hearing *see* Hearing Assessment, Diagnostic Audiology F13
Mental health *see* Psychological Tests
Muscle function, electromyography (EMG) *see* Measurement, Musculoskeletal 4A0F
Muscle function, manual *see* Motor Function Assessment, Rehabilitation F01
Neurophysiologic monitoring, intra-operative *see* Monitoring, Physiological Systems 4A1
Range of motion *see* Motor Function Assessment, Rehabilitation F01
Vestibular function *see* Vestibular Assessment, Diagnostic Audiology F15
Thalamectomy
see Excision, Thalamus 00B9
Thalamotomy
see Drainage, Thalamus 0099
Thenar muscle
use Hand Muscle, Right
use Hand Muscle, Left
Therapeutic massage
Musculoskeletal System 8E0KX1Z
Reproductive System
Prostate 8E0VX1C
Rectum 8E0VX1D
Therapeutic occlusion coil(s)
use Intraluminal Device
Thermography 4A0ZXKZ
Thermotherapy, prostate
see Destruction, Prostate 0V50
Third cranial nerve
use Oculomotor Nerve
Third occipital nerve
use Cervical Nerve
Third ventricle
use Cerebral Ventricle
Thoracectomy
see Excision, Anatomical Regions, General 0WB
Thoracentesis
see Drainage, Anatomical Regions, General 0W9
Thoracic aortic plexus
use Thoracic Sympathetic Nerve
Thoracic esophagus
use Esophagus, Middle
Thoracic facet joint
use Thoracic Vertebral Joint
Thoracic ganglion
use Thoracic Sympathetic Nerve
Thoracoacromial artery
use Axillary Artery, Right
use Axillary Artery, Left
Thoracocentesis
see Drainage, Anatomical Regions, General 0W9
Thoracolumbar facet joint
use Thoracolumbar Vertebral Joint
Thoracoplasty
see Repair, Anatomical Regions, General 0WQ
see Supplement, Anatomical Regions, General 0WU
Thoracostomy tube
use Drainage Device
Thoracostomy, for lung collapse
see Drainage, Respiratory System 0B9
Thoracotomy
see Drainage, Anatomical Regions, General 0W9
Thoratec® IVAD (Implantable Ventricular Assist Device)
use Implantable Heart Assist System in Heart and Great Vessels
Thoratec Paracorporeal Ventricular Assist Device
use Short-term External Heart Assist System in Heart and Great Vessels
Thrombectomy
see Extirpation
Thymectomy
see Excision, Lymphatic and Hemic Systems 07B
see Resection, Lymphatic and Hemic Systems 07T
Thymopexy
see Repair, Lymphatic and Hemic Systems 07Q
see Reposition, Lymphatic and Hemic Systems 07S
Thymus gland
use Thymus
Thyroarytenoid muscle
use Neck Muscle, Right
use Neck Muscle, Left
Thyrocervical trunk
use Thyroid Artery, Right
use Thyroid Artery, Left
Thyroid cartilage
use Larynx
Thyroidectomy
see Excision, Endocrine System 0GB
see Resection, Endocrine System 0GT
Thyroidorrhaphy
see Repair, Endocrine System 0GQ
Thyroidoscopy 0GJK4ZZ
Thyroidotomy
see Drainage, Endocrine System 0G9
Tibial insert
use Liner in Lower Joints
Tibialis anterior muscle
use Lower Leg Muscle, Right
use Lower Leg Muscle, Left
Tibialis posterior muscle
use Lower Leg Muscle, Right
use Lower Leg Muscle, Left
Tibiofemoral joint
use Knee Joint, Right
use Knee Joint, Left
use Knee Joint, Tibial Surface, Right
use Knee Joint, Tibial Surface, Left
Tisagenlecleucel
use Engineered Autologous Chimeric Antigen Receptor T-cell Immunotherapy
Tissue bank graft
use Nonautologous Tissue Substitute

Tissue expander
- Insertion of device in
  - Breast
    - Bilateral 0HHV
    - Left 0HHU
    - Right 0HHT
  - Nipple
    - Left 0HHX
    - Right 0HHW
  - Subcutaneous Tissue and Fascia
    - Abdomen 0JH8
    - Back 0JH7
    - Buttock 0JH9
    - Chest 0JH6
    - Face 0JH1
    - Foot
      - Left 0JHR
      - Right 0JHQ
    - Hand
      - Left 0JHK
      - Right 0JHJ
    - Lower Arm
      - Left 0JHH
      - Right 0JHG
    - Lower Leg
      - Left 0JHP
      - Right 0JHN
    - Neck
      - Left 0JH5
      - Right 0JH4
    - Pelvic Region 0JHC
    - Perineum 0JHB
    - Scalp 0JH0
    - Upper Arm
      - Left 0JHF
      - Right 0JHD
    - Upper Leg
      - Left 0JHM
      - Right 0JHL
- Removal of device from
  - Breast
    - Left 0HPU
    - Right 0HPT
  - Subcutaneous Tissue and Fascia
    - Head and Neck 0JPS
    - Lower Extremity 0JPW
    - Trunk 0JPT
    - Upper Extremity 0JPV
- Revision of device in
  - Breast
    - Left 0HWU
    - Right 0HWT
  - Subcutaneous Tissue and Fascia
    - Head and Neck 0JWS
    - Lower Extremity 0JWW
    - Trunk 0JWT
    - Upper Extremity 0JWV

Tissue expander (inflatable)(injectable)
- *use* Tissue Expander in Skin and Breast
- *use* Tissue Expander in Subcutaneous Tissue and Fascia

Tissue plasminogen activator (tPA)(r-tPA)
- *use* Other Thrombolytic

Titanium sternal fixation system (TSFS)
- *use* Internal Fixation Device, Rigid Plate in 0PH
- *use* Internal Fixation Device, Rigid Plate in 0PS

Tomographic (Tomo) nuclear medicine imaging
- Abdomen CW20
- Abdomen and Chest CW24
- Abdomen and Pelvis CW21
- Anatomical Regions, Multiple CW2YYZZ
- Bladder, Kidneys and Ureters CT23
- Brain C020
- Breast CH2YYZZ
  - Bilateral CH22

Tomographic (Tomo) nuclear medicine imaging — *continued*
- Breast — *continued*
  - Left CH21
  - Right CH20
- Bronchi and Lungs CB22
- Central Nervous System C02YYZZ
- Cerebrospinal Fluid C025
- Chest CW23
- Chest and Abdomen CW24
- Chest and Neck CW26
- Digestive System CD2YYZZ
- Endocrine System CG2YYZZ
- Extremity
  - Lower CW2D
    - Bilateral CP2F
    - Left CP2D
    - Right CP2C
  - Upper CW2M
    - Bilateral CP2B
    - Left CP29
    - Right CP28
- Gallbladder CF24
- Gastrointestinal Tract CD27
- Gland, Parathyroid CG21
- Head and Neck CW2B
- Heart C22YYZZ
  - Right and Left C226
- Hepatobiliary System and Pancreas CF2YYZZ
- Kidneys, Ureters and Bladder CT23
- Liver CF25
- Liver and Spleen CF26
- Lungs and Bronchi CB22
- Lymphatics and Hematologic System C72YYZZ
- Musculoskeletal System, Other CP2YYZZ
- Myocardium C22G
- Neck and Chest CW26
- Neck and Head CW2B
- Pancreas and Hepatobiliary System CF2YYZZ
- Pelvic Region CW2J
- Pelvis CP26
- Pelvis and Abdomen CW21
- Pelvis and Spine CP27
- Respiratory System CB2YYZZ
- Skin CH2YYZZ
- Skull CP21
- Skull and Cervical Spine CP23
- Spine
  - Cervical CP22
  - Cervical and Skull CP23
  - Lumbar CP2H
  - Thoracic CP2G
  - Thoracolumbar CP2J
- Spine and Pelvis CP27
- Spleen C722
- Spleen and Liver CF26
- Subcutaneous Tissue CH2YYZZ
- Thorax CP24
- Ureters, Kidneys and Bladder CT23
- Urinary System CT2YYZZ

Tomography, computerized
- *see* Computerized Tomography (CT Scan)

Tongue, base of
- *use* Pharynx

Tonometry 4A07XBZ

Tonsillectomy
- *see* Excision, Mouth and Throat 0CB
- *see* Resection, Mouth and Throat 0CT

Tonsillotomy
- *see* Drainage, Mouth and Throat 0C9

Total anomalous pulmonary venous return (TAPVR) repair
- *see* Bypass, Atrium, Left 0217
- *see* Bypass, Vena Cava, Superior 021V

Total artificial (replacement) heart
- *use* Synthetic Substitute

Total parenteral nutrition (TPN)
- *see* Introduction of Nutritional Substance

Trachectomy
- *see* Excision, Trachea 0BB1
- *see* Resection, Trachea 0BT1

Trachelectomy
- *see* Excision, Cervix 0UBC
- *see* Resection, Cervix 0UTC

Trachelopexy
- *see* Repair, Cervix 0UQC
- *see* Reposition, Cervix 0USC

Tracheloplasty
- *see* Repair, Cervix 0UQC

Trachelorrhaphy
- *see* Repair, Cervix 0UQC

Trachelotomy
- *see* Drainage, Cervix 0U9C

Tracheobronchial lymph node
- *use* Lymphatic, Thorax

Tracheoesophageal fistulization 0B110D6

Tracheolysis
- *see* Release, Respiratory System 0BN

Tracheoplasty
- *see* Repair, Respiratory System 0BQ
- *see* Supplement, Respiratory System 0BU

Tracheorrhaphy
- *see* Repair, Respiratory System 0BQ

Tracheoscopy 0BJ18ZZ

Tracheostomy
- *see* Bypass, Respiratory System 0B1

Tracheostomy device
- Bypass, Trachea 0B11
- Change device in, Trachea 0B21XFZ
- Removal of device from, Trachea 0BP1
- Revision of device in, Trachea 0BW1

Tracheostomy tube
- *use* Tracheostomy Device in Respiratory System

Tracheotomy
- *see* Drainage, Respiratory System 0B9

Traction
- Abdominal Wall 2W63X
- Arm
  - Lower
    - Left 2W6DX
    - Right 2W6CX
  - Upper
    - Left 2W6BX
    - Right 2W6AX
- Back 2W65X
- Chest Wall 2W64X
- Extremity
  - Lower
    - Left 2W6MX
    - Right 2W6LX
  - Upper
    - Left 2W69X
    - Right 2W68X
- Face 2W61X
- Finger
  - Left 2W6KX
  - Right 2W6JX
- Foot
  - Left 2W6TX
  - Right 2W6SX
- Hand
  - Left 2W6FX
  - Right 2W6EX
- Head 2W60X
- Inguinal Region
  - Left 2W67X
  - Right 2W66X
- Leg
  - Lower
    - Left 2W6RX

Traction — *continued*
Leg — *continued*
Right 2W6QX
Upper
Left 2W6PX
Right 2W6NX
Neck 2W62X
Thumb
Left 2W6HX
Right 2W6GX
Toe
Left 2W6VX
Right 2W6UX
Tractotomy
see Division, Central Nervous System and Cranial Nerves 008
Tragus
use External Ear, Right
use External Ear, Left
use External Ear, Bilateral
Training, caregiver
see Caregiver Training
TRAM (transverse rectus abdominis myocutaneous) flap reconstruction
Free *see* Replacement, Skin and Breast 0HR
Pedicled *see* Transfer, Muscles 0KX
Transection
see Division
Transfer
Buccal Mucosa 0CX4
Bursa and Ligament
Abdomen
Left 0MXJ
Right 0MXH
Ankle
Left 0MXR
Right 0MXQ
Elbow
Left 0MX4
Right 0MX3
Foot
Left 0MXT
Right 0MXS
Hand
Left 0MX8
Right 0MX7
Head and Neck 0MX0
Hip
Left 0MXM
Right 0MXL
Knee
Left 0MXP
Right 0MXN
Lower Extremity
Left 0MXW
Right 0MXV
Perineum 0MXK
Rib(s) 0MXG
Shoulder
Left 0MX2
Right 0MX1
Spine
Lower 0MXD
Upper 0MXC
Sternum 0MXF
Upper Extremity
Left 0MXB
Right 0MX9
Wrist
Left 0MX6
Right 0MX5
Finger
Left 0XXP0ZM
Right 0XXN0ZL
Gingiva
Lower 0CX6
Upper 0CX5
Transfer — *continued*
Intestine
Large 0DXE
Small 0DX8
Lip
Lower 0CX1
Upper 0CX0
Muscle
Abdomen
Left 0KXL
Right 0KXK
Extraocular
Left 08XM
Right 08XL
Facial 0KX1
Foot
Left 0KXW
Right 0KXV
Hand
Left 0KXD
Right 0KXC
Head 0KX0
Hip
Left 0KXP
Right 0KXN
Lower Arm and Wrist
Left 0KXB
Right 0KX9
Lower Leg
Left 0KXT
Right 0KXS
Neck
Left 0KX3
Right 0KX2
Perineum 0KXM
Shoulder
Left 0KX6
Right 0KX5
Thorax
Left 0KXJ
Right 0KXH
Tongue, Palate, Pharynx 0KX4
Trunk
Left 0KXG
Right 0KXF
Upper Arm
Left 0KX8
Right 0KX7
Upper Leg
Left 0KXR
Right 0KXQ
Nerve
Abducens 00XL
Accessory 00XR
Acoustic 00XN
Cervical 01X1
Facial 00XM
Femoral 01XD
Glossopharyngeal 00XP
Hypoglossal 00XS
Lumbar 01XB
Median 01X5
Oculomotor 00XH
Olfactory 00XF
Optic 00XG
Peroneal 01XH
Phrenic 01X2
Pudendal 01XC
Radial 01X6
Sciatic 01XF
Thoracic 01X8
Tibial 01XG
Trigeminal 00XK
Trochlear 00XJ
Ulnar 01X4
Vagus 00XQ
Palate, Soft 0CX3
Transfer — *continued*
Prepuce 0VXT
Skin
Abdomen 0HX7XZZ
Back 0HX6XZZ
Buttock 0HX8XZZ
Chest 0HX5XZZ
Ear
Left 0HX3XZZ
Right 0HX2XZZ
Face 0HX1XZZ
Foot
Left 0HXNXZZ
Right 0HXMXZZ
Hand
Left 0HXGXZZ
Right 0HXFXZZ
Inguinal 0HXAXZZ
Lower Arm
Left 0HXEXZZ
Right 0HXDXZZ
Lower Leg
Left 0HXLXZZ
Right 0HXKXZZ
Neck 0HX4XZZ
Perineum 0HX9XZZ
Scalp 0HX0XZZ
Upper Arm
Left 0HXCXZZ
Right 0HXBXZZ
Upper Leg
Left 0HXJXZZ
Right 0HXHXZZ
Stomach 0DX6
Subcutaneous Tissue and Fascia
Abdomen 0JX8
Back 0JX7
Buttock 0JX9
Chest 0JX6
Face 0JX1
Foot
Left 0JXR
Right 0JXQ
Hand
Left 0JXK
Right 0JXJ
Lower Arm
Left 0JXH
Right 0JXG
Lower Leg
Left 0JXP
Right 0JXN
Neck
Left 0JX5
Right 0JX4
Pelvic Region 0JXC
Perineum 0JXB
Scalp 0JX0
Upper Arm
Left 0JXF
Right 0JXD
Upper Leg
Left 0JXM
Right 0JXL
Tendon
Abdomen
Left 0LXG
Right 0LXF
Ankle
Left 0LXT
Right 0LXS
Foot
Left 0LXW
Right 0LXV
Hand
Left 0LX8
Right 0LX7

Transfer — *continued*
- Tendon — *continued*
  - Head and Neck 0LX0
  - Hip
    - Left 0LXK
    - Right 0LXJ
  - Knee
    - Left 0LXR
    - Right 0LXQ
  - Lower Arm and Wrist
    - Left 0LX6
    - Right 0LX5
  - Lower Leg
    - Left 0LXP
    - Right 0LXN
  - Perineum 0LXH
  - Shoulder
    - Left 0LX2
    - Right 0LX1
  - Thorax
    - Left 0LXD
    - Right 0LXC
  - Trunk
    - Left 0LXB
    - Right 0LX9
  - Upper Arm
    - Left 0LX4
    - Right 0LX3
  - Upper Leg
    - Left 0LXM
    - Right 0LXL
- Tongue 0CX7

Transfusion
- Artery
  - Central
    - Antihemophilic Factors 3026
    - Blood
      - Platelets 3026
      - Red Cells 3026
        - Frozen 3026
      - White Cells 3026
      - Whole 3026
    - Bone Marrow 3026
    - Factor IX 3026
    - Fibrinogen 3026
    - Globulin 3026
    - Plasma
      - Fresh 3026
      - Frozen 3026
    - Plasma Cryoprecipitate 3026
    - Serum Albumin 3026
    - Stem Cells
      - Cord Blood 3026
      - Hematopoietic 3026
  - Peripheral
    - Antihemophilic Factors 3025
    - Blood
      - Platelets 3025
      - Red Cells 3025
        - Frozen 3025
      - White Cells 3025
      - Whole 3025
    - Bone Marrow 3025
    - Factor IX 3025
    - Fibrinogen 3025
    - Globulin 3025
    - Plasma
      - Fresh 3025
      - Frozen 3025
    - Plasma Cryoprecipitate 3025
    - Serum Albumin 3025
    - Stem Cells
      - Cord Blood 3025
      - Hematopoietic 3025
- Products of Conception
  - Antihemophilic Factors 3027
  - Blood

Transfusion — *continued*
- Products of Conception — *continued*
    - Platelets 3027
    - Red Cells 3027
      - Frozen 3027
    - White Cells 3027
    - Whole 3027
  - Factor IX 3027
  - Fibrinogen 3027
  - Globulin 3027
  - Plasma
    - Fresh 3027
    - Frozen 3027
  - Plasma Cryoprecipitate 3027
  - Serum Albumin 3027
- Vein
  - 4-Factor Prothrombin Complex Concentrate 3028
  - Central
    - Antihemophilic Factors 3024
    - Blood
      - Platelets 3024
      - Red Cells 3024
        - Frozen 3024
      - White Cells 3024
      - Whole 3024
    - Bone Marrow 3024
    - Factor IX 3024
    - Fibrinogen 3024
    - Globulin 3024
    - Plasma
      - Fresh 3024
      - Frozen 3024
    - Plasma Cryoprecipitate 3024
    - Serum Albumin 3024
    - Stem Cells
      - Cord Blood 3024
      - Embryonic 3024
      - Hematopoietic 3024
  - Peripheral
    - Antihemophilic Factors 3023
    - Blood
      - Platelets 3023
      - Red Cells 3023
        - Frozen 3023
      - White Cells 3023
      - Whole 3023
    - Bone Marrow 3023
    - Factor IX 3023
    - Fibrinogen 3023
    - Globulin 3023
    - Plasma
      - Fresh 3023
      - Frozen 3023
    - Plasma Cryoprecipitate 3023
    - Serum Albumin 3023
    - Stem Cells
      - Cord Blood 3023
      - Embryonic 3023
      - Hematopoietic 3023

Transplant
- *see* Transplantation

Transplantation
- Bone marrow *see* Transfusion, Circulatory 302
- Esophagus 0DY50Z
- Face 0WY20Z
- Hand
  - Left 0XYK0Z
  - Right 0XYJ0Z
- Heart 02YA0Z
- Hematopoietic cell *see* Transfusion, Circulatory 302
- Intestine
  - Large 0DYE0Z
  - Small 0DY80Z

Transplantation — *continued*
- Kidney
  - Left 0TY10Z
  - Right 0TY00Z
- Liver 0FY00Z
- Lung
  - Bilateral 0BYM0Z
  - Left 0BYL0Z
  - Lower Lobe
    - Left 0BYJ0Z
    - Right 0BYF0Z
  - Middle Lobe, Right 0BYD0Z
  - Right 0BYK0Z
  - Upper Lobe
    - Left 0BYG0Z
    - Right 0BYC0Z
- Lung Lingula 0BYH0Z
- Ovary
  - Left 0UY10Z
  - Right 0UY00Z
- Pancreas 0FYG0Z
- Products of Conception 10Y0
- Spleen 07YP0Z
- Stem cell *see* Transfusion, Circulatory 302
- Stomach 0DY60Z
- Thymus 07YM0Z
- Uterus 0UY90Z

Transposition
- *see* Bypass
- *see* Reposition
- *see* Transfer

Transversalis fascia
- *use* Subcutaneous Tissue and Fascia, Trunk

Transverse (cutaneous) cervical nerve
- *use* Cervical Plexus

Transverse acetabular ligament
- *use* Hip Bursa and Ligament, Right
- *use* Hip Bursa and Ligament, Left

Transverse facial artery
- *use* Temporal Artery, Right
- *use* Temporal Artery, Left

Transverse foramen
- *use* Cervical Vertebra

Transverse humeral ligament
- *use* Shoulder Bursa and Ligament, Right
- *use* Shoulder Bursa and Ligament, Left

Transverse ligament of atlas
- *use* Head and Neck Bursa and Ligament

Transverse process
- *use* Cervical Vertebra
- *use* Thoracic Vertebra
- *use* Lumbar Vertebra

Transverse rectus abdominis myocutaneous flap
- Replacement
  - Bilateral 0HRV076
  - Left 0HRU076
  - Right 0HRT076
- Transfer
  - Left 0KXL
  - Right 0KXK

Transverse scapular ligament
- *use* Shoulder Bursa and Ligament, Right
- *use* Shoulder Bursa and Ligament, Left

Transverse thoracis muscle
- *use* Thorax Muscle, Right
- *use* Thorax Muscle, Left

Transversospinalis muscle
- *use* Trunk Muscle, Right
- *use* Trunk Muscle, Left

Transversus abdominis muscle
- *use* Abdomen Muscle, Right
- *use* Abdomen Muscle, Left

Trapezium bone
- *use* Carpal, Right
- *use* Carpal, Left

- **Trapezius muscle**
  - *use* Trunk Muscle, Right
  - *use* Trunk Muscle, Left
- **Trapezoid bone**
  - *use* Carpal, Right
  - *use* Carpal, Left
- **Triceps brachii muscle**
  - *use* Upper Arm Muscle, Right
  - *use* Upper Arm Muscle, Left
- **Tricuspid annulus**
  - *use* Tricuspid Valve
- **Trifacial nerve**
  - *use* Trigeminal Nerve
- **Trifecta™ Valve (aortic)**
  - *use* Zooplastic Tissue in Heart and Great Vessels
- **Trigone of bladder**
  - *use* Bladder
- **Trimming, excisional**
  - *see* Excision
- **Triquetral bone**
  - *use* Carpal, Right
  - *use* Carpal, Left
- **Trochanteric bursa**
  - *use* Hip Bursa and Ligament, Right
  - *use* Hip Bursa and Ligament, Left
- **TUMT (transurethral microwave thermotherapy of prostate)** 0V507ZZ
- **TUNA (transurethral needle ablation of prostate)** 0V507ZZ
- **Tunneled central venous catheter**
  - *use* Vascular Access Device, Tunneled in Subcutaneous Tissue and Fascia
- **Tunneled spinal (intrathecal) catheter**
  - *use* Infusion Device
- **Turbinectomy**
  - *see* Excision, Ear, Nose, Sinus 09B
  - *see* Resection, Ear, Nose, Sinus 09T
- **Turbinoplasty**
  - *see* Repair, Ear, Nose, Sinus 09Q
  - *see* Replacement, Ear, Nose, Sinus 09R
  - *see* Supplement, Ear, Nose, Sinus 09U
- **Turbinotomy**
  - *see* Division, Ear, Nose, Sinus 098
  - *see* Drainage, Ear, Nose, Sinus 099
- **TURP (transurethral resection of prostate)**
  - *see* Excision, Prostate 0VB0
  - *see* Resection, Prostate 0VT0
- **Twelfth cranial nerve**
  - *use* Hypoglossal Nerve
- **Two lead pacemaker**
  - *use* Pacemaker, Dual Chamber in 0JH
- **Tympanic cavity**
  - *use* Middle Ear, Right
  - *use* Middle Ear, Left
- **Tympanic nerve**
  - *use* Glossopharyngeal Nerve
- **Tympanic part of temporal bone**
  - *use* Temporal Bone, Right
  - *use* Temporal Bone, Left
- **Tympanogram**
  - *see* Hearing Assessment, Diagnostic Audiology F13
- **Tympanoplasty**
  - *see* Repair, Ear, Nose, Sinus 09Q
  - *see* Replacement, Ear, Nose, Sinus 09R
  - *see* Supplement, Ear, Nose, Sinus 09U
- **Tympanosympathectomy**
  - *see* Excision, Nerve, Head and Neck Sympathetic 01BK
- **Tympanotomy**
  - *see* Drainage, Ear, Nose, Sinus 099

U

- **Ulnar collateral carpal ligament**
  - *use* Wrist Bursa and Ligament, Right
  - *use* Wrist Bursa and Ligament, Left
- **Ulnar collateral ligament**
  - *use* Elbow Bursa and Ligament, Right
  - *use* Elbow Bursa and Ligament, Left
- **Ulnar notch**
  - *use* Radius, Right
  - *use* Radius, Left
- **Ulnar vein**
  - *use* Brachial Vein, Right
  - *use* Brachial Vein, Left
- **Ultrafiltration**
  - Hemodialysis *see* Performance, Urinary 5A1D
  - Therapeutic plasmapheresis *see* Pheresis, Circulatory 6A55
- **Ultraflex™ Precision Colonic Stent System**
  - *use* Intraluminal Device
- **ULTRAPRO® Hernia System (UHS)**
  - *use* Synthetic Substitute
- **ULTRAPRO® Partially Absorbable Lightweight Mesh**
  - *use* Synthetic Substitute
- **ULTRAPRO® Plug**
  - *use* Synthetic Substitute
- **Ultrasonic osteogenic stimulator**
  - *use* Bone Growth Stimulator in Head and Facial Bones
  - *use* Bone Growth Stimulator in Upper Bones
  - *use* Bone Growth Stimulator in Lower Bones
- **Ultrasonography**
  - Abdomen BW40ZZZ
  - Abdomen and Pelvis BW41ZZZ
  - Abdominal Wall BH49ZZZ
  - Aorta
    - Abdominal, Intravascular B440ZZ3
    - Thoracic, Intravascular B340ZZ3
  - Appendix BD48ZZZ
  - Artery
    - Brachiocephalic-Subclavian, Right, Intravascular B341ZZ3
    - Celiac and Mesenteric, Intravascular B44KZZ3
    - Common Carotid
      - Bilateral, Intravascular B345ZZ3
      - Left, Intravascular B344ZZ3
      - Right, Intravascular B343ZZ3
    - Coronary
      - Multiple B241YZZ
        - Intravascular B241ZZ3
        - Transesophageal B241ZZ4
      - Single B240YZZ
        - Intravascular B240ZZ3
        - Transesophageal B240ZZ4
    - Femoral, Intravascular B44LZZ3
    - Inferior Mesenteric, Intravascular B445ZZ3
    - Internal Carotid
      - Bilateral, Intravascular B348ZZ3
      - Left, Intravascular B347ZZ3
      - Right, Intravascular B346ZZ3
    - Intra-Abdominal, Other, Intravascular B44BZZ3
    - Intracranial, Intravascular B34RZZ3
    - Lower Extremity
      - Bilateral, Intravascular B44HZZ3
      - Left, Intravascular B44GZZ3
      - Right, Intravascular B44FZZ3
    - Mesenteric and Celiac, Intravascular B44KZZ3
    - Ophthalmic, Intravascular B34VZZ3

Ultrasonography — *continued*

  - Artery — *continued*
    - Penile, Intravascular B44NZZ3
    - Pulmonary
      - Left, Intravascular B34TZZ3
      - Right, Intravascular B34SZZ3
    - Renal
      - Bilateral, Intravascular B448ZZ3
      - Left, Intravascular B447ZZ3
      - Right, Intravascular B446ZZ3
    - Subclavian, Left, Intravascular B342ZZ3
    - Superior Mesenteric, Intravascular B444ZZ3
    - Upper Extremity
      - Bilateral, Intravascular B34KZZ3
      - Left, Intravascular B34JZZ3
      - Right, Intravascular B34HZZ3
  - Bile Duct BF40ZZZ
  - Bile Duct and Gallbladder BF43ZZZ
  - Bladder BT40ZZZ
    - and Kidney BT4JZZZ
  - Brain B040ZZZ
  - Breast
    - Bilateral BH42ZZZ
    - Left BH41ZZZ
    - Right BH40ZZZ
  - Chest Wall BH4BZZZ
  - Coccyx BR4FZZZ
  - Connective Tissue
    - Lower Extremity BL41ZZZ
    - Upper Extremity BL40ZZZ
  - Duodenum BD49ZZZ
  - Elbow
    - Left, Densitometry BP4HZZ1
    - Right, Densitometry BP4GZZ1
  - Esophagus BD41ZZZ
  - Extremity
    - Lower BH48ZZZ
    - Upper BH47ZZZ
  - Eye
    - Bilateral B847ZZZ
    - Left B846ZZZ
    - Right B845ZZZ
  - Fallopian Tube
    - Bilateral BU42
    - Left BU41
    - Right BU40
  - Fetal Umbilical Cord BY47ZZZ
  - Fetus
    - First Trimester, Multiple Gestation BY4BZZZ
    - Second Trimester, Multiple Gestation BY4DZZZ
    - Single
      - First Trimester BY49ZZZ
      - Second Trimester BY4CZZZ
      - Third Trimester BY4FZZZ
    - Third Trimester, Multiple Gestation BY4GZZZ
  - Gallbladder BF42ZZZ
  - Gallbladder and Bile Duct BF43ZZZ
  - Gastrointestinal Tract BD47ZZZ
  - Gland
    - Adrenal
      - Bilateral BG42ZZZ
      - Left BG41ZZZ
      - Right BG40ZZZ
    - Parathyroid BG43ZZZ
    - Thyroid BG44ZZZ
  - Hand
    - Left, Densitometry BP4PZZ1
    - Right, Densitometry BP4NZZ1
  - Head and Neck BH4CZZZ
  - Heart
    - Left B245YZZ
      - Intravascular B245ZZ3
      - Transesophageal B245ZZ4

Ultrasonography — *continued*
Heart — *continued*
Pediatric B24DYZZ
Intravascular B24DZZ3
Transesophageal B24DZZ4
Right B244YZZ
Intravascular B244ZZ3
Transesophageal B244ZZ4
Right and Left B246YZZ
Intravascular B246ZZ3
Transesophageal B246ZZ4
Heart with Aorta B24BYZZ
Intravascular B24BZZ3
Transesophageal B24BZZ4
Hepatobiliary System, All BF4CZZZ
Hip
Bilateral BQ42ZZZ
Left BQ41ZZZ
Right BQ40ZZZ
Kidney
and Bladder BT4JZZZ
Bilateral BT43ZZZ
Left BT42ZZZ
Right BT41ZZZ
Transplant BT49ZZZ
Knee
Bilateral BQ49ZZZ
Left BQ48ZZZ
Right BQ47ZZZ
Liver BF45ZZZ
Liver and Spleen BF46ZZZ
Mediastinum BB4CZZZ
Neck BW4FZZZ
Ovary
Bilateral BU45
Left BU44
Right BU43
Ovary and Uterus BU4C
Pancreas BF47ZZZ
Pelvic Region BW4GZZZ
Pelvis and Abdomen BW41ZZZ
Penis BV4BZZZ
Pericardium B24CYZZ
Intravascular B24CZZ3
Transesophageal B24CZZ4
Placenta BY48ZZZ
Pleura BB4BZZZ
Prostate and Seminal Vesicle BV49ZZZ
Rectum BD4CZZZ
Sacrum BR4FZZZ
Scrotum BV44ZZZ
Seminal Vesicle and Prostate BV49ZZZ
Shoulder
Left, Densitometry BP49ZZ1
Right, Densitometry BP48ZZ1
Spinal Cord B04BZZZ
Spine
Cervical BR40ZZZ
Lumbar BR49ZZZ
Thoracic BR47ZZZ
Spleen and Liver BF46ZZZ
Stomach BD42ZZZ
Tendon
Lower Extremity BL43ZZZ
Upper Extremity BL42ZZZ
Ureter
Bilateral BT48ZZZ
Left BT47ZZZ
Right BT46ZZZ
Urethra BT45ZZZ
Uterus BU46
Uterus and Ovary BU4C
Vein
Jugular
Left, Intravascular B544ZZ3
Right, Intravascular B543ZZ3

Ultrasonography — *continued*
Vein — *continued*
Lower Extremity
Bilateral, Intravascular B54DZZ3
Left, Intravascular B54CZZ3
Right, Intravascular B54BZZ3
Portal, Intravascular B54TZZ3
Renal
Bilateral, Intravascular B54LZZ3
Left, Intravascular B54KZZ3
Right, Intravascular B54JZZ3
Splanchnic, Intravascular B54TZZ3
Subclavian
Left, Intravascular B547ZZ3
Right, Intravascular B546ZZ3
Upper Extremity
Bilateral, Intravascular B54PZZ3
Left, Intravascular B54NZZ3
Right, Intravascular B54MZZ3
Vena Cava
Inferior, Intravascular B549ZZ3
Superior, Intravascular B548ZZ3
Wrist
Left, Densitometry BP4MZZ1
Right, Densitometry BP4LZZ1
Ultrasound bone healing system
use Bone Growth Stimulator in Head and Facial Bones
use Bone Growth Stimulator in Upper Bones
use Bone Growth Stimulator in Lower Bones
Ultrasound therapy
Heart 6A75
No Qualifier 6A75
Vessels
Head and Neck 6A75
Other 6A75
Peripheral 6A75
Ultraviolet light therapy, skin 6A80
Umbilical artery
use Internal Iliac Artery, Right
use Internal Iliac Artery, Left
use Lower Artery
Uniplanar external fixator
use External Fixation Device, Monoplanar in 0PH
use External Fixation Device, Monoplanar in 0PS
use External Fixation Device, Monoplanar in 0QH
use External Fixation Device, Monoplanar in 0QS
Upper GI series
see Fluoroscopy, Gastrointestinal, Upper BD15
Ureteral orifice
use Ureter, Right
use Ureter, Left
use Ureters, Bilateral
use Ureter
Ureterectomy
see Excision, Urinary System 0TB
see Resection, Urinary System 0TT
Ureterocolostomy
see Bypass, Urinary System 0T1
Ureterocystostomy
see Bypass, Urinary System 0T1
Ureteroenterostomy
see Bypass, Urinary System 0T1
Ureteroileostomy
see Bypass, Urinary System 0T1
Ureterolithotomy
see Extirpation, Urinary System 0TC
Ureterolysis
see Release, Urinary System 0TN

Ureteroneocystostomy
see Bypass, Urinary System 0T1
see Reposition, Urinary System 0TS
Ureteropelvic junction (UPJ)
use Kidney Pelvis, Right
use Kidney Pelvis, Left
Ureteropexy
see Repair, Urinary System 0TQ
see Reposition, Urinary System 0TS
Ureteroplasty
see Repair, Urinary System 0TQ
see Replacement, Urinary System 0TR
see Supplement, Urinary System 0TU
Ureteroplication
see Restriction, Urinary System 0TV
Ureteropyelography
see Fluoroscopy, Urinary System BT1
Ureterorrhaphy
see Repair, Urinary System 0TQ
Ureteroscopy 0TJ98ZZ
Ureterostomy
see Bypass, Urinary System 0T1
see Drainage, Urinary System 0T9
Ureterotomy
see Drainage, Urinary System 0T9
Ureteroureterostomy
see Bypass, Urinary System 0T1
Ureterovesical orifice
use Ureter, Right
use Ureter, Left
use Ureters, Bilateral
use Ureter
Urethral catheterization, indwelling 0T9B70Z
Urethrectomy
see Excision, Urethra 0TBD
see Resection, Urethra 0TTD
Urethrolithotomy
see Extirpation, Urethra 0TCD
Urethrolysis
see Release, Urethra 0TND
Urethropexy
see Repair, Urethra 0TQD
see Reposition, Urethra 0TSD
Urethroplasty
see Repair, Urethra 0TQD
see Replacement, Urethra 0TRD
see Supplement, Urethra 0TUD
Urethrorrhaphy
see Repair, Urethra 0TQD
Urethroscopy 0TJD8ZZ
Urethrotomy
see Drainage, Urethra 0T9D
Uridine triacetate XW0DX82
Urinary incontinence stimulator lead
use Stimulator Lead in Urinary System
Urography
see Fluoroscopy, Urinary System BT1
Ustekinumab
use Other New Technology Therapeutic Substance
Uterine artery
use Internal Iliac Artery, Right
use Internal Iliac Artery, Left
Uterine artery embolization (UAE)
see Occlusion, Lower Arteries 04L
Uterine cornu
use Uterus
Uterine tube
use Fallopian Tube, Right
use Fallopian Tube, Left
Uterine vein
use Hypogastric Vein, Right
use Hypogastric Vein, Left
Uvulectomy
see Excision, Uvula 0CBN
see Resection, Uvula 0CTN

Uvulorrhaphy
see Repair, Uvula 0CQN
Uvulotomy
see Drainage, Uvula 0C9N

V

Vaccination
see Introduction of Serum, Toxoid, and Vaccine
Vacuum extraction, obstetric 10D07Z6
Vaginal artery
use Internal Iliac Artery, Right
use Internal Iliac Artery, Left
Vaginal pessary
use Intraluminal Device, Pessary in Female Reproductive System
Vaginal vein
use Hypogastric Vein, Right
use Hypogastric Vein, Left
Vaginectomy
see Excision, Vagina 0UBG
see Resection, Vagina 0UTG
Vaginofixation
see Repair, Vagina 0UQG
see Reposition, Vagina 0USG
Vaginoplasty
see Repair, Vagina 0UQG
see Supplement, Vagina 0UUG
Vaginorrhaphy
see Repair, Vagina 0UQG
Vaginoscopy 0UJH8ZZ
Vaginotomy
see Drainage, Female Reproductive System 0U9
Vagotomy
see Division, Nerve, Vagus 008Q
Valiant® Thoracic Stent Graft
use Intraluminal Device
Valvotomy, valvulotomy
see Division, Heart and Great Vessels 028
see Release, Heart and Great Vessels 02N
Valvuloplasty
see Repair, Heart and Great Vessels 02Q
see Replacement, Heart and Great Vessels 02R
see Supplement, Heart and Great Vessels 02U
Valvuloplasty, Alfieri stitch
see Restriction, Valve, Mitral 02VG
Vascular access device
Totally Implantable
Insertion of device in
Abdomen 0JH8
Chest 0JH6
Lower Arm
Left 0JHH
Right 0JHG
Lower Leg
Left 0JHP
Right 0JHN
Upper Arm
Left 0JHF
Right 0JHD
Upper Leg
Left 0JHM
Right 0JHL
Removal of device from
Lower Extremity 0JPW
Trunk 0JPT
Upper Extremity 0JPV
Revision of device in
Lower Extremity 0JWW
Trunk 0JWT
Upper Extremity 0JWV
Vascular access device — *continued*
Tunneled
Insertion of device in
Abdomen 0JH8
Chest 0JH6
Lower Arm
Left 0JHH
Right 0JHG
Lower Leg
Left 0JHP
Right 0JHN
Upper Arm
Left 0JHF
Right 0JHD
Upper Leg
Left 0JHM
Right 0JHL
Removal of device from
Lower Extremity 0JPW
Trunk 0JPT
Upper Extremity 0JPV
Revision of device in
Lower Extremity 0JWW
Trunk 0JWT
Upper Extremity 0JWV
Vasectomy
see Excision, Male Reproductive System 0VB
Vasography
see Plain Radiography, Male Reproductive System BV0
see Fluoroscopy, Male Reproductive System BV1
Vasoligation
see Occlusion, Male Reproductive System 0VL
Vasorrhaphy
see Repair, Male Reproductive System 0VQ
Vasostomy
see Bypass, Male Reproductive System 0V1
Vasotomy
Drainage *see* Drainage, Male Reproductive System 0V9
With ligation *see* Occlusion, Male Reproductive System 0VL
Vasovasostomy
see Repair, Male Reproductive System 0VQ
Vastus intermedius muscle
use Upper Leg Muscle, Right
use Upper Leg Muscle, Left
Vastus lateralis muscle
use Upper Leg Muscle, Right
use Upper Leg Muscle, Left
Vastus medialis muscle
use Upper Leg Muscle, Right
use Upper Leg Muscle, Left
VCG (vectorcardiogram)
see Measurement, Cardiac 4A02
Vectra® Vascular Access Graft
use Vascular Access Device, Tunneled in Subcutaneous Tissue and Fascia
Venectomy
see Excision, Upper Veins 05B
see Excision, Lower Veins 06B
Venography
see Plain Radiography, Veins B50
see Fluoroscopy, Veins B51
Venorrhaphy
see Repair, Upper Veins 05Q
see Repair, Lower Veins 06Q
Venotripsy
see Occlusion, Upper Veins 05L
see Occlusion, Lower Veins 06L
Ventricular fold
use Larynx
Ventriculoatriostomy
see Bypass, Central Nervous System and Cranial Nerves 001
Ventriculocisternostomy
see Bypass, Central Nervous System and Cranial Nerves 001
Ventriculogram, cardiac
Combined left and right heart *see* Fluoroscopy, Heart, Right and Left B216
Left ventricle *see* Fluoroscopy, Heart, Left B215
Right ventricle *see* Fluoroscopy, Heart, Right B214
Ventriculopuncture, through previously implanted catheter 8C01X6J
Ventriculoscopy 00J04ZZ
Ventriculostomy
External drainage *see* Drainage, Cerebral Ventricle 0096
Internal shunt *see* Bypass, Cerebral Ventricle 0016
Ventriculovenostomy
see Bypass, Cerebral Ventricle 0016
Ventrio™ Hernia Patch
use Synthetic Substitute
VEP (visual evoked potential) 4A07X0Z
Vermiform appendix
use Appendix
Vermilion border
use Upper Lip
use Lower Lip
Versa®
use Pacemaker, Dual Chamber in 0JH
Version, obstetric
External 10S0XZZ
Internal 10S07ZZ
Vertebral arch
use Cervical Vertebra
use Thoracic Vertebra
use Lumbar Vertebra
Vertebral body
use Cervical Vertebra
use Thoracic Vertebra
use Lumbar Vertebra
Vertebral canal
use Spinal Canal
Vertebral foramen
use Cervical Vertebra
use Thoracic Vertebra
use Lumbar Vertebra
Vertebral lamina
use Cervical Vertebra
use Thoracic Vertebra
use Lumbar Vertebra
Vertebral pedicle
use Cervical Vertebra
use Thoracic Vertebra
use Lumbar Vertebra
Vesical vein
use Hypogastric Vein, Right
use Hypogastric Vein, Left
Vesicotomy
see Drainage, Urinary System 0T9
Vesiculectomy
see Excision, Male Reproductive System 0VB
see Resection, Male Reproductive System 0VT
Vesiculogram, seminal
see Plain Radiography, Male Reproductive System BV0
Vesiculotomy
see Drainage, Male Reproductive System 0V9
Vestibular (Scarpa's) ganglion
use Acoustic Nerve
Vestibular assessment F15Z
Vestibular nerve
use Acoustic Nerve
Vestibular treatment F0C

Vestibulocochlear nerve
use Acoustic Nerve
VH-IVUS (virtual histology intravascular ultrasound)
see Ultrasonography, Heart B24
Virchow's (supraclavicular) lymph node
use Lymphatic, Right Neck
use Lymphatic, Left Neck
Virtuoso® (II) (DR) (VR)
use Defibrillator Generator in 0JH
Vistogard®
use Uridine Triacetate
Vitrectomy
see Excision, Eye 08B
see Resection, Eye 08T
Vitreous body
use Vitreous, Right
use Vitreous, Left
Viva™ (XT)(S)
use Cardiac Resynchronization Defibrillator Pulse Generator in 0JH
Vocal fold
use Vocal Cord, Right
use Vocal Cord, Left
Vocational
Assessment *see* Activities of Daily Living Assessment, Rehabilitation F02
Retraining *see* Activities of Daily Living Treatment, Rehabilitation F08
Volar (palmar) digital vein
use Hand Vein, Right
use Hand Vein, Left
Volar (palmar) metacarpal vein
use Hand Vein, Right
use Hand Vein, Left
Vomer bone
use Nasal Septum
Vomer of nasal septum
use Nasal Bone
Voraxaze®
use Glucarpidase
Vulvectomy
see Excision, Female Reproductive System 0UB
see Resection, Female Reproductive System 0UT
VYXEOS™
use Cytarabine and Daunorubicin Liposome Antineoplastic

W

WALLSTENT® Endoprosthesis
use Intraluminal Device
Washing
see Irrigation
Wedge resection, pulmonary
see Excision, Respiratory System 0BB
Window
see Drainage
Wiring, dental 2W31X9Z

X-ray
see Plain Radiography
X-STOP® Spacer
use Spinal Stabilization Device, Interspinous Process in 0RH
use Spinal Stabilization Device, Interspinous Process in 0SH
Xact® Carotid Stent System
use Intraluminal Device
Xenograft
use Zooplastic Tissue in Heart and Great Vessels
XIENCE™ Everolimus Eluting Coronary Stent System
use Intraluminal Device, Drug-eluting in Heart and Great Vessels
Xiphoid process
use Sternum
XLIF® System
use Interbody Fusion Device in Lower Joints

Yoga therapy 8E0ZXY4

Z

Z-plasty, skin for scar contracture
see Release, Skin and Breast 0HN
Zenith® AAA Endovascular Graft
use Intraluminal Device, Branched or Fenestrated, One or Two Arteries in 04V
use Intraluminal Device, Branched or Fenestrated, Three or More Arteries in 04V
use Intraluminal Device
Zenith Flex® AAA Endovascular Graft
use Intraluminal Device
Zenith TX2® TAA Endovascular Graft
use Intraluminal Device
Zenith® Renu™ AAA Ancillary Graft
use Intraluminal Device
Zilver® PTX® (paclitaxel) Drug-eluting Peripheral Stent
use Intraluminal Device, Drug-eluting in Upper Arteries
use Intraluminal Device, Drug-eluting in Lower Arteries
Zimmer® NexGen® LPS Mobile Bearing Knee
use Synthetic Substitute
Zimmer® NexGen® LPS-Flex Mobile Knee
use Synthetic Substitute
ZINPLAVA™
use Bezlotoxumab Monoclonal Antibody
Zonule of Zinn
use Lens, Right
use Lens, Left
Zooplastic tissue, rapid deployment Technique, Replacement X2RF
Zotarolimus-eluting coronary stent
use Intraluminal Device, Drug-eluting in Heart and Great Vessels
Zygomatic process of frontal bone
use Frontal Bone
Zygomatic process of temporal bone
use Temporal Bone, Right
use Temporal Bone, Left
Zygomaticus muscle
use Facial Muscle
Zyvox®
use Oxazolidinones

ICD-10-PCS Tables

Medical and Surgical 001-0YW

Central Nervous System and Cranial Nerves 001-00X

0 Medical and Surgical
0 Central Nervous System and Cranial Nerves
1 Bypass: Altering the route of passage of the contents of a tubular body part

Body Part Character 4	Approach Character 5	Device Character 6	Qualifier Character 7
6 Cerebral Ventricle	**0** Open **3** Percutaneous **4** Percutaneous Endoscopic	**7** Autologous Tissue Substitute **J** Synthetic Substitute **K** Nonautologous Tissue Substitute	**0** Nasopharynx **1** Mastoid Sinus **2** Atrium **3** Blood Vessel **4** Pleural Cavity **5** Intestine **6** Peritoneal Cavity **7** Urinary Tract **8** Bone Marrow **B** Cerebral Cisterns
6 Cerebral Ventricle	**0** Open **3** Percutaneous **4** Percutaneous Endoscopic	**Z** No Device	**B** Cerebral Cisterns
U Spinal Canal ♀	**0** Open **3** Percutaneous **4** Percutaneous Endoscopic	**7** Autologous Tissue Substitute **J** Synthetic Substitute **K** Nonautologous Tissue Substitute	**2** Atrium **4** Pleural Cavity **6** Peritoneal Cavity **7** Urinary Tract **9** Fallopian Tube

♀ 001U479 001U4J9 001U4K9

0 Medical and Surgical
0 Central Nervous System and Cranial Nerves
2 Change: Taking out or off a device from a body part and putting back an identical or similar device in or on the same body part without cutting or puncturing the skin or a mucous membrane

Body Part Character 4	Approach Character 5	Device Character 6	Qualifier Character 7
0 Brain **E** Cranial Nerve **U** Spinal Canal	**X** External	**0** Drainage Device **Y** Other Device	**Z** No Qualifier

0 Medical and Surgical
0 Central Nervous System and Cranial Nerves
5 Destruction: Physical eradication of all or a portion of a body part by the direct use of energy, force, or a destructive agent

Body Part Character 4	Approach Character 5	Device Character 6	Qualifier Character 7
0 Brain **1** Cerebral Meninges **2** Dura Mater **6** Cerebral Ventricle **7** Cerebral Hemisphere **8** Basal Ganglia **9** Thalamus **A** Hypothalamus **B** Pons **C** Cerebellum **D** Medulla Oblongata **F** Olfactory Nerve **G** Optic Nerve **H** Oculomotor Nerve **J** Trochlear Nerve **K** Trigeminal Nerve **L** Abducens Nerve **M** Facial Nerve **N** Acoustic Nerve **P** Glossopharyngeal Nerve **Q** Vagus Nerve **R** Accessory Nerve **S** Hypoglossal Nerve **T** Spinal Meninges **W** Cervical Spinal Cord **X** Thoracic Spinal Cord **Y** Lumbar Spinal Cord	**0** Open **3** Percutaneous **4** Percutaneous Endoscopic	**Z** No Device	**Z** No Qualifier

0 Medical and Surgical
0 Central Nervous System and Cranial Nerves
7 Dilation: Expanding an orifice or the lumen of a tubular body part

Body Part Character 4	Approach Character 5	Device Character 6	Qualifier Character 7
6 Cerebral Ventricle	**0** Open **3** Percutaneous **4** Percutaneous Endoscopic	**Z** No Device	**Z** No Qualifier

0 Medical and Surgical
0 Central Nervous System and Cranial Nerves
8 Division: Cutting into a body part, without draining fluids and/or gases from the body part, in order to separate or transect a body part

Body Part Character 4	Approach Character 5	Device Character 6	Qualifier Character 7
0 Brain **7** Cerebral Hemisphere **8** Basal Ganglia **F** Olfactory Nerve **G** Optic Nerve **H** Oculomotor Nerve **J** Trochlear Nerve **K** Trigeminal Nerve **L** Abducens Nerve **M** Facial Nerve **N** Acoustic Nerve **P** Glossopharyngeal Nerve **Q** Vagus Nerve **R** Accessory Nerve **S** Hypoglossal Nerve **W** Cervical Spinal Cord **X** Thoracic Spinal Cord **Y** Lumbar Spinal Cord	**0** Open **3** Percutaneous **4** Percutaneous Endoscopic	**Z** No Device	**Z** No Qualifier

0 **Medical and Surgical**
0 **Central Nervous System and Cranial Nerves**
9 **Drainage:** Taking or letting out fluids and/or gases from a body part

Body Part Character 4	Approach Character 5	Device Character 6	Qualifier Character 7
0 Brain **1** Cerebral Meninges **2** Dura Mater **3** Epidural Space, Intracranial **4** Subdural Space, Intracranial **5** Subarachnoid Space, Intracranial **6** Cerebral Ventricle **7** Cerebral Hemisphere **8** Basal Ganglia **9** Thalamus **A** Hypothalamus **B** Pons **C** Cerebellum **D** Medulla Oblongata **F** Olfactory Nerve **G** Optic Nerve **H** Oculomotor Nerve **J** Trochlear Nerve **K** Trigeminal Nerve **L** Abducens Nerve **M** Facial Nerve **N** Acoustic Nerve **P** Glossopharyngeal Nerve **Q** Vagus Nerve **R** Accessory Nerve **S** Hypoglossal Nerve **T** Spinal Meninges **U** Spinal Canal **W** Cervical Spinal Cord **X** Thoracic Spinal Cord **Y** Lumbar Spinal Cord	**0** Open **3** Percutaneous **4** Percutaneous Endoscopic	**0** Drainage Device	**Z** No Qualifier
0 Brain **1** Cerebral Meninges **2** Dura Mater **3** Epidural Space, Intracranial **4** Subdural Space, Intracranial **5** Subarachnoid Space, Intracranial **6** Cerebral Ventricle **7** Cerebral Hemisphere **8** Basal Ganglia **9** Thalamus **A** Hypothalamus **B** Pons **C** Cerebellum **D** Medulla Oblongata **F** Olfactory Nerve **G** Optic Nerve **H** Oculomotor Nerve **J** Trochlear Nerve **K** Trigeminal Nerve **L** Abducens Nerve **M** Facial Nerve **N** Acoustic Nerve **P** Glossopharyngeal Nerve **Q** Vagus Nerve **R** Accessory Nerve **S** Hypoglossal Nerve **T** Spinal Meninges **U** Spinal Canal **W** Cervical Spinal Cord **X** Thoracic Spinal Cord **Y** Lumbar Spinal Cord	**0** Open **3** Percutaneous **4** Percutaneous Endoscopic	**Z** No Device	**X** Diagnostic **Z** No Qualifier

0 Medical and Surgical
0 Central Nervous System and Cranial Nerves
B Excision: Cutting out or off, without replacement, a portion of a body part

Body Part Character 4	Approach Character 5	Device Character 6	Qualifier Character 7
0 Brain **1** Cerebral Meninges **2** Dura Mater **6** Cerebral Ventricle **7** Cerebral Hemisphere **8** Basal Ganglia **9** Thalamus **A** Hypothalamus **B** Pons **C** Cerebellum **D** Medulla Oblongata **F** Olfactory Nerve **G** Optic Nerve **H** Oculomotor Nerve **J** Trochlear Nerve **K** Trigeminal Nerve **L** Abducens Nerve **M** Facial Nerve **N** Acoustic Nerve **P** Glossopharyngeal Nerve **Q** Vagus Nerve **R** Accessory Nerve **S** Hypoglossal Nerve **T** Spinal Meninges **W** Cervical Spinal Cord **X** Thoracic Spinal Cord **Y** Lumbar Spinal Cord	**0** Open **3** Percutaneous **4** Percutaneous Endoscopic	**Z** No Device	**X** Diagnostic **Z** No Qualifier

0 Medical and Surgical
0 Central Nervous System and Cranial Nerves
C Extirpation: Taking or cutting out solid matter from a body part

Body Part Character 4	Approach Character 5	Device Character 6	Qualifier Character 7
0 Brain **1** Cerebral Meninges **2** Dura Mater **3** Epidural Space, Intracranial **4** Subdural Space, Intracranial **5** Subarachnoid Space, Intracranial **6** Cerebral Ventricle **7** Cerebral Hemisphere **8** Basal Ganglia **9** Thalamus **A** Hypothalamus **B** Pons **C** Cerebellum **D** Medulla Oblongata **F** Olfactory Nerve **G** Optic Nerve **H** Oculomotor Nerve **J** Trochlear Nerve **K** Trigeminal Nerve **L** Abducens Nerve **M** Facial Nerve **N** Acoustic Nerve **P** Glossopharyngeal Nerve **Q** Vagus Nerve **R** Accessory Nerve **S** Hypoglossal Nerve **T** Spinal Meninges **U** Spinal Canal **W** Cervical Spinal Cord **X** Thoracic Spinal Cord **Y** Lumbar Spinal Cord	**0** Open **3** Percutaneous **4** Percutaneous Endoscopic	**Z** No Device	**Z** No Qualifier

0 Medical and Surgical
0 Central Nervous System and Cranial Nerves
D Extraction: Pulling or stripping out or off all or a portion of a body part by the use of force

Body Part Character 4	Approach Character 5	Device Character 6	Qualifier Character 7
1 Cerebral Meninges **2** Dura Mater **F** Olfactory Nerve **G** Optic Nerve **H** Oculomotor Nerve **J** Trochlear Nerve **K** Trigeminal Nerve **L** Abducens Nerve **M** Facial Nerve **N** Acoustic Nerve **P** Glossopharyngeal Nerve **Q** Vagus Nerve **R** Accessory Nerve **S** Hypoglossal Nerve **T** Spinal Meninges	**0** Open **3** Percutaneous **4** Percutaneous Endoscopic	**Z** No Device	**Z** No Qualifier

0 Medical and Surgical
0 Central Nervous System and Cranial Nerves
F Fragmentation: Breaking solid matter in a body part into pieces

Body Part Character 4	Approach Character 5	Device Character 6	Qualifier Character 7
3 Epidural Space, Intracranial NC **4** Subdural Space, Intracranial NC **5** Subarachnoid Space, Intracranial NC **6** Cerebral Ventricle NC **U** Spinal Canal	**0** Open **3** Percutaneous **4** Percutaneous Endoscopic **X** External	**Z** No Device	**Z** No Qualifier

NC 00F3XZZ 00F4XZZ 00F5XZZ 00F6XZZ

0 Medical and Surgical
0 Central Nervous System and Cranial Nerves
H Insertion: Putting in a nonbiological appliance that monitors, assists, performs, or prevents a physiological function but does not physically take the place of a body part

Body Part Character 4	Approach Character 5	Device Character 6	Qualifier Character 7
0 Brain CC DRG	**0** Open	**2** Monitoring Device **3** Infusion Device **4** Radioactive Element, Cesium-131 Collagen Implant **M** Neurostimulator Lead **Y** Other Device	**Z** No Qualifier
0 Brain CC	**3** Percutaneous **4** Percutaneous Endoscopic	**2** Monitoring Device **3** Infusion Device **M** Neurostimulator Lead **Y** Other Device	**Z** No Qualifier
6 Cerebral Ventricle CC **E** Cranial Nerve CC **U** Spinal Canal CC **V** Spinal Cord CC	**0** Open **3** Percutaneous **4** Percutaneous Endoscopic	**2** Monitoring Device **3** Infusion Device **M** Neurostimulator Lead **Y** Other Device	**Z** No Qualifier

CC 00H00MZ 00H03MZ 00H04MZ 00H60MZ 00H63MZ 00H64MZ 00HE0MZ 00HE3MZ 00HE4MZ 00HU0MZ 00HU3MZ 00HU4MZ 00HV0MZ 00HV3MZ 00HV4MZ

DRG 00H004Z

0 Medical and Surgical
0 Central Nervous System and Cranial Nerves
J Inspection: Visually and/or manually exploring a body part

Body Part Character 4	Approach Character 5	Device Character 6	Qualifier Character 7
0 Brain **E** Cranial Nerve **U** Spinal Canal **V** Spinal Cord	**0** Open **3** Percutaneous **4** Percutaneous Endoscopic	**Z** No Device	**Z** No Qualifier

0 Medical and Surgical
0 Central Nervous System and Cranial Nerves
K Map: Locating the route of passage of electrical impulses and/or locating functional areas in a body part

Body Part Character 4	Approach Character 5	Device Character 6	Qualifier Character 7
0 Brain **7** Cerebral Hemisphere **8** Basal Ganglia **9** Thalamus **A** Hypothalamus **B** Pons **C** Cerebellum **D** Medulla Oblongata	**0** Open **3** Percutaneous **4** Percutaneous Endoscopic	**Z** No Device	**Z** No Qualifier

0 Medical and Surgical
0 Central Nervous System and Cranial Nerves
N Release: Freeing a body part from an abnormal physical constraint by cutting or by the use of force

Body Part Character 4	Approach Character 5	Device Character 6	Qualifier Character 7
0 Brain **1** Cerebral Meninges **2** Dura Mater **6** Cerebral Ventricle **7** Cerebral Hemisphere **8** Basal Ganglia **9** Thalamus **A** Hypothalamus **B** Pons **C** Cerebellum **D** Medulla Oblongata **F** Olfactory Nerve **G** Optic Nerve **H** Oculomotor Nerve **J** Trochlear Nerve **K** Trigeminal Nerve **L** Abducens Nerve **M** Facial Nerve **N** Acoustic Nerve **P** Glossopharyngeal Nerve **Q** Vagus Nerve **R** Accessory Nerve **S** Hypoglossal Nerve **T** Spinal Meninges **W** Cervical Spinal Cord **X** Thoracic Spinal Cord **Y** Lumbar Spinal Cord	**0** Open **3** Percutaneous **4** Percutaneous Endoscopic	**Z** No Device	**Z** No Qualifier

0 Medical and Surgical
0 Central Nervous System and Cranial Nerves
P Removal: Taking out or off a device from a body part

Body Part	Approach	Device	Qualifier
Character 4	Character 5	Character 6	Character 7
0 Brain **V** Spinal Cord	**0** Open **3** Percutaneous **4** Percutaneous Endoscopic	**0** Drainage Device **2** Monitoring Device **3** Infusion Device **7** Autologous Tissue Substitute **J** Synthetic Substitute **K** Nonautologous Tissue Substitute **M** Neurostimulator Lead **Y** Other Device	**Z** No Qualifier
0 Brain **V** Spinal Cord	**X** External	**0** Drainage Device **2** Monitoring Device **3** Infusion Device **M** Neurostimulator Lead	**Z** No Qualifier
6 Cerebral Ventricle **U** Spinal Canal	**0** Open **3** Percutaneous **4** Percutaneous Endoscopic	**0** Drainage Device **2** Monitoring Device **3** Infusion Device **J** Synthetic Substitute **M** Neurostimulator Lead **Y** Other Device	**Z** No Qualifier
6 Cerebral Ventricle **U** Spinal Canal	**X** External	**0** Drainage Device **2** Monitoring Device **3** Infusion Device **M** Neurostimulator Lead	**Z** No Qualifier
E Cranial Nerve	**0** Open **3** Percutaneous **4** Percutaneous Endoscopic	**0** Drainage Device **2** Monitoring Device **3** Infusion Device **7** Autologous Tissue Substitute **M** Neurostimulator Lead **Y** Other Device	**Z** No Qualifier
E Cranial Nerve	**X** External	**0** Drainage Device **2** Monitoring Device **3** Infusion Device **M** Neurostimulator Lead	**Z** No Qualifier

0 Medical and Surgical
0 Central Nervous System and Cranial Nerves
Q Repair: Restoring, to the extent possible, a body part to its normal anatomic structure and function

Body Part Character 4	Approach Character 5	Device Character 6	Qualifier Character 7
0 Brain **1** Cerebral Meninges **2** Dura Mater **6** Cerebral Ventricle **7** Cerebral Hemisphere **8** Basal Ganglia **9** Thalamus **A** Hypothalamus **B** Pons **C** Cerebellum **D** Medulla Oblongata **F** Olfactory Nerve **G** Optic Nerve **H** Oculomotor Nerve **J** Trochlear Nerve **K** Trigeminal Nerve **L** Abducens Nerve **M** Facial Nerve **N** Acoustic Nerve **P** Glossopharyngeal Nerve **Q** Vagus Nerve **R** Accessory Nerve **S** Hypoglossal Nerve **T** Spinal Meninges **W** Cervical Spinal Cord **X** Thoracic Spinal Cord **Y** Lumbar Spinal Cord	**0** Open **3** Percutaneous **4** Percutaneous Endoscopic	**Z** No Device	**Z** No Qualifier

0 Medical and Surgical
0 Central Nervous System and Cranial Nerves
R Replacement: Putting in or on biological or synthetic material that physically takes the place and/or function of all or a portion of a body part

Body Part Character 4	Approach Character 5	Device Character 6	Qualifier Character 7
1 Cerebral Meninges **2** Dura Mater **6** Cerebral Ventricle **F** Olfactory Nerve **G** Optic Nerve **H** Oculomotor Nerve **J** Trochlear Nerve **K** Trigeminal Nerve **L** Abducens Nerve **M** Facial Nerve **N** Acoustic Nerve **P** Glossopharyngeal Nerve **Q** Vagus Nerve **R** Accessory Nerve **S** Hypoglossal Nerve **T** Spinal Meninges	**0** Open **4** Percutaneous Endoscopic	**7** Autologous Tissue Substitute **J** Synthetic Substitute **K** Nonautologous Tissue Substitute	**Z** No Qualifier

0 Medical and Surgical
0 Central Nervous System and Cranial Nerves
S Reposition: Moving to its normal location, or other suitable location, all or a portion of a body part

Body Part Character 4	Approach Character 5	Device Character 6	Qualifier Character 7
F Olfactory Nerve **G** Optic Nerve **H** Oculomotor Nerve **J** Trochlear Nerve **K** Trigeminal Nerve **L** Abducens Nerve **M** Facial Nerve **N** Acoustic Nerve **P** Glossopharyngeal Nerve **Q** Vagus Nerve **R** Accessory Nerve **S** Hypoglossal Nerve **W** Cervical Spinal Cord **X** Thoracic Spinal Cord **Y** Lumbar Spinal Cord	**0** Open **3** Percutaneous **4** Percutaneous Endoscopic	**Z** No Device	**Z** No Qualifier

0 Medical and Surgical
0 Central Nervous System and Cranial Nerves
T Resection: Cutting out or off, without replacement, all of a body part

Body Part Character 4	Approach Character 5	Device Character 6	Qualifier Character 7
7 Cerebral Hemisphere	**0** Open **3** Percutaneous **4** Percutaneous Endoscopic	**Z** No Device	**Z** No Qualifier

0 Medical and Surgical
0 Central Nervous System and Cranial Nerves
U Supplement: Putting in or on biological or synthetic material that physically reinforces and/or augments the function of a portion of a body part

Body Part Character 4	Approach Character 5	Device Character 6	Qualifier Character 7
1 Cerebral Meninges **2** Dura Mater **6** Cerebral Ventricle **F** Olfactory Nerve **G** Optic Nerve **H** Oculomotor Nerve **J** Trochlear Nerve **K** Trigeminal Nerve **L** Abducens Nerve **M** Facial Nerve **N** Acoustic Nerve **P** Glossopharyngeal Nerve **Q** Vagus Nerve **R** Accessory Nerve **S** Hypoglossal Nerve **T** Spinal Meninges	**0** Open **3** Percutaneous **4** Percutaneous Endoscopic	**7** Autologous Tissue Substitute **J** Synthetic Substitute **K** Nonautologous Tissue Substitute	**Z** No Qualifier

0 Medical and Surgical
0 Central Nervous System and Cranial Nerves
W Revision: Correcting, to the extent possible, a portion of a malfunctioning device or the position of a displaced device

Body Part Character 4	Approach Character 5	Device Character 6	Qualifier Character 7
0 Brain **V** Spinal Cord	**0** Open **3** Percutaneous **4** Percutaneous Endoscopic	**0** Drainage Device **2** Monitoring Device **3** Infusion Device **7** Autologous Tissue Substitute **J** Synthetic Substitute **K** Nonautologous Tissue Substitute **M** Neurostimulator Lead **Y** Other Device	**Z** No Qualifier
0 Brain **V** Spinal Cord	**X** External	**0** Drainage Device **2** Monitoring Device **3** Infusion Device **7** Autologous Tissue Substitute **J** Synthetic Substitute **K** Nonautologous Tissue Substitute **M** Neurostimulator Lead	**Z** No Qualifier
6 Cerebral Ventricle **U** Spinal Canal	**0** Open **3** Percutaneous **4** Percutaneous Endoscopic	**0** Drainage Device **2** Monitoring Device **3** Infusion Device **J** Synthetic Substitute **M** Neurostimulator Lead **Y** Other Device	**Z** No Qualifier
6 Cerebral Ventricle **U** Spinal Canal	**X** External	**0** Drainage Device **2** Monitoring Device **3** Infusion Device **J** Synthetic Substitute **M** Neurostimulator Lead	**Z** No Qualifier
E Cranial Nerve	**0** Open **3** Percutaneous **4** Percutaneous Endoscopic	**0** Drainage Device **2** Monitoring Device **3** Infusion Device **7** Autologous Tissue Substitute **M** Neurostimulator Lead **Y** Other Device	**Z** No Qualifier
E Cranial Nerve	**X** External	**0** Drainage Device **2** Monitoring Device **3** Infusion Device **7** Autologous Tissue Substitute **M** Neurostimulator Lead	**Z** No Qualifier

0 Medical and Surgical
0 Central Nervous System and Cranial Nerves
X Transfer: Moving, without taking out, all or a portion of a body part to another location to take over the function of all or a portion of a body part

Body Part Character 4	Approach Character 5	Device Character 6	Qualifier Character 7
F Olfactory Nerve **G** Optic Nerve **H** Oculomotor Nerve **J** Trochlear Nerve **K** Trigeminal Nerve **L** Abducens Nerve **M** Facial Nerve **N** Acoustic Nerve **P** Glossopharyngeal Nerve **Q** Vagus Nerve **R** Accessory Nerve **S** Hypoglossal Nerve	**0** Open **4** Percutaneous Endoscopic	**Z** No Device	**F** Olfactory Nerve **G** Optic Nerve **H** Oculomotor Nerve **J** Trochlear Nerve **K** Trigeminal Nerve **L** Abducens Nerve **M** Facial Nerve **N** Acoustic Nerve **P** Glossopharyngeal Nerve **Q** Vagus Nerve **R** Accessory Nerve **S** Hypoglossal Nerve

NOTES

Peripheral Nervous System 012-01X

0 Medical and Surgical
1 Peripheral Nervous System
2 Change: Taking out or off a device from a body part and putting back an identical or similar device in or on the same body part without cutting or puncturing the skin or a mucous membrane

Body Part	Approach	Device	Qualifier
Character 4	**Character 5**	**Character 6**	**Character 7**
Y Peripheral Nerve	**X** External	**0** Drainage Device **Y** Other Device	**Z** No Qualifier

0 Medical and Surgical
1 Peripheral Nervous System
5 Destruction: Physical eradication of all or a portion of a body part by the direct use of energy, force, or a destructive agent

Body Part	Approach	Device	Qualifier
Character 4	**Character 5**	**Character 6**	**Character 7**
0 Cervical Plexus **1** Cervical Nerve **2** Phrenic Nerve **3** Brachial Plexus **4** Ulnar Nerve **5** Median Nerve **6** Radial Nerve **8** Thoracic Nerve **9** Lumbar Plexus **A** Lumbosacral Plexus **B** Lumbar Nerve **C** Pudendal Nerve **D** Femoral Nerve **F** Sciatic Nerve **G** Tibial Nerve **H** Peroneal Nerve **K** Head and Neck Sympathetic Nerve **L** Thoracic Sympathetic Nerve **M** Abdominal Sympathetic Nerve **N** Lumbar Sympathetic Nerve **P** Sacral Sympathetic Nerve **Q** Sacral Plexus **R** Sacral Nerve	**0** Open **3** Percutaneous **4** Percutaneous Endoscopic	**Z** No Device	**Z** No Qualifier

0 Medical and Surgical
1 Peripheral Nervous System
8 Division: Cutting into a body part, without draining fluids and/or gases from the body part, in order to separate or transect a body part

Body Part Character 4	Approach Character 5	Device Character 6	Qualifier Character 7
0 Cervical Plexus **1** Cervical Nerve **2** Phrenic Nerve **3** Brachial Plexus **4** Ulnar Nerve **5** Median Nerve **6** Radial Nerve **8** Thoracic Nerve **9** Lumbar Plexus **A** Lumbosacral Plexus **B** Lumbar Nerve **C** Pudendal Nerve **D** Femoral Nerve **F** Sciatic Nerve **G** Tibial Nerve **H** Peroneal Nerve **K** Head and Neck Sympathetic Nerve **L** Thoracic Sympathetic Nerve **M** Abdominal Sympathetic Nerve **N** Lumbar Sympathetic Nerve **P** Sacral Sympathetic Nerve **Q** Sacral Plexus **R** Sacral Nerve	**0** Open **3** Percutaneous **4** Percutaneous Endoscopic	**Z** No Device	**Z** No Qualifier

0 Medical and Surgical
1 Peripheral Nervous System
9 Drainage: Taking or letting out fluids and/or gases from a body part

Body Part Character 4	Approach Character 5	Device Character 6	Qualifier Character 7
0 Cervical Plexus **1** Cervical Nerve **2** Phrenic Nerve **3** Brachial Plexus **4** Ulnar Nerve **5** Median Nerve **6** Radial Nerve **8** Thoracic Nerve **9** Lumbar Plexus **A** Lumbosacral Plexus **B** Lumbar Nerve **C** Pudendal Nerve **D** Femoral Nerve **F** Sciatic Nerve **G** Tibial Nerve **H** Peroneal Nerve **K** Head and Neck Sympathetic Nerve **L** Thoracic Sympathetic Nerve **M** Abdominal Sympathetic Nerve **N** Lumbar Sympathetic Nerve **P** Sacral Sympathetic Nerve **Q** Sacral Plexus **R** Sacral Nerve	**0** Open **3** Percutaneous **4** Percutaneous Endoscopic	**0** Drainage Device	**Z** No Qualifier

019 continued on next page

0 Medical and Surgical
1 Peripheral Nervous System
9 Drainage: Taking or letting out fluids and/or gases from a body part

019 continued from previous page

Body Part Character 4	Approach Character 5	Device Character 6	Qualifier Character 7
0 Cervical Plexus **1** Cervical Nerve **2** Phrenic Nerve **3** Brachial Plexus **4** Ulnar Nerve **5** Median Nerve **6** Radial Nerve **8** Thoracic Nerve **9** Lumbar Plexus **A** Lumbosacral Plexus **B** Lumbar Nerve **C** Pudendal Nerve **D** Femoral Nerve **F** Sciatic Nerve **G** Tibial Nerve **H** Peroneal Nerve **K** Head and Neck Sympathetic Nerve **L** Thoracic Sympathetic Nerve **M** Abdominal Sympathetic Nerve **N** Lumbar Sympathetic Nerve **P** Sacral Sympathetic Nerve **Q** Sacral Plexus **R** Sacral Nerve	**0** Open **3** Percutaneous **4** Percutaneous Endoscopic	**Z** No Device	**X** Diagnostic **Z** No Qualifier

0 Medical and Surgical
1 Peripheral Nervous System
B Excision: Cutting out or off, without replacement, a portion of a body part

Body Part Character 4	Approach Character 5	Device Character 6	Qualifier Character 7
0 Cervical Plexus **1** Cervical Nerve **2** Phrenic Nerve **3** Brachial Plexus CC **4** Ulnar Nerve **5** Median Nerve **6** Radial Nerve **8** Thoracic Nerve **9** Lumbar Plexus **A** Lumbosacral Plexus **B** Lumbar Nerve **C** Pudendal Nerve **D** Femoral Nerve **F** Sciatic Nerve **G** Tibial Nerve **H** Peroneal Nerve **K** Head and Neck Sympathetic Nerve **L** Thoracic Sympathetic Nerve CC **M** Abdominal Sympathetic Nerve **N** Lumbar Sympathetic Nerve **P** Sacral Sympathetic Nerve **Q** Sacral Plexus **R** Sacral Nerve	**0** Open **3** Percutaneous **4** Percutaneous Endoscopic	**Z** No Device	**X** Diagnostic **Z** No Qualifier

CC 01B30ZZ 01BL0ZZ

LC Limited Coverage NC Noncovered HAC HAC-associated Procedure CC Combination Cluster - See Appendix G for code lists
DRG Non-OR-Affecting MS-DRG Assignment New/Revised Text in **Orange** ♂ Male ♀ Female

0 Medical and Surgical
1 Peripheral Nervous System
C Extirpation: Taking or cutting out solid matter from a body part

Body Part Character 4	Approach Character 5	Device Character 6	Qualifier Character 7
0 Cervical Plexus **1** Cervical Nerve **2** Phrenic Nerve **3** Brachial Plexus **4** Ulnar Nerve **5** Median Nerve **6** Radial Nerve **8** Thoracic Nerve **9** Lumbar Plexus **A** Lumbosacral Plexus **B** Lumbar Nerve **C** Pudendal Nerve **D** Femoral Nerve **F** Sciatic Nerve **G** Tibial Nerve **H** Peroneal Nerve **K** Head and Neck Sympathetic Nerve **L** Thoracic Sympathetic Nerve **M** Abdominal Sympathetic Nerve **N** Lumbar Sympathetic Nerve **P** Sacral Sympathetic Nerve **Q** Sacral Plexus **R** Sacral Nerve	**0** Open **3** Percutaneous **4** Percutaneous Endoscopic	**Z** No Device	**Z** No Qualifier

0 Medical and Surgical
1 Peripheral Nervous System
D Extraction: Pulling or stripping out or off all or a portion of a body part by the use of force

Body Part Character 4	Approach Character 5	Device Character 6	Qualifier Character 7
0 Cervical Plexus **1** Cervical Nerve **2** Phrenic Nerve **3** Brachial Plexus **4** Ulnar Nerve **5** Median Nerve **6** Radial Nerve **8** Thoracic Nerve **9** Lumbar Plexus **A** Lumbosacral Plexus **B** Lumbar Nerve **C** Pudendal Nerve **D** Femoral Nerve **F** Sciatic Nerve **G** Tibial Nerve **H** Peroneal Nerve **K** Head and Neck Sympathetic Nerve **L** Thoracic Sympathetic Nerve **M** Abdominal Sympathetic Nerve **N** Lumbar Sympathetic Nerve **P** Sacral Sympathetic Nerve **Q** Sacral Plexus **R** Sacral Nerve	**0** Open **3** Percutaneous **4** Percutaneous Endoscopic	**Z** No Device	**Z** No Qualifier

0 Medical and Surgical
1 Peripheral Nervous System
H Insertion: Putting in a nonbiological appliance that monitors, assists, performs, or prevents a physiological function but does not physically take the place of a body part

Body Part Character 4	Approach Character 5	Device Character 6	Qualifier Character 7
Y Peripheral Nerve CC	**0** Open **3** Percutaneous **4** Percutaneous Endoscopic	**2** Monitoring Device **M** Neurostimulator Lead **Y** Other Device	**Z** No Qualifier

CC 01HY0MZ 01HY3MZ 01HY4MZ

0 Medical and Surgical
1 Peripheral Nervous System
J Inspection: Visually and/or manually exploring a body part

Body Part Character 4	Approach Character 5	Device Character 6	Qualifier Character 7
Y Peripheral Nerve	**0** Open **3** Percutaneous **4** Percutaneous Endoscopic	**Z** No Device	**Z** No Qualifier

0 Medical and Surgical
1 Peripheral Nervous System
N Release: Freeing a body part from an abnormal physical constraint by cutting or by the use of force

Body Part Character 4	Approach Character 5	Device Character 6	Qualifier Character 7
0 Cervical Plexus **1** Cervical Nerve **2** Phrenic Nerve **3** Brachial Plexus **4** Ulnar Nerve **5** Median Nerve **6** Radial Nerve **8** Thoracic Nerve **9** Lumbar Plexus **A** Lumbosacral Plexus **B** Lumbar Nerve **C** Pudendal Nerve **D** Femoral Nerve **F** Sciatic Nerve **G** Tibial Nerve **H** Peroneal Nerve **K** Head and Neck Sympathetic Nerve **L** Thoracic Sympathetic Nerve **M** Abdominal Sympathetic Nerve **N** Lumbar Sympathetic Nerve **P** Sacral Sympathetic Nerve **Q** Sacral Plexus **R** Sacral Nerve	**0** Open **3** Percutaneous **4** Percutaneous Endoscopic	**Z** No Device	**Z** No Qualifier

0 Medical and Surgical
1 Peripheral Nervous System
P Removal: Taking out or off a device from a body part

Body Part Character 4	Approach Character 5	Device Character 6	Qualifier Character 7
Y Peripheral Nerve	**0** Open **3** Percutaneous **4** Percutaneous Endoscopic	**0** Drainage Device **2** Monitoring Device **7** Autologous Tissue Substitute **M** Neurostimulator Lead **Y** Other Device	**Z** No Qualifier
Y Peripheral Nerve	**X** External	**0** Drainage Device **2** Monitoring Device **M** Neurostimulator Lead	**Z** No Qualifier

LC Limited Coverage NC Noncovered HAC HAC-associated Procedure CC Combination Cluster - See Appendix G for code lists
DRG Non-OR-Affecting MS-DRG Assignment New/Revised Text in **Orange** ♂ Male ♀ Female

0 Medical and Surgical
1 Peripheral Nervous System
Q Repair: Restoring, to the extent possible, a body part to its normal anatomic structure and function

Body Part Character 4	Approach Character 5	Device Character 6	Qualifier Character 7
0 Cervical Plexus **1** Cervical Nerve **2** Phrenic Nerve **3** Brachial Plexus **4** Ulnar Nerve **5** Median Nerve **6** Radial Nerve **8** Thoracic Nerve **9** Lumbar Plexus **A** Lumbosacral Plexus **B** Lumbar Nerve **C** Pudendal Nerve **D** Femoral Nerve **F** Sciatic Nerve **G** Tibial Nerve **H** Peroneal Nerve **K** Head and Neck Sympathetic Nerve **L** Thoracic Sympathetic Nerve **M** Abdominal Sympathetic Nerve **N** Lumbar Sympathetic Nerve **P** Sacral Sympathetic Nerve **Q** Sacral Plexus **R** Sacral Nerve	**0** Open **3** Percutaneous **4** Percutaneous Endoscopic	**Z** No Device	**Z** No Qualifier

0 Medical and Surgical
1 Peripheral Nervous System
R Replacement: Putting in or on biological or synthetic material that physically takes the place and/or function of all or a portion of a body part

Body Part Character 4	Approach Character 5	Device Character 6	Qualifier Character 7
1 Cervical Nerve **2** Phrenic Nerve **4** Ulnar Nerve **5** Median Nerve **6** Radial Nerve **8** Thoracic Nerve **B** Lumbar Nerve **C** Pudendal Nerve **D** Femoral Nerve **F** Sciatic Nerve **G** Tibial Nerve **H** Peroneal Nerve **R** Sacral Nerve	**0** Open **4** Percutaneous Endoscopic	**7** Autologous Tissue Substitute **J** Synthetic Substitute **K** Nonautologous Tissue Substitute	**Z** No Qualifier

LC Limited Coverage NC Noncovered HAC HAC-associated Procedure CC Combination Cluster - See Appendix G for code lists
DRG Non-OR-Affecting MS-DRG Assignment New/Revised Text in **Orange** ♂ Male ♀ Female

0 Medical and Surgical
1 Peripheral Nervous System
S Reposition: Moving to its normal location, or other suitable location, all or a portion of a body part

Body Part Character 4	Approach Character 5	Device Character 6	Qualifier Character 7
0 Cervical Plexus **1** Cervical Nerve **2** Phrenic Nerve **3** Brachial Plexus **4** Ulnar Nerve **5** Median Nerve **6** Radial Nerve **8** Thoracic Nerve **9** Lumbar Plexus **A** Lumbosacral Plexus **B** Lumbar Nerve **C** Pudendal Nerve **D** Femoral Nerve **F** Sciatic Nerve **G** Tibial Nerve **H** Peroneal Nerve **Q** Sacral Plexus **R** Sacral Nerve	**0** Open **3** Percutaneous **4** Percutaneous Endoscopic	**Z** No Device	**Z** No Qualifier

0 Medical and Surgical
1 Peripheral Nervous System
U Supplement: Putting in or on biological or synthetic material that physically reinforces and/or augments the function of a portion of a body part

Body Part Character 4	Approach Character 5	Device Character 6	Qualifier Character 7
1 Cervical Nerve **2** Phrenic Nerve **4** Ulnar Nerve **5** Median Nerve **6** Radial Nerve **8** Thoracic Nerve **B** Lumbar Nerve **C** Pudendal Nerve **D** Femoral Nerve **F** Sciatic Nerve **G** Tibial Nerve **H** Peroneal Nerve **R** Sacral Nerve	**0** Open **3** Percutaneous **4** Percutaneous Endoscopic	**7** Autologous Tissue Substitute **J** Synthetic Substitute **K** Nonautologous Tissue Substitute	**Z** No Qualifier

0 Medical and Surgical
1 Peripheral Nervous System
W Revision: Correcting, to the extent possible, a portion of a malfunctioning device or the position of a displaced device

Body Part Character 4	Approach Character 5	Device Character 6	Qualifier Character 7
Y Peripheral Nerve	**0** Open **3** Percutaneous **4** Percutaneous Endoscopic	**0** Drainage Device **2** Monitoring Device **7** Autologous Tissue Substitute **M** Neurostimulator Lead **Y** Other Device	**Z** No Qualifier
Y Peripheral Nerve	**X** External	**0** Drainage Device **2** Monitoring Device **7** Autologous Tissue Substitute **M** Neurostimulator Lead	**Z** No Qualifier

0 Medical and Surgical
1 Peripheral Nervous System
X Transfer: Moving, without taking out, all or a portion of a body part to another location to take over the function of all or a portion of a body part

Body Part	Approach	Device	Qualifier
Character 4	**Character 5**	**Character 6**	**Character 7**
1 Cervical Nerve **2** Phrenic Nerve	**0** Open **4** Percutaneous Endoscopic	**Z** No Device	**1** Cervical Nerve **2** Phrenic Nerve
4 Ulnar Nerve **5** Median Nerve **6** Radial Nerve	**0** Open **4** Percutaneous Endoscopic	**Z** No Device	**4** Ulnar Nerve **5** Median Nerve **6** Radial Nerve
8 Thoracic Nerve	**0** Open **4** Percutaneous Endoscopic	**Z** No Device	**8** Thoracic Nerve
B Lumbar Nerve **C** Pudendal Nerve	**0** Open **4** Percutaneous Endoscopic	**Z** No Device	**B** Lumbar Nerve **C** Perineal Nerve
D Femoral Nerve **F** Sciatic Nerve **G** Tibial Nerve **H** Peroneal Nerve	**0** Open **4** Percutaneous Endoscopic	**Z** No Device	**D** Femoral Nerve **F** Sciatic Nerve **G** Tibial Nerve **H** Peroneal Nerve

NOTES

NOTES

Heart and Great Vessels 021-02Y

0 Medical and Surgical
2 Heart and Great Vessels
1 Bypass: Altering the route of passage of the contents of a tubular body part

Body Part Character 4	Approach Character 5	Device Character 6	Qualifier Character 7
0 Coronary Artery, One Artery HAC **1** Coronary Artery, Two Arteries HAC **2** Coronary Artery, Three Arteries HAC **3** Coronary Artery, Four or More Arteries HAC	**0** Open	**8** Zooplastic Tissue **9** Autologous Venous Tissue **A** Autologous Arterial Tissue **J** Synthetic Substitute **K** Nonautologous Tissue Substitute	**3** Coronary Artery **8** Internal Mammary, Right **9** Internal Mammary, Left **C** Thoracic Artery **F** Abdominal Artery **W** Aorta
0 Coronary Artery, One Artery HAC **1** Coronary Artery, Two Arteries HAC **2** Coronary Artery, Three Arteries HAC **3** Coronary Artery, Four or More Arteries HAC	**0** Open	**Z** No Device	**3** Coronary Artery **8** Internal Mammary, Right **9** Internal Mammary, Left **C** Thoracic Artery **F** Abdominal Artery
0 Coronary Artery, One Artery **1** Coronary Artery, Two Arteries **2** Coronary Artery, Three Arteries **3** Coronary Artery, Four or More Arteries	**3** Percutaneous	**4** Intraluminal Device, Drug-eluting **D** Intraluminal Device	**4** Coronary Vein
0 Coronary Artery, One Artery **1** Coronary Artery, Two Arteries **2** Coronary Artery, Three Arteries **3** Coronary Artery, Four or More Arteries	**4** Percutaneous Endoscopic	**4** Intraluminal Device, Drug-eluting **D** Intraluminal Device	**4** Coronary Vein
0 Coronary Artery, One Artery HAC **1** Coronary Artery, Two Arteries HAC **2** Coronary Artery, Three Arteries HAC **3** Coronary Artery, Four or More Arteries HAC	**4** Percutaneous Endoscopic	**8** Zooplastic Tissue **9** Autologous Venous Tissue **A** Autologous Arterial Tissue **J** Synthetic Substitute **K** Nonautologous Tissue Substitute	**3** Coronary Artery **8** Internal Mammary, Right **9** Internal Mammary, Left **C** Thoracic Artery **F** Abdominal Artery **W** Aorta
0 Coronary Artery, One Artery HAC **1** Coronary Artery, Two Arteries HAC **2** Coronary Artery, Three Arteries HAC **3** Coronary Artery, Four or More Arteries HAC	**4** Percutaneous Endoscopic	**Z** No Device	**3** Coronary Artery **8** Internal Mammary, Right **9** Internal Mammary, Left **C** Thoracic Artery **F** Abdominal Artery
6 Atrium, Right	**0** Open **4** Percutaneous Endoscopic	**8** Zooplastic Tissue **9** Autologous Venous Tissue **A** Autologous Arterial Tissue **J** Synthetic Substitute **K** Nonautologous Tissue Substitute	**P** Pulmonary Trunk **Q** Pulmonary Artery, Right **R** Pulmonary Artery, Left
6 Atrium, Right	**0** Open **4** Percutaneous Endoscopic	**Z** No Device	**7** Atrium, Left **P** Pulmonary Trunk **Q** Pulmonary Artery, Right **R** Pulmonary Artery, Left

021 continued on next page

021 continued from previous page

0 Medical and Surgical
2 Heart and Great Vessels
1 Bypass: Altering the route of passage of the contents of a tubular body part

Body Part Character 4	Approach Character 5	Device Character 6	Qualifier Character 7
6 Atrium, Right	**3** Percutaneous	**Z** No Device	**7** Atrium, Left
7 Atrium, Left CC **V** Superior Vena Cava	**0** Open **4** Percutaneous Endoscopic	**8** Zooplastic Tissue **9** Autologous Venous Tissue **A** Autologous Arterial Tissue **J** Synthetic Substitute **K** Nonautologous Tissue Substitute **Z** No Device	**P** Pulmonary Trunk **Q** Pulmonary Artery, Right **R** Pulmonary Artery, Left **S** Pulmonary Vein, Right **T** Pulmonary Vein, Left **U** Pulmonary Vein, Confluence
K Ventricle, Right **L** Ventricle, Left	**0** Open **4** Percutaneous Endoscopic	**8** Zooplastic Tissue **9** Autologous Venous Tissue **A** Autologous Arterial Tissue **J** Synthetic Substitute **K** Nonautologous Tissue Substitute	**P** Pulmonary Trunk **Q** Pulmonary Artery, Right **R** Pulmonary Artery, Left
K Ventricle, Right **L** Ventricle, Left	**0** Open **4** Percutaneous Endoscopic	**Z** No Device	**5** Coronary Circulation **8** Internal Mammary, Right **9** Internal Mammary, Left **C** Thoracic Artery **F** Abdominal Artery **P** Pulmonary Trunk **Q** Pulmonary Artery, Right **R** Pulmonary Artery, Left **W** Aorta
P Pulmonary Trunk **Q** Pulmonary Artery, Right **R** Pulmonary Artery, Left	**0** Open **4** Percutaneous Endoscopic	**8** Zooplastic Tissue **9** Autologous Venous Tissue **A** Autologous Arterial Tissue **J** Synthetic Substitute **K** Nonautologous Tissue Substitute **Z** No Device	**A** Innominate Artery **B** Subclavian **D** Carotid
W Thoracic Aorta, Descending	**0** Open	**8** Zooplastic Tissue **9** Autologous Venous Tissue **A** Autologous Arterial Tissue **J** Synthetic Substitute **K** Nonautologous Tissue Substitute	**B** Subclavian **D** Carotid **F** Abdominal Artery **G** Axillary Artery **H** Brachial Artery **P** Pulmonary Trunk **Q** Pulmonary Artery, Right **R** Pulmonary Artery, Left **V** Lower Extremity Artery
W Thoracic Aorta, Descending	**0** Open	**Z** No Device	**B** Subclavian **D** Carotid **P** Pulmonary Trunk **Q** Pulmonary Artery, Right **R** Pulmonary Artery, Left
W Thoracic Aorta, Descending	**4** Percutaneous Endoscopic	**8** Zooplastic Tissue **9** Autologous Venous Tissue **A** Autologous Arterial Tissue **J** Synthetic Substitute **K** Nonautologous Tissue Substitute **Z** No Device	**B** Subclavian **D** Carotid **P** Pulmonary Trunk **Q** Pulmonary Artery, Right **R** Pulmonary Artery, Left

021 continued on next page

0 Medical and Surgical

2 Heart and Great Vessels

1 Bypass: Altering the route of passage of the contents of a tubular body part

021 continued from previous page

Body Part Character 4	Approach Character 5	Device Character 6	Qualifier Character 7
X Thoracic Aorta, Ascending/Arch	**0** Open **4** Percutaneous Endoscopic	**8** Zooplastic Tissue **9** Autologous Venous Tissue **A** Autologous Arterial Tissue **J** Synthetic Substitute **K** Nonautologous Tissue Substitute **Z** No Device	**B** Subclavian **D** Carotid **P** Pulmonary Trunk **Q** Pulmonary Artery, Right **R** Pulmonary Artery, Left

HAC 0210083 0210088 0210089 021008C 021008F 021008W 0210093 0210098 0210099 021009C 021009F 021009W 02100A3 02100A8 02100A9 02100AC 02100AF 02100AW 02100J3 02100J8 02100J9 02100JC 02100JF 02100JW 02100K3 02100K8 02100K9 02100KC 02100KF 02100KW 02100Z3 02100Z8 02100Z9 02100ZC 02100ZF 0210483 0210488 0210489 021048C 021048F 021048W 0210493 0210498 0210499 021049C 021049F 021049W 02104A3 02104A8 02104A9 02104AC 02104AF 02104AW 02104J3 02104J8 02104J9 02104JC 02104JF 02104JW 02104K3 02104K8 02104K9 02104KC 02104KF 02104KW 02104Z3 02104Z8 02104Z9 02104ZC 02104ZF 0211083 0211088 0211089 021108C 021108F 021108W 0211093 0211098 0211099 021109C 021109F 021109W 02110A3 02110A8 02110A9 02110AC 02110AF 02110AW 02110J3 02110J8 02110J9 02110JC 02110JF 02110JW 02110K3 02110K8 02110K9 02110KC 02110KF 02110KW 02110Z3 02110Z8 02110Z9 02110ZC 02110ZF 0211483 0211488 0211489 021148C 021148F 021148W 0211493 0211498 0211499 021149C 021149F 021149W 02114A3 02114A8 02114A9 02114AC 02114AF 02114AW 02114J3 02114J8 02114J9 02114JC 02114JF 02114JW 02114K3 02114K8 02114K9 02114KC 02114KF 02114KW 02114Z3 02114Z8 02114Z9 02114ZC 02114ZF 0212083 0212088 0212089 021208C 021208F 021208W 0212093 0212098 0212099 021209C 021209F 021209W 02120A3 02120A8 02120A9 02120AC 02120AF 02120AW 02120J3 02120J8 02120J9 02120JC 02120JF 02120JW 02120K3 02120K8 02120K9 02120KC 02120KF 02120KW 02120Z3 02120Z8 02120Z9 02120ZC 02120ZF 0212483 0212488 0212489 021248C 021248F 021248W 0212493 0212498 0212499 021249C 021249F 021249W 02124A3 02124A8 02124A9 02124AC 02124AF 02124AW 02124J3 02124J8 02124J9 02124JC 02124JF 02124JW 02124K3 02124K8 02124K9 02124KC 02124KF 02124KW 02124Z3 02124Z8 02124Z9 02124ZC 02124ZF 0213083 0213088 0213089 021308C 021308F 021308W 0213093 0213098 0213099 021309C 021309F 021309W 02130A3 02130A8 02130A9 02130AC 02130AF 02130AW 02130J3 02130J8 02130J9 02130JC 02130JF 02130JW 02130K3 02130K8 02130K9 02130KC 02130KF 02130KW 02130Z3 02130Z8 02130Z9 02130ZC 02130ZF 0213483 0213488 0213489 021348C 021348F 021348W 0213493 0213498 0213499 021349C 021349F 021349W 02134A3 02134A8 02134A9 02134AC 02134AF 02134AW 02134J3 02134J8 02134J9 02134JC 02134JF 02134JW 02134K3 02134K8 02134K9 02134KC 02134KF 02134KW 02134Z3 02134Z8 02134Z9 02134ZC 02134ZF

Surgical site infection, mediastinitis, following coronary artery bypass graft (CABG) and secondary diagnosis J98.51, J98.59.

CC 02170ZP 02170ZQ 02170ZR

0 Medical and Surgical

2 Heart and Great Vessels

4 Creation: Putting in or on biological or synthetic material to form a new body part that to the extent possible replicates the anatomic structure or function of an absent body part

Body Part Character 4	Approach Character 5	Device Character 6	Qualifier Character 7
F Aortic Valve	**0** Open	**7** Autologous Tissue Substitute **8** Zooplastic Tissue **J** Synthetic Substitute **K** Nonautologous Tissue Substitute	**J** Truncal Valve
G Mitral Valve **J** Tricuspid Valve	**0** Open	**7** Autologous Tissue Substitute **8** Zooplastic Tissue **J** Synthetic Substitute **K** Nonautologous Tissue Substitute	**2** Common Atrioventricular Valve

0 Medical and Surgical
2 Heart and Great Vessels
5 Destruction: Physical eradication of all or a portion of a body part by the direct use of energy, force, or a destructive agent

Body Part Character 4	Approach Character 5	Device Character 6	Qualifier Character 7
4 Coronary Vein **5** Atrial Septum **6** Atrium, Right **8** Conduction Mechanism **9** Chordae Tendineae **D** Papillary Muscle **F** Aortic Valve **G** Mitral Valve **H** Pulmonary Valve **J** Tricuspid Valve **K** Ventricle, Right **L** Ventricle, Left **M** Ventricular Septum **N** Pericardium **P** Pulmonary Trunk **Q** Pulmonary Artery, Right **R** Pulmonary Artery, Left **S** Pulmonary Vein, Right **T** Pulmonary Vein, Left **V** Superior Vena Cava **W** Thoracic Aorta, Descending **X** Thoracic Aorta, Ascending/Arch	**0** Open **3** Percutaneous **4** Percutaneous Endoscopic	**Z** No Device	**Z** No Qualifier
7 Atrium, Left	**0** Open **3** Percutaneous **4** Percutaneous Endoscopic	**Z** No Device	**K** Left Atrial Appendage **Z** No Qualifier

0 Medical and Surgical
2 Heart and Great Vessels
7 Dilation: Expanding an orifice or the lumen of a tubular body part

Body Part Character 4	Approach Character 5	Device Character 6	Qualifier Character 7
0 Coronary Artery, One Artery **1** Coronary Artery, Two Arteries **2** Coronary Artery, Three Arteries **3** Coronary Artery, Four or More Arteries	**0** Open **3** Percutaneous **4** Percutaneous Endoscopic	**4** Intraluminal Device, Drug-eluting **5** Intraluminal Device, Drug-eluting, Two **6** Intraluminal Device, Drug-eluting, Three **7** Intraluminal Device, Drug-eluting, Four or More **D** Intraluminal Device **E** Intraluminal Device, Two **F** Intraluminal Device, Three **G** Intraluminal Device, Four or More **T** Intraluminal Device, Radioactive **Z** No Device	**6** Bifurcation **Z** No Qualifier
F Aortic Valve **G** Mitral Valve **H** Pulmonary Valve **J** Tricuspid Valve **K** Ventricle, Right **L** Ventricle, Left **P** Pulmonary Trunk **Q** Pulmonary Artery, Right **S** Pulmonary Vein, Right **T** Pulmonary Vein, Left **V** Superior Vena Cava **W** Thoracic Aorta, Descending **X** Thoracic Aorta, Ascending/Arch	**0** Open **3** Percutaneous **4** Percutaneous Endoscopic	**4** Intraluminal Device, Drug-eluting **D** Intraluminal Device **Z** No Device	**Z** No Qualifier
R Pulmonary Artery, Left	**0** Open **3** Percutaneous **4** Percutaneous Endoscopic	**4** Intraluminal Device, Drug-eluting **D** Intraluminal Device **Z** No Device	**T** Ductus Arteriosus **Z** No Qualifier

0 Medical and Surgical
2 Heart and Great Vessels
8 Division: Cutting into a body part, without draining fluids and/or gases from the body part, in order to separate or transect a body part

Body Part Character 4	Approach Character 5	Device Character 6	Qualifier Character 7
8 Conduction Mechanism **9** Chordae Tendineae **D** Papillary Muscle	**0** Open **3** Percutaneous **4** Percutaneous Endoscopic	**Z** No Device	**Z** No Qualifier

0 Medical and Surgical
2 Heart and Great Vessels
B Excision: Cutting out or off, without replacement, a portion of a body part

Body Part Character 4	Approach Character 5	Device Character 6	Qualifier Character 7
4 Coronary Vein **5** Atrial Septum **6** Atrium, Right **8** Conduction Mechanism **9** Chordae Tendineae **D** Papillary Muscle **F** Aortic Valve **G** Mitral Valve **H** Pulmonary Valve **J** Tricuspid Valve **K** Ventricle, Right NC CC **L** Ventricle, Left NC **M** Ventricular Septum **N** Pericardium **P** Pulmonary Trunk **Q** Pulmonary Artery, Right **R** Pulmonary Artery, Left **S** Pulmonary Vein, Right **T** Pulmonary Vein, Left **V** Superior Vena Cava **W** Thoracic Aorta, Descending **X** Thoracic Aorta, Ascending/Arch	**0** Open **3** Percutaneous **4** Percutaneous Endoscopic	**Z** No Device	**X** Diagnostic **Z** No Qualifier
7 Atrium, Left DRG	**0** Open **3** Percutaneous **4** Percutaneous Endoscopic	**Z** No Device	**K** Left Atrial Appendage **X** Diagnostic **Z** No Qualifier

NC 02BK0ZZ 02BK3ZZ 02BK4ZZ 02BL0ZZ 02BL3ZZ 02BL4ZZ

CC 02BK0ZZ

DRG 02B70ZK 02B73ZK 02B74ZK

0 Medical and Surgical
2 Heart and Great Vessels
C Extirpation: Taking or cutting out solid matter from a body part

Body Part Character 4	Approach Character 5	Device Character 6	Qualifier Character 7
0 Coronary Artery, One Artery **1** Coronary Artery, Two Arteries **2** Coronary Artery, Three Arteries **3** Coronary Artery, Four or More Arteries	**0** Open **3** Percutaneous **4** Percutaneous Endoscopic	**Z** No Device	**6** Bifurcation **Z** No Qualifier
4 Coronary Vein **5** Atrial Septum **6** Atrium, Right **7** Atrium, Left **8** Conduction Mechanism **9** Chordae Tendineae **D** Papillary Muscle **F** Aortic Valve **G** Mitral Valve **H** Pulmonary Valve **J** Tricuspid Valve **K** Ventricle, Right **L** Ventricle, Left **M** Ventricular Septum **N** Pericardium **P** Pulmonary Trunk **Q** Pulmonary Artery, Right **R** Pulmonary Artery, Left **S** Pulmonary Vein, Right **T** Pulmonary Vein, Left **V** Superior Vena Cava **W** Thoracic Aorta, Descending **X** Thoracic Aorta, Ascending/Arch	**0** Open **3** Percutaneous **4** Percutaneous Endoscopic	**Z** No Device	**Z** No Qualifier

0 Medical and Surgical
2 Heart and Great Vessels
F Fragmentation: Breaking solid matter in a body part into pieces

Body Part Character 4	Approach Character 5	Device Character 6	Qualifier Character 7
N Pericardium NC	**0** Open **3** Percutaneous **4** Percutaneous Endoscopic **X** External	**Z** No Device	**Z** No Qualifier

NC 02FNXZZ

0 Medical and Surgical
2 Heart and Great Vessels
H Insertion: Putting in a nonbiological appliance that monitors, assists, performs, or prevents a physiological function but does not physically take the place of a body part

Body Part	Approach	Device	Qualifier
Character 4	**Character 5**	**Character 6**	**Character 7**
4 Coronary Vein CC HAC **6** Atrium, Right CC HAC **7** Atrium, Left CC HAC **K** Ventricle, Right CC HAC **L** Ventricle, Left CC HAC	**0** Open **3** Percutaneous **4** Percutaneous Endoscopic	**0** Monitoring Device, Pressure Sensor **2** Monitoring Device **3** Infusion Device **D** Intraluminal Device **J** Cardiac Lead, Pacemaker **K** Cardiac Lead, Defibrillator **M** Cardiac Lead **N** Intracardiac Pacemaker **Y** Other Device	**Z** No Qualifier
A Heart NC LC	**0** Open **3** Percutaneous **4** Percutaneous Endoscopic	**Q** Implantable Heart Assist System **Y** Other Device	**Z** No Qualifier
A Heart CC	**0** Open **3** Percutaneous **4** Percutaneous Endoscopic	**R** Short term External Heart Assist System	**J** Intraoperative **S** Biventricular **Z** No Qualifier
N Pericardium CC HAC	**0** Open **3** Percutaneous **4** Percutaneous Endoscopic	**0** Monitoring Device, Pressure Sensor **2** Monitoring Device **J** Cardiac Lead, Pacemaker **K** Cardiac Lead, Defibrillator **M** Cardiac Lead **Y** Other Device	**Z** No Qualifier
P Pulmonary Trunk **Q** Pulmonary Artery, Right **R** Pulmonary Artery, Left **S** Pulmonary Vein, Right HAC **T** Pulmonary Vein, Left HAC **V** Superior Vena Cava HAC **W** Thoracic Aorta, Descending	**0** Open **3** Percutaneous **4** Percutaneous Endoscopic	**0** Monitoring Device, Pressure Sensor **2** Monitoring Device **3** Infusion Device **D** Intraluminal Device **Y** Other Device	**Z** No Qualifier
X Thoracic Aorta, Ascending/Arch	**0** Open **3** Percutaneous **4** Percutaneous Endoscopic	**0** Monitoring Device, Pressure Sensor **2** Monitoring Device **3** Infusion Device **D** Intraluminal Device	**Z** No Qualifier

LC 02HA0QZ

NC 02HA3QZ 02HA4QZ

HAC 02H633Z 02HK33Z 02HS33Z 02HS43Z 02HT33Z 02HT43Z 02HV33Z 02HV43Z
Iatrogenic pneumothorax w/ venous catheterization procedures and secondary diagnosis J95.811.

HAC 02H43JZ 02H43KZ 02H43MZ 02H63JZ 02H63MZ 02H73JZ 02H73MZ 02HK3JZ 02HL3JZ 02HN0JZ 02HN0MZ 02HN3JZ 02HN3MZ 02HN4JZ 02HN4MZ
Surgical site infection (SSI) following cardiac implantable electronic device (CIED) procedures and secondary diagnosis K68.11, T81.4XXA, T82.6XXA, T82.7XXA.

CC 02H40JZ 02H40KZ 02H40MZ 02H43JZ 02H43KZ 02H43MZ 02H44JZ 02H44KZ 02H44MZ 02H60JZ 02H60KZ 02H60MZ 02H63JZ 02H63KZ 02H63MZ 02H64JZ 02H64KZ 02H64MZ 02H70JZ 02H70KZ 02H70MZ 02H73JZ 02H73KZ 02H73MZ 02H74JZ 02H74KZ 02H74MZ 02HA0RS 02HA0RZ 02HA3RS 02HA4RS 02HA4RZ 02HK00Z 02HK02Z 02HK0JZ 02HK0KZ 02HK0MZ 02HK30Z 02HK32Z 02HK3JZ 02HK3KZ 02HK3MZ 02HK40Z 02HK42Z 02HK4JZ 02HK4KZ 02HK4MZ 02HL0JZ 02HL0KZ 02HL0MZ 02HL3JZ 02HL3KZ 02HL3MZ 02HL4JZ 02HL4KZ 02HL4MZ 02HN0JZ 02HN0KZ 02HN0MZ 02HN3JZ 02HN3KZ 02HN3MZ 02HN4JZ 02HN4KZ 02HN4MZ

0 Medical and Surgical
2 Heart and Great Vessels
J Inspection: Visually and/or manually exploring a body part

Body Part	Approach	Device	Qualifier
Character 4	**Character 5**	**Character 6**	**Character 7**
A Heart **Y** Great Vessel	**0** Open **3** Percutaneous **4** Percutaneous Endoscopic	**Z** No Device	**Z** No Qualifier

0 Medical and Surgical
2 Heart and Great Vessels
K Map: Locating the route of passage of electrical impulses and/or locating functional areas in a body part

Body Part	Approach	Device	Qualifier
Character 4	Character 5	Character 6	Character 7
8 Conduction Mechanism	0 Open 3 Percutaneous 4 Percutaneous Endoscopic	Z No Device	Z No Qualifier

0 Medical and Surgical
2 Heart and Great Vessels
L Occlusion: Completely closing an orifice or the lumen of a tubular body part

Body Part	Approach	Device	Qualifier
Character 4	Character 5	Character 6	Character 7
7 Atrium, Left	0 Open 3 Percutaneous 4 Percutaneous Endoscopic	C Extraluminal Device D Intraluminal Device Z No Device	K Left Atrial Appendage
H Pulmonary Valve P Pulmonary Trunk Q Pulmonary Artery, Right S Pulmonary Vein, Right CC T Pulmonary Vein, Left CC V Superior Vena Cava	0 Open 3 Percutaneous 4 Percutaneous Endoscopic	C Extraluminal Device D Intraluminal Device Z No Device	Z No Qualifier
R Pulmonary Artery, Left CC	0 Open 3 Percutaneous 4 Percutaneous Endoscopic	C Extraluminal Device D Intraluminal Device Z No Device	T Ductus Arteriosus Z No Qualifier
W Thoracic Aorta, Descending	3 Percutaneous	D Intraluminal Device	J Temporary

CC 02LR0ZT 02LS0ZZ 02LT0ZZ

0 Medical and Surgical
2 Heart and Great Vessels
N Release: Freeing a body part from an abnormal physical constraint by cutting or by the use of force

Body Part	Approach	Device	Qualifier
Character 4	Character 5	Character 6	Character 7
0 Coronary Artery, One Artery 1 Coronary Artery, Two Arteries 2 Coronary Artery, Three Arteries 3 Coronary Artery, Four or More Arteries 4 Coronary Vein 5 Atrial Septum 6 Atrium, Right 7 Atrium, Left 8 Conduction Mechanism 9 Chordae Tendineae D Papillary Muscle F Aortic Valve G Mitral Valve H Pulmonary Valve CC J Tricuspid Valve K Ventricle, Right L Ventricle, Left M Ventricular Septum N Pericardium P Pulmonary Trunk Q Pulmonary Artery, Right R Pulmonary Artery, Left S Pulmonary Vein, Right T Pulmonary Vein, Left V Superior Vena Cava W Thoracic Aorta, Descending X Thoracic Aorta, Ascending/Arch	0 Open 3 Percutaneous 4 Percutaneous Endoscopic	Z No Device	Z No Qualifier

CC 02NH0ZZ

0 Medical and Surgical
2 Heart and Great Vessels
P Removal: Taking out or off a device from a body part

Body Part Character 4	Approach Character 5	Device Character 6	Qualifier Character 7
A Heart HAC CC	**0** Open **3** Percutaneous **4** Percutaneous Endoscopic	**2** Monitoring Device **3** Infusion Device **7** Autologous Tissue Substitute **8** Zooplastic Tissue **C** Extraluminal Device **D** Intraluminal Device **J** Synthetic Substitute **K** Nonautologous Tissue Substitute **M** Cardiac Lead **N** Intracardiac Pacemaker **Q** Implantable Heart Assist System **Y** Other Device	**Z** No Qualifier
A Heart CC	**0** Open **3** Percutaneous **4** Percutaneous Endoscopic	**R** Short-term External Heart Assist System	**S** Biventricular **Z** No Qualifier
A Heart HAC CC	**X** External	**2** Monitoring Device **3** Infusion Device **D** Intraluminal Device **M** Cardiac Lead	**Z** No Qualifier
Y Great Vessel	**0** Open **3** Percutaneous **4** Percutaneous Endoscopic	**2** Monitoring Device **3** Infusion Device **7** Autologous Tissue Substitute **8** Zooplastic Tissue **C** Extraluminal Device **D** Intraluminal Device **J** Synthetic Substitute **K** Nonautologous Tissue Substitute **Y** Other Device	**Z** No Qualifier
Y Great Vessel	**X** External	**2** Monitoring Device **3** Infusion Device **D** Intraluminal Device	**Z** No Qualifier

HAC 02PA0MZ 02PA3MZ 02PA4MZ 02PAXMZ
Surgical site infection (SSI) following cardiac implantable electronic device (CIED) procedures and secondary diagnosis K68.11, T81.4XXA, T82.6XXA, T82.7XXA.

CC 02PA0MZ 02PA0RZ 02PA3MZ 02PA3RZ 02PA4MZ 02PA4RZ 02PAXMZ

0 Medical and Surgical
2 Heart and Great Vessels
Q Repair: Restoring, to the extent possible, a body part to its normal anatomic structure and function

Body Part Character 4	Approach Character 5	Device Character 6	Qualifier Character 7
0 Coronary Artery, One Artery **1** Coronary Artery, Two Arteries **2** Coronary Artery, Three Arteries **3** Coronary Artery, Four or More Arteries **4** Coronary Vein **5** Atrial Septum **6** Atrium, Right **7** Atrium, Left **8** Conduction Mechanism **9** Chordae Tendineae **A** Heart **B** Heart, Right **C** Heart, Left **D** Papillary Muscle **H** Pulmonary Valve **K** Ventricle, Right **L** Ventricle, Left **M** Ventricular Septum **N** Pericardium **P** Pulmonary Trunk **Q** Pulmonary Artery, Right **R** Pulmonary Artery, Left **S** Pulmonary Vein, Right **T** Pulmonary Vein, Left **V** Superior Vena Cava **W** Thoracic Aorta, Descending **X** Thoracic Aorta, Ascending/Arch	**0** Open **3** Percutaneous **4** Percutaneous Endoscopic	**Z** No Device	**Z** No Qualifier
F Aortic Valve	**0** Open **3** Percutaneous **4** Percutaneous Endoscopic	**Z** No Device	**J** Truncal Valve **Z** No Qualifier
G Mitral Valve	**0** Open **3** Percutaneous **4** Percutaneous Endoscopic	**Z** No Device	**E** Atrioventricular Valve, Left **Z** No Qualifier
J Tricuspid Valve	**0** Open **3** Percutaneous **4** Percutaneous Endoscopic	**Z** No Device	**G** Atrioventricular Valve, Right **Z** No Qualifier

0 Medical and Surgical
2 Heart and Great Vessels
R Replacement: Putting in or on biological or synthetic material that physically takes the place and/or function of all or a portion of a body part

Body Part	Approach	Device	Qualifier
Character 4	Character 5	Character 6	Character 7
5 Atrial Septum **6** Atrium, Right **7** Atrium, Left **9** Chordae Tendineae **D** Papillary Muscle **K** Ventricle, Right NC LC CC **L** Ventricle, Left NC LC CC **M** Ventricular Septum CC **N** Pericardium **P** Pulmonary Trunk CC **Q** Pulmonary Artery, Right CC **R** Pulmonary Artery, Left CC **S** Pulmonary Vein, Right **T** Pulmonary Vein, Left **V** Superior Vena Cava **W** Thoracic Aorta, Descending **X** Thoracic Aorta, Ascending/Arch	**0** Open **4** Percutaneous Endoscopic	**7** Autologous Tissue Substitute **8** Zooplastic Tissue **J** Synthetic Substitute **K** Nonautologous Tissue Substitute	**Z** No Qualifier
F Aortic Valve **G** Mitral Valve **H** Pulmonary Valve **J** Tricuspid Valve	**0** Open **4** Percutaneous Endoscopic	**7** Autologous Tissue Substitute **8** Zooplastic Tissue **J** Synthetic Substitute **K** Nonautologous Tissue Substitute	**Z** No Qualifier
F Aortic Valve **G** Mitral Valve **H** Pulmonary Valve **J** Tricuspid Valve	**3** Percutaneous	**7** Autologous Tissue Substitute **8** Zooplastic Tissue **J** Synthetic Substitute **K** Nonautologous Tissue Substitute	**H** Transapical **Z** No Qualifier

LC 02RK0JZ with 02RL0JZ
Limited coverage when combined with diagnosis code Z00.6.

NC 02RK0JZ or 02RL0JZ with 02RL0JZ
Noncovered except when combined with diagnosis code Z00.6.

CC 02RK0JZ 02RL0JZ 02RM0JZ 02RP0JZ 02RQ07Z 02RQ0JZ 02RR07Z 02RR0JZ

0 Medical and Surgical
2 Heart and Great Vessels
S Reposition: Moving to its normal location, or other suitable location, all or a portion of a body part

Body Part	Approach	Device	Qualifier
Character 4	Character 5	Character 6	Character 7
0 Coronary Artery, One Artery **1** Coronary Artery, Two Arteries **P** Pulmonary Trunk CC **Q** Pulmonary Artery, Right **R** Pulmonary Artery, Left **S** Pulmonary Vein, Right **T** Pulmonary Vein, Left **V** Superior Vena Cava **W** Thoracic Aorta, Descending CC **X** Thoracic Aorta, Ascending/Arch	**0** Open	**Z** No Device	**Z** No Qualifier

CC 02SP0ZZ 02SW0ZZ

0 Medical and Surgical
2 Heart and Great Vessels
T Resection: Cutting out or off, without replacement, all of a body part

Body Part Character 4	Approach Character 5	Device Character 6	Qualifier Character 7
5 Atrial Septum **8** Conduction Mechanism **9** Chordae Tendineae **D** Papillary Muscle **H** Pulmonary Valve **M** Ventricular Septum **N** Pericardium	**0** Open **3** Percutaneous **4** Percutaneous Endoscopic	**Z** No Device	**Z** No Qualifier

0 Medical and Surgical
2 Heart and Great Vessels
U Supplement: Putting in or on biological or synthetic material that physically reinforces and/or augments the function of a portion of a body part

Body Part Character 4	Approach Character 5	Device Character 6	Qualifier Character 7
5 Atrial Septum **6** Atrium, Right **7** Atrium, Left CC **9** Chordae Tendineae **A** Heart **D** Papillary Muscle **H** Pulmonary Valve **K** Ventricle, Right **L** Ventricle, Left **M** Ventricular Septum **N** Pericardium **P** Pulmonary Trunk **Q** Pulmonary Artery, Right **R** Pulmonary Artery, Left **S** Pulmonary Vein, Right **T** Pulmonary Vein, Left **V** Superior Vena Cava **W** Thoracic Aorta, Descending **X** Thoracic Aorta, Ascending/Arch	**0** Open **3** Percutaneous **4** Percutaneous Endoscopic	**7** Autologous Tissue Substitute **8** Zooplastic Tissue **J** Synthetic Substitute **K** Nonautologous Tissue Substitute	**Z** No Qualifier
F Aortic Valve	**0** Open **3** Percutaneous **4** Percutaneous Endoscopic	**7** Autologous Tissue Substitute **8** Zooplastic Tissue **J** Synthetic Substitute **K** Nonautologous Tissue Substitute	**J** Truncal Valve **Z** No Qualifier
G Mitral Valve	**0** Open **3** Percutaneous **4** Percutaneous Endoscopic	**7** Autologous Tissue Substitute **8** Zooplastic Tissue **J** Synthetic Substitute **K** Nonautologous Tissue Substitute	**E** Atrioventricular Valve, Left **Z** No Qualifier
J Tricuspid Valve	**0** Open **3** Percutaneous **4** Percutaneous Endoscopic	**7** Autologous Tissue Substitute **8** Zooplastic Tissue **J** Synthetic Substitute **K** Nonautologous Tissue Substitute	**G** Atrioventricular Valve, Right **Z** No Qualifier

CC 02U70JZ

0 Medical and Surgical
2 Heart and Great Vessels
V Restriction: Partially closing an orifice or the lumen of a tubular body part

Body Part Character 4	Approach Character 5	Device Character 6	Qualifier Character 7
A Heart	**0** Open **3** Percutaneous **4** Percutaneous Endoscopic	**C** Extraluminal Device **Z** No Device	**Z** No Qualifier
G Mitral Valve	**0** Open **3** Percutaneous **4** Percutaneous Endoscopic	**Z** No Device	**Z** No Qualifier
P Pulmonary Trunk **Q** Pulmonary Artery, Right **S** Pulmonary Vein, Right **T** Pulmonary Vein, Left **V** Superior Vena Cava	**0** Open **3** Percutaneous **4** Percutaneous Endoscopic	**C** Extraluminal Device **D** Intraluminal Device **Z** No Device	**Z** No Qualifier
R Pulmonary Artery, Left CC	**0** Open **3** Percutaneous **4** Percutaneous Endoscopic	**C** Extraluminal Device **D** Intraluminal Device **Z** No Device	**T** Ductus Arteriosus **Z** No Qualifier
W Thoracic Aorta, Descending **X** Thoracic Aorta, Ascending/Arch	**0** Open **3** Percutaneous **4** Percutaneous Endoscopic	**C** Extraluminal Device **D** Intraluminal Device **E** Intraluminal Device, Branched or Fenestrated, One or Two Arteries **F** Intraluminal Device, Branched or Fenestrated, Three or More Arteries **Z** No Device	**Z** No Qualifier

CC 02VR0ZT

0 Medical and Surgical
2 Heart and Great Vessels
W Revision: Correcting, to the extent possible, a portion of a malfunctioning device or the position of a displaced device

Body Part Character 4	Approach Character 5	Device Character 6	Qualifier Character 7
5 Atrial Septum **M** Ventricular Septum	**0** Open **4** Percutaneous Endoscopic	**J** Synthetic Substitute	**Z** No Qualifier
A Heart NC CC HAC LC	**0** Open **3** Percutaneous **4** Percutaneous Endoscopic	**2** Monitoring Device **3** Infusion Device **7** Autologous Tissue Substitute **8** Zooplastic Tissue **C** Extraluminal Device **D** Intraluminal Device **J** Synthetic Substitute **K** Nonautologous Tissue Substitute **M** Cardiac Lead **N** Intracardiac Pacemaker **Q** Implantable Heart Assist System **Y** Other Device	**Z** No Qualifier
A Heart CC	**0** Open **3** Percutaneous **4** Percutaneous Endoscopic	**R** Short-term External Heart Assist System	**S** Biventricular **Z** No Qualifier
A Heart	**X** External	**2** Monitoring Device **3** Infusion Device **7** Autologous Tissue Substitute **8** Zooplastic Tissue **C** Extraluminal Device **D** Intraluminal Device **J** Synthetic Substitute **K** Nonautologous Tissue Substitute **M** Cardiac Lead **N** Intracardiac Pacemaker **Q** Implantable Heart Assist System	**Z** No Qualifier

02W continued on next page

0 Medical and Surgical
2 Heart and Great Vessels
W Revision: Correcting, to the extent possible, a portion of a malfunctioning device or the position of a displaced device

02W continued from previous page

Body Part	Approach	Device	Qualifier
Character 4	Character 5	Character 6	Character 7
A Heart	X External	R Short-term External Heart Assist System	S Biventricular Z No Qualifier
F Aortic Valve G Mitral Valve H Pulmonary Valve J Tricuspid Valve	0 Open 3 Percutaneous 4 Percutaneous Endoscopic	7 Autologous Tissue Substitute 8 Zooplastic Tissue J Synthetic Substitute K Nonautologous Tissue Substitute	Z No Qualifier
Y Great Vessel	0 Open 3 Percutaneous 4 Percutaneous Endoscopic	2 Monitoring Device 3 Infusion Device 7 Autologous Tissue Substitute 8 Zooplastic Tissue C Extraluminal Device D Intraluminal Device J Synthetic Substitute K Nonautologous Tissue Substitute Y Other Device	Z No Qualifier
Y Great Vessel	X External	2 Monitoring Device 3 Infusion Device 7 Autologous Tissue Substitute 8 Zooplastic Tissue C Extraluminal Device D Intraluminal Device J Synthetic Substitute K Nonautologous Tissue Substitute	Z No Qualifier

LC 02WA0JZ 02WA0QZ
NC 02WA3QZ 02WA4QZ
HAC 02WA0MZ 02WA3MZ 02WA4MZ
Surgical site infection (SSI) following cardiac implantable electronic device (CIED) procedures and secondary diagnosis K68.11, T81.4XXA, T82.6XXA, T82.7XXA.
CC 02WA0QZ 02WA0RZ 02WA3QZ 02WA3RZ 02WA4QZ 02WA4RZ

0 Medical and Surgical
2 Heart and Great Vessels
Y Transplantation: Putting in or on all or a portion of a living body part taken from another individual or animal to physically take the place and/or function of all or a portion of a similar body part

Body Part	Approach	Device	Qualifier
Character 4	Character 5	Character 6	Character 7
A Heart LC	0 Open	Z No Device	0 Allogeneic 1 Syngeneic 2 Zooplastic

LC 02YA0Z0 02YA0Z1 02YA0Z2

NOTES

Upper Arteries 031-03W

0 Medical and Surgical
3 Upper Arteries
1 Bypass: Altering the route of passage of the contents of a tubular body part

Body Part	Approach	Device	Qualifier
Character 4	**Character 5**	**Character 6**	**Character 7**
2 Innominate Artery	0 Open	9 Autologous Venous Tissue A Autologous Arterial Tissue J Synthetic Substitute K Nonautologous Tissue Substitute Z No Device	0 Upper Arm Artery, Right 1 Upper Arm Artery, Left 2 Upper Arm Artery, Bilateral 3 Lower Arm Artery, Right 4 Lower Arm Artery, Left 5 Lower Arm Artery, Bilateral 6 Upper Leg Artery, Right 7 Upper Leg Artery, Left 8 Upper Leg Artery, Bilateral 9 Lower Leg Artery, Right B Lower Leg Artery, Left C Lower Leg Artery, Bilateral D Upper Arm Vein F Lower Arm Vein J Extracranial Artery, Right K Extracranial Artery, Left
3 Subclavian Artery, Right 4 Subclavian Artery, Left	0 Open	9 Autologous Venous Tissue A Autologous Arterial Tissue J Synthetic Substitute K Nonautologous Tissue Substitute Z No Device	0 Upper Arm Artery, Right 1 Upper Arm Artery, Left 2 Upper Arm Artery, Bilateral 3 Lower Arm Artery, Right 4 Lower Arm Artery, Left 5 Lower Arm Artery, Bilateral 6 Upper Leg Artery, Right 7 Upper Leg Artery, Left 8 Upper Leg Artery, Bilateral 9 Lower Leg Artery, Right B Lower Leg Artery, Left C Lower Leg Artery, Bilateral D Upper Arm Vein F Lower Arm Vein J Extracranial Artery, Right K Extracranial Artery, Left M Pulmonary Artery, Right N Pulmonary Artery, Left
5 Axillary Artery, Right 6 Axillary Artery, Left	0 Open	9 Autologous Venous Tissue A Autologous Arterial Tissue J Synthetic Substitute K Nonautologous Tissue Substitute Z No Device	0 Upper Arm Artery, Right 1 Upper Arm Artery, Left 2 Upper Arm Artery, Bilateral 3 Lower Arm Artery, Right 4 Lower Arm Artery, Left 5 Lower Arm Artery, Bilateral 6 Upper Leg Artery, Right 7 Upper Leg Artery, Left 8 Upper Leg Artery, Bilateral 9 Lower Leg Artery, Right B Lower Leg Artery, Left C Lower Leg Artery, Bilateral D Upper Arm Vein F Lower Arm Vein J Extracranial Artery, Right K Extracranial Artery, Left T Abdominal Artery V Superior Vena Cava

031 continued on next page

0 Medical and Surgical
3 Upper Arteries
1 Bypass: Altering the route of passage of the contents of a tubular body part

031 continued from previous page

Body Part Character 4	Approach Character 5	Device Character 6	Qualifier Character 7
7 Brachial Artery, Right	**0** Open	**9** Autologous Venous Tissue **A** Autologous Arterial Tissue **J** Synthetic Substitute **K** Nonautologous Tissue Substitute **Z** No Device	**0** Upper Arm Artery, Right **3** Lower Arm Artery, Right **D** Upper Arm Vein **F** Lower Arm Vein **V** Superior Vena Cava
8 Brachial Artery, Left	**0** Open	**9** Autologous Venous Tissue **A** Autologous Arterial Tissue **J** Synthetic Substitute **K** Nonautologous Tissue Substitute **Z** No Device	**1** Upper Arm Artery, Left **4** Lower Arm Artery, Left **D** Upper Arm Vein **F** Lower Arm Vein **V** Superior Vena Cava
9 Ulnar Artery, Right **B** Radial Artery, Right CC	**0** Open	**9** Autologous Venous Tissue **A** Autologous Arterial Tissue **J** Synthetic Substitute **K** Nonautologous Tissue Substitute **Z** No Device	**3** Lower Arm Artery, Right **F** Lower Arm Vein
A Ulnar Artery, Left **C** Radial Artery, Left CC	**0** Open	**9** Autologous Venous Tissue **A** Autologous Arterial Tissue **J** Synthetic Substitute **K** Nonautologous Tissue Substitute **Z** No Device	**4** Lower Arm Artery, Left **F** Lower Arm Vein
G Intracranial Artery **S** Temporal Artery, Right NC **T** Temporal Artery, Left NC	**0** Open	**9** Autologous Venous Tissue **A** Autologous Arterial Tissue **J** Synthetic Substitute **K** Nonautologous Tissue Substitute **Z** No Device	**G** Intracranial Artery
H Common Carotid Artery, Right NC **J** Common Carotid Artery, Left NC	**0** Open	**9** Autologous Venous Tissue **A** Autologous Arterial Tissue **J** Synthetic Substitute **K** Nonautologous Tissue Substitute **Z** No Device	**G** Intracranial Artery **J** Extracranial Artery, Right **K** Extracranial Artery, Left **Y** Upper Artery
K Internal Carotid Artery, Right **L** Internal Carotid Artery, Left **M** External Carotid Artery, Right **N** External Carotid Artery, Left	**0** Open	**9** Autologous Venous Tissue **A** Autologous Arterial Tissue **J** Synthetic Substitute **K** Nonautologous Tissue Substitute **Z** No Device	**J** Extracranial Artery, Right **K** Extracranial Artery, Left

NC 031H09G 031H0AG 031H0JG 031H0KG 031H0ZG 031J09G 031J0AG 031J0JG 031J0KG 031J0ZG 031S09G 031S0AG 031S0JG 031S0KG 031S0ZG 031T09G 031T0AG 031T0JG 031T0KG 031T0ZG

CC 031B0JF 031C0JF

0 Medical and Surgical
3 Upper Arteries
5 Destruction: Physical eradication of all or a portion of a body part by the direct use of energy, force, or a destructive agent

Body Part Character 4	Approach Character 5	Device Character 6	Qualifier Character 7
0 Internal Mammary Artery, Right **1** Internal Mammary Artery, Left **2** Innominate Artery **3** Subclavian Artery, Right **4** Subclavian Artery, Left **5** Axillary Artery, Right **6** Axillary Artery, Left **7** Brachial Artery, Right **8** Brachial Artery, Left **9** Ulnar Artery, Right **A** Ulnar Artery, Left **B** Radial Artery, Right **C** Radial Artery, Left **D** Hand Artery, Right **F** Hand Artery, Left **G** Intracranial Artery **H** Common Carotid Artery, Right **J** Common Carotid Artery, Left **K** Internal Carotid Artery, Right **L** Internal Carotid Artery, Left **M** External Carotid Artery, Right **N** External Carotid Artery, Left **P** Vertebral Artery, Right **Q** Vertebral Artery, Left **R** Face Artery **S** Temporal Artery, Right **T** Temporal Artery, Left **U** Thyroid Artery, Right **V** Thyroid Artery, Left **Y** Upper Artery	**0** Open **3** Percutaneous **4** Percutaneous Endoscopic	**Z** No Device	**Z** No Qualifier

0 Medical and Surgical
3 Upper Arteries
7 Dilation: Expanding an orifice or the lumen of a tubular body part

Body Part Character 4	Approach Character 5	Device Character 6	Qualifier Character 7
0 Internal Mammary Artery, Right **1** Internal Mammary Artery, Left **2** Innominate Artery **3** Subclavian Artery, Right **4** Subclavian Artery, Left **5** Axillary Artery, Right **6** Axillary Artery, Left **7** Brachial Artery, Right **8** Brachial Artery, Left **9** Ulnar Artery, Right **A** Ulnar Artery, Left **B** Radial Artery, Right **C** Radial Artery, Left	**0** Open **3** Percutaneous **4** Percutaneous Endoscopic	**4** Intraluminal Device, Drug-eluting **5** Intraluminal Device, Drug-eluting, Two **6** Intraluminal Device, Drug-eluting, Three **7** Intraluminal Device, Drug-eluting, Four or More **E** Intraluminal Device, Two **F** Intraluminal Device, Three **G** Intraluminal Device, Four or More	**6** Bifurcation **Z** No Qualifier
0 Internal Mammary Artery, Right **1** Internal Mammary Artery, Left **2** Innominate Artery **3** Subclavian Artery, Right **4** Subclavian Artery, Left **5** Axillary Artery, Right **6** Axillary Artery, Left **7** Brachial Artery, Right **8** Brachial Artery, Left **9** Ulnar Artery, Right **A** Ulnar Artery, Left **B** Radial Artery, Right **C** Radial Artery, Left	**0** Open **3** Percutaneous **4** PercutaneousEndoscopic	**D** Intraluminal Device **Z** No Device	**1** Drug-Coated Balloon **6** Bifurcation **Z** No Qualifier
D Hand Artery, Right **F** Hand Artery, Left **G** Intracranial Artery NC **H** Common Carotid Artery, Right **J** Common Carotid Artery, Left **K** Internal Carotid Artery, Right **L** Internal Carotid Artery, Left **M** External Carotid Artery, Right **N** External Carotid Artery, Left **P** Vertebral Artery, Right **Q** Vertebral Artery, Left **R** Face Artery **S** Temporal Artery, Right **T** Temporal Artery, Left **U** Thyroid Artery, Right **V** Thyroid Artery, Left **Y** Upper Artery	**0** Open **3** Percutaneous **4** PercutaneousEndoscopic	**4** Intraluminal Device, Drug-eluting **5** Intraluminal Device, Drug-eluting, Two **6** Intraluminal Device, Drug-eluting, Three **7** Intraluminal Device, Drug-eluting, Four or More **D** Intraluminal Device **E** Intraluminal Device, Two **F** Intraluminal Device, Three **G** Intraluminal Device, Four or More **Z** No Device	**6** Bifurcation **Z** No Qualifier

NC 037G3Z6 037G3ZZ 037G4Z6 037G4ZZ

0 Medical and Surgical
3 Upper Arteries
9 Drainage: Taking or letting out fluids and/or gases from a body part

Body Part Character 4	Approach Character 5	Device Character 6	Qualifier Character 7
0 Internal Mammary Artery, Right **1** Internal Mammary Artery, Left **2** Innominate Artery **3** Subclavian Artery, Right **4** Subclavian Artery, Left **5** Axillary Artery, Right **6** Axillary Artery, Left **7** Brachial Artery, Right **8** Brachial Artery, Left **9** Ulnar Artery, Right **A** Ulnar Artery, Left **B** Radial Artery, Right **C** Radial Artery, Left **D** Hand Artery, Right **F** Hand Artery, Left **G** Intracranial Artery **H** Common Carotid Artery, Right **J** Common Carotid Artery, Left **K** Internal Carotid Artery, Right **L** Internal Carotid Artery, Left **M** External Carotid Artery, Right **N** External Carotid Artery, Left **P** Vertebral Artery, Right **Q** Vertebral Artery, Left **R** Face Artery **S** Temporal Artery, Right **T** Temporal Artery, Left **U** Thyroid Artery, Right **V** Thyroid Artery, Left **Y** Upper Artery	**0** Open **3** Percutaneous **4** Percutaneous Endoscopic	**0** Drainage Device	**Z** No Qualifier
0 Internal Mammary Artery, Right **1** Internal Mammary Artery, Left **2** Innominate Artery **3** Subclavian Artery, Right **4** Subclavian Artery, Left **5** Axillary Artery, Right **6** Axillary Artery, Left **7** Brachial Artery, Right **8** Brachial Artery, Left **9** Ulnar Artery, Right **A** Ulnar Artery, Left **B** Radial Artery, Right **C** Radial Artery, Left **D** Hand Artery, Right **F** Hand Artery, Left **G** Intracranial Artery **H** Common Carotid Artery, Right **J** Common Carotid Artery, Left **K** Internal Carotid Artery, Right **L** Internal Carotid Artery, Left **M** External Carotid Artery, Right **N** External Carotid Artery, Left **P** Vertebral Artery, Right **Q** Vertebral Artery, Left **R** Face Artery **S** Temporal Artery, Right **T** Temporal Artery, Left **U** Thyroid Artery, Right **V** Thyroid Artery, Left **Y** Upper Artery	**0** Open **3** Percutaneous **4** Percutaneous Endoscopic	**Z** No Device	**X** Diagnostic **Z** No Qualifier

0 Medical and Surgical
3 Upper Arteries
B Excision: Cutting out or off, without replacement, a portion of a body part

Body Part	Approach	Device	Qualifier
Character 4	Character 5	Character 6	Character 7
0 Internal Mammary Artery, Right **1** Internal Mammary Artery, Left **2** Innominate Artery **3** Subclavian Artery, Right **4** Subclavian Artery, Left **5** Axillary Artery, Right **6** Axillary Artery, Left **7** Brachial Artery, Right **8** Brachial Artery, Left **9** Ulnar Artery, Right **A** Ulnar Artery, Left **B** Radial Artery, Right **C** Radial Artery, Left **D** Hand Artery, Right **F** Hand Artery, Left **G** Intracranial Artery **H** Common Carotid Artery, Right **J** Common Carotid Artery, Left **K** Internal Carotid Artery, Right **L** Internal Carotid Artery, Left **M** External Carotid Artery, Right **N** External Carotid Artery, Left **P** Vertebral Artery, Right **Q** Vertebral Artery, Left **R** Face Artery **S** Temporal Artery, Right **T** Temporal Artery, Left **U** Thyroid Artery, Right **V** Thyroid Artery, Left **Y** Upper Artery	**0** Open **3** Percutaneous **4** Percutaneous Endoscopic	**Z** No Device	**X** Diagnostic **Z** No Qualifier

0 Medical and Surgical
3 Upper Arteries
C Extirpation: Taking or cutting out solid matter from a body part

Body Part Character 4	Approach Character 5	Device Character 6	Qualifier Character 7
0 Internal Mammary Artery, Right **1** Internal Mammary Artery, Left **2** Innominate Artery **3** Subclavian Artery, Right **4** Subclavian Artery, Left **5** Axillary Artery, Right **6** Axillary Artery, Left **7** Brachial Artery, Right **8** Brachial Artery, Left **9** Ulnar Artery, Right **A** Ulnar Artery, Left **B** Radial Artery, Right **C** Radial Artery, Left **D** Hand Artery, Right **F** Hand Artery, Left **R** Face Artery **S** Temporal Artery, Right **T** Temporal Artery, Left **U** Thyroid Artery, Right **V** Thyroid Artery, Left **Y** Upper Artery	**0** Open **3** Percutaneous **4** Percutaneous Endoscopic	**Z** No Device	**6** Bifurcation **Z** No Qualifier
G Intracranial Artery **H** Common Carotid Artery, Right **J** Common Carotid Artery, Left **K** Internal Carotid Artery, Right **L** Internal Carotid Artery, Left **M** External Carotid Artery, Right **N** External Carotid Artery, Left **P** Vertebral Artery, Right **Q** Vertebral Artery, Left	**0** Open **4** PercutaneousEndoscopic	**Z** No Device	**6** Bifurcation **Z** No Qualifier
G Intracranial Artery **H** Common Carotid Artery, Right **J** Common Carotid Artery, Left **K** Internal Carotid Artery, Right **L** Internal Carotid Artery, Left **M** External Carotid Artery, Right **N** External Carotid Artery, Left **P** Vertebral Artery, Right **Q** Vertebral Artery, Left	**3** Percutaneous	**Z** No Device	**6** Bifurcation **7** Stent Retriever **Z** No Qualifier

0 Medical and Surgical
3 Upper Arteries
H Insertion: Putting in a nonbiological appliance that monitors, assists, performs, or prevents a physiological function but does not physically take the place of a body part

Body Part Character 4	Approach Character 5	Device Character 6	Qualifier Character 7
0 Internal Mammary Artery, Right **1** Internal Mammary Artery, Left **2** Innominate Artery **3** Subclavian Artery, Right **4** Subclavian Artery, Left **5** Axillary Artery, Right **6** Axillary Artery, Left **7** Brachial Artery, Right **8** Brachial Artery, Left **9** Ulnar Artery, Right **A** Ulnar Artery, Left **B** Radial Artery, Right **C** Radial Artery, Left **D** Hand Artery, Right **F** Hand Artery, Left **G** Intracranial Artery **H** Common Carotid Artery, Right **J** Common Carotid Artery, Left **M** External Carotid Artery, Right **N** External Carotid Artery, Left **P** Vertebral Artery, Right **Q** Vertebral Artery, Left **R** Face Artery **S** Temporal Artery, Right **T** Temporal Artery, Left **U** Thyroid Artery, Right **V** Thyroid Artery, Left	**0** Open **3** Percutaneous **4** Percutaneous Endoscopic	**3** Infusion Device **D** Intraluminal Device	**Z** No Qualifier
K Internal Carotid Artery, Right CC **L** Internal Carotid Artery, Left	**0** Open **3** Percutaneous **4** Percutaneous Endoscopic	**3** Infusion Device **D** Intraluminal Device **M** Stimulator Lead	**Z** No Qualifier
Y Upper Artery CC	**0** Open **3** Percutaneous **4** Percutaneous Endoscopic	**2** Monitoring Device **3** Infusion Device **D** Intraluminal Device **Y** Other Device	**Z** No Qualifier

CC 03HK0MZ 03HK3MZ 03HK4MZ 03HL0MZ 03HL3MZ 03HL4MZ

0 Medical and Surgical
3 Upper Arteries
J Inspection: Visually and/or manually exploring a body part

Body Part Character 4	Approach Character 5	Device Character 6	Qualifier Character 7
Y Upper Artery	**0** Open **3** Percutaneous **4** Percutaneous Endoscopic **X** External	**Z** No Device	**Z** No Qualifier

0 Medical and Surgical
3 Upper Arteries
L Occlusion: Completely closing an orifice or the lumen of a tubular body part

Body Part Character 4	Approach Character 5	Device Character 6	Qualifier Character 7
0 Internal Mammary Artery, Right **1** Internal Mammary Artery, Left **2** Innominate Artery **3** Subclavian Artery, Right **4** Subclavian Artery, Left **5** Axillary Artery, Right **6** Axillary Artery, Left **7** Brachial Artery, Right **8** Brachial Artery, Left **9** Ulnar Artery, Right **A** Ulnar Artery, Left **B** Radial Artery, Right **C** Radial Artery, Left **D** Hand Artery, Right **F** Hand Artery, Left **R** Face Artery **S** Temporal Artery, Right **T** Temporal Artery, Left **U** Thyroid Artery, Right **V** Thyroid Artery, Left **Y** Upper Artery	**0** Open **3** Percutaneous **4** Percutaneous Endoscopic	**C** Extraluminal Device **D** Intraluminal Device **Z** No Device	**Z** No Qualifier
G Intracranial Artery **H** Common Carotid Artery, Right **J** Common Carotid Artery, Left **K** Internal Carotid Artery, Right **L** Internal Carotid Artery, Left **M** External Carotid Artery, Right **N** External Carotid Artery, Left **P** Vertebral Artery, Right **Q** Vertebral Artery, Left	**0** Open **3** Percutaneous **4** Percutaneous Endoscopic	**B** Intraluminal Device, Bioactive **C** Extraluminal Device **D** Intraluminal Device **Z** No Device	**Z** No Qualifier

0 Medical and Surgical
3 Upper Arteries
N Release: Freeing a body part from an abnormal physical constraint by cutting or by the use of force

Body Part Character 4	Approach Character 5	Device Character 6	Qualifier Character 7
0 Internal Mammary Artery, Right 1 Internal Mammary Artery, Left 2 Innominate Artery 3 Subclavian Artery, Right 4 Subclavian Artery, Left 5 Axillary Artery, Right 6 Axillary Artery, Left 7 Brachial Artery, Right 8 Brachial Artery, Left 9 Ulnar Artery, Right A Ulnar Artery, Left B Radial Artery, Right C Radial Artery, Left D Hand Artery, Right F Hand Artery, Left G Intracranial Artery H Common Carotid Artery, Right J Common Carotid Artery, Left K Internal Carotid Artery, Right L Internal Carotid Artery, Left M External Carotid Artery, Right N External Carotid Artery, Left P Vertebral Artery, Right Q Vertebral Artery, Left R Face Artery S Temporal Artery, Right T Temporal Artery, Left U Thyroid Artery, Right V Thyroid Artery, Left Y Upper Artery	0 Open 3 Percutaneous 4 Percutaneous Endoscopic	Z No Device	Z No Qualifier

0 Medical and Surgical
3 Upper Arteries
P Removal: Taking out or off a device from a body part

Body Part Character 4	Approach Character 5	Device Character 6	Qualifier Character 7
Y Upper Artery CC	0 Open 3 Percutaneous 4 Percutaneous Endoscopic	0 Drainage Device 2 Monitoring Device 3 Infusion Device 7 Autologous Tissue Substitute C Extraluminal Device D Intraluminal Device J Synthetic Substitute K Nonautologous Tissue Substitute M Stimulator Lead Y Other Device	Z No Qualifier
Y Upper Artery	X External	0 Drainage Device 2 Monitoring Device 3 Infusion Device D Intraluminal Device M Stimulator Lead	Z No Qualifier

CC 03PY0JZ 03PY0MZ 03PY3JZ 03PY3MZ 03PY4JZ 03PY4MZ

0 Medical and Surgical
3 Upper Arteries
Q Repair: Restoring, to the extent possible, a body part to its normal anatomic structure and function

Body Part Character 4	Approach Character 5	Device Character 6	Qualifier Character 7
0 Internal Mammary Artery, Right **1** Internal Mammary Artery, Left **2** Innominate Artery **3** Subclavian Artery, Right **4** Subclavian Artery, Left **5** Axillary Artery, Right **6** Axillary Artery, Left **7** Brachial Artery, Right **8** Brachial Artery, Left **9** Ulnar Artery, Right **A** Ulnar Artery, Left **B** Radial Artery, Right **C** Radial Artery, Left **D** Hand Artery, Right **F** Hand Artery, Left **G** Intracranial Artery **H** Common Carotid Artery, Right **J** Common Carotid Artery, Left **K** Internal Carotid Artery, Right **L** Internal Carotid Artery, Left **M** External Carotid Artery, Right **N** External Carotid Artery, Left **P** Vertebral Artery, Right **Q** Vertebral Artery, Left **R** Face Artery **S** Temporal Artery, Right **T** Temporal Artery, Left **U** Thyroid Artery, Right **V** Thyroid Artery, Left **Y** Upper Artery	**0** Open **3** Percutaneous **4** Percutaneous Endoscopic	**Z** No Device	**Z** No Qualifier

0 Medical and Surgical
3 Upper Arteries
R Replacement: Putting in or on biological or synthetic material that physically takes the place and/or function of all or a portion of a body part

Body Part	Approach	Device	Qualifier
Character 4	Character 5	Character 6	Character 7
0 Internal Mammary Artery, Right **1** Internal Mammary Artery, Left **2** Innominate Artery **3** Subclavian Artery, Right **4** Subclavian Artery, Left **5** Axillary Artery, Right **6** Axillary Artery, Left **7** Brachial Artery, Right **8** Brachial Artery, Left **9** Ulnar Artery, Right **A** Ulnar Artery, Left **B** Radial Artery, Right **C** Radial Artery, Left **D** Hand Artery, Right **F** Hand Artery, Left **G** Intracranial Artery **H** Common Carotid Artery, Right **J** Common Carotid Artery, Left **K** Internal Carotid Artery, Right **L** Internal Carotid Artery, Left **M** External Carotid Artery, Right **N** External Carotid Artery, Left **P** Vertebral Artery, Right **Q** Vertebral Artery, Left **R** Face Artery **S** Temporal Artery, Right **T** Temporal Artery, Left **U** Thyroid Artery, Right **V** Thyroid Artery, Left **Y** Upper Artery	**0** Open **4** Percutaneous Endoscopic	**7** Autologous Tissue Substitute **J** Synthetic Substitute **K** Nonautologous Tissue Substitute	**Z** No Qualifier

0 Medical and Surgical
3 Upper Arteries
S Reposition: Moving to its normal location, or other suitable location, all or a portion of a body part

Body Part Character 4	Approach Character 5	Device Character 6	Qualifier Character 7
0 Internal Mammary Artery, Right **1** Internal Mammary Artery, Left **2** Innominate Artery **3** Subclavian Artery, Right **4** Subclavian Artery, Left **5** Axillary Artery, Right **6** Axillary Artery, Left **7** Brachial Artery, Right **8** Brachial Artery, Left **9** Ulnar Artery, Right **A** Ulnar Artery, Left **B** Radial Artery, Right **C** Radial Artery, Left **D** Hand Artery, Right **F** Hand Artery, Left **G** Intracranial Artery **H** Common Carotid Artery, Right **J** Common Carotid Artery, Left **K** Internal Carotid Artery, Right **L** Internal Carotid Artery, Left **M** External Carotid Artery, Right **N** External Carotid Artery, Left **P** Vertebral Artery, Right **Q** Vertebral Artery, Left **R** Face Artery **S** Temporal Artery, Right **T** Temporal Artery, Left **U** Thyroid Artery, Right **V** Thyroid Artery, Left **Y** Upper Artery	**0** Open **3** Percutaneous **4** Percutaneous Endoscopic	**Z** No Device	**Z** No Qualifier

0 Medical and Surgical
3 Upper Arteries
U Supplement: Putting in or on biological or synthetic material that physically reinforces and/or augments the function of a portion of a body part

Body Part	Approach	Device	Qualifier
Character 4	**Character 5**	**Character 6**	**Character 7**
0 Internal Mammary Artery, Right **1** Internal Mammary Artery, Left **2** Innominate Artery **3** Subclavian Artery, Right **4** Subclavian Artery, Left **5** Axillary Artery, Right **6** Axillary Artery, Left **7** Brachial Artery, Right **8** Brachial Artery, Left **9** Ulnar Artery, Right **A** Ulnar Artery, Left **B** Radial Artery, Right **C** Radial Artery, Left **D** Hand Artery, Right **F** Hand Artery, Left **G** Intracranial Artery **H** Common Carotid Artery, Right **J** Common Carotid Artery, Left **K** Internal Carotid Artery, Right **L** Internal Carotid Artery, Left **M** External Carotid Artery, Right **N** External Carotid Artery, Left **P** Vertebral Artery, Right **Q** Vertebral Artery, Left **R** Face Artery **S** Temporal Artery, Right **T** Temporal Artery, Left **U** Thyroid Artery, Right **V** Thyroid Artery, Left **Y** Upper Artery	**0** Open **3** Percutaneous **4** Percutaneous Endoscopic	**7** Autologous Tissue Substitute **J** Synthetic Substitute **K** Nonautologous Tissue Substitute	**Z** No Qualifier

0 Medical and Surgical
3 Upper Arteries
V Restriction: Partially closing an orifice or the lumen of a tubular body part

Body Part Character 4	Approach Character 5	Device Character 6	Qualifier Character 7
0 Internal Mammary Artery, Right **1** Internal Mammary Artery, Left **2** Innominate Artery **3** Subclavian Artery, Right **4** Subclavian Artery, Left **5** Axillary Artery, Right **6** Axillary Artery, Left **7** Brachial Artery, Right **8** Brachial Artery, Left **9** Ulnar Artery, Right **A** Ulnar Artery, Left **B** Radial Artery, Right **C** Radial Artery, Left **D** Hand Artery, Right **F** Hand Artery, Left **R** Face Artery **S** Temporal Artery, Right **T** Temporal Artery, Left **U** Thyroid Artery, Right **V** Thyroid Artery, Left **Y** Upper Artery	**0** Open **3** Percutaneous **4** Percutaneous Endoscopic	**C** Extraluminal Device **D** Intraluminal Device **Z** No Device	**Z** No Qualifier
G Intracranial Artery **H** Common Carotid Artery, Right **J** Common Carotid Artery, Left **K** Internal Carotid Artery, Right **L** Internal Carotid Artery, Left **M** External Carotid Artery, Right **N** External Carotid Artery, Left **P** Vertebral Artery, Right **Q** Vertebral Artery, Left	**0** Open **3** Percutaneous **4** Percutaneous Endoscopic	**B** Intraluminal Device, Bioactive **C** Extraluminal Device **D** Intraluminal Device **Z** No Device	**Z** No Qualifier

0 Medical and Surgical
3 Upper Arteries
W Revision: Correcting, to the extent possible, a portion of a malfunctioning device or the position of a displaced device

Body Part Character 4	Approach Character 5	Device Character 6	Qualifier Character 7
Y Upper Artery	**0** Open **3** Percutaneous **4** Percutaneous Endoscopic	**0** Drainage Device **2** Monitoring Device **3** Infusion Device **7** Autologous Tissue Substitute **C** Extraluminal Device **D** Intraluminal Device **J** Synthetic Substitute **K** Nonautologous Tissue Substitute **M** Stimulator Lead **Y** Other Device	**Z** No Qualifier
Y Upper Artery	**X** External	**0** Drainage Device **2** Monitoring Device **3** Infusion Device **7** Autologous Tissue Substitute **C** Extraluminal Device **D** Intraluminal Device **J** Synthetic Substitute **K** Nonautologous Tissue Substitute **M** Stimulator Lead	**Z** No Qualifier

NOTES

Lower Arteries 041-04W

0 Medical and Surgical
4 Lower Arteries
1 Bypass: Altering the route of passage of the contents of a tubular body part

Body Part Character 4	Approach Character 5	Device Character 6	Qualifier Character 7
0 Abdominal Aorta **C** Common Iliac Artery, Right **D** Common Iliac Artery, Left	**0** Open **4** Percutaneous Endoscopic	**9** Autologous Venous Tissue **A** Autologous Arterial Tissue **J** Synthetic Substitute **K** Nonautologous Tissue Substitute **Z** No Device	**0** Abdominal Aorta **1** Celiac Artery **2** Mesenteric Artery **3** Renal Artery, Right **4** Renal Artery, Left **5** Renal Artery, Bilateral **6** Common Iliac Artery, Right **7** Common Iliac Artery, Left **8** Common Iliac Arteries, Bilateral **9** Internal Iliac Artery, Right **B** Internal Iliac Artery, Left **C** Internal Iliac Arteries, Bilateral **D** External Iliac Artery, Right **F** External Iliac Artery, Left **G** External Iliac Arteries, Bilateral **H** Femoral Artery, Right **J** Femoral Artery, Left **K** Femoral Arteries, Bilateral **Q** Lower Extremity Artery **R** Lower Artery
3 Hepatic Artery **4** Splenic Artery	**0** Open **4** Percutaneous Endoscopic	**9** Autologous Venous Tissue **A** Autologous Arterial Tissue **J** Synthetic Substitute **K** Nonautologous Tissue Substitute **Z** No Device	**3** Renal Artery, Right **4** Renal Artery, Left **5** Renal Artery, Bilateral
E Internal Iliac Artery, Right **F** Internal Iliac Artery, Left **H** External Iliac Artery, Right **J** External Iliac Artery, Left	**0** Open **4** Percutaneous Endoscopic	**9** Autologous Venous Tissue **A** Autologous Arterial Tissue **J** Synthetic Substitute **K** Nonautologous Tissue Substitute **Z** No Device	**9** Internal Iliac Artery, Right **B** Internal Iliac Artery, Left **C** Internal Iliac Arteries, Bilateral **D** External Iliac Artery, Right **F** External Iliac Artery, Left **G** External Iliac Arteries, Bilateral **H** Femoral Artery, Right **J** Femoral Artery, Left **K** Femoral Arteries, Bilateral **P** Foot Artery **Q** Lower Extremity Artery
K Femoral Artery, Right **L** Femoral Artery, Left	**0** Open **4** Percutaneous Endoscopic	**9** Autologous Venous Tissue **A** Autologous Arterial Tissue **J** Synthetic Substitute **K** Nonautologous Tissue Substitute **Z** No Device	**H** Femoral Artery, Right **J** Femoral Artery, Left **K** Femoral Arteries, Bilateral **L** Popliteal Artery **M** Peroneal Artery **N** Posterior Tibial Artery **P** Foot Artery **Q** Lower Extremity Artery **S** Lower Extremity Vein
K Femoral Artery, Right **L** Femoral Artery, Left	**3** Percutaneous	**J** Synthetic Substitute	**Q** Lower Extremity Artery **S** Lower Extremity Vein
M Popliteal Artery, Right **N** Popliteal Artery, Left	**0** Open **4** Percutaneous Endoscopic	**9** Autologous Venous Tissue **A** Autologous Arterial Tissue **J** Synthetic Substitute **K** Nonautologous Tissue Substitute **Z** No Device	**L** Popliteal Artery **M** Peroneal Artery **P** Foot Artery **Q** Lower Extremity Artery **S** Lower Extremity Vein
M Popliteal Artery, Right **N** Popliteal Artery, Left	**3** Percutaneous	**J** Synthetic Substitute	**Q** Lower Extremity Artery **S** Lower Extremity Vein

041 continued on next page

0 Medical and Surgical
4 Lower Arteries
1 Bypass: Altering the route of passage of the contents of a tubular body part

041 continued from previous page

Body Part Character 4	Approach Character 5	Device Character 6	Qualifier Character 7
P Anterior Tibial Artery, Right Q Anterior Tibial Artery, Left R Posterior Tibial Artery, Right S Posterior Tibial Artery	0 Open 3 Percutaneous 4 Percutaneous Endoscopic	J Synthetic Substitute	Q Lower Extremity Artery S Lower Extremity Vein
T Peroneal Artery, Right U Peroneal Artery, Left V Foot Artery, Right W Foot Artery, Left	0 Open 4 Percutaneous Endoscopic	9 Autologous Venous Tissue A Autologous Arterial Tissue J Synthetic Substitute K Nonautologous Tissue Substitute Z No Device	P Foot Artery Q Lower Extremity Artery S Lower Extremity Vein
T Peroneal Artery, Right U Peroneal Artery, Left V Foot Artery, Right W Foot Artery, Left	3 Percutaneous	J Synthetic Substitute	Q Lower Extremity Artery S Lower Extremity Vein

0 Medical and Surgical
4 Lower Arteries
5 Destruction: Physical eradication of all or a portion of a body part by the direct use of energy, force, or a destructive agent

Body Part Character 4	Approach Character 5	Device Character 6	Qualifier Character 7
0 Abdominal Aorta 1 Celiac Artery 2 Gastric Artery 3 Hepatic Artery 4 Splenic Artery 5 Superior Mesenteric Artery 6 Colic Artery, Right 7 Colic Artery, Left 8 Colic Artery, Middle 9 Renal Artery, Right A Renal Artery, Left B Inferior Mesenteric Artery C Common Iliac Artery, Right D Common Iliac Artery, Left E Internal Iliac Artery, Right F Internal Iliac Artery, Left H External Iliac Artery, Right J External Iliac Artery, Left K Femoral Artery, Right L Femoral Artery, Left M Popliteal Artery, Right N Popliteal Artery, Left P Anterior Tibial Artery, Right Q Anterior Tibial Artery, Left R Posterior Tibial Artery, Right S Posterior Tibial Artery, Left T Peroneal Artery, Right U Peroneal Artery, Left V Foot Artery, Right W Foot Artery, Left Y Lower Artery	0 Open 3 Percutaneous 4 Percutaneous Endoscopic	Z No Device	Z No Qualifier

0 Medical and Surgical
4 Lower Arteries
7 Dilation: Expanding an orifice or the lumen of a tubular body part

Body Part Character 4	Approach Character 5	Device Character 6	Qualifier Character 7
0 Abdominal Aorta **1** Celiac Artery **2** Gastric Artery **3** Hepatic Artery **4** Splenic Artery **5** Superior Mesenteric Artery **6** Colic Artery, Right **7** Colic Artery, Left **8** Colic Artery, Middle **9** Renal Artery, Right **A** Renal Artery, Left **B** Inferior Mesenteric Artery **C** Common Iliac Artery, Right **D** Common Iliac Artery, Left **E** Internal Iliac Artery, Right **F** Internal Iliac Artery, Left **H** External Iliac Artery, Right **J** External Iliac Artery, Left **K** Femoral Artery, Right **L** Femoral Artery, Left **M** Popliteal Artery, Right **N** Popliteal Artery, Left **P** Anterior Tibial Artery, Right **Q** Anterior Tibial Artery, Left **R** Posterior Tibial Artery, Right **S** Posterior Tibial Artery, Left **T** Peroneal Artery, Right **U** Peroneal Artery, Left **V** Foot Artery, Right **W** Foot Artery, Left **Y** Lower Artery	**0** Open **3** Percutaneous **4** Percutaneous Endoscopic	**4** Intraluminal Device, Drug-eluting **D** Intraluminal Device **Z** No Device	**1** Drug-Coated Balloon **6** Bifurcation **Z** No Qualifier
0 Abdominal Aorta **1** Celiac Artery **2** Gastric Artery **3** Hepatic Artery **4** Splenic Artery **5** Superior Mesenteric Artery **6** Colic Artery, Right **7** Colic Artery, Left **8** Colic Artery, Middle **9** Renal Artery, Right **A** Renal Artery, Left **B** Inferior Mesenteric Artery **C** Common Iliac Artery, Right **D** Common Iliac Artery, Left **E** Internal Iliac Artery, Right **F** Internal Iliac Artery, Left **H** External Iliac Artery, Right **J** External Iliac Artery, Left **K** Femoral Artery, Right **L** Femoral Artery, Left **M** Popliteal Artery, Right **N** Popliteal Artery, Left **P** Anterior Tibial Artery, Right **Q** Anterior Tibial Artery, Left **R** Posterior Tibial Artery, Right **S** Posterior Tibial Artery, Left **T** Peroneal Artery, Right **U** Peroneal Artery, Left **V** Foot Artery, Right **W** Foot Artery, Left **Y** Lower Artery	**0** Open **3** Percutaneous **4** Percutaneous Endoscopic	**5** Intraluminal Device, Drug-eluting, Two **6** Intraluminal Device, Drug-eluting, Three **7** Intraluminal Device, Drug-eluting, Four or More **E** Intraluminal Device, Two **F** Intraluminal Device, Three **G** Intraluminal Device, Four or More	**6** Bifurcation **Z** No Qualifier

LC Limited Coverage NC Noncovered HAC HAC-associated Procedure CC Combination Cluster - See Appendix G for code lists
DRG Non-OR-Affecting MS-DRG Assignment New/Revised Text in **Orange** ♂ Male ♀ Female

0 Medical and Surgical
4 Lower Arteries
9 Drainage: Taking or letting out fluids and/or gases from a body part

Body Part Character 4	Approach Character 5	Device Character 6	Qualifier Character 7
0 Abdominal Aorta **1** Celiac Artery **2** Gastric Artery **3** Hepatic Artery **4** Splenic Artery **5** Superior Mesenteric Artery **6** Colic Artery, Right **7** Colic Artery, Left **8** Colic Artery, Middle **9** Renal Artery, Right **A** Renal Artery, Left **B** Inferior Mesenteric Artery **C** Common Iliac Artery, Right **D** Common Iliac Artery, Left **E** Internal Iliac Artery, Right **F** Internal Iliac Artery, Left **H** External Iliac Artery, Right **J** External Iliac Artery, Left **K** Femoral Artery, Right **L** Femoral Artery, Left **M** Popliteal Artery, Right **N** Popliteal Artery, Left **P** Anterior Tibial Artery, Right **Q** Anterior Tibial Artery, Left **R** Posterior Tibial Artery, Right **S** Posterior Tibial Artery, Left **T** Peroneal Artery, Right **U** Peroneal Artery, Left **V** Foot Artery, Right **W** Foot Artery, Left **Y** Lower Artery	**0** Open **3** Percutaneous **4** Percutaneous Endoscopic	**0** Drainage Device	**Z** No Qualifier
0 Abdominal Aorta **1** Celiac Artery **2** Gastric Artery **3** Hepatic Artery **4** Splenic Artery **5** Superior Mesenteric Artery **6** Colic Artery, Right **7** Colic Artery, Left **8** Colic Artery, Middle **9** Renal Artery, Right **A** Renal Artery, Left **B** Inferior Mesenteric Artery **C** Common Iliac Artery, Right **D** Common Iliac Artery, Left **E** Internal Iliac Artery, Right **F** Internal Iliac Artery, Left **H** External Iliac Artery, Right **J** External Iliac Artery, Left **K** Femoral Artery, Right **L** Femoral Artery, Left **M** Popliteal Artery, Right **N** Popliteal Artery, Left **P** Anterior Tibial Artery, Right **Q** Anterior Tibial Artery, Left **R** Posterior Tibial Artery, Right **S** Posterior Tibial Artery, Left **T** Peroneal Artery, Right **U** Peroneal Artery, Left **V** Foot Artery, Right **W** Foot Artery, Left **Y** Lower Artery	**0** Open **3** Percutaneous **4** Percutaneous Endoscopic	**Z** No Device	**X** Diagnostic **Z** No Qualifier

0 Medical and Surgical
4 Lower Arteries
B Excision: Cutting out or off, without replacement, a portion of a body part

Body Part Character 4	Approach Character 5	Device Character 6	Qualifier Character 7
0 Abdominal Aorta **1** Celiac Artery **2** Gastric Artery **3** Hepatic Artery **4** Splenic Artery **5** Superior Mesenteric Artery **6** Colic Artery, Right **7** Colic Artery, Left **8** Colic Artery, Middle **9** Renal Artery, Right **A** Renal Artery, Left **B** Inferior Mesenteric Artery **C** Common Iliac Artery, Right **D** Common Iliac Artery, Left **E** Internal Iliac Artery, Right **F** Internal Iliac Artery, Left **H** External Iliac Artery, Right **J** External Iliac Artery, Left **K** Femoral Artery, Right **L** Femoral Artery, Left **M** Popliteal Artery, Right **N** Popliteal Artery, Left **P** Anterior Tibial Artery, Right **Q** Anterior Tibial Artery, Left **R** Posterior Tibial Artery, Right **S** Posterior Tibial Artery, Left **T** Peroneal Artery, Right **U** Peroneal Artery, Left **V** Foot Artery, Right **W** Foot Artery, Left **Y** Lower Artery	**0** Open **3** Percutaneous **4** Percutaneous Endoscopic	**Z** No Device	**X** Diagnostic **Z** No Qualifier

0 Medical and Surgical
4 Lower Arteries
C Extirpation: Taking or cutting out solid matter from a body part

Body Part Character 4	Approach Character 5	Device Character 6	Qualifier Character 7
0 Abdominal Aorta **1** Celiac Artery **2** Gastric Artery **3** Hepatic Artery **4** Splenic Artery **5** Superior Mesenteric Artery **6** Colic Artery, Right **7** Colic Artery, Left **8** Colic Artery, Middle **9** Renal Artery, Right **A** Renal Artery, Left **B** Inferior Mesenteric Artery **C** Common Iliac Artery, Right **D** Common Iliac Artery, Left **E** Internal Iliac Artery, Right **F** Internal Iliac Artery, Left **H** External Iliac Artery, Right **J** External Iliac Artery, Left **K** Femoral Artery, Right **L** Femoral Artery, Left **M** Popliteal Artery, Right **N** Popliteal Artery, Left **P** Anterior Tibial Artery, Right **Q** Anterior Tibial Artery, Left **R** Posterior Tibial Artery, Right **S** Posterior Tibial Artery, Left **T** Peroneal Artery, Right **U** Peroneal Artery, Left **V** Foot Artery, Right **W** Foot Artery, Left **Y** Lower Artery	**0** Open **3** Percutaneous **4** Percutaneous Endoscopic	**Z** No Device	**6** Bifurcation **Z** No Qualifier

0 Medical and Surgical
4 Lower Arteries
H Insertion: Putting in a nonbiological appliance that monitors, assists, performs, or prevents a physiological function but does not physically take the place of a body part

Body Part	Approach	Device	Qualifier
Character 4	Character 5	Character 6	Character 7
0 Abdominal Aorta	**0** Open **3** Percutaneous **4** Percutaneous Endoscopic	**2** Monitoring Device **3** Infusion Device **D** Intraluminal Device	**Z** No Qualifier
1 Celiac Artery **2** Gastric Artery **3** Hepatic Artery **4** Splenic Artery **5** Superior Mesenteric Artery **6** Colic Artery, Right **7** Colic Artery, Left **8** Colic Artery, Middle **9** Renal Artery, Right **A** Renal Artery, Left **B** Inferior Mesenteric Artery **C** Common Iliac Artery, Right **D** Common Iliac Artery, Left **E** Internal Iliac Artery, Right **F** Internal Iliac Artery, Left **H** External Iliac Artery, Right **J** External Iliac Artery, Left **K** Femoral Artery, Right **L** Femoral Artery, Left **M** Popliteal Artery, Right **N** Popliteal Artery, Left **P** Anterior Tibial Artery, Right **Q** Anterior Tibial Artery, Left **R** Posterior Tibial Artery, Right **S** Posterior Tibial Artery, Left **T** Peroneal Artery, Right **U** Peroneal Artery, Left **V** Foot Artery, Right **W** Foot Artery, Left	**0** Open **3** Percutaneous **4** Percutaneous Endoscopic	**3** Infusion Device **D** Intraluminal Device	**Z** No Qualifier
Y Lower Artery	**0** Open **3** Percutaneous **4** Percutaneous Endoscopic	**2** Monitoring Device **3** Infusion Device **D** Intraluminal Device **Y** Other Device	**Z** No Qualifier

0 Medical and Surgical
4 Lower Arteries
J Inspection: Visually and/or manually exploring a body part

Body Part	Approach	Device	Qualifier
Character 4	Character 5	Character 6	Character 7
Y Lower Artery	**0** Open **3** Percutaneous **4** Percutaneous Endoscopic **X** External	**Z** No Device	**Z** No Qualifier

0 Medical and Surgical
4 Lower Arteries
L Occlusion: Completely closing an orifice or the lumen of a tubular body part

Body Part Character 4	Approach Character 5	Device Character 6	Qualifier Character 7
0 Abdominal Aorta	**0** Open **4** Percutaneous Endoscopic	**C** Extraluminal Device **D** Intraluminal Device **Z** No Device	**Z** No Qualifier
0 Abdominal Aorta	**3** Percutaneous	**C** Extraluminal Device **Z** No Device	**Z** No Qualifier
0 Abdominal Aorta	**3** Percutaneous	**D** Intraluminal Device	**J** Temporary **Z** No Qualifier
1 Celiac Artery **2** Gastric Artery **3** Hepatic Artery **4** Splenic Artery **5** Superior Mesenteric Artery **6** Colic Artery, Right **7** Colic Artery, Left **8** Colic Artery, Middle **9** Renal Artery, Right **A** Renal Artery, Left **B** Inferior Mesenteric Artery **C** Common Iliac Artery, Right **D** Common Iliac Artery, Left **H** External Iliac Artery, Right **J** External Iliac Artery, Left **K** Femoral Artery, Right **L** Femoral Artery, Left **M** Popliteal Artery, Right **N** Popliteal Artery, Left **P** Anterior Tibial Artery, Right **Q** Anterior Tibial Artery, Left **R** Posterior Tibial Artery, Right **S** Posterior Tibial Artery, Left **T** Peroneal Artery, Right **U** Peroneal Artery, Left **V** Foot Artery, Right **W** Foot Artery, Left **Y** Lower Artery	**0** Open **3** Percutaneous **4** Percutaneous Endoscopic	**C** Extraluminal Device **D** Intraluminal Device **Z** No Device	**Z** No Qualifier
E Internal Iliac Artery, Right ♀	**0** Open **3** Percutaneous **4** Percutaneous Endoscopic	**C** Extraluminal Device **D** Intraluminal Device **Z** No Device	**T** Uterine Artery, Right **Z** No Qualifier
F Internal Iliac Artery, Left ♀	**0** Open **3** Percutaneous **4** Percutaneous Endoscopic	**C** Extraluminal Device **D** Intraluminal Device **Z** No Device	**U** Uterine Artery, Left **Z** No Qualifier

♀ 04LE0CT 04LE0DT 04LE0ZT 04LE3CT 04LE3DT 04LE3ZT 04LE4CT 04LE4DT 04LE4ZT 04LF0CU 04LF0DU 04LF0ZU 04LF3CU 04LF3DU 04LF3ZU 04LF4CU 04LF4DU 04LF4ZU

0 Medical and Surgical
4 Lower Arteries
N Release: Freeing a body part from an abnormal physical constraint by cutting or by the use of force

Body Part Character 4	Approach Character 5	Device Character 6	Qualifier Character 7
0 Abdominal Aorta **1** Celiac Artery **2** Gastric Artery **3** Hepatic Artery **4** Splenic Artery **5** Superior Mesenteric Artery **6** Colic Artery, Right **7** Colic Artery, Left **8** Colic Artery, Middle **9** Renal Artery, Right **A** Renal Artery, Left **B** Inferior Mesenteric Artery **C** Common Iliac Artery, Right **D** Common Iliac Artery, Left **E** Internal Iliac Artery, Right **F** Internal Iliac Artery, Left **H** External Iliac Artery, Right **J** External Iliac Artery, Left **K** Femoral Artery, Right **L** Femoral Artery, Left **M** Popliteal Artery, Right **N** Popliteal Artery, Left **P** Anterior Tibial Artery, Right **Q** Anterior Tibial Artery, Left **R** Posterior Tibial Artery, Right **S** Posterior Tibial Artery, Left **T** Peroneal Artery, Right **U** Peroneal Artery, Left **V** Foot Artery, Right **W** Foot Artery, Left **Y** Lower Artery	**0** Open **3** Percutaneous **4** Percutaneous Endoscopic	**Z** No Device	**Z** No Qualifier

0 Medical and Surgical
4 Lower Arteries
P Removal: Taking out or off a device from a body part

Body Part Character 4	Approach Character 5	Device Character 6	Qualifier Character 7
Y Lower Artery	**0** Open **3** Percutaneous **4** Percutaneous Endoscopic	**0** Drainage Device **2** Monitoring Device **3** Infusion Device **7** Autologous Tissue Substitute **C** Extraluminal Device **D** Intraluminal Device **J** Synthetic Substitute **K** Nonautologous Tissue Substitute **Y** Other Device	**Z** No Qualifier
Y Lower Artery	**X** External	**0** Drainage Device **1** Radioactive Element **2** Monitoring Device **3** Infusion Device **D** Intraluminal Device	**Z** No Qualifier

0 Medical and Surgical
4 Lower Arteries
Q Repair: Restoring, to the extent possible, a body part to its normal anatomic structure and function

Body Part Character 4	Approach Character 5	Device Character 6	Qualifier Character 7
0 Abdominal Aorta **1** Celiac Artery **2** Gastric Artery **3** Hepatic Artery **4** Splenic Artery **5** Superior Mesenteric Artery **6** Colic Artery, Right **7** Colic Artery, Left **8** Colic Artery, Middle **9** Renal Artery, Right **A** Renal Artery, Left **B** Inferior Mesenteric Artery **C** Common Iliac Artery, Right **D** Common Iliac Artery, Left **E** Internal Iliac Artery, Right **F** Internal Iliac Artery, Left **H** External Iliac Artery, Right **J** External Iliac Artery, Left **K** Femoral Artery, Right **L** Femoral Artery, Left **M** Popliteal Artery, Right **N** Popliteal Artery, Left **P** Anterior Tibial Artery, Right **Q** Anterior Tibial Artery, Left **R** Posterior Tibial Artery, Right **S** Posterior Tibial Artery, Left **T** Peroneal Artery, Right **U** Peroneal Artery, Left **V** Foot Artery, Right **W** Foot Artery, Left **Y** Lower Artery	**0** Open **3** Percutaneous **4** Percutaneous Endoscopic	**Z** No Device	**Z** No Qualifier

0 Medical and Surgical
4 Lower Arteries
R Replacement: Putting in or on biological or synthetic material that physically takes the place and/or function of all or a portion of a body part

Body Part Character 4	Approach Character 5	Device Character 6	Qualifier Character 7
0 Abdominal Aorta **1** Celiac Artery **2** Gastric Artery **3** Hepatic Artery **4** Splenic Artery **5** Superior Mesenteric Artery **6** Colic Artery, Right **7** Colic Artery, Left **8** Colic Artery, Middle **9** Renal Artery, Right **A** Renal Artery, Left **B** Inferior Mesenteric Artery **C** Common Iliac Artery, Right **D** Common Iliac Artery, Left **E** Internal Iliac Artery, Right **F** Internal Iliac Artery, Left **H** External Iliac Artery, Right **J** External Iliac Artery, Left **K** Femoral Artery, Right **L** Femoral Artery, Left **M** Popliteal Artery, Right **N** Popliteal Artery, Left **P** Anterior Tibial Artery, Right **Q** Anterior Tibial Artery, Left **R** Posterior Tibial Artery, Right **S** Posterior Tibial Artery, Left **T** Peroneal Artery, Right **U** Peroneal Artery, Left **V** Foot Artery, Right **W** Foot Artery, Left **Y** Lower Artery	**0** Open **4** Percutaneous Endoscopic	**7** Autologous Tissue Substitute **J** Synthetic Substitute **K** Nonautologous Tissue Substitute	**Z** No Qualifier

0 Medical and Surgical
4 Lower Arteries
S Reposition: Moving to its normal location, or other suitable location, all or a portion of a body part

Body Part Character 4	Approach Character 5	Device Character 6	Qualifier Character 7
0 Abdominal Aorta **1** Celiac Artery **2** Gastric Artery **3** Hepatic Artery **4** Splenic Artery **5** Superior Mesenteric Artery **6** Colic Artery, Right **7** Colic Artery, Left **8** Colic Artery, Middle **9** Renal Artery, Right **A** Renal Artery, Left **B** Inferior Mesenteric Artery **C** Common Iliac Artery, Right **D** Common Iliac Artery, Left **E** Internal Iliac Artery, Right **F** Internal Iliac Artery, Left **H** External Iliac Artery, Right **J** External Iliac Artery, Left **K** Femoral Artery, Right **L** Femoral Artery, Left **M** Popliteal Artery, Right **N** Popliteal Artery, Left **P** Anterior Tibial Artery, Right **Q** Anterior Tibial Artery, Left **R** Posterior Tibial Artery, Right **S** Posterior Tibial Artery, Left **T** Peroneal Artery, Right **U** Peroneal Artery, Left **V** Foot Artery, Right **W** Foot Artery, Left **Y** Lower Artery	**0** Open **3** Percutaneous **4** Percutaneous Endoscopic	**Z** No Device	**Z** No Qualifier

0 Medical and Surgical
4 Lower Arteries
U Supplement: Putting in or on biological or synthetic material that physically reinforces and/or augments the function of a portion of a body part

Body Part Character 4	Approach Character 5	Device Character 6	Qualifier Character 7
0 Abdominal Aorta **1** Celiac Artery **2** Gastric Artery **3** Hepatic Artery **4** Splenic Artery **5** Superior Mesenteric Artery **6** Colic Artery, Right **7** Colic Artery, Left **8** Colic Artery, Middle **9** Renal Artery, Right **A** Renal Artery, Left **B** Inferior Mesenteric Artery **C** Common Iliac Artery, Right **D** Common Iliac Artery, Left **E** Internal Iliac Artery, Right **F** Internal Iliac Artery, Left **H** External Iliac Artery, Right **J** External Iliac Artery, Left **K** Femoral Artery, Right **L** Femoral Artery, Left **M** Popliteal Artery, Right **N** Popliteal Artery, Left **P** Anterior Tibial Artery, Right **Q** Anterior Tibial Artery, Left **R** Posterior Tibial Artery, Right **S** Posterior Tibial Artery, Left **T** Peroneal Artery, Right **U** Peroneal Artery, Left **V** Foot Artery, Right **W** Foot Artery, Left **Y** Lower Artery	**0** Open **3** Percutaneous **4** Percutaneous Endoscopic	**7** Autologous Tissue Substitute **J** Synthetic Substitute **K** Nonautologous Tissue Substitute	**Z** No Qualifier

0 Medical and Surgical
4 Lower Arteries
V Restriction: Partially closing an orifice or the lumen of a tubular body part

Body Part Character 4	Approach Character 5	Device Character 6	Qualifier Character 7
0 Abdominal Aorta	**0** Open **3** Percutaneous **4** Percutaneous Endoscopic	**C** Extraluminal Device **E** Intraluminal Device, Branched or Fenestrated, One or Two Arteries **F** Intraluminal Device, Branched or Fenestrated, Three or More Arteries **Z** No Device	**6** Bifurcation **Z** No Qualifier
0 Abdominal Aorta	**0** Open **3** Percutaneous **4** Percutaneous Endoscopic	**D** Intraluminal Device	**6** Bifurcation **J** Temporary **Z** No Qualifier
1 Celiac Artery **2** Gastric Artery **3** Hepatic Artery **4** Splenic Artery **5** Superior Mesenteric Artery **6** Colic Artery, Right **7** Colic Artery, Left **8** Colic Artery, Middle **9** Renal Artery, Right **A** Renal Artery, Left **B** Inferior Mesenteric Artery **E** Internal Iliac Artery, Right **F** Internal Iliac Artery, Left **H** External Iliac Artery, Right **J** External Iliac Artery, Left **K** Femoral Artery, Right **L** Femoral Artery, Left **M** Popliteal Artery, Right **N** Popliteal Artery, Left **P** Anterior Tibial Artery, Right **Q** Anterior Tibial Artery, Left **R** Posterior Tibial Artery, Right **S** Posterior Tibial Artery, Left **T** Peroneal Artery, Right **U** Peroneal Artery, Left **V** Foot Artery, Right **W** Foot Artery, Left **Y** Lower Artery	**0** Open **3** Percutaneous **4** Percutaneous Endoscopic	**C** Extraluminal Device **D** Intraluminal Device **Z** No Device	**Z** No Qualifier
C Common Iliac Artery, Right **D** Common Iliac Artery, Left	**0** Open **3** Percutaneous **4** Percutaneous Endoscopic	**C** Extraluminal Device **D** Intraluminal Device **E** Intraluminal Device, Branched or Fenestrated, One or Two Arteries **Z** No Device	**Z** No Qualifier

0 Medical and Surgical
4 Lower Arteries
W Revision: Correcting, to the extent possible, a portion of a malfunctioning device or the position of a displaced device

Body Part	Approach	Device	Qualifier
Character 4	Character 5	Character 6	Character 7
Y Lower Artery	**0** Open **3** Percutaneous **4** Percutaneous Endoscopic	**0** Drainage Device **2** Monitoring Device **3** Infusion Device **7** Autologous Tissue Substitute **C** Extraluminal Device **D** Intraluminal Device **J** Synthetic Substitute **K** Nonautologous Tissue Substitute **Y** Other Device	**Z** No Qualifier
Y Lower Artery	**X** External	**0** Drainage Device **2** Monitoring Device **3** Infusion Device **7** Autologous Tissue Substitute **C** Extraluminal Device **D** Intraluminal Device **J** Synthetic Substitute **K** Nonautologous Tissue Substitute	**Z** No Qualifier

NOTES

Upper Veins 051-05W

0 Medical and Surgical
5 Upper Veins
1 Bypass: Altering the route of passage of the contents of a tubular body part

Body Part Character 4	Approach Character 5	Device Character 6	Qualifier Character 7
0 Azygos Vein **1** Hemiazygos Vein **3** Innominate Vein, Right **4** Innominate Vein, Left **5** Subclavian Vein, Right **6** Subclavian Vein, Left **7** Axillary Vein, Right **8** Axillary Vein, Left **9** Brachial Vein, Right **A** Brachial Vein, Left **B** Basilic Vein, Right **C** Basilic Vein, Left **D** Cephalic Vein, Right **F** Cephalic Vein, Left **G** Hand Vein, Right **H** Hand Vein, Left **L** Intracranial Vein **M** Internal Jugular Vein, Right **N** Internal Jugular Vein, Left **P** External Jugular Vein, Right **Q** External Jugular Vein, Left **R** Vertebral Vein, Right **S** Vertebral Vein, Left **T** Face Vein, Right **V** Face Vein, Left	**0** Open **4** Percutaneous Endoscopic	**7** Autologous Tissue Substitute **9** Autologous Venous Tissue **A** Autologous Arterial Tissue **J** Synthetic Substitute **K** Nonautologous Tissue Substitute **Z** No Device	**Y** Upper Vein

0 Medical and Surgical
5 Upper Veins
5 Destruction: Physical eradication of all or a portion of a body part by the direct use of energy, force, or a destructive agent

Body Part Character 4	Approach Character 5	Device Character 6	Qualifier Character 7
0 Azygos Vein 1 Hemiazygos Vein 3 Innominate Vein, Right 4 Innominate Vein, Left 5 Subclavian Vein, Right 6 Subclavian Vein, Left 7 Axillary Vein, Right 8 Axillary Vein, Left 9 Brachial Vein, Right A Brachial Vein, Left B Basilic Vein, Right C Basilic Vein, Left D Cephalic Vein, Right F Cephalic Vein, Left G Hand Vein, Right H Hand Vein, Left L Intracranial Vein M Internal Jugular Vein, Right N Internal Jugular Vein, Left P External Jugular Vein, Right Q External Jugular Vein, Left R Vertebral Vein, Right S Vertebral Vein, Left T Face Vein, Right V Face Vein, Left Y Upper Vein	0 Open 3 Percutaneous 4 Percutaneous Endoscopic	Z No Device	Z No Qualifier

0 Medical and Surgical
5 Upper Veins
7 Dilation: Expanding an orifice or the lumen of a tubular body part

Body Part Character 4	Approach Character 5	Device Character 6	Qualifier Character 7
0 Azygos Vein 1 Hemiazygos Vein G Hand Vein, Right H Hand Vein, Left L Intracranial Vein NC M Internal Jugular Vein, Right N Internal Jugular Vein, Left P External Jugular Vein, Right Q External Jugular Vein, Left R Vertebral Vein, Right S Vertebral Vein, Left T Face Vein, Right V Face Vein, Left Y Upper Vein	0 Open 3 Percutaneous 4 Percutaneous Endoscopic	D Intraluminal Device Z No Device	Z No Qualifier
3 Innominate Vein, Right 4 Innominate Vein, Left 5 Subclavian Vein, Right 6 Subclavian Vein, Left 7 Axillary Vein, Right 8 Axillary Vein, Left 9 Brachial Vein, Right A Brachial Vein, Left B Basilic Vein, Right C Basilic Vein, Left D Cephalic Vein, Right F Cephalic Vein, Left	0 Open 3 Percutaneous 4 Percutaneous Endoscopic	D Intraluminal Device Z No Device	1 Drug-Coated Balloon Z No Qualifier

NC 057L3ZZ 057L4ZZ

0 Medical and Surgical
5 Upper Veins
9 Drainage: Taking or letting out fluids and/or gases from a body part

Body Part Character 4	Approach Character 5	Device Character 6	Qualifier Character 7
0 Azygos Vein **1** Hemiazygos Vein **3** Innominate Vein, Right **4** Innominate Vein, Left **5** Subclavian Vein, Right **6** Subclavian Vein, Left **7** Axillary Vein, Right **8** Axillary Vein, Left **9** Brachial Vein, Right **A** Brachial Vein, Left **B** Basilic Vein, Right **C** Basilic Vein, Left **D** Cephalic Vein, Right **F** Cephalic Vein, Left **G** Hand Vein, Right **H** Hand Vein, Left **L** Intracranial Vein **M** Internal Jugular Vein, Right **N** Internal Jugular Vein, Left **P** External Jugular Vein, Right **Q** External Jugular Vein, Left **R** Vertebral Vein, Right **S** Vertebral Vein, Left **T** Face Vein, Right **V** Face Vein, Left **Y** Upper Vein	**0** Open **3** Percutaneous **4** Percutaneous Endoscopic	**0** Drainage Device	**Z** No Qualifier
0 Azygos Vein **1** Hemiazygos Vein **3** Innominate Vein, Right **4** Innominate Vein, Left **5** Subclavian Vein, Right **6** Subclavian Vein, Left **7** Axillary Vein, Right **8** Axillary Vein, Left **9** Brachial Vein, Right **A** Brachial Vein, Left **B** Basilic Vein, Right **C** Basilic Vein, Left **D** Cephalic Vein, Right **F** Cephalic Vein, Left **G** Hand Vein, Right **H** Hand Vein, Left **L** Intracranial Vein **M** Internal Jugular Vein, Right **N** Internal Jugular Vein, Left **P** External Jugular Vein, Right **Q** External Jugular Vein, Left **R** Vertebral Vein, Right **S** Vertebral Vein, Left **T** Face Vein, Right **V** Face Vein, Left **Y** Upper Vein	**0** Open **3** Percutaneous **4** Percutaneous Endoscopic	**Z** No Device	**X** Diagnostic **Z** No Qualifier

0 Medical and Surgical
5 Upper Veins
B Excision: Cutting out or off, without replacement, a portion of a body part

Body Part Character 4	Approach Character 5	Device Character 6	Qualifier Character 7
0 Azygos Vein	**0** Open	**Z** No Device	**X** Diagnostic
1 Hemiazygos Vein	**3** Percutaneous		**Z** No Qualifier
3 Innominate Vein, Right	**4** Percutaneous Endoscopic		
4 Innominate Vein, Left			
5 Subclavian Vein, Right			
6 Subclavian Vein, Left			
7 Axillary Vein, Right			
8 Axillary Vein, Left			
9 Brachial Vein, Right			
A Brachial Vein, Left			
B Basilic Vein, Right			
C Basilic Vein, Left			
D Cephalic Vein, Right			
F Cephalic Vein, Left			
G Hand Vein, Right			
H Hand Vein, Left			
L Intracranial Vein			
M Internal Jugular Vein, Right			
N Internal Jugular Vein, Left			
P External Jugular Vein, Right			
Q External Jugular Vein, Left			
R Vertebral Vein, Right			
S Vertebral Vein, Left			
T Face Vein, Right			
V Face Vein, Left			
Y Upper Vein			

0 Medical and Surgical
5 Upper Veins
C Extirpation: Taking or cutting out solid matter from a body part

Body Part Character 4	Approach Character 5	Device Character 6	Qualifier Character 7
0 Azygos Vein	**0** Open	**Z** No Device	**Z** No Qualifier
1 Hemiazygos Vein	**3** Percutaneous		
3 Innominate Vein, Right	**4** Percutaneous Endoscopic		
4 Innominate Vein, Left			
5 Subclavian Vein, Right			
6 Subclavian Vein, Left			
7 Axillary Vein, Right			
8 Axillary Vein, Left			
9 Brachial Vein, Right			
A Brachial Vein, Left			
B Basilic Vein, Right			
C Basilic Vein, Left			
D Cephalic Vein, Right			
F Cephalic Vein, Left			
G Hand Vein, Right			
H Hand Vein, Left			
L Intracranial Vein			
M Internal Jugular Vein, Right			
N Internal Jugular Vein, Left			
P External Jugular Vein, Right			
Q External Jugular Vein, Left			
R Vertebral Vein, Right			
S Vertebral Vein, Left			
T Face Vein, Right			
V Face Vein, Left			
Y Upper Vein			

0 Medical and Surgical
5 Upper Veins
D Extraction: Pulling or stripping out or off all or a portion of a body part by the use of force

Body Part	Approach	Device	Qualifier
Character 4	Character 5	Character 6	Character 7
9 Brachial Vein, Right A Brachial Vein, Left B Basilic Vein, Right C Basilic Vein, Left D Cephalic Vein, Right F Cephalic Vein, Left G Hand Vein, Right H Hand Vein, Left Y Upper Vein	0 Open 3 Percutaneous	Z No Device	Z No Qualifier

0 Medical and Surgical
5 Upper Veins
H Insertion: Putting in a nonbiological appliance that monitors, assists, performs, or prevents a physiological function but does not physically take the place of a body part

Body Part	Approach	Device	Qualifier
Character 4	Character 5	Character 6	Character 7
0 Azygos Vein HAC	0 Open 3 Percutaneous 4 Percutaneous Endoscopic	2 Monitoring Device 3 Infusion Device D Intraluminal Device M Neurostimulator Lead	Z No Qualifier
1 Hemiazygos Vein HAC 5 Subclavian Vein, Right CC HAC 6 Subclavian Vein, Left CC HAC 7 Axillary Vein, Right 8 Axillary Vein, Left 9 Brachial Vein, Right A Brachial Vein, Left B Basilic Vein, Right C Basilic Vein, Left D Cephalic Vein, Right F Cephalic Vein, Left G Hand Vein, Right H Hand Vein, Left L Intracranial Vein M Internal Jugular Vein, Right CC HAC N Internal Jugular Vein, Left CC HAC P External Jugular Vein, Right CC HAC Q External Jugular Vein, Left CC HAC R Vertebral Vein, Right S Vertebral Vein, Left T Face Vein, Right V Face Vein, Left	0 Open 3 Percutaneous 4 Percutaneous Endoscopic	3 Infusion Device D Intraluminal Device	Z No Qualifier
3 Innominate Vein, Right HAC 4 Innominate Vein, Left HAC	0 Open 3 Percutaneous 4 Percutaneous Endoscopic	3 Infusion Device D Intraluminal Device M Neurostimulator Lead	Z No Qualifier
Y Upper Vein	0 Open 3 Percutaneous 4 Percutaneous Endoscopic	2 Monitoring Device 3 Infusion Device D Intraluminal Device Y Other Device	Z No Qualifier

HAC 05H033Z 05H043Z 05H133Z 05H143Z 05H333Z 05H343Z 05H433Z 05H443Z 05H533Z 05H543Z 05H633Z 05H643Z 05HM33Z 05HN33Z 05HP33Z 05HQ33Z
Iatrogenic pneumothorax w/ venous catheterization procedures and secondary diagnosis J95.811.
CC 05H533Z 05H633Z 05HM33Z 05HN33Z 05HP33Z 05HQ33Z

LC Limited Coverage NC Noncovered HAC HAC-associated Procedure CC Combination Cluster - See Appendix G for code lists
DRG Non-OR-Affecting MS-DRG Assignment New/Revised Text in Orange ♂ Male ♀ Female

0 Medical and Surgical
5 Upper Veins
J Inspection: Visually and/or manually exploring a body part

Body Part Character 4	Approach Character 5	Device Character 6	Qualifier Character 7
Y Upper Vein	**0** Open **3** Percutaneous **4** Percutaneous Endoscopic **X** External	**Z** No Device	**Z** No Qualifier

0 Medical and Surgical
5 Upper Veins
L Occlusion: Completely closing an orifice or the lumen of a tubular body part

Body Part Character 4	Approach Character 5	Device Character 6	Qualifier Character 7
0 Azygos Vein **1** Hemiazygos Vein **3** Innominate Vein, Right **4** Innominate Vein, Left **5** Subclavian Vein, Right **6** Subclavian Vein, Left **7** Axillary Vein, Right **8** Axillary Vein, Left **9** Brachial Vein, Right **A** Brachial Vein, Left **B** Basilic Vein, Right **C** Basilic Vein, Left **D** Cephalic Vein, Right **F** Cephalic Vein, Left **G** Hand Vein, Right **H** Hand Vein, Left **L** Intracranial Vein **M** Internal Jugular Vein, Right **N** Internal Jugular Vein, Left **P** External Jugular Vein, Right **Q** External Jugular Vein, Left **R** Vertebral Vein, Right **S** Vertebral Vein, Left **T** Face Vein, Right **V** Face Vein, Left **Y** Upper Vein	**0** Open **3** Percutaneous **4** Percutaneous Endoscopic	**C** Extraluminal Device **D** Intraluminal Device **Z** No Device	**Z** No Qualifier

0 Medical and Surgical
5 Upper Veins
N Release: Freeing a body part from an abnormal physical constraint by cutting or by the use of force

Body Part Character 4	Approach Character 5	Device Character 6	Qualifier Character 7
0 Azygos Vein **1** Hemiazygos Vein **3** Innominate Vein, Right **4** Innominate Vein, Left **5** Subclavian Vein, Right **6** Subclavian Vein, Left **7** Axillary Vein, Right **8** Axillary Vein, Left **9** Brachial Vein, Right **A** Brachial Vein, Left **B** Basilic Vein, Right **C** Basilic Vein, Left **D** Cephalic Vein, Right **F** Cephalic Vein, Left **G** Hand Vein, Right **H** Hand Vein, Left **L** Intracranial Vein **M** Internal Jugular Vein, Right **N** Internal Jugular Vein, Left **P** External Jugular Vein, Right **Q** External Jugular Vein, Left **R** Vertebral Vein, Right **S** Vertebral Vein, Left **T** Face Vein, Right **V** Face Vein, Left **Y** Upper Vein	**0** Open **3** Percutaneous **4** Percutaneous Endoscopic	**Z** No Device	**Z** No Qualifier

0 Medical and Surgical
5 Upper Veins
P Removal: Taking out or off a device from a body part

Body Part Character 4	Approach Character 5	Device Character 6	Qualifier Character 7
0 Azygos Vein	**0** Open **3** Percutaneous **4** Percutaneous Endoscopic **X** External	**2** Monitoring Device **M** Neurostimulator Lead	**Z** No Qualifier
3 Innominate Vein, Right **4** Innominate Vein, Left	**0** Open **3** Percutaneous **4** Percutaneous Endoscopic **X** External	**M** Neurostimulator Lead	**Z** No Qualifier
Y Upper Vein	**0** Open **3** Percutaneous **4** Percutaneous Endoscopic	**0** Drainage Device **2** Monitoring Device **3** Infusion Device **7** Autologous Tissue Substitute **C** Extraluminal Device **D** Intraluminal Device **J** Synthetic Substitute **K** Nonautologous Tissue Substitute **Y** Other Device	**Z** No Qualifier
Y Upper Vein	**X** External	**0** Drainage Device **2** Monitoring Device **3** Infusion Device **D** Intraluminal Device	**Z** No Qualifier

0 Medical and Surgical
5 Upper Veins
Q Repair: Restoring, to the extent possible, a body part to its normal anatomic structure and function

Body Part Character 4	Approach Character 5	Device Character 6	Qualifier Character 7
0 Azygos Vein **1** Hemiazygos Vein **3** Innominate Vein, Right **4** Innominate Vein, Left **5** Subclavian Vein, Right **6** Subclavian Vein, Left **7** Axillary Vein, Right **8** Axillary Vein, Left **9** Brachial Vein, Right **A** Brachial Vein, Left **B** Basilic Vein, Right **C** Basilic Vein, Left **D** Cephalic Vein, Right **F** Cephalic Vein, Left **G** Hand Vein, Right **H** Hand Vein, Left **L** Intracranial Vein **M** Internal Jugular Vein, Right **N** Internal Jugular Vein, Left **P** External Jugular Vein, Right **Q** External Jugular Vein, Left **R** Vertebral Vein, Right **S** Vertebral Vein, Left **T** Face Vein, Right **V** Face Vein, Left **Y** Upper Vein	**0** Open **3** Percutaneous **4** Percutaneous Endoscopic	**Z** No Device	**Z** No Qualifier

0 Medical and Surgical
5 Upper Veins
R Replacement: Putting in or on biological or synthetic material that physically takes the place and/or function of all or a portion of a body part

Body Part Character 4	Approach Character 5	Device Character 6	Qualifier Character 7
0 Azygos Vein **1** Hemiazygos Vein **3** Innominate Vein, Right **4** Innominate Vein, Left **5** Subclavian Vein, Right **6** Subclavian Vein, Left **7** Axillary Vein, Right **8** Axillary Vein, Left **9** Brachial Vein, Right **A** Brachial Vein, Left **B** Basilic Vein, Right **C** Basilic Vein, Left **D** Cephalic Vein, Right **F** Cephalic Vein, Left **G** Hand Vein, Right **H** Hand Vein, Left **L** Intracranial Vein **M** Internal Jugular Vein, Right **N** Internal Jugular Vein, Left **P** External Jugular Vein, Right **Q** External Jugular Vein, Left **R** Vertebral Vein, Right **S** Vertebral Vein, Left **T** Face Vein, Right **V** Face Vein, Left **Y** Upper Vein	**0** Open **4** Percutaneous Endoscopic	**7** Autologous Tissue Substitute **J** Synthetic Substitute **K** Nonautologous Tissue Substitute	**Z** No Qualifier

0 Medical and Surgical
5 Upper Veins
S Reposition: Moving to its normal location, or other suitable location, all or a portion of a body part

Body Part Character 4	Approach Character 5	Device Character 6	Qualifier Character 7
0 Azygos Vein **1** Hemiazygos Vein **3** Innominate Vein, Right **4** Innominate Vein, Left **5** Subclavian Vein, Right **6** Subclavian Vein, Left **7** Axillary Vein, Right **8** Axillary Vein, Left **9** Brachial Vein, Right **A** Brachial Vein, Left **B** Basilic Vein, Right **C** Basilic Vein, Left **D** Cephalic Vein, Right **F** Cephalic Vein, Left **G** Hand Vein, Right **H** Hand Vein, Left **L** Intracranial Vein **M** Internal Jugular Vein, Right **N** Internal Jugular Vein, Left **P** External Jugular Vein, Right **Q** External Jugular Vein, Left **R** Vertebral Vein, Right **S** Vertebral Vein, Left **T** Face Vein, Right **V** Face Vein, Left **Y** Upper Vein	**0** Open **3** Percutaneous **4** Percutaneous Endoscopic	**Z** No Device	**Z** No Qualifier

0 Medical and Surgical
5 Upper Veins
U Supplement: Putting in or on biological or synthetic material that physically reinforces and/or augments the function of a portion of a body part

Body Part Character 4	Approach Character 5	Device Character 6	Qualifier Character 7
0 Azygos Vein **1** Hemiazygos Vein **3** Innominate Vein, Right **4** Innominate Vein, Left **5** Subclavian Vein, Right **6** Subclavian Vein, Left **7** Axillary Vein, Right **8** Axillary Vein, Left **9** Brachial Vein, Right **A** Brachial Vein, Left **B** Basilic Vein, Right **C** Basilic Vein, Left **D** Cephalic Vein, Right **F** Cephalic Vein, Left **G** Hand Vein, Right **H** Hand Vein, Left **L** Intracranial Vein **M** Internal Jugular Vein, Right **N** Internal Jugular Vein, Left **P** External Jugular Vein, Right **Q** External Jugular Vein, Left **R** Vertebral Vein, Right **S** Vertebral Vein, Left **T** Face Vein, Right **V** Face Vein, Left **Y** Upper Vein	**0** Open **3** Percutaneous **4** Percutaneous Endoscopic	**7** Autologous Tissue Substitute **J** Synthetic Substitute **K** Nonautologous Tissue Substitute	**Z** No Qualifier

0 Medical and Surgical
5 Upper Veins
V Restriction: Partially closing an orifice or the lumen of a tubular body part

Body Part Character 4	Approach Character 5	Device Character 6	Qualifier Character 7
0 Azygos Vein **1** Hemiazygos Vein **3** Innominate Vein, Right **4** Innominate Vein, Left **5** Subclavian Vein, Right **6** Subclavian Vein, Left **7** Axillary Vein, Right **8** Axillary Vein, Left **9** Brachial Vein, Right **A** Brachial Vein, Left **B** Basilic Vein, Right **C** Basilic Vein, Left **D** Cephalic Vein, Right **F** Cephalic Vein, Left **G** Hand Vein, Right **H** Hand Vein, Left **L** Intracranial Vein **M** Internal Jugular Vein, Right **N** Internal Jugular Vein, Left **P** External Jugular Vein, Right **Q** External Jugular Vein, Left **R** Vertebral Vein, Right **S** Vertebral Vein, Left **T** Face Vein, Right **V** Face Vein, Left **Y** Upper Vein	**0** Open **3** Percutaneous **4** Percutaneous Endoscopic	**C** Extraluminal Device **D** Intraluminal Device **Z** No Device	**Z** No Qualifier

0 Medical and Surgical
5 Upper Veins
W Revision: Correcting, to the extent possible, a portion of a malfunctioning device or the position of a displaced device

Body Part Character 4	Approach Character 5	Device Character 6	Qualifier Character 7
0 Azygos Vein	**0** Open **3** Percutaneous **4** Percutaneous Endoscopic **X** External	**2** Monitoring Device **M** Neurostimulator Lead	**Z** No Qualifier
3 Innominate Vein, Right **4** Innominate Vein, Left	**0** Open **3** Percutaneous **4** Percutaneous Endoscopic **X** External	**M** Neurostimulator Lead	**Z** No Qualifier
Y Upper Vein	**0** Open **3** Percutaneous **4** Percutaneous Endoscopic	**0** Drainage Device **2** Monitoring Device **3** Infusion Device **7** Autologous Tissue Substitute **C** Extraluminal Device **D** Intraluminal Device **J** Synthetic Substitute **K** Nonautologous Tissue Substitute **Y** Other Device	**Z** No Qualifier
Y Upper Vein	**X** External	**0** Drainage Device **2** Monitoring Device **3** Infusion Device **7** Autologous Tissue Substitute **C** Extraluminal Device **D** Intraluminal Device **J** Synthetic Substitute **K** Nonautologous Tissue Substitute	**Z** No Qualifier

NOTES

NOTES

Lower Veins 061-06W

0 Medical and Surgical
6 Lower Veins
1 Bypass: Altering the route of passage of the contents of a tubular body part

Body Part	Approach	Device	Qualifier
Character 4	**Character 5**	**Character 6**	**Character 7**
0 Inferior Vena Cava	**0** Open **4** Percutaneous Endoscopic	**7** Autologous Tissue Substitute **9** Autologous Venous Tissue **A** Autologous Arterial Tissue **J** Synthetic Substitute **K** Nonautologous Tissue Substitute **Z** No Device	**5** Superior Mesenteric Vein **6** Inferior Mesenteric Vein **P** Pulmonary Trunk **Q** Pulmonary Artery, Right **R** Pulmonary Artery, Left **Y** Lower Vein
1 Splenic Vein	**0** Open **4** Percutaneous Endoscopic	**7** Autologous Tissue Substitute **9** Autologous Venous Tissue **A** Autologous Arterial Tissue **J** Synthetic Substitute **K** Nonautologous Tissue Substitute **Z** No Device	**9** Renal Vein, Right **B** Renal Vein, Left **Y** Lower Vein
2 Gastric Vein **3** Esophageal Vein **4** Hepatic Vein **5** Superior Mesenteric Vein **6** Inferior Mesenteric Vein **7** Colic Vein **9** Renal Vein, Right **B** Renal Vein, Left **C** Common Iliac Vein, Right **D** Common Iliac Vein, Left **F** External Iliac Vein, Right **G** External Iliac Vein, Left **H** Hypogastric Vein, Right **J** Hypogastric Vein, Left **M** Femoral Vein, Right **N** Femoral Vein, Left **P** Saphenous Vein, Right **Q** Saphenous Vein, Left **T** Foot Vein, Right **V** Foot Vein, Left	**0** Open **4** Percutaneous Endoscopic	**7** Autologous Tissue Substitute **9** Autologous Venous Tissue **A** Autologous Arterial Tissue **J** Synthetic Substitute **K** Nonautologous Tissue Substitute **Z** No Device	**Y** Lower Vein
8 Portal Vein	**0** Open	**7** Autologous Tissue Substitute **9** Autologous Venous Tissue **A** Autologous Arterial Tissue **J** Synthetic Substitute **K** Nonautologous Tissue Substitute **Z** No Device	**9** Renal Vein, Right **B** Renal Vein, Left **Y** Lower Vein
8 Portal Vein	**3** Percutaneous	**J** Synthetic Substitute	**4** Hepatic Vein **Y** Lower Vein
8 Portal Vein	**4** Percutaneous Endoscopic	**7** Autologous Tissue Substitute **9** Autologous Venous Tissue **A** Autologous Arterial Tissue **K** Nonautologous Tissue Substitute **Z** No Device	**9** Renal Vein, Right **B** Renal Vein, Left **Y** Lower Vein
8 Portal Vein	**4** Percutaneous Endoscopic	**J** Synthetic Substitute	**4** Hepatic Vein **9** Renal Vein, Right **B** Renal Vein, Left **Y** Lower Vein

0 Medical and Surgical
6 Lower Veins
5 Destruction: Physical eradication of all or a portion of a body part by the direct use of energy, force, or a destructive agent

Body Part Character 4	Approach Character 5	Device Character 6	Qualifier Character 7
0 Inferior Vena Cava **1** Splenic Vein **2** Gastric Vein **3** Esophageal Vein **4** Hepatic Vein **5** Superior Mesenteric Vein **6** Inferior Mesenteric Vein **7** Colic Vein **8** Portal Vein **9** Renal Vein, Right **B** Renal Vein, Left **C** Common Iliac Vein, Right **D** Common Iliac Vein, Left **F** External Iliac Vein, Right **G** External Iliac Vein, Left **H** Hypogastric Vein, Right **J** Hypogastric Vein, Left **M** Femoral Vein, Right **N** Femoral Vein, Left **P** Saphenous Vein, Right **Q** Saphenous Vein, Left **T** Foot Vein, Right **V** Foot Vein, Left	**0** Open **3** Percutaneous **4** Percutaneous Endoscopic	**Z** No Device	**Z** No Qualifier
Y Lower Vein	**0** Open **3** Percutaneous **4** Percutaneous Endoscopic	**Z** No Device	**C** Hemorrhoidal Plexus **Z** No Qualifier

0 Medical and Surgical
6 Lower Veins
7 Dilation: Expanding an orifice or the lumen of a tubular body part

Body Part Character 4	Approach Character 5	Device Character 6	Qualifier Character 7
0 Inferior Vena Cava **1** Splenic Vein **2** Gastric Vein **3** Esophageal Vein **4** Hepatic Vein **5** Superior Mesenteric Vein **6** Inferior Mesenteric Vein **7** Colic Vein **8** Portal Vein **9** Renal Vein, Right **B** Renal Vein, Left **C** Common Iliac Vein, Right **D** Common Iliac Vein, Left **F** External Iliac Vein, Right **G** External Iliac Vein, Left **H** Hypogastric Vein, Right **J** Hypogastric Vein, Left **M** Femoral Vein, Right **N** Femoral Vein, Left **P** Saphenous Vein, Right **Q** Saphenous Vein, Left **T** Foot Vein, Right **V** Foot Vein, Left **Y** Lower Vein	**0** Open **3** Percutaneous **4** Percutaneous Endoscopic	**D** Intraluminal Device **Z** No Device	**Z** No Qualifier

0 Medical and Surgical
6 Lower Veins
9 Drainage: Taking or letting out fluids and/or gases from a body part

Body Part Character 4	Approach Character 5	Device Character 6	Qualifier Character 7
0 Inferior Vena Cava **1** Splenic Vein **2** Gastric Vein **3** Esophageal Vein **4** Hepatic Vein **5** Superior Mesenteric Vein **6** Inferior Mesenteric Vein **7** Colic Vein **8** Portal Vein **9** Renal Vein, Right **B** Renal Vein, Left **C** Common Iliac Vein, Right **D** Common Iliac Vein, Left **F** External Iliac Vein, Right **G** External Iliac Vein, Left **H** Hypogastric Vein, Right **J** Hypogastric Vein, Left **M** Femoral Vein, Right **N** Femoral Vein, Left **P** Saphenous Vein, Right **Q** Saphenous Vein, Left **T** Foot Vein, Right **V** Foot Vein, Left **Y** Lower Vein	**0** Open **3** Percutaneous **4** Percutaneous Endoscopic	**0** Drainage Device	**Z** No Qualifier
0 Inferior Vena Cava **1** Splenic Vein **2** Gastric Vein **3** Esophageal Vein **4** Hepatic Vein **5** Superior Mesenteric Vein **6** Inferior Mesenteric Vein **7** Colic Vein **8** Portal Vein **9** Renal Vein, Right **B** Renal Vein, Left **C** Common Iliac Vein, Right **D** Common Iliac Vein, Left **F** External Iliac Vein, Right **G** External Iliac Vein, Left **H** Hypogastric Vein, Right **J** Hypogastric Vein, Left **M** Femoral Vein, Right **N** Femoral Vein, Left **P** Saphenous Vein, Right **Q** Saphenous Vein, Left **T** Foot Vein, Right **V** Foot Vein, Left **Y** Lower Vein	**0** Open **3** Percutaneous **4** Percutaneous Endoscopic	**Z** No Device	**X** Diagnostic **Z** No Qualifier

0 Medical and Surgical
6 Lower Veins
B Excision: Cutting out or off, without replacement, a portion of a body part

Body Part	Approach	Device	Qualifier
Character 4	Character 5	Character 6	Character 7
0 Inferior Vena Cava **1** Splenic Vein **2** Gastric Vein **3** Esophageal Vein **4** Hepatic Vein **5** Superior Mesenteric Vein **6** Inferior Mesenteric Vein **7** Colic Vein **8** Portal Vein **9** Renal Vein, Right **B** Renal Vein, Left **C** Common Iliac Vein, Right **D** Common Iliac Vein, Left **F** External Iliac Vein, Right **G** External Iliac Vein, Left **H** Hypogastric Vein, Right **J** Hypogastric Vein, Left **M** Femoral Vein, Right **N** Femoral Vein, Left **P** Saphenous Vein, Right **Q** Saphenous Vein, Left **T** Foot Vein, Right **V** Foot Vein, Left	**0** Open **3** Percutaneous **4** Percutaneous Endoscopic	**Z** No Device	**X** Diagnostic **Z** No Qualifier
Y Lower Vein	**0** Open **3** Percutaneous **4** Percutaneous Endoscopic	**Z** No Device	**C** Hemorrhoidal Plexus **X** Diagnostic **Z** No Qualifier

0 Medical and Surgical
6 Lower Veins
C Extirpation: Taking or cutting out solid matter from a body part

Body Part	Approach	Device	Qualifier
Character 4	Character 5	Character 6	Character 7
0 Inferior Vena Cava **1** Splenic Vein **2** Gastric Vein **3** Esophageal Vein **4** Hepatic Vein **5** Superior Mesenteric Vein **6** Inferior Mesenteric Vein **7** Colic Vein **8** Portal Vein **9** Renal Vein, Right **B** Renal Vein, Left **C** Common Iliac Vein, Right **D** Common Iliac Vein, Left **F** External Iliac Vein, Right **G** External Iliac Vein, Left **H** Hypogastric Vein, Right **J** Hypogastric Vein, Left **M** Femoral Vein, Right **N** Femoral Vein, Left **P** Saphenous Vein, Right **Q** Saphenous Vein, Left **T** Foot Vein, Right **V** Foot Vein, Left **Y** Lower Vein	**0** Open **3** Percutaneous **4** Percutaneous Endoscopic	**Z** No Device	**Z** No Qualifier

0 Medical and Surgical
6 Lower Veins
D Extraction: Pulling or stripping out or off all or a portion of a body part by the use of force

Body Part Character 4	Approach Character 5	Device Character 6	Qualifier Character 7
M Femoral Vein, Right **N** Femoral Vein, Left **P** Saphenous Vein, Right **Q** Saphenous Vein, Left **T** Foot Vein, Right **V** Foot Vein, Left **Y** Lower Vein	**0** Open **3** Percutaneous **4** Percutaneous Endoscopic	**Z** No Device	**Z** No Qualifier

0 Medical and Surgical
6 Lower Veins
H Insertion: Putting in a nonbiological appliance that monitors, assists, performs, or prevents a physiological function but does not physically take the place of a body part

Body Part Character 4	Approach Character 5	Device Character 6	Qualifier Character 7
0 Inferior Vena Cava	**0** Open **3** Percutaneous	**3** Infusion Device	**T** Via Umbilical Vein **Z** No Qualifier
0 Inferior Vena Cava	**0** Open **3** Percutaneous	**D** Intraluminal Device	**Z** No Qualifier
0 Inferior Vena Cava	**4** Percutaneous Endoscopic	**3** Infusion Device **D** Intraluminal Device	**Z** No Qualifier
1 Splenic Vein **2** Gastric Vein **3** Esophageal Vein **4** Hepatic Vein **5** Superior Mesenteric Vein **6** Inferior Mesenteric Vein **7** Colic Vein **8** Portal Vein **9** Renal Vein, Right **B** Renal Vein, Left **C** Common Iliac Vein, Right **D** Common Iliac Vein, Left **F** External Iliac Vein, Right **G** External Iliac Vein, Left **H** Hypogastric Vein, Right **J** Hypogastric Vein, Left **M** Femoral Vein, Right CC **N** Femoral Vein, Left CC **P** Saphenous Vein, Right **Q** Saphenous Vein, Left **T** Foot Vein, Right **V** Foot Vein, Left	**0** Open **3** Percutaneous **4** Percutaneous Endoscopic	**3** Infusion Device **D** Intraluminal Device	**Z** No Qualifier
Y Lower Vein	**0** Open **3** Percutaneous **4** Percutaneous Endoscopic	**2** Monitoring Device **3** Infusion Device **D** Intraluminal Device **Y** Other Device	**Z** No Qualifier

CC 06HM33Z 06HN33Z

LC Limited Coverage NC Noncovered HAC HAC-associated Procedure CC Combination Cluster - See Appendix G for code lists
DRG Non-OR-Affecting MS-DRG Assignment New/Revised Text in Orange ♂ Male ♀ Female

0 Medical and Surgical
6 Lower Veins
J Inspection: Visually and/or manually exploring a body part

Body Part Character 4	Approach Character 5	Device Character 6	Qualifier Character 7
Y Lower Vein	**0** Open **3** Percutaneous **4** Percutaneous Endoscopic **X** External	**Z** No Device	**Z** No Qualifier

0 Medical and Surgical
6 Lower Veins
L Occlusion: Completely closing an orifice or the lumen of a tubular body part

Body Part Character 4	Approach Character 5	Device Character 6	Qualifier Character 7
0 Inferior Vena Cava **1** Splenic Vein **2** Gastric Vein **4** Hepatic Vein **5** Superior Mesenteric Vein **6** Inferior Mesenteric Vein **7** Colic Vein **8** Portal Vein **9** Renal Vein, Right **B** Renal Vein, Left **C** Common Iliac Vein, Right **D** Common Iliac Vein, Left **F** External Iliac Vein, Right **G** External Iliac Vein, Left **H** Hypogastric Vein, Right **J** Hypogastric Vein, Left **M** Femoral Vein, Right **N** Femoral Vein, Left **P** Saphenous Vein, Right **Q** Saphenous Vein, Left **T** Foot Vein, Right **V** Foot Vein, Left	**0** Open **3** Percutaneous **4** Percutaneous Endoscopic	**C** Extraluminal Device **D** Intraluminal Device **Z** No Device	**Z** No Qualifier
3 Esophageal Vein	**0** Open **3** Percutaneous **4** Percutaneous Endoscopic **7** Via Natural or Artificial Opening **8** Via Natural or Artificial Opening Endoscopic	**C** Extraluminal Device **D** Intraluminal Device **Z** No Device	**Z** No Qualifier
Y Lower Vein	**0** Open **3** Percutaneous **4** Percutaneous Endoscopic	**C** Extraluminal Device **D** Intraluminal Device **Z** No Device	**C** Hemorrhoidal Plexus **Z** No Qualifier

0 Medical and Surgical
6 Lower Veins
N Release: Freeing a body part from an abnormal physical constraint by cutting or by the use of force

Body Part Character 4	Approach Character 5	Device Character 6	Qualifier Character 7
0 Inferior Vena Cava **1** Splenic Vein **2** Gastric Vein **3** Esophageal Vein **4** Hepatic Vein **5** Superior Mesenteric Vein **6** Inferior Mesenteric Vein **7** Colic Vein **8** Portal Vein **9** Renal Vein, Right **B** Renal Vein, Left **C** Common Iliac Vein, Right **D** Common Iliac Vein, Left **F** External Iliac Vein, Right **G** External Iliac Vein, Left **H** Hypogastric Vein, Right **J** Hypogastric Vein, Left **M** Femoral Vein, Right **N** Femoral Vein, Left **P** Saphenous Vein, Right **Q** Saphenous Vein, Left **T** Foot Vein, Right **V** Foot Vein, Left **Y** Lower Vein	**0** Open **3** Percutaneous **4** Percutaneous Endoscopic	**Z** No Device	**Z** No Qualifier

0 Medical and Surgical
6 Lower Veins
P Removal: Taking out or off a device from a body part

Body Part Character 4	Approach Character 5	Device Character 6	Qualifier Character 7
Y Lower Vein	**0** Open **3** Percutaneous **4** Percutaneous Endoscopic	**0** Drainage Device **2** Monitoring Device **3** Infusion Device **7** Autologous Tissue Substitute **C** Extraluminal Device **D** Intraluminal Device **J** Synthetic Substitute **K** Nonautologous Tissue Substitute **Y** Other Device	**Z** No Qualifier
Y Lower Vein	**X** External	**0** Drainage Device **2** Monitoring Device **3** Infusion Device **D** Intraluminal Device	**Z** No Qualifier

0 Medical and Surgical
6 Lower Veins
Q Repair: Restoring, to the extent possible, a body part to its normal anatomic structure and function

Body Part Character 4	Approach Character 5	Device Character 6	Qualifier Character 7
0 Inferior Vena Cava **1** Splenic Vein **2** Gastric Vein **3** Esophageal Vein **4** Hepatic Vein **5** Superior Mesenteric Vein **6** Inferior Mesenteric Vein **7** Colic Vein **8** Portal Vein **9** Renal Vein, Right **B** Renal Vein, Left **C** Common Iliac Vein, Right **D** Common Iliac Vein, Left **F** External Iliac Vein, Right **G** External Iliac Vein, Left **H** Hypogastric Vein, Right **J** Hypogastric Vein, Left **M** Femoral Vein, Right **N** Femoral Vein, Left **P** Saphenous Vein, Right **Q** Saphenous Vein, Left **T** Foot Vein, Right **V** Foot Vein, Left **Y** Lower Vein	**0** Open **3** Percutaneous **4** Percutaneous Endoscopic	**Z** No Device	**Z** No Qualifier

0 Medical and Surgical
6 Lower Veins
R Replacement: Putting in or on biological or synthetic material that physically takes the place and/or function of all or a portion of a body part

Body Part Character 4	Approach Character 5	Device Character 6	Qualifier Character 7
0 Inferior Vena Cava **1** Splenic Vein **2** Gastric Vein **3** Esophageal Vein **4** Hepatic Vein **5** Superior Mesenteric Vein **6** Inferior Mesenteric Vein **7** Colic Vein **8** Portal Vein **9** Renal Vein, Right **B** Renal Vein, Left **C** Common Iliac Vein, Right **D** Common Iliac Vein, Left **F** External Iliac Vein, Right **G** External Iliac Vein, Left **H** Hypogastric Vein, Right **J** Hypogastric Vein, Left **M** Femoral Vein, Right **N** Femoral Vein, Left **P** Saphenous Vein, Right **Q** Saphenous Vein, Left **T** Foot Vein, Right **V** Foot Vein, Left **Y** Lower Vein	**0** Open **4** Percutaneous Endoscopic	**7** Autologous Tissue Substitute **J** Synthetic Substitute **K** Nonautologous Tissue Substitute	**Z** No Qualifier

0 Medical and Surgical
6 Lower Veins
S Reposition: Moving to its normal location, or other suitable location, all or a portion of a body part

Body Part Character 4	Approach Character 5	Device Character 6	Qualifier Character 7
0 Inferior Vena Cava **1** Splenic Vein **2** Gastric Vein **3** Esophageal Vein **4** Hepatic Vein **5** Superior Mesenteric Vein **6** Inferior Mesenteric Vein **7** Colic Vein **8** Portal Vein **9** Renal Vein, Right **B** Renal Vein, Left **C** Common Iliac Vein, Right **D** Common Iliac Vein, Left **F** External Iliac Vein, Right **G** External Iliac Vein, Left **H** Hypogastric Vein, Right **J** Hypogastric Vein, Left **M** Femoral Vein, Right **N** Femoral Vein, Left **P** Saphenous Vein, Right **Q** Saphenous Vein, Left **T** Foot Vein, Right **V** Foot Vein, Left **Y** Lower Vein	**0** Open **3** Percutaneous **4** Percutaneous Endoscopic	**Z** No Device	**Z** No Qualifier

0 Medical and Surgical
6 Lower Veins
U Supplement: Putting in or on biological or synthetic material that physically reinforces and/or augments the function of a portion of a body part

Body Part Character 4	Approach Character 5	Device Character 6	Qualifier Character 7
0 Inferior Vena Cava **1** Splenic Vein **2** Gastric Vein **3** Esophageal Vein **4** Hepatic Vein **5** Superior Mesenteric Vein **6** Inferior Mesenteric Vein **7** Colic Vein **8** Portal Vein **9** Renal Vein, Right **B** Renal Vein, Left **C** Common Iliac Vein, Right **D** Common Iliac Vein, Left **F** External Iliac Vein, Right **G** External Iliac Vein, Left **H** Hypogastric Vein, Right **J** Hypogastric Vein, Left **M** Femoral Vein, Right **N** Femoral Vein, Left **P** Saphenous Vein, Right **Q** Saphenous Vein, Left **T** Foot Vein, Right **V** Foot Vein, Left **Y** Lower Vein	**0** Open **3** Percutaneous **4** Percutaneous Endoscopic	**7** Autologous Tissue Substitute **J** Synthetic Substitute **K** Nonautologous Tissue Substitute	**Z** No Qualifier

0 Medical and Surgical
6 Lower Veins
V Restriction: Partially closing an orifice or the lumen of a tubular body part

Body Part Character 4	Approach Character 5	Device Character 6	Qualifier Character 7
0 Inferior Vena Cava **1** Splenic Vein **2** Gastric Vein **3** Esophageal Vein **4** Hepatic Vein **5** Superior Mesenteric Vein **6** Inferior Mesenteric Vein **7** Colic Vein **8** Portal Vein **9** Renal Vein, Right **B** Renal Vein, Left **C** Common Iliac Vein, Right **D** Common Iliac Vein, Left **F** External Iliac Vein, Right **G** External Iliac Vein, Left **H** Hypogastric Vein, Right **J** Hypogastric Vein, Left **M** Femoral Vein, Right **N** Femoral Vein, Left **P** Saphenous Vein, Right **Q** Saphenous Vein, Left **T** Foot Vein, Right **V** Foot Vein, Left **Y** Lower Vein	**0** Open **3** Percutaneous **4** Percutaneous Endoscopic	**C** Extraluminal Device **D** Intraluminal Device **Z** No Device	**Z** No Qualifier

0 Medical and Surgical
6 Lower Veins
W Revision: Correcting, to the extent possible, a portion of a malfunctioning device or the position of a displaced device

Body Part Character 4	Approach Character 5	Device Character 6	Qualifier Character 7
Y Lower Vein	**0** Open **3** Percutaneous **4** Percutaneous Endoscopic	**0** Drainage Device **2** Monitoring Device **3** Infusion Device **7** Autologous Tissue Substitute **C** Extraluminal Device **D** Intraluminal Device **J** Synthetic Substitute **K** Nonautologous Tissue Substitute **Y** Other Device	**Z** No Qualifier
Y Lower Vein	**X** External	**0** Drainage Device **2** Monitoring Device **3** Infusion Device **7** Autologous Tissue Substitute **C** Extraluminal Device **D** Intraluminal Device **J** Synthetic Substitute **K** Nonautologous Tissue Substitute	**Z** No Qualifier

NOTES

NOTES

Lymphatic and Hemic Systems 072-07Y

0 Medical and Surgical
7 Lymphatic and Hemic Systems
2 Change: Taking out or off a device from a body part and putting back an identical or similar device in or on the same body part without cutting or puncturing the skin or a mucous membrane

Body Part Character 4	Approach Character 5	Device Character 6	Qualifier Character 7
K Thoracic Duct **L** Cisterna Chyli **M** Thymus **N** Lymphatic **P** Spleen **T** Bone Marrow	**X** External	**0** Drainage Device **Y** Other Device	**Z** No Qualifier

0 Medical and Surgical
7 Lymphatic and Hemic Systems
5 Destruction: Physical eradication of all or a portion of a body part by the direct use of energy, force, or a destructive agent

Body Part Character 4	Approach Character 5	Device Character 6	Qualifier Character 7
0 Lymphatic, Head **1** Lymphatic, Right Neck **2** Lymphatic, Left Neck **3** Lymphatic, Right Upper Extremity **4** Lymphatic, Left Upper Extremity **5** Lymphatic, Right Axillary **6** Lymphatic, Left Axillary **7** Lymphatic, Thorax **8** Lymphatic, Internal Mammary, Right **9** Lymphatic, Internal Mammary, Left **B** Lymphatic, Mesenteric **C** Lymphatic, Pelvis **D** Lymphatic, Aortic **F** Lymphatic, Right Lower Extremity **G** Lymphatic, Left Lower Extremity **H** Lymphatic, Right Inguinal **J** Lymphatic, Left Inguinal **K** Thoracic Duct **L** Cisterna Chyli **M** Thymus **P** Spleen	**0** Open **3** Percutaneous **4** Percutaneous Endoscopic	**Z** No Device	**Z** No Qualifier

0 Medical and Surgical
7 Lymphatic and Hemic Systems
9 Drainage: Taking or letting out fluids and/or gases from a body part

Body Part Character 4	Approach Character 5	Device Character 6	Qualifier Character 7
0 Lymphatic, Head **1** Lymphatic, Right Neck **2** Lymphatic, Left Neck **3** Lymphatic, Right Upper Extremity **4** Lymphatic, Left Upper Extremity **5** Lymphatic, Right Axillary **6** Lymphatic, Left Axillary **7** Lymphatic, Thorax **8** Lymphatic, Internal Mammary, Right **9** Lymphatic, Internal Mammary, Left **B** Lymphatic, Mesenteric **C** Lymphatic, Pelvis **D** Lymphatic, Aortic **F** Lymphatic, Right Lower Extremity **G** Lymphatic, Left Lower Extremity **H** Lymphatic, Right Inguinal **J** Lymphatic, Left Inguinal **K** Thoracic Duct **L** Cisterna Chyli	**0** Open **3** Percutaneous **4** Percutaneous Endoscopic **8** Via Natural or Artificial Opening Endoscopic	**0** Drainage Device	**Z** No Qualifier
0 Lymphatic, Head **1** Lymphatic, Right Neck **2** Lymphatic, Left Neck **3** Lymphatic, Right Upper Extremity **4** Lymphatic, Left Upper Extremity **5** Lymphatic, Right Axillary **6** Lymphatic, Left Axillary **7** Lymphatic, Thorax **8** Lymphatic, Internal Mammary, Right **9** Lymphatic, Internal Mammary, Left **B** Lymphatic, Mesenteric **C** Lymphatic, Pelvis **D** Lymphatic, Aortic **F** Lymphatic, Right Lower Extremity **G** Lymphatic, Left Lower Extremity **H** Lymphatic, Right Inguinal **J** Lymphatic, Left Inguinal **K** Thoracic Duct **L** Cisterna Chyli	**0** Open **3** Percutaneous **4** Percutaneous Endoscopic **8** Via Natural or Artificial Opening Endoscopic	**Z** No Device	**X** Diagnostic **Z** No Qualifier
M Thymus **P** Spleen **T** Bone Marrow	**0** Open **3** Percutaneous **4** Percutaneous Endoscopic	**0** Drainage Device	**Z** No Qualifier
M Thymus **P** Spleen **T** Bone Marrow	**0** Open **3** Percutaneous **4** Percutaneous Endoscopic	**Z** No Device	**X** Diagnostic **Z** No Qualifier

0 Medical and Surgical
7 Lymphatic and Hemic Systems
B Excision: Cutting out or off, without replacement, a portion of a body part

Body Part Character 4	Approach Character 5	Device Character 6	Qualifier Character 7
0 Lymphatic, Head 1 Lymphatic, Right Neck 2 Lymphatic, Left Neck 3 Lymphatic, Right Upper Extremity 4 Lymphatic, Left Upper Extremity 5 Lymphatic, Right Axillary 6 Lymphatic, Left Axillary 7 Lymphatic, Thorax 8 Lymphatic, Internal Mammary, Right 9 Lymphatic, Internal Mammary, Left B Lymphatic, Mesenteric C Lymphatic, Pelvis D Lymphatic, Aortic F Lymphatic, Right Lower Extremity G Lymphatic, Left Lower Extremity H Lymphatic, Right Inguinal CC J Lymphatic, Left Inguinal CC K Thoracic Duct L Cisterna Chyli M Thymus P Spleen	0 Open 3 Percutaneous 4 Percutaneous Endoscopic	Z No Device	X Diagnostic Z No Qualifier

CC 07BH0ZZ 07BH4ZZ 07BJ0ZZ 07BJ4ZZ

0 Medical and Surgical
7 Lymphatic and Hemic Systems
C Extirpation: Taking or cutting out solid matter from a body part

Body Part Character 4	Approach Character 5	Device Character 6	Qualifier Character 7
0 Lymphatic, Head 1 Lymphatic, Right Neck 2 Lymphatic, Left Neck 3 Lymphatic, Right Upper Extremity 4 Lymphatic, Left Upper Extremity 5 Lymphatic, Right Axillary 6 Lymphatic, Left Axillary 7 Lymphatic, Thorax 8 Lymphatic, Internal Mammary, Right 9 Lymphatic, Internal Mammary, Left B Lymphatic, Mesenteric C Lymphatic, Pelvis D Lymphatic, Aortic F Lymphatic, Right Lower Extremity G Lymphatic, Left Lower Extremity H Lymphatic, Right Inguinal J Lymphatic, Left Inguinal K Thoracic Duct L Cisterna Chyli M Thymus P Spleen	0 Open 3 Percutaneous 4 Percutaneous Endoscopic	Z No Device	Z No Qualifier

0 Medical and Surgical
7 Lymphatic and Hemic Systems
D Extraction: Pulling or stripping out or off all or a portion of a body part by the use of force

Body Part Character 4	Approach Character 5	Device Character 6	Qualifier Character 7
0 Lymphatic, Head **1** Lymphatic, Right Neck **2** Lymphatic, Left Neck **3** Lymphatic, Right Upper Extremity **4** Lymphatic, Left Upper Extremity **5** Lymphatic, Right Axillary **6** Lymphatic, Left Axillary **7** Lymphatic, Thorax **8** Lymphatic, Internal Mammary, Right **9** Lymphatic, Internal Mammary, Left **B** Lymphatic, Mesenteric **C** Lymphatic, Pelvis **D** Lymphatic, Aortic **F** Lymphatic, Right Lower Extremity **G** Lymphatic, Left Lower Extremity **H** Lymphatic, Right Inguinal **J** Lymphatic, Left Inguinal **K** Thoracic Duct **L** Cisterna Chyli	**3** Percutaneous **4** Percutaneous Endoscopic **8** Via Natural or Artificial Opening Endoscopic	**Z** No Device	**X** Diagnostic
M Thymus **P** Spleen	**3** Percutaneous **4** Percutaneous Endoscopic	**Z** No Device	**X** Diagnostic
Q Bone Marrow, Sternum **R** Bone Marrow, Iliac **S** Bone Marrow, Vertebral	**0** Open **3** Percutaneous	**Z** No Device	**X** Diagnostic **Z** No Qualifier

0 Medical and Surgical
7 Lymphatic and Hemic Systems
H Insertion: Putting in a nonbiological appliance that monitors, assists, performs, or prevents a physiological function but does not physically take the place of a body part

Body Part Character 4	Approach Character 5	Device Character 6	Qualifier Character 7
K Thoracic Duct **L** Cisterna Chyli **M** Thymus **N** Lymphatic **P** Spleen	**0** Open **3** Percutaneous **4** Percutaneous Endoscopic	**3** Infusion Device **Y** Other Device	**Z** No Qualifier

0 Medical and Surgical
7 Lymphatic and Hemic Systems
J Inspection: Visually and/or manually exploring a body part

Body Part Character 4	Approach Character 5	Device Character 6	Qualifier Character 7
K Thoracic Duct **L** Cisterna Chyli **M** Thymus **T** Bone Marrow	**0** Open **3** Percutaneous **4** Percutaneous Endoscopic	**Z** No Device	**Z** No Qualifier
N Lymphatic	**0** Open **3** Percutaneous **4** Percutaneous Endoscopic **8** Via Natural or Artificial Opening Endoscopic **X** External	**Z** No Device	**Z** No Qualifier
P Spleen	**0** Open **3** Percutaneous **4** Percutaneous Endoscopic **X** External	**Z** No Device	**Z** No Qualifier

0 Medical and Surgical
7 Lymphatic and Hemic Systems
L Occlusion: Completely closing an orifice or the lumen of a tubular body part

Body Part Character 4	Approach Character 5	Device Character 6	Qualifier Character 7
0 Lymphatic, Head **1** Lymphatic, Right Neck **2** Lymphatic, Left Neck **3** Lymphatic, Right Upper Extremity **4** Lymphatic, Left Upper Extremity **5** Lymphatic, Right Axillary **6** Lymphatic, Left Axillary **7** Lymphatic, Thorax **8** Lymphatic, Internal Mammary, Right **9** Lymphatic, Internal Mammary, Left **B** Lymphatic, Mesenteric **C** Lymphatic, Pelvis **D** Lymphatic, Aortic **F** Lymphatic, Right Lower Extremity **G** Lymphatic, Left Lower Extremity **H** Lymphatic, Right Inguinal **J** Lymphatic, Left Inguinal **K** Thoracic Duct **L** Cisterna Chyli	**0** Open **3** Percutaneous **4** Percutaneous Endoscopic	**C** Extraluminal Device **D** Intraluminal Device **Z** No Device	**Z** No Qualifier

0 Medical and Surgical
7 Lymphatic and Hemic Systems
N Release: Freeing a body part from an abnormal physical constraint by cutting or by the use of force

Body Part Character 4	Approach Character 5	Device Character 6	Qualifier Character 7
0 Lymphatic, Head **1** Lymphatic, Right Neck **2** Lymphatic, Left Neck **3** Lymphatic, Right Upper Extremity **4** Lymphatic, Left Upper Extremity **5** Lymphatic, Right Axillary **6** Lymphatic, Left Axillary **7** Lymphatic, Thorax **8** Lymphatic, Internal Mammary, Right **9** Lymphatic, Internal Mammary, Left **B** Lymphatic, Mesenteric **C** Lymphatic, Pelvis **D** Lymphatic, Aortic **F** Lymphatic, Right Lower Extremity **G** Lymphatic, Left Lower Extremity **H** Lymphatic, Right Inguinal **J** Lymphatic, Left Inguinal **K** Thoracic Duct **L** Cisterna Chyli **M** Thymus **P** Spleen	**0** Open **3** Percutaneous **4** Percutaneous Endoscopic	**Z** No Device	**Z** No Qualifier

0 Medical and Surgical
7 Lymphatic and Hemic Systems
P Removal: Taking out or off a device from a body part

Body Part Character 4	Approach Character 5	Device Character 6	Qualifier Character 7
K Thoracic Duct **L** Cisterna Chyli **N** Lymphatic	**0** Open **3** Percutaneous **4** Percutaneous Endoscopic	**0** Drainage Device **3** Infusion Device **7** Autologous Tissue Substitute **C** Extraluminal Device **D** Intraluminal Device **J** Synthetic Substitute **K** Nonautologous Tissue Substitute **Y** Other Device	**Z** No Qualifier
K Thoracic Duct **L** Cisterna Chyli **N** Lymphatic	**X** External	**0** Drainage Device **3** Infusion Device **D** Intraluminal Device	**Z** No Qualifier
M Thymus **P** Spleen	**0** Open **3** Percutaneous **4** Percutaneous Endoscopic	**0** Drainage Device **3** Infusion Device **Y** Other Device	**Z** No Qualifier
M Thymus **P** Spleen	**X** External	**0** Drainage Device **3** Infusion Device	**Z** No Qualifier
T Bone Marrow	**0** Open **3** Percutaneous **4** Percutaneous Endoscopic **X** External	**0** Drainage Device	**Z** No Qualifier

0 Medical and Surgical
7 Lymphatic and Hemic Systems
Q Repair: Restoring, to the extent possible, a body part to its normal anatomic structure and function

Body Part Character 4	Approach Character 5	Device Character 6	Qualifier Character 7
0 Lymphatic, Head **1** Lymphatic, Right Neck **2** Lymphatic, Left Neck **3** Lymphatic, Right Upper Extremity **4** Lymphatic, Left Upper Extremity **5** Lymphatic, Right Axillary **6** Lymphatic, Left Axillary **7** Lymphatic, Thorax **8** Lymphatic, Internal Mammary, Right **9** Lymphatic, Internal Mammary, Left **B** Lymphatic, Mesenteric **C** Lymphatic, Pelvis **D** Lymphatic, Aortic **F** Lymphatic, Right Lower Extremity **G** Lymphatic, Left Lower Extremity **H** Lymphatic, Right Inguinal **J** Lymphatic, Left Inguinal **K** Thoracic Duct **L** Cisterna Chyli	**0** Open **3** Percutaneous **4** Percutaneous Endoscopic **8** Via Natural or Artificial Opening Endoscopic	**Z** No Device	**Z** No Qualifier
M Thymus **P** Spleen	**0** Open **3** Percutaneous **4** Percutaneous Endoscopic	**Z** No Device	**Z** No Qualifier

0 Medical and Surgical
7 Lymphatic and Hemic Systems
S Reposition: Moving to its normal location, or other suitable location, all or a portion of a body part

Body Part Character 4	Approach Character 5	Device Character 6	Qualifier Character 7
M Thymus **P** Spleen	**0** Open	**Z** No Device	**Z** No Qualifier

0 Medical and Surgical
7 Lymphatic and Hemic Systems
T Resection: Cutting out or off, without replacement, all of a body part

Body Part Character 4	Approach Character 5	Device Character 6	Qualifier Character 7
0 Lymphatic, Head **1** Lymphatic, Right Neck **2** Lymphatic, Left Neck **3** Lymphatic, Right Upper Extremity **4** Lymphatic, Left Upper Extremity **5** Lymphatic, Right Axillary CC **6** Lymphatic, Left Axillary CC **7** Lymphatic, Thorax CC **8** Lymphatic, Internal Mammary, Right CC **9** Lymphatic, Internal Mammary, Left CC **B** Lymphatic, Mesenteric **C** Lymphatic, Pelvis **D** Lymphatic, Aortic **F** Lymphatic, Right Lower Extremity **G** Lymphatic, Left Lower Extremity **H** Lymphatic, Right Inguinal **J** Lymphatic, Left Inguinal **K** Thoracic Duct **L** Cisterna Chyli **M** Thymus **P** Spleen	**0** Open **4** Percutaneous Endoscopic	**Z** No Device	**Z** No Qualifier

CC 07T50ZZ 07T60ZZ 07T70ZZ 07T80ZZ 07T90ZZ

0 Medical and Surgical
7 Lymphatic and Hemic Systems
U Supplement: Putting in or on biological or synthetic material that physically reinforces and/or augments the function of a portion of a body part

Body Part Character 4	Approach Character 5	Device Character 6	Qualifier Character 7
0 Lymphatic, Head **1** Lymphatic, Right Neck **2** Lymphatic, Left Neck **3** Lymphatic, Right Upper Extremity **4** Lymphatic, Left Upper Extremity **5** Lymphatic, Right Axillary **6** Lymphatic, Left Axillary **7** Lymphatic, Thorax **8** Lymphatic, Internal Mammary, Right **9** Lymphatic, Internal Mammary, Left **B** Lymphatic, Mesenteric **C** Lymphatic, Pelvis **D** Lymphatic, Aortic **F** Lymphatic, Right Lower Extremity **G** Lymphatic, Left Lower Extremity **H** Lymphatic, Right Inguinal **J** Lymphatic, Left Inguinal **K** Thoracic Duct **L** Cisterna Chyli	**0** Open **4** Percutaneous Endoscopic	**7** Autologous Tissue Substitute **J** Synthetic Substitute **K** Nonautologous Tissue Substitute	**Z** No Qualifier

0 Medical and Surgical
7 Lymphatic and Hemic Systems
V Restriction: Partially closing an orifice or the lumen of a tubular body part

Body Part Character 4	Approach Character 5	Device Character 6	Qualifier Character 7
0 Lymphatic, Head 1 Lymphatic, Right Neck 2 Lymphatic, Left Neck 3 Lymphatic, Right Upper Extremity 4 Lymphatic, Left Upper Extremity 5 Lymphatic, Right Axillary 6 Lymphatic, Left Axillary 7 Lymphatic, Thorax 8 Lymphatic, Internal Mammary, Right 9 Lymphatic, Internal Mammary, Left B Lymphatic, Mesenteric C Lymphatic, Pelvis D Lymphatic, Aortic F Lymphatic, Right Lower Extremity G Lymphatic, Left Lower Extremity H Lymphatic, Right Inguinal J Lymphatic, Left Inguinal K Thoracic Duct L Cisterna Chyli	0 Open 3 Percutaneous 4 Percutaneous Endoscopic	C Extraluminal Device D Intraluminal Device Z No Device	Z No Qualifier

0 Medical and Surgical
7 Lymphatic and Hemic Systems
W Revision: Correcting, to the extent possible, a portion of a malfunctioning device or the position of a displaced device

Body Part Character 4	Approach Character 5	Device Character 6	Qualifier Character 7
K Thoracic Duct L Cisterna Chyli N Lymphatic	0 Open 3 Percutaneous 4 Percutaneous Endoscopic	0 Drainage Device 3 Infusion Device 7 Autologous Tissue Substitute C Extraluminal Device D Intraluminal Device J Synthetic Substitute K Nonautologous Tissue Substitute Y Other Device	Z No Qualifier
K Thoracic Duct L Cisterna Chyli N Lymphatic	X External	0 Drainage Device 3 Infusion Device 7 Autologous Tissue Substitute C Extraluminal Device D Intraluminal Device J Synthetic Substitute K Nonautologous Tissue Substitute	Z No Qualifier
M Thymus P Spleen	0 Open 3 Percutaneous 4 Percutaneous Endoscopic	0 Drainage Device 3 Infusion Device Y Other Device	Z No Qualifier
M Thymus P Spleen	X External	0 Drainage Device 3 Infusion Device	Z No Qualifier
T Bone Marrow	0 Open 3 Percutaneous 4 Percutaneous Endoscopic X External	0 Drainage Device	Z No Qualifier

0 Medical and Surgical
7 Lymphatic and Hemic Systems
Y Transplantation: Putting in or on all or a portion of a living body part taken from another individual or animal to physically take the place and/or function of all or a portion of a similar body part

Body Part Character 4	Approach Character 5	Device Character 6	Qualifier Character 7
M Thymus **P** Spleen	**0** Open	**Z** No Device	**0** Allogeneic **1** Syngeneic **2** Zooplastic

NOTES

NOTES

Eye 080-08X

0 Medical and Surgical
8 Eye
0 Alteration: Modifying the anatomic structure of a body part without affecting the function of the body part

Body Part	Approach	Device	Qualifier
Character 4	**Character 5**	**Character 6**	**Character 7**
N Upper Eyelid, Right **P** Upper Eyelid, Left **Q** Lower Eyelid, Right **R** Lower Eyelid, Left	**0** Open **3** Percutaneous **X** External	**7** Autologous Tissue Substitute **J** Synthetic Substitute **K** Nonautologous Tissue Substitute **Z** No Device	**Z** No Qualifier

0 Medical and Surgical
8 Eye
1 Bypass: Altering the route of passage of the contents of a tubular body part

Body Part	Approach	Device	Qualifier
Character 4	**Character 5**	**Character 6**	**Character 7**
2 Anterior Chamber, Right **3** Anterior Chamber, Left	**3** Percutaneous	**J** Synthetic Substitute **K** Nonautologous Tissue Substitute **Z** No Device	**4** Sclera
X Lacrimal Duct, Right **Y** Lacrimal Duct, Left	**0** Open **3** Percutaneous	**J** Synthetic Substitute **K** Nonautologous Tissue Substitute **Z** No Device	**3** Nasal Cavity

0 Medical and Surgical
8 Eye
2 Change: Taking out or off a device from a body part and putting back an identical or similar device in or on the same body part without cutting or puncturing the skin or a mucous membrane

Body Part	Approach	Device	Qualifier
Character 4	**Character 5**	**Character 6**	**Character 7**
0 Eye, Right **1** Eye, Left	**X** External	**0** Drainage Device **Y** Other Device	**Z** No Qualifier

0 Medical and Surgical
8 Eye
5 Destruction: Physical eradication of all or a portion of a body part by the direct use of energy, force, or a destructive agent

Body Part Character 4	Approach Character 5	Device Character 6	Qualifier Character 7
0 Eye, Right **1** Eye, Left **6** Sclera, Right **7** Sclera, Left **8** Cornea, Right **9** Cornea, Left **S** Conjunctiva, Right **T** Conjunctiva, Left	**X** External	**Z** No Device	**Z** No Qualifier
2 Anterior Chamber, Right **3** Anterior Chamber, Left **4** Vitreous, Right **5** Vitreous, Left **C** Iris, Right **D** Iris, Left **E** Retina, Right **F** Retina, Left **G** Retinal Vessel, Right **H** Retinal Vessel, Left **J** Lens, Right **K** Lens, Left	**3** Percutaneous	**Z** No Device	**Z** No Qualifier
A Choroid, Right **B** Choroid, Left **L** Extraocular Muscle, Right **M** Extraocular Muscle, Left **V** Lacrimal Gland, Right **W** Lacrimal Gland, Left	**0** Open **3** Percutaneous	**Z** No Device	**Z** No Qualifier
N Upper Eyelid, Right **P** Upper Eyelid, Left **Q** Lower Eyelid, Right **R** Lower Eyelid, Left	**0** Open **3** Percutaneous **X** External	**Z** No Device	**Z** No Qualifier
X Lacrimal Duct, Right **Y** Lacrimal Duct, Left	**0** Open **3** Percutaneous **7** Via Natural or Artificial Opening **8** Via Natural or Artificial Opening Endoscopic	**Z** No Device	**Z** No Qualifier

0 Medical and Surgical
8 Eye
7 Dilation: Expanding an orifice or the lumen of a tubular body part

Body Part Character 4	Approach Character 5	Device Character 6	Qualifier Character 7
X Lacrimal Duct, Right **Y** Lacrimal Duct, Left	**0** Open **3** Percutaneous **7** Via Natural or Artificial Opening **8** Via Natural or Artificial Opening Endoscopic	**D** Intraluminal Device **Z** No Device	**Z** No Qualifier

0 Medical and Surgical
8 Eye
9 Drainage: Taking or letting out fluids and/or gases from a body part

Body Part	Approach	Device	Qualifier
Character 4	Character 5	Character 6	Character 7
0 Eye, Right **1** Eye, Left **6** Sclera, Right **7** Sclera, Left **8** Cornea, Right **9** Cornea, Left **S** Conjunctiva, Right **T** Conjunctiva, Left	**X** External	**0** Drainage Device	**Z** No Qualifier
0 Eye, Right **1** Eye, Left **6** Sclera, Right **7** Sclera, Left **8** Cornea, Right **9** Cornea, Left **S** Conjunctiva, Right **T** Conjunctiva, Left	**X** External	**Z** No Device	**X** Diagnostic **Z** No Qualifier
2 Anterior Chamber, Right **3** Anterior Chamber, Left **4** Vitreous, Right **5** Vitreous, Left **C** Iris, Right **D** Iris, Left **E** Retina, Right **F** Retina, Left **G** Retinal Vessel, Right **H** Retinal Vessel, Left **J** Lens, Right **K** Lens, Left	**3** Percutaneous	**0** Drainage Device	**Z** No Qualifier
2 Anterior Chamber, Right **3** Anterior Chamber, Left **4** Vitreous, Right **5** Vitreous, Left **C** Iris, Right **D** Iris, Left **E** Retina, Right **F** Retina, Left **G** Retinal Vessel, Right **H** Retinal Vessel, Left **J** Lens, Right **K** Lens, Left	**3** Percutaneous	**Z** No Device	**X** Diagnostic **Z** No Qualifier
A Choroid, Right **B** Choroid, Left **L** Extraocular Muscle, Right **M** Extraocular Muscle, Left **V** Lacrimal Gland, Right **W** Lacrimal Gland, Left	**0** Open **3** Percutaneous	**0** Drainage Device	**Z** No Qualifier
A Choroid, Right **B** Choroid, Left **L** Extraocular Muscle, Right **M** Extraocular Muscle, Left **V** Lacrimal Gland, Right **W** Lacrimal Gland, Left	**0** Open **3** Percutaneous	**Z** No Device	**X** Diagnostic **Z** No Qualifier
N Upper Eyelid, Right **P** Upper Eyelid, Left **Q** Lower Eyelid, Right **R** Lower Eyelid, Left	**0** Open **3** Percutaneous **X** External	**0** Drainage Device	**Z** No Qualifier

089 continued on next page

089 continued from previous page

0 Medical and Surgical
8 Eye
9 Drainage: Taking or letting out fluids and/or gases from a body part

Body Part Character 4	Approach Character 5	Device Character 6	Qualifier Character 7
N Upper Eyelid, Right **P** Upper Eyelid, Left **Q** Lower Eyelid, Right **R** Lower Eyelid, Left	**0** Open **3** Percutaneous **X** External	**Z** No Device	**X** Diagnostic **Z** No Qualifier
X Lacrimal Duct, Right **Y** Lacrimal Duct, Left	**0** Open **3** Percutaneous **7** Via Natural or Artificial Opening **8** Via Natural or Artificial Opening Endoscopic	**0** Drainage Device	**Z** No Qualifier
X Lacrimal Duct, Right **Y** Lacrimal Duct, Left	**0** Open **3** Percutaneous **7** Via Natural or Artificial Opening **8** Via Natural or Artificial Opening Endoscopic	**Z** No Device	**X** Diagnostic **Z** No Qualifier

0 Medical and Surgical
8 Eye
B Excision: Cutting out or off, without replacement, a portion of a body part

Body Part Character 4	Approach Character 5	Device Character 6	Qualifier Character 7
0 Eye, Right **1** Eye, Left **N** Upper Eyelid, Right **P** Upper Eyelid, Left **Q** Lower Eyelid, Right **R** Lower Eyelid, Left	**0** Open **3** Percutaneous **X** External	**Z** No Device	**X** Diagnostic **Z** No Qualifier
4 Vitreous, Right **5** Vitreous, Left **C** Iris, Right CC **D** Iris, Left CC **E** Retina, Right **F** Retina, Left **J** Lens, Right **K** Lens, Left	**3** Percutaneous	**Z** No Device	**X** Diagnostic **Z** No Qualifier
6 Sclera, Right CC **7** Sclera, Left CC **8** Cornea, Right **9** Cornea, Left **S** Conjunctiva, Right **T** Conjunctiva, Left	**X** External	**Z** No Device	**X** Diagnostic **Z** No Qualifier
A Choroid, Right **B** Choroid, Left **L** Extraocular Muscle, Right **M** Extraocular Muscle, Left **V** Lacrimal Gland, Right **W** Lacrimal Gland, Left	**0** Open **3** Percutaneous	**Z** No Device	**X** Diagnostic **Z** No Qualifier
X Lacrimal Duct, Right **Y** Lacrimal Duct, Left	**0** Open **3** Percutaneous **7** Via Natural or Artificial Opening **8** Via Natural or Artificial Opening Endoscopic	**Z** No Device	**X** Diagnostic **Z** No Qualifier

CC 08B6XZZ 08B7XZZ 08BC3ZZ 08BD3ZZ

0 Medical and Surgical
8 Eye
C Extirpation: Taking or cutting out solid matter from a body part

Body Part Character 4	Approach Character 5	Device Character 6	Qualifier Character 7
0 Eye, Right **1** Eye, Left **6** Sclera, Right **7** Sclera, Left **8** Cornea, Right **9** Cornea, Left **S** Conjunctiva, Right **T** Conjunctiva, Left	**X** External	**Z** No Device	**Z** No Qualifier
2 Anterior Chamber, Right **3** Anterior Chamber, Left **4** Vitreous, Right **5** Vitreous, Left **C** Iris, Right **D** Iris, Left **E** Retina, Right **F** Retina, Left **G** Retinal Vessel, Right **H** Retinal Vessel, Left **J** Lens, Right **K** Lens, Left	**3** Percutaneous **X** External	**Z** No Device	**Z** No Qualifier
A Choroid, Right **B** Choroid, Left **L** Extraocular Muscle, Right **M** Extraocular Muscle, Left **N** Upper Eyelid, Right **P** Upper Eyelid, Left **Q** Lower Eyelid, Right **R** Lower Eyelid, Left **V** Lacrimal Gland, Right **W** Lacrimal Gland, Left	**0** Open **3** Percutaneous **X** External	**Z** No Device	**Z** No Qualifier
X Lacrimal Duct, Right **Y** Lacrimal Duct, Left	**0** Open **3** Percutaneous **7** Via Natural or Artificial Opening **8** Via Natural or Artificial Opening Endoscopic	**Z** No Device	**Z** No Qualifier

0 Medical and Surgical
8 Eye
D Extraction: Pulling or stripping out or off all or a portion of a body part by the use of force

Body Part Character 4	Approach Character 5	Device Character 6	Qualifier Character 7
8 Cornea, Right **9** Cornea, Left	**X** External	**Z** No Device	**X** Diagnostic **Z** No Qualifier
J Lens, Right **K** Lens, Left	**3** Percutaneous	**Z** No Device	**Z** No Qualifier

0 Medical and Surgical
8 Eye
F Fragmentation: Breaking solid matter in a body part into pieces

Body Part Character 4	Approach Character 5	Device Character 6	Qualifier Character 7
4 Vitreous, Right NC **5** Vitreous, Left NC	**3** Percutaneous **X** External	**Z** No Device	**Z** No Qualifier

NC 08F4XZZ 08F5XZZ

0 Medical and Surgical
8 Eye
H Insertion: Putting in a nonbiological appliance that monitors, assists, performs, or prevents a physiological function but does not physically take the place of a body part

Body Part	Approach	Device	Qualifier
Character 4	**Character 5**	**Character 6**	**Character 7**
0 Eye, Right **1** Eye, Left	**0** Open	**5** Epiretinal Visual Prosthesis **Y** Other Device	**Z** No Qualifier
0 Eye, Right **1** Eye, Left	**3** Percutaneous	**1** Radioactive Element **3** Infusion Device **Y** Other Device	**Z** No Qualifier
0 Eye, Right **1** Eye, Left	**7** Via Natural or Artificial Opening **8** Via Natural or Artificial Opening Endoscopic	**Y** Other Device	**Z** No Qualifier
0 Eye, Right **1** Eye, Left	**X** External	**1** Radioactive Element **3** Infusion Device	**Z** No Qualifier

0 Medical and Surgical
8 Eye
J Inspection: Visually and/or manually exploring a body part

Body Part	Approach	Device	Qualifier
Character 4	**Character 5**	**Character 6**	**Character 7**
0 Eye, Right **1** Eye, Left **J** Lens, Right **K** Lens, Left	**X** External	**Z** No Device	**Z** No Qualifier
L Extraocular Muscle, Right **M** Extraocular Muscle, Left	**0** Open **X** External	**Z** No Device	**Z** No Qualifier

0 Medical and Surgical
8 Eye
L Occlusion: Completely closing an orifice or the lumen of a tubular body part

Body Part	Approach	Device	Qualifier
Character 4	**Character 5**	**Character 6**	**Character 7**
X Lacrimal Duct, Right **Y** Lacrimal Duct, Left	**0** Open **3** Percutaneous	**C** Extraluminal Device **D** Intraluminal Device **Z** No Device	**Z** No Qualifier
X Lacrimal Duct, Right **Y** Lacrimal Duct, Left	**7** Via Natural or Artificial Opening **8** Via Natural or Artificial Opening Endoscopic	**D** Intraluminal Device **Z** No Device	**Z** No Qualifier

0 Medical and Surgical
8 Eye
M Reattachment: Putting back in or on all or a portion of a separated body part to its normal location or other suitable location

Body Part	Approach	Device	Qualifier
Character 4	**Character 5**	**Character 6**	**Character 7**
N Upper Eyelid, Right **P** Upper Eyelid, Left **Q** Lower Eyelid, Right **R** Lower Eyelid, Left	**X** External	**Z** No Device	**Z** No Qualifier

LC Limited Coverage NC Noncovered HAC HAC-associated Procedure CC Combination Cluster - See Appendix G for code lists
DRG Non-OR-Affecting MS-DRG Assignment New/Revised Text in **Orange** ♂ Male ♀ Female

0 Medical and Surgical
8 Eye
N Release: Freeing a body part from an abnormal physical constraint by cutting or by the use of force

Body Part Character 4	Approach Character 5	Device Character 6	Qualifier Character 7
0 Eye, Right **1** Eye, Left **6** Sclera, Right **7** Sclera, Left **8** Cornea, Right **9** Cornea, Left **S** Conjunctiva, Right **T** Conjunctiva, Left	**X** External	**Z** No Device	**Z** No Qualifier
2 Anterior Chamber, Right **3** Anterior Chamber, Left **4** Vitreous, Right **5** Vitreous, Left **C** Iris, Right **D** Iris, Left **E** Retina, Right **F** Retina, Left **G** Retinal Vessel, Right **H** Retinal Vessel, Left **J** Lens, Right **K** Lens, Left	**3** Percutaneous	**Z** No Device	**Z** No Qualifier
A Choroid, Right **B** Choroid, Left **L** Extraocular Muscle, Right **M** Extraocular Muscle, Left **V** Lacrimal Gland, Right **W** Lacrimal Gland, Left	**0** Open **3** Percutaneous	**Z** No Device	**Z** No Qualifier
N Upper Eyelid, Right **P** Upper Eyelid, Left **Q** Lower Eyelid, Right **R** Lower Eyelid, Left	**0** Open **3** Percutaneous **X** External	**Z** No Device	**Z** No Qualifier
X Lacrimal Duct, Right **Y** Lacrimal Duct, Left	**0** Open **3** Percutaneous **7** Via Natural or Artificial Opening **8** Via Natural or Artificial Opening Endoscopic	**Z** No Device	**Z** No Qualifier

0 Medical and Surgical
8 Eye
P Removal: Taking out or off a device from a body part

Body Part Character 4	Approach Character 5	Device Character 6	Qualifier Character 7
0 Eye, Right **1** Eye, Left	**0** Open **3** Percutaneous **7** Via Natural or Artificial Opening **8** Via Natural or Artificial Opening Endoscopic	**0** Drainage Device **1** Radioactive Element **3** Infusion Device **7** Autologous Tissue Substitute **C** Extraluminal Device **D** Intraluminal Device **J** Synthetic Substitute **K** Nonautologous Tissue Substitute **Y** Other Device	**Z** No Qualifier
0 Eye, Right **1** Eye, Left	**X** External	**0** Drainage Device **1** Radioactive Element **3** Infusion Device **7** Autologous Tissue Substitute **C** Extraluminal Device **D** Intraluminal Device **J** Synthetic Substitute **K** Nonautologous Tissue Substitute	**Z** No Qualifier
J Lens, Right **K** Lens, Left	**3** Percutaneous	**J** Synthetic Substitute **Y** Other Device	**Z** No Qualifier
L Extraocular Muscle, Right **M** Extraocular Muscle, Left	**0** Open **3** Percutaneous	**0** Drainage Device **7** Autologous Tissue Substitute **J** Synthetic Substitute **K** Nonautologous Tissue Substitute **Y** Other Device	**Z** No Qualifier

0 Medical and Surgical
8 Eye
Q Repair: Restoring, to the extent possible, a body part to its normal anatomic structure and function

Body Part Character 4	Approach Character 5	Device Character 6	Qualifier Character 7
0 Eye, Right **1** Eye, Left **6** Sclera, Right **7** Sclera, Left **8** Cornea, Right NC **9** Cornea, Left NC **S** Conjunctiva, Right **T** Conjunctiva, Left	**X** External	**Z** No Device	**Z** No Qualifier
2 Anterior Chamber, Right **3** Anterior Chamber, Left **4** Vitreous, Right **5** Vitreous, Left **C** Iris, Right **D** Iris, Left **E** Retina, Right **F** Retina, Left **G** Retinal Vessel, Right **H** Retinal Vessel, Left **J** Lens, Right **K** Lens, Left	**3** Percutaneous	**Z** No Device	**Z** No Qualifier
A Choroid, Right **B** Choroid, Left **L** Extraocular Muscle, Right **M** Extraocular Muscle, Left **V** Lacrimal Gland, Right **W** Lacrimal Gland, Left	**0** Open **3** Percutaneous	**Z** No Device	**Z** No Qualifier
N Upper Eyelid, Right **P** Upper Eyelid, Left **Q** Lower Eyelid, Right **R** Lower Eyelid, Left	**0** Open **3** Percutaneous **X** External	**Z** No Device	**Z** No Qualifier
X Lacrimal Duct, Right **Y** Lacrimal Duct, Left	**0** Open **3** Percutaneous **7** Via Natural or Artificial Opening **8** Via Natural or Artificial Opening Endoscopic	**Z** No Device	**Z** No Qualifier

NC 08Q8XZZ 08Q9XZZ

0 Medical and Surgical
8 Eye
R Replacement: Putting in or on biological or synthetic material that physically takes the place and/or function of all or a portion of a body part

Body Part Character 4	Approach Character 5	Device Character 6	Qualifier Character 7
0 Eye, Right **1** Eye, Left **A** Choroid, Right **B** Choroid, Left	**0** Open **3** Percutaneous	**7** Autologous Tissue Substitute **J** Synthetic Substitute **K** Nonautologous Tissue Substitute	**Z** No Qualifier
4 Vitreous, Right **5** Vitreous, Left **C** Iris, Right **D** Iris, Left **G** Retinal Vessel, Right **H** Retinal Vessel, Left	**3** Percutaneous	**7** Autologous Tissue Substitute **J** Synthetic Substitute **K** Nonautologous Tissue Substitute	**Z** No Qualifier
6 Sclera, Right **7** Sclera, Left **S** Conjunctiva, Right **T** Conjunctiva, Left	**X** External	**7** Autologous Tissue Substitute **J** Synthetic Substitute **K** Nonautologous Tissue Substitute	**Z** No Qualifier
8 Cornea, Right **9** Cornea, Left	**3** Percutaneous **X** External	**7** Autologous Tissue Substitute **J** Synthetic Substitute **K** Nonautologous Tissue Substitute	**Z** No Qualifier
J Lens, Right **K** Lens, Left	**3** Percutaneous	**0** Synthetic Substitute, Intraocular Telescope **7** Autologous Tissue Substitute **J** Synthetic Substitute **K** Nonautologous Tissue Substitute	**Z** No Qualifier
N Upper Eyelid, Right **P** Upper Eyelid, Left **Q** Lower Eyelid, Right **R** Lower Eyelid, Left	**0** Open **3** Percutaneous **X** External	**7** Autologous Tissue Substitute **J** Synthetic Substitute **K** Nonautologous Tissue Substitute	**Z** No Qualifier
X Lacrimal Duct, Right **Y** Lacrimal Duct, Left	**0** Open **3** Percutaneous **7** Via Natural or Artificial Opening **8** Via Natural or Artificial Opening Endoscopic	**7** Autologous Tissue Substitute **J** Synthetic Substitute **K** Nonautologous Tissue Substitute	**Z** No Qualifier

0 Medical and Surgical
8 Eye
S Reposition: Moving to its normal location, or other suitable location, all or a portion of a body part

Body Part Character 4	Approach Character 5	Device Character 6	Qualifier Character 7
C Iris, Right **D** Iris, Left **G** Retinal Vessel, Right **H** Retinal Vessel, Left **J** Lens, Right **K** Lens, Left	**3** Percutaneous	**Z** No Device	**Z** No Qualifier
L Extraocular Muscle, Right **M** Extraocular Muscle, Left **V** Lacrimal Gland, Right **W** Lacrimal Gland, Left	**0** Open **3** Percutaneous	**Z** No Device	**Z** No Qualifier
N Upper Eyelid, Right CC **P** Upper Eyelid, Left CC **Q** Lower Eyelid, Right CC **R** Lower Eyelid, Left CC	**0** Open **3** Percutaneous **X** External	**Z** No Device	**Z** No Qualifier
X Lacrimal Duct, Right **Y** Lacrimal Duct, Left	**0** Open **3** Percutaneous **7** Via Natural or Artificial Opening **8** Via Natural or Artificial Opening Endoscopic	**Z** No Device	**Z** No Qualifier

CC 08SN0ZZ 08SN3ZZ 08SNXZZ 08SP0ZZ 08SP3ZZ 08SPXZZ 08SQ0ZZ 08SQ3ZZ 08SQXZZ 08SR0ZZ 08SR3ZZ 08SRXZZ

0 Medical and Surgical
8 Eye
T Resection: Cutting out or off, without replacement, all of a body part

Body Part Character 4	Approach Character 5	Device Character 6	Qualifier Character 7
0 Eye, Right CC **1** Eye, Left CC **8** Cornea, Right **9** Cornea, Left	**X** External	**Z** No Device	**Z** No Qualifier
4 Vitreous, Right **5** Vitreous, Left **C** Iris, Right **D** Iris, Left **J** Lens, Right **K** Lens, Left	**3** Percutaneous	**Z** No Device	**Z** No Qualifier
L Extraocular Muscle, Right **M** Extraocular Muscle, Left **V** Lacrimal Gland, Right **W** Lacrimal Gland, Left	**0** Open **3** Percutaneous	**Z** No Device	**Z** No Qualifier
N Upper Eyelid, Right **P** Upper Eyelid, Left **Q** Lower Eyelid, Right **R** Lower Eyelid, Left	**0** Open **X** External	**Z** No Device	**Z** No Qualifier
X Lacrimal Duct, Right **Y** Lacrimal Duct, Left	**0** Open **3** Percutaneous **7** Via Natural or Artificial Opening **8** Via Natural or Artificial Opening Endoscopic	**Z** No Device	**Z** No Qualifier

CC 08T0XZZ 08T1XZZ

0 Medical and Surgical
8 Eye
U Supplement: Putting in or on biological or synthetic material that physically reinforces and/or augments the function of a portion of a body part

Body Part Character 4	Approach Character 5	Device Character 6	Qualifier Character 7
0 Eye, Right **1** Eye, Left **C** Iris, Right **D** Iris, Left **E** Retina, Right **F** Retina, Left **G** Retinal Vessel, Right **H** Retinal Vessel, Left **L** Extraocular Muscle, Right **M** Extraocular Muscle, Left	**0** Open **3** Percutaneous	**7** Autologous Tissue Substitute **J** Synthetic Substitute **K** Nonautologous Tissue Substitute	**Z** No Qualifier
8 Cornea, Right NC **9** Cornea, Left NC **N** Upper Eyelid, Right **P** Upper Eyelid, Left **Q** Lower Eyelid, Right **R** Lower Eyelid, Left	**0** Open **3** Percutaneous **X** External	**7** Autologous Tissue Substitute **J** Synthetic Substitute **K** Nonautologous Tissue Substitute	**Z** No Qualifier
X Lacrimal Duct, Right **Y** Lacrimal Duct, Left	**0** Open **3** Percutaneous **7** Via Natural or Artificial Opening **8** Via Natural or Artificial Opening Endoscopic	**7** Autologous Tissue Substitute **J** Synthetic Substitute **K** Nonautologous Tissue Substitute	**Z** No Qualifier

NC 08U80KZ 08U83KZ 08U8XKZ 08U90KZ 08U93KZ 08U9XKZ

0 Medical and Surgical
8 Eye
V Restriction: Partially closing an orifice or the lumen of a tubular body part

Body Part Character 4	Approach Character 5	Device Character 6	Qualifier Character 7
X Lacrimal Duct, Right **Y** Lacrimal Duct, Left	**0** Open **3** Percutaneous	**C** Extraluminal Device **D** Intraluminal Device **Z** No Device	**Z** No Qualifier
X Lacrimal Duct, Right **Y** Lacrimal Duct, Left	**7** Via Natural or Artificial Opening **8** Via Natural or Artificial Opening Endoscopic	**D** Intraluminal Device **Z** No Device	**Z** No Qualifier

0 **Medical and Surgical**
8 **Eye**
W **Revision:** Correcting, to the extent possible, a portion of a malfunctioning device or the position of a displaced device

Body Part Character 4	Approach Character 5	Device Character 6	Qualifier Character 7
0 Eye, Right **1** Eye, Left	**0** Open **3** Percutaneous **7** Via Natural or Artificial Opening **8** Via Natural or Artificial Opening Endoscopic	**0** Drainage Device **3** Infusion Device **7** Autologous Tissue Substitute **C** Extraluminal Device **D** Intraluminal Device **J** Synthetic Substitute **K** Nonautologous Tissue Substitute **Y** Other Device	**Z** No Qualifier
0 Eye, Right **1** Eye, Left	**X** External	**0** Drainage Device **3** Infusion Device **7** Autologous Tissue Substitute **C** Extraluminal Device **D** Intraluminal Device **J** Synthetic Substitute **K** Nonautologous Tissue Substitute	**Z** No Qualifier
J Lens, Right **K** Lens, Left	**3** Percutaneous	**J** Synthetic Substitute **Y** Other Device	**Z** No Qualifier
J Lens, Right **K** Lens, Left	**X** External	**J** Synthetic Substitute	**Z** No Qualifier
L Extraocular Muscle, Right **M** Extraocular Muscle, Left	**0** Open **3** Percutaneous	**0** Drainage Device **7** Autologous Tissue Substitute **J** Synthetic Substitute **K** Nonautologous Tissue Substitute **Y** Other Device	**Z** No Qualifier

0 **Medical and Surgical**
8 **Eye**
X **Transfer:** Moving, without taking out, all or a portion of a body part to another location to take over the function of all or a portion of a body part

Body Part Character 4	Approach Character 5	Device Character 6	Qualifier Character 7
L Extraocular Muscle, Right **M** Extraocular Muscle, Left	**0** Open **3** Percutaneous	**Z** No Device	**Z** No Qualifier

NOTES

Ear, Nose, Sinus 090-09W

0 Medical and Surgical
9 Ear, Nose, Sinus
0 Alteration: Modifying the anatomic structure of a body part without affecting the function of the body part

Body Part	Approach	Device	Qualifier
Character 4	Character 5	Character 6	Character 7
0 External Ear, Right 1 External Ear, Left 2 External Ear, Bilateral K Nasal Mucosa and Soft Tissue	0 Open 3 Percutaneous 4 Percutaneous Endoscopic X External	7 Autologous Tissue Substitute J Synthetic Substitute K Nonautologous Tissue Substitute Z No Device	Z No Qualifier

0 Medical and Surgical
9 Ear, Nose, Sinus
1 Bypass: Altering the route of passage of the contents of a tubular body part

Body Part	Approach	Device	Qualifier
Character 4	Character 5	Character 6	Character 7
D Inner Ear, Right E Inner Ear, Left	0 Open	7 Autologous Tissue Substitute J Synthetic Substitute K Nonautologous Tissue Substitute Z No Device	0 Endolymphatic

0 Medical and Surgical
9 Ear, Nose, Sinus
2 Change: Taking out or off a device from a body part and putting back an identical or similar device in or on the same body part without cutting or puncturing the skin or a mucous membrane

Body Part	Approach	Device	Qualifier
Character 4	Character 5	Character 6	Character 7
H Ear, Right J Ear, Left K Nasal Mucosa and Soft Tissue Y Sinus	X External	0 Drainage Device Y Other Device	Z No Qualifier

0 Medical and Surgical
9 Ear, Nose, Sinus
3 Control: Stopping, or attempting to stop, postprocedural or other acute bleeding

Body Part	Approach	Device	Qualifier
Character 4	Character 5	Character 6	Character 7
K Nasal Mucosa and Soft Tissue	7 Via Natural or Artificial Opening 8 Via Natural or Artificial Opening Endoscopic	Z No Device	Z No Qualifier

0 Medical and Surgical
9 Ear, Nose, Sinus
5 Destruction: Physical eradication of all or a portion of a body part by the direct use of energy, force, or a destructive agent

Body Part Character 4	Approach Character 5	Device Character 6	Qualifier Character 7
0 External Ear, Right **1** External Ear, Left	**0** Open **3** Percutaneous **4** Percutaneous Endoscopic **X** External	**Z** No Device	**Z** No Qualifier
3 External Auditory Canal, Right **4** External Auditory Canal, Left	**0** Open **3** Percutaneous **4** Percutaneous Endoscopic **7** Via Natural or Artificial Opening **8** Via Natural or Artificial Opening Endoscopic **X** External	**Z** No Device	**Z** No Qualifier
5 Middle Ear, Right **6** Middle Ear, Left **9** Auditory Ossicle, Right **A** Auditory Ossicle, Left **D** Inner Ear, Right **E** Inner Ear, Left	**0** Open **8** Via Natural or Artificial Opening Endoscopic	**Z** No Device	**Z** No Qualifier
7 Tympanic Membrane, Right **8** Tympanic Membrane, Left **F** Eustachian Tube, Right **G** Eustachian Tube, Left **L** Nasal Turbinate **N** Nasopharynx	**0** Open **3** Percutaneous **4** Percutaneous Endoscopic **7** Via Natural or Artificial Opening **8** Via Natural or Artificial Opening Endoscopic	**Z** No Device	**Z** No Qualifier
B Mastoid Sinus, Right **C** Mastoid Sinus, Left **M** Nasal Septum **P** Accessory Sinus **Q** Maxillary Sinus, Right **R** Maxillary Sinus, Left **S** Frontal Sinus, Right **T** Frontal Sinus, Left **U** Ethmoid Sinus, Right **V** Ethmoid Sinus, Left **W** Sphenoid Sinus, Right **X** Sphenoid Sinus, Left	**0** Open **3** Percutaneous **4** Percutaneous Endoscopic **8** Via Natural or Artificial Opening Endoscopic	**Z** No Device	**Z** No Qualifier
K Nasal Mucosa and Soft Tissue	**0** Open **3** Percutaneous **4** Percutaneous Endoscopic **8** Via Natural or Artificial Opening Endoscopic **X** External	**Z** No Device	**Z** No Qualifier

0 Medical and Surgical
9 Ear, Nose, Sinus
7 Dilation: Expanding an orifice or the lumen of a tubular body part

Body Part Character 4	Approach Character 5	Device Character 6	Qualifier Character 7
F Eustachian Tube, Right **G** Eustachian Tube, Left	**0** Open **7** Via Natural or Artificial Opening **8** Via Natural or Artificial Opening Endoscopic	**D** Intraluminal Device **Z** No Device	**Z** No Qualifier
F Eustachian Tube, Right **G** Eustachian Tube, Left	**3** Percutaneous **4** Percutaneous Endoscopic	**Z** No Device	**Z** No Qualifier

0 Medical and Surgical
9 Ear, Nose, Sinus
8 Division: Cutting into a body part, without draining fluids and/or gases from the body part, in order to separate or transect a body part

Body Part Character 4	Approach Character 5	Device Character 6	Qualifier Character 7
L Nasal Turbinate	0 Open 3 Percutaneous 4 Percutaneous Endoscopic 7 Via Natural or Artificial Opening 8 Via Natural or Artificial Opening Endoscopic	Z No Device	Z No Qualifier

0 Medical and Surgical
9 Ear, Nose, Sinus
9 Drainage: Taking or letting out fluids and/or gases from a body part

Body Part Character 4	Approach Character 5	Device Character 6	Qualifier Character 7
0 External Ear, Right 1 External Ear, Left	0 Open 3 Percutaneous 4 Percutaneous Endoscopic X External	0 Drainage Device	Z No Qualifier
0 External Ear, Right 1 External Ear, Left	0 Open 3 Percutaneous 4 Percutaneous Endoscopic X External	Z No Device	X Diagnostic Z No Qualifier
3 External Auditory Canal, Right 4 External Auditory Canal, Left K Nasal Mucosa and Soft Tissue	0 Open 3 Percutaneous 4 Percutaneous Endoscopic 7 Via Natural or Artificial Opening 8 Via Natural or Artificial Opening Endoscopic X External	0 Drainage Device	Z No Qualifier
3 External Auditory Canal, Right 4 External Auditory Canal, Left K Nasal Mucosa and Soft Tissue	0 Open 3 Percutaneous 4 Percutaneous Endoscopic 7 Via Natural or Artificial Opening 8 Via Natural or Artificial Opening Endoscopic X External	Z No Device	X Diagnostic Z No Qualifier
5 Middle Ear, Right 6 Middle Ear, Left 9 Auditory Ossicle, Right A Auditory Ossicle, Left D Inner Ear, Right E Inner Ear, Left	0 Open 7 Via Natural or Artificial Opening 8 Via Natural or Artificial Opening Endoscopic	0 Drainage Device	Z No Qualifier
5 Middle Ear, Right 6 Middle Ear, Left 9 Auditory Ossicle, Right A Auditory Ossicle, Left D Inner Ear, Right E Inner Ear, Left	0 Open 7 Via Natural or Artificial Opening 8 Via Natural or Artificial Opening Endoscopic	Z No Device	X Diagnostic Z No Qualifier

099 continued on next page

0 Medical and Surgical
9 Ear, Nose, Sinus
9 Drainage: Taking or letting out fluids and/or gases from a body part

099 continued from previous page

Body Part Character 4	Approach Character 5	Device Character 6	Qualifier Character 7
7 Tympanic Membrane, Right **8** Tympanic Membrane, Left **B** Mastoid Sinus, Right **C** Mastoid Sinus, Left **F** Eustachian Tube, Right **G** Eustachian Tube, Left **L** Nasal Turbinate **M** Nasal Septum **N** Nasopharynx **P** Accessory Sinus **Q** Maxillary Sinus, Right **R** Maxillary Sinus, Left **S** Frontal Sinus, Right **T** Frontal Sinus, Left **U** Ethmoid Sinus, Right **V** Ethmoid Sinus, Left **W** Sphenoid Sinus, Right **X** Sphenoid Sinus, Left	**0** Open **3** Percutaneous **4** Percutaneous Endoscopic **7** Via Natural or Artificial Opening **8** Via Natural or Artificial Opening Endoscopic	**0** Drainage Device	**Z** No Qualifier
7 Tympanic Membrane, Right **8** Tympanic Membrane, Left **B** Mastoid Sinus, Right **C** Mastoid Sinus, Left **F** Eustachian Tube, Right **G** Eustachian Tube, Left **L** Nasal Turbinate **M** Nasal Septum **N** Nasopharynx **P** Accessory Sinus **Q** Maxillary Sinus, Right **R** Maxillary Sinus, Left **S** Frontal Sinus, Right **T** Frontal Sinus, Left **U** Ethmoid Sinus, Right **V** Ethmoid Sinus, Left **W** Sphenoid Sinus, Right **X** Sphenoid Sinus, Left	**0** Open **3** Percutaneous **4** Percutaneous Endoscopic **7** Via Natural or Artificial Opening **8** Via Natural or Artificial Opening Endoscopic	**Z** No Device	**X** Diagnostic **Z** No Qualifier

0 Medical and Surgical
9 Ear, Nose, Sinus
B Excision: Cutting out or off, without replacement, a portion of a body part

Body Part Character 4	Approach Character 5	Device Character 6	Qualifier Character 7
0 External Ear, Right **1** External Ear, Left	**0** Open **3** Percutaneous **4** Percutaneous Endoscopic **X** External	**Z** No Device	**X** Diagnostic **Z** No Qualifier
3 External Auditory Canal, Right **4** External Auditory Canal, Left	**0** Open **3** Percutaneous **4** Percutaneous Endoscopic **7** Via Natural or Artificial Opening **8** Via Natural or Artificial Opening Endoscopic **X** External	**Z** No Device	**X** Diagnostic **Z** No Qualifier
5 Middle Ear, Right **6** Middle Ear, Left **9** Auditory Ossicle, Right **A** Auditory Ossicle, Left **D** Inner Ear, Right **E** Inner Ear, Left	**0** Open **8** Via Natural or Artificial Opening Endoscopic	**Z** No Device	**X** Diagnostic **Z** No Qualifier
7 Tympanic Membrane, Right **8** Tympanic Membrane, Left **F** Eustachian Tube, Right **G** Eustachian Tube, Left **L** Nasal Turbinate **N** Nasopharynx	**0** Open **3** Percutaneous **4** Percutaneous Endoscopic **7** Via Natural or Artificial Opening **8** Via Natural or Artificial Opening Endoscopic	**Z** No Device	**X** Diagnostic **Z** No Qualifier
B Mastoid Sinus, Right **C** Mastoid Sinus, Left **M** Nasal Septum **P** Accessory Sinus **Q** Maxillary Sinus, Right **R** Maxillary Sinus, Left **S** Frontal Sinus, Right **T** Frontal Sinus, Left **U** Ethmoid Sinus, Right **V** Ethmoid Sinus, Left **W** Sphenoid Sinus, Right **X** Sphenoid Sinus, Left	**0** Open **3** Percutaneous **4** Percutaneous Endoscopic **8** Via Natural or Artificial Opening Endoscopic	**Z** No Device	**X** Diagnostic **Z** No Qualifier
K Nasal Mucosa and Soft Tissue	**0** Open **3** Percutaneous **4** Percutaneous Endoscopic **8** Via Natural or Artificial Opening Endoscopic **X** External	**Z** No Device	**X** Diagnostic **Z** No Qualifier

0 Medical and Surgical
9 Ear, Nose, Sinus
C Extirpation: Taking or cutting out solid matter from a body part

Body Part Character 4	Approach Character 5	Device Character 6	Qualifier Character 7
0 External Ear, Right **1** External Ear, Left	**0** Open **3** Percutaneous **4** Percutaneous Endoscopic **X** External	**Z** No Device	**Z** No Qualifier
3 External Auditory Canal, Right **4** External Auditory Canal, Left	**0** Open **3** Percutaneous **4** Percutaneous Endoscopic **7** Via Natural or Artificial Opening **8** Via Natural or Artificial Opening Endoscopic **X** External	**Z** No Device	**Z** No Qualifier
5 Middle Ear, Right **6** Middle Ear, Left **9** Auditory Ossicle, Right **A** Auditory Ossicle, Left **D** Inner Ear, Right **E** Inner Ear, Left	**0** Open **8** Via Natural or Artificial Opening Endoscopic	**Z** No Device	**Z** No Qualifier
7 Tympanic Membrane, Right **8** Tympanic Membrane, Left **F** Eustachian Tube, Right **G** Eustachian Tube, Left **L** Nasal Turbinate **N** Nasopharynx	**0** Open **3** Percutaneous **4** Percutaneous Endoscopic **7** Via Natural or Artificial Opening **8** Via Natural or Artificial Opening Endoscopic	**Z** No Device	**Z** No Qualifier
B Mastoid Sinus, Right **C** Mastoid Sinus, Left **M** Nasal Septum **P** Accessory Sinus **Q** Maxillary Sinus, Right **R** Maxillary Sinus, Left **S** Frontal Sinus, Right **T** Frontal Sinus, Left **U** Ethmoid Sinus, Right **V** Ethmoid Sinus, Left **W** Sphenoid Sinus, Right **X** Sphenoid Sinus, Left	**0** Open **3** Percutaneous **4** Percutaneous Endoscopic **8** Via Natural or Artificial Opening Endoscopic	**Z** No Device	**Z** No Qualifier
K Nasal Mucosa and Soft Tissue	**0** Open **3** Percutaneous **4** Percutaneous Endoscopic **8** Via Natural or Artificial Opening Endoscopic **X** External	**Z** No Device	**Z** No Qualifier

0 Medical and Surgical
9 Ear, Nose, Sinus
D Extraction: Pulling or stripping out or off all or a portion of a body part by the use of force

Body Part	Approach	Device	Qualifier
Character 4	**Character 5**	**Character 6**	**Character 7**
7 Tympanic Membrane, Right **8** Tympanic Membrane, Left **L** Nasal Turbinate	**0** Open **3** Percutaneous **4** Percutaneous Endoscopic **7** Via Natural or Artificial Opening **8** Via Natural or Artificial Opening Endoscopic	**Z** No Device	**Z** No Qualifier
9 Auditory Ossicle, Right **A** Auditory Ossicle, Left	**0** Open	**Z** No Device	**Z** No Qualifier
B Mastoid Sinus, Right **C** Mastoid Sinus, Left **M** Nasal Septum **P** Accessory Sinus **Q** Maxillary Sinus, Right **R** Maxillary Sinus, Left **S** Frontal Sinus, Right **T** Frontal Sinus, Left **U** Ethmoid Sinus, Right **V** Ethmoid Sinus, Left **W** Sphenoid Sinus, Right **X** Sphenoid Sinus, Left	**0** Open **3** Percutaneous **4** Percutaneous Endoscopic	**Z** No Device	**Z** No Qualifier

0 Medical and Surgical
9 Ear, Nose, Sinus
H Insertion: Putting in a nonbiological appliance that monitors, assists, performs, or prevents a physiological function but does not physically take the place of a body part

Body Part	Approach	Device	Qualifier
Character 4	**Character 5**	**Character 6**	**Character 7**
D Inner Ear, Right **E** Inner Ear, Left	**0** Open **3** Percutaneous **4** Percutaneous Endoscopic	**4** Hearing Device, Bone Conduction **5** Hearing Device, Single Channel Cochlear Prosthesis **6** Hearing Device, Multiple Channel Cochlear Prosthesis **S** Hearing Device	**Z** No Qualifier
H Ear, Right **J** Ear, Left **K** Nasal Mucosa and Soft Tissue **Y** Sinus	**0** Open **3** Percutaneous **4** Percutaneous Endoscopic **7** Via Natural or Artificial Opening **8** Via Natural or Artificial Opening Endoscopic	**Y** Other Device	**Z** No Qualifier
N Nasopharynx	**7** Via Natural or Artificial Opening **8** Via Natural or Artificial Opening Endoscopic	**B** Intraluminal Device, Airway	**Z** No Qualifier

0 Medical and Surgical
9 Ear, Nose, Sinus
J Inspection: Visually and/or manually exploring a body part

Body Part	Approach	Device	Qualifier
Character 4	**Character 5**	**Character 6**	**Character 7**
7 Tympanic Membrane, Right **8** Tympanic Membrane, Left **H** Ear, Right **J** Ear, Left	**0** Open **3** Percutaneous **4** Percutaneous Endoscopic **7** Via Natural or Artificial Opening **8** Via Natural or Artificial Opening Endoscopic **X** External	**Z** No Device	**Z** No Qualifier
D Inner Ear, Right **E** Inner Ear, Left **K** Nasal Mucosa and Soft tissue **Y** Sinus	**0** Open **3** Percutaneous **4** Percutaneous Endoscopic **8** Via Natural or Artificial Opening Endoscopic **X** External	**Z** No Device	**Z** No Qualifier

0 Medical and Surgical
9 Ear, Nose, Sinus
M Reattachment: Putting back in or on all or a portion of a separated body part to its normal location or other suitable location

Body Part Character 4	Approach Character 5	Device Character 6	Qualifier Character 7
0 External Ear, Right **1** External Ear, Left **K** Nasal Mucosa and Soft Tissue	**X** External	**Z** No Device	**Z** No Qualifier

0 Medical and Surgical
9 Ear, Nose, Sinus
N Release: Freeing a body part from an abnormal physical constraint by cutting or by the use of force

Body Part Character 4	Approach Character 5	Device Character 6	Qualifier Character 7
0 External Ear, Right **1** External Ear, Left	**0** Open **3** Percutaneous **4** Percutaneous Endoscopic **X** External	**Z** No Device	**Z** No Qualifier
3 External Auditory Canal, Right **4** External Auditory Canal, Left	**0** Open **3** Percutaneous **4** Percutaneous Endoscopic **7** Via Natural or Artificial Opening **8** Via Natural or Artificial Opening Endoscopic **X** External	**Z** No Device	**Z** No Qualifier
5 Middle Ear, Right **6** Middle Ear, Left **9** Auditory Ossicle, Right **A** Auditory Ossicle, Left **D** Inner Ear, Right **E** Inner Ear, Left	**0** Open **8** Via Natural or Artificial Opening Endoscopic	**Z** No Device	**Z** No Qualifier
7 Tympanic Membrane, Right **8** Tympanic Membrane, Left **F** Eustachian Tube, Right **G** Eustachian Tube, Left **L** Nasal Turbinate **N** Nasopharynx	**0** Open **3** Percutaneous **4** Percutaneous Endoscopic **7** Via Natural or Artificial Opening **8** Via Natural or Artificial Opening Endoscopic	**Z** No Device	**Z** No Qualifier
B Mastoid Sinus, Right **C** Mastoid Sinus, Left **M** Nasal Septum **P** Accessory Sinus **Q** Maxillary Sinus, Right **R** Maxillary Sinus, Left **S** Frontal Sinus, Right **T** Frontal Sinus, Left **U** Ethmoid Sinus, Right **V** Ethmoid Sinus, Left **W** Sphenoid Sinus, Right **X** Sphenoid Sinus, Left	**0** Open **3** Percutaneous **4** Percutaneous Endoscopic **8** Via Natural or Artificial Opening Endoscopic	**Z** No Device	**Z** No Qualifier
K Nasal Mucosa and Soft Tissue	**0** Open **3** Percutaneous **4** Percutaneous Endoscopic **8** Via Natural or Artificial Opening Endoscopic **X** External	**Z** No Device	**Z** No Qualifier

0 Medical and Surgical
9 Ear, Nose, Sinus
P Removal: Taking out or off a device from a body part

Body Part Character 4	Approach Character 5	Device Character 6	Qualifier Character 7
7 Tympanic Membrane, Right **8** Tympanic Membrane, Left	**0** Open **7** Via Natural or Artificial Opening **8** Via Natural or Artificial Opening Endoscopic **X** External	**0** Drainage Device	**Z** No Qualifier
D Inner Ear, Right **E** Inner Ear, Left	**0** Open **7** Via Natural or Artificial Opening **8** Via Natural or Artificial Opening Endoscopic	**S** Hearing Device	**Z** No Qualifier
H Ear, Right **J** Ear, Left **K** Nasal Mucosa and Soft Tissue	**0** Open **3** Percutaneous **4** Percutaneous Endoscopic **7** Via Natural or Artificial Opening **8** Via Natural or Artificial Opening Endoscopic	**0** Drainage Device **7** Autologous Tissue Substitute **D** Intraluminal Device **J** Synthetic Substitute **K** Nonautologous Tissue Substitute **Y** Other Device	**Z** No Qualifier
H Ear, Right **J** Ear, Left **K** Nasal Mucosa and Soft Tissue	**X** External	**0** Drainage Device **7** Autologous Tissue Substitute **D** Intraluminal Device **J** Synthetic Substitute **K** Nonautologous Tissue Substitute	**Z** No Qualifier
Y Sinus	**0** Open **3** Percutaneous **4** Percutaneous Endoscopic	**0** Drainage Device **Y** Other Device	**Z** No Qualifier
Y Sinus	**7** Via Natural or Artificial Opening **8** Via Natural or Artificial Opening Endoscopic	**Y** Other Device	**Z** No Qualifier
Y Sinus	**X** External	**0** Drainage Device	**Z** No Qualifier

0 Medical and Surgical
9 Ear, Nose, Sinus
Q Repair: Restoring, to the extent possible, a body part to its normal anatomic structure and function

Body Part Character 4	Approach Character 5	Device Character 6	Qualifier Character 7
0 External Ear, Right **1** External Ear, Left **2** External Ear, Bilateral	**0** Open **3** Percutaneous **4** Percutaneous Endoscopic **X** External	**Z** No Device	**Z** No Qualifier
3 External Auditory Canal, Right **4** External Auditory Canal, Left **F** Eustachian Tube, Right **G** Eustachian Tube, Left	**0** Open **3** Percutaneous **4** Percutaneous Endoscopic **7** Via Natural or Artificial Opening **8** Via Natural or Artificial Opening Endoscopic **X** External	**Z** No Device	**Z** No Qualifier
5 Middle Ear, Right **6** Middle Ear, Left **9** Auditory Ossicle, Right **A** Auditory Ossicle, Left **D** Inner Ear, Right **E** Inner Ear, Left	**0** Open **8** Via Natural or Artificial Opening Endoscopic	**Z** No Device	**Z** No Qualifier
7 Tympanic Membrane, Right **8** Tympanic Membrane, Left **L** Nasal Turbinate **N** Nasopharynx	**0** Open **3** Percutaneous **4** Percutaneous Endoscopic **7** Via Natural or Artificial Opening **8** Via Natural or Artificial Opening Endoscopic	**Z** No Device	**Z** No Qualifier
B Mastoid Sinus, Right **C** Mastoid Sinus, Left **M** Nasal Septum **P** Accessory Sinus **Q** Maxillary Sinus, Right CC **R** Maxillary Sinus, Left **S** Frontal Sinus, Right **T** Frontal Sinus, Left **U** Ethmoid Sinus, Right **V** Ethmoid Sinus, Left **W** Sphenoid Sinus, Right **X** Sphenoid Sinus, Left	**0** Open **3** Percutaneous **4** Percutaneous Endoscopic **8** Via Natural or Artificial Opening Endoscopic	**Z** No Device	**Z** No Qualifier
K Nasal Mucosa and Soft Tissue CC	**0** Open **3** Percutaneous **4** Percutaneous Endoscopic **8** Via Natural or Artificial Opening Endoscopic **X** External	**Z** No Device	**Z** No Qualifier

CC 09QK0ZZ 09QK3ZZ 09QK4ZZ 09QQ0ZZ 09QQ3ZZ 09QQ4ZZ

0 Medical and Surgical
9 Ear, Nose, Sinus
R Replacement: Putting in or on biological or synthetic material that physically takes the place and/or function of all or a portion of a body part

Body Part Character 4	Approach Character 5	Device Character 6	Qualifier Character 7
0 External Ear, Right **1** External Ear, Left **2** External Ear, Bilateral **K** Nasal Mucosa and Soft Tissue	**0** Open **X** External	**7** Autologous Tissue Substitute **J** Synthetic Substitute **K** Nonautologous Tissue Substitute	**Z** No Qualifier
5 Middle Ear, Right **6** Middle Ear, Left **9** Auditory Ossicle, Right **A** Auditory Ossicle, Left **D** Inner Ear, Right **E** Inner Ear, Left	**0** Open	**7** Autologous Tissue Substitute **J** Synthetic Substitute **K** Nonautologous Tissue Substitute	**Z** No Qualifier
7 Tympanic Membrane, Right **8** Tympanic Membrane, Left **N** Nasopharynx	**0** Open **7** Via Natural or Artificial Opening **8** Via Natural or Artificial Opening Endoscopic	**7** Autologous Tissue Substitute **J** Synthetic Substitute **K** Nonautologous Tissue Substitute	**Z** No Qualifier
L Nasal Turbinate	**0** Open **3** Percutaneous **4** Percutaneous Endoscopic **7** Via Natural or Artificial Opening **8** Via Natural or Artificial Opening Endoscopic	**7** Autologous Tissue Substitute **J** Synthetic Substitute **K** Nonautologous Tissue Substitute	**Z** No Qualifier
M Nasal Septum	**0** Open **3** Percutaneous **4** Percutaneous Endoscopic	**7** Autologous Tissue Substitute **J** Synthetic Substitute **K** Nonautologous Tissue Substitute	**Z** No Qualifier

0 Medical and Surgical
9 Ear, Nose, Sinus
S Reposition: Moving to its normal location, or other suitable location, all or a portion of a body part

Body Part Character 4	Approach Character 5	Device Character 6	Qualifier Character 7
0 External Ear, Right **1** External Ear, Left **2** External Ear, Bilateral **K** Nasal Mucosa and Soft Tissue	**0** Open **4** Percutaneous Endoscopic **X** External	**Z** No Device	**Z** No Qualifier
7 Tympanic Membrane, Right **8** Tympanic Membrane, Left **F** Eustachian Tube, Right **G** Eustachian Tube, Left **L** Nasal Turbinate	**0** Open **4** Percutaneous Endoscopic **7** Via Natural or Artificial Opening **8** Via Natural or Artificial Opening Endoscopic	**Z** No Device	**Z** No Qualifier
9 Auditory Ossicle, Right **A** Auditory Ossicle, Left **M** Nasal Septum	**0** Open **4** Percutaneous Endoscopic	**Z** No Device	**Z** No Qualifier

0 Medical and Surgical
9 Ear, Nose, Sinus
T Resection: Cutting out or off, without replacement, all of a body part

Body Part Character 4	Approach Character 5	Device Character 6	Qualifier Character 7
0 External Ear, Right **1** External Ear, Left	**0** Open **4** Percutaneous Endoscopic **X** External	**Z** No Device	**Z** No Qualifier
5 Middle Ear, Right **6** Middle Ear, Left **9** Auditory Ossicle, Right **A** Auditory Ossicle, Left **D** Inner Ear, Right **E** Inner Ear, Left	**0** Open **8** Via Natural or Artificial Opening Endoscopic	**Z** No Device	**Z** No Qualifier
7 Tympanic Membrane, Right **8** Tympanic Membrane, Left **F** Eustachian Tube, Right **G** Eustachian Tube, Left **L** Nasal Turbinate **N** Nasopharynx	**0** Open **4** Percutaneous Endoscopic **7** Via Natural or Artificial Opening **8** Via Natural or Artificial Opening Endoscopic	**Z** No Device	**Z** No Qualifier
B Mastoid Sinus, Right **C** Mastoid Sinus, Left **M** Nasal Septum **P** Accessory Sinus **Q** Maxillary Sinus, Right **R** Maxillary Sinus, Left **S** Frontal Sinus, Right **T** Frontal Sinus, Left **U** Ethmoid Sinus, Right **V** Ethmoid Sinus, Left **W** Sphenoid Sinus, Right **X** Sphenoid Sinus, Left	**0** Open **4** Percutaneous Endoscopic **8** Via Natural or Artificial Opening Endoscopic	**Z** No Device	**Z** No Qualifier
K Nasal Mucosa and Soft Tissue	**0** Open **4** Percutaneous Endoscopic **8** Via Natural or Artificial Opening Endoscopic **X** External	**Z** No Device	**Z** No Qualifier

0 Medical and Surgical
9 Ear, Nose, Sinus
U Supplement: Putting in or on biological or synthetic material that physically reinforces and/or augments the function of a portion of a body part

Body Part	Approach	Device	Qualifier
Character 4	Character 5	Character 6	Character 7
0 External Ear, Right **1** External Ear, Left **2** External Ear, Bilateral	**0** Open **X** External	**7** Autologous Tissue Substitute **J** Synthetic Substitute **K** Nonautologous Tissue Substitute	**Z** No Qualifier
5 Middle Ear, Right **6** Middle Ear, Left **9** Auditory Ossicle, Right **A** Auditory Ossicle, Left **D** Inner Ear, Right **E** Inner Ear, Left	**0** Open **8** Via Natural or Artificial Opening Endoscopic	**7** Autologous Tissue Substitute **J** Synthetic Substitute **K** Nonautologous Tissue Substitute	**Z** No Qualifier
7 Tympanic Membrane, Right **8** Tympanic Membrane, Left **N** Nasopharynx	**0** Open **7** Via Natural or Artificial Opening **8** Via Natural or Artificial Opening Endoscopic	**7** Autologous Tissue Substitute **J** Synthetic Substitute **K** Nonautologous Tissue Substitute	**Z** No Qualifier
K Nasal Mucosa and Soft Tissue	**0** Open **8** Via Natural or Artificial Opening Endoscopic **X** External	**7** Autologous Tissue Substitute **J** Synthetic Substitute **K** Nonautologous Tissue Substitute	**Z** No Qualifier
L Nasal Turbinate	**0** Open **3** Percutaneous **4** Percutaneous Endoscopic **7** Via Natural or Artificial Opening **8** Via Natural or Artificial Opening Endoscopic	**7** Autologous Tissue Substitute **J** Synthetic Substitute **K** Nonautologous Tissue Substitute	**Z** No Qualifier
M Nasal Septum	**0** Open **3** Percutaneous **4** Percutaneous Endoscopic **8** Via Natural or Artificial Opening Endoscopic	**7** Autologous Tissue Substitute **J** Synthetic Substitute **K** Nonautologous Tissue Substitute	**Z** No Qualifier

0 Medical and Surgical
9 Ear, Nose, Sinus
W Revision: Correcting, to the extent possible, a portion of a malfunctioning device or the position of a displaced device

Body Part Character 4	Approach Character 5	Device Character 6	Qualifier Character 7
7 Tympanic Membrane, Right **8** Tympanic Membrane, Left **9** Auditory Ossicle, Right **A** Auditory Ossicle, Left	**0** Open **7** Via Natural or Artificial Opening **8** Via Natural or Artificial Opening Endoscopic	**7** Autologous Tissue Substitute **J** Synthetic Substitute **K** Nonautologous Tissue Substitute	**Z** No Qualifier
D Inner Ear, Right **E** Inner Ear, Left	**0** Open **7** Via Natural or Artificial Opening **8** Via Natural or Artificial Opening Endoscopic	**S** Hearing Device	**Z** No Qualifier
H Ear, Right **J** Ear, Left **K** Nasal Mucosa and Soft Tissue	**0** Open **3** Percutaneous **4** Percutaneous Endoscopic **7** Via Natural or Artificial Opening **8** Via Natural or Artificial Opening Endoscopic	**0** Drainage Device **7** Autologous Tissue Substitute **D** Intraluminal Device **J** Synthetic Substitute **K** Nonautologous Tissue Substitute **Y** Other Device	**Z** No Qualifier
H Ear, Right **J** Ear, Left **K** Nasal Mucosa and Soft Tissue	**X** External	**0** Drainage Device **7** Autologous Tissue Substitute **D** Intraluminal Device **J** Synthetic Substitute **K** Nonautologous Tissue Substitute	**Z** No Qualifier
Y Sinus	**0** Open **3** Percutaneous **4** Percutaneous Endoscopic	**0** Drainage Device **Y** Other Device	**Z** No Qualifier
Y Sinus	**7** Via Natural or Artificial Opening **8** Via Natural or Artificial Opening Endoscopic	**Y** Other Device	**Z** No Qualifier
Y Sinus	**X** External	**0** Drainage Device	**Z** No Qualifier

NOTES

NOTES

Respiratory System 0B1-0BY

0 Medical and Surgical
B Respiratory System
1 Bypass: Altering the route of passage of the contents of a tubular body part

Body Part Character 4	Approach Character 5	Device Character 6	Qualifier Character 7
1 Trachea	**0** Open	**D** Intraluminal Device	**6** Esophagus
1 Trachea	**0** Open	**F** Tracheostomy Device **Z** No Device	**4** Cutaneous
1 Trachea	**3** Percutaneous **4** Percutaneous Endoscopic	**F** Tracheostomy Device **Z** No Device	**4** Cutaneous

0 Medical and Surgical
B Respiratory System
2 Change: Taking out or off a device from a body part and putting back an identical or similar device in or on the same body part without cutting or puncturing the skin or a mucous membrane

Body Part Character 4	Approach Character 5	Device Character 6	Qualifier Character 7
0 Tracheobronchial Tree **K** Lung, Right **L** Lung, Left **Q** Pleura **T** Diaphragm	**X** External	**0** Drainage Device **Y** Other Device	**Z** No Qualifier
1 Trachea	**X** External	**0** Drainage Device **E** Intraluminal Device, Endotracheal Airway **F** Tracheostomy Device **Y** Other Device	**Z** No Qualifier

0 Medical and Surgical
B Respiratory System
5 Destruction: Physical eradication of all or a portion of a body part by the direct use of energy, force, or a destructive agent

Body Part Character 4	Approach Character 5	Device Character 6	Qualifier Character 7
1 Trachea **2** Carina **3** Main Bronchus, Right **4** Upper Lobe Bronchus, Right **5** Middle Lobe Bronchus, Right **6** Lower Lobe Bronchus, Right **7** Main Bronchus, Left **8** Upper Lobe Bronchus, Left **9** Lingula Bronchus **B** Lower Lobe Bronchus, Left **C** Upper Lung Lobe, Right **D** Middle Lung Lobe, Right **F** Lower Lung Lobe, Right **G** Upper Lung Lobe, Left **H** Lung Lingula **J** Lower Lung Lobe, Left **K** Lung, Right **L** Lung, Left **M** Lungs, Bilateral	**0** Open **3** Percutaneous **4** Percutaneous Endoscopic **7** Via Natural or Artificial Opening **8** Via Natural or Artificial Opening Endoscopic	**Z** No Device	**Z** No Qualifier
N Pleura, Right **P** Pleura, Left **T** Diaphragm	**0** Open **3** Percutaneous **4** Percutaneous Endoscopic	**Z** No Device	**Z** No Qualifier

0 Medical and Surgical
B Respiratory System
7 Dilation: Expanding an orifice or the lumen of a tubular body part

Body Part Character 4	Approach Character 5	Device Character 6	Qualifier Character 7
1 Trachea **2** Carina **3** Main Bronchus, Right **4** Upper Lobe Bronchus, Right **5** Middle Lobe Bronchus, Right **6** Lower Lobe Bronchus, Right **7** Main Bronchus, Left **8** Upper Lobe Bronchus, Left **9** Lingula Bronchus **B** Lower Lobe Bronchus, Left	**0** Open **3** Percutaneous **4** Percutaneous Endoscopic **7** Via Natural or Artificial Opening **8** Via Natural or Artificial Opening Endoscopic	**D** Intraluminal Device **Z** No Device	**Z** No Qualifier

0 Medical and Surgical
B Respiratory System
9 Drainage: Taking or letting out fluids and/or gases from a body part

Body Part Character 4	Approach Character 5	Device Character 6	Qualifier Character 7
1 Trachea **2** Carina **3** Main Bronchus, Right **4** Upper Lobe Bronchus, Right **5** Middle Lobe Bronchus, Right **6** Lower Lobe Bronchus, Right **7** Main Bronchus, Left **8** Upper Lobe Bronchus, Left **9** Lingula Bronchus **B** Lower Lobe Bronchus, Left **C** Upper Lung Lobe, Right **D** Middle Lung Lobe, Right **F** Lower Lung Lobe, Right **G** Upper Lung Lobe, Left **H** Lung Lingula **J** Lower Lung Lobe, Left **K** Lung, Right **L** Lung, Left **M** Lungs, Bilateral	**0** Open **3** Percutaneous **4** Percutaneous Endoscopic **7** Via Natural or Artificial Opening **8** Via Natural or Artificial Opening Endoscopic	**0** Drainage Device	**Z** No Qualifier
1 Trachea **2** Carina **3** Main Bronchus, Right **4** Upper Lobe Bronchus, Right **5** Middle Lobe Bronchus, Right **6** Lower Lobe Bronchus, Right **7** Main Bronchus, Left **8** Upper Lobe Bronchus, Left **9** Lingula Bronchus **B** Lower Lobe Bronchus, Left **C** Upper Lung Lobe, Right **D** Middle Lung Lobe, Right **F** Lower Lung Lobe, Right **G** Upper Lung Lobe, Left **H** Lung Lingula **J** Lower Lung Lobe, Left **K** Lung, Right **L** Lung, Left **M** Lungs, Bilateral	**0** Open **3** Percutaneous **4** Percutaneous Endoscopic **7** Via Natural or Artificial Opening **8** Via Natural or Artificial Opening Endoscopic	**Z** No Device	**X** Diagnostic **Z** No Qualifier

0B9 continued on next page

0B9 continued from previous page

0 Medical and Surgical
B Respiratory System
9 Drainage: Taking or letting out fluids and/or gases from a body part

Body Part Character 4	Approach Character 5	Device Character 6	Qualifier Character 7
N Pleura, Right **P** Pleura, Left	**0** Open **3** Percutaneous **4** Percutaneous Endoscopic **8** Via Natural or Artificial Opening Endoscopic	**0** Drainage Device	**Z** No Qualifier
N Pleura, Right **P** Pleura, Left	**0** Open **3** Percutaneous **4** Percutaneous Endoscopic **8** Via Natural or Artificial Opening Endoscopic	**Z** No Device	**X** Diagnostic **Z** No Qualifier
T Diaphragm	**0** Open **3** Percutaneous **4** Percutaneous Endoscopic	**0** Drainage Device	**Z** No Qualifier
T Diaphragm	**0** Open **3** Percutaneous **4** Percutaneous Endoscopic	**Z** No Device	**X** Diagnostic **Z** No Qualifier

0 Medical and Surgical
B Respiratory System
B Excision: Cutting out or off, without replacement, a portion of a body part

Body Part Character 4	Approach Character 5	Device Character 6	Qualifier Character 7
1 Trachea **2** Carina **3** Main Bronchus, Right **4** Upper Lobe Bronchus, Right **5** Middle Lobe Bronchus, Right **6** Lower Lobe Bronchus, Right **7** Main Bronchus, Left **8** Upper Lobe Bronchus, Left **9** Lingula Bronchus **B** Lower Lobe Bronchus, Left **C** Upper Lung Lobe, Right **D** Middle Lung Lobe, Right **F** Lower Lung Lobe, Right **G** Upper Lung Lobe, Left **H** Lung Lingula **J** Lower Lung Lobe, Left **K** Lung, Right **L** Lung, Left **M** Lungs, Bilateral	**0** Open **3** Percutaneous **4** Percutaneous Endoscopic **7** Via Natural or Artificial Opening **8** Via Natural or Artificial Opening Endoscopic	**Z** No Device	**X** Diagnostic **Z** No Qualifier
N Pleura, Right **P** Pleura, Left	**0** Open **3** Percutaneous **4** Percutaneous Endoscopic **8** Via Natural or Artificial Opening Endoscopic	**Z** No Device	**X** Diagnostic **Z** No Qualifier
T Diaphragm	**0** Open **3** Percutaneous **4** Percutaneous Endoscopic	**Z** No Device	**X** Diagnostic **Z** No Qualifier

0 Medical and Surgical
B Respiratory System
C Extirpation: Taking or cutting out solid matter from a body part

Body Part	Approach	Device	Qualifier
Character 4	Character 5	Character 6	Character 7
1 Trachea **2** Carina **3** Main Bronchus, Right **4** Upper Lobe Bronchus, Right **5** Middle Lobe Bronchus, Right **6** Lower Lobe Bronchus, Right **7** Main Bronchus, Left **8** Upper Lobe Bronchus, Left **9** Lingula Bronchus **B** Lower Lobe Bronchus, Left **C** Upper Lung Lobe, Right **D** Middle Lung Lobe, Right **F** Lower Lung Lobe, Right **G** Upper Lung Lobe, Left **H** Lung Lingula **J** Lower Lung Lobe, Left **K** Lung, Right **L** Lung, Left **M** Lungs, Bilateral	**0** Open **3** Percutaneous **4** Percutaneous Endoscopic **7** Via Natural or Artificial Opening **8** Via Natural or Artificial Opening Endoscopic	**Z** No Device	**Z** No Qualifier
N Pleura, Right **P** Pleura, Left **T** Diaphragm	**0** Open **3** Percutaneous **4** Percutaneous Endoscopic	**Z** No Device	**Z** No Qualifier

0 Medical and Surgical
B Respiratory System
D Extraction: Pulling or stripping out or off all or a portion of a body part by the use of force

Body Part	Approach	Device	Qualifier
Character 4	Character 5	Character 6	Character 7
1 Trachea **2** Carina **3** Main Bronchus, Right **4** Upper Lobe Bronchus, Right **5** Middle Lobe Bronchus, Right **6** Lower Lobe Bronchus, Right **7** Main Bronchus, Left **8** Upper Lobe Bronchus, Left **9** Lingula Bronchus **B** Lower Lobe Bronchus, Left **C** Upper Lung Lobe, Right **D** Middle Lung Lobe, Right **F** Lower Lung Lobe, Right **G** Upper Lung Lobe, Left **H** Lung Lingula **J** Lower Lung Lobe, Left **K** Lung, Right **L** Lung, Left **M** Lungs, Bilateral	**4** Percutaneous Endoscopic **8** Via Natural or Artificial Opening Endoscopic	**Z** No Device	**X** Diagnostic
N Pleura, Right **P** Pleura, Left	**0** Open **3** Percutaneous **4** Percutaneous Endoscopic	**Z** No Device	**X** Diagnostic **Z** No Qualifier

LC Limited Coverage NC Noncovered HAC HAC-associated Procedure CC Combination Cluster - See Appendix G for code lists
DRG Non-OR-Affecting MS-DRG Assignment New/Revised Text in Orange ♂ Male ♀ Female

0 Medical and Surgical
B Respiratory System
F Fragmentation: Breaking solid matter in a body part into pieces

Body Part Character 4	Approach Character 5	Device Character 6	Qualifier Character 7
1 Trachea NC 2 Carina NC 3 Main Bronchus, Right NC 4 Upper Lobe Bronchus, Right NC 5 Middle Lobe Bronchus, Right NC 6 Lower Lobe Bronchus, Right NC 7 Main Bronchus, Left NC 8 Upper Lobe Bronchus, Left NC 9 Lingula Bronchus NC B Lower Lobe Bronchus, Left NC	0 Open 3 Percutaneous 4 Percutaneous Endoscopic 7 Via Natural or Artificial Opening 8 Via Natural or Artificial Opening Endoscopic X External	Z No Device	Z No Qualifier

NC 0BF1XZZ 0BF2XZZ 0BF3XZZ 0BF4XZZ 0BF5XZZ 0BF6XZZ 0BF7XZZ 0BF8XZZ 0BF9XZZ 0BFBXZZ

0 Medical and Surgical
B Respiratory System
H Insertion: Putting in a nonbiological appliance that monitors, assists, performs, or prevents a physiological function but does not physically take the place of a body part

Body Part Character 4	Approach Character 5	Device Character 6	Qualifier Character 7
0 Tracheobronchial Tree	0 Open 3 Percutaneous 4 Percutaneous Endoscopic 7 Via Natural or Artificial Opening 8 Via Natural or Artificial Opening Endoscopic	1 Radioactive Element 2 Monitoring Device 3 Infusion Device D Intraluminal Device Y Other Device	Z No Qualifier
1 Trachea	0 Open	2 Monitoring Device D Intraluminal Device Y Other Device	Z No Qualifier
1 Trachea	3 Percutaneous	D Intraluminal Device E Intraluminal Device, Endotracheal Airway Y Other Device	Z No Qualifier
1 Trachea	4 Percutaneous Endoscopic	D Intraluminal Device Y Other Device	Z No Qualifier
1 Trachea	7 Via Natural or Artificial Opening 8 Via Natural or Artificial Opening Endoscopic	2 Monitoring Device D Intraluminal Device E Intraluminal Device, Endotracheal Airway Y Other Device	Z No Qualifier
3 Main Bronchus, Right 4 Upper Lobe Bronchus, Right 5 Middle Lobe Bronchus, Right 6 Lower Lobe Bronchus, Right 7 Main Bronchus, Left 8 Upper Lobe Bronchus, Left 9 Lingula Bronchus B Lower Lobe Bronchus, Left	0 Open 3 Percutaneous 4 Percutaneous Endoscopic 7 Via Natural or Artificial Opening 8 Via Natural or Artificial Opening Endoscopic	G Intraluminal Device, Endobronchial Valve	Z No Qualifier
K Lung, Right L Lung, Left	0 Open 3 Percutaneous 4 Percutaneous Endoscopic 7 Via Natural or Artificial Opening 8 Via Natural or Artificial Opening Endoscopic	1 Radioactive Element 2 Monitoring Device 3 Infusion Device Y Other Device	Z No Qualifier

0BH continued on next page

0 Medical and Surgical
B Respiratory System
H Insertion: Putting in a nonbiological appliance that monitors, assists, performs, or prevents a physiological function but does not physically take the place of a body part

0BH continued from previous page

Body Part Character 4	Approach Character 5	Device Character 6	Qualifier Character 7
Q Pleura	**0** Open **3** Percutaneous **4** Percutaneous Endoscopic **7** Via Natural or Artificial Opening **8** Via Natural or Artificial Opening Endoscopic	**Y** Other Device	**Z** No Qualifier
T Diaphragm	**0** Open **3** Percutaneous **4** Percutaneous Endoscopic	**2** Monitoring Device **M** Diaphragmatic Pacemaker Lead **Y** Other Device	**Z** No Qualifier
T Diaphragm	**7** Via Natural or Artificial Opening **8** Via Natural or Artificial Opening Endoscopic	**Y** Other Device	**Z** No Qualifier

0 Medical and Surgical
B Respiratory System
J Inspection: Visually and/or manually exploring a body part

Body Part Character 4	Approach Character 5	Device Character 6	Qualifier Character 7
0 Tracheobronchial Tree **1** Trachea **K** Lung, Right **L** Lung, Left **Q** Pleura **T** Diaphragm	**0** Open **3** Percutaneous **4** Percutaneous Endoscopic **7** Via Natural or Artificial Opening **8** Via Natural or Artificial Opening Endoscopic **X** External	**Z** No Device	**Z** No Qualifier

0 Medical and Surgical
B Respiratory System
L Occlusion: Completely closing an orifice or the lumen of a tubular body part

Body Part Character 4	Approach Character 5	Device Character 6	Qualifier Character 7
1 Trachea **2** Carina **3** Main Bronchus, Right **4** Upper Lobe Bronchus, Right **5** Middle Lobe Bronchus, Right **6** Lower Lobe Bronchus, Right **7** Main Bronchus, Left **8** Upper Lobe Bronchus, Left **9** Lingula Bronchus **B** Lower Lobe Bronchus, Left	**0** Open **3** Percutaneous **4** Percutaneous Endoscopic	**C** Extraluminal Device **D** Intraluminal Device **Z** No Device	**Z** No Qualifier
1 Trachea **2** Carina **3** Main Bronchus, Right **4** Upper Lobe Bronchus, Right **5** Middle Lobe Bronchus, Right **6** Lower Lobe Bronchus, Right **7** Main Bronchus, Left **8** Upper Lobe Bronchus, Left **9** Lingula Bronchus **B** Lower Lobe Bronchus, Left	**7** Via Natural or Artificial Opening **8** Via Natural or Artificial Opening Endoscopic	**D** Intraluminal Device **Z** No Device	**Z** No Qualifier

0 Medical and Surgical
B Respiratory System
M Reattachment: Putting back in or on all or a portion of a separated body part to its normal location or other suitable location

Body Part Character 4	Approach Character 5	Device Character 6	Qualifier Character 7
1 Trachea **2** Carina **3** Main Bronchus, Right **4** Upper Lobe Bronchus, Right **5** Middle Lobe Bronchus, Right **6** Lower Lobe Bronchus, Right **7** Main Bronchus, Left **8** Upper Lobe Bronchus, Left **9** Lingula Bronchus **B** Lower Lobe Bronchus, Left **C** Upper Lung Lobe, Right **D** Middle Lung Lobe, Right **F** Lower Lung Lobe, Right **G** Upper Lung Lobe, Left **H** Lung Lingula **J** Lower Lung Lobe, Left **K** Lung, Right **L** Lung, Left **T** Diaphragm	**0** Open	**Z** No Device	**Z** No Qualifier

0 Medical and Surgical
B Respiratory System
N Release: Freeing a body part from an abnormal physical constraint by cutting or by the use of force

Body Part Character 4	Approach Character 5	Device Character 6	Qualifier Character 7
1 Trachea **2** Carina **3** Main Bronchus, Right **4** Upper Lobe Bronchus, Right **5** Middle Lobe Bronchus, Right **6** Lower Lobe Bronchus, Right **7** Main Bronchus, Left **8** Upper Lobe Bronchus, Left **9** Lingula Bronchus **B** Lower Lobe Bronchus, Left **C** Upper Lung Lobe, Right **D** Middle Lung Lobe, Right **F** Lower Lung Lobe, Right **G** Upper Lung Lobe, Left **H** Lung Lingula **J** Lower Lung Lobe, Left **K** Lung, Right **L** Lung, Left **M** Lungs, Bilateral	**0** Open **3** Percutaneous **4** Percutaneous Endoscopic **7** Via Natural or Artificial Opening **8** Via Natural or Artificial Opening Endoscopic	**Z** No Device	**Z** No Qualifier
N Pleura, Right **P** Pleura, Left **T** Diaphragm	**0** Open **3** Percutaneous **4** Percutaneous Endoscopic	**Z** No Device	**Z** No Qualifier

0 Medical and Surgical
B Respiratory System
P Removal: Taking out or off a device from a body part

Body Part Character 4	Approach Character 5	Device Character 6	Qualifier Character 7
0 Tracheobronchial Tree	**0** Open **3** Percutaneous **4** Percutaneous Endoscopic **7** Via Natural or Artificial Opening **8** Via Natural or Artificial Opening Endoscopic	**0** Drainage Device **1** Radioactive Element **2** Monitoring Device **3** Infusion Device **7** Autologous Tissue Substitute **C** Extraluminal Device **D** Intraluminal Device **J** Synthetic Substitute **K** Nonautologous Tissue Substitute **Y** Other Device	**Z** No Qualifier
0 Tracheobronchial Tree	**X** External	**0** Drainage Device **1** Radioactive Element **2** Monitoring Device **3** Infusion Device **D** Intraluminal Device	**Z** No Qualifier
1 Trachea	**0** Open **3** Percutaneous **4** Percutaneous Endoscopic **7** Via Natural or Artificial Opening **8** Via Natural or Artificial Opening Endoscopic	**0** Drainage Device **2** Monitoring Device **7** Autologous Tissue Substitute **C** Extraluminal Device **D** Intraluminal Device **F** Tracheostomy Device **J** Synthetic Substitute **K** Nonautologous Tissue Substitute	**Z** No Qualifier
1 Trachea	**X** External	**0** Drainage Device **2** Monitoring Device **D** Intraluminal Device **F** Tracheostomy Device	**Z** No Qualifier
K Lung, Right **L** Lung, Left	**0** Open **3** Percutaneous **4** Percutaneous Endoscopic **7** Via Natural or Artificial Opening **8** Via Natural or Artificial Opening Endoscopic	**0** Drainage Device **1** Radioactive Element **2** Monitoring Device **3** Infusion Device **Y** Other Device	**Z** No Qualifier
K Lung, Right **L** Lung, Left	**X** External	**0** Drainage Device **1** Radioactive Element **2** Monitoring Device **3** Infusion Device	**Z** No Qualifier
Q Pleura	**0** Open **3** Percutaneous **4** Percutaneous Endoscopic **7** Via Natural or Artificial Opening **8** Via Natural or Artificial Opening Endoscopic	**0** Drainage Device **1** Radioactive Element **2** Monitoring Device **Y** Other Device	**Z** No Qualifier
Q Pleura	**X** External	**0** Drainage Device **1** Radioactive Element **2** Monitoring Device	**Z** No Qualifier
T Diaphragm	**0** Open **3** Percutaneous **4** Percutaneous Endoscopic **7** Via Natural or Artificial Opening **8** Via Natural or Artificial Opening Endoscopic	**0** Drainage Device **2** Monitoring Device **7** Autologous Tissue Substitute **J** Synthetic Substitute **K** Nonautologous Tissue Substitute **M** Diaphragmatic Pacemaker Lead **Y** Other Device	**Z** No Qualifier
T Diaphragm	**X** External	**0** Drainage Device **2** Monitoring Device **M** Diaphragmatic Pacemaker Lead	**Z** No Qualifier

0 Medical and Surgical
B Respiratory System
Q Repair: Restoring, to the extent possible, a body part to its normal anatomic structure and function

Body Part Character 4	Approach Character 5	Device Character 6	Qualifier Character 7
1 Trachea CC **2** Carina **3** Main Bronchus, Right CC **4** Upper Lobe Bronchus, Right CC **5** Middle Lobe Bronchus, Right CC **6** Lower Lobe Bronchus, Right CC **7** Main Bronchus, Left CC **8** Upper Lobe Bronchus, Left CC **9** Lingula Bronchus CC **B** Lower Lobe Bronchus, Left CC **C** Upper Lung Lobe, Right **D** Middle Lung Lobe, Right **F** Lower Lung Lobe, Right **G** Upper Lung Lobe, Left **H** Lung Lingula **J** Lower Lung Lobe, Left **K** Lung, Right CC **L** Lung, Left CC **M** Lungs, Bilateral CC	**0** Open **3** Percutaneous **4** Percutaneous Endoscopic **7** Via Natural or Artificial Opening **8** Via Natural or Artificial Opening Endoscopic	**Z** No Device	**Z** No Qualifier
N Pleura, Right CC **P** Pleura, Left CC **T** Diaphragm	**0** Open **3** Percutaneous **4** Percutaneous Endoscopic	**Z** No Device	**Z** No Qualifier

CC 0BQ10ZZ 0BQ13ZZ 0BQ14ZZ 0BQ17ZZ 0BQ18ZZ 0BQ30ZZ 0BQ33ZZ 0BQ34ZZ 0BQ37ZZ 0BQ38ZZ 0BQ40ZZ 0BQ43ZZ 0BQ44ZZ 0BQ47ZZ 0BQ48ZZ 0BQ50ZZ 0BQ53ZZ 0BQ54ZZ 0BQ57ZZ 0BQ58ZZ 0BQ60ZZ 0BQ63ZZ 0BQ64ZZ 0BQ67ZZ 0BQ68ZZ 0BQ70ZZ 0BQ73ZZ 0BQ74ZZ 0BQ77ZZ 0BQ78ZZ 0BQ80ZZ 0BQ83ZZ 0BQ84ZZ 0BQ87ZZ 0BQ88ZZ 0BQ90ZZ 0BQ93ZZ 0BQ94ZZ 0BQ97ZZ 0BQ98ZZ 0BQB0ZZ 0BQB3ZZ 0BQB4ZZ 0BQB7ZZ 0BQB8ZZ 0BQK0ZZ 0BQK3ZZ 0BQK4ZZ 0BQK7ZZ 0BQK8ZZ 0BQL0ZZ 0BQL3ZZ 0BQL4ZZ 0BQL7ZZ 0BQL8ZZ 0BQM0ZZ 0BQM3ZZ 0BQM4ZZ 0BQM7ZZ 0BQM8ZZ 0BQN0ZZ 0BQN3ZZ 0BQN4ZZ 0BQP0ZZ 0BQP3ZZ 0BQP4ZZ

0 Medical and Surgical
B Respiratory System
R Replacement: Putting in or on biological or synthetic material that physically takes the place and/or function of all or a portion of a body part

Body Part Character 4	Approach Character 5	Device Character 6	Qualifier Character 7
1 Trachea **2** Carina **3** Main Bronchus, Right **4** Upper Lobe Bronchus, Right **5** Middle Lobe Bronchus, Right **6** Lower Lobe Bronchus, Right **7** Main Bronchus, Left **8** Upper Lobe Bronchus, Left **9** Lingula Bronchus **B** Lower Lobe Bronchus, Left **T** Diaphragm	**0** Open **4** Percutaneous Endoscopic	**7** Autologous Tissue Substitute **J** Synthetic Substitute **K** Nonautologous Tissue Substitute	**Z** No Qualifier

0 Medical and Surgical
B Respiratory System
S Reposition: Moving to its normal location, or other suitable location, all or a portion of a body part

Body Part Character 4	Approach Character 5	Device Character 6	Qualifier Character 7
1 Trachea **2** Carina **3** Main Bronchus, Right **4** Upper Lobe Bronchus, Right **5** Middle Lobe Bronchus, Right **6** Lower Lobe Bronchus, Right **7** Main Bronchus, Left **8** Upper Lobe Bronchus, Left **9** Lingula Bronchus **B** Lower Lobe Bronchus, Left **C** Upper Lung Lobe, Right **D** Middle Lung Lobe, Right **F** Lower Lung Lobe, Right **G** Upper Lung Lobe, Left **H** Lung Lingula **J** Lower Lung Lobe, Left **K** Lung, Right **L** Lung, Left **T** Diaphragm	**0** Open	**Z** No Device	**Z** No Qualifier

0 Medical and Surgical
B Respiratory System
T Resection: Cutting out or off, without replacement, all of a body part

Body Part Character 4	Approach Character 5	Device Character 6	Qualifier Character 7
1 Trachea **2** Carina **3** Main Bronchus, Right **4** Upper Lobe Bronchus, Right **5** Middle Lobe Bronchus, Right **6** Lower Lobe Bronchus, Right **7** Main Bronchus, Left **8** Upper Lobe Bronchus, Left **9** Lingula Bronchus **B** Lower Lobe Bronchus, Left **C** Upper Lung Lobe, Right **D** Middle Lung Lobe, Right **F** Lower Lung Lobe, Right **G** Upper Lung Lobe, Left **H** Lung Lingula **J** Lower Lung Lobe, Left **K** Lung, Right CC **L** Lung, Left CC **M** Lungs, Bilateral CC **T** Diaphragm	**0** Open **4** Percutaneous Endoscopic	**Z** No Device	**Z** No Qualifier

CC 0BTK0ZZ 0BTL0ZZ 0BTM0ZZ

0 Medical and Surgical
B Respiratory System
U Supplement: Putting in or on biological or synthetic material that physically reinforces and/or augments the function of a portion of a body part

Body Part Character 4	Approach Character 5	Device Character 6	Qualifier Character 7
1 Trachea **2** Carina **3** Main Bronchus, Right **4** Upper Lobe Bronchus, Right **5** Middle Lobe Bronchus, Right **6** Lower Lobe Bronchus, Right **7** Main Bronchus, Left **8** Upper Lobe Bronchus, Left **9** Lingula Bronchus **B** Lower Lobe Bronchus, Left	**0** Open **4** Percutaneous Endoscopic **8** Via Natural or Artificial Opening Endoscopic	**7** Autologous Tissue Substitute **J** Synthetic Substitute **K** Nonautologous Tissue Substitute	**Z** No Qualifier
T Diaphragm	**0** Open **4** Percutaneous Endoscopic	**7** Autologous Tissue Substitute **J** Synthetic Substitute **K** Nonautologous Tissue Substitute	**Z** No Qualifier

0 Medical and Surgical
B Respiratory System
V Restriction: Partially closing an orifice or the lumen of a tubular body part

Body Part Character 4	Approach Character 5	Device Character 6	Qualifier Character 7
1 Trachea **2** Carina **3** Main Bronchus, Right **4** Upper Lobe Bronchus, Right **5** Middle Lobe Bronchus, Right **6** Lower Lobe Bronchus, Right **7** Main Bronchus, Left **8** Upper Lobe Bronchus, Left **9** Lingula Bronchus **B** Lower Lobe Bronchus, Left	**0** Open **3** Percutaneous **4** Percutaneous Endoscopic	**C** Extraluminal Device **D** Intraluminal Device **Z** No Device	**Z** No Qualifier
1 Trachea **2** Carina **3** Main Bronchus, Right **4** Upper Lobe Bronchus, Right **5** Middle Lobe Bronchus, Right **6** Lower Lobe Bronchus, Right **7** Main Bronchus, Left **8** Upper Lobe Bronchus, Left **9** Lingula Bronchus **B** Lower Lobe Bronchus, Left	**7** Via Natural or Artificial Opening **8** Via Natural or Artificial Opening Endoscopic	**D** Intraluminal Device **Z** No Device	**Z** No Qualifier

0 Medical and Surgical
B Respiratory System
W Revision: Correcting, to the extent possible, a portion of a malfunctioning device or the position of a displaced device

Body Part Character 4	Approach Character 5	Device Character 6	Qualifier Character 7
0 Tracheobronchial Tree	**0** Open **3** Percutaneous **4** Percutaneous Endoscopic **7** Via Natural or Artificial Opening **8** Via Natural or Artificial Opening Endoscopic	**0** Drainage Device **2** Monitoring Device **3** Infusion Device **7** Autologous Tissue Substitute **C** Extraluminal Device **D** Intraluminal Device **J** Synthetic Substitute **K** Nonautologous Tissue Substitute **Y** Other Device	**Z** No Qualifier
0 Tracheobronchial Tree	**X** External	**0** Drainage Device **2** Monitoring Device **3** Infusion Device **7** Autologous Tissue Substitute **C** Extraluminal Device **D** Intraluminal Device **J** Synthetic Substitute **K** Nonautologous Tissue Substitute	**Z** No Qualifier
1 Trachea	**0** Open **3** Percutaneous **4** Percutaneous Endoscopic **7** Via Natural or Artificial Opening **8** Via Natural or Artificial Opening Endoscopic **X** External	**0** Drainage Device **2** Monitoring Device **7** Autologous Tissue Substitute **C** Extraluminal Device **D** Intraluminal Device **F** Tracheostomy Device **J** Synthetic Substitute **K** Nonautologous Tissue Substitute	**Z** No Qualifier
K Lung, Right **L** Lung, Left	**0** Open **3** Percutaneous **4** Percutaneous Endoscopic **7** Via Natural or Artificial Opening **8** Via Natural or Artificial Opening Endoscopic	**0** Drainage Device **2** Monitoring Device **3** Infusion Device **Y** Other Device	**Z** No Qualifier
K Lung, Right **L** Lung, Left	**X** External	**0** Drainage Device **2** Monitoring Device **3** Infusion Device	**Z** No Qualifier
Q Pleura	**0** Open **3** Percutaneous **4** Percutaneous Endoscopic **7** Via Natural or Artificial Opening **8** Via Natural or Artificial Opening Endoscopic	**0** Drainage Device **2** Monitoring Device **Y** Other Device	**Z** No Qualifier
Q Pleura	**X** External	**0** Drainage Device **2** Monitoring Device	**Z** No Qualifier
T Diaphragm	**0** Open **3** Percutaneous **4** Percutaneous Endoscopic **7** Via Natural or Artificial Opening **8** Via Natural or Artificial Opening Endoscopic	**0** Drainage Device **2** Monitoring Device **7** Autologous Tissue Substitute **J** Synthetic Substitute **K** Nonautologous Tissue Substitute **M** Diaphragmatic Pacemaker Lead **Y** Other Device	**Z** No Qualifier
T Diaphragm	**X** External	**0** Drainage Device **2** Monitoring Device **7** Autologous Tissue Substitute **J** Synthetic Substitute **K** Nonautologous Tissue Substitute **M** Diaphragmatic Pacemaker Lead	**Z** No Qualifier

0 Medical and Surgical
B Respiratory System
Y Transplantation: Putting in or on all or a portion of a living body part taken from another individual or animal to physically take the place and/or function of all or a portion of a similar body part

Body Part Character 4	Approach Character 5	Device Character 6	Qualifier Character 7
C Upper Lung Lobe, Right LC **D** Middle Lung Lobe, Right LC **F** Lower Lung Lobe, Right LC **G** Upper Lung Lobe, Left LC **H** Lung Lingula LC **J** Lower Lung Lobe, Left LC **K** Lung, Right LC **L** Lung, Left LC **M** Lungs, Bilateral LC	**0** Open	**Z** No Device	**0** Allogeneic **1** Syngeneic **2** Zooplastic

LC 0BYC0Z0 0BYC0Z1 0BYC0Z2 0BYD0Z0 0BYD0Z1 0BYD0Z2 0BYF0Z0 0BYF0Z1 0BYF0Z2 0BYG0Z0 0BYG0Z1 0BYG0Z2 0BYH0Z0 0BYH0Z1 0BYH0Z2 0BYJ0Z0 0BYJ0Z1 0BYJ0Z2 0BYK0Z0 0BYK0Z1 0BYK0Z2 0BYL0Z0 0BYL0Z1 0BYL0Z2 0BYM0Z0 0BYM0Z1 0BYM0Z2

NOTES

Mouth and Throat 0C0-0CX

0 Medical and Surgical
C Mouth and Throat
0 Alteration: Modifying the anatomic structure of a body part without affecting the function of the body part

Body Part Character 4	Approach Character 5	Device Character 6	Qualifier Character 7
0 Upper Lip **1** Lower Lip	**X** External	**7** Autologous Tissue Substitute **J** Synthetic Substitute **K** Nonautologous Tissue Substitute **Z** No Device	**Z** No Qualifier

0 Medical and Surgical
C Mouth and Throat
2 Change: Taking out or off a device from a body part and putting back an identical or similar device in or on the same body part without cutting or puncturing the skin or a mucous membrane

Body Part Character 4	Approach Character 5	Device Character 6	Qualifier Character 7
A Salivary Gland **S** Larynx **Y** Mouth and Throat	**X** External	**0** Drainage Device **Y** Other Device	**Z** No Qualifier

0 Medical and Surgical
C Mouth and Throat
5 Destruction: Physical eradication of all or a portion of a body part by the direct use of energy, force, or a destructive agent

Body Part Character 4	Approach Character 5	Device Character 6	Qualifier Character 7
0 Upper Lip **1** Lower Lip **2** Hard Palate **3** Soft Palate **4** Buccal Mucosa **5** Upper Gingiva **6** Lower Gingiva **7** Tongue **N** Uvula **P** Tonsils **Q** Adenoids	**0** Open **3** Percutaneous **X** External	**Z** No Device	**Z** No Qualifier
8 Parotid Gland, Right **9** Parotid Gland, Left **B** Parotid Duct, Right **C** Parotid Duct, Left **D** Sublingual Gland, Right **F** Sublingual Gland, Left **G** Submaxillary Gland, Right **H** Submaxillary Gland, Left **J** Minor Salivary Gland	**0** Open **3** Percutaneous	**Z** No Device	**Z** No Qualifier
M Pharynx **R** Epiglottis **S** Larynx **T** Vocal Cord, Right **V** Vocal Cord, Left	**0** Open **3** Percutaneous **4** Percutaneous Endoscopic **7** Via Natural or Artificial Opening **8** Via Natural or Artificial Opening Endoscopic	**Z** No Device	**Z** No Qualifier
W Upper Tooth **X** Lower Tooth	**0** Open **X** External	**Z** No Device	**0** Single **1** Multiple **2** All

0 Medical and Surgical
C Mouth and Throat
7 Dilation: Expanding an orifice or the lumen of a tubular body part

Body Part Character 4	Approach Character 5	Device Character 6	Qualifier Character 7
B Parotid Duct, Right **C** Parotid Duct, Left	**0** Open **3** Percutaneous **7** Via Natural or Artificial Opening	**D** Intraluminal Device **Z** No Device	**Z** No Qualifier
M Pharynx	**7** Via Natural or Artificial Opening **8** Via Natural or Artificial Opening Endoscopic	**D** Intraluminal Device **Z** No Device	**Z** No Qualifier
S Larynx CC	**0** Open **3** Percutaneous **4** Percutaneous Endoscopic **7** Via Natural or Artificial Opening **8** Via Natural or Artificial Opening Endoscopic	**D** Intraluminal Device **Z** No Device	**Z** No Qualifier

CC 0C7S0DZ 0C7S3DZ 0C7S4DZ 0C7S7DZ 0C7S8DZ

0 Medical and Surgical
C Mouth and Throat
9 Drainage: Taking or letting out fluids and/or gases from a body part

Body Part Character 4	Approach Character 5	Device Character 6	Qualifier Character 7
0 Upper Lip **1** Lower Lip **2** Hard Palate **3** Soft Palate **4** Buccal Mucosa **5** Upper Gingiva **6** Lower Gingiva **7** Tongue **N** Uvula **P** Tonsils **Q** Adenoids	**0** Open **3** Percutaneous **X** External	**0** Drainage Device	**Z** No Qualifier
0 Upper Lip **1** Lower Lip **2** Hard Palate **3** Soft Palate **4** Buccal Mucosa **5** Upper Gingiva **6** Lower Gingiva **7** Tongue **N** Uvula **P** Tonsils **Q** Adenoids	**0** Open **3** Percutaneous **X** External	**Z** No Device	**X** Diagnostic **Z** No Qualifier
8 Parotid Gland, Right **9** Parotid Gland, Left **B** Parotid Duct, Right **C** Parotid Duct, Left **D** Sublingual Gland, Right **F** Sublingual Gland, Left **G** Submaxillary Gland, Right **H** Submaxillary Gland, Left **J** Minor Salivary Gland	**0** Open **3** Percutaneous	**0** Drainage Device	**Z** No Qualifier

0C9 continued on next page

0C9 continued from previous page

0 Medical and Surgical
C Mouth and Throat
9 Drainage: Taking or letting out fluids and/or gases from a body part

Body Part	Approach	Device	Qualifier
Character 4	**Character 5**	**Character 6**	**Character 7**
8 Parotid Gland, Right **9** Parotid Gland, Left **B** Parotid Duct, Right **C** Parotid Duct, Left **D** Sublingual Gland, Right **F** Sublingual Gland, Left **G** Submaxillary Gland, Right **H** Submaxillary Gland, Left **J** Minor Salivary Gland	**0** Open **3** Percutaneous	**Z** No Device	**X** Diagnostic **Z** No Qualifier
M Pharynx **R** Epiglottis **S** Larynx **T** Vocal Cord, Right **V** Vocal Cord, Left	**0** Open **3** Percutaneous **4** Percutaneous Endoscopic **7** Via Natural or Artificial Opening **8** Via Natural or Artificial Opening Endoscopic	**0** Drainage Device	**Z** No Qualifier
M Pharynx **R** Epiglottis **S** Larynx **T** Vocal Cord, Right **V** Vocal Cord, Left	**0** Open **3** Percutaneous **4** Percutaneous Endoscopic **7** Via Natural or Artificial Opening **8** Via Natural or Artificial Opening Endoscopic	**Z** No Device	**X** Diagnostic **Z** No Qualifier
W Upper Tooth **X** Lower Tooth	**0** Open **X** External	**0** Drainage Device **Z** No Device	**0** Single **1** Multiple **2** All

0 Medical and Surgical
C Mouth and Throat
B Excision: Cutting out or off, without replacement, a portion of a body part

Body Part	Approach	Device	Qualifier
Character 4	**Character 5**	**Character 6**	**Character 7**
0 Upper Lip **1** Lower Lip **2** Hard Palate **3** Soft Palate **4** Buccal Mucosa **5** Upper Gingiva **6** Lower Gingiva **7** Tongue **N** Uvula **P** Tonsils **Q** Adenoids	**0** Open **3** Percutaneous **X** External	**Z** No Device	**X** Diagnostic **Z** No Qualifier
8 Parotid Gland, Right **9** Parotid Gland, Left **B** Parotid Duct, Right **C** Parotid Duct, Left **D** Sublingual Gland, Right **F** Sublingual Gland, Left **G** Submaxillary Gland, Right **H** Submaxillary Gland, Left **J** Minor Salivary Gland	**0** Open **3** Percutaneous	**Z** No Device	**X** Diagnostic **Z** No Qualifier
M Pharynx **R** Epiglottis **S** Larynx **T** Vocal Cord, Right **V** Vocal Cord, Left	**0** Open **3** Percutaneous **4** Percutaneous Endoscopic **7** Via Natural or Artificial Opening **8** Via Natural or Artificial Opening Endoscopic	**Z** No Device	**X** Diagnostic **Z** No Qualifier
W Upper Tooth **X** Lower Tooth	**0** Open **X** External	**Z** No Device	**0** Single **1** Multiple **2** All

0 Medical and Surgical
C Mouth and Throat
C Extirpation: Taking or cutting out solid matter from a body part

Body Part Character 4	Approach Character 5	Device Character 6	Qualifier Character 7
0 Upper Lip **1** Lower Lip **2** Hard Palate **3** Soft Palate **4** Buccal Mucosa **5** Upper Gingiva **6** Lower Gingiva **7** Tongue **N** Uvula **P** Tonsils **Q** Adenoids	**0** Open **3** Percutaneous **X** External	**Z** No Device	**Z** No Qualifier
8 Parotid Gland, Right **9** Parotid Gland, Left **B** Parotid Duct, Right **C** Parotid Duct, Left **D** Sublingual Gland, Right **F** Sublingual Gland, Left **G** Submaxillary Gland, Right **H** Submaxillary Gland, Left **J** Minor Salivary Gland	**0** Open **3** Percutaneous	**Z** No Device	**Z** No Qualifier
M Pharynx **R** Epiglottis **S** Larynx **T** Vocal Cord, Right **V** Vocal Cord, Left	**0** Open **3** Percutaneous **4** Percutaneous Endoscopic **7** Via Natural or Artificial Opening **8** Via Natural or Artificial Opening Endoscopic	**Z** No Device	**Z** No Qualifier
W Upper Tooth **X** Lower Tooth	**0** Open **X** External	**Z** No Device	**0** Single **1** Multiple **2** All

0 Medical and Surgical
C Mouth and Throat
D Extraction: Pulling or stripping out or off all or a portion of a body part by the use of force

Body Part Character 4	Approach Character 5	Device Character 6	Qualifier Character 7
T Vocal Cord, Right **V** Vocal Cord, Left	**0** Open **3** Percutaneous **4** Percutaneous Endoscopic **7** Via Natural or Artificial Opening **8** Via Natural or Artificial Opening Endoscopic	**Z** No Device	**Z** No Qualifier
W Upper Tooth **X** Lower Tooth	**X** External	**Z** No Device	**0** Single **1** Multiple **2** All

0 Medical and Surgical
C Mouth and Throat
F Fragmentation: Breaking solid matter in a body part into pieces

Body Part Character 4	Approach Character 5	Device Character 6	Qualifier Character 7
B Parotid Duct, Right NC **C** Parotid Duct, Left NC	**0** Open **3** Percutaneous **7** Via Natural or Artificial Opening **X** External	**Z** No Device	**Z** No Qualifier

NC 0CFBXZZ 0CFCXZZ

0 Medical and Surgical
C Mouth and Throat
H Insertion: Putting in a nonbiological appliance that monitors, assists, performs, or prevents a physiological function but does not physically take the place of a body part

Body Part Character 4	Approach Character 5	Device Character 6	Qualifier Character 7
7 Tongue	**0** Open **3** Percutaneous **X** External	**1** Radioactive Element	**Z** No Qualifier
A Salivary Gland **S** Larynx	**0** Open **3** Percutaneous **7** Via Natural or Artificial Opening **8** Via Natural or Artificial Opening Endoscopic	**Y** Other Device	**Z** No Qualifier
Y Mouth and Throat	**0** Open **3** Percutaneous	**Y** Other Device	**Z** No Qualifier
Y Mouth and Throat	**7** Via Natural or Artificial Opening **8** Via Natural or Artificial Opening Endoscopic	**B** Intraluminal Device, Airway **Y** Other Device	**Z** No Qualifier

0 Medical and Surgical
C Mouth and Throat
J Inspection: Visually and/or manually exploring a body part

Body Part Character 4	Approach Character 5	Device Character 6	Qualifier Character 7
A Salivary Gland	**0** Open **3** Percutaneous **X** External	**Z** No Device	**Z** No Qualifier
S Larynx **Y** Mouth and Throat	**0** Open **3** Percutaneous **4** Percutaneous Endoscopic **7** Via Natural or Artificial Opening **8** Via Natural or Artificial Opening Endoscopic **X** External	**Z** No Device	**Z** No Qualifier

0 Medical and Surgical
C Mouth and Throat
L Occlusion: Completely closing an orifice or the lumen of a tubular body part

Body Part Character 4	Approach Character 5	Device Character 6	Qualifier Character 7
B Parotid Duct, Right **C** Parotid Duct, Left	**0** Open **3** Percutaneous **4** Percutaneous Endoscopic	**C** Extraluminal Device **D** Intraluminal Device **Z** No Device	**Z** No Qualifier
B Parotid Duct, Right **C** Parotid Duct, Left	**7** Via Natural or Artificial Opening **8** Via Natural or Artificial Opening Endoscopic	**D** Intraluminal Device **Z** No Device	**Z** No Qualifier

0 Medical and Surgical
C Mouth and Throat
M Reattachment: Putting back in or on all or a portion of a separated body part to its normal location or other suitable location

Body Part Character 4	Approach Character 5	Device Character 6	Qualifier Character 7
0 Upper Lip **1** Lower Lip **3** Soft Palate **7** Tongue **N** Uvula	**0** Open	**Z** No Device	**Z** No Qualifier
W Upper Tooth **X** Lower Tooth	**0** Open **X** External	**Z** No Device	**0** Single **1** Multiple **2** All

0 Medical and Surgical
C Mouth and Throat
N Release: Freeing a body part from an abnormal physical constraint by cutting or by the use of force

Body Part Character 4	Approach Character 5	Device Character 6	Qualifier Character 7
0 Upper Lip **1** Lower Lip **2** Hard Palate **3** Soft Palate **4** Buccal Mucosa **5** Upper Gingiva **6** Lower Gingiva **7** Tongue **N** Uvula **P** Tonsils **Q** Adenoids	**0** Open **3** Percutaneous **X** External	**Z** No Device	**Z** No Qualifier
8 Parotid Gland, Right **9** Parotid Gland, Left **B** Parotid Duct, Right **C** Parotid Duct, Left **D** Sublingual Gland, Right **F** Sublingual Gland, Left **G** Submaxillary Gland, Right **H** Submaxillary Gland, Left **J** Minor Salivary Gland	**0** Open **3** Percutaneous	**Z** No Device	**Z** No Qualifier
M Pharynx **R** Epiglottis **S** Larynx **T** Vocal Cord, Right **V** Vocal Cord, Left	**0** Open **3** Percutaneous **4** Percutaneous Endoscopic **7** Via Natural or Artificial Opening **8** Via Natural or Artificial Opening Endoscopic	**Z** No Device	**Z** No Qualifier
W Upper Tooth **X** Lower Tooth	**0** Open **X** External	**Z** No Device	**0** Single **1** Multiple **2** All

0 Medical and Surgical
C Mouth and Throat
P Removal: Taking out or off a device from a body part

Body Part Character 4	Approach Character 5	Device Character 6	Qualifier Character 7
A Salivary Gland	**0** Open **3** Percutaneous	**0** Drainage Device **C** Extraluminal Device **Y** Other Device	**Z** No Qualifier
A Salivary Gland	**7** Via Natural or Artificial Opening **8** Via Natural or Artificial Opening Endoscopic	**Y** Other Device	**Z** No Qualifier
S Larynx CC	**0** Open **3** Percutaneous **7** Via Natural or Artificial Opening **8** Via Natural or Artificial Opening Endoscopic	**0** Drainage Device **7** Autologous Tissue Substitute **D** Intraluminal Device **J** Synthetic Substitute **K** Nonautologous Tissue Substitute **Y** Other Device	**Z** No Qualifier
S Larynx	**X** External	**0** Drainage Device **7** Autologous Tissue Substitute **D** Intraluminal Device **J** Synthetic Substitute **K** Nonautologous Tissue Substitute	**Z** No Qualifier

0CP continued on next page

0 Medical and Surgical
C Mouth and Throat
P Removal: Taking out or off a device from a body part

0CP continued from previous page

Body Part Character 4	Approach Character 5	Device Character 6	Qualifier Character 7
Y Mouth and Throat	**0** Open **3** Percutaneous **7** Via Natural or Artificial Opening **8** Via Natural or Artificial Opening Endoscopic	**0** Drainage Device **1** Radioactive Element **7** Autologous Tissue Substitute **D** Intraluminal Device **J** Synthetic Substitute **K** Nonautologous Tissue Substitute **Y** Other Device	**Z** No Qualifier
Y Mouth and Throat	**X** External	**0** Drainage Device **1** Radioactive Element **7** Autologous Tissue Substitute **D** Intraluminal Device **J** Synthetic Substitute **K** Nonautologous Tissue Substitute	**Z** No Qualifier

CC 0CPS0DZ 0CPS3DZ 0CPS7DZ 0CPS8DZ

0 Medical and Surgical
C Mouth and Throat
Q Repair: Restoring, to the extent possible, a body part to its normal anatomic structure and function

Body Part Character 4	Approach Character 5	Device Character 6	Qualifier Character 7
0 Upper Lip CC **1** Lower Lip CC **2** Hard Palate **3** Soft Palate **4** Buccal Mucosa CC **5** Upper Gingiva **6** Lower Gingiva **7** Tongue **N** Uvula **P** Tonsils **Q** Adenoids	**0** Open **3** Percutaneous **X** External	**Z** No Device	**Z** No Qualifier
8 Parotid Gland, Right **9** Parotid Gland, Left **B** Parotid Duct, Right **C** Parotid Duct, Left **D** Sublingual Gland, Right **F** Sublingual Gland, Left **G** Submaxillary Gland, Right **H** Submaxillary Gland, Left **J** Minor Salivary Gland	**0** Open **3** Percutaneous	**Z** No Device	**Z** No Qualifier
M Pharynx CC **R** Epiglottis **S** Larynx **T** Vocal Cord, Right **V** Vocal Cord, Left	**0** Open **3** Percutaneous **4** Percutaneous Endoscopic **7** Via Natural or Artificial Opening **8** Via Natural or Artificial Opening Endoscopic	**Z** No Device	**Z** No Qualifier
W Upper Tooth **X** Lower Tooth	**0** Open **X** External	**Z** No Device	**0** Single **1** Multiple **2** All

CC 0CQ00ZZ 0CQ03ZZ 0CQ10ZZ 0CQ13ZZ 0CQ40ZZ 0CQ43ZZ 0CQ4XZZ 0CQM0ZZ 0CQM3ZZ 0CQM4ZZ 0CQM7ZZ 0CQM8ZZ

0 Medical and Surgical
C Mouth and Throat
R Replacement: Putting in or on biological or synthetic material that physically takes the place and/or function of all or a portion of a body part

Body Part Character 4	Approach Character 5	Device Character 6	Qualifier Character 7
0 Upper Lip **1** Lower Lip **2** Hard Palate **3** Soft Palate **4** Buccal Mucosa **5** Upper Gingiva **6** Lower Gingiva **7** Tongue **N** Uvula	**0** Open **3** Percutaneous **X** External	**7** Autologous Tissue Substitute **J** Synthetic Substitute **K** Nonautologous Tissue Substitute	**Z** No Qualifier
B Parotid Duct, Right **C** Parotid Duct, Left	**0** Open **3** Percutaneous	**7** Autologous Tissue Substitute **J** Synthetic Substitute **K** Nonautologous Tissue Substitute	**Z** No Qualifier
M Pharynx **R** Epiglottis **S** Larynx CC **T** Vocal Cord, Right **V** Vocal Cord, Left	**0** Open **7** Via Natural or Artificial Opening **8** Via Natural or Artificial Opening Endoscopic	**7** Autologous Tissue Substitute **J** Synthetic Substitute **K** Nonautologous Tissue Substitute	**Z** No Qualifier
W Upper Tooth **X** Lower Tooth	**0** Open **X** External	**7** Autologous Tissue Substitute **J** Synthetic Substitute **K** Nonautologous Tissue Substitute	**0** Single **1** Multiple **2** All

CC 0CRS0JZ 0CRS7JZ 0CRS8JZ

0 Medical and Surgical
C Mouth and Throat
S Reposition: Moving to its normal location, or other suitable location, all or a portion of a body part

Body Part Character 4	Approach Character 5	Device Character 6	Qualifier Character 7
0 Upper Lip **1** Lower Lip **2** Hard Palate **3** Soft Palate **7** Tongue **N** Uvula	**0** Open **X** External	**Z** No Device	**Z** No Qualifier
B Parotid Duct, Right **C** Parotid Duct, Left	**0** Open **3** Percutaneous	**Z** No Device	**Z** No Qualifier
R Epiglottis **T** Vocal Cord, Right **V** Vocal Cord, Left	**0** Open **7** Via Natural or Artificial Opening **8** Via Natural or Artificial Opening Endoscopic	**Z** No Device	**Z** No Qualifier
W Upper Tooth **X** Lower Tooth	**0** Open **X** External	**5** External Fixation Device **Z** No Device	**0** Single **1** Multiple **2** All

0 Medical and Surgical
C Mouth and Throat
T Resection: Cutting out or off, without replacement, all of a body part

Body Part Character 4	Approach Character 5	Device Character 6	Qualifier Character 7
0 Upper Lip **1** Lower Lip **2** Hard Palate **3** Soft Palate **7** Tongue **N** Uvula **P** Tonsils CC **Q** Adenoids CC	**0** Open **X** External	**Z** No Device	**Z** No Qualifier
8 Parotid Gland, Right **9** Parotid Gland, Left **B** Parotid Duct, Right **C** Parotid Duct, Left **D** Sublingual Gland, Right **F** Sublingual Gland, Left **G** Submaxillary Gland, Right **H** Submaxillary Gland, Left **J** Minor Salivary Gland	**0** Open	**Z** No Device	**Z** No Qualifier
M Pharynx **R** Epiglottis **S** Larynx **T** Vocal Cord, Right **V** Vocal Cord, Left	**0** Open **4** Percutaneous Endoscopic **7** Via Natural or Artificial Opening **8** Via Natural or Artificial Opening Endoscopic	**Z** No Device	**Z** No Qualifier
W Upper Tooth **X** Lower Tooth	**0** Open	**Z** No Device	**0** Single **1** Multiple **2** All

CC 0CTP0ZZ 0CTPXZZ 0CTQ0ZZ 0CTQXZZ

0 Medical and Surgical
C Mouth and Throat
U Supplement: Putting in or on biological or synthetic material that physically reinforces and/or augments the function of a portion of a body part

Body Part Character 4	Approach Character 5	Device Character 6	Qualifier Character 7
0 Upper Lip **1** Lower Lip **2** Hard Palate **3** Soft Palate **4** Buccal Mucosa **5** Upper Gingiva **6** Lower Gingiva **7** Tongue **N** Uvula	**0** Open **3** Percutaneous **X** External	**7** Autologous Tissue Substitute **J** Synthetic Substitute **K** Nonautologous Tissue Substitute	**Z** No Qualifier
M Pharynx **R** Epiglottis **S** Larynx CC **T** Vocal Cord, Right **V** Vocal Cord, Left	**0** Open **7** Via Natural or Artificial Opening **8** Via Natural or Artificial Opening Endoscopic	**7** Autologous Tissue Substitute **J** Synthetic Substitute **K** Nonautologous Tissue Substitute	**Z** No Qualifier

CC 0CUS0JZ 0CUS7JZ 0CUS8JZ

0 Medical and Surgical
C Mouth and Throat
V Restriction: Partially closing an orifice or the lumen of a tubular body part

Body Part Character 4	Approach Character 5	Device Character 6	Qualifier Character 7
B Parotid Duct, Right **C** Parotid Duct, Left	**0** Open **3** Percutaneous	**C** Extraluminal Device **D** Intraluminal Device **Z** No Device	**Z** No Qualifier
B Parotid Duct, Right **C** Parotid Duct, Left	**7** Via Natural or Artificial Opening **8** Via Natural or Artificial Opening Endoscopic	**D** Intraluminal Device **Z** No Device	**Z** No Qualifier

0 Medical and Surgical
C Mouth and Throat
W Revision: Correcting, to the extent possible, a portion of a malfunctioning device or the position of a displaced device

Body Part Character 4	Approach Character 5	Device Character 6	Qualifier Character 7
A Salivary Gland	**0** Open **3** Percutaneous	**0** Drainage Device **C** Extraluminal Device **Y** Other Device	**Z** No Qualifier
A Salivary Gland	**7** Via Natural or Artificial Opening **8** Via Natural or Artificial Opening Endoscopic	**Y** Other Device	**Z** No Qualifier
A Salivary Gland	**X** External	**0** Drainage Device **C** Extraluminal Device	**Z** No Qualifier
S Larynx	**0** Open **3** Percutaneous **7** Via Natural or Artificial Opening **8** Via Natural or Artificial Opening Endoscopic	**0** Drainage Device **7** Autologous Tissue Substitute **D** Intraluminal Device **J** Synthetic Substitute **K** Nonautologous Tissue Substitute **Y** Other Device	**Z** No Qualifier
S Larynx	**X** External	**0** Drainage Device **7** Autologous Tissue Substitute **D** Intraluminal Device **J** Synthetic Substitute **K** Nonautologous Tissue Substitute	**Z** No Qualifier
Y Mouth and Throat	**0** Open **3** Percutaneous **7** Via Natural or Artificial Opening **8** Via Natural or Artificial Opening Endoscopic	**0** Drainage Device **1** Radioactive Element **7** Autologous Tissue Substitute **D** Intraluminal Device **J** Synthetic Substitute **K** Nonautologous Tissue Substitute **Y** Other Device	**Z** No Qualifier
Y Mouth and Throat	**X** External	**0** Drainage Device **1** Radioactive Element **7** Autologous Tissue Substitute **D** Intraluminal Device **J** Synthetic Substitute **K** Nonautologous Tissue Substitute	**Z** No Qualifier

0 Medical and Surgical
C Mouth and Throat
X Transfer: Moving, without taking out, all or a portion of a body part to another location to take over the function of all or a portion of a body part

Body Part Character 4	Approach Character 5	Device Character 6	Qualifier Character 7
0 Upper Lip **1** Lower Lip **3** Soft Palate **4** Buccal Mucosa **5** Upper Gingiva **6** Lower Gingiva **7** Tongue	**0** Open **X** External	**Z** No Device	**Z** No Qualifier

NOTES

NOTES

Gastrointestinal System 0D1-0DY

0 Medical and Surgical
D Gastrointestinal System
1 Bypass: Altering the route of passage of the contents of a tubular body part

Body Part Character 4	Approach Character 5	Device Character 6	Qualifier Character 7
1 Esophagus, Upper **2** Esophagus, Middle **3** Esophagus, Lower **5** Esophagus	**0** Open **4** Percutaneous Endoscopic **8** Via Natural or Artificial Opening Endoscopic	**7** Autologous Tissue Substitute **J** Synthetic Substitute **K** Nonautologous Tissue Substitute **Z** No Device	**4** Cutaneous **6** Stomach **9** Duodenum **A** Jejunum **B** Ileum
1 Esophagus, Upper **2** Esophagus, Middle **3** Esophagus, Lower **5** Esophagus	**3** Percutaneous	**J** Synthetic Substitute	**4** Cutaneous
6 Stomach HAC CC **9** Duodenum	**0** Open **4** Percutaneous Endoscopic **8** Via Natural or Artificial Opening Endoscopic	**7** Autologous Tissue Substitute **J** Synthetic Substitute **K** Nonautologous Tissue Substitute **Z** No Device	**4** Cutaneous **9** Duodenum **A** Jejunum **B** Ileum **L** Transverse Colon
6 Stomach **9** Duodenum	**3** Percutaneous	**J** Synthetic Substitute	**4** Cutaneous
A Jejunum	**0** Open **4** Percutaneous Endoscopic **8** Via Natural or Artificial Opening Endoscopic	**7** Autologous Tissue Substitute **J** Synthetic Substitute **K** Nonautologous Tissue Substitute **Z** No Device	**4** Cutaneous **A** Jejunum **B** Ileum **H** Cecum **K** Ascending Colon **L** Transverse Colon **M** Descending Colon **N** Sigmoid Colon **P** Rectum **Q** Anus
A Jejunum	**3** Percutaneous	**J** Synthetic Substitute	**4** Cutaneous
B Ileum	**0** Open **4** Percutaneous Endoscopic **8** Via Natural or Artificial Opening Endoscopic	**7** Autologous Tissue Substitute **J** Synthetic Substitute **K** Nonautologous Tissue Substitute **Z** No Device	**4** Cutaneous **B** Ileum **H** Cecum **K** Ascending Colon **L** Transverse Colon **M** Descending Colon **N** Sigmoid Colon **P** Rectum **Q** Anus
B Ileum	**3** Percutaneous	**J** Synthetic Substitute	**4** Cutaneous
H Cecum	**0** Open **4** Percutaneous Endoscopic **8** Via Natural or Artificial Opening Endoscopic	**7** Autologous Tissue Substitute **J** Synthetic Substitute **K** Nonautologous Tissue Substitute **Z** No Device	**4** Cutaneous **H** Cecum **K** Ascending Colon **L** Transverse Colon **M** Descending Colon **N** Sigmoid Colon **P** Rectum
H Cecum	**3** Percutaneous	**J** Synthetic Substitute	**4** Cutaneous
K Ascending Colon	**0** Open **4** Percutaneous Endoscopic **8** Via Natural or Artificial Opening Endoscopic	**7** Autologous Tissue Substitute **J** Synthetic Substitute **K** Nonautologous Tissue Substitute **Z** No Device	**4** Cutaneous **K** Ascending Colon **L** Transverse Colon **M** Descending Colon **N** Sigmoid Colon **P** Rectum
K Ascending Colon	**3** Percutaneous	**J** Synthetic Substitute	**4** Cutaneous

0D1 continued on next page

0 Medical and Surgical
D Gastrointestinal System
1 Bypass: Altering the route of passage of the contents of a tubular body part

0D1 continued from previous page

Body Part Character 4	Approach Character 5	Device Character 6	Qualifier Character 7
L Transverse Colon	0 Open 4 Percutaneous Endoscopic 8 Via Natural or Artificial Opening Endoscopic	7 Autologous Tissue Substitute J Synthetic Substitute K Nonautologous Tissue Substitute Z No Device	4 Cutaneous L Transverse Colon M Descending Colon N Sigmoid Colon P Rectum
L Transverse Colon	3 Percutaneous	J Synthetic Substitute	4 Cutaneous
M Descending Colon	0 Open 4 Percutaneous Endoscopic 8 Via Natural or Artificial Opening Endoscopic	7 Autologous Tissue Substitute J Synthetic Substitute K Nonautologous Tissue Substitute Z No Device	4 Cutaneous M Descending Colon N Sigmoid Colon P Rectum
M Descending Colon	3 Percutaneous	J Synthetic Substitute	4 Cutaneous
N Sigmoid Colon CC	0 Open 4 Percutaneous Endoscopic 8 Via Natural or Artificial Opening Endoscopic	7 Autologous Tissue Substitute J Synthetic Substitute K Nonautologous Tissue Substitute Z No Device	4 Cutaneous N Sigmoid Colon P Rectum
N Sigmoid Colon	3 Percutaneous	J Synthetic Substitute	4 Cutaneous

HAC 0D16079 0D1607A 0D1607B 0D1607L 0D160J9 0D160JA 0D160JB 0D160JL 0D160K9 0D160KA 0D160KB 0D160KL 0D160Z9 0D160ZA 0D160ZB 0D160ZL 0D16479 0D1647A 0D1647B 0D1647L 0D164J9 0D164JA 0D164JB 0D164JL 0D164K9 0D164KA 0D164KB 0D164KL 0D164Z9 0D164ZA 0D164ZB 0D164ZL 0D16879 0D1687A 0D1687B 0D1687L 0D168J9 0D168JA 0D168JB 0D168JL 0D168K9 0D168KA 0D168KB 0D168KL 0D168Z9 0D168ZA 0D168ZB 0D168ZL
Surgical site infection following bariatric surgery procedures and principal diagnoses E66.01 and secondary diagnoses K68.11, K95.01, K95.81, T81.4XXA.

CC 0D1607A 0D160JA 0D160KA 0D160ZA 0D160ZB 0D1N0Z4 0D1N4Z4

0 Medical and Surgical
D Gastrointestinal System
2 Change: Taking out or off a device from a body part and putting back an identical or similar device in or on the same body part without cutting or puncturing the skin or a mucous membrane

Body Part Character 4	Approach Character 5	Device Character 6	Qualifier Character 7
0 Upper Intestinal Tract D Lower Intestinal Tract	X External	0 Drainage Device U Feeding Device Y Other Device	Z No Qualifier
U Omentum V Mesentery W Peritoneum	X External	0 Drainage Device Y Other Device	Z No Qualifier

0 Medical and Surgical
D Gastrointestinal System
5 Destruction: Physical eradication of all or a portion of a body part by the direct use of energy, force, or a destructive agent

Body Part Character 4	Approach Character 5	Device Character 6	Qualifier Character 7
1 Esophagus, Upper **2** Esophagus, Middle **3** Esophagus, Lower **4** Esophagogastric Junction **5** Esophagus **6** Stomach **7** Stomach, Pylorus **8** Small Intestine **9** Duodenum **A** Jejunum **B** Ileum **C** Ileocecal Valve **E** Large Intestine **F** Large Intestine, Right **G** Large Intestine, Left **H** Cecum **J** Appendix **K** Ascending Colon **L** Transverse Colon **M** Descending Colon **N** Sigmoid Colon **P** Rectum	**0** Open **3** Percutaneous **4** Percutaneous Endoscopic **7** Via Natural or Artificial Opening **8** Via Natural or Artificial Opening Endoscopic	**Z** No Device	**Z** No Qualifier
Q Anus	**0** Open **3** Percutaneous **4** Percutaneous Endoscopic **7** Via Natural or Artificial Opening **8** Via Natural or Artificial Opening Endoscopic **X** External	**Z** No Device	**Z** No Qualifier
R Anal Sphincter **U** Omentum **V** Mesentery **W** Peritoneum	**0** Open **3** Percutaneous **4** Percutaneous Endoscopic	**Z** No Device	**Z** No Qualifier

0 Medical and Surgical
D Gastrointestinal System
7 Dilation: Expanding an orifice or the lumen of a tubular body part

Body Part Character 4	Approach Character 5	Device Character 6	Qualifier Character 7
1 Esophagus, Upper **2** Esophagus, Middle **3** Esophagus, Lower **4** Esophagogastric Junction **5** Esophagus **6** Stomach **7** Stomach, Pylorus **8** Small Intestine **9** Duodenum **A** Jejunum **B** Ileum **C** Ileocecal Valve **E** Large Intestine **F** Large Intestine, Right **G** Large Intestine, Left **H** Cecum **K** Ascending Colon **L** Transverse Colon **M** Descending Colon **N** Sigmoid Colon **P** Rectum **Q** Anus	**0** Open **3** Percutaneous **4** Percutaneous Endoscopic **7** Via Natural or Artificial Opening **8** Via Natural or Artificial Opening Endoscopic	**D** Intraluminal Device **Z** No Device	**Z** No Qualifier

0 Medical and Surgical
D Gastrointestinal System
8 Division: Cutting into a body part, without draining fluids and/or gases from the body part, in order to separate or transect a body part

Body Part Character 4	Approach Character 5	Device Character 6	Qualifier Character 7
4 Esophagogastric Junction **7** Stomach, Pylorus	**0** Open **3** Percutaneous **4** Percutaneous Endoscopic **7** Via Natural or Artificial Opening **8** Via Natural or Artificial Opening Endoscopic	**Z** No Device	**Z** No Qualifier
R Anal Sphincter	**0** Open **3** Percutaneous	**Z** No Device	**Z** No Qualifier

0 Medical and Surgical
D Gastrointestinal System
9 Drainage: Taking or letting out fluids and/or gases from a body part

Body Part Character 4	Approach Character 5	Device Character 6	Qualifier Character 7
1 Esophagus, Upper **2** Esophagus, Middle **3** Esophagus, Lower **4** Esophagogastric Junction **5** Esophagus **6** Stomach **7** Stomach, Pylorus **8** Small Intestine **9** Duodenum **A** Jejunum **B** Ileum **C** Ileocecal Valve **E** Large Intestine **F** Large Intestine, Right **G** Large Intestine, Left **H** Cecum **J** Appendix **K** Ascending Colon **L** Transverse Colon **M** Descending Colon **N** Sigmoid Colon **P** Rectum	**0** Open **3** Percutaneous **4** Percutaneous Endoscopic **7** Via Natural or Artificial Opening **8** Via Natural or Artificial Opening Endoscopic	**0** Drainage Device	**Z** No Qualifier
1 Esophagus, Upper **2** Esophagus, Middle **3** Esophagus, Lower **4** Esophagogastric Junction **5** Esophagus **6** Stomach **7** Stomach, Pylorus **8** Small Intestine **9** Duodenum **A** Jejunum **B** Ileum **C** Ileocecal Valve **E** Large Intestine **F** Large Intestine, Right **G** Large Intestine, Left **H** Cecum **J** Appendix **K** Ascending Colon **L** Transverse Colon **M** Descending Colon **N** Sigmoid Colon **P** Rectum	**0** Open **3** Percutaneous **4** Percutaneous Endoscopic **7** Via Natural or Artificial Opening **8** Via Natural or Artificial Opening Endoscopic	**Z** No Device	**X** Diagnostic **Z** No Qualifier
Q Anus	**0** Open **3** Percutaneous **4** Percutaneous Endoscopic **7** Via Natural or Artificial Opening **8** Via Natural or Artificial Opening Endoscopic **X** External	**0** Drainage Device	**Z** No Qualifier
Q Anus	**0** Open **3** Percutaneous **4** Percutaneous Endoscopic **7** Via Natural or Artificial Opening **8** Via Natural or Artificial Opening Endoscopic **X** External	**Z** No Device	**X** Diagnostic **Z** No Qualifier

0D9 continued on next page

0D9 continued from previous page

0 Medical and Surgical
D Gastrointestinal System
9 Drainage: Taking or letting out fluids and/or gases from a body part

Body Part Character 4	Approach Character 5	Device Character 6	Qualifier Character 7
R Anal Sphincter **U** Omentum **V** Mesentery **W** Peritoneum	**0** Open **3** Percutaneous **4** Percutaneous Endoscopic	**0** Drainage Device	**Z** No Qualifier
R Anal Sphincter **U** Omentum **V** Mesentery **W** Peritoneum	**0** Open **3** Percutaneous **4** Percutaneous Endoscopic	**Z** No Device	**X** Diagnostic **Z** No Qualifier

0 Medical and Surgical
D Gastrointestinal System
B Excision: Cutting out or off, without replacement, a portion of a body part

Body Part Character 4	Approach Character 5	Device Character 6	Qualifier Character 7
1 Esophagus, Upper **2** Esophagus, Middle **3** Esophagus, Lower **4** Esophagogastric Junction **5** Esophagus **7** Stomach, Pylorus **8** Small Intestine CC **9** Duodenum CC **A** Jejunum **B** Ileum CC **C** Ileocecal Valve **E** Large Intestine CC **F** Large Intestine, Right **H** Cecum **J** Appendix **K** Ascending Colon **P** Rectum	**0** Open **3** Percutaneous **4** Percutaneous Endoscopic **7** Via Natural or Artificial Opening **8** Via Natural or Artificial Opening Endoscopic	**Z** No Device	**X** Diagnostic **Z** No Qualifier
6 Stomach	**0** Open **3** Percutaneous **4** Percutaneous Endoscopic **7** Via Natural or Artificial Opening **8** Via Natural or Artificial Opening Endoscopic	**Z** No Device	**3** Vertical **X** Diagnostic **Z** No Qualifier
G Large Intestine, Left **L** Transverse Colon **M** Descending Colon **N** Sigmoid Colon CC	**0** Open **3** Percutaneous **4** Percutaneous Endoscopic **7** Via Natural or Artificial Opening **8** Via Natural or Artificial Opening Endoscopic	**Z** No Device	**X** Diagnostic **Z** No Qualifier
G Large Intestine, Left **L** Transverse Colon **M** Descending Colon **N** Sigmoid Colon	**F** Via Natural or Artificial Opening With Percutaneous Endoscopic Assistance	**Z** No Device	**Z** No Qualifier
Q Anus	**0** Open **3** Percutaneous **4** Percutaneous Endoscopic **7** Via Natural or Artificial Opening **8** Via Natural or Artificial Opening Endoscopic **X** External	**Z** No Device	**X** Diagnostic **Z** No Qualifier

0DB continued on next page

0DB continued from previous page

0 Medical and Surgical
D Gastrointestinal System
B Excision: Cutting out or off, without replacement, a portion of a body part

Body Part Character 4	Approach Character 5	Device Character 6	Qualifier Character 7
R Anal Sphincter **U** Omentum **V** Mesentery **W** Peritoneum	**0** Open **3** Percutaneous **4** Percutaneous Endoscopic	**Z** No Device	**X** Diagnostic **Z** No Qualifier

CC 0DB80ZZ 0DB90ZZ 0DBB0ZZ 0DBE0ZZ 0DBN0ZZ

0 Medical and Surgical
D Gastrointestinal System
C Extirpation: Taking or cutting out solid matter from a body part

Body Part Character 4	Approach Character 5	Device Character 6	Qualifier Character 7
1 Esophagus, Upper **2** Esophagus, Middle **3** Esophagus, Lower **4** Esophagogastric Junction **5** Esophagus **6** Stomach **7** Stomach, Pylorus **8** Small Intestine **9** Duodenum **A** Jejunum **B** Ileum **C** Ileocecal Valve **E** Large Intestine **F** Large Intestine, Right **G** Large Intestine, Left **H** Cecum **J** Appendix **K** Ascending Colon **L** Transverse Colon **M** Descending Colon **N** Sigmoid Colon **P** Rectum	**0** Open **3** Percutaneous **4** Percutaneous Endoscopic **7** Via Natural or Artificial Opening **8** Via Natural or Artificial Opening Endoscopic	**Z** No Device	**Z** No Qualifier
Q Anus	**0** Open **3** Percutaneous **4** Percutaneous Endoscopic **7** Via Natural or Artificial Opening **8** Via Natural or Artificial Opening Endoscopic **X** External	**Z** No Device	**Z** No Qualifier
R Anal Sphincter **U** Omentum **V** Mesentery **W** Peritoneum	**0** Open **3** Percutaneous **4** Percutaneous Endoscopic	**Z** No Device	**Z** No Qualifier

0 Medical and Surgical
D Gastrointestinal System
D Extraction: Pulling or stripping out or off all or a portion of a body part by the use of force

Body Part	Approach	Device	Qualifier
Character 4	Character 5	Character 6	Character 7
1 Esophagus, Upper **2** Esophagus, Middle **3** Esophagus, Lower **4** Esophagogastric Junction **5** Esophagus **6** Stomach **7** Stomach, Pylorus **8** Small Intestine **9** Duodenum **A** Jejunum **B** Ileum **C** Ileocecal Valve **E** Large Intestine **F** Large Intestine, Right **G** Large Intestine, Left **H** Cecum **J** Appendix **K** Ascending Colon **L** Transverse Colon **M** Descending Colon **N** Sigmoid Colon **P** Rectum	**3** Percutaneous **4** Percutaneous Endoscopic **8** Via Natural or Artificial Opening Endoscopic	**Z** No Device	**X** Diagnostic
Q Anus	**3** Percutaneous **4** Percutaneous Endoscopic **8** Via Natural or Artificial Opening Endoscopic **X** External	**Z** No Device	**X** Diagnostic

0 Medical and Surgical
D Gastrointestinal System
F Fragmentation: Breaking solid matter in a body part into pieces

Body Part	Approach	Device	Qualifier
Character 4	Character 5	Character 6	Character 7
5 Esophagus NC **6** Stomach NC **8** Small Intestine NC **9** Duodenum NC **A** Jejunum NC **B** Ileum NC **E** Large Intestine NC **F** Large Intestine, Right NC **G** Large Intestine, Left NC **H** Cecum NC **J** Appendix NC **K** Ascending Colon NC **L** Transverse Colon NC **M** Descending Colon NC **N** Sigmoid Colon NC **P** Rectum NC **Q** Anus NC	**0** Open **3** Percutaneous **4** Percutaneous Endoscopic **7** Via Natural or Artificial Opening **8** Via Natural or Artificial Opening Endoscopic **X** External	**Z** No Device	**Z** No Qualifier

NC 0DF5XZZ 0DF6XZZ 0DF8XZZ 0DF9XZZ 0DFAXZZ 0DFBXZZ 0DFEXZZ 0DFFXZZ 0DFGXZZ 0DFHXZZ 0DFJXZZ 0DFKXZZ 0DFLXZZ 0DFMXZZ 0DFNXZZ 0DFPXZZ 0DFQXZZ

0 Medical and Surgical
D Gastrointestinal System
H Insertion: Putting in a nonbiological appliance that monitors, assists, performs, or prevents a physiological function but does not physically take the place of a body part

Body Part	Approach	Device	Qualifier
Character 4	Character 5	Character 6	Character 7
0 Upper Intestinal Tract **D** Lower Intestinal Tract	**0** Open **3** Percutaneous **4** Percutaneous Endoscopic **7** Via Natural or Artificial Opening **8** Via Natural or Artificial Opening Endoscopic	**Y** Other Device	**Z** No Qualifier
5 Esophagus	**0** Open **3** Percutaneous **4** Percutaneous Endoscopic	**1** Radioactive Element **2** Monitoring Device **3** Infusion Device **D** Intraluminal Device **U** Feeding Device **Y** Other Device	**Z** No Qualifier
5 Esophagus	**7** Via Natural or Artificial Opening **8** Via Natural or Artificial Opening Endoscopic	**1** Radioactive Element **2** Monitoring Device **3** Infusion Device **B** Intraluminal Device, Airway **D** Intraluminal Device **U** Feeding Device **Y** Other Device	**Z** No Qualifier
6 Stomach CC	**0** Open **3** Percutaneous **4** Percutaneous Endoscopic	**2** Monitoring Device **3** Infusion Device **D** Intraluminal Device **M** Stimulator Lead **U** Feeding Device **Y** Other Device	**Z** No Qualifier
6 Stomach	**7** Via Natural or Artificial Opening **8** Via Natural or Artificial Opening Endoscopic	**2** Monitoring Device **3** Infusion Device **D** Intraluminal Device **U** Feeding Device **Y** Other Device	**Z** No Qualifier
8 Small Intestine **9** Duodenum **A** Jejunum **B** Ileum	**0** Open **3** Percutaneous **4** Percutaneous Endoscopic **7** Via Natural or Artificial Opening **8** Via Natural or Artificial Opening Endoscopic	**2** Monitoring Device **3** Infusion Device **D** Intraluminal Device **U** Feeding Device	**Z** No Qualifier
E Large Intestine	**0** Open **3** Percutaneous **4** Percutaneous Endoscopic **7** Via Natural or Artificial Opening **8** Via Natural or Artificial Opening Endoscopic	**D** Intraluminal Device	**Z** No Qualifier
P Rectum	**0** Open **3** Percutaneous **4** Percutaneous Endoscopic **7** Via Natural or Artificial Opening **8** Via Natural or Artificial Opening Endoscopic	**1** Radioactive Element **D** Intraluminal Device	**Z** No Qualifier
Q Anus	**0** Open **3** Percutaneous **4** Percutaneous Endoscopic	**D** Intraluminal Device **L** Artificial Sphincter	**Z** No Qualifier
Q Anus	**7** Via Natural or Artificial Opening **8** Via Natural or Artificial Opening Endoscopic	**D** Intraluminal Device	**Z** No Qualifier
R Anal Sphincter	**0** Open **3** Percutaneous **4** Percutaneous Endoscopic	**M** Stimulator Lead	**Z** No Qualifier

CC 0DH60MZ 0DH63MZ 0DH64MZ

LC Limited Coverage NC Noncovered HAC HAC-associated Procedure CC Combination Cluster - See Appendix G for code lists
DRG Non-OR-Affecting MS-DRG Assignment New/Revised Text in **Orange** ♂ Male ♀ Female

0 Medical and Surgical
D Gastrointestinal System
J Inspection: Visually and/or manually exploring a body part

Body Part Character 4	Approach Character 5	Device Character 6	Qualifier Character 7
0 Upper Intestinal Tract **6** Stomach **D** Lower Intestinal Tract	**0** Open **3** Percutaneous **4** Percutaneous Endoscopic **7** Via Natural or Artificial Opening **8** Via Natural or Artificial Opening Endoscopic **X** External	**Z** No Device	**Z** No Qualifier
U Omentum **V** Mesentery **W** Peritoneum	**0** Open **3** Percutaneous **4** Percutaneous Endoscopic **X** External	**Z** No Device	**Z** No Qualifier

0 Medical and Surgical
D Gastrointestinal System
L Occlusion: Completely closing an orifice or the lumen of a tubular body part

Body Part Character 4	Approach Character 5	Device Character 6	Qualifier Character 7
1 Esophagus, Upper **2** Esophagus, Middle **3** Esophagus, Lower **4** Esophagogastric Junction **5** Esophagus **6** Stomach **7** Stomach, Pylorus **8** Small Intestine **9** Duodenum **A** Jejunum **B** Ileum **C** Ileocecal Valve **E** Large Intestine **F** Large Intestine, Right **G** Large Intestine, Left **H** Cecum **K** Ascending Colon **L** Transverse Colon **M** Descending Colon **N** Sigmoid Colon **P** Rectum	**0** Open **3** Percutaneous **4** Percutaneous Endoscopic	**C** Extraluminal Device **D** Intraluminal Device **Z** No Device	**Z** No Qualifier
1 Esophagus, Upper **2** Esophagus, Middle **3** Esophagus, Lower **4** Esophagogastric Junction **5** Esophagus **6** Stomach **7** Stomach, Pylorus **8** Small Intestine **9** Duodenum **A** Jejunum **B** Ileum **C** Ileocecal Valve **E** Large Intestine **F** Large Intestine, Right **G** Large Intestine, Left **H** Cecum **K** Ascending Colon **L** Transverse Colon **M** Descending Colon **N** Sigmoid Colon **P** Rectum	**7** Via Natural or Artificial Opening **8** Via Natural or Artificial Opening Endoscopic	**D** Intraluminal Device **Z** No Device	**Z** No Qualifier

0DL continued on next page

0DL continued from previous page

0 Medical and Surgical
D Gastrointestinal System
L Occlusion: Completely closing an orifice or the lumen of a tubular body part

Body Part Character 4	Approach Character 5	Device Character 6	Qualifier Character 7
Q Anus	**0** Open **3** Percutaneous **4** Percutaneous Endoscopic **X** External	**C** Extraluminal Device **D** Intraluminal Device **Z** No Device	**Z** No Qualifier
Q Anus	**7** Via Natural or Artificial Opening **8** Via Natural or Artificial Opening Endoscopic	**D** Intraluminal Device **Z** No Device	**Z** No Qualifier

0 Medical and Surgical
D Gastrointestinal System
M Reattachment: Putting back in or on all or a portion of a separated body part to its normal location or other suitable location

Body Part Character 4	Approach Character 5	Device Character 6	Qualifier Character 7
5 Esophagus **6** Stomach **8** Small Intestine **9** Duodenum **A** Jejunum **B** Ileum **E** Large Intestine **F** Large Intestine, Right **G** Large Intestine, Left **H** Cecum **K** Ascending Colon **L** Transverse Colon **M** Descending Colon **N** Sigmoid Colon **P** Rectum	**0** Open **4** Percutaneous Endoscopic	**Z** No Device	**Z** No Qualifier

0 Medical and Surgical
D Gastrointestinal System
N Release: Freeing a body part from an abnormal physical constraint by cutting or by the use of force

Body Part Character 4	Approach Character 5	Device Character 6	Qualifier Character 7
1 Esophagus, Upper **2** Esophagus, Middle **3** Esophagus, Lower **4** Esophagogastric Junction **5** Esophagus **6** Stomach **7** Stomach, Pylorus **8** Small Intestine **9** Duodenum **A** Jejunum **B** Ileum **C** Ileocecal Valve **E** Large Intestine **F** Large Intestine, Right **G** Large Intestine, Left **H** Cecum **J** Appendix **K** Ascending Colon **L** Transverse Colon **M** Descending Colon **N** Sigmoid Colon **P** Rectum	**0** Open **3** Percutaneous **4** Percutaneous Endoscopic **7** Via Natural or Artificial Opening **8** Via Natural or Artificial Opening Endoscopic	**Z** No Device	**Z** No Qualifier

0DN continued on next page

0DN continued from previous page

0 Medical and Surgical
D Gastrointestinal System
N Release: Freeing a body part from an abnormal physical constraint by cutting or by the use of force

Body Part Character 4	Approach Character 5	Device Character 6	Qualifier Character 7
Q Anus	**0** Open **3** Percutaneous **4** Percutaneous Endoscopic **7** Via Natural or Artificial Opening **8** Via Natural or Artificial Opening Endoscopic **X** External	**Z** No Device	**Z** No Qualifier
R Anal Sphincter **U** Omentum **V** Mesentery **W** Peritoneum	**0** Open **3** Percutaneous **4** Percutaneous Endoscopic	**Z** No Device	**Z** No Qualifier

0 Medical and Surgical
D Gastrointestinal System
P Removal: Taking out or off a device from a body part

Body Part Character 4	Approach Character 5	Device Character 6	Qualifier Character 7
0 Upper Intestinal Tract **D** Lower Intestinal Tract	**0** Open **3** Percutaneous **4** Percutaneous Endoscopic **7** Via Natural or Artificial Opening **8** Via Natural or Artificial Opening Endoscopic	**0** Drainage Device **2** Monitoring Device **3** Infusion Device **7** Autologous Tissue Substitute **C** Extraluminal Device **D** Intraluminal Device **J** Synthetic Substitute **K** Nonautologous Tissue Substitute **U** Feeding Device **Y** Other Device	**Z** No Qualifier
0 Upper Intestinal Tract **D** Lower Intestinal Tract	**X** External	**0** Drainage Device **2** Monitoring Device **3** Infusion Device **D** Intraluminal Device **U** Feeding Device	**Z** No Qualifier
5 Esophagus	**0** Open **3** Percutaneous **4** Percutaneous Endoscopic	**1** Radioactive Element **2** Monitoring Device **3** Infusion Device **U** Feeding Device **Y** Other Device	**Z** No Qualifier
5 Esophagus	**7** Via Natural or Artificial Opening **8** Via Natural or Artificial Opening Endoscopic	**1** Radioactive Element **D** Intraluminal Device **Y** Other Device	**Z** No Qualifier
5 Esophagus	**X** External	**1** Radioactive Element **2** Monitoring Device **3** Infusion Device **D** Intraluminal Device **U** Feeding Device	**Z** No Qualifier
6 Stomach	**0** Open **3** Percutaneous **4** Percutaneous Endoscopic	**0** Drainage Device **2** Monitoring Device **3** Infusion Device **7** Autologous Tissue Substitute **C** Extraluminal Device **D** Intraluminal Device **J** Synthetic Substitute **K** Nonautologous Tissue Substitute **M** Stimulator Lead **U** Feeding Device **Y** Other Device	**Z** No Qualifier

0DP continued on next page

0 Medical and Surgical
D Gastrointestinal System
P Removal: Taking out or off a device from a body part

0DP continued from previous page

Body Part Character 4	Approach Character 5	Device Character 6	Qualifier Character 7
6 Stomach	**7** Via Natural or Artificial Opening **8** Via Natural or Artificial Opening Endoscopic	**0** Drainage Device **2** Monitoring Device **3** Infusion Device **7** Autologous Tissue Substitute **C** Extraluminal Device **D** Intraluminal Device **J** Synthetic Substitute **K** Nonautologous Tissue Substitute **U** Feeding Device **Y** Other Device	**Z** No Qualifier
6 Stomach	**X** External	**0** Drainage Device **2** Monitoring Device **3** Infusion Device **D** Intraluminal Device **U** Feeding Device	**Z** No Qualifier
P Rectum	**0** Open **3** Percutaneous **4** Percutaneous Endoscopic **7** Via Natural or Artificial Opening **8** Via Natural or Artificial Opening Endoscopic **X** External	**1** Radioactive Element	**Z** No Qualifier
Q Anus	**0** Open **3** Percutaneous **4** Percutaneous Endoscopic **7** Via Natural or Artificial Opening **8** Via Natural or Artificial Opening Endoscopic	**L** Artificial Sphincter	**Z** No Qualifier
R Anal Sphincter	**0** Open **3** Percutaneous **4** Percutaneous Endoscopic	**M** Stimulator Lead	**Z** No Qualifier
U Omentum **V** Mesentery **W** Peritoneum	**0** Open **3** Percutaneous **4** Percutaneous Endoscopic	**0** Drainage Device **1** Radioactive Element **7** Autologous Tissue Substitute **J** Synthetic Substitute **K** Nonautologous Tissue Substitute	**Z** No Qualifier

0 Medical and Surgical
D Gastrointestinal System
Q Repair: Restoring, to the extent possible, a body part to its normal anatomic structure and function

Body Part Character 4	Approach Character 5	Device Character 6	Qualifier Character 7
1 Esophagus, Upper **2** Esophagus, Middle **3** Esophagus, Lower **4** Esophagogastric Junction **5** Esophagus CC **6** Stomach CC **7** Stomach, Pylorus **8** Small Intestine CC **9** Duodenum CC **A** Jejunum CC **B** Ileum CC **C** Ileocecal Valve **E** Large Intestine CC **F** Large Intestine, Right CC **G** Large Intestine, Left CC **H** Cecum CC **J** Appendix CC **K** Ascending Colon CC **L** Transverse Colon CC **M** Descending Colon CC **N** Sigmoid Colon CC **P** Rectum CC	**0** Open **3** Percutaneous **4** Percutaneous Endoscopic **7** Via Natural or Artificial Opening **8** Via Natural or Artificial Opening Endoscopic	**Z** No Device	**Z** No Qualifier
Q Anus CC	**0** Open **3** Percutaneous **4** Percutaneous Endoscopic **7** Via Natural or Artificial Opening **8** Via Natural or Artificial Opening Endoscopic **X** External	**Z** No Device	**Z** No Qualifier
R Anal Sphincter **U** Omentum **V** Mesentery **W** Peritoneum CC	**0** Open **3** Percutaneous **4** Percutaneous Endoscopic	**Z** No Device	**Z** No Qualifier

CC 0DQ50ZZ 0DQ53ZZ 0DQ54ZZ 0DQ57ZZ 0DQ58ZZ 0DQ60ZZ 0DQ63ZZ 0DQ64ZZ 0DQ67ZZ 0DQ68ZZ 0DQ80ZZ 0DQ90ZZ 0DQA0ZZ 0DQB0ZZ 0DQE0ZZ 0DQF0ZZ 0DQG0ZZ 0DQH0ZZ 0DQJ0ZZ 0DQJ3ZZ 0DQJ4ZZ 0DQJ7ZZ 0DQJ8ZZ 0DQK0ZZ 0DQL0ZZ 0DQM0ZZ 0DQN0ZZ 0DQN3ZZ 0DQN4ZZ 0DQN7ZZ 0DQN8ZZ 0DQP0ZZ 0DQP3ZZ 0DQP4ZZ 0DQP7ZZ 0DQP8ZZ 0DQQ0ZZ 0DQQ3ZZ 0DQQ4ZZ 0DQQ7ZZ 0DQQ8ZZ 0DQW0ZZ 0DQW3ZZ 0DQW4ZZ

0 Medical and Surgical
D Gastrointestinal System
R Replacement: Putting in or on biological or synthetic material that physically takes the place and/or function of all or a portion of a body part

Body Part Character 4	Approach Character 5	Device Character 6	Qualifier Character 7
5 Esophagus	**0** Open **4** Percutaneous Endoscopic **7** Via Natural or Artificial Opening **8** Via Natural or Artificial Opening Endoscopic	**7** Autologous Tissue Substitute **J** Synthetic Substitute **K** Nonautologous Tissue Substitute	**Z** No Qualifier
R Anal Sphincter **U** Omentum **V** Mesentery **W** Peritoneum	**0** Open **4** Percutaneous Endoscopic	**7** Autologous Tissue Substitute **J** Synthetic Substitute **K** Nonautologous Tissue Substitute	**Z** No Qualifier

0 Medical and Surgical
D Gastrointestinal System
S Reposition: Moving to its normal location, or other suitable location, all or a portion of a body part

Body Part Character 4	Approach Character 5	Device Character 6	Qualifier Character 7
5 Esophagus **6** Stomach **9** Duodenum **A** Jejunum **B** Ileum **H** Cecum **K** Ascending Colon **L** Transverse Colon **M** Descending Colon **N** Sigmoid Colon **P** Rectum **Q** Anus	**0** Open **4** Percutaneous Endoscopic **7** Via Natural or Artificial Opening **8** Via Natural or Artificial Opening Endoscopic **X** External	**Z** No Device	**Z** No Qualifier
8 Small Intestine **E** Large Intestine	**0** Open **4** Percutaneous Endoscopic **7** Via Natural or Artificial Opening **8** Via Natural or Artificial Opening Endoscopic	**Z** No Device	**Z** No Qualifier

0 Medical and Surgical
D Gastrointestinal System
T Resection: Cutting out or off, without replacement, all of a body part

Body Part Character 4	Approach Character 5	Device Character 6	Qualifier Character 7
1 Esophagus, Upper **2** Esophagus, Middle **3** Esophagus, Lower **4** Esophagogastric Junction **5** Esophagus **6** Stomach **7** Stomach, Pylorus **8** Small Intestine **9** Duodenum CC **A** Jejunum **B** Ileum **C** Ileocecal Valve **E** Large Intestine **F** Large Intestine, Right **H** Cecum **J** Appendix **K** Ascending Colon **P** Rectum CC **Q** Anus	**0** Open **4** Percutaneous Endoscopic **7** Via Natural or Artificial Opening **8** Via Natural or Artificial Opening Endoscopic	**Z** No Device	**Z** No Qualifier
G Large Intestine, Left **L** Transverse Colon **M** Descending Colon **N** Sigmoid Colon CC	**0** Open **4** Percutaneous Endoscopic **7** Via Natural or Artificial Opening **8** Via Natural or Artificial Opening Endoscopic **F** Via Natural or Artificial Opening With Percutaneous Endoscopic Assistance	**Z** No Device	**Z** No Qualifier
R Anal Sphincter **U** Omentum	**0** Open **4** Percutaneous Endoscopic	**Z** No Device	**Z** No Qualifier

CC 0DT90ZZ 0DTN0ZZ 0DTN4ZZ 0DTP0ZZ 0DTP4ZZ 0DTP7ZZ 0DTP8ZZ

0 Medical and Surgical
D Gastrointestinal System
U Supplement: Putting in or on biological or synthetic material that physically reinforces and/or augments the function of a portion of a body part

Body Part Character 4	Approach Character 5	Device Character 6	Qualifier Character 7
1 Esophagus, Upper **2** Esophagus, Middle **3** Esophagus, Lower **4** Esophagogastric Junction **5** Esophagus **6** Stomach **7** Stomach, Pylorus **8** Small Intestine **9** Duodenum **A** Jejunum **B** Ileum **C** Ileocecal Valve **E** Large Intestine **F** Large Intestine, Right **G** Large Intestine, Left **H** Cecum **K** Ascending Colon **L** Transverse Colon **M** Descending Colon **N** Sigmoid Colon **P** Rectum	**0** Open **4** Percutaneous Endoscopic **7** Via Natural or Artificial Opening **8** Via Natural or Artificial Opening Endoscopic	**7** Autologous Tissue Substitute **J** Synthetic Substitute **K** Nonautologous Tissue Substitute	**Z** No Qualifier
Q Anus	**0** Open **4** Percutaneous Endoscopic **7** Via Natural or Artificial Opening **8** Via Natural or Artificial Opening Endoscopic **X** External	**7** Autologous Tissue Substitute **J** Synthetic Substitute **K** Nonautologous Tissue Substitute	**Z** No Qualifier
R Anal Sphincter **U** Omentum **V** Mesentery **W** Peritoneum	**0** Open **4** Percutaneous Endoscopic	**7** Autologous Tissue Substitute **J** Synthetic Substitute **K** Nonautologous Tissue Substitute	**Z** No Qualifier

0 Medical and Surgical
D Gastrointestinal System
V Restriction: Partially closing an orifice or the lumen of a tubular body part

Body Part Character 4	Approach Character 5	Device Character 6	Qualifier Character 7
1 Esophagus, Upper **2** Esophagus, Middle **3** Esophagus, Lower **4** Esophagogastric Junction **5** Esophagus **6** Stomach HAC **7** Stomach, Pylorus **8** Small Intestine **9** Duodenum **A** Jejunum **B** Ileum **C** Ileocecal Valve **E** Large Intestine **F** Large Intestine, Right **G** Large Intestine, Left **H** Cecum **K** Ascending Colon **L** Transverse Colon **M** Descending Colon **N** Sigmoid Colon **P** Rectum	**0** Open **3** Percutaneous **4** Percutaneous Endoscopic	**C** Extraluminal Device **D** Intraluminal Device **Z** No Device	**Z** No Qualifier

0DV continued on next page

0 Medical and Surgical
D Gastrointestinal System
V Restriction: Partially closing an orifice or the lumen of a tubular body part

0DV continued from previous page

Body Part Character 4	Approach Character 5	Device Character 6	Qualifier Character 7
1 Esophagus, Upper 2 Esophagus, Middle 3 Esophagus, Lower 4 Esophagogastric Junction 5 Esophagus 6 Stomach NC 7 Stomach, Pylorus 8 Small Intestine 9 Duodenum A Jejunum B Ileum C Ileocecal Valve E Large Intestine F Large Intestine, Right G Large Intestine, Left H Cecum K Ascending Colon L Transverse Colon M Descending Colon N Sigmoid Colon P Rectum	7 Via Natural or Artificial Opening 8 Via Natural or Artificial Opening Endoscopic	D Intraluminal Device Z No Device	Z No Qualifier
Q Anus	0 Open 3 Percutaneous 4 Percutaneous Endoscopic X External	C Extraluminal Device D Intraluminal Device Z No Device	Z No Qualifier
Q Anus	7 Via Natural or Artificial Opening 8 Via Natural or Artificial Opening Endoscopic	D Intraluminal Device Z No Device	Z No Qualifier

NC 0DV67DZ 0DV68DZ
HAC 0DV64CZ
Surgical A1:E1309 infection following bariatric surgery procedures and principal diagnoses E66.01 and secondary diagnoses K68.11, K95.01, K95.81, T81.4XXA.

0 Medical and Surgical
D Gastrointestinal System
W Revision: Correcting, to the extent possible, a portion of a malfunctioning device or the position of a displaced device

Body Part Character 4	Approach Character 5	Device Character 6	Qualifier Character 7
0 Upper Intestinal Tract D Lower Intestinal Tract	0 Open 3 Percutaneous 4 Percutaneous Endoscopic 7 Via Natural or Artificial Opening 8 Via Natural or Artificial Opening Endoscopic	0 Drainage Device 2 Monitoring Device 3 Infusion Device 7 Autologous Tissue Substitute C Extraluminal Device D Intraluminal Device J Synthetic Substitute K Nonautologous Tissue Substitute U Feeding Device Y Other Device	Z No Qualifier
0 Upper Intestinal Tract D Lower Intestinal Tract	X External	0 Drainage Device 2 Monitoring Device 3 Infusion Device 7 Autologous Tissue Substitute C Extraluminal Device D Intraluminal Device J Synthetic Substitute K Nonautologous Tissue Substitute U Feeding Device	Z No Qualifier

0DW continued on next page

0 Medical and Surgical
D Gastrointestinal System
W Revision: Correcting, to the extent possible, a portion of a malfunctioning device or the position of a displaced device

0DW continued from previous page

Body Part Character 4	Approach Character 5	Device Character 6	Qualifier Character 7
5 Esophagus	**0** Open **3** Percutaneous **4** Percutaneous Endoscopic	**Y** Other Device	**Z** No Qualifier
5 Esophagus	**7** Via Natural or Artificial Opening **8** Via Natural or Artificial Opening Endoscopic	**D** Intraluminal Device **Y** Other Device	**Z** No Qualifier
5 Esophagus	**X** External	**D** Intraluminal Device	**Z** No Qualifier
6 Stomach	**0** Open **3** Percutaneous **4** Percutaneous Endoscopic	**0** Drainage Device **2** Monitoring Device **3** Infusion Device **7** Autologous Tissue Substitute **C** Extraluminal Device **D** Intraluminal Device **J** Synthetic Substitute **K** Nonautologous Tissue Substitute **M** Stimulator Lead **U** Feeding Device **Y** Other Device	**Z** No Qualifier
6 Stomach	**7** Via Natural or Artificial Opening **8** Via Natural or Artificial Opening Endoscopic	**0** Drainage Device **2** Monitoring Device **3** Infusion Device **7** Autologous Tissue Substitute **C** Extraluminal Device **D** Intraluminal Device **J** Synthetic Substitute **K** Nonautologous Tissue Substitute **U** Feeding Device **Y** Other Device	**Z** No Qualifier
6 Stomach	**X** External	**0** Drainage Device **2** Monitoring Device **3** Infusion Device **7** Autologous Tissue Substitute **C** Extraluminal Device **D** Intraluminal Device **J** Synthetic Substitute **K** Nonautologous Tissue Substitute **U** Feeding Device	**Z** No Qualifier
8 Small Intestine **E** Large Intestine	**0** Open **4** Percutaneous Endoscopic **7** Via Natural or Artificial Opening **8** Via Natural or Artificial Opening Endoscopic	**7** Autologous Tissue Substitute **J** Synthetic Substitute **K** Nonautologous Tissue Substitute	**Z** No Qualifier
Q Anus	**0** Open **3** Percutaneous **4** Percutaneous Endoscopic **7** Via Natural or Artificial Opening **8** Via Natural or Artificial Opening Endoscopic	**L** Artificial Sphincter	**Z** No Qualifier
R Anal Sphincter	**0** Open **3** Percutaneous **4** Percutaneous Endoscopic	**M** Stimulator Lead	**Z** No Qualifier
U Omentum **V** Mesentery **W** Peritoneum	**0** Open **3** Percutaneous **4** Percutaneous Endoscopic	**0** Drainage Device **7** Autologous Tissue Substitute **J** Synthetic Substitute **K** Nonautologous Tissue Substitute	**Z** No Qualifier

0 Medical and Surgical
D Gastrointestinal System
X Transfer: Moving, without taking out, all or a portion of a body part to another location to take over the function of all or a portion of a body part

Body Part Character 4	Approach Character 5	Device Character 6	Qualifier Character 7
6 Stomach **8** Small Intestine **E** Large Intestine	**0** Open **4** Percutaneous Endoscopic	**Z** No Device	**5** Esophagus

0 Medical and Surgical
D Gastrointestinal System
Y Transplantation: Putting in or on all or a portion of a living body part taken from another individual or animal to physically take the place and/or function of all or a portion of a similar body part

Body Part Character 4	Approach Character 5	Device Character 6	Qualifier Character 7
5 Esophagus **6** Stomach **8** Small Intestine LC **E** Large Intestine LC	**0** Open	**Z** No Device	**0** Allogeneic **1** Syngeneic **2** Zooplastic

LC 0DY80Z0 0DY80Z1 0DY80Z2 0DYE0Z0 0DYE0Z1 0DYE0Z2

NOTES

Hepatobiliary System and Pancreas 0F1-0FY

0 Medical and Surgical
F Hepatobiliary System and Pancreas
1 Bypass: Altering the route of passage of the contents of a tubular body part

Body Part Character 4	Approach Character 5	Device Character 6	Qualifier Character 7
4 Gallbladder **5** Hepatic Duct, Right **6** Hepatic Duct, Left **7** Hepatic Duct, Common **8** Cystic Duct **9** Common Bile Duct CC	**0** Open **4** Percutaneous Endoscopic	**D** Intraluminal Device **Z** No Device	**3** Duodenum **4** Stomach **5** Hepatic Duct, Right **6** Hepatic Duct, Left **7** Hepatic Duct, Caudate **8** Cystic Duct **9** Common Bile Duct **B** Small Intestine
D Pancreatic Duct **F** Pancreatic Duct, Accessory **G** Pancreas CC	**0** Open **4** Percutaneous Endoscopic	**D** Intraluminal Device **Z** No Device	**3** Duodenum **B** Small Intestine **C** Large Intestine

CC 0F190Z3 0F1G0ZC

0 Medical and Surgical
F Hepatobiliary System and Pancreas
2 Change: Taking out or off a device from a body part and putting back an identical or similar device in or on the same body part without cutting or puncturing the skin or a mucous membrane

Body Part Character 4	Approach Character 5	Device Character 6	Qualifier Character 7
0 Liver **4** Gallbladder **B** Hepatobiliary Duct **D** Pancreatic Duct **G** Pancreas	**X** External	**0** Drainage Device **Y** Other Device	**Z** No Qualifier

0 Medical and Surgical
F Hepatobiliary System and Pancreas
5 Destruction: Physical eradication of all or a portion of a body part by the direct use of energy, force, or a destructive agent

Body Part Character 4	Approach Character 5	Device Character 6	Qualifier Character 7
0 Liver **1** Liver, Right Lobe **2** Liver, Left Lobe	**0** Open **3** Percutaneous **4** Percutaneous Endoscopic	**Z** No Device	**F** Irreversible Electroporation **Z** No Qualifier
4 Gallbladder	**0** Open **3** Percutaneous **4** Percutaneous Endoscopic **8** Via Natural or Artificial Opening Endoscopic	**Z** No Device	**Z** No Qualifier
5 Hepatic Duct, Right **6** Hepatic Duct, Left **7** Hepatic Duct, Common **8** Cystic Duct **9** Common Bile Duct **C** Ampulla of Vater **D** Pancreatic Duct **F** Pancreatic Duct, Accessory	**0** Open **3** Percutaneous **4** Percutaneous Endoscopic **7** Via Natural or Artificial Opening **8** Via Natural or Artificial Opening Endoscopic	**Z** No Device	**Z** No Qualifier
G Pancreas	**0** Open **3** Percutaneous **4** Percutaneous Endoscopic	**Z** No Device	**F** Irreversible Electroporation **Z** No Qualifier
G Pancreas	**8** Via Natural or Artificial Opening Endoscopic	**Z** No Device	**Z** No Qualifier

0 Medical and Surgical
F Hepatobiliary System and Pancreas
7 Dilation: Expanding an orifice or the lumen of a tubular body part

Body Part Character 4	Approach Character 5	Device Character 6	Qualifier Character 7
5 Hepatic Duct, Right CC **6** Hepatic Duct, Left CC **7** Hepatic Duct, Common **8** Cystic Duct CC **9** Common Bile Duct CC **C** Ampulla of Vater **D** Pancreatic Duct CC **F** Pancreatic Duct, Accessory	**0** Open **3** Percutaneous **4** Percutaneous Endoscopic **7** Via Natural or Artificial Opening **8** Via Natural or Artificial Opening Endoscopic	**D** Intraluminal Device **Z** No Device	**Z** No Qualifier

CC 0F757DZ 0F758DZ 0F767DZ 0F768DZ 0F787DZ 0F788DZ 0F797DZ 0F798DZ 0F7D7DZ 0F7D8DZ

0 Medical and Surgical
F Hepatobiliary System and Pancreas
8 Division: Cutting into a body part, without draining fluids and/or gases from the body part, in order to separate or transect a body part

Body Part Character 4	Approach Character 5	Device Character 6	Qualifier Character 7
G Pancreas	**0** Open **3** Percutaneous **4** Percutaneous Endoscopic	**Z** No Device	**Z** No Qualifier

0 Medical and Surgical
F Hepatobiliary System and Pancreas
9 Drainage: Taking or letting out fluids and/or gases from a body part

Body Part Character 4	Approach Character 5	Device Character 6	Qualifier Character 7
0 Liver **1** Liver, Right Lobe **2** Liver, Left Lobe	**0** Open **3** Percutaneous **4** Percutaneous Endoscopic	**0** Drainage Device	**Z** No Qualifier
0 Liver **1** Liver, Right Lobe **2** Liver, Left Lobe	**0** Open **3** Percutaneous **4** Percutaneous Endoscopic	**Z** No Device	**X** Diagnostic **Z** No Qualifier
4 Gallbladder **G** Pancreas	**0** Open **3** Percutaneous **4** Percutaneous Endoscopic **8** Via Natural or Artificial Opening Endoscopic	**0** Drainage Device	**Z** No Qualifier
4 Gallbladder **G** Pancreas	**0** Open **3** Percutaneous **4** Percutaneous Endoscopic **8** Via Natural or Artificial Opening Endoscopic	**Z** No Device	**X** Diagnostic **Z** No Qualifier
5 Hepatic Duct, Right **6** Hepatic Duct, Left **7** Hepatic Duct, Common **8** Cystic Duct **9** Common Bile Duct **C** Ampulla of Vater **D** Pancreatic Duct **F** Pancreatic Duct, Accessory	**0** Open **3** Percutaneous **4** Percutaneous Endoscopic **7** Via Natural or Artificial Opening **8** Via Natural or Artificial Opening Endoscopic	**0** Drainage Device	**Z** No Qualifier
5 Hepatic Duct, Right **6** Hepatic Duct, Left **7** Hepatic Duct, Common **8** Cystic Duct **9** Common Bile Duct **C** Ampulla of Vater **D** Pancreatic Duct **F** Pancreatic Duct, Accessory	**0** Open **3** Percutaneous **4** Percutaneous Endoscopic **7** Via Natural or Artificial Opening **8** Via Natural or Artificial Opening Endoscopic	**Z** No Device	**X** Diagnostic **Z** No Qualifier

0 Medical and Surgical
F Hepatobiliary System and Pancreas
B Excision: Cutting out or off, without replacement, a portion of a body part

Body Part Character 4	Approach Character 5	Device Character 6	Qualifier Character 7
0 Liver 1 Liver, Right Lobe 2 Liver, Left Lobe	0 Open 3 Percutaneous 4 Percutaneous Endoscopic	Z No Device	X Diagnostic Z No Qualifier
4 Gallbladder G Pancreas	0 Open 3 Percutaneous 4 Percutaneous Endoscopic 8 Via Natural or Artificial Opening Endoscopic	Z No Device	X Diagnostic Z No Qualifier
5 Hepatic Duct, Right 6 Hepatic Duct, Left 7 Hepatic Duct, Common 8 Cystic Duct 9 Common Bile Duct C Ampulla of Vater D Pancreatic Duct F Pancreatic Duct, Accessory	0 Open 3 Percutaneous 4 Percutaneous Endoscopic 7 Via Natural or Artificial Opening 8 Via Natural or Artificial Opening Endoscopic	Z No Device	X Diagnostic Z No Qualifier

0 Medical and Surgical
F Hepatobiliary System and Pancreas
C Extirpation: Taking or cutting out solid matter from a body part

Body Part Character 4	Approach Character 5	Device Character 6	Qualifier Character 7
0 Liver 1 Liver, Right Lobe 2 Liver, Left Lobe	0 Open 3 Percutaneous 4 Percutaneous Endoscopic	Z No Device	Z No Qualifier
4 Gallbladder G Pancreas	0 Open 3 Percutaneous 4 Percutaneous Endoscopic 8 Via Natural or Artificial Opening Endoscopic	Z No Device	Z No Qualifier
5 Hepatic Duct, Right 6 Hepatic Duct, Left 7 Hepatic Duct, Common 8 Cystic Duct 9 Common Bile Duct C Ampulla of Vater D Pancreatic Duct F Pancreatic Duct, Accessory	0 Open 3 Percutaneous 4 Percutaneous Endoscopic 7 Via Natural or Artificial Opening 8 Via Natural or Artificial Opening Endoscopic	Z No Device	Z No Qualifier

0 Medical and Surgical
F Hepatobiliary System and Pancreas
D Extraction: Pulling or stripping out or off all or a portion of a body part by the use of force

Body Part Character 4	Approach Character 5	Device Character 6	Qualifier Character 7
0 Liver 1 Liver, Right Lobe 2 Liver, Left Lobe	3 Percutaneous 4 Percutaneous Endoscopic	Z No Device	X Diagnostic
4 Gallbladder 5 Hepatic Duct, Right 6 Hepatic Duct, Left 7 Hepatic Duct, Common 8 Cystic Duct 9 Common Bile Duct C Ampulla of Vater D Pancreatic Duct F Pancreatic Duct, Accessory G Pancreas	3 Percutaneous 4 Percutaneous Endoscopic 8 Via Natural or Artificial Opening Endoscopic	Z No Device	X Diagnostic

LC Limited Coverage NC Noncovered HAC HAC-associated Procedure CC Combination Cluster - See Appendix G for code lists
DRG Non-OR-Affecting MS-DRG Assignment New/Revised Text in **Orange** ♂ Male ♀ Female

0 Medical and Surgical
F Hepatobiliary System and Pancreas
F Fragmentation: Breaking solid matter in a body part into pieces

Body Part Character 4	Approach Character 5	Device Character 6	Qualifier Character 7
4 Gallbladder NC 5 Hepatic Duct, Right NC 6 Hepatic Duct, Left NC 7 Hepatic Duct, Common 8 Cystic Duct NC 9 Common Bile Duct NC C Ampulla of Vater NC D Pancreatic Duct NC F Pancreatic Duct, Accessory NC	0 Open 3 Percutaneous 4 Percutaneous Endoscopic 7 Via Natural or Artificial Opening 8 Via Natural or Artificial Opening Endoscopic X External	Z No Device	Z No Qualifier

NC 0FF4XZZ 0FF5XZZ 0FF6XZZ 0FF8XZZ 0FF9XZZ 0FFCXZZ 0FFDXZZ 0FFFXZZ

0 Medical and Surgical
F Hepatobiliary System and Pancreas
H Insertion: Putting in a nonbiological appliance that monitors, assists, performs, or prevents a physiological function but does not physically take the place of a body part

Body Part Character 4	Approach Character 5	Device Character 6	Qualifier Character 7
0 Liver 4 Gallbladder G Pancreas	0 Open 3 Percutaneous 4 Percutaneous Endoscopic	2 Monitoring Device 3 Infusion Device Y Other Device	Z No Qualifier
1 Liver, Right Lobe 2 Liver, Left Lobe	0 Open 3 Percutaneous 4 Percutaneous Endoscopic	2 Monitoring Device 3 Infusion Device	Z No Qualifier
B Hepatobiliary Duct CC D Pancreatic Duct	0 Open 3 Percutaneous 4 Percutaneous Endoscopic 7 Via Natural or Artificial Opening 8 Via Natural or Artificial Opening Endoscopic	1 Radioactive Element 2 Monitoring Device 3 Infusion Device D Intraluminal Device Y Other Device	Z No Qualifier

CC 0FHB7DZ 0FHB8DZ

0 Medical and Surgical
F Hepatobiliary System and Pancreas
J Inspection: Visually and/or manually exploring a body part

Body Part Character 4	Approach Character 5	Device Character 6	Qualifier Character 7
0 Liver	0 Open 3 Percutaneous 4 Percutaneous Endoscopic X External	Z No Device	Z No Qualifier
4 Gallbladder G Pancreas	0 Open 3 Percutaneous 4 Percutaneous Endoscopic 8 Via Natural or Artificial Opening Endoscopic X External	Z No Device	Z No Qualifier
B Hepatobiliary Duct D Pancreatic Duct	0 Open 3 Percutaneous 4 Percutaneous Endoscopic 7 Via Natural or Artificial Opening 8 Via Natural or Artificial Opening Endoscopic	Z No Device	Z No Qualifier

0 Medical and Surgical
F Hepatobiliary System and Pancreas
L Occlusion: Completely closing an orifice or the lumen of a tubular body part

Body Part Character 4	Approach Character 5	Device Character 6	Qualifier Character 7
5 Hepatic Duct, Right **6** Hepatic Duct, Left **7** Hepatic Duct, Common **8** Cystic Duct **9** Common Bile Duct **C** Ampulla of Vater **D** Pancreatic Duct **F** Pancreatic Duct, Accessory	**0** Open **3** Percutaneous **4** Percutaneous Endoscopic	**C** Extraluminal Device **D** Intraluminal Device **Z** No Device	**Z** No Qualifier
5 Hepatic Duct, Right **6** Hepatic Duct, Left **7** Hepatic Duct, Common **8** Cystic Duct **9** Common Bile Duct **C** Ampulla of Vater **D** Pancreatic Duct **F** Pancreatic Duct, Accessory	**7** Via Natural or Artificial Opening **8** Via Natural or Artificial Opening Endoscopic	**D** Intraluminal Device **Z** No Device	**Z** No Qualifier

0 Medical and Surgical
F Hepatobiliary System and Pancreas
M Reattachment: Putting back in or on all or a portion of a separated body part to its normal location or other suitable location

Body Part Character 4	Approach Character 5	Device Character 6	Qualifier Character 7
0 Liver **1** Liver, Right Lobe **2** Liver, Left Lobe **4** Gallbladder **5** Hepatic Duct, Right **6** Hepatic Duct, Left **7** Hepatic Duct, Common **8** Cystic Duct **9** Common Bile Duct **C** Ampulla of Vater **D** Pancreatic Duct **F** Pancreatic Duct, Accessory **G** Pancreas	**0** Open **4** Percutaneous Endoscopic	**Z** No Device	**Z** No Qualifier

0 Medical and Surgical
F Hepatobiliary System and Pancreas
N Release: Freeing a body part from an abnormal physical constraint by cutting or by the use of force

Body Part Character 4	Approach Character 5	Device Character 6	Qualifier Character 7
0 Liver **1** Liver, Right Lobe **2** Liver, Left Lobe	**0** Open **3** Percutaneous **4** Percutaneous Endoscopic	**Z** No Device	**Z** No Qualifier
4 Gallbladder **G** Pancreas	**0** Open **3** Percutaneous **4** Percutaneous Endoscopic **8** Via Natural or Artificial Opening Endoscopic	**Z** No Device	**Z** No Qualifier
5 Hepatic Duct, Right **6** Hepatic Duct, Left **7** Hepatic Duct, Common **8** Cystic Duct **9** Common Bile Duct **C** Ampulla of Vater **D** Pancreatic Duct **F** Pancreatic Duct, Accessory	**0** Open **3** Percutaneous **4** Percutaneous Endoscopic **7** Via Natural or Artificial Opening **8** Via Natural or Artificial Opening Endoscopic	**Z** No Device	**Z** No Qualifier

0 Medical and Surgical
F Hepatobiliary System and Pancreas
P Removal: Taking out or off a device from a body part

Body Part Character 4	Approach Character 5	Device Character 6	Qualifier Character 7
0 Liver	**0** Open **3** Percutaneous **4** Percutaneous Endoscopic	**0** Drainage Device **2** Monitoring Device **3** Infusion Device **Y** Other Device	**Z** No Qualifier
0 Liver	**X** External	**0** Drainage Device **2** Monitoring Device **3** Infusion Device	**Z** No Qualifier
4 Gallbladder **G** Pancreas	**0** Open **3** Percutaneous **4** Percutaneous Endoscopic	**0** Drainage Device **2** Monitoring Device **3** Infusion Device **D** Intraluminal Device **Y** Other Device	**Z** No Qualifier
4 Gallbladder **G** Pancreas	**X** External	**0** Drainage Device **2** Monitoring Device **3** Infusion Device **D** Intraluminal Device	**Z** No Qualifier
B Hepatobiliary Duct CC **D** Pancreatic Duct CC	**0** Open **3** Percutaneous **4** Percutaneous Endoscopic **7** Via Natural or Artificial Opening **8** Via Natural or Artificial Opening Endoscopic	**0** Drainage Device **1** Radioactive Element **2** Monitoring Device **3** Infusion Device **7** Autologous Tissue Substitute **C** Extraluminal Device **D** Intraluminal Device **J** Synthetic Substitute **K** Nonautologous Tissue Substitute **Y** Other Device	**Z** No Qualifier
B Hepatobiliary Duct CC **D** Pancreatic Duct CC	**X** External	**0** Drainage Device **1** Radioactive Element **2** Monitoring Device **3** Infusion Device **D** Intraluminal Device	**Z** No Qualifier

CC 0FPB7DZ 0FPB8DZ 0FPBXDZ 0FPD7DZ 0FPD8DZ 0FPDXDZ

0 Medical and Surgical
F Hepatobiliary System and Pancreas
Q Repair: Restoring, to the extent possible, a body part to its normal anatomic structure and function

Body Part Character 4	Approach Character 5	Device Character 6	Qualifier Character 7
0 Liver CC **1** Liver, Right Lobe **2** Liver, Left Lobe	**0** Open **3** Percutaneous **4** Percutaneous Endoscopic	**Z** No Device	**Z** No Qualifier
4 Gallbladder CC **G** Pancreas	**0** Open **3** Percutaneous **4** Percutaneous Endoscopic **8** Via Natural or Artificial Opening Endoscopic	**Z** No Device	**Z** No Qualifier
5 Hepatic Duct, Right **6** Hepatic Duct, Left **7** Hepatic Duct, Common **8** Cystic Duct **9** Common Bile Duct **C** Ampulla of Vater **D** Pancreatic Duct **F** Pancreatic Duct, Accessory	**0** Open **3** Percutaneous **4** Percutaneous Endoscopic **7** Via Natural or Artificial Opening **8** Via Natural or Artificial Opening Endoscopic	**Z** No Device	**Z** No Qualifier

CC 0FQ00ZZ 0FQ03ZZ 0FQ04ZZ 0FQ40ZZ 0FQ43ZZ 0FQ44ZZ

0 Medical and Surgical
F Hepatobiliary System and Pancreas
R Replacement: Putting in or on biological or synthetic material that physically takes the place and/or function of all or a portion of a body part

Body Part Character 4	Approach Character 5	Device Character 6	Qualifier Character 7
5 Hepatic Duct, Right **6** Hepatic Duct, Left **7** Hepatic Duct, Common **8** Cystic Duct **9** Common Bile Duct **C** Ampulla of Vater **D** Pancreatic Duct **F** Pancreatic Duct, Accessory	**0** Open **4** Percutaneous Endoscopic **8** Via Natural or Artificial Opening Endoscopic	**7** Autologous Tissue Substitute **J** Synthetic Substitute **K** Nonautologous Tissue Substitute	**Z** No Qualifier

0 Medical and Surgical
F Hepatobiliary System and Pancreas
S Reposition: Moving to its normal location, or other suitable location, all or a portion of a body part

Body Part Character 4	Approach Character 5	Device Character 6	Qualifier Character 7
0 Liver **4** Gallbladder **5** Hepatic Duct, Right **6** Hepatic Duct, Left **7** Hepatic Duct, Common **8** Cystic Duct **9** Common Bile Duct **C** Ampulla of Vater **D** Pancreatic Duct **F** Pancreatic Duct, Accessory **G** Pancreas	**0** Open **4** Percutaneous Endoscopic	**Z** No Device	**Z** No Qualifier

0 Medical and Surgical
F Hepatobiliary System and Pancreas
T Resection: Cutting out or off, without replacement, all of a body part

Body Part Character 4	Approach Character 5	Device Character 6	Qualifier Character 7
0 Liver **1** Liver, Right Lobe **2** Liver, Left Lobe **4** Gallbladder **G** Pancreas CC	**0** Open **4** Percutaneous Endoscopic	**Z** No Device	**Z** No Qualifier
5 Hepatic Duct, Right **6** Hepatic Duct, Left **7** Hepatic Duct, Common **8** Cystic Duct **9** Common Bile Duct **C** Ampulla of Vater **D** Pancreatic Duct **F** Pancreatic Duct, Accessory	**0** Open **4** Percutaneous Endoscopic **7** Via Natural or Artificial Opening **8** Via Natural or Artificial Opening Endoscopic	**Z** No Device	**Z** No Qualifier

CC 0FTG0ZZ

0 Medical and Surgical
F Hepatobiliary System and Pancreas
U Supplement: Putting in or on biological or synthetic material that physically reinforces and/or augments the function of a portion of a body part

Body Part Character 4	Approach Character 5	Device Character 6	Qualifier Character 7
5 Hepatic Duct, Right **6** Hepatic Duct, Left **7** Hepatic Duct, Common **8** Cystic Duct **9** Common Bile Duct **C** Ampulla of Vater **D** Pancreatic Duct **F** Pancreatic Duct, Accessory	**0** Open **3** Percutaneous **4** Percutaneous Endoscopic **8** Via Natural or Artificial Opening Endoscopic	**7** Autologous Tissue Substitute **J** Synthetic Substitute **K** Nonautologous Tissue Substitute	**Z** No Qualifier

0 Medical and Surgical
F Hepatobiliary System and Pancreas
V Restriction: Partially closing an orifice or the lumen of a tubular body part

Body Part Character 4	Approach Character 5	Device Character 6	Qualifier Character 7
5 Hepatic Duct, Right **6** Hepatic Duct, Left **7** Hepatic Duct, Common **8** Cystic Duct **9** Common Bile Duct **C** Ampulla of Vater **D** Pancreatic Duct **F** Pancreatic Duct, Accessory	**0** Open **3** Percutaneous **4** Percutaneous Endoscopic	**C** Extraluminal Device **D** Intraluminal Device **Z** No Device	**Z** No Qualifier
5 Hepatic Duct, Right **6** Hepatic Duct, Left **7** Hepatic Duct, Common **8** Cystic Duct **9** Common Bile Duct **C** Ampulla of Vater **D** Pancreatic Duct **F** Pancreatic Duct, Accessory	**7** Via Natural or Artificial Opening **8** Via Natural or Artificial Opening Endoscopic	**D** Intraluminal Device **Z** No Device	**Z** No Qualifier

0 Medical and Surgical
F Hepatobiliary System and Pancreas
W Revision: Correcting, to the extent possible, a portion of a malfunctioning device or the position of a displaced device

Body Part Character 4	Approach Character 5	Device Character 6	Qualifier Character 7
0 Liver	**0** Open **3** Percutaneous **4** Percutaneous Endoscopic	**0** Drainage Device **2** Monitoring Device **3** Infusion Device **Y** Other Device	**Z** No Qualifier
0 Liver	**X** External	**0** Drainage Device **2** Monitoring Device **3** Infusion Device	**Z** No Qualifier
4 Gallbladder **G** Pancreas	**0** Open **3** Percutaneous **4** Percutaneous Endoscopic	**0** Drainage Device **2** Monitoring Device **3** Infusion Device **D** Intraluminal Device **Y** Other Device	**Z** No Qualifier
4 Gallbladder **G** Pancreas	**X** External	**0** Drainage Device **2** Monitoring Device **3** Infusion Device **D** Intraluminal Device	**Z** No Qualifier

0FW continued on next page

0 Medical and Surgical
F Hepatobiliary System and Pancreas
W Revision: Correcting, to the extent possible, a portion of a malfunctioning device or the position of a displaced device

0FW continued from previous page

Body Part Character 4	Approach Character 5	Device Character 6	Qualifier Character 7
B Hepatobiliary Duct **D** Pancreatic Duct	**0** Open **3** Percutaneous **4** Percutaneous Endoscopic **7** Via Natural or Artificial Opening **8** Via Natural or Artificial Opening Endoscopic	**0** Drainage Device **2** Monitoring Device **3** Infusion Device **7** Autologous Tissue Substitute **C** Extraluminal Device **D** Intraluminal Device **J** Synthetic Substitute **K** Nonautologous Tissue Substitute **Y** Other Device	**Z** No Qualifier
B Hepatobiliary Duct **D** Pancreatic Duct	**X** External	**0** Drainage Device **2** Monitoring Device **3** Infusion Device **7** Autologous Tissue Substitute **C** Extraluminal Device **D** Intraluminal Device **J** Synthetic Substitute **K** Nonautologous Tissue Substitute	**Z** No Qualifier

0 Medical and Surgical
F Hepatobiliary System and Pancreas
Y Transplantation: Putting in or on all or a portion of a living body part taken from another individual or animal to physically take the place and/or function of all or a portion of a similar body part

Body Part Character 4	Approach Character 5	Device Character 6	Qualifier Character 7
0 Liver LC **G** Pancreas NC LC CC	**0** Open	**Z** No Device	**0** Allogeneic **1** Syngeneic **2** Zooplastic

LC 0FY00Z0 0FY00Z1 0FY00Z2 0FYG0Z0 0FYG0Z1
NC 0FYG0Z2
NC 0FYG0Z0 0FYG0Z1
The procedure identified is a noncovered procedure except when combined with procedures codes 0TY00Z0, 0TY00Z1, 0TY00Z2, 0TY10Z0, 0TY10Z1, 0TY10Z2 and with diagnosis codes: E10.10, E10.11, E10.21, E10.22, E10.29, E10.311, E10.319, E10.3211, E10.3212, E10.3213, E10.3219, E10.3291, E10.3292, E10.3293, E10.3299, E10.3311, E10.3312, E10.3313, E10.3319, E10.3391, E10.3392, E10.3393, E10.3399, E10.3411, E10.3412, E10.3413, E10.3419, E10.3491, E10.3492, E10.3493, E10.3499, E10.3511, E10.3512, E10.3513, E10.3519, E10.3521, E10.3522, E10.3523, E10.3529, E10.3531, E10.3532, E10.3533, E10.3539, E10.3541, E10.3542, E10.3543, E10.3549, E10.3551, E10.3552, E10.3553, E10.3559, E10.3591, E10.3592, E10.3593, E10.3599, E10.36, E10.37X1, E10.37X2, E10.37X3, E10.37X9, E10.39, E10.40, E10.41, E10.42, E10.43, E10.44, E10.49, E10.51, E10.52, E10.59, E10.610, E10.618, E10.620, E10.621, E10.622, E10.628, E10.630, E10.638, E10.641, E10.649, E10.65, E10.69, E10.8, E10.9, E89.1.
CC 0FYG0Z0 0FYG0Z1 0FYG0Z2

NOTES

Endocrine System 0G2-0GW

0 Medical and Surgical
G Endocrine System
2 Change: Taking out or off a device from a body part and putting back an identical or similar device in or on the same body part without cutting or puncturing the skin or a mucous membrane

Body Part Character 4	Approach Character 5	Device Character 6	Qualifier Character 7
0 Pituitary Gland **1** Pineal Body **5** Adrenal Gland **K** Thyroid Gland **R** Parathyroid Gland **S** Endocrine Gland	**X** External	**0** Drainage Device **Y** Other Device	**Z** No Qualifier

0 Medical and Surgical
G Endocrine System
5 Destruction: Physical eradication of all or a portion of a body part by the direct use of energy, force, or a destructive agent

Body Part Character 4	Approach Character 5	Device Character 6	Qualifier Character 7
0 Pituitary Gland **1** Pineal Body **2** Adrenal Gland, Left **3** Adrenal Gland, Right **4** Adrenal Glands, Bilateral **6** Carotid Body, Left **7** Carotid Body, Right **8** Carotid Bodies, Bilateral **9** Para-aortic Body **B** Coccygeal Glomus **C** Glomus Jugulare **D** Aortic Body **F** Paraganglion Extremity **G** Thyroid Gland Lobe, Left **H** Thyroid Gland Lobe, Right **K** Thyroid Gland **L** Superior Parathyroid Gland, Right **M** Superior Parathyroid Gland, Left **N** Inferior Parathyroid Gland, Right **P** Inferior Parathyroid Gland, Left **Q** Parathyroid Glands, Multiple **R** Parathyroid Gland	**0** Open **3** Percutaneous **4** Percutaneous Endoscopic	**Z** No Device	**Z** No Qualifier

0 Medical and Surgical
G Endocrine System
8 Division: Cutting into a body part, without draining fluids and/or gases from the body part, in order to separate or transect a body part

Body Part Character 4	Approach Character 5	Device Character 6	Qualifier Character 7
0 Pituitary Gland **J** Thyroid Gland Isthmus	**0** Open **3** Percutaneous **4** Percutaneous Endoscopic	**Z** No Device	**Z** No Qualifier

0 Medical and Surgical
G Endocrine System
9 Drainage: Taking or letting out fluids and/or gases from a body part

Body Part Character 4	Approach Character 5	Device Character 6	Qualifier Character 7
0 Pituitary Gland 1 Pineal Body 2 Adrenal Gland, Left 3 Adrenal Gland, Right 4 Adrenal Glands, Bilateral 6 Carotid Body, Left 7 Carotid Body, Right 8 Carotid Bodies, Bilateral 9 Para-aortic Body B Coccygeal Glomus C Glomus Jugulare D Aortic Body F Paraganglion Extremity G Thyroid Gland Lobe, Left H Thyroid Gland Lobe, Right K Thyroid Gland L Superior Parathyroid Gland, Right M Superior Parathyroid Gland, Left N Inferior Parathyroid Gland, Right P Inferior Parathyroid Gland, Left Q Parathyroid Glands, Multiple R Parathyroid Gland	0 Open 3 Percutaneous 4 Percutaneous Endoscopic	0 Drainage Device	Z No Qualifier
0 Pituitary Gland 1 Pineal Body 2 Adrenal Gland, Left 3 Adrenal Gland, Right 4 Adrenal Glands, Bilateral 6 Carotid Body, Left 7 Carotid Body, Right 8 Carotid Bodies, Bilateral 9 Para-aortic Body B Coccygeal Glomus C Glomus Jugulare D Aortic Body F Paraganglion Extremity G Thyroid Gland Lobe, Left H Thyroid Gland Lobe, Right K Thyroid Gland L Superior Parathyroid Gland, Right M Superior Parathyroid Gland, Left N Inferior Parathyroid Gland, Right P Inferior Parathyroid Gland, Left Q Parathyroid Glands, Multiple R Parathyroid Gland	0 Open 3 Percutaneous 4 Percutaneous Endoscopic	Z No Device	X Diagnostic Z No Qualifier

0 Medical and Surgical
G Endocrine System
B Excision: Cutting out or off, without replacement, a portion of a body part

Body Part Character 4	Approach Character 5	Device Character 6	Qualifier Character 7
0 Pituitary Gland **1** Pineal Body **2** Adrenal Gland, Left **3** Adrenal Gland, Right **4** Adrenal Glands, Bilateral **6** Carotid Body, Left **7** Carotid Body, Right **8** Carotid Bodies, Bilateral **9** Para-aortic Body **B** Coccygeal Glomus **C** Glomus Jugulare **D** Aortic Body **F** Paraganglion Extremity **G** Thyroid Gland Lobe, Left **H** Thyroid Gland Lobe, Right **J** Thyroid Gland Isthmus **L** Superior Parathyroid Gland, Right **M** Superior Parathyroid Gland, Left **N** Inferior Parathyroid Gland, Right **P** Inferior Parathyroid Gland, Left **Q** Parathyroid Glands, Multiple **R** Parathyroid Gland	**0** Open **3** Percutaneous **4** Percutaneous Endoscopic	**Z** No Device	**X** Diagnostic **Z** No Qualifier

0 Medical and Surgical
G Endocrine System
C Extirpation: Taking or cutting out solid matter from a body part

Body Part Character 4	Approach Character 5	Device Character 6	Qualifier Character 7
0 Pituitary Gland **1** Pineal Body **2** Adrenal Gland, Left **3** Adrenal Gland, Right **4** Adrenal Glands, Bilateral **6** Carotid Body, Left **7** Carotid Body, Right **8** Carotid Bodies, Bilateral **9** Para-aortic Body **B** Coccygeal Glomus **C** Glomus Jugulare **D** Aortic Body **F** Paraganglion Extremity **G** Thyroid Gland Lobe, Left **H** Thyroid Gland Lobe, Right **K** Thyroid Gland **L** Superior Parathyroid Gland, Right **M** Superior Parathyroid Gland, Left **N** Inferior Parathyroid Gland, Right **P** Inferior Parathyroid Gland, Left **Q** Parathyroid Glands, Multiple **R** Parathyroid Gland	**0** Open **3** Percutaneous **4** Percutaneous Endoscopic	**Z** No Device	**Z** No Qualifier

0 Medical and Surgical
G Endocrine System
H Insertion: Putting in a nonbiological appliance that monitors, assists, performs, or prevents a physiological function but does not physically take the place of a body part

Body Part	Approach	Device	Qualifier
Character 4	**Character 5**	**Character 6**	**Character 7**
S Endocrine Gland	**0** Open **3** Percutaneous **4** Percutaneous Endoscopic	**2** Monitoring Device **3** Infusion Device **Y** Other Device	**Z** No Qualifier

0 Medical and Surgical
G Endocrine System
J Inspection: Visually and/or manually exploring a body part

Body Part	Approach	Device	Qualifier
Character 4	**Character 5**	**Character 6**	**Character 7**
0 Pituitary Gland **1** Pineal Body **5** Adrenal Gland **K** Thyroid Gland **R** Parathyroid Gland **S** Endocrine Gland	**0** Open **3** Percutaneous **4** Percutaneous Endoscopic	**Z** No Device	**Z** No Qualifier

0 Medical and Surgical
G Endocrine System
M Reattachment: Putting back in or on all or a portion of a separated body part to its normal location or other suitable location

Body Part	Approach	Device	Qualifier
Character 4	**Character 5**	**Character 6**	**Character 7**
2 Adrenal Gland, Left **3** Adrenal Gland, Right **G** Thyroid Gland Lobe, Left **H** Thyroid Gland Lobe, Right **L** Superior Parathyroid Gland, Right **M** Superior Parathyroid Gland, Left **N** Inferior Parathyroid Gland, Right **P** Inferior Parathyroid Gland, Left **Q** Parathyroid Glands, Multiple **R** Parathyroid Gland	**0** Open **4** Percutaneous Endoscopic	**Z** No Device	**Z** No Qualifier

0 Medical and Surgical
G Endocrine System
N Release: Freeing a body part from an abnormal physical constraint by cutting or by the use of force

Body Part Character 4	Approach Character 5	Device Character 6	Qualifier Character 7
0 Pituitary Gland **1** Pineal Body **2** Adrenal Gland, Left **3** Adrenal Gland, Right **4** Adrenal Glands, Bilateral **6** Carotid Body, Left **7** Carotid Body, Right **8** Carotid Bodies, Bilateral **9** Para-aortic Body **B** Coccygeal Glomus **C** Glomus Jugulare **D** Aortic Body **F** Paraganglion Extremity **G** Thyroid Gland Lobe, Left **H** Thyroid Gland Lobe, Right **K** Thyroid Gland **L** Superior Parathyroid Gland, Right **M** Superior Parathyroid Gland, Left **N** Inferior Parathyroid Gland, Right **P** Inferior Parathyroid Gland, Left **Q** Parathyroid Glands, Multiple **R** Parathyroid Gland	**0** Open **3** Percutaneous **4** Percutaneous Endoscopic	**Z** No Device	**Z** No Qualifier

0 Medical and Surgical
G Endocrine System
P Removal: Taking out or off a device from a body part

Body Part Character 4	Approach Character 5	Device Character 6	Qualifier Character 7
0 Pituitary Gland **1** Pineal Body **5** Adrenal Gland **K** Thyroid Gland **R** Parathyroid Gland	**0** Open **3** Percutaneous **4** Percutaneous Endoscopic **X** External	**0** Drainage Device	**Z** No Qualifier
S Endocrine Gland	**0** Open **3** Percutaneous **4** Percutaneous Endoscopic	**0** Drainage Device **2** Monitoring Device **3** Infusion Device **Y** Other Device	**Z** No Qualifier
S Endocrine Gland	**X** External	**0** Drainage Device **2** Monitoring Device **3** Infusion Device	**Z** No Qualifier

0 Medical and Surgical
G Endocrine System
Q Repair: Restoring, to the extent possible, a body part to its normal anatomic structure and function

Body Part Character 4	Approach Character 5	Device Character 6	Qualifier Character 7
0 Pituitary Gland **1** Pineal Body **2** Adrenal Gland, Left **3** Adrenal Gland, Right **4** Adrenal Glands, Bilateral **6** Carotid Body, Left **7** Carotid Body, Right **8** Carotid Bodies, Bilateral **9** Para-aortic Body **B** Coccygeal Glomus **C** Glomus Jugulare **D** Aortic Body **F** Paraganglion Extremity **G** Thyroid Gland Lobe, Left **H** Thyroid Gland Lobe, Right **J** Thyroid Gland Isthmus **K** Thyroid Gland **L** Superior Parathyroid Gland, Right **M** Superior Parathyroid Gland, Left **N** Inferior Parathyroid Gland, Right **P** Inferior Parathyroid Gland, Left **Q** Parathyroid Glands, Multiple **R** Parathyroid Gland	**0** Open **3** Percutaneous **4** Percutaneous Endoscopic	**Z** No Device	**Z** No Qualifier

0 Medical and Surgical
G Endocrine System
S Reposition: Moving to its normal location, or other suitable location, all or a portion of a body part

Body Part Character 4	Approach Character 5	Device Character 6	Qualifier Character 7
2 Adrenal Gland, Left **3** Adrenal Gland, Right **G** Thyroid Gland Lobe, Left **H** Thyroid Gland Lobe, Right **L** Superior Parathyroid Gland, Right **M** Superior Parathyroid Gland, Left **N** Inferior Parathyroid Gland, Right **P** Inferior Parathyroid Gland, Left **Q** Parathyroid Glands, Multiple **R** Parathyroid Gland	**0** Open **4** Percutaneous Endoscopic	**Z** No Device	**Z** No Qualifier

0 Medical and Surgical
G Endocrine System
T Resection: Cutting out or off, without replacement, all of a body part

Body Part Character 4	Approach Character 5	Device Character 6	Qualifier Character 7
0 Pituitary Gland **1** Pineal Body **2** Adrenal Gland, Left **3** Adrenal Gland, Right **4** Adrenal Glands, Bilateral **6** Carotid Body, Left **7** Carotid Body, Right **8** Carotid Bodies, Bilateral **9** Para-aortic Body **B** Coccygeal Glomus **C** Glomus Jugulare **D** Aortic Body **F** Paraganglion Extremity **G** Thyroid Gland Lobe, Left **H** Thyroid Gland Lobe, Right **J** Thyroid Gland Isthmus **K** Thyroid Gland **L** Superior Parathyroid Gland, Right **M** Superior Parathyroid Gland, Left **N** Inferior Parathyroid Gland, Right **P** Inferior Parathyroid Gland, Left **Q** Parathyroid Glands, Multiple **R** Parathyroid Gland	**0** Open **4** Percutaneous Endoscopic	**Z** No Device	**Z** No Qualifier

0 Medical and Surgical
G Endocrine System
W Revision: Correcting, to the extent possible, a portion of a malfunctioning device or the position of a displaced device

Body Part Character 4	Approach Character 5	Device Character 6	Qualifier Character 7
0 Pituitary Gland **1** Pineal Body **5** Adrenal Gland **K** Thyroid Gland **R** Parathyroid Gland	**0** Open **3** Percutaneous **4** Percutaneous Endoscopic **X** External	**0** Drainage Device	**Z** No Qualifier
S Endocrine Gland	**0** Open **3** Percutaneous **4** Percutaneous Endoscopic	**0** Drainage Device **2** Monitoring Device **3** Infusion Device **Y** Other Device	**Z** No Qualifier
S Endocrine Gland	**X** External	**0** Drainage Device **2** Monitoring Device **3** Infusion Device	**Z** No Qualifier

NOTES

Skin and Breast 0H0-0HX

0 Medical and Surgical
H Skin and Breast
0 Alteration: Modifying the anatomic structure of a body part without affecting the function of the body part

Body Part Character 4	Approach Character 5	Device Character 6	Qualifier Character 7
T Breast, Right **U** Breast, Left **V** Breast, Bilateral	**0** Open **3** Percutaneous **X** External	**7** Autologous Tissue Substitute **J** Synthetic Substitute **K** Nonautologous Tissue Substitute **Z** No Device	**Z** No Qualifier

0 Medical and Surgical
H Skin and Breast
2 Change: Taking out or off a device from a body part and putting back an identical or similar device in or on the same body part without cutting or puncturing the skin or a mucous membrane

Body Part Character 4	Approach Character 5	Device Character 6	Qualifier Character 7
P Skin **T** Breast, Right **U** Breast, Left	**X** External	**0** Drainage Device **Y** Other Device	**Z** No Qualifier

0 Medical and Surgical
H Skin and Breast
5 Destruction: Physical eradication of all or a portion of a body part by the direct use of energy, force, or a destructive agent

Body Part Character 4	Approach Character 5	Device Character 6	Qualifier Character 7
0 Skin, Scalp **1** Skin, Face **2** Skin, Right Ear **3** Skin, Left Ear **4** Skin, Neck **5** Skin, Chest **6** Skin, Back **7** Skin, Abdomen **8** Skin, Buttock **9** Skin, Perineum **A** Skin, Inguinal **B** Skin, Right Upper Arm **C** Skin, Left Upper Arm **D** Skin, Right Lower Arm **E** Skin, Left Lower Arm **F** Skin, Right Hand **G** Skin, Left Hand **H** Skin, Right Upper Leg **J** Skin, Left Upper Leg **K** Skin, Right Lower Leg **L** Skin, Left Lower Leg **M** Skin, Right Foot **N** Skin, Left Foot	**X** External	**Z** No Device	**D** Multiple **Z** No Qualifier
Q Finger Nail **R** Toe Nail	**X** External	**Z** No Device	**Z** No Qualifier
T Breast, Right **U** Breast, Left **V** Breast, Bilateral **W** Nipple, Right **X** Nipple, Left	**0** Open **3** Percutaneous **7** Via Natural or Artificial Opening **8** Via Natural or Artificial Opening Endoscopic **X** External	**Z** No Device	**Z** No Qualifier

0 Medical and Surgical
H Skin and Breast
8 Division: Cutting into a body part, without draining fluids and/or gases from the body part, in order to separate or transect a body part

Body Part Character 4	Approach Character 5	Device Character 6	Qualifier Character 7
0 Skin, Scalp 1 Skin, Face 2 Skin, Right Ear 3 Skin, Left Ear 4 Skin, Neck 5 Skin, Chest 6 Skin, Back 7 Skin, Abdomen 8 Skin, Buttock 9 Skin, Perineum A Skin, Inguinal B Skin, Right Upper Arm C Skin, Left Upper Arm D Skin, Right Lower Arm E Skin, Left Lower Arm F Skin, Right Hand G Skin, Left Hand H Skin, Right Upper Leg J Skin, Left Upper Leg K Skin, Right Lower Leg L Skin, Left Lower Leg M Skin, Right Foot N Skin, Left Foot	X External	Z No Device	Z No Qualifier

0 Medical and Surgical
H Skin and Breast
9 Drainage: Taking or letting out fluids and/or gases from a body part

Body Part Character 4	Approach Character 5	Device Character 6	Qualifier Character 7
0 Skin, Scalp 1 Skin, Face 2 Skin, Right Ear 3 Skin, Left Ear 4 Skin, Neck 5 Skin, Chest 6 Skin, Back 7 Skin, Abdomen 8 Skin, Buttock 9 Skin, Perineum A Skin, Inguinal B Skin, Right Upper Arm C Skin, Left Upper Arm D Skin, Right Lower Arm E Skin, Left Lower Arm F Skin, Right Hand G Skin, Left Hand H Skin, Right Upper Leg J Skin, Left Upper Leg K Skin, Right Lower Leg L Skin, Left Lower Leg M Skin, Right Foot N Skin, Left Foot Q Finger Nail R Toe Nail	X External	0 Drainage Device	Z No Qualifier

0H9 continued on next page

0 Medical and Surgical
H Skin and Breast
9 Drainage: Taking or letting out fluids and/or gases from a body part

0H9 continued from previous page

Body Part Character 4	Approach Character 5	Device Character 6	Qualifier Character 7
0 Skin, Scalp **1** Skin, Face **2** Skin, Right Ear **3** Skin, Left Ear **4** Skin, Neck **5** Skin, Chest **6** Skin, Back **7** Skin, Abdomen **8** Skin, Buttock **9** Skin, Perineum **A** Skin, Inguinal **B** Skin, Right Upper Arm **C** Skin, Left Upper Arm **D** Skin, Right Lower Arm **E** Skin, Left Lower Arm **F** Skin, Right Hand **G** Skin, Left Hand **H** Skin, Right Upper Leg **J** Skin, Left Upper Leg **K** Skin, Right Lower Leg **L** Skin, Left Lower Leg **M** Skin, Right Foot **N** Skin, Left Foot **Q** Finger Nail **R** Toe Nail	**X** External	**Z** No Device	**X** Diagnostic **Z** No Qualifier
T Breast, Right **U** Breast, Left **V** Breast, Bilateral **W** Nipple, Right **X** Nipple, Left	**0** Open **3** Percutaneous **7** Via Natural or Artificial Opening **8** Via Natural or Artificial Opening Endoscopic **X** External	**0** Drainage Device	**Z** No Qualifier
T Breast, Right **U** Breast, Left **V** Breast, Bilateral **W** Nipple, Right **X** Nipple, Left	**0** Open **3** Percutaneous **7** Via Natural or Artificial Opening **8** Via Natural or Artificial Opening Endoscopic **X** External	**Z** No Device	**X** Diagnostic **Z** No Qualifier

0 Medical and Surgical
H Skin and Breast
B Excision: Cutting out or off, without replacement, a portion of a body part

Body Part Character 4	Approach Character 5	Device Character 6	Qualifier Character 7
0 Skin, Scalp **1** Skin, Face **2** Skin, Right Ear **3** Skin, Left Ear **4** Skin, Neck **5** Skin, Chest **6** Skin, Back **7** Skin, Abdomen **8** Skin, Buttock **9** Skin, Perineum **A** Skin, Inguinal **B** Skin, Right Upper Arm **C** Skin, Left Upper Arm **D** Skin, Right Lower Arm **E** Skin, Left Lower Arm **F** Skin, Right Hand **G** Skin, Left Hand **H** Skin, Right Upper Leg **J** Skin, Left Upper Leg **K** Skin, Right Lower Leg **L** Skin, Left Lower Leg **M** Skin, Right Foot **N** Skin, Left Foot **Q** Finger Nail **R** Toe Nail	**X** External	**Z** No Device	**X** Diagnostic **Z** No Qualifier
T Breast, Right **U** Breast, Left **V** Breast, Bilateral **W** Nipple, Right **X** Nipple, Left **Y** Supernumerary Breast	**0** Open **3** Percutaneous **7** Via Natural or Artificial Opening **8** Via Natural or Artificial Opening Endoscopic **X** External	**Z** No Device	**X** Diagnostic **Z** No Qualifier

0 Medical and Surgical
H Skin and Breast
C Extirpation: Taking or cutting out solid matter from a body part

Body Part Character 4	Approach Character 5	Device Character 6	Qualifier Character 7
0 Skin, Scalp **1** Skin, Face **2** Skin, Right Ear **3** Skin, Left Ear **4** Skin, Neck **5** Skin, Chest **6** Skin, Back **7** Skin, Abdomen **8** Skin, Buttock **9** Skin, Perineum **A** Skin, Inguinal **B** Skin, Right Upper Arm **C** Skin, Left Upper Arm **D** Skin, Right Lower Arm **E** Skin, Left Lower Arm **F** Skin, Right Hand **G** Skin, Left Hand **H** Skin, Right Upper Leg **J** Skin, Left Upper Leg **K** Skin, Right Lower Leg **L** Skin, Left Lower Leg **M** Skin, Right Foot **N** Skin, Left Foot **Q** Finger Nail **R** Toe Nail	**X** External	**Z** No Device	**Z** No Qualifier
T Breast, Right **U** Breast, Left **V** Breast, Bilateral **W** Nipple, Right **X** Nipple, Left	**0** Open **3** Percutaneous **7** Via Natural or Artificial Opening **8** Via Natural or Artificial Opening Endoscopic **X** External	**Z** No Device	**Z** No Qualifier

0 Medical and Surgical
H Skin and Breast
D Extraction: Pulling or stripping out or off all or a portion of a body part by the use of force

Body Part Character 4	Approach Character 5	Device Character 6	Qualifier Character 7
0 Skin, Scalp **1** Skin, Face **2** Skin, Right Ear **3** Skin, Left Ear **4** Skin, Neck **5** Skin, Chest **6** Skin, Back **7** Skin, Abdomen **8** Skin, Buttock **9** Skin, Perineum **A** Skin, Inguinal **B** Skin, Right Upper Arm **C** Skin, Left Upper Arm **D** Skin, Right Lower Arm **E** Skin, Left Lower Arm **F** Skin, Right Hand **G** Skin, Left Hand **H** Skin, Right Upper Leg **J** Skin, Left Upper Leg **K** Skin, Right Lower Leg **L** Skin, Left Lower Leg **M** Skin, Right Foot **N** Skin, Left Foot **Q** Finger Nail **R** Toe Nail **S** Hair	**X** External	**Z** No Device	**Z** No Qualifier

0 Medical and Surgical
H Skin and Breast
H Insertion: Putting in a nonbiological appliance that monitors, assists, performs, or prevents a physiological function but does not physically take the place of a body part

Body Part Character 4	Approach Character 5	Device Character 6	Qualifier Character 7
P Skin	**X** External	**Y** Other Device	**Z** No Qualifier
T Breast, Right **U** Breast, Left	**0** Open **3** Percutaneous **7** Via Natural or Artificial Opening **8** Via Natural or Artificial Opening Endoscopic	**1** Radioactive Element **N** Tissue Expander **Y** Other Device	**Z** No Qualifier
T Breast, Right **U** Breast, Left	**X** External	**1** Radioactive Element	**Z** No Qualifier
V Breast, Bilateral **W** Nipple, Right **X** Nipple, Left	**0** Open **3** Percutaneous **7** Via Natural or Artificial Opening **8** Via Natural or Artificial Opening Endoscopic	**1** Radioactive Element **N** Tissue Expander	**Z** No Qualifier
V Breast, Bilateral **W** Nipple, Right **X** Nipple, Left	**X** External	**1** Radioactive Element	**Z** No Qualifier

0 Medical and Surgical
H Skin and Breast
J Inspection: Visually and/or manually exploring a body part

Body Part	Approach	Device	Qualifier
Character 4	Character 5	Character 6	Character 7
P Skin Q Finger Nail R Toe Nail	X External	Z No Device	Z No Qualifier
T Breast, Right U Breast, Left	0 Open 3 Percutaneous 7 Via Natural or Artificial Opening 8 Via Natural or Artificial Opening Endoscopic X External	Z No Device	Z No Qualifier

0 Medical and Surgical
H Skin and Breast
M Reattachment: Putting back in or on all or a portion of a separated body part to its normal location or other suitable location

Body Part	Approach	Device	Qualifier
Character 4	Character 5	Character 6	Character 7
0 Skin, Scalp 1 Skin, Face 2 Skin, Right Ear 3 Skin, Left Ear 4 Skin, Neck 5 Skin, Chest 6 Skin, Back 7 Skin, Abdomen 8 Skin, Buttock 9 Skin, Perineum A Skin, Inguinal B Skin, Right Upper Arm C Skin, Left Upper Arm D Skin, Right Lower Arm E Skin, Left Lower Arm F Skin, Right Hand G Skin, Left Hand H Skin, Right Upper Leg J Skin, Left Upper Leg K Skin, Right Lower Leg L Skin, Left Lower Leg M Skin, Right Foot N Skin, Left Foot T Breast, Right U Breast, Left V Breast, Bilateral W Nipple, Right X Nipple, Left	X External	Z No Device	Z No Qualifier

0 Medical and Surgical
H Skin and Breast
N Release: Freeing a body part from an abnormal physical constraint by cutting or by the use of force

Body Part Character 4	Approach Character 5	Device Character 6	Qualifier Character 7
0 Skin, Scalp **1** Skin, Face **2** Skin, Right Ear **3** Skin, Left Ear **4** Skin, Neck **5** Skin, Chest **6** Skin, Back **7** Skin, Abdomen **8** Skin, Buttock **9** Skin, Perineum **A** Skin, Inguinal **B** Skin, Right Upper Arm **C** Skin, Left Upper Arm **D** Skin, Right Lower Arm **E** Skin, Left Lower Arm **F** Skin, Right Hand **G** Skin, Left Hand **H** Skin, Right Upper Leg **J** Skin, Left Upper Leg **K** Skin, Right Lower Leg **L** Skin, Left Lower Leg **M** Skin, Right Foot **N** Skin, Left Foot **Q** Finger Nail **R** Toe Nail	**X** External	**Z** No Device	**Z** No Qualifier
T Breast, Right **U** Breast, Left **V** Breast, Bilateral **W** Nipple, Right **X** Nipple, Left	**0** Open **3** Percutaneous **7** Via Natural or Artificial Opening **8** Via Natural or Artificial Opening Endoscopic **X** External	**Z** No Device	**Z** No Qualifier

0 Medical and Surgical
H Skin and Breast
P Removal: Taking out or off a device from a body part

Body Part Character 4	Approach Character 5	Device Character 6	Qualifier Character 7
P Skin	**X** External	**0** Drainage Device **7** Autologous Tissue Substitute **J** Synthetic Substitute **K** Nonautologous Tissue Substitute **Y** Other Device	**Z** No Qualifier
Q Finger Nail **R** Toe Nail	**X** External	**0** Drainage Device **7** Autologous Tissue Substitute **J** Synthetic Substitute **K** Nonautologous Tissue Substitute	**Z** No Qualifier
S Hair	**X** External	**7** Autologous Tissue Substitute **J** Synthetic Substitute **K** Nonautologous Tissue Substitute	**Z** No Qualifier
T Breast, Right **U** Breast, Left	**0** Open **3** Percutaneous **7** Via Natural or Artificial Opening **8** Via Natural or Artificial Opening Endoscopic	**0** Drainage Device **1** Radioactive Element **7** Autologous Tissue Substitute **J** Synthetic Substitute **K** Nonautologous Tissue Substitute **N** Tissue Expander **Y** Other Device	**Z** No Qualifier

0HP continued on next page

0HP continued from previous page

0 Medical and Surgical
H Skin and Breast
P Removal: Taking out or off a device from a body part

Body Part Character 4	Approach Character 5	Device Character 6	Qualifier Character 7
T Breast, Right **U** Breast, Left	**X** External	**0** Drainage Device **1** Radioactive Element **7** Autologous Tissue Substitute **J** Synthetic Substitute **K** Nonautologous Tissue Substitute	**Z** No Qualifier

0 Medical and Surgical
H Skin and Breast
Q Repair: Restoring, to the extent possible, a body part to its normal anatomic structure and function

Body Part Character 4	Approach Character 5	Device Character 6	Qualifier Character 7
0 Skin, Scalp **1** Skin, Face **2** Skin, Right Ear **3** Skin, Left Ear **4** Skin, Neck **5** Skin, Chest **6** Skin, Back **7** Skin, Abdomen **8** Skin, Buttock **9** Skin, Perineum CC **A** Skin, Inguinal **B** Skin, Right Upper Arm **C** Skin, Left Upper Arm **D** Skin, Right Lower Arm **E** Skin, Left Lower Arm **F** Skin, Right Hand **G** Skin, Left Hand **H** Skin, Right Upper Leg **J** Skin, Left Upper Leg **K** Skin, Right Lower Leg **L** Skin, Left Lower Leg **M** Skin, Right Foot **N** Skin, Left Foot **Q** Finger Nail **R** Toe Nail	**X** External	**Z** No Device	**Z** No Qualifier
T Breast, Right **U** Breast, Left **V** Breast, Bilateral **W** Nipple, Right **X** Nipple, Left **Y** Supernumerary Breast	**0** Open **3** Percutaneous **7** Via Natural or Artificial Opening **8** Via Natural or Artificial Opening Endoscopic **X** External	**Z** No Device	**Z** No Qualifier

CC 0HQ9XZZ

0 Medical and Surgical
H Skin and Breast
R Replacement: Putting in or on biological or synthetic material that physically takes the place and/or function of all or a portion of a body part

Body Part Character 4	Approach Character 5	Device Character 6	Qualifier Character 7
0 Skin, Scalp **1** Skin, Face **2** Skin, Right Ear **3** Skin, Left Ear **4** Skin, Neck **5** Skin, Chest **6** Skin, Back **7** Skin, Abdomen **8** Skin, Buttock **9** Skin, Perineum **A** Skin, Inguinal **B** Skin, Right Upper Arm **C** Skin, Left Upper Arm **D** Skin, Right Lower Arm **E** Skin, Left Lower Arm **F** Skin, Right Hand **G** Skin, Left Hand **H** Skin, Right Upper Leg **J** Skin, Left Upper Leg **K** Skin, Right Lower Leg **L** Skin, Left Lower Leg **M** Skin, Right Foot **N** Skin, Left Foot	**X** External	**7** Autologous Tissue Substitute **K** Nonautologous Tissue Substitute	**3** Full Thickness **4** Partial Thickness
0 Skin, Scalp **1** Skin, Face **2** Skin, Right Ear **3** Skin, Left Ear **4** Skin, Neck **5** Skin, Chest **6** Skin, Back **7** Skin, Abdomen **8** Skin, Buttock **9** Skin, Perineum **A** Skin, Inguinal **B** Skin, Right Upper Arm **C** Skin, Left Upper Arm **D** Skin, Right Lower Arm **E** Skin, Left Lower Arm **F** Skin, Right Hand **G** Skin, Left Hand **H** Skin, Right Upper Leg **J** Skin, Left Upper Leg **K** Skin, Right Lower Leg **L** Skin, Left Lower Leg **M** Skin, Right Foot **N** Skin, Left Foot	**X** External	**J** Synthetic Substitute	**3** Full Thickness **4** Partial Thickness **Z** No Qualifier
Q Finger Nail **R** Toe Nail **S** Hair	**X** External	**7** Autologous Tissue Substitute **J** Synthetic Substitute **K** Nonautologous Tissue Substitute	**Z** No Qualifier
T Breast, Right **U** Breast, Left **V** Breast, Bilateral	**0** Open	**7** Autologous Tissue Substitute	**5** Latissimus Dorsi Myocutaneous Flap **6** Transverse Rectus Abdominis Myocutaneous Flap **7** Deep Inferior Epigastric Artery Perforator Flap **8** Superficial Inferior Epigastric Artery Flap **9** Gluteal Artery Perforator Flap **Z** No Qualifier

0HR continued on next page

0HR continued from previous page

0 Medical and Surgical
H Skin and Breast
R Replacement: Putting in or on biological or synthetic material that physically takes the place and/or function of all or a portion of a body part

Body Part Character 4	Approach Character 5	Device Character 6	Qualifier Character 7
T Breast, Right **U** Breast, Left **V** Breast, Bilateral	**0** Open	**J** Synthetic Substitute **K** Nonautologous Tissue Substitute	**Z** No Qualifier
T Breast, Right CC **U** Breast, Left CC **V** Breast, Bilateral CC	**3** Percutaneous **X** External	**7** Autologous Tissue Substitute **J** Synthetic Substitute **K** Nonautologous Tissue Substitute	**Z** No Qualifier
W Nipple, Right **X** Nipple, Left	**0** Open **3** Percutaneous **X** External	**7** Autologous Tissue Substitute **J** Synthetic Substitute **K** Nonautologous Tissue Substitute	**Z** No Qualifier

CC 0HRT37Z 0HRU37Z 0HRV37Z

0 Medical and Surgical
H Skin and Breast
S Reposition: Moving to its normal location, or other suitable location, all or a portion of a body part

Body Part Character 4	Approach Character 5	Device Character 6	Qualifier Character 7
S Hair **W** Nipple, Right **X** Nipple, Left	**X** External	**Z** No Device	**Z** No Qualifier
T Breast, Right **U** Breast, Left **V** Breast, Bilateral	**0** Open	**Z** No Device	**Z** No Qualifier

0 Medical and Surgical
H Skin and Breast
T Resection: Cutting out or off, without replacement, all of a body part

Body Part Character 4	Approach Character 5	Device Character 6	Qualifier Character 7
Q Finger Nail **R** Toe Nail **W** Nipple, Right **X** Nipple, Left	**X** External	**Z** No Device	**Z** No Qualifier
T Breast, Right CC **U** Breast, Left CC **V** Breast, Bilateral CC **Y** Supernumerary Breast	**0** Open	**Z** No Device	**Z** No Qualifier

CC 0HTT0ZZ 0HTU0ZZ 0HTV0ZZ

0 Medical and Surgical
H Skin and Breast
U Supplement: Putting in or on biological or synthetic material that physically reinforces and/or augments the function of a portion of a body part

Body Part Character 4	Approach Character 5	Device Character 6	Qualifier Character 7
T Breast, Right **U** Breast, Left **V** Breast, Bilateral **W** Nipple, Right **X** Nipple, Left	**0** Open **3** Percutaneous **7** Via Natural or Artificial Opening **8** Via Natural or Artificial Opening Endoscopic **X** External	**7** Autologous Tissue Substitute **J** Synthetic Substitute **K** Nonautologous Tissue Substitute	**Z** No Qualifier

0 Medical and Surgical
H Skin and Breast
W Revision: Correcting, to the extent possible, a portion of a malfunctioning device or the position of a displaced device

Body Part Character 4	Approach Character 5	Device Character 6	Qualifier Character 7
P Skin	**X** External	**0** Drainage Device **7** Autologous Tissue Substitute **J** Synthetic Substitute **K** Nonautologous Tissue Substitute **Y** Other Device	**Z** No Qualifier
Q Finger Nail **R** Toe Nail	**X** External	**0** Drainage Device **7** Autologous Tissue Substitute **J** Synthetic Substitute **K** Nonautologous Tissue Substitute	**Z** No Qualifier
S Hair	**X** External	**7** Autologous Tissue Substitute **J** Synthetic Substitute **K** Nonautologous Tissue Substitute	**Z** No Qualifier
T Breast, Right **U** Breast, Left	**0** Open **3** Percutaneous **7** Via Natural or Artificial Opening **8** Via Natural or Artificial Opening Endoscopic	**0** Drainage Device **7** Autologous Tissue Substitute **J** Synthetic Substitute **K** Nonautologous Tissue Substitute **N** Tissue Expander **Y** Other Device	**Z** No Qualifier
T Breast, Right **U** Breast, Left	**X** External	**0** Drainage Device **7** Autologous Tissue Substitute **J** Synthetic Substitute **K** Nonautologous Tissue Substitute	**Z** No Qualifier

0 Medical and Surgical
H Skin and Breast
X Transfer: Moving, without taking out, all or a portion of a body part to another location to take over the function of all or a portion of a body part

Body Part	Approach	Device	Qualifier
Character 4	**Character 5**	**Character 6**	**Character 7**
0 Skin, Scalp **1** Skin, Face **2** Skin, Right Ear **3** Skin, Left Ear **4** Skin, Neck **5** Skin, Chest **6** Skin, Back **7** Skin, Abdomen **8** Skin, Buttock **9** Skin, Perineum **A** Skin, Inguinal **B** Skin, Right Upper Arm **C** Skin, Left Upper Arm **D** Skin, Right Lower Arm **E** Skin, Left Lower Arm **F** Skin, Right Hand **G** Skin, Left Hand **H** Skin, Right Upper Leg **J** Skin, Left Upper Leg **K** Skin, Right Lower Leg **L** Skin, Left Lower Leg **M** Skin, Right Foot **N** Skin, Left Foot	**X** External	**Z** No Device	**Z** No Qualifier

NOTES

Subcutaneous Tissue and Fascia 0J0-0JX

0 Medical and Surgical
J Subcutaneous Tissue and Fascia
0 Alteration: Modifying the anatomic structure of a body part without affecting the function of the body part

Body Part Character 4	Approach Character 5	Device Character 6	Qualifier Character 7
1 Subcutaneous Tissue and Fascia, Face **4** Subcutaneous Tissue and Fascia, Right Neck **5** Subcutaneous Tissue and Fascia, Left Neck **6** Subcutaneous Tissue and Fascia, Chest **7** Subcutaneous Tissue and Fascia, Back **8** Subcutaneous Tissue and Fascia, Abdomen **9** Subcutaneous Tissue and Fascia, Buttock **D** Subcutaneous Tissue and Fascia, Right Upper Arm **F** Subcutaneous Tissue and Fascia, Left Upper Arm **G** Subcutaneous Tissue and Fascia, Right Lower Arm **H** Subcutaneous Tissue and Fascia, Left Lower Arm **L** Subcutaneous Tissue and Fascia, Right Upper Leg **M** Subcutaneous Tissue and Fascia, Left Upper Leg **N** Subcutaneous Tissue and Fascia, Right Lower Leg **P** Subcutaneous Tissue and Fascia, Left Lower Leg	**0** Open **3** Percutaneous	**Z** No Device	**Z** No Qualifier

0 Medical and Surgical
J Subcutaneous Tissue and Fascia
2 Change: Taking out or off a device from a body part and putting back an identical or similar device in or on the same body part without cutting or puncturing the skin or a mucous membrane

Body Part Character 4	Approach Character 5	Device Character 6	Qualifier Character 7
S Subcutaneous Tissue and Fascia, Head and Neck **T** Subcutaneous Tissue and Fascia, Trunk **V** Subcutaneous Tissue and Fascia, Upper Extremity **W** Subcutaneous Tissue and Fascia, Lower Extremity	**X** External	**0** Drainage Device **Y** Other Device	**Z** No Qualifier

0 Medical and Surgical
J Subcutaneous Tissue and Fascia
5 Destruction: Physical eradication of all or a portion of a body part by the direct use of energy, force, or a destructive agent

Body Part Character 4	Approach Character 5	Device Character 6	Qualifier Character 7
0 Subcutaneous Tissue and Fascia, Scalp **1** Subcutaneous Tissue and Fascia, Face **4** Subcutaneous Tissue and Fascia, Right Neck **5** Subcutaneous Tissue and Fascia, Left Neck **6** Subcutaneous Tissue and Fascia, Chest **7** Subcutaneous Tissue and Fascia, Back **8** Subcutaneous Tissue and Fascia, Abdomen **9** Subcutaneous Tissue and Fascia, Buttock **B** Subcutaneous Tissue and Fascia, Perineum **C** Subcutaneous Tissue and Fascia, Pelvic Region **D** Subcutaneous Tissue and Fascia, Right Upper Arm **F** Subcutaneous Tissue and Fascia, Left Upper Arm **G** Subcutaneous Tissue and Fascia, Right Lower Arm **H** Subcutaneous Tissue and Fascia, Left Lower Arm **J** Subcutaneous Tissue and Fascia, Right Hand **K** Subcutaneous Tissue and Fascia, Left Hand **L** Subcutaneous Tissue and Fascia, Right Upper Leg **M** Subcutaneous Tissue and Fascia, Left Upper Leg **N** Subcutaneous Tissue and Fascia, Right Lower Leg **P** Subcutaneous Tissue and Fascia, Left Lower Leg **Q** Subcutaneous Tissue and Fascia, Right Foot **R** Subcutaneous Tissue and Fascia, Left Foot	**0** Open **3** Percutaneous	**Z** No Device	**Z** No Qualifier

0 Medical and Surgical
J Subcutaneous Tissue and Fascia
8 Division: Cutting into a body part, without draining fluids and/or gases from the body part, in order to separate or transect a body part

Body Part Character 4	Approach Character 5	Device Character 6	Qualifier Character 7
0 Subcutaneous Tissue and Fascia, Scalp **1** Subcutaneous Tissue and Fascia, Face **4** Subcutaneous Tissue and Fascia, Right Neck **5** Subcutaneous Tissue and Fascia, Left Neck **6** Subcutaneous Tissue and Fascia, Chest **7** Subcutaneous Tissue and Fascia, Back **8** Subcutaneous Tissue and Fascia, Abdomen **9** Subcutaneous Tissue and Fascia, Buttock **B** Subcutaneous Tissue and Fascia, Perineum **C** Subcutaneous Tissue and Fascia, Pelvic Region **D** Subcutaneous Tissue and Fascia, Right Upper Arm **F** Subcutaneous Tissue and Fascia, Left Upper Arm **G** Subcutaneous Tissue and Fascia, Right Lower Arm **H** Subcutaneous Tissue and Fascia, Left Lower Arm **J** Subcutaneous Tissue and Fascia, Right Hand **K** Subcutaneous Tissue and Fascia, Left Hand **L** Subcutaneous Tissue and Fascia, Right Upper Leg **M** Subcutaneous Tissue and Fascia, Left Upper Leg **N** Subcutaneous Tissue and Fascia, Right Lower Leg **P** Subcutaneous Tissue and Fascia, Left Lower Leg **Q** Subcutaneous Tissue and Fascia, Right Foot **R** Subcutaneous Tissue and Fascia, Left Foot **S** Subcutaneous Tissue and Fascia, Head and Neck **T** Subcutaneous Tissue and Fascia, Trunk **V** Subcutaneous Tissue and Fascia, Upper Extremity **W** Subcutaneous Tissue and Fascia, Lower Extremity	**0** Open **3** Percutaneous	**Z** No Device	**Z** No Qualifier

0 Medical and Surgical
J Subcutaneous Tissue and Fascia
9 Drainage: Taking or letting out fluids and/or gases from a body part

Body Part Character 4	Approach Character 5	Device Character 6	Qualifier Character 7
0 Subcutaneous Tissue and Fascia, Scalp **1** Subcutaneous Tissue and Fascia, Face **4** Subcutaneous Tissue and Fascia, Right Neck **5** Subcutaneous Tissue and Fascia, Left Neck **6** Subcutaneous Tissue and Fascia, Chest **7** Subcutaneous Tissue and Fascia, Back **8** Subcutaneous Tissue and Fascia, Abdomen **9** Subcutaneous Tissue and Fascia, Buttock **B** Subcutaneous Tissue and Fascia, Perineum **C** Subcutaneous Tissue and Fascia, Pelvic Region **D** Subcutaneous Tissue and Fascia, Right Upper Arm **F** Subcutaneous Tissue and Fascia, Left Upper Arm **G** Subcutaneous Tissue and Fascia, Right Lower Arm **H** Subcutaneous Tissue and Fascia, Left Lower Arm **J** Subcutaneous Tissue and Fascia, Right Hand **K** Subcutaneous Tissue and Fascia, Left Hand **L** Subcutaneous Tissue and Fascia, Right Upper Leg **M** Subcutaneous Tissue and Fascia, Left Upper Leg **N** Subcutaneous Tissue and Fascia, Right Lower Leg **P** Subcutaneous Tissue and Fascia, Left Lower Leg **Q** Subcutaneous Tissue and Fascia, Right Foot **R** Subcutaneous Tissue and Fascia, Left Foot	**0** Open **3** Percutaneous	**0** Drainage Device	**Z** No Qualifier

0J9 continued on next page

0J9 continued from previous page

0 Medical and Surgical
J Subcutaneous Tissue and Fascia
9 Drainage: Taking or letting out fluids and/or gases from a body part

Body Part Character 4	Approach Character 5	Device Character 6	Qualifier Character 7
0 Subcutaneous Tissue and Fascia, Scalp **1** Subcutaneous Tissue and Fascia, Face **4** Subcutaneous Tissue and Fascia, Right Neck **5** Subcutaneous Tissue and Fascia, Left Neck **6** Subcutaneous Tissue and Fascia, Chest **7** Subcutaneous Tissue and Fascia, Back **8** Subcutaneous Tissue and Fascia, Abdomen **9** Subcutaneous Tissue and Fascia, Buttock **B** Subcutaneous Tissue and Fascia, Perineum **C** Subcutaneous Tissue and Fascia, Pelvic Region **D** Subcutaneous Tissue and Fascia, Right Upper Arm **F** Subcutaneous Tissue and Fascia, Left Upper Arm **G** Subcutaneous Tissue and Fascia, Right Lower Arm **H** Subcutaneous Tissue and Fascia, Left Lower Arm **J** Subcutaneous Tissue and Fascia, Right Hand **K** Subcutaneous Tissue and Fascia, Left Hand **L** Subcutaneous Tissue and Fascia, Right Upper Leg **M** Subcutaneous Tissue and Fascia, Left Upper Leg **N** Subcutaneous Tissue and Fascia, Right Lower Leg **P** Subcutaneous Tissue and Fascia, Left Lower Leg **Q** Subcutaneous Tissue and Fascia, Right Foot **R** Subcutaneous Tissue and Fascia, Left Foot	**0** Open **3** Percutaneous	**Z** No Device	**X** Diagnostic **Z** No Qualifier

0 Medical and Surgical
J Subcutaneous Tissue and Fascia
B Excision: Cutting out or off, without replacement, a portion of a body part

Body Part Character 4	Approach Character 5	Device Character 6	Qualifier Character 7
0 Subcutaneous Tissue and Fascia, Scalp DRG 1 Subcutaneous Tissue and Fascia, Face 4 Subcutaneous Tissue and Fascia, Right Neck DRG 5 Subcutaneous Tissue and Fascia, Left Neck DRG 6 Subcutaneous Tissue and Fascia, Chest DRG 7 Subcutaneous Tissue and Fascia, Back DRG 8 Subcutaneous Tissue and Fascia, Abdomen DRG 9 Subcutaneous Tissue and Fascia, Buttock DRG B Subcutaneous Tissue and Fascia, Perineum DRG C Subcutaneous Tissue and Fascia, Pelvic Region DRG D Subcutaneous Tissue and Fascia, Right Upper Arm DRG F Subcutaneous Tissue and Fascia, Left Upper Arm DRG G Subcutaneous Tissue and Fascia, Right Lower Arm DRG H Subcutaneous Tissue and Fascia, Left Lower Arm DRG J Subcutaneous Tissue and Fascia, Right Hand K Subcutaneous Tissue and Fascia, Left Hand L Subcutaneous Tissue and Fascia, Right Upper Leg DRG CC M Subcutaneous Tissue and Fascia, Left Upper Leg DRG CC N Subcutaneous Tissue and Fascia, Right Lower Leg DRG P Subcutaneous Tissue and Fascia, Left Lower Leg DRG Q Subcutaneous Tissue and Fascia, Right Foot DRG R Subcutaneous Tissue and Fascia, Left Foot	0 Open 3 Percutaneous	Z No Device	X Diagnostic Z No Qualifier

DRG 0JB03ZZ 0JB43ZZ 0JB53ZZ 0JB63ZZ 0JB73ZZ 0JB83ZZ 0JB93ZZ 0JBB3ZZ 0JBC3ZZ 0JBD3ZZ 0JBF3ZZ 0JBG3ZZ 0JBH3ZZ 0JBL3ZZ 0JBM3ZZ 0JBN3ZZ 0JBP3ZZ 0JBQ3ZZ

CC 0JBL0ZZ 0JBM0ZZ

0 Medical and Surgical
J Subcutaneous Tissue and Fascia
C Extirpation: Taking or cutting out solid matter from a body part

Body Part Character 4	Approach Character 5	Device Character 6	Qualifier Character 7
0 Subcutaneous Tissue and Fascia, Scalp **1** Subcutaneous Tissue and Fascia, Face **4** Subcutaneous Tissue and Fascia, Right Neck **5** Subcutaneous Tissue and Fascia, Left Neck **6** Subcutaneous Tissue and Fascia, Chest **7** Subcutaneous Tissue and Fascia, Back **8** Subcutaneous Tissue and Fascia, Abdomen **9** Subcutaneous Tissue and Fascia, Buttock **B** Subcutaneous Tissue and Fascia, Perineum **C** Subcutaneous Tissue and Fascia, Pelvic Region **D** Subcutaneous Tissue and Fascia, Right Upper Arm **F** Subcutaneous Tissue and Fascia, Left Upper Arm **G** Subcutaneous Tissue and Fascia, Right Lower Arm **H** Subcutaneous Tissue and Fascia, Left Lower Arm **J** Subcutaneous Tissue and Fascia, Right Hand **K** Subcutaneous Tissue and Fascia, Left Hand **L** Subcutaneous Tissue and Fascia, Right Upper Leg **M** Subcutaneous Tissue and Fascia, Left Upper Leg **N** Subcutaneous Tissue and Fascia, Right Lower Leg **P** Subcutaneous Tissue and Fascia, Left Lower Leg **Q** Subcutaneous Tissue and Fascia, Right Foot **R** Subcutaneous Tissue and Fascia, Left Foot	**0** Open **3** Percutaneous	**Z** No Device	**Z** No Qualifier

0 Medical and Surgical
J Subcutaneous Tissue and Fascia
D Extraction: Pulling or stripping out or off all or a portion of a body part by the use of force

Body Part Character 4	Approach Character 5	Device Character 6	Qualifier Character 7
0 Subcutaneous Tissue and Fascia, Scalp **1** Subcutaneous Tissue and Fascia, Face **4** Subcutaneous Tissue and Fascia, Right Neck **5** Subcutaneous Tissue and Fascia, Left Neck **6** Subcutaneous Tissue and Fascia, Chest CC **7** Subcutaneous Tissue and Fascia, Back CC **8** Subcutaneous Tissue and Fascia, Abdomen CC **9** Subcutaneous Tissue and Fascia, Buttock CC **B** Subcutaneous Tissue and Fascia, Perineum **C** Subcutaneous Tissue and Fascia, Pelvic Region **D** Subcutaneous Tissue and Fascia, Right Upper Arm **F** Subcutaneous Tissue and Fascia, Left Upper Arm **G** Subcutaneous Tissue and Fascia, Right Lower Arm **H** Subcutaneous Tissue and Fascia, Left Lower Arm **J** Subcutaneous Tissue and Fascia, Right Hand **K** Subcutaneous Tissue and Fascia, Left Hand **L** Subcutaneous Tissue and Fascia, Right Upper Leg CC **M** Subcutaneous Tissue and Fascia, Left Upper Leg CC **N** Subcutaneous Tissue and Fascia, Right Lower Leg **P** Subcutaneous Tissue and Fascia, Left Lower Leg **Q** Subcutaneous Tissue and Fascia, Right Foot **R** Subcutaneous Tissue and Fascia, Left Foot	**0** Open **3** Percutaneous	**Z** No Device	**Z** No Qualifier

CC 0JD63ZZ 0JD73ZZ 0JD83ZZ 0JD93ZZ 0JDL3ZZ 0JDM3ZZ

0 Medical and Surgical
J Subcutaneous Tissue and Fascia
H Insertion: Putting in a nonbiological appliance that monitors, assists, performs, or prevents a physiological function but does not physically take the place of a body part

Body Part	Approach	Device	Qualifier
Character 4	Character 5	Character 6	Character 7
0 Subcutaneous Tissue and Fascia, Scalp 1 Subcutaneous Tissue and Fascia, Face 4 Subcutaneous Tissue and Fascia, Right Neck 5 Subcutaneous Tissue and Fascia, Left Neck 9 Subcutaneous Tissue and Fascia, Buttock B Subcutaneous Tissue and Fascia, Perineum C Subcutaneous Tissue and Fascia, Pelvic Region J Subcutaneous Tissue and Fascia, Right Hand K Subcutaneous Tissue and Fascia, Left Hand Q Subcutaneous Tissue and Fascia, Right Foot R Subcutaneous Tissue and Fascia, Left Foot	0 Open 3 Percutaneous	N Tissue Expander	Z No Qualifier
6 Subcutaneous Tissue and Fascia, Chest CC HAC 8 Subcutaneous Tissue and Fascia, Abdomen NC CC HAC	0 Open 3 Percutaneous	0 Monitoring Device, Hemodynamic 2 Monitoring Device 4 Pacemaker, Single Chamber 5 Pacemaker, Single Chamber Rate Responsive 6 Pacemaker, Dual Chamber 7 Cardiac Resynchronization Pacemaker Pulse Generator 8 Defibrillator Generator 9 Cardiac Resynchronization Defibrillator Pulse Generator A Contractility Modulation Device B Stimulator Generator, Single Array C Stimulator Generator, Single Array Rechargeable D Stimulator Generator, Multiple Array E Stimulator Generator, Multiple Array Rechargeable H Contraceptive Device M Stimulator Generator N Tissue Expander P Cardiac Rhythm Related Device V Infusion Device, Pump W Vascular Access Device, Totally Implantable X Vascular Access Device, Tunneled	Z No Qualifier

0JH continued on next page

0JH continued from previous page

0 Medical and Surgical
J Subcutaneous Tissue and Fascia
H Insertion: Putting in a nonbiological appliance that monitors, assists, performs, or prevents a physiological function but does not physically take the place of a body part

Body Part Character 4	Approach Character 5	Device Character 6	Qualifier Character 7
7 Subcutaneous Tissue and Fascia, Back NC CC	**0** Open **3** Percutaneous	**B** Stimulator Generator, Single Array **C** Stimulator Generator, Single Array Rechargeable **D** Stimulator Generator, Multiple Array **E** Stimulator Generator, Multiple Array Rechargeable **M** Stimulator Generator **N** Tissue Expander **V** Infusion Device, Pump	**Z** No Qualifier
D Subcutaneous Tissue and Fascia, Right Upper Arm **F** Subcutaneous Tissue and Fascia, Left Upper Arm **G** Subcutaneous Tissue and Fascia, Right Lower Arm **H** Subcutaneous Tissue and Fascia, Left Lower Arm **L** Subcutaneous Tissue and Fascia, Right Upper Leg DRG **M** Subcutaneous Tissue and Fascia, Left Upper Leg DRG **N** Subcutaneous Tissue and Fascia, Right Lower Leg DRG **P** Subcutaneous Tissue and Fascia, Left Lower Leg DRG	**0** Open **3** Percutaneous	**H** Contraceptive Device **N** Tissue Expander **V** Infusion Device, Pump **W** Vascular Access Device, Totally Implantable **X** Vascular Access Device, Tunneled	**Z** No Qualifier
S Subcutaneous Tissue and Fascia, Head and Neck **V** Subcutaneous Tissue and Fascia, Upper Extremity **W** Subcutaneous Tissue and Fascia, Lower Extremity	**0** Open **3** Percutaneous	**1** Radioactive Element **3** Infusion Device **Y** Other Device	**Z** No Qualifier
T Subcutaneous Tissue and Fascia, Trunk	**0** Open **3** Percutaneous	**1** Radioactive Element **3** Infusion Device **V** Infusion Device, Pump **Y** Other Device	**Z** No Qualifier

NC 0JH70MZ 0JH73MZ 0JH80MZ 0JH83MZ

CC 0JH600Z 0JH604Z 0JH605Z 0JH606Z 0JH607Z 0JH608Z 0JH609Z 0JH60AZ 0JH60BZ 0JH60CZ 0JH60DZ 0JH60EZ 0JH60MZ 0JH60PZ 0JH630Z 0JH634Z 0JH635Z 0JH636Z 0JH637Z 0JH638Z 0JH639Z 0JH63AZ 0JH63BZ 0JH63CZ 0JH63DZ 0JH63EZ 0JH63MZ 0JH63PZ 0JH70BZ 0JH70CZ 0JH70DZ 0JH70EZ 0JH70MZ 0JH73BZ 0JH73CZ 0JH73DZ 0JH73EZ 0JH73MZ 0JH800Z 0JH804Z 0JH805Z 0JH806Z 0JH807Z 0JH808Z 0JH809Z 0JH80AZ 0JH80BZ 0JH80CZ 0JH80DZ 0JH80EZ 0JH80MZ 0JH80PZ 0JH830Z 0JH834Z 0JH835Z 0JH836Z 0JH837Z 0JH838Z 0JH839Z 0JH83AZ 0JH83BZ 0JH83CZ 0JH83DZ 0JH83EZ 0JH83MZ 0JH83PZ

HAC 0JH604Z 0JH605Z 0JH606Z 0JH607Z 0JH608Z 0JH609Z 0JH60PZ 0JH634Z 0JH635Z 0JH636Z 0JH637Z 0JH638Z 0JH639Z 0JH63PZ 0JH804Z 0JH805Z 0JH806Z 0JH807Z 0JH808Z 0JH809Z 0JH80PZ 0JH834Z 0JH835Z 0JH836Z 0JH837Z 0JH838Z 0JH839Z 0JH83PZ

Surgical site infection (SSI) following cardiac implantable electronic device (CIED) procedures and secondary diagnosis K68.11, T81.4XXA, T82.6XXA, T82.7XXA.

HAC 0JH63XZ

Iatrogenic pneumothorax w/ venous catheterization procedures and secondary diagnosis J95.811.

DRG 0JHL0WZ 0JHL0XZ 0JHL3WZ 0JHL3XZ 0JHM0WZ 0JHM0XZ 0JHM3WZ 0JHM3XZ 0JHN0WZ 0JHN0XZ 0JHN3HZ 0JHN3WZ 0JHN3XZ 0JHP0HZ 0JHP0WZ 0JHP0XZ 0JHP3HZ 0JHP3WZ 0JHP3XZ

0 Medical and Surgical
J Subcutaneous Tissue and Fascia
J Inspection: Visually and/or manually exploring a body part

Body Part Character 4	Approach Character 5	Device Character 6	Qualifier Character 7
S Subcutaneous Tissue and Fascia, Head and Neck **T** Subcutaneous Tissue and Fascia, Trunk **V** Subcutaneous Tissue and Fascia, Upper Extremity **W** Subcutaneous Tissue and Fascia, Lower Extremity	**0** Open **3** Percutaneous **X** External	**Z** No Device	**Z** No Qualifier

0 Medical and Surgical
J Subcutaneous Tissue and Fascia
N Release: Freeing a body part from an abnormal physical constraint by cutting or by the use of force

Body Part Character 4	Approach Character 5	Device Character 6	Qualifier Character 7
0 Subcutaneous Tissue and Fascia, Scalp **1** Subcutaneous Tissue and Fascia, Face **4** Subcutaneous Tissue and Fascia, Right Neck **5** Subcutaneous Tissue and Fascia, Left Neck **6** Subcutaneous Tissue and Fascia, Chest **7** Subcutaneous Tissue and Fascia, Back **8** Subcutaneous Tissue and Fascia, Abdomen **9** Subcutaneous Tissue and Fascia, Buttock **B** Subcutaneous Tissue and Fascia, Perineum **C** Subcutaneous Tissue and Fascia, Pelvic Region **D** Subcutaneous Tissue and Fascia, Right Upper Arm **F** Subcutaneous Tissue and Fascia, Left Upper Arm **G** Subcutaneous Tissue and Fascia, Right Lower Arm **H** Subcutaneous Tissue and Fascia, Left Lower Arm **J** Subcutaneous Tissue and Fascia, Right Hand **K** Subcutaneous Tissue and Fascia, Left Hand **L** Subcutaneous Tissue and Fascia, Right Upper Leg **M** Subcutaneous Tissue and Fascia, Left Upper Leg **N** Subcutaneous Tissue and Fascia, Right Lower Leg **P** Subcutaneous Tissue and Fascia, Left Lower Leg **Q** Subcutaneous Tissue and Fascia, Right Foot **R** Subcutaneous Tissue and Fascia, Left Foot	**0** Open **3** Percutaneous **X** External	**Z** No Device	**Z** No Qualifier

0 Medical and Surgical
J Subcutaneous Tissue and Fascia
P Removal: Taking out or off a device from a body part

Body Part Character 4	Approach Character 5	Device Character 6	Qualifier Character 7
S Subcutaneous Tissue and Fascia, Head and Neck	**0** Open **3** Percutaneous	**0** Drainage Device **1** Radioactive Element **3** Infusion Device **7** Autologous Tissue Substitute **J** Synthetic Substitute **K** Nonautologous Tissue Substitute **N** Tissue Expander **Y** Other Device	**Z** No Qualifier
S Subcutaneous Tissue and Fascia, Head and Neck	**X** External	**0** Drainage Device **1** Radioactive Element **3** Infusion Device	**Z** No Qualifier
T Subcutaneous Tissue and Fascia, Trunk HAC CC	**0** Open **3** Percutaneous	**0** Drainage Device **1** Radioactive Element **2** Monitoring Device **3** Infusion Device **7** Autologous Tissue Substitute **H** Contraceptive Device **J** Synthetic Substitute **K** Nonautologous Tissue Substitute **M** Stimulator Generator **N** Tissue Expander **P** Cardiac Rhythm Related Device **V** Infusion Device, Pump **W** Vascular Access Device, Totally Implantable **X** Vascular Access Device, Tunneled **Y** Other Device	**Z** No Qualifier
T Subcutaneous Tissue and Fascia, Trunk	**X** External	**0** Drainage Device **1** Radioactive Element **2** Monitoring Device **3** Infusion Device **H** Contraceptive Device **V** Infusion Device, Pump **X** Vascular Access Device, Tunneled	**Z** No Qualifier
V Subcutaneous Tissue and Fascia, Upper Extremity **W** Subcutaneous Tissue and Fascia, Lower Extremity	**0** Open **3** Percutaneous	**0** Drainage Device **1** Radioactive Element **3** Infusion Device **7** Autologous Tissue Substitute **H** Contraceptive Device **J** Synthetic Substitute **K** Nonautologous Tissue Substitute **N** Tissue Expander **V** Infusion Device, Pump **W** Vascular Access Device, Totally Implantable **X** Vascular Access Device, Tunneled **Y** Other Device	**Z** No Qualifier
V Subcutaneous Tissue and Fascia, Upper Extremity **W** Subcutaneous Tissue and Fascia, Lower Extremity	**X** External	**0** Drainage Device **1** Radioactive Element **3** Infusion Device **H** Contraceptive Device **V** Infusion Device, Pump **X** Vascular Access Device, Tunneled	**Z** No Qualifier

HAC 0JPT0PZ 0JPT3PZ
Surgical site infection (SSI) following cardiac implantable electronic device (CIED) procedures and secondary diagnosis K68.11, T81.4XXA, T82.6XXA, T82.7XXA.

CC 0JPT0PZ 0JPT3PZ

0 Medical and Surgical
J Subcutaneous Tissue and Fascia
Q Repair: Restoring, to the extent possible, a body part to its normal anatomic structure and function

Body Part Character 4	Approach Character 5	Device Character 6	Qualifier Character 7
0 Subcutaneous Tissue and Fascia, Scalp **1** Subcutaneous Tissue and Fascia, Face **4** Subcutaneous Tissue and Fascia, Right Neck **5** Subcutaneous Tissue and Fascia, Left Neck **6** Subcutaneous Tissue and Fascia, Chest **7** Subcutaneous Tissue and Fascia, Back **8** Subcutaneous Tissue and Fascia, Abdomen **9** Subcutaneous Tissue and Fascia, Buttock **B** Subcutaneous Tissue and Fascia, Perineum **C** Subcutaneous Tissue and Fascia, Pelvic Region **D** Subcutaneous Tissue and Fascia, Right Upper Arm **F** Subcutaneous Tissue and Fascia, Left Upper Arm **G** Subcutaneous Tissue and Fascia, Right Lower Arm **H** Subcutaneous Tissue and Fascia, Left Lower Arm **J** Subcutaneous Tissue and Fascia, Right Hand **K** Subcutaneous Tissue and Fascia, Left Hand **L** Subcutaneous Tissue and Fascia, Right Upper Leg **M** Subcutaneous Tissue and Fascia, Left Upper Leg **N** Subcutaneous Tissue and Fascia, Right Lower Leg **P** Subcutaneous Tissue and Fascia, Left Lower Leg **Q** Subcutaneous Tissue and Fascia, Right Foot **R** Subcutaneous Tissue and Fascia, Left Foot	**0** Open **3** Percutaneous	**Z** No Device	**Z** No Qualifier

0 Medical and Surgical
J Subcutaneous Tissue and Fascia
R Replacement: Putting in or on biological or synthetic material that physically takes the place and/or function of all or a portion of a body part

Body Part Character 4	Approach Character 5	Device Character 6	Qualifier Character 7
0 Subcutaneous Tissue and Fascia, Scalp **1** Subcutaneous Tissue and Fascia, Face **4** Subcutaneous Tissue and Fascia, Right Neck **5** Subcutaneous Tissue and Fascia, Left Neck **6** Subcutaneous Tissue and Fascia, Chest **7** Subcutaneous Tissue and Fascia, Back **8** Subcutaneous Tissue and Fascia, Abdomen **9** Subcutaneous Tissue and Fascia, Buttock **B** Subcutaneous Tissue and Fascia, Perineum **C** Subcutaneous Tissue and Fascia, Pelvic Region **D** Subcutaneous Tissue and Fascia, Right Upper Arm **F** Subcutaneous Tissue and Fascia, Left Upper Arm **G** Subcutaneous Tissue and Fascia, Right Lower Arm **H** Subcutaneous Tissue and Fascia, Left Lower Arm **J** Subcutaneous Tissue and Fascia, Right Hand **K** Subcutaneous Tissue and Fascia, Left Hand **L** Subcutaneous Tissue and Fascia, Right Upper Leg **M** Subcutaneous Tissue and Fascia, Left Upper Leg **N** Subcutaneous Tissue and Fascia, Right Lower Leg **P** Subcutaneous Tissue and Fascia, Left Lower Leg **Q** Subcutaneous Tissue and Fascia, Right Foot **R** Subcutaneous Tissue and Fascia, Left Foot	**0** Open **3** Percutaneous	**7** Autologous Tissue Substitute **J** Synthetic Substitute **K** Nonautologous Tissue Substitute	**Z** No Qualifier

0 Medical and Surgical
J Subcutaneous Tissue and Fascia
U Supplement: Putting in or on biological or synthetic material that physically reinforces and/or augments the function of a portion of a body part

Body Part Character 4	Approach Character 5	Device Character 6	Qualifier Character 7
0 Subcutaneous Tissue and Fascia, Scalp **1** Subcutaneous Tissue and Fascia, Face **4** Subcutaneous Tissue and Fascia, Right Neck **5** Subcutaneous Tissue and Fascia, Left Neck **6** Subcutaneous Tissue and Fascia, Chest **7** Subcutaneous Tissue and Fascia, Back **8** Subcutaneous Tissue and Fascia, Abdomen **9** Subcutaneous Tissue and Fascia, Buttock **B** Subcutaneous Tissue and Fascia, Perineum **C** Subcutaneous Tissue and Fascia, Pelvic Region **D** Subcutaneous Tissue and Fascia, Right Upper Arm **F** Subcutaneous Tissue and Fascia, Left Upper Arm **G** Subcutaneous Tissue and Fascia, Right Lower Arm **H** Subcutaneous Tissue and Fascia, Left Lower Arm **J** Subcutaneous Tissue and Fascia, Right Hand **K** Subcutaneous Tissue and Fascia, Left Hand **L** Subcutaneous Tissue and Fascia, Right Upper Leg **M** Subcutaneous Tissue and Fascia, Left Upper Leg **N** Subcutaneous Tissue and Fascia, Right Lower Leg **P** Subcutaneous Tissue and Fascia, Left Lower Leg **Q** Subcutaneous Tissue and Fascia, Right Foot **R** Subcutaneous Tissue and Fascia, Left Foot	**0** Open **3** Percutaneous	**7** Autologous Tissue Substitute **J** Synthetic Substitute **K** Nonautologous Tissue Substitute	**Z** No Qualifier

0 Medical and Surgical
J Subcutaneous Tissue and Fascia
W Revision: Correcting, to the extent possible, a portion of a malfunctioning device or the position of a displaced device

Body Part Character 4	Approach Character 5	Device Character 6	Qualifier Character 7
S Subcutaneous Tissue and Fascia, Head and Neck DRG	**0** Open **3** Percutaneous	**0** Drainage Device **3** Infusion Device **7** Autologous Tissue Substitute **J** Synthetic Substitute **K** Nonautologous Tissue Substitute **N** Tissue Expander **Y** Other Device	**Z** No Qualifier

0JW continued on next page

0JW continued from previous page

0 Medical and Surgical
J Subcutaneous Tissue and Fascia
W Revision: Correcting, to the extent possible, a portion of a malfunctioning device or the position of a displaced device

Body Part Character 4	Approach Character 5	Device Character 6	Qualifier Character 7
S Subcutaneous Tissue and Fascia, Head and Neck	**X** External	**0** Drainage Device **3** Infusion Device **7** Autologous Tissue Substitute **J** Synthetic Substitute **K** Nonautologous Tissue Substitute **N** Tissue Expander	**Z** No Qualifier
T Subcutaneous Tissue and Fascia, Trunk HAC DRG	**0** Open **3** Percutaneous	**0** Drainage Device **2** Monitoring Device **3** Infusion Device **7** Autologous Tissue Substitute **H** Contraceptive Device **J** Synthetic Substitute **K** Nonautologous Tissue Substitute **M** Stimulator Generator **N** Tissue Expander **P** Cardiac Rhythm Related Device **V** Infusion Device, Pump **W** Vascular Access Device, Totally Implantable **X** Vascular Access Device, Tunneled **Y** Other Device	**Z** No Qualifier
T Subcutaneous Tissue and Fascia, Trunk DRG	**X** External	**0** Drainage Device **2** Monitoring Device **3** Infusion Device **7** Autologous Tissue Substitute **H** Contraceptive Device **J** Synthetic Substitute **K** Nonautologous Tissue Substitute **M** Stimulator Generator **N** Tissue Expander **P** Cardiac Rhythm Related Device **V** Infusion Device, Pump **W** Vascular Access Device, Totally Implantable **X** Vascular Access Device, Tunneled	**Z** No Qualifier
V Subcutaneous Tissue and Fascia, Upper Extremity DRG **W** Subcutaneous Tissue and Fascia, Lower Extremity DRG	**0** Open **3** Percutaneous	**0** Drainage Device **3** Infusion Device **7** Autologous Tissue Substitute **H** Contraceptive Device **J** Synthetic Substitute **K** Nonautologous Tissue Substitute **N** Tissue Expander **V** Infusion Device, Pump **W** Vascular Access Device, Totally Implantable **X** Vascular Access Device, Tunneled **Y** Other Device	**Z** No Qualifier
V Subcutaneous Tissue and Fascia, Upper Extremity **W** Subcutaneous Tissue and Fascia, Lower Extremity	**X** External	**0** Drainage Device **3** Infusion Device **7** Autologous Tissue Substitute **H** Contraceptive Device **J** Synthetic Substitute **K** Nonautologous Tissue Substitute **N** Tissue Expander **V** Infusion Device, Pump **W** Vascular Access Device, Totally Implantable **X** Vascular Access Device, Tunneled	**Z** No Qualifier

0JW continued on next page

0JW continued from previous page

HAC 0JWT0PZ 0JWT3PZ
Surgical site infection (SSI) following cardiac implantable electronic device (CIED) procedures and secondary diagnosis K68.11, T81.4XXA, T82.6XXA, T82.7XXA.

DRG 0JWS00Z 0JWS03Z 0JWS07Z 0JWS0JZ 0JWS0KZ 0JWS0NZ 0JWS0YZ 0JWS30Z 0JWS33Z 0JWS37Z 0JWS3JZ 0JWS3KZ 0JWS3NZ 0JWS3YZ 0JWT00Z 0JWT03Z 0JWT07Z 0JWT0HZ 0JWT0JZ 0JWT0KZ 0JWT0MZ 0JWT0NZ 0JWT0VZ 0JWT0WZ 0JWT0XZ 0JWT30Z 0JWT33Z 0JWT37Z 0JWT3HZ 0JWT3JZ 0JWT3KZ 0JWT3MZ 0JWT3NZ 0JWT3VZ 0JWT3WZ 0JWT3XZ 0JWTXMZ 0JWV00Z 0JWV03Z 0JWV07Z 0JWV0HZ 0JWV0JZ 0JWV0KZ 0JWV0NZ 0JWV0VZ 0JWV0WZ 0JWV0XZ 0JWV0YZ 0JWV30Z 0JWV33Z 0JWV37Z 0JWV3HZ 0JWV3JZ 0JWV3KZ 0JWV3NZ 0JWV3VZ 0JWV3WZ 0JWV3XZ 0JWV3YZ 0JWW00Z 0JWW03Z 0JWW07Z 0JWW0HZ 0JWW0JZ 0JWW0KZ 0JWW0NZ 0JWW0VZ 0JWW0WZ 0JWW0XZ 0JWW0YZ 0JWW30Z 0JWW33Z 0JWW37Z 0JWW3HZ 0JWW3JZ 0JWW3KZ 0JWW3NZ 0JWW3VZ 0JWW3WZ 0JWW3XZ 0JWW3YZ

0 Medical and Surgical
J Subcutaneous Tissue and Fascia
X Transfer: Moving, without taking out, all or a portion of a body part to another location to take over the function of all or a portion of a body part

Body Part Character 4	Approach Character 5	Device Character 6	Qualifier Character 7
0 Subcutaneous Tissue and Fascia, Scalp **1** Subcutaneous Tissue and Fascia, Face **4** Subcutaneous Tissue and Fascia, Right Neck **5** Subcutaneous Tissue and Fascia, Left Neck **6** Subcutaneous Tissue and Fascia, Chest **7** Subcutaneous Tissue and Fascia, Back **8** Subcutaneous Tissue and Fascia, Abdomen **9** Subcutaneous Tissue and Fascia, Buttock **B** Subcutaneous Tissue and Fascia, Perineum **C** Subcutaneous Tissue and Fascia, Pelvic Region **D** Subcutaneous Tissue and Fascia, Right Upper Arm **F** Subcutaneous Tissue and Fascia, Left Upper Arm **G** Subcutaneous Tissue and Fascia, Right Lower Arm **H** Subcutaneous Tissue and Fascia, Left Lower Arm **J** Subcutaneous Tissue and Fascia, Right Hand **K** Subcutaneous Tissue and Fascia, Left Hand **L** Subcutaneous Tissue and Fascia, Right Upper Leg **M** Subcutaneous Tissue and Fascia, Left Upper Leg **N** Subcutaneous Tissue and Fascia, Right Lower Leg **P** Subcutaneous Tissue and Fascia, Left Lower Leg **Q** Subcutaneous Tissue and Fascia, Right Foot **R** Subcutaneous Tissue and Fascia, Left Foot	**0** Open **3** Percutaneous	**Z** No Device	**B** Skin and Subcutaneous Tissue **C** Skin, Subcutaneous Tissue and Fascia **Z** No Qualifier

NOTES

Muscles 0K2-0KX

0 Medical and Surgical
K Muscles
2 Change: Taking out or off a device from a body part and putting back an identical or similar device in or on the same body part without cutting or puncturing the skin or a mucous membrane

Body Part Character 4	Approach Character 5	Device Character 6	Qualifier Character 7
X Upper Muscle **Y** Lower Muscle	**X** External	**0** Drainage Device **Y** Other Device	**Z** No Qualifier

0 Medical and Surgical
K Muscles
5 Destruction: Physical eradication of all or a portion of a body part by the direct use of energy, force, or a destructive agent

Body Part Character 4	Approach Character 5	Device Character 6	Qualifier Character 7
0 Head Muscle **1** Facial Muscle **2** Neck Muscle, Right **3** Neck Muscle, Left **4** Tongue, Palate, Pharynx Muscle **5** Shoulder Muscle, Right **6** Shoulder Muscle, Left **7** Upper Arm Muscle, Right **8** Upper Arm Muscle, Left **9** Lower Arm and Wrist Muscle, Right **B** Lower Arm and Wrist Muscle, Left **C** Hand Muscle, Right **D** Hand Muscle, Left **F** Trunk Muscle, Right **G** Trunk Muscle, Left **H** Thorax Muscle, Right **J** Thorax Muscle, Left **K** Abdomen Muscle, Right **L** Abdomen Muscle, Left **M** Perineum Muscle **N** Hip Muscle, Right **P** Hip Muscle, Left **Q** Upper Leg Muscle, Right **R** Upper Leg Muscle, Left **S** Lower Leg Muscle, Right **T** Lower Leg Muscle, Left **V** Foot Muscle, Right **W** Foot Muscle, Left	**0** Open **3** Percutaneous **4** Percutaneous Endoscopic	**Z** No Device	**Z** No Qualifier

0 Medical and Surgical
K Muscles
8 Division: Cutting into a body part, without draining fluids and/or gases from the body part, in order to separate or transect a body part

Body Part Character 4	Approach Character 5	Device Character 6	Qualifier Character 7
0 Head Muscle **1** Facial Muscle **2** Neck Muscle, Right **3** Neck Muscle, Left **4** Tongue, Palate, Pharynx Muscle **5** Shoulder Muscle, Right **6** Shoulder Muscle, Left **7** Upper Arm Muscle, Right **8** Upper Arm Muscle, Left **9** Lower Arm and Wrist Muscle, Right **B** Lower Arm and Wrist Muscle, Left **C** Hand Muscle, Right **D** Hand Muscle, Left **F** Trunk Muscle, Right **G** Trunk Muscle, Left **H** Thorax Muscle, Right **J** Thorax Muscle, Left **K** Abdomen Muscle, Right **L** Abdomen Muscle, Left **M** Perineum Muscle **N** Hip Muscle, Right **P** Hip Muscle, Left **Q** Upper Leg Muscle, Right **R** Upper Leg Muscle, Left **S** Lower Leg Muscle, Right **T** Lower Leg Muscle, Left **V** Foot Muscle, Right **W** Foot Muscle, Left	**0** Open **3** Percutaneous **4** Percutaneous Endoscopic	**Z** No Device	**Z** No Qualifier

0 Medical and Surgical
K Muscles
9 Drainage: Taking or letting out fluids and/or gases from a body part

Body Part Character 4	Approach Character 5	Device Character 6	Qualifier Character 7
0 Head Muscle **1** Facial Muscle **2** Neck Muscle, Right **3** Neck Muscle, Left **4** Tongue, Palate, Pharynx Muscle **5** Shoulder Muscle, Right **6** Shoulder Muscle, Left **7** Upper Arm Muscle, Right **8** Upper Arm Muscle, Left **9** Lower Arm and Wrist Muscle, Right **B** Lower Arm and Wrist Muscle, Left **C** Hand Muscle, Right **D** Hand Muscle, Left **F** Trunk Muscle, Right **G** Trunk Muscle, Left **H** Thorax Muscle, Right **J** Thorax Muscle, Left **K** Abdomen Muscle, Right **L** Abdomen Muscle, Left **M** Perineum Muscle **N** Hip Muscle, Right **P** Hip Muscle, Left **Q** Upper Leg Muscle, Right **R** Upper Leg Muscle, Left **S** Lower Leg Muscle, Right **T** Lower Leg Muscle, Left **V** Foot Muscle, Right **W** Foot Muscle, Left	**0** Open **3** Percutaneous **4** Percutaneous Endoscopic	**0** Drainage Device	**Z** No Qualifier
0 Head Muscle **1** Facial Muscle **2** Neck Muscle, Right **3** Neck Muscle, Left **4** Tongue, Palate, Pharynx Muscle **5** Shoulder Muscle, Right **6** Shoulder Muscle, Left **7** Upper Arm Muscle, Right **8** Upper Arm Muscle, Left **9** Lower Arm and Wrist Muscle, Right **B** Lower Arm and Wrist Muscle, Left **C** Hand Muscle, Right **D** Hand Muscle, Left **F** Trunk Muscle, Right **G** Trunk Muscle, Left **H** Thorax Muscle, Right **J** Thorax Muscle, Left **K** Abdomen Muscle, Right **L** Abdomen Muscle, Left **M** Perineum Muscle **N** Hip Muscle, Right **P** Hip Muscle, Left **Q** Upper Leg Muscle, Right **R** Upper Leg Muscle, Left **S** Lower Leg Muscle, Right **T** Lower Leg Muscle, Left **V** Foot Muscle, Right **W** Foot Muscle, Left	**0** Open **3** Percutaneous **4** Percutaneous Endoscopic	**Z** No Device	**X** Diagnostic **Z** No Qualifier

0 **Medical and Surgical**
K **Muscles**
B **Excision:** Cutting out or off, without replacement, a portion of a body part

Body Part Character 4	Approach Character 5	Device Character 6	Qualifier Character 7
0 Head Muscle **1** Facial Muscle **2** Neck Muscle, Right **3** Neck Muscle, Left **4** Tongue, Palate, Pharynx Muscle **5** Shoulder Muscle, Right **6** Shoulder Muscle, Left **7** Upper Arm Muscle, Right **8** Upper Arm Muscle, Left **9** Lower Arm and Wrist Muscle, Right **B** Lower Arm and Wrist Muscle, Left **C** Hand Muscle, Right **D** Hand Muscle, Left **F** Trunk Muscle, Right **G** Trunk Muscle, Left **H** Thorax Muscle, Right **J** Thorax Muscle, Left **K** Abdomen Muscle, Right **L** Abdomen Muscle, Left **M** Perineum Muscle **N** Hip Muscle, Right **P** Hip Muscle, Left **Q** Upper Leg Muscle, Right **R** Upper Leg Muscle, Left **S** Lower Leg Muscle, Right **T** Lower Leg Muscle, Left **V** Foot Muscle, Right **W** Foot Muscle, Left	**0** Open **3** Percutaneous **4** Percutaneous Endoscopic	**Z** No Device	**X** Diagnostic **Z** No Qualifier

0 **Medical and Surgical**
K **Muscles**
C **Extirpation:** Taking or cutting out solid matter from a body part

Body Part Character 4	Approach Character 5	Device Character 6	Qualifier Character 7
0 Head Muscle **1** Facial Muscle **2** Neck Muscle, Right **3** Neck Muscle, Left **4** Tongue, Palate, Pharynx Muscle **5** Shoulder Muscle, Right **6** Shoulder Muscle, Left **7** Upper Arm Muscle, Right **8** Upper Arm Muscle, Left **9** Lower Arm and Wrist Muscle, Right **B** Lower Arm and Wrist Muscle, Left **C** Hand Muscle, Right **D** Hand Muscle, Left **F** Trunk Muscle, Right **G** Trunk Muscle, Left **H** Thorax Muscle, Right **J** Thorax Muscle, Left **K** Abdomen Muscle, Right **L** Abdomen Muscle, Left **M** Perineum Muscle **N** Hip Muscle, Right **P** Hip Muscle, Left **Q** Upper Leg Muscle, Right **R** Upper Leg Muscle, Left **S** Lower Leg Muscle, Right **T** Lower Leg Muscle, Left **V** Foot Muscle, Right **W** Foot Muscle, Left	**0** Open **3** Percutaneous **4** Percutaneous Endoscopic	**Z** No Device	**Z** No Qualifier

0 Medical and Surgical
K Muscles
D Extraction: Pulling or stripping out or off all or a portion of a body part by the use of force

Body Part Character 4	Approach Character 5	Device Character 6	Qualifier Character 7
0 Head Muscle **1** Facial Muscle **2** Neck Muscle, Right **3** Neck Muscle, Left **4** Tongue, Palate, Pharynx Muscle **5** Shoulder Muscle, Right **6** Shoulder Muscle, Left **7** Upper Arm Muscle, Right **8** Upper Arm Muscle, Left **9** Lower Arm and Wrist Muscle, Right **B** Lower Arm and Wrist Muscle, Left **C** Hand Muscle, Right **D** Hand Muscle, Left **F** Trunk Muscle, Right **G** Trunk Muscle, Left **H** Thorax Muscle, Right **J** Thorax Muscle, Left **K** Abdomen Muscle, Right **L** Abdomen Muscle, Left **M** Perineum Muscle **N** Hip Muscle, Right **P** Hip Muscle, Left **Q** Upper Leg Muscle, Right **R** Upper Leg Muscle, Left **S** Lower Leg Muscle, Right **T** Lower Leg Muscle, Left **V** Foot Muscle, Right **W** Foot Muscle, Left	**0** Open	**Z** No Device	**Z** No Qualifier

0 Medical and Surgical
K Muscles
H Insertion: Putting in a nonbiological appliance that monitors, assists, performs, or prevents a physiological function but does not physically take the place of a body part

Body Part Character 4	Approach Character 5	Device Character 6	Qualifier Character 7
X Upper Muscle **Y** Lower Muscle	**0** Open **3** Percutaneous **4** Percutaneous Endoscopic	**M** Stimulator Lead **Y** Other Device	**Z** No Qualifier

0 Medical and Surgical
K Muscles
J Inspection: Visually and/or manually exploring a body part

Body Part Character 4	Approach Character 5	Device Character 6	Qualifier Character 7
X Upper Muscle **Y** Lower Muscle	**0** Open **3** Percutaneous **4** Percutaneous Endoscopic **X** External	**Z** No Device	**Z** No Qualifier

0 Medical and Surgical
K Muscles
M Reattachment: Putting back in or on all or a portion of a separated body part to its normal location or other suitable location

Body Part Character 4	Approach Character 5	Device Character 6	Qualifier Character 7
0 Head Muscle **1** Facial Muscle **2** Neck Muscle, Right **3** Neck Muscle, Left **4** Tongue, Palate, Pharynx Muscle **5** Shoulder Muscle, Right **6** Shoulder Muscle, Left **7** Upper Arm Muscle, Right **8** Upper Arm Muscle, Left **9** Lower Arm and Wrist Muscle, Right **B** Lower Arm and Wrist Muscle, Left **C** Hand Muscle, Right **D** Hand Muscle, Left **F** Trunk Muscle, Right **G** Trunk Muscle, Left **H** Thorax Muscle, Right **J** Thorax Muscle, Left **K** Abdomen Muscle, Right **L** Abdomen Muscle, Left **M** Perineum Muscle **N** Hip Muscle, Right **P** Hip Muscle, Left **Q** Upper Leg Muscle, Right **R** Upper Leg Muscle, Left **S** Lower Leg Muscle, Right **T** Lower Leg Muscle, Left **V** Foot Muscle, Right **W** Foot Muscle, Left	**0** Open **4** Percutaneous Endoscopic	**Z** No Device	**Z** No Qualifier

0 Medical and Surgical
K Muscles
N Release: Freeing a body part from an abnormal physical constraint by cutting or by the use of force

Body Part	Approach	Device	Qualifier
Character 4	**Character 5**	**Character 6**	**Character 7**
0 Head Muscle **1** Facial Muscle **2** Neck Muscle, Right **3** Neck Muscle, Left **4** Tongue, Palate, Pharynx Muscle **5** Shoulder Muscle, Right **6** Shoulder Muscle, Left **7** Upper Arm Muscle, Right **8** Upper Arm Muscle, Left **9** Lower Arm and Wrist Muscle, Right **B** Lower Arm and Wrist Muscle, Left **C** Hand Muscle, Right **D** Hand Muscle, Left **F** Trunk Muscle, Right **G** Trunk Muscle, Left **H** Thorax Muscle, Right **J** Thorax Muscle, Left **K** Abdomen Muscle, Right **L** Abdomen Muscle, Left **M** Perineum Muscle **N** Hip Muscle, Right **P** Hip Muscle, Left **Q** Upper Leg Muscle, Right **R** Upper Leg Muscle, Left **S** Lower Leg Muscle, Right **T** Lower Leg Muscle, Left **V** Foot Muscle, Right **W** Foot Muscle, Left	**0** Open **3** Percutaneous **4** Percutaneous Endoscopic **X** External	**Z** No Device	**Z** No Qualifier

0 Medical and Surgical
K Muscles
P Removal: Taking out or off a device from a body part

Body Part	Approach	Device	Qualifier
Character 4	**Character 5**	**Character 6**	**Character 7**
X Upper Muscle **Y** Lower Muscle	**0** Open **3** Percutaneous **4** Percutaneous Endoscopic	**0** Drainage Device **7** Autologous Tissue Substitute **J** Synthetic Substitute **K** Nonautologous Tissue Substitute **M** Stimulator Lead **Y** Other Device	**Z** No Qualifier
X Upper Muscle **Y** Lower Muscle	**X** External	**0** Drainage Device **M** Stimulator Lead	**Z** No Qualifier

0 Medical and Surgical
K Muscles
Q Repair: Restoring, to the extent possible, a body part to its normal anatomic structure and function

Body Part	Approach	Device	Qualifier
Character 4	**Character 5**	**Character 6**	**Character 7**
0 Head Muscle **1** Facial Muscle **2** Neck Muscle, Right **3** Neck Muscle, Left **4** Tongue, Palate, Pharynx Muscle **5** Shoulder Muscle, Right **6** Shoulder Muscle, Left **7** Upper Arm Muscle, Right **8** Upper Arm Muscle, Left **9** Lower Arm and Wrist Muscle, Right **B** Lower Arm and Wrist Muscle, Left **C** Hand Muscle, Right **D** Hand Muscle, Left **F** Trunk Muscle, Right **G** Trunk Muscle, Left **H** Thorax Muscle, Right **J** Thorax Muscle, Left **K** Abdomen Muscle, Right **L** Abdomen Muscle, Left **M** Perineum Muscle **N** Hip Muscle, Right **P** Hip Muscle, Left **Q** Upper Leg Muscle, Right **R** Upper Leg Muscle, Left **S** Lower Leg Muscle, Right **T** Lower Leg Muscle, Left **V** Foot Muscle, Right **W** Foot Muscle, Left	**0** Open **3** Percutaneous **4** Percutaneous Endoscopic	**Z** No Device	**Z** No Qualifier

0 Medical and Surgical
K Muscles
R Replacement: Putting in or on biological or synthetic material that physically takes the place and/or function of all or a portion of a body part

Body Part	Approach	Device	Qualifier
Character 4	**Character 5**	**Character 6**	**Character 7**
0 Head Muscle **1** Facial Muscle **2** Neck Muscle, Right **3** Neck Muscle, Left **4** Tongue, Palate, Pharynx Muscle **5** Shoulder Muscle, Right **6** Shoulder Muscle, Left **7** Upper Arm Muscle, Right **8** Upper Arm Muscle, Left **9** Lower Arm and Wrist Muscle, Right **B** Lower Arm and Wrist Muscle, Left **C** Hand Muscle, Right **D** Hand Muscle, Left **F** Trunk Muscle, Right **G** Trunk Muscle, Left **H** Thorax Muscle, Right **J** Thorax Muscle, Left **K** Abdomen Muscle, Right **L** Abdomen Muscle, Left **M** Perineum Muscle **N** Hip Muscle, Right **P** Hip Muscle, Left **Q** Upper Leg Muscle, Right **R** Upper Leg Muscle, Left **S** Lower Leg Muscle, Right **T** Lower Leg Muscle, Left **V** Foot Muscle, Right **W** Foot Muscle, Left	**0** Open **4** Percutaneous Endoscopic	**7** Autologous Tissue Substitute **J** Synthetic Substitute **K** Nonautologous Tissue Substitute	**Z** No Qualifier

0 Medical and Surgical
K Muscles
S Reposition: Moving to its normal location, or other suitable location, all or a portion of a body part

Body Part Character 4	Approach Character 5	Device Character 6	Qualifier Character 7
0 Head Muscle **1** Facial Muscle **2** Neck Muscle, Right **3** Neck Muscle, Left **4** Tongue, Palate, Pharynx Muscle **5** Shoulder Muscle, Right **6** Shoulder Muscle, Left **7** Upper Arm Muscle, Right **8** Upper Arm Muscle, Left **9** Lower Arm and Wrist Muscle, Right **B** Lower Arm and Wrist Muscle, Left **C** Hand Muscle, Right **D** Hand Muscle, Left **F** Trunk Muscle, Right **G** Trunk Muscle, Left **H** Thorax Muscle, Right **J** Thorax Muscle, Left **K** Abdomen Muscle, Right **L** Abdomen Muscle, Left **M** Perineum Muscle **N** Hip Muscle, Right **P** Hip Muscle, Left **Q** Upper Leg Muscle, Right **R** Upper Leg Muscle, Left **S** Lower Leg Muscle, Right **T** Lower Leg Muscle, Left **V** Foot Muscle, Right **W** Foot Muscle, Left	**0** Open **4** Percutaneous Endoscopic	**Z** No Device	**Z** No Qualifier

0 Medical and Surgical
K Muscles
T Resection: Cutting out or off, without replacement, all of a body part

Body Part Character 4	Approach Character 5	Device Character 6	Qualifier Character 7
0 Head Muscle **1** Facial Muscle **2** Neck Muscle, Right **3** Neck Muscle, Left **4** Tongue, Palate, Pharynx Muscle **5** Shoulder Muscle, Right **6** Shoulder Muscle, Left **7** Upper Arm Muscle, Right **8** Upper Arm Muscle, Left **9** Lower Arm and Wrist Muscle, Right **B** Lower Arm and Wrist Muscle, Left **C** Hand Muscle, Right **D** Hand Muscle, Left **F** Trunk Muscle, Right **G** Trunk Muscle, Left **H** Thorax Muscle, Right CC **J** Thorax Muscle, Left CC **K** Abdomen Muscle, Right **L** Abdomen Muscle, Left **M** Perineum Muscle **N** Hip Muscle, Right **P** Hip Muscle, Left **Q** Upper Leg Muscle, Right **R** Upper Leg Muscle, Left **S** Lower Leg Muscle, Right **T** Lower Leg Muscle, Left **V** Foot Muscle, Right **W** Foot Muscle, Left	**0** Open **4** Percutaneous Endoscopic	**Z** No Device	**Z** No Qualifier

CC 0KTH0ZZ 0KTJ0ZZ

LC Limited Coverage NC Noncovered HAC HAC-associated Procedure CC Combination Cluster - See Appendix G for code lists
DRG Non-OR-Affecting MS-DRG Assignment New/Revised Text in **Orange** ♂ Male ♀ Female

0 Medical and Surgical
K Muscles
U Supplement: Putting in or on biological or synthetic material that physically reinforces and/or augments the function of a portion of a body part

Body Part	Approach	Device	Qualifier
Character 4	Character 5	Character 6	Character 7
0 Head Muscle **1** Facial Muscle **2** Neck Muscle, Right **3** Neck Muscle, Left **4** Tongue, Palate, Pharynx Muscle **5** Shoulder Muscle, Right **6** Shoulder Muscle, Left **7** Upper Arm Muscle, Right **8** Upper Arm Muscle, Left **9** Lower Arm and Wrist Muscle, Right **B** Lower Arm and Wrist Muscle, Left **C** Hand Muscle, Right **D** Hand Muscle, Left **F** Trunk Muscle, Right **G** Trunk Muscle, Left **H** Thorax Muscle, Right **J** Thorax Muscle, Left **K** Abdomen Muscle, Right **L** Abdomen Muscle, Left **M** Perineum Muscle **N** Hip Muscle, Right **P** Hip Muscle, Left **Q** Upper Leg Muscle, Right **R** Upper Leg Muscle, Left **S** Lower Leg Muscle, Right **T** Lower Leg Muscle, Left **V** Foot Muscle, Right **W** Foot Muscle, Left	**0** Open **4** Percutaneous Endoscopic	**7** Autologous Tissue Substitute **J** Synthetic Substitute **K** Nonautologous Tissue Substitute	**Z** No Qualifier

0 Medical and Surgical
K Muscles
W Revision: Correcting, to the extent possible, a portion of a malfunctioning device or the position of a displaced device

Body Part	Approach	Device	Qualifier
Character 4	Character 5	Character 6	Character 7
X Upper Muscle **Y** Lower Muscle	**0** Open **3** Percutaneous **4** Percutaneous Endoscopic	**0** Drainage Device **7** Autologous Tissue Substitute **J** Synthetic Substitute **K** Nonautologous Tissue Substitute **M** Stimulator Lead **Y** Other Device	**Z** No Qualifier
X Upper Muscle **Y** Lower Muscle	**X** External	**0** Drainage Device **7** Autologous Tissue Substitute **J** Synthetic Substitute **K** Nonautologous Tissue Substitute **M** Stimulator Lead	**Z** No Qualifier

0 **Medical and Surgical**
K **Muscles**
X **Transfer:** Moving, without taking out, all or a portion of a body part to another location to take over the function of all or a portion of a body part

Body Part Character 4	Approach Character 5	Device Character 6	Qualifier Character 7
0 Head Muscle **1** Facial Muscle CC **2** Neck Muscle, Right **3** Neck Muscle, Left **4** Tongue, Palate, Pharynx Muscle **5** Shoulder Muscle, Right **6** Shoulder Muscle, Left **7** Upper Arm Muscle, Right **8** Upper Arm Muscle, Left **9** Lower Arm and Wrist Muscle, Right **B** Lower Arm and Wrist Muscle, Left **C** Hand Muscle, Right **D** Hand Muscle, Left **H** Thorax Muscle, Right **J** Thorax Muscle, Left **M** Perineum Muscle **N** Hip Muscle, Right **P** Hip Muscle, Left **Q** Upper Leg Muscle, Right **R** Upper Leg Muscle, Left **S** Lower Leg Muscle, Right CC **T** Lower Leg Muscle, Left CC **V** Foot Muscle, Right **W** Foot Muscle, Left	**0** Open **4** Percutaneous Endoscopic	**Z** No Device	**0** Skin **1** Subcutaneous Tissue **2** Skin and Subcutaneous Tissue **Z** No Qualifier
F Trunk Muscle, Right **G** Trunk Muscle, Left	**0** Open **4** Percutaneous Endoscopic	**Z** No Device	**0** Skin **1** Subcutaneous Tissue **2** Skin and Subcutaneous Tissue **5** Latissimus Dorsi Myocutaneous Flap **7** Deep Inferior Epigastric Artery Perforator Flap **8** Superficial Inferior Epigastric Artery Flap **9** Gluteal Artery Perforator Flap **Z** No Qualifier
K Abdomen Muscle, Right **L** Abdomen Muscle, Left	**0** Open **4** Percutaneous Endoscopic	**Z** No Device	**0** Skin **1** Subcutaneous Tissue **2** Skin and Subcutaneous Tissue **6** Transverse Rectus Abdominis Myocutaneous Flap **Z** No Qualifier

CC 0KX10ZZ 0KX14ZZ 0KXS0ZZ 0KXS4ZZ 0KXT0ZZ 0KXT4ZZ

NOTES

Tendons 0L2-0LX

0 Medical and Surgical
L Tendons
2 Change: Taking out or off a device from a body part and putting back an identical or similar device in or on the same body part without cutting or puncturing the skin or a mucous membrane

Body Part	Approach	Device	Qualifier
Character 4	Character 5	Character 6	Character 7
X Upper Tendon **Y** Lower Tendon	**X** External	**0** Drainage Device **Y** Other Device	**Z** No Qualifier

0 Medical and Surgical
L Tendons
5 Destruction: Physical eradication of all or a portion of a body part by the direct use of energy, force, or a destructive agent

Body Part	Approach	Device	Qualifier
Character 4	Character 5	Character 6	Character 7
0 Head and Neck Tendon **1** Shoulder Tendon, Right **2** Shoulder Tendon, Left **3** Upper Arm Tendon, Right **4** Upper Arm Tendon, Left **5** Lower Arm and Wrist Tendon, Right **6** Lower Arm and Wrist Tendon, Left **7** Hand Tendon, Right **8** Hand Tendon, Left **9** Trunk Tendon, Right **B** Trunk Tendon, Left **C** Thorax Tendon, Right **D** Thorax Tendon, Left **F** Abdomen Tendon, Right **G** Abdomen Tendon, Left **H** Perineum Tendon **J** Hip Tendon, Right **K** Hip Tendon, Left **L** Upper Leg Tendon, Right **M** Upper Leg Tendon, Left **N** Lower Leg Tendon, Right **P** Lower Leg Tendon, Left **Q** Knee Tendon, Right **R** Knee Tendon, Left **S** Ankle Tendon, Right **T** Ankle Tendon, Left **V** Foot Tendon, Right **W** Foot Tendon, Left	**0** Open **3** Percutaneous **4** Percutaneous Endoscopic	**Z** No Device	**Z** No Qualifier

0 Medical and Surgical
L Tendons
8 Division: Cutting into a body part, without draining fluids and/or gases from the body part, in order to separate or transect a body part

Body Part Character 4	Approach Character 5	Device Character 6	Qualifier Character 7
0 Head and Neck Tendon **1** Shoulder Tendon, Right **2** Shoulder Tendon, Left **3** Upper Arm Tendon, Right **4** Upper Arm Tendon, Left **5** Lower Arm and Wrist Tendon, Right **6** Lower Arm and Wrist Tendon, Left **7** Hand Tendon, Right **8** Hand Tendon, Left **9** Trunk Tendon, Right **B** Trunk Tendon, Left **C** Thorax Tendon, Right **D** Thorax Tendon, Left **F** Abdomen Tendon, Right **G** Abdomen Tendon, Left **H** Perineum Tendon **J** Hip Tendon, Right **K** Hip Tendon, Left **L** Upper Leg Tendon, Right **M** Upper Leg Tendon, Left **N** Lower Leg Tendon, Right **P** Lower Leg Tendon, Left **Q** Knee Tendon, Right **R** Knee Tendon, Left **S** Ankle Tendon, Right **T** Ankle Tendon, Left **V** Foot Tendon, Right **W** Foot Tendon, Left	**0** Open **3** Percutaneous **4** Percutaneous Endoscopic	**Z** No Device	**Z** No Qualifier

0 Medical and Surgical
L Tendons
9 Drainage: Taking or letting out fluids and/or gases from a body part

Body Part Character 4	Approach Character 5	Device Character 6	Qualifier Character 7
0 Head and Neck Tendon **1** Shoulder Tendon, Right **2** Shoulder Tendon, Left **3** Upper Arm Tendon, Right **4** Upper Arm Tendon, Left **5** Lower Arm and Wrist Tendon, Right **6** Lower Arm and Wrist Tendon, Left **7** Hand Tendon, Right **8** Hand Tendon, Left **9** Trunk Tendon, Right **B** Trunk Tendon, Left **C** Thorax Tendon, Right **D** Thorax Tendon, Left **F** Abdomen Tendon, Right **G** Abdomen Tendon, Left **H** Perineum Tendon **J** Hip Tendon, Right **K** Hip Tendon, Left **L** Upper Leg Tendon, Right **M** Upper Leg Tendon, Left **N** Lower Leg Tendon, Right **P** Lower Leg Tendon, Left **Q** Knee Tendon, Right **R** Knee Tendon, Left **S** Ankle Tendon, Right **T** Ankle Tendon, Left **V** Foot Tendon, Right **W** Foot Tendon, Left	**0** Open **3** Percutaneous **4** Percutaneous Endoscopic	**0** Drainage Device	**Z** No Qualifier
0 Head and Neck Tendon **1** Shoulder Tendon, Right **2** Shoulder Tendon, Left **3** Upper Arm Tendon, Right **4** Upper Arm Tendon, Left **5** Lower Arm and Wrist Tendon, Right **6** Lower Arm and Wrist Tendon, Left **7** Hand Tendon, Right **8** Hand Tendon, Left **9** Trunk Tendon, Right **B** Trunk Tendon, Left **C** Thorax Tendon, Right **D** Thorax Tendon, Left **F** Abdomen Tendon, Right **G** Abdomen Tendon, Left **H** Perineum Tendon **J** Hip Tendon, Right **K** Hip Tendon, Left **L** Upper Leg Tendon, Right **M** Upper Leg Tendon, Left **N** Lower Leg Tendon, Right **P** Lower Leg Tendon, Left **Q** Knee Tendon, Right **R** Knee Tendon, Left **S** Ankle Tendon, Right **T** Ankle Tendon, Left **V** Foot Tendon, Right **W** Foot Tendon, Left	**0** Open **3** Percutaneous **4** Percutaneous Endoscopic	**Z** No Device	**X** Diagnostic **Z** No Qualifier

0 Medical and Surgical
L Tendons
B Excision: Cutting out or off, without replacement, a portion of a body part

Body Part Character 4	Approach Character 5	Device Character 6	Qualifier Character 7
0 Head and Neck Tendon **1** Shoulder Tendon, Right **2** Shoulder Tendon, Left **3** Upper Arm Tendon, Right **4** Upper Arm Tendon, Left **5** Lower Arm and Wrist Tendon, Right **6** Lower Arm and Wrist Tendon, Left **7** Hand Tendon, Right **8** Hand Tendon, Left **9** Trunk Tendon, Right **B** Trunk Tendon, Left **C** Thorax Tendon, Right **D** Thorax Tendon, Left **F** Abdomen Tendon, Right **G** Abdomen Tendon, Left **H** Perineum Tendon **J** Hip Tendon, Right **K** Hip Tendon, Left **L** Upper Leg Tendon, Right **M** Upper Leg Tendon, Left **N** Lower Leg Tendon, Right **P** Lower Leg Tendon, Left **Q** Knee Tendon, Right **R** Knee Tendon, Left **S** Ankle Tendon, Right **T** Ankle Tendon, Left **V** Foot Tendon, Right **W** Foot Tendon, Left	**0** Open **3** Percutaneous **4** Percutaneous Endoscopic	**Z** No Device	**X** Diagnostic **Z** No Qualifier

0 Medical and Surgical
L Tendons
C Extirpation: Taking or cutting out solid matter from a body part

Body Part Character 4	Approach Character 5	Device Character 6	Qualifier Character 7
0 Head and Neck Tendon **1** Shoulder Tendon, Right **2** Shoulder Tendon, Left **3** Upper Arm Tendon, Right **4** Upper Arm Tendon, Left **5** Lower Arm and Wrist Tendon, Right **6** Lower Arm and Wrist Tendon, Left **7** Hand Tendon, Right **8** Hand Tendon, Left **9** Trunk Tendon, Right **B** Trunk Tendon, Left **C** Thorax Tendon, Right **D** Thorax Tendon, Left **F** Abdomen Tendon, Right **G** Abdomen Tendon, Left **H** Perineum Tendon **J** Hip Tendon, Right **K** Hip Tendon, Left **L** Upper Leg Tendon, Right **M** Upper Leg Tendon, Left **N** Lower Leg Tendon, Right **P** Lower Leg Tendon, Left **Q** Knee Tendon, Right **R** Knee Tendon, Left **S** Ankle Tendon, Right **T** Ankle Tendon, Left **V** Foot Tendon, Right **W** Foot Tendon, Left	**0** Open **3** Percutaneous **4** Percutaneous Endoscopic	**Z** No Device	**Z** No Qualifier

0 Medical and Surgical
L Tendons
D Extraction: Pulling or stripping out or off all or a portion of a body part by the use of force

Body Part Character 4	Approach Character 5	Device Character 6	Qualifier Character 7
0 Head and Neck Tendon **1** Shoulder Tendon, Right **2** Shoulder Tendon, Left **3** Upper Arm Tendon, Right **4** Upper Arm Tendon, Left **5** Lower Arm and Wrist Tendon, Right **6** Lower Arm and Wrist Tendon, Left **7** Hand Tendon, Right **8** Hand Tendon, Left **9** Trunk Tendon, Right **B** Trunk Tendon, Left **C** Thorax Tendon, Right **D** Thorax Tendon, Left **F** Abdomen Tendon, Right **G** Abdomen Tendon, Left **H** Perineum Tendon **J** Hip Tendon, Right **K** Hip Tendon, Left **L** Upper Leg Tendon, Right **M** Upper Leg Tendon, Left **N** Lower Leg Tendon, Right **P** Lower Leg Tendon, Left **Q** Knee Tendon, Right **R** Knee Tendon, Left **S** Ankle Tendon, Right **T** Ankle Tendon, Left **V** Foot Tendon, Right **W** Foot Tendon, Left	**0** Open	**Z** No Device	**Z** No Qualifier

0 Medical and Surgical
L Tendons
H Insertion: Putting in a nonbiological appliance that monitors, assists, performs, or prevents a physiological function but does not physically take the place of a body part

Body Part Character 4	Approach Character 5	Device Character 6	Qualifier Character 7
X Upper Tendon **Y** Lower Tendon	**0** Open **3** Percutaneous **4** Percutaneous Endoscopic	**Y** Other Device	**Z** No Qualifier

0 Medical and Surgical
L Tendons
J Inspection: Visually and/or manually exploring a body part

Body Part Character 4	Approach Character 5	Device Character 6	Qualifier Character 7
X Upper Tendon **Y** Lower Tendon	**0** Open **3** Percutaneous **4** Percutaneous Endoscopic **X** External	**Z** No Device	**Z** No Qualifier

0 Medical and Surgical
L Tendons
M Reattachment: Putting back in or on all or a portion of a separated body part to its normal location or other suitable location

Body Part Character 4	Approach Character 5	Device Character 6	Qualifier Character 7
0 Head and Neck Tendon **1** Shoulder Tendon, Right **2** Shoulder Tendon, Left **3** Upper Arm Tendon, Right **4** Upper Arm Tendon, Left **5** Lower Arm and Wrist Tendon, Right **6** Lower Arm and Wrist Tendon, Left **7** Hand Tendon, Right **8** Hand Tendon, Left **9** Trunk Tendon, Right **B** Trunk Tendon, Left **C** Thorax Tendon, Right **D** Thorax Tendon, Left **F** Abdomen Tendon, Right **G** Abdomen Tendon, Left **H** Perineum Tendon **J** Hip Tendon, Right **K** Hip Tendon, Left **L** Upper Leg Tendon, Right **M** Upper Leg Tendon, Left **N** Lower Leg Tendon, Right **P** Lower Leg Tendon, Left **Q** Knee Tendon, Right **R** Knee Tendon, Left **S** Ankle Tendon, Right **T** Ankle Tendon, Left **V** Foot Tendon, Right **W** Foot Tendon, Left	**0** Open **4** Percutaneous Endoscopic	**Z** No Device	**Z** No Qualifier

0 Medical and Surgical
L Tendons
N Release: Freeing a body part from an abnormal physical constraint by cutting or by the use of force

Body Part Character 4	Approach Character 5	Device Character 6	Qualifier Character 7
0 Head and Neck Tendon **1** Shoulder Tendon, Right **2** Shoulder Tendon, Left **3** Upper Arm Tendon, Right **4** Upper Arm Tendon, Left **5** Lower Arm and Wrist Tendon, Right **6** Lower Arm and Wrist Tendon, Left **7** Hand Tendon, Right **8** Hand Tendon, Left **9** Trunk Tendon, Right **B** Trunk Tendon, Left **C** Thorax Tendon, Right **D** Thorax Tendon, Left **F** Abdomen Tendon, Right **G** Abdomen Tendon, Left **H** Perineum Tendon **J** Hip Tendon, Right **K** Hip Tendon, Left **L** Upper Leg Tendon, Right **M** Upper Leg Tendon, Left **N** Lower Leg Tendon, Right **P** Lower Leg Tendon, Left **Q** Knee Tendon, Right **R** Knee Tendon, Left **S** Ankle Tendon, Right **T** Ankle Tendon, Left **V** Foot Tendon, Right **W** Foot Tendon, Left	**0** Open **3** Percutaneous **4** Percutaneous Endoscopic **X** External	**Z** No Device	**Z** No Qualifier

0 Medical and Surgical
L Tendons
P Removal: Taking out or off a device from a body part

Body Part Character 4	Approach Character 5	Device Character 6	Qualifier Character 7
X Upper Tendon **Y** Lower Tendon	**0** Open **3** Percutaneous **4** Percutaneous Endoscopic	**0** Drainage Device **7** Autologous Tissue Substitute **J** Synthetic Substitute **K** Nonautologous Tissue Substitute **Y** Other Device	**Z** No Qualifier
X Upper Tendon **Y** Lower Tendon	**X** External	**0** Drainage Device	**Z** No Qualifier

0 Medical and Surgical
L Tendons
Q Repair: Restoring, to the extent possible, a body part to its normal anatomic structure and function

Body Part Character 4	Approach Character 5	Device Character 6	Qualifier Character 7
0 Head and Neck Tendon **1** Shoulder Tendon, Right **2** Shoulder Tendon, Left **3** Upper Arm Tendon, Right **4** Upper Arm Tendon, Left **5** Lower Arm and Wrist Tendon, Right **6** Lower Arm and Wrist Tendon, Left **7** Hand Tendon, Right **8** Hand Tendon, Left **9** Trunk Tendon, Right **B** Trunk Tendon, Left **C** Thorax Tendon, Right **D** Thorax Tendon, Left **F** Abdomen Tendon, Right **G** Abdomen Tendon, Left **H** Perineum Tendon **J** Hip Tendon, Right **K** Hip Tendon, Left **L** Upper Leg Tendon, Right **M** Upper Leg Tendon, Left **N** Lower Leg Tendon, Right **P** Lower Leg Tendon, Left **Q** Knee Tendon, Right **R** Knee Tendon, Left **S** Ankle Tendon, Right **T** Ankle Tendon, Left **V** Foot Tendon, Right **W** Foot Tendon, Left	**0** Open **3** Percutaneous **4** Percutaneous Endoscopic	**Z** No Device	**Z** No Qualifier

0 Medical and Surgical
L Tendons
R Replacement: Putting in or on biological or synthetic material that physically takes the place and/or function of all or a portion of a body part

Body Part Character 4	Approach Character 5	Device Character 6	Qualifier Character 7
0 Head and Neck Tendon **1** Shoulder Tendon, Right **2** Shoulder Tendon, Left **3** Upper Arm Tendon, Right **4** Upper Arm Tendon, Left **5** Lower Arm and Wrist Tendon, Right **6** Lower Arm and Wrist Tendon, Left **7** Hand Tendon, Right **8** Hand Tendon, Left **9** Trunk Tendon, Right **B** Trunk Tendon, Left **C** Thorax Tendon, Right **D** Thorax Tendon, Left **F** Abdomen Tendon, Right **G** Abdomen Tendon, Left **H** Perineum Tendon **J** Hip Tendon, Right **K** Hip Tendon, Left **L** Upper Leg Tendon, Right **M** Upper Leg Tendon, Left **N** Lower Leg Tendon, Right **P** Lower Leg Tendon, Left **Q** Knee Tendon, Right **R** Knee Tendon, Left **S** Ankle Tendon, Right **T** Ankle Tendon, Left **V** Foot Tendon, Right **W** Foot Tendon, Left	**0** Open **4** Percutaneous Endoscopic	**7** Autologous Tissue Substitute **J** Synthetic Substitute **K** Nonautologous Tissue Substitute	**Z** No Qualifier

0 Medical and Surgical
L Tendons
S Reposition: Moving to its normal location, or other suitable location, all or a portion of a body part

Body Part Character 4	Approach Character 5	Device Character 6	Qualifier Character 7
0 Head and Neck Tendon **1** Shoulder Tendon, Right **2** Shoulder Tendon, Left **3** Upper Arm Tendon, Right **4** Upper Arm Tendon, Left **5** Lower Arm and Wrist Tendon, Right **6** Lower Arm and Wrist Tendon, Left **7** Hand Tendon, Right **8** Hand Tendon, Left **9** Trunk Tendon, Right **B** Trunk Tendon, Left **C** Thorax Tendon, Right **D** Thorax Tendon, Left **F** Abdomen Tendon, Right **G** Abdomen Tendon, Left **H** Perineum Tendon **J** Hip Tendon, Right **K** Hip Tendon, Left **L** Upper Leg Tendon, Right **M** Upper Leg Tendon, Left **N** Lower Leg Tendon, Right **P** Lower Leg Tendon, Left **Q** Knee Tendon, Right CC **R** Knee Tendon, Left CC **S** Ankle Tendon, Right **T** Ankle Tendon, Left **V** Foot Tendon, Right **W** Foot Tendon, Left	**0** Open **4** Percutaneous Endoscopic	**Z** No Device	**Z** No Qualifier

CC 0LSQ0ZZ 0LSQ4ZZ 0LSR0ZZ 0LSR4ZZ

0 Medical and Surgical
L Tendons
T Resection: Cutting out or off, without replacement, all of a body part

Body Part Character 4	Approach Character 5	Device Character 6	Qualifier Character 7
0 Head and Neck Tendon **1** Shoulder Tendon, Right **2** Shoulder Tendon, Left **3** Upper Arm Tendon, Right **4** Upper Arm Tendon, Left **5** Lower Arm and Wrist Tendon, Right **6** Lower Arm and Wrist Tendon, Left **7** Hand Tendon, Right **8** Hand Tendon, Left **9** Trunk Tendon, Right **B** Trunk Tendon, Left **C** Thorax Tendon, Right **D** Thorax Tendon, Left **F** Abdomen Tendon, Right **G** Abdomen Tendon, Left **H** Perineum Tendon **J** Hip Tendon, Right **K** Hip Tendon, Left **L** Upper Leg Tendon, Right **M** Upper Leg Tendon, Left **N** Lower Leg Tendon, Right **P** Lower Leg Tendon, Left **Q** Knee Tendon, Right **R** Knee Tendon, Left **S** Ankle Tendon, Right **T** Ankle Tendon, Left **V** Foot Tendon, Right **W** Foot Tendon, Left	**0** Open **4** Percutaneous Endoscopic	**Z** No Device	**Z** No Qualifier

LC Limited Coverage NC Noncovered HAC HAC-associated Procedure CC Combination Cluster - See Appendix G for code lists
DRG Non-OR-Affecting MS-DRG Assignment New/Revised Text in **Orange** ♂ Male ♀ Female

0 Medical and Surgical
L Tendons
U Supplement: Putting in or on biological or synthetic material that physically reinforces and/or augments the function of a portion of a body part

Body Part Character 4	Approach Character 5	Device Character 6	Qualifier Character 7
0 Head and Neck Tendon **1** Shoulder Tendon, Right **2** Shoulder Tendon, Left **3** Upper Arm Tendon, Right **4** Upper Arm Tendon, Left **5** Lower Arm and Wrist Tendon, Right **6** Lower Arm and Wrist Tendon, Left **7** Hand Tendon, Right **8** Hand Tendon, Left **9** Trunk Tendon, Right **B** Trunk Tendon, Left **C** Thorax Tendon, Right **D** Thorax Tendon, Left **F** Abdomen Tendon, Right **G** Abdomen Tendon, Left **H** Perineum Tendon **J** Hip Tendon, Right **K** Hip Tendon, Left **L** Upper Leg Tendon, Right **M** Upper Leg Tendon, Left **N** Lower Leg Tendon, Right **P** Lower Leg Tendon, Left **Q** Knee Tendon, Right **R** Knee Tendon, Left **S** Ankle Tendon, Right **T** Ankle Tendon, Left **V** Foot Tendon, Right **W** Foot Tendon, Left	**0** Open **4** Percutaneous Endoscopic	**7** Autologous Tissue Substitute **J** Synthetic Substitute **K** Nonautologous Tissue Substitute	**Z** No Qualifier

0 Medical and Surgical
L Tendons
W Revision: Correcting, to the extent possible, a portion of a malfunctioning device or the position of a displaced device

Body Part Character 4	Approach Character 5	Device Character 6	Qualifier Character 7
X Upper Tendon **Y** Lower Tendon	**0** Open **3** Percutaneous **4** Percutaneous Endoscopic	**0** Drainage Device **7** Autologous Tissue Substitute **J** Synthetic Substitute **K** Nonautologous Tissue Substitute **Y** Other Device	**Z** No Qualifier
X Upper Tendon **Y** Lower Tendon	**X** External	**0** Drainage Device **7** Autologous Tissue Substitute **J** Synthetic Substitute **K** Nonautologous Tissue Substitute	**Z** No Qualifier

0 Medical and Surgical
L Tendons
X Transfer: Moving, without taking out, all or a portion of a body part to another location to take over the function of all or a portion of a body part

Body Part Character 4	Approach Character 5	Device Character 6	Qualifier Character 7
0 Head and Neck Tendon **1** Shoulder Tendon, Right **2** Shoulder Tendon, Left **3** Upper Arm Tendon, Right **4** Upper Arm Tendon, Left **5** Lower Arm and Wrist Tendon, Right **6** Lower Arm and Wrist Tendon, Left **7** Hand Tendon, Right **8** Hand Tendon, Left **9** Trunk Tendon, Right **B** Trunk Tendon, Left **C** Thorax Tendon, Right **D** Thorax Tendon, Left **F** Abdomen Tendon, Right **G** Abdomen Tendon, Left **H** Perineum Tendon **J** Hip Tendon, Right **K** Hip Tendon, Left **L** Upper Leg Tendon, Right **M** Upper Leg Tendon, Left **N** Lower Leg Tendon, Right **P** Lower Leg Tendon, Left **Q** Knee Tendon, Right **R** Knee Tendon, Left **S** Ankle Tendon, Right **T** Ankle Tendon, Left **V** Foot Tendon, Right **W** Foot Tendon, Left	**0** Open **4** Percutaneous Endoscopic	**Z** No Device	**Z** No Qualifier

NOTES

Bursae and Ligaments 0M2-0MX

0 Medical and Surgical
M Bursae and Ligaments
2 Change: Taking out or off a device from a body part and putting back an identical or similar device in or on the same body part without cutting or puncturing the skin or a mucous membrane

Body Part	Approach	Device	Qualifier
Character 4	**Character 5**	**Character 6**	**Character 7**
X Upper Bursa and Ligament **Y** Lower Bursa and Ligament	**X** External	**0** Drainage Device **Y** Other Device	**Z** No Qualifier

0 Medical and Surgical
M Bursae and Ligaments
5 Destruction: Physical eradication of all or a portion of a body part by the direct use of energy, force, or a destructive agent

Body Part	Approach	Device	Qualifier
Character 4	**Character 5**	**Character 6**	**Character 7**
0 Head and Neck Bursa and Ligament **1** Shoulder Bursa and Ligament, Right **2** Shoulder Bursa and Ligament, Left **3** Elbow Bursa and Ligament, Right **4** Elbow Bursa and Ligament, Left **5** Wrist Bursa and Ligament, Right **6** Wrist Bursa and Ligament, Left **7** Hand Bursa and Ligament, Right **8** Hand Bursa and Ligament, Left **9** Upper Extremity Bursa and Ligament, Right **B** Upper Extremity Bursa and Ligament, Left **C** Upper Spine Bursa and Ligament **D** Lower Spine Bursa and Ligament **F** Sternum Bursa and Ligament **G** Rib(s) Bursa and Ligament **H** Abdomen Bursa and Ligament, Right **J** Abdomen Bursa and Ligament, Left **K** Perineum Bursa and Ligament **L** Hip Bursa and Ligament, Right **M** Hip Bursa and Ligament, Left **N** Knee Bursa and Ligament, Right **P** Knee Bursa and Ligament, Left **Q** Ankle Bursa and Ligament, Right **R** Ankle Bursa and Ligament, Left **S** Foot Bursa and Ligament, Right **T** Foot Bursa and Ligament, Left **V** Lower Extremity Bursa and Ligament, Right **W** Lower Extremity Bursa and Ligament, Left	**0** Open **3** Percutaneous **4** Percutaneous Endoscopic	**Z** No Device	**Z** No Qualifier

0 Medical and Surgical
M Bursae and Ligaments
8 Division: Cutting into a body part, without draining fluids and/or gases from the body part, in order to separate or transect a body part

Body Part Character 4	Approach Character 5	Device Character 6	Qualifier Character 7
0 Head and Neck Bursa and Ligament **1** Shoulder Bursa and Ligament, Right **2** Shoulder Bursa and Ligament, Left **3** Elbow Bursa and Ligament, Right **4** Elbow Bursa and Ligament, Left **5** Wrist Bursa and Ligament, Right **6** Wrist Bursa and Ligament, Left **7** Hand Bursa and Ligament, Right **8** Hand Bursa and Ligament, Left **9** Upper Extremity Bursa and Ligament, Right **B** Upper Extremity Bursa and Ligament, Left **C** Upper Spine Bursa and Ligament **D** Lower Spine Bursa and Ligament **F** Sternum Bursa and Ligament **G** Rib(s) Bursa and Ligament **H** Abdomen Bursa and Ligament, Right **J** Abdomen Bursa and Ligament, Left **K** Perineum Bursa and Ligament **L** Hip Bursa and Ligament, Right **M** Hip Bursa and Ligament, Left **N** Knee Bursa and Ligament, Right **P** Knee Bursa and Ligament, Left **Q** Ankle Bursa and Ligament, Right **R** Ankle Bursa and Ligament, Left **S** Foot Bursa and Ligament, Right **T** Foot Bursa and Ligament, Left **V** Lower Extremity Bursa and Ligament, Right **W** Lower Extremity Bursa and Ligament, Left	**0** Open **3** Percutaneous **4** Percutaneous Endoscopic	**Z** No Device	**Z** No Qualifier

0 Medical and Surgical
M Bursae and Ligaments
9 Drainage: Taking or letting out fluids and/or gases from a body part

Body Part Character 4	Approach Character 5	Device Character 6	Qualifier Character 7
0 Head and Neck Bursa and Ligament **1** Shoulder Bursa and Ligament, Right **2** Shoulder Bursa and Ligament, Left **3** Elbow Bursa and Ligament, Right **4** Elbow Bursa and Ligament, Left **5** Wrist Bursa and Ligament, Right **6** Wrist Bursa and Ligament, Left **7** Hand Bursa and Ligament, Right **8** Hand Bursa and Ligament, Left **9** Upper Extremity Bursa and Ligament, Right **B** Upper Extremity Bursa and Ligament, Left **C** Upper Spine Bursa and Ligament **D** Lower Spine Bursa and Ligament **F** Sternum Bursa and Ligament **G** Rib(s) Bursa and Ligament **H** Abdomen Bursa and Ligament, Right **J** Abdomen Bursa and Ligament, Left **K** Perineum Bursa and Ligament **L** Hip Bursa and Ligament, Right **M** Hip Bursa and Ligament, Left **N** Knee Bursa and Ligament, Right **P** Knee Bursa and Ligament, Left **Q** Ankle Bursa and Ligament, Right **R** Ankle Bursa and Ligament, Left **S** Foot Bursa and Ligament, Right **T** Foot Bursa and Ligament, Left **V** Lower Extremity Bursa and Ligament, Right **W** Lower Extremity Bursa and Ligament, Left	**0** Open **3** Percutaneous **4** Percutaneous Endoscopic	**0** Drainage Device	**Z** No Qualifier

0M9 continued on next page

0 Medical and Surgical
M Bursae and Ligaments
9 Drainage: Taking or letting out fluids and/or gases from a body part

0M9 continued from previous page

Body Part Character 4	Approach Character 5	Device Character 6	Qualifier Character 7
0 Head and Neck Bursa and Ligament 1 Shoulder Bursa and Ligament, Right 2 Shoulder Bursa and Ligament, Left 3 Elbow Bursa and Ligament, Right 4 Elbow Bursa and Ligament, Left 5 Wrist Bursa and Ligament, Right 6 Wrist Bursa and Ligament, Left 7 Hand Bursa and Ligament, Right 8 Hand Bursa and Ligament, Left 9 Upper Extremity Bursa and Ligament, Right B Upper Extremity Bursa and Ligament, Left C Upper Spine Bursa and Ligament D Lower Spine Bursa and Ligament F Sternum Bursa and Ligament G Rib(s) Bursa and Ligament H Abdomen Bursa and Ligament, Right J Abdomen Bursa and Ligament, Left K Perineum Bursa and Ligament L Hip Bursa and Ligament, Right M Hip Bursa and Ligament, Left N Knee Bursa and Ligament, Right P Knee Bursa and Ligament, Left Q Ankle Bursa and Ligament, Right R Ankle Bursa and Ligament, Left S Foot Bursa and Ligament, Right T Foot Bursa and Ligament, Left V Lower Extremity Bursa and Ligament, Right W Lower Extremity Bursa and Ligament, Left	0 Open 3 Percutaneous 4 Percutaneous Endoscopic	Z No Device	X Diagnostic Z No Qualifier

0 Medical and Surgical
M Bursae and Ligaments
B Excision: Cutting out or off, without replacement, a portion of a body part

Body Part Character 4	Approach Character 5	Device Character 6	Qualifier Character 7
0 Head and Neck Bursa and Ligament **1** Shoulder Bursa and Ligament, Right **2** Shoulder Bursa and Ligament, Left **3** Elbow Bursa and Ligament, Right **4** Elbow Bursa and Ligament, Left **5** Wrist Bursa and Ligament, Right **6** Wrist Bursa and Ligament, Left **7** Hand Bursa and Ligament, Right **8** Hand Bursa and Ligament, Left **9** Upper Extremity Bursa and Ligament, Right **B** Upper Extremity Bursa and Ligament, Left **C** Upper Spine Bursa and Ligament **D** Lower Spine Bursa and Ligament **F** Sternum Bursa and Ligament **G** Rib(s) Bursa and Ligament **H** Abdomen Bursa and Ligament, Right **J** Abdomen Bursa and Ligament, Left **K** Perineum Bursa and Ligament **L** Hip Bursa and Ligament, Right **M** Hip Bursa and Ligament, Left **N** Knee Bursa and Ligament, Right **P** Knee Bursa and Ligament, Left **Q** Ankle Bursa and Ligament, Right **R** Ankle Bursa and Ligament, Left **S** Foot Bursa and Ligament, Right **T** Foot Bursa and Ligament, Left **V** Lower Extremity Bursa and Ligament, Right **W** Lower Extremity Bursa and Ligament, Left	**0** Open **3** Percutaneous **4** Percutaneous Endoscopic	**Z** No Device	**X** Diagnostic **Z** No Qualifier

0 Medical and Surgical
M Bursae and Ligaments
C Extirpation: Taking or cutting out solid matter from a body part

Body Part Character 4	Approach Character 5	Device Character 6	Qualifier Character 7
0 Head and Neck Bursa and Ligament **1** Shoulder Bursa and Ligament, Right **2** Shoulder Bursa and Ligament, Left **3** Elbow Bursa and Ligament, Right **4** Elbow Bursa and Ligament, Left **5** Wrist Bursa and Ligament, Right **6** Wrist Bursa and Ligament, Left **7** Hand Bursa and Ligament, Right **8** Hand Bursa and Ligament, Left **9** Upper Extremity Bursa and Ligament, Right **B** Upper Extremity Bursa and Ligament, Left **C** Upper Spine Bursa and Ligament **D** Lower Spine Bursa and Ligament **F** Sternum Bursa and Ligament **G** Rib(s) Bursa and Ligament **H** Abdomen Bursa and Ligament, Right **J** Abdomen Bursa and Ligament, Left **K** Perineum Bursa and Ligament **L** Hip Bursa and Ligament, Right **M** Hip Bursa and Ligament, Left **N** Knee Bursa and Ligament, Right **P** Knee Bursa and Ligament, Left **Q** Ankle Bursa and Ligament, Right **R** Ankle Bursa and Ligament, Left **S** Foot Bursa and Ligament, Right **T** Foot Bursa and Ligament, Left **V** Lower Extremity Bursa and Ligament, Right **W** Lower Extremity Bursa and Ligament, Left	**0** Open **3** Percutaneous **4** Percutaneous Endoscopic	**Z** No Device	**Z** No Qualifier

LC Limited Coverage NC Noncovered HAC HAC-associated Procedure CC Combination Cluster - See Appendix G for code lists
DRG Non-OR-Affecting MS-DRG Assignment New/Revised Text in **Orange** ♂ Male ♀ Female

0 Medical and Surgical
M Bursae and Ligaments
D Extraction: Pulling or stripping out or off all or a portion of a body part by the use of force

Body Part Character 4	Approach Character 5	Device Character 6	Qualifier Character 7
0 Head and Neck Bursa and Ligament **1** Shoulder Bursa and Ligament, Right **2** Shoulder Bursa and Ligament, Left **3** Elbow Bursa and Ligament, Right **4** Elbow Bursa and Ligament, Left **5** Wrist Bursa and Ligament, Right **6** Wrist Bursa and Ligament, Left **7** Hand Bursa and Ligament, Right **8** Hand Bursa and Ligament, Left **9** Upper Extremity Bursa and Ligament, Right **B** Upper Extremity Bursa and Ligament, Left **C** Upper Spine Bursa and Ligament **D** Lower Spine Bursa and Ligament **F** Sternum Bursa and Ligament **G** Rib(s) Bursa and Ligament **H** Abdomen Bursa and Ligament, Right **J** Abdomen Bursa and Ligament, Left **K** Perineum Bursa and Ligament **L** Hip Bursa and Ligament, Right **M** Hip Bursa and Ligament, Left **N** Knee Bursa and Ligament, Right **P** Knee Bursa and Ligament, Left **Q** Ankle Bursa and Ligament, Right **R** Ankle Bursa and Ligament, Left **S** Foot Bursa and Ligament, Right **T** Foot Bursa and Ligament, Left **V** Lower Extremity Bursa and Ligament, Right **W** Lower Extremity Bursa and Ligament, Left	**0** Open **3** Percutaneous **4** Percutaneous Endoscopic	**Z** No Device	**Z** No Qualifier

0 Medical and Surgical
M Bursae and Ligaments
H Insertion: Putting in a nonbiological appliance that monitors, assists, performs, or prevents a physiological function but does not physically take the place of a body part

Body Part Character 4	Approach Character 5	Device Character 6	Qualifier Character 7
X Upper Bursa and Ligament **Y** Lower Bursa and Ligament	**0** Open **3** Percutaneous **4** Percutaneous Endoscopic	**Y** Other Device	**Z** No Qualifier

0 Medical and Surgical
M Bursae and Ligaments
J Inspection: Visually and/or manually exploring a body part

Body Part	Approach	Device	Qualifier
Character 4	**Character 5**	**Character 6**	**Character 7**
X Upper Bursa and Ligament **Y** Lower Bursa and Ligament	**0** Open **3** Percutaneous **4** Percutaneous Endoscopic **X** External	**Z** No Device	**Z** No Qualifier

0 Medical and Surgical
M Bursae and Ligaments
M Reattachment: Putting back in or on all or a portion of a separated body part to its normal location or other suitable location

Body Part	Approach	Device	Qualifier
Character 4	**Character 5**	**Character 6**	**Character 7**
0 Head and Neck Bursa and Ligament **1** Shoulder Bursa and Ligament, Right **2** Shoulder Bursa and Ligament, Left **3** Elbow Bursa and Ligament, Right **4** Elbow Bursa and Ligament, Left **5** Wrist Bursa and Ligament, Right **6** Wrist Bursa and Ligament, Left **7** Hand Bursa and Ligament, Right **8** Hand Bursa and Ligament, Left **9** Upper Extremity Bursa and Ligament, Right **B** Upper Extremity Bursa and Ligament, Left **C** Upper Spine Bursa and Ligament **D** Lower Spine Bursa and Ligament **F** Sternum Bursa and Ligament **G** Rib(s) Bursa and Ligament **H** Abdomen Bursa and Ligament, Right **J** Abdomen Bursa and Ligament, Left **K** Perineum Bursa and Ligament **L** Hip Bursa and Ligament, Right **M** Hip Bursa and Ligament, Left **N** Knee Bursa and Ligament, Right **P** Knee Bursa and Ligament, Left **Q** Ankle Bursa and Ligament, Right **R** Ankle Bursa and Ligament, Left **S** Foot Bursa and Ligament, Right **T** Foot Bursa and Ligament, Left **V** Lower Extremity Bursa and Ligament, Right **W** Lower Extremity Bursa and Ligament, Left	**0** Open **4** Percutaneous Endoscopic	**Z** No Device	**Z** No Qualifier

0 Medical and Surgical
M Bursae and Ligaments
N Release: Freeing a body part from an abnormal physical constraint by cutting or by the use of force

Body Part Character 4	Approach Character 5	Device Character 6	Qualifier Character 7
0 Head and Neck Bursa and Ligament **1** Shoulder Bursa and Ligament, Right **2** Shoulder Bursa and Ligament, Left **3** Elbow Bursa and Ligament, Right **4** Elbow Bursa and Ligament, Left **5** Wrist Bursa and Ligament, Right **6** Wrist Bursa and Ligament, Left **7** Hand Bursa and Ligament, Right **8** Hand Bursa and Ligament, Left **9** Upper Extremity Bursa and Ligament, Right **B** Upper Extremity Bursa and Ligament, Left **C** Upper Spine Bursa and Ligament **D** Lower Spine Bursa and Ligament **F** Sternum Bursa and Ligament **G** Rib(s) Bursa and Ligament **H** Abdomen Bursa and Ligament, Right **J** Abdomen Bursa and Ligament, Left **K** Perineum Bursa and Ligament **L** Hip Bursa and Ligament, Right **M** Hip Bursa and Ligament, Left **N** Knee Bursa and Ligament, Right **P** Knee Bursa and Ligament, Left **Q** Ankle Bursa and Ligament, Right **R** Ankle Bursa and Ligament, Left **S** Foot Bursa and Ligament, Right **T** Foot Bursa and Ligament, Left **V** Lower Extremity Bursa and Ligament, Right **W** Lower Extremity Bursa and Ligament, Left	**0** Open **3** Percutaneous **4** Percutaneous Endoscopic **X** External	**Z** No Device	**Z** No Qualifier

0 Medical and Surgical
M Bursae and Ligaments
P Removal: Taking out or off a device from a body part

Body Part Character 4	Approach Character 5	Device Character 6	Qualifier Character 7
X Upper Bursa and Ligament **Y** Lower Bursa and Ligament	**0** Open **3** Percutaneous **4** Percutaneous Endoscopic	**0** Drainage Device **7** Autologous Tissue Substitute **J** Synthetic Substitute **K** Nonautologous Tissue Substitute **Y** Other Device	**Z** No Qualifier
X Upper Bursa and Ligament **Y** Lower Bursa and Ligament	**X** External	**0** Drainage Device	**Z** No Qualifier

0 Medical and Surgical
M Bursae and Ligaments
Q Repair: Restoring, to the extent possible, a body part to its normal anatomic structure and function

Body Part Character 4	Approach Character 5	Device Character 6	Qualifier Character 7
0 Head and Neck Bursa and Ligament **1** Shoulder Bursa and Ligament, Right **2** Shoulder Bursa and Ligament, Left **3** Elbow Bursa and Ligament, Right **4** Elbow Bursa and Ligament, Left **5** Wrist Bursa and Ligament, Right **6** Wrist Bursa and Ligament, Left **7** Hand Bursa and Ligament, Right **8** Hand Bursa and Ligament, Left **9** Upper Extremity Bursa and Ligament, Right **B** Upper Extremity Bursa and Ligament, Left **C** Upper Spine Bursa and Ligament **D** Lower Spine Bursa and Ligament **F** Sternum Bursa and Ligament **G** Rib(s) Bursa and Ligament **H** Abdomen Bursa and Ligament, Right **J** Abdomen Bursa and Ligament, Left **K** Perineum Bursa and Ligament **L** Hip Bursa and Ligament, Right **M** Hip Bursa and Ligament, Left **N** Knee Bursa and Ligament, Right CC **P** Knee Bursa and Ligament, Left CC **Q** Ankle Bursa and Ligament, Right **R** Ankle Bursa and Ligament, Left **S** Foot Bursa and Ligament, Right CC **T** Foot Bursa and Ligament, Left CC **V** Lower Extremity Bursa and Ligament, Right **W** Lower Extremity Bursa and Ligament, Left	**0** Open **3** Percutaneous **4** Percutaneous Endoscopic	**Z** No Device	**Z** No Qualifier

CC 0MQN0ZZ 0MQN3ZZ 0MQN4ZZ 0MQP0ZZ 0MQP3ZZ 0MQP4ZZ 0MQS0ZZ 0MQS3ZZ 0MQS4ZZ 0MQT0ZZ 0MQT3ZZ 0MQT4ZZ

0 Medical and Surgical
M Bursae and Ligaments
R Replacement: Putting in or on biological or synthetic material that physically takes the place and/or function of all or a portion of a body part

Body Part Character 4	Approach Character 5	Device Character 6	Qualifier Character 7
0 Head and Neck Bursa and Ligament **1** Shoulder Bursa and Ligament, Right **2** Shoulder Bursa and Ligament, Left **3** Elbow Bursa and Ligament, Right **4** Elbow Bursa and Ligament, Left **5** Wrist Bursa and Ligament, Right **6** Wrist Bursa and Ligament, Left **7** Hand Bursa and Ligament, Right **8** Hand Bursa and Ligament, Left **9** Upper Extremity Bursa and Ligament, Right **B** Upper Extremity Bursa and Ligament, Left **C** Upper Spine Bursa and Ligament **D** Lower Spine Bursa and Ligament **F** Sternum Bursa and Ligament **G** Rib(s) Bursa and Ligament **H** Abdomen Bursa and Ligament, Right **J** Abdomen Bursa and Ligament, Left **K** Perineum Bursa and Ligament **L** Hip Bursa and Ligament, Right **M** Hip Bursa and Ligament, Left **N** Knee Bursa and Ligament, Right **P** Knee Bursa and Ligament, Left **Q** Ankle Bursa and Ligament, Right **R** Ankle Bursa and Ligament, Left **S** Foot Bursa and Ligament, Right **T** Foot Bursa and Ligament, Left **V** Lower Extremity Bursa and Ligament, Right **W** Lower Extremity Bursa and Ligament, Left	**0** Open **4** Percutaneous Endoscopic	**7** Autologous Tissue Substitute **J** Synthetic Substitute **K** Nonautologous Tissue Substitute	**Z** No Qualifier

0 Medical and Surgical
M Bursae and Ligaments
S Reposition: Moving to its normal location, or other suitable location, all or a portion of a body part

Body Part	Approach	Device	Qualifier
Character 4	**Character 5**	**Character 6**	**Character 7**
0 Head and Neck Bursa and Ligament **1** Shoulder Bursa and Ligament, Right **2** Shoulder Bursa and Ligament, Left **3** Elbow Bursa and Ligament, Right **4** Elbow Bursa and Ligament, Left **5** Wrist Bursa and Ligament, Right **6** Wrist Bursa and Ligament, Left **7** Hand Bursa and Ligament, Right **8** Hand Bursa and Ligament, Left **9** Upper Extremity Bursa and Ligament, Right **B** Upper Extremity Bursa and Ligament, Left **C** Upper Spine Bursa and Ligament **D** Lower Spine Bursa and Ligament **F** Sternum Bursa and Ligament **G** Rib(s) Bursa and Ligament **H** Abdomen Bursa and Ligament, Right **J** Abdomen Bursa and Ligament, Left **K** Perineum Bursa and Ligament **L** Hip Bursa and Ligament, Right **M** Hip Bursa and Ligament, Left **N** Knee Bursa and Ligament, Right **P** Knee Bursa and Ligament, Left **Q** Ankle Bursa and Ligament, Right **R** Ankle Bursa and Ligament, Left **S** Foot Bursa and Ligament, Right **T** Foot Bursa and Ligament, Left **V** Lower Extremity Bursa and Ligament, Right **W** Lower Extremity Bursa and Ligament, Left	**0** Open **4** Percutaneous Endoscopic	**Z** No Device	**Z** No Qualifier

0 Medical and Surgical
M Bursae and Ligaments
T Resection: Cutting out or off, without replacement, all of a body part

Body Part Character 4	Approach Character 5	Device Character 6	Qualifier Character 7
0 Head and Neck Bursa and Ligament **1** Shoulder Bursa and Ligament, Right **2** Shoulder Bursa and Ligament, Left **3** Elbow Bursa and Ligament, Right **4** Elbow Bursa and Ligament, Left **5** Wrist Bursa and Ligament, Right **6** Wrist Bursa and Ligament, Left **7** Hand Bursa and Ligament, Right **8** Hand Bursa and Ligament, Left **9** Upper Extremity Bursa and Ligament, Right **B** Upper Extremity Bursa and Ligament, Left **C** Upper Spine Bursa and Ligament **D** Lower Spine Bursa and Ligament **F** Sternum Bursa and Ligament **G** Rib(s) Bursa and Ligament **H** Abdomen Bursa and Ligament, Right **J** Abdomen Bursa and Ligament, Left **K** Perineum Bursa and Ligament **L** Hip Bursa and Ligament, Right **M** Hip Bursa and Ligament, Left **N** Knee Bursa and Ligament, Right **P** Knee Bursa and Ligament, Left **Q** Ankle Bursa and Ligament, Right **R** Ankle Bursa and Ligament, Left **S** Foot Bursa and Ligament, Right **T** Foot Bursa and Ligament, Left **V** Lower Extremity Bursa and Ligament, Right **W** Lower Extremity Bursa and Ligament, Left	**0** Open **4** Percutaneous Endoscopic	**Z** No Device	**Z** No Qualifier

0 Medical and Surgical
M Bursae and Ligaments
U Supplement: Putting in or on biological or synthetic material that physically reinforces and/or augments the function of a portion of a body part

Body Part Character 4	Approach Character 5	Device Character 6	Qualifier Character 7
0 Head and Neck Bursa and Ligament **1** Shoulder Bursa and Ligament, Right **2** Shoulder Bursa and Ligament, Left **3** Elbow Bursa and Ligament, Right **4** Elbow Bursa and Ligament, Left **5** Wrist Bursa and Ligament, Right **6** Wrist Bursa and Ligament, Left **7** Hand Bursa and Ligament, Right **8** Hand Bursa and Ligament, Left **9** Upper Extremity Bursa and Ligament, Right **B** Upper Extremity Bursa and Ligament, Left **C** Upper Spine Bursa and Ligament **D** Lower Spine Bursa and Ligament **F** Sternum Bursa and Ligament **G** Rib(s) Bursa and Ligament **H** Abdomen Bursa and Ligament, Right **J** Abdomen Bursa and Ligament, Left **K** Perineum Bursa and Ligament **L** Hip Bursa and Ligament, Right **M** Hip Bursa and Ligament, Left **N** Knee Bursa and Ligament, Right **P** Knee Bursa and Ligament, Left **Q** Ankle Bursa and Ligament, Right **R** Ankle Bursa and Ligament, Left **S** Foot Bursa and Ligament, Right **T** Foot Bursa and Ligament, Left **V** Lower Extremity Bursa and Ligament, Right **W** Lower Extremity Bursa and Ligament, Left	**0** Open **4** Percutaneous Endoscopic	**7** Autologous Tissue Substitute **J** Synthetic Substitute **K** Nonautologous Tissue Substitute	**Z** No Qualifier

0 Medical and Surgical
M Bursae and Ligaments
W Revision: Correcting, to the extent possible, a portion of a malfunctioning device or the position of a displaced device

Body Part Character 4	Approach Character 5	Device Character 6	Qualifier Character 7
X Upper Bursa and Ligament **Y** Lower Bursa and Ligament	**0** Open **3** Percutaneous **4** Percutaneous Endoscopic	**0** Drainage Device **7** Autologous Tissue Substitute **J** Synthetic Substitute **K** Nonautologous Tissue Substitute **Y** Other Device	**Z** No Qualifier
X Upper Bursa and Ligament **Y** Lower Bursa and Ligament	**X** External	**0** Drainage Device **7** Autologous Tissue Substitute **J** Synthetic Substitute **K** Nonautologous Tissue Substitute	**Z** No Qualifier

0 Medical and Surgical
M Bursae and Ligaments
X Transfer: Moving, without taking out, all or a portion of a body part to another location to take over the function of all or a portion of a body part

Body Part Character 4	Approach Character 5	Device Character 6	Qualifier Character 7
0 Head and Neck Bursa and Ligament **1** Shoulder Bursa and Ligament, Right **2** Shoulder Bursa and Ligament, Left **3** Elbow Bursa and Ligament, Right **4** Elbow Bursa and Ligament, Left **5** Wrist Bursa and Ligament, Right **6** Wrist Bursa and Ligament, Left **7** Hand Bursa and Ligament, Right **8** Hand Bursa and Ligament, Left **9** Upper Extremity Bursa and Ligament, Right **B** Upper Extremity Bursa and Ligament, Left **C** Upper Spine Bursa and Ligament **D** Lower Spine Bursa and Ligament **F** Sternum Bursa and Ligament **G** Rib(s) Bursa and Ligament **H** Abdomen Bursa and Ligament, Right **J** Abdomen Bursa and Ligament, Left **K** Perineum Bursa and Ligament **L** Hip Bursa and Ligament, Right **M** Hip Bursa and Ligament, Left **N** Knee Bursa and Ligament, Right **P** Knee Bursa and Ligament, Left **Q** Ankle Bursa and Ligament, Right **R** Ankle Bursa and Ligament, Left **S** Foot Bursa and Ligament, Right **T** Foot Bursa and Ligament, Left **V** Lower Extremity Bursa and Ligament, Right **W** Lower Extremity Bursa and Ligament, Left	**0** Open **4** Percutaneous Endoscopic	**Z** No Device	**Z** No Qualifier

NOTES

Head and Facial Bones 0N2-0NW

0 Medical and Surgical
N Head and Facial Bones
2 Change: Taking out or off a device from a body part and putting back an identical or similar device in or on the same body part without cutting or puncturing the skin or a mucous membrane

Body Part Character 4	Approach Character 5	Device Character 6	Qualifier Character 7
0 Skull **B** Nasal Bone **W** Facial Bone	**X** External	**0** Drainage Device **Y** Other Device	**Z** No Qualifier

0 Medical and Surgical
N Head and Facial Bones
5 Destruction: Physical eradication of all or a portion of a body part by the direct use of energy, force, or a destructive agent

Body Part Character 4	Approach Character 5	Device Character 6	Qualifier Character 7
0 Skull **1** Frontal Bone **3** Parietal Bone, Right **4** Parietal Bone, Left **5** Temporal Bone, Right **6** Temporal Bone, Left **7** Occipital Bone **B** Nasal Bone **C** Sphenoid Bone **F** Ethmoid Bone, Right **G** Ethmoid Bone, Left **H** Lacrimal Bone, Right **J** Lacrimal Bone, Left **K** Palatine Bone, Right **L** Palatine Bone, Left **M** Zygomatic Bone, Right **N** Zygomatic Bone, Left **P** Orbit, Right **Q** Orbit, Left **R** Maxilla **T** Mandible, Right **V** Mandible, Left **X** Hyoid Bone	**0** Open **3** Percutaneous **4** Percutaneous Endoscopic	**Z** No Device	**Z** No Qualifier

0 Medical and Surgical
N Head and Facial Bones
8 Division: Cutting into a body part, without draining fluids and/or gases from the body part, in order to separate or transect a body part

Body Part Character 4	Approach Character 5	Device Character 6	Qualifier Character 7
0 Skull **1** Frontal Bone **3** Parietal Bone, Right **4** Parietal Bone, Left **5** Temporal Bone, Right **6** Temporal Bone, Left **7** Occipital Bone **B** Nasal Bone **C** Sphenoid Bone **F** Ethmoid Bone, Right **G** Ethmoid Bone, Left **H** Lacrimal Bone, Right **J** Lacrimal Bone, Left **K** Palatine Bone, Right **L** Palatine Bone, Left **M** Zygomatic Bone, Right **N** Zygomatic Bone, Left **P** Orbit, Right **Q** Orbit, Left **R** Maxilla **T** Mandible, Right **V** Mandible, Left **X** Hyoid Bone	**0** Open **3** Percutaneous **4** Percutaneous Endoscopic	**Z** No Device	**Z** No Qualifier

0 Medical and Surgical
N Head and Facial Bones
9 Drainage: Taking or letting out fluids and/or gases from a body part

Body Part Character 4	Approach Character 5	Device Character 6	Qualifier Character 7
0 Skull **1** Frontal Bone **3** Parietal Bone, Right **4** Parietal Bone, Left **5** Temporal Bone, Right **6** Temporal Bone, Left **7** Occipital Bone **B** Nasal Bone **C** Sphenoid Bone **F** Ethmoid Bone, Right **G** Ethmoid Bone, Left **H** Lacrimal Bone, Right **J** Lacrimal Bone, Left **K** Palatine Bone, Right **L** Palatine Bone, Left **M** Zygomatic Bone, Right **N** Zygomatic Bone, Left **P** Orbit, Right **Q** Orbit, Left **R** Maxilla **T** Mandible, Right **V** Mandible, Left **X** Hyoid Bone	**0** Open **3** Percutaneous **4** Percutaneous Endoscopic	**0** Drainage Device	**Z** No Qualifier
0 Skull **1** Frontal Bone **3** Parietal Bone, Right **4** Parietal Bone, Left **5** Temporal Bone, Right **6** Temporal Bone, Left **7** Occipital Bone **B** Nasal Bone **C** Sphenoid Bone **F** Ethmoid Bone, Right **G** Ethmoid Bone, Left **H** Lacrimal Bone, Right **J** Lacrimal Bone, Left **K** Palatine Bone, Right **L** Palatine Bone, Left **M** Zygomatic Bone, Right **N** Zygomatic Bone, Left **P** Orbit, Right **Q** Orbit, Left **R** Maxilla **T** Mandible, Right **V** Mandible, Left **X** Hyoid Bone	**0** Open **3** Percutaneous **4** Percutaneous Endoscopic	**Z** No Device	**X** Diagnostic **Z** No Qualifier

0 Medical and Surgical
N Head and Facial Bones
B Excision: Cutting out or off, without replacement, a portion of a body part

Body Part Character 4	Approach Character 5	Device Character 6	Qualifier Character 7
0 Skull	**0** Open	**Z** No Device	**X** Diagnostic
1 Frontal Bone	**3** Percutaneous		**Z** No Qualifier
3 Parietal Bone, Right	**4** Percutaneous Endoscopic		
4 Parietal Bone, Left			
5 Temporal Bone, Right			
6 Temporal Bone, Left			
7 Occipital Bone			
B Nasal Bone			
C Sphenoid Bone			
F Ethmoid Bone, Right			
G Ethmoid Bone, Left			
H Lacrimal Bone, Right			
J Lacrimal Bone, Left			
K Palatine Bone, Right			
L Palatine Bone, Left			
M Zygomatic Bone, Right			
N Zygomatic Bone, Left			
P Orbit, Right CC			
Q Orbit, Left CC			
R Maxilla CC			
T Mandible, Right			
V Mandible, Left			
X Hyoid Bone			

CC 0NBP0ZZ 0NBP3ZZ 0NBP4ZZ 0NBQ0ZZ 0NBQ3ZZ 0NBQ4ZZ 0NBR0ZZ 0NBR4ZZ 0NBS0ZZ 0NBS4ZZ

0 Medical and Surgical
N Head and Facial Bones
C Extirpation: Taking or cutting out solid matter from a body part

Body Part Character 4	Approach Character 5	Device Character 6	Qualifier Character 7
1 Frontal Bone	**0** Open	**Z** No Device	**Z** No Qualifier
3 Parietal Bone, Right	**3** Percutaneous		
4 Parietal Bone, Left	**4** Percutaneous Endoscopic		
5 Temporal Bone, Right			
6 Temporal Bone, Left			
7 Occipital Bone			
B Nasal Bone			
C Sphenoid Bone			
F Ethmoid Bone, Right			
G Ethmoid Bone, Left			
H Lacrimal Bone, Right			
J Lacrimal Bone, Left			
K Palatine Bone, Right			
L Palatine Bone, Left			
M Zygomatic Bone, Right			
N Zygomatic Bone, Left			
P Orbit, Right			
Q Orbit, Left			
R Maxilla			
T Mandible, Right			
V Mandible, Left			
X Hyoid Bone			

0 Medical and Surgical
N Head and Facial Bones
D Extraction: Pulling or stripping out or off all or a portion of a body part by the use of force

Body Part Character 4	Approach Character 5	Device Character 6	Qualifier Character 7
0 Skull **1** Frontal Bone **3** Parietal Bone, Right **4** Parietal Bone, Left **5** Temporal Bone, Right **6** Temporal Bone, Left **7** Occipital Bone **B** Nasal Bone **C** Sphenoid Bone **F** Ethmoid Bone, Right **G** Ethmoid Bone, Left **H** Lacrimal Bone, Right **J** Lacrimal Bone, Left **K** Palatine Bone, Right **L** Palatine Bone, Left **M** Zygomatic Bone, Right **N** Zygomatic Bone, Left **P** Orbit, Right **Q** Orbit, Left **R** Maxilla **T** Mandible, Right **V** Mandible, Left **X** Hyoid Bone	**0** Open	**Z** No Device	**Z** No Qualifier

0 Medical and Surgical
N Head and Facial Bones
H Insertion: Putting in a nonbiological appliance that monitors, assists, performs, or prevents a physiological function but does not physically take the place of a body part

Body Part Character 4	Approach Character 5	Device Character 6	Qualifier Character 7
0 Skull CC	**0** Open	**4** Internal Fixation Device **5** External Fixation Device **M** Bone Growth Stimulator **N** Neurostimulator Generator	**Z** No Qualifier
0 Skull	**3** Percutaneous **4** Percutaneous Endoscopic	**4** Internal Fixation Device **5** External Fixation Device **M** Bone Growth Stimulator	**Z** No Qualifier
1 Frontal Bone **3** Parietal Bone, Right **4** Parietal Bone, Left **7** Occipital Bone **C** Sphenoid Bone **F** Ethmoid Bone, Right **G** Ethmoid Bone, Left **H** Lacrimal Bone, Right **J** Lacrimal Bone, Left **K** Palatine Bone, Right **L** Palatine Bone, Left **M** Zygomatic Bone, Right **N** Zygomatic Bone, Left **P** Orbit, Right **Q** Orbit, Left **X** Hyoid Bone	**0** Open **3** Percutaneous **4** Percutaneous Endoscopic	**4** Internal Fixation Device	**Z** No Qualifier
5 Temporal Bone, Right **6** Temporal Bone, Left	**0** Open **3** Percutaneous **4** Percutaneous Endoscopic	**4** Internal Fixation Device **S** Hearing Device	**Z** No Qualifier
B Nasal Bone	**0** Open **3** Percutaneous **4** Percutaneous Endoscopic	**4** Internal Fixation Device **M** Bone Growth Stimulator	**Z** No Qualifier
R Maxilla **T** Mandible, Right **V** Mandible, Left	**0** Open **3** Percutaneous **4** Percutaneous Endoscopic	**4** Internal Fixation Device **5** External Fixation Device	**Z** No Qualifier
W Facial Bone	**0** Open **3** Percutaneous **4** Percutaneous Endoscopic	**M** Bone Growth Stimulator	**Z** No Qualifier

CC 0NH00NZ

0 Medical and Surgical
N Head and Facial Bones
J Inspection: Visually and/or manually exploring a body part

Body Part Character 4	Approach Character 5	Device Character 6	Qualifier Character 7
0 Skull **B** Nasal Bone **W** Facial Bone	**0** Open **3** Percutaneous **4** Percutaneous Endoscopic **X** External	**Z** No Device	**Z** No Qualifier

0 Medical and Surgical
N Head and Facial Bones
N Release: Freeing a body part from an abnormal physical constraint by cutting or by the use of force

Body Part Character 4	Approach Character 5	Device Character 6	Qualifier Character 7
1 Frontal Bone **3** Parietal Bone, Right **4** Parietal Bone, Left **5** Temporal Bone, Right **6** Temporal Bone, Left **7** Occipital Bone **B** Nasal Bone **C** Sphenoid Bone **F** Ethmoid Bone, Right **G** Ethmoid Bone, Left **H** Lacrimal Bone, Right **J** Lacrimal Bone, Left **K** Palatine Bone, Right **L** Palatine Bone, Left **M** Zygomatic Bone, Right **N** Zygomatic Bone, Left **P** Orbit, Right **Q** Orbit, Left **R** Maxilla **T** Mandible, Right **V** Mandible, Left **X** Hyoid Bone	**0** Open **3** Percutaneous **4** Percutaneous Endoscopic	**Z** No Device	**Z** No Qualifier

0 Medical and Surgical
N Head and Facial Bones
P Removal: Taking out or off a device from a body part

Body Part Character 4	Approach Character 5	Device Character 6	Qualifier Character 7
0 Skull	**0** Open	**0** Drainage Device **4** Internal Fixation Device **5** External Fixation Device **7** Autologous Tissue Substitute **J** Synthetic Substitute **K** Nonautologous Tissue Substitute **M** Bone Growth Stimulator **N** Neurostimulator Generator **S** Hearing Device	**Z** No Qualifier
0 Skull	**3** Percutaneous **4** Percutaneous Endoscopic	**0** Drainage Device **4** Internal Fixation Device **5** External Fixation Device **7** Autologous Tissue Substitute **J** Synthetic Substitute **K** Nonautologous Tissue Substitute **M** Bone Growth Stimulator **S** Hearing Device	**Z** No Qualifier
0 Skull	**X** External	**0** Drainage Device **4** Internal Fixation Device **5** External Fixation Device **M** Bone Growth Stimulator **S** Hearing Device	**Z** No Qualifier
B Nasal Bone **W** Facial Bone	**0** Open **3** Percutaneous **4** Percutaneous Endoscopic	**0** Drainage Device **4** Internal Fixation Device **7** Autologous Tissue Substitute **J** Synthetic Substitute **K** Nonautologous Tissue Substitute **M** Bone Growth Stimulator	**Z** No Qualifier
B Nasal Bone **W** Facial Bone	**X** External	**0** Drainage Device **4** Internal Fixation Device **M** Bone Growth Stimulator	**Z** No Qualifier

0 Medical and Surgical
N Head and Facial Bones
Q Repair: Restoring, to the extent possible, a body part to its normal anatomic structure and function

Body Part Character 4	Approach Character 5	Device Character 6	Qualifier Character 7
0 Skull **1** Frontal Bone **3** Parietal Bone, Right **4** Parietal Bone, Left **5** Temporal Bone, Right **6** Temporal Bone, Left **7** Occipital Bone **B** Nasal Bone **C** Sphenoid Bone **F** Ethmoid Bone, Right **G** Ethmoid Bone, Left **H** Lacrimal Bone, Right **J** Lacrimal Bone, Left **K** Palatine Bone, Right **L** Palatine Bone, Left **M** Zygomatic Bone, Right **N** Zygomatic Bone, Left **P** Orbit, Right **Q** Orbit, Left **R** Maxilla **T** Mandible, Right **V** Mandible, Left **X** Hyoid Bone	**0** Open **3** Percutaneous **4** Percutaneous Endoscopic **X** External	**Z** No Device	**Z** No Qualifier

0 Medical and Surgical
N Head and Facial Bones
R Replacement: Putting in or on biological or synthetic material that physically takes the place and/or function of all or a portion of a body part

Body Part Character 4	Approach Character 5	Device Character 6	Qualifier Character 7
0 Skull **1** Frontal Bone **3** Parietal Bone, Right **4** Parietal Bone, Left **5** Temporal Bone, Right **6** Temporal Bone, Left **7** Occipital Bone **B** Nasal Bone **C** Sphenoid Bone **F** Ethmoid Bone, Right **G** Ethmoid Bone, Left **H** Lacrimal Bone, Right **J** Lacrimal Bone, Left **K** Palatine Bone, Right **L** Palatine Bone, Left **M** Zygomatic Bone, Right **N** Zygomatic Bone, Left **P** Orbit, Right **Q** Orbit, Left **R** Maxilla **T** Mandible, Right **V** Mandible, Left **X** Hyoid Bone	**0** Open **3** Percutaneous **4** Percutaneous Endoscopic	**7** Autologous Tissue Substitute **J** Synthetic Substitute **K** Nonautologous Tissue Substitute	**Z** No Qualifier

0 Medical and Surgical
N Head and Facial Bones
S Reposition: Moving to its normal location, or other suitable location, all or a portion of a body part

Body Part Character 4	Approach Character 5	Device Character 6	Qualifier Character 7
0 Skull **R** Maxilla **T** Mandible, Right **V** Mandible, Left	**0** Open **3** Percutaneous **4** Percutaneous Endoscopic	**4** Internal Fixation Device **5** External Fixation Device **Z** No Device	**Z** No Qualifier
0 Skull **R** Maxilla **T** Mandible, Right **V** Mandible, Left	**X** External	**Z** No Device	**Z** No Qualifier
1 Frontal Bone **3** Parietal Bone, Right **4** Parietal Bone, Left **5** Temporal Bone, Right **6** Temporal Bone, Left **7** Occipital Bone **B** Nasal Bone **C** Sphenoid Bone **F** Ethmoid Bone, Right **G** Ethmoid Bone, Left **H** Lacrimal Bone, Right **J** Lacrimal Bone, Left **K** Palatine Bone, Right **L** Palatine Bone, Left **M** Zygomatic Bone, Right **N** Zygomatic Bone, Left **P** Orbit, Right **Q** Orbit, Left **X** Hyoid Bone	**0** Open **3** Percutaneous **4** Percutaneous Endoscopic	**4** Internal Fixation Device **Z** No Device	**Z** No Qualifier
1 Frontal Bone **3** Parietal Bone, Right **4** Parietal Bone, Left **5** Temporal Bone, Right **6** Temporal Bone, Left **7** Occipital Bone **B** Nasal Bone **C** Sphenoid Bone **F** Ethmoid Bone, Right **G** Ethmoid Bone, Left **H** Lacrimal Bone, Right **J** Lacrimal Bone, Left **K** Palatine Bone, Right **L** Palatine Bone, Left **M** Zygomatic Bone, Right **N** Zygomatic Bone, Left **P** Orbit, Right **Q** Orbit, Left **X** Hyoid Bone	**X** External	**Z** No Device	**Z** No Qualifier

0 Medical and Surgical
N Head and Facial Bones
T Resection: Cutting out or off, without replacement, all of a body part

Body Part	Approach	Device	Qualifier
Character 4	**Character 5**	**Character 6**	**Character 7**
1 Frontal Bone **3** Parietal Bone, Right **4** Parietal Bone, Left **5** Temporal Bone, Right **6** Temporal Bone, Left **7** Occipital Bone **B** Nasal Bone **C** Sphenoid Bone **F** Ethmoid Bone, Right **G** Ethmoid Bone, Left **H** Lacrimal Bone, Right **J** Lacrimal Bone, Left **K** Palatine Bone, Right **L** Palatine Bone, Left **M** Zygomatic Bone, Right **N** Zygomatic Bone, Left **P** Orbit, Right **Q** Orbit, Left **R** Maxilla **T** Mandible, Right **V** Mandible, Left **X** Hyoid Bone	**0** Open	**Z** No Device	**Z** No Qualifier

0 Medical and Surgical
N Head and Facial Bones
U Supplement: Putting in or on biological or synthetic material that physically reinforces and/or augments the function of a portion of a body part

Body Part	Approach	Device	Qualifier
Character 4	**Character 5**	**Character 6**	**Character 7**
0 Skull **1** Frontal Bone **3** Parietal Bone, Right **4** Parietal Bone, Left **5** Temporal Bone, Right **6** Temporal Bone, Left **7** Occipital Bone **B** Nasal Bone **C** Sphenoid Bone **F** Ethmoid Bone, Right **G** Ethmoid Bone, Left **H** Lacrimal Bone, Right **J** Lacrimal Bone, Left **K** Palatine Bone, Right **L** Palatine Bone, Left **M** Zygomatic Bone, Right **N** Zygomatic Bone, Left **P** Orbit, Right **Q** Orbit, Left **R** Maxilla **T** Mandible, Right **V** Mandible, Left **X** Hyoid Bone	**0** Open **3** Percutaneous **4** Percutaneous Endoscopic	**7** Autologous Tissue Substitute **J** Synthetic Substitute **K** Nonautologous Tissue Substitute	**Z** No Qualifier

0 Medical and Surgical
N Head and Facial Bones
W Revision: Correcting, to the extent possible, a portion of a malfunctioning device or the position of a displaced device

Body Part	Approach	Device	Qualifier
Character 4	**Character 5**	**Character 6**	**Character 7**
0 Skull	**0** Open	**0** Drainage Device **4** Internal Fixation Device **5** External Fixation Device **7** Autologous Tissue Substitute **J** Synthetic Substitute **K** Nonautologous Tissue Substitute **M** Bone Growth Stimulator **N** Neurostimulator Generator **S** Hearing Device	**Z** No Qualifier
0 Skull	**3** Percutaneous **4** Percutaneous Endoscopic **X** External	**0** Drainage Device **4** Internal Fixation Device **5** External Fixation Device **7** Autologous Tissue Substitute **J** Synthetic Substitute **K** Nonautologous Tissue Substitute **M** Bone Growth Stimulator **S** Hearing Device	**Z** No Qualifier
B Nasal Bone **W** Facial Bone	**0** Open **3** Percutaneous **4** Percutaneous Endoscopic **X** External	**0** Drainage Device **4** Internal Fixation Device **7** Autologous Tissue Substitute **J** Synthetic Substitute **K** Nonautologous Tissue Substitute **M** Bone Growth Stimulator	**Z** No Qualifier

NOTES

Upper Bones 0P2-0PW

0 Medical and Surgical
P Upper Bones
2 Change: Taking out or off a device from a body part and putting back an identical or similar device in or on the same body part without cutting or puncturing the skin or a mucous membrane

Body Part	Approach	Device	Qualifier
Character 4	**Character 5**	**Character 6**	**Character 7**
Y Upper Bone	**X** External	**0** Drainage Device **Y** Other Device	**Z** No Qualifier

0 Medical and Surgical
P Upper Bones
5 Destruction: Physical eradication of all or a portion of a body part by the direct use of energy, force, or a destructive agent

Body Part	Approach	Device	Qualifier
Character 4	**Character 5**	**Character 6**	**Character 7**
0 Sternum **1** Ribs, 1 to 2 **2** Ribs, 3 or More **3** Cervical Vertebra **4** Thoracic Vertebra **5** Scapula, Right **6** Scapula, Left **7** Glenoid Cavity, Right **8** Glenoid Cavity, Left **9** Clavicle, Right **B** Clavicle, Left **C** Humeral Head, Right **D** Humeral Head, Left **F** Humeral Shaft, Right **G** Humeral Shaft, Left **H** Radius, Right **J** Radius, Left **K** Ulna, Right **L** Ulna, Left **M** Carpal, Right **N** Carpal, Left **P** Metacarpal, Right **Q** Metacarpal, Left **R** Thumb Phalanx, Right **S** Thumb Phalanx, Left **T** Finger Phalanx, Right **V** Finger Phalanx, Left	**0** Open **3** Percutaneous **4** Percutaneous Endoscopic	**Z** No Device	**Z** No Qualifier

0 Medical and Surgical
P Upper Bones
8 Division: Cutting into a body part, without draining fluids and/or gases from the body part, in order to separate or transect a body part

Body Part Character 4	Approach Character 5	Device Character 6	Qualifier Character 7
0 Sternum **1** Ribs, 1 to 2 **2** Ribs, 3 or More **3** Cervical Vertebra **4** Thoracic Vertebra **5** Scapula, Right **6** Scapula, Left **7** Glenoid Cavity, Right **8** Glenoid Cavity, Left **9** Clavicle, Right **B** Clavicle, Left **C** Humeral Head, Right **D** Humeral Head, Left **F** Humeral Shaft, Right CC **G** Humeral Shaft, Left CC **H** Radius, Right CC **J** Radius, Left CC **K** Ulna, Right CC **L** Ulna, Left CC **M** Carpal, Right CC **N** Carpal, Left CC **P** Metacarpal, Right CC **Q** Metacarpal, Left CC **R** Thumb Phalanx, Right **S** Thumb Phalanx, Left **T** Finger Phalanx, Right CC **V** Finger Phalanx, Left CC	**0** Open **3** Percutaneous **4** Percutaneous Endoscopic	**Z** No Device	**Z** No Qualifier

CC 0P8F0ZZ 0P8F3ZZ 0P8F4ZZ 0P8G0ZZ 0P8G3ZZ 0P8G4ZZ 0P8H0ZZ 0P8H3ZZ 0P8H4ZZ 0P8J0ZZ 0P8J3ZZ 0P8J4ZZ 0P8K0ZZ 0P8K3ZZ 0P8K4ZZ 0P8L0ZZ 0P8L3ZZ 0P8L4ZZ 0P8M0ZZ 0P8M3ZZ 0P8M4ZZ 0P8N0ZZ 0P8N3ZZ 0P8N4ZZ 0P8P0ZZ 0P8P3ZZ 0P8P4ZZ 0P8Q0ZZ 0P8Q3ZZ 0P8Q4ZZ 0P8T0ZZ 0P8T3ZZ 0P8T4ZZ 0P8V0ZZ 0P8V3ZZ 0P8V4ZZ

0 Medical and Surgical
P Upper Bones
9 Drainage: Taking or letting out fluids and/or gases from a body part

Body Part Character 4	Approach Character 5	Device Character 6	Qualifier Character 7
0 Sternum **1** Ribs, 1 to 2 **2** Ribs, 3 or More **3** Cervical Vertebra **4** Thoracic Vertebra **5** Scapula, Right **6** Scapula, Left **7** Glenoid Cavity, Right **8** Glenoid Cavity, Left **9** Clavicle, Right **B** Clavicle, Left **C** Humeral Head, Right **D** Humeral Head, Left **F** Humeral Shaft, Right **G** Humeral Shaft, Left **H** Radius, Right **J** Radius, Left **K** Ulna, Right **L** Ulna, Left **M** Carpal, Right **N** Carpal, Left **P** Metacarpal, Right **Q** Metacarpal, Left **R** Thumb Phalanx, Right **S** Thumb Phalanx, Left **T** Finger Phalanx, Right **V** Finger Phalanx, Left	**0** Open **3** Percutaneous **4** Percutaneous Endoscopic	**0** Drainage Device	**Z** No Qualifier
0 Sternum **1** Ribs, 1 to 2 **2** Ribs, 3 or More **3** Cervical Vertebra **4** Thoracic Vertebra **5** Scapula, Right **6** Scapula, Left **7** Glenoid Cavity, Right **8** Glenoid Cavity, Left **9** Clavicle, Right **B** Clavicle, Left **C** Humeral Head, Right **D** Humeral Head, Left **F** Humeral Shaft, Right **G** Humeral Shaft, Left **H** Radius, Right **J** Radius, Left **K** Ulna, Right **L** Ulna, Left **M** Carpal, Right **N** Carpal, Left **P** Metacarpal, Right **Q** Metacarpal, Left **R** Thumb Phalanx, Right **S** Thumb Phalanx, Left **T** Finger Phalanx, Right **V** Finger Phalanx, Left	**0** Open **3** Percutaneous **4** Percutaneous Endoscopic	**Z** No Device	**X** Diagnostic **Z** No Qualifier

0 Medical and Surgical
P Upper Bones
B Excision: Cutting out or off, without replacement, a portion of a body part

Body Part Character 4	Approach Character 5	Device Character 6	Qualifier Character 7
0 Sternum 1 Ribs, 1 to 2 CC 2 Ribs, 3 or More CC 3 Cervical Vertebra 4 Thoracic Vertebra 5 Scapula, Right 6 Scapula, Left 7 Glenoid Cavity, Right 8 Glenoid Cavity, Left 9 Clavicle, Right B Clavicle, Left C Humeral Head, Right D Humeral Head, Left F Humeral Shaft, Right G Humeral Shaft, Left H Radius, Right J Radius, Left K Ulna, Right L Ulna, Left M Carpal, Right N Carpal, Left P Metacarpal, Right Q Metacarpal, Left R Thumb Phalanx, Right S Thumb Phalanx, Left T Finger Phalanx, Right V Finger Phalanx, Left	0 Open 3 Percutaneous 4 Percutaneous Endoscopic	Z No Device	X Diagnostic Z No Qualifier

CC 0PB10ZZ 0PB20ZZ

0 Medical and Surgical
P Upper Bones
C Extirpation: Taking or cutting out solid matter from a body part

Body Part Character 4	Approach Character 5	Device Character 6	Qualifier Character 7
0 Sternum 1 Ribs, 1 to 2 2 Ribs, 3 or More 3 Cervical Vertebra 4 Thoracic Vertebra 5 Scapula, Right 6 Scapula, Left 7 Glenoid Cavity, Right 8 Glenoid Cavity, Left 9 Clavicle, Right B Clavicle, Left C Humeral Head, Right D Humeral Head, Left F Humeral Shaft, Right G Humeral Shaft, Left H Radius, Right J Radius, Left K Ulna, Right L Ulna, Left M Carpal, Right N Carpal, Left P Metacarpal, Right Q Metacarpal, Left R Thumb Phalanx, Right S Thumb Phalanx, Left T Finger Phalanx, Right V Finger Phalanx, Left	0 Open 3 Percutaneous 4 Percutaneous Endoscopic	Z No Device	Z No Qualifier

0 Medical and Surgical
P Upper Bones
D Extraction: Pulling or stripping out or off all or a portion of a body part by the use of force

Body Part Character 4	Approach Character 5	Device Character 6	Qualifier Character 7
0 Sternum **1** Ribs, 1 to 2 **2** Ribs, 3 or More **3** Cervical Vertebra **4** Thoracic Vertebra **5** Scapula, Right **6** Scapula, Left **7** Glenoid Cavity, Right **8** Glenoid Cavity, Left **9** Clavicle, Right **B** Clavicle, Left **C** Humeral Head, Right **D** Humeral Head, Left **F** Humeral Shaft, Right **G** Humeral Shaft, Left **H** Radius, Right **J** Radius, Left **K** Ulna, Right **L** Ulna, Left **M** Carpal, Right **N** Carpal, Left **P** Metacarpal, Right **Q** Metacarpal, Left **R** Thumb Phalanx, Right **S** Thumb Phalanx, Left **T** Finger Phalanx, Right **V** Finger Phalanx, Left	**0** Open	**Z** No Device	**Z** No Qualifier

0 Medical and Surgical
P Upper Bones
H Insertion: Putting in a nonbiological appliance that monitors, assists, performs, or prevents a physiological function but does not physically take the place of a body part

Body Part Character 4	Approach Character 5	Device Character 6	Qualifier Character 7
0 Sternum	**0** Open **3** Percutaneous **4** Percutaneous Endoscopic	**0** Internal Fixation Device, Rigid Plate **4** Internal Fixation Device	**Z** No Qualifier
1 Ribs, 1 to 2 **2** Ribs, 3 or More **3** Cervical Vertebra **4** Thoracic Vertebra **5** Scapula, Right **6** Scapula, Left **7** Glenoid Cavity, Right **8** Glenoid Cavity, Left **9** Clavicle, Right **B** Clavicle, Left	**0** Open **3** Percutaneous **4** Percutaneous Endoscopic	**4** Internal Fixation Device	**Z** No Qualifier
C Humeral Head, Right **D** Humeral Head, Left **F** Humeral Shaft, Right **G** Humeral Shaft, Left **H** Radius, Right **J** Radius, Left **K** Ulna, Right **L** Ulna, Left	**0** Open **3** Percutaneous **4** Percutaneous Endoscopic	**4** Internal Fixation Device **5** External Fixation Device **6** Internal Fixation Device, Intramedullary **8** External Fixation Device, Limb Lengthening **B** External Fixation Device, Monoplanar **C** External Fixation Device, Ring **D** External Fixation Device, Hybrid	**Z** No Qualifier
M Carpal, Right **N** Carpal, Left **P** Metacarpal, Right **Q** Metacarpal, Left **R** Thumb Phalanx, Right **S** Thumb Phalanx, Left **T** Finger Phalanx, Right **V** Finger Phalanx, Left	**0** Open **3** Percutaneous **4** Percutaneous Endoscopic	**4** Internal Fixation Device **5** External Fixation Device	**Z** No Qualifier
Y Upper Bone	**0** Open **3** Percutaneous **4** Percutaneous Endoscopic	**M** Bone Growth Stimulator	**Z** No Qualifier

0 Medical and Surgical
P Upper Bones
J Inspection: Visually and/or manually exploring a body part

Body Part Character 4	Approach Character 5	Device Character 6	Qualifier Character 7
Y Upper Bone	**0** Open **3** Percutaneous **4** Percutaneous Endoscopic **X** External	**Z** No Device	**Z** No Qualifier

0 Medical and Surgical
P Upper Bones
N Release: Freeing a body part from an abnormal physical constraint by cutting or by the use of force

Body Part Character 4	Approach Character 5	Device Character 6	Qualifier Character 7
0 Sternum **1** Ribs, 1 to 2 **2** Ribs, 3 or More **3** Cervical Vertebra **4** Thoracic Vertebra **5** Scapula, Right **6** Scapula, Left **7** Glenoid Cavity, Right **8** Glenoid Cavity, Left **9** Clavicle, Right **B** Clavicle, Left **C** Humeral Head, Right **D** Humeral Head, Left **F** Humeral Shaft, Right **G** Humeral Shaft, Left **H** Radius, Right **J** Radius, Left **K** Ulna, Right **L** Ulna, Left **M** Carpal, Right **N** Carpal, Left **P** Metacarpal, Right **Q** Metacarpal, Left **R** Thumb Phalanx, Right **S** Thumb Phalanx, Left **T** Finger Phalanx, Right **V** Finger Phalanx, Left	**0** Open **3** Percutaneous **4** Percutaneous Endoscopic	**Z** No Device	**Z** No Qualifier

0 Medical and Surgical
P Upper Bones
P Removal: Taking out or off a device from a body part

Body Part Character 4	Approach Character 5	Device Character 6	Qualifier Character 7
0 Sternum **1** Ribs, 1 to 2 **2** Ribs, 3 or More **3** Cervical Vertebra **4** Thoracic Vertebra **5** Scapula, Right **6** Scapula, Left **7** Glenoid Cavity, Right **8** Glenoid Cavity, Left **9** Clavicle, Right **B** Clavicle, Left	**0** Open **3** Percutaneous **4** Percutaneous Endoscopic	**4** Internal Fixation Device **7** Autologous Tissue Substitute **J** Synthetic Substitute **K** Nonautologous Tissue Substitute	**Z** No Qualifier
0 Sternum **1** Ribs, 1 to 2 **2** Ribs, 3 or More **3** Cervical Vertebra **4** Thoracic Vertebra **5** Scapula, Right **6** Scapula, Left **7** Glenoid Cavity, Right **8** Glenoid Cavity, Left **9** Clavicle, Right **B** Clavicle, Left	**X** External	**4** Internal Fixation Device	**Z** No Qualifier

0PP continued on next page

0PP continued from previous page

0 Medical and Surgical
P Upper Bones
P Removal: Taking out or off a device from a body part

Body Part	Approach	Device	Qualifier
Character 4	**Character 5**	**Character 6**	**Character 7**
C Humeral Head, Right **D** Humeral Head, Left **F** Humeral Shaft, Right **G** Humeral Shaft, Left **H** Radius, Right **J** Radius, Left **K** Ulna, Right **L** Ulna, Left **M** Carpal, Right **N** Carpal, Left **P** Metacarpal, Right **Q** Metacarpal, Left **R** Thumb Phalanx, Right **S** Thumb Phalanx, Left **T** Finger Phalanx, Right **V** Finger Phalanx, Left	**0** Open **3** Percutaneous **4** Percutaneous Endoscopic	**4** Internal Fixation Device **5** External Fixation Device **7** Autologous Tissue Substitute **J** Synthetic Substitute **K** Nonautologous Tissue Substitute	**Z** No Qualifier
C Humeral Head, Right **D** Humeral Head, Left **F** Humeral Shaft, Right **G** Humeral Shaft, Left **H** Radius, Right **J** Radius, Left **K** Ulna, Right **L** Ulna, Left **M** Carpal, Right **N** Carpal, Left **P** Metacarpal, Right **Q** Metacarpal, Left **R** Thumb Phalanx, Right **S** Thumb Phalanx, Left **T** Finger Phalanx, Right **V** Finger Phalanx, Left	**X** External	**4** Internal Fixation Device **5** External Fixation Device	**Z** No Qualifier
Y Upper Bone	**0** Open **3** Percutaneous **4** Percutaneous Endoscopic **X** External	**0** Drainage Device **M** Bone Growth Stimulator	**Z** No Qualifier

0 Medical and Surgical
P Upper Bones
Q Repair: Restoring, to the extent possible, a body part to its normal anatomic structure and function

Body Part	Approach	Device	Qualifier
Character 4	Character 5	Character 6	Character 7
0 Sternum 1 Ribs, 1 to 2 2 Ribs, 3 or More 3 Cervical Vertebra 4 Thoracic Vertebra 5 Scapula, Right 6 Scapula, Left 7 Glenoid Cavity, Right 8 Glenoid Cavity, Left 9 Clavicle, Right B Clavicle, Left C Humeral Head, Right D Humeral Head, Left F Humeral Shaft, Right G Humeral Shaft, Left H Radius, Right J Radius, Left K Ulna, Right L Ulna, Left M Carpal, Right N Carpal, Left P Metacarpal, Right Q Metacarpal, Left R Thumb Phalanx, Right S Thumb Phalanx, Left T Finger Phalanx, Right V Finger Phalanx, Left	0 Open 3 Percutaneous 4 Percutaneous Endoscopic X External	Z No Device	Z No Qualifier

0 Medical and Surgical
P Upper Bones
R Replacement: Putting in or on biological or synthetic material that physically takes the place and/or function of all or a portion of a body part

Body Part	Approach	Device	Qualifier
Character 4	Character 5	Character 6	Character 7
0 Sternum 1 Ribs, 1 to 2 2 Ribs, 3 or More 3 Cervical Vertebra 4 Thoracic Vertebra 5 Scapula, Right 6 Scapula, Left 7 Glenoid Cavity, Right 8 Glenoid Cavity, Left 9 Clavicle, Right B Clavicle, Left C Humeral Head, Right D Humeral Head, Left F Humeral Shaft, Right G Humeral Shaft, Left H Radius, Right J Radius, Left K Ulna, Right L Ulna, Left M Carpal, Right N Carpal, Left P Metacarpal, Right Q Metacarpal, Left R Thumb Phalanx, Right S Thumb Phalanx, Left T Finger Phalanx, Right V Finger Phalanx, Left	0 Open 3 Percutaneous 4 Percutaneous Endoscopic	7 Autologous Tissue Substitute J Synthetic Substitute K Nonautologous Tissue Substitute	Z No Qualifier

0 Medical and Surgical
P Upper Bones
S Reposition: Moving to its normal location, or other suitable location, all or a portion of a body part

Body Part Character 4	Approach Character 5	Device Character 6	Qualifier Character 7
0 Sternum	**0** Open **3** Percutaneous **4** Percutaneous Endoscopic	**0** Internal Fixation Device, Rigid Plate **4** Internal Fixation Device **Z** No Device	**Z** No Qualifier
0 Sternum	**X** External	**Z** No Device	**Z** No Qualifier
1 Ribs, 1 to 2 **2** Ribs, 3 or More **3** Cervical Vertebra CC **4** Thoracic Vertebra CC **5** Scapula, Right **6** Scapula, Left **7** Glenoid Cavity, Right **8** Glenoid Cavity, Left **9** Clavicle, Right **B** Clavicle, Left	**0** Open **3** Percutaneous **4** Percutaneous Endoscopic	**4** Internal Fixation Device **Z** No Device	**Z** No Qualifier
1 Ribs, 1 to 2 **2** Ribs, 3 or More **3** Cervical Vertebra **4** Thoracic Vertebra **5** Scapula, Right **6** Scapula, Left **7** Glenoid Cavity, Right **8** Glenoid Cavity, Left **9** Clavicle, Right **B** Clavicle, Left	**X** External	**Z** No Device	**Z** No Qualifier
C Humeral Head, Right **D** Humeral Head, Left **F** Humeral Shaft, Right **G** Humeral Shaft, Left **H** Radius, Right **J** Radius, Left **K** Ulna, Right **L** Ulna, Left	**0** Open **3** Percutaneous **4** Percutaneous Endoscopic	**4** Internal Fixation Device **5** External Fixation Device **6** Internal Fixation Device, Intramedullary **B** External Fixation Device, Monoplanar **C** External Fixation Device, Ring **D** External Fixation Device, Hybrid **Z** No Device	**Z** No Qualifier
C Humeral Head, Right **D** Humeral Head, Left **F** Humeral Shaft, Right **G** Humeral Shaft, Left **H** Radius, Right **J** Radius, Left **K** Ulna, Right **L** Ulna, Left	**X** External	**Z** No Device	**Z** No Qualifier
M Carpal, Right **N** Carpal, Left **P** Metacarpal, Right **Q** Metacarpal, Left **R** Thumb Phalanx, Right **S** Thumb Phalanx, Left **T** Finger Phalanx, Right **V** Finger Phalanx, Left	**0** Open **3** Percutaneous **4** Percutaneous Endoscopic	**4** Internal Fixation Device **5** External Fixation Device **Z** No Device	**Z** No Qualifier
M Carpal, Right **N** Carpal, Left **P** Metacarpal, Right **Q** Metacarpal, Left **R** Thumb Phalanx, Right **S** Thumb Phalanx, Left **T** Finger Phalanx, Right **V** Finger Phalanx, Left	**X** External	**Z** No Device	**Z** No Qualifier

CC 0PS33ZZ 0PS43ZZ

0 Medical and Surgical
P Upper Bones
T Resection: Cutting out or off, without replacement, all of a body part

Body Part Character 4	Approach Character 5	Device Character 6	Qualifier Character 7
0 Sternum 1 Ribs, 1 to 2 2 Ribs, 3 or More 5 Scapula, Right 6 Scapula, Left 7 Glenoid Cavity, Right 8 Glenoid Cavity, Left 9 Clavicle, Right B Clavicle, Left C Humeral Head, Right CC D Humeral Head, Left CC F Humeral Shaft, Right CC G Humeral Shaft, Left CC H Radius, Right J Radius, Left K Ulna, Right L Ulna, Left M Carpal, Right N Carpal, Left P Metacarpal, Right Q Metacarpal, Left R Thumb Phalanx, Right S Thumb Phalanx, Left T Finger Phalanx, Right V Finger Phalanx, Left	0 Open	Z No Device	Z No Qualifier

CC 0PTC0ZZ 0PTD0ZZ 0PTF0ZZ 0PTG0ZZ

0 Medical and Surgical
P Upper Bones
U Supplement: Putting in or on biological or synthetic material that physically reinforces and/or augments the function of a portion of a body part

Body Part Character 4	Approach Character 5	Device Character 6	Qualifier Character 7
0 Sternum 1 Ribs, 1 to 2 2 Ribs, 3 or More 3 Cervical Vertebra CC 4 Thoracic Vertebra CC 5 Scapula, Right 6 Scapula, Left 7 Glenoid Cavity, Right 8 Glenoid Cavity, Left 9 Clavicle, Right B Clavicle, Left C Humeral Head, Right D Humeral Head, Left F Humeral Shaft, Right CC G Humeral Shaft, Left CC H Radius, Right CC J Radius, Left CC K Ulna, Right CC L Ulna, Left CC M Carpal, Right CC N Carpal, Left CC P Metacarpal, Right CC Q Metacarpal, Left CC R Thumb Phalanx, Right S Thumb Phalanx, Left T Finger Phalanx, Right CC V Finger Phalanx, Left CC	0 Open 3 Percutaneous 4 Percutaneous Endoscopic	7 Autologous Tissue Substitute J Synthetic Substitute K Nonautologous Tissue Substitute	Z No Qualifier

0PU continued on next page

0PU continued from previous page

CC 0PU33JZ 0PU43JZ 0PUF07Z 0PUF0KZ 0PUF37Z 0PUF3KZ 0PUF47Z 0PUF4KZ 0PUG07Z 0PUG0KZ 0PUG37Z 0PUG3KZ 0PUG47Z 0PUG4KZ 0PUH07Z 0PUH0KZ 0PUH37Z 0PUH3KZ 0PUH47Z 0PUH4KZ 0PUJ07Z 0PUJ0KZ 0PUJ37Z 0PUJ3KZ 0PUJ47Z 0PUJ4KZ 0PUK07Z 0PUK0KZ 0PUK37Z 0PUK3KZ 0PUK47Z 0PUK4KZ 0PUL07Z 0PUL0KZ 0PUL37Z 0PUL3KZ 0PUL47Z 0PUL4KZ 0PUM07Z 0PUM0KZ 0PUM37Z 0PUM3KZ 0PUM47Z 0PUM4KZ 0PUN07Z 0PUN0KZ 0PUN37Z 0PUN3KZ 0PUN47Z 0PUN4KZ 0PUP07Z 0PUP0KZ 0PUP37Z 0PUP3KZ 0PUP47Z 0PUP4KZ 0PUQ07Z 0PUQ0KZ 0PUQ37Z 0PUQ3KZ 0PUQ47Z 0PUQ4KZ 0PUT07Z 0PUT0KZ 0PUT37Z 0PUT3KZ 0PUT47Z 0PUT4KZ 0PUV07Z 0PUV0KZ 0PUV37Z 0PUV3KZ 0PUV47Z 0PUV4KZ

0 Medical and Surgical
P Upper Bones
W Revision: Correcting, to the extent possible, a portion of a malfunctioning device or the position of a displaced device

Body Part Character 4	Approach Character 5	Device Character 6	Qualifier Character 7
0 Sternum **1** Ribs, 1 to 2 **2** Ribs, 3 or More **3** Cervical Vertebra **4** Thoracic Vertebra **5** Scapula, Right **6** Scapula, Left **7** Glenoid Cavity, Right **8** Glenoid Cavity, Left **9** Clavicle, Right **B** Clavicle, Left	**0** Open **3** Percutaneous **4** Percutaneous Endoscopic **X** External	**4** Internal Fixation Device **7** Autologous Tissue Substitute **J** Synthetic Substitute **K** Nonautologous Tissue Substitute	**Z** No Qualifier
C Humeral Head, Right **D** Humeral Head, Left **F** Humeral Shaft, Right **G** Humeral Shaft, Left **H** Radius, Right **J** Radius, Left **K** Ulna, Right **L** Ulna, Left **M** Carpal, Right **N** Carpal, Left **P** Metacarpal, Right **Q** Metacarpal, Left **R** Thumb Phalanx, Right **S** Thumb Phalanx, Left **T** Finger Phalanx, Right **V** Finger Phalanx, Left	**0** Open **3** Percutaneous **4** Percutaneous Endoscopic **X** External	**4** Internal Fixation Device **5** External Fixation Device **7** Autologous Tissue Substitute **J** Synthetic Substitute **K** Nonautologous Tissue Substitute	**Z** No Qualifier
Y Upper Bone	**0** Open **3** Percutaneous **4** Percutaneous Endoscopic **X** External	**0** Drainage Device **M** Bone Growth Stimulator	**Z** No Qualifier

NOTES

NOTES

Lower Bones 0Q2-0QW

0 Medical and Surgical
Q Lower Bones
2 Change: Taking out or off a device from a body part and putting back an identical or similar device in or on the same body part without cutting or puncturing the skin or a mucous membrane

Body Part	Approach	Device	Qualifier
Character 4	**Character 5**	**Character 6**	**Character 7**
Y Lower Bone	**X** External	**0** Drainage Device **Y** Other Device	**Z** No Qualifier

0 Medical and Surgical
Q Lower Bones
5 Destruction: Physical eradication of all or a portion of a body part by the direct use of energy, force, or a destructive agent

Body Part	Approach	Device	Qualifier
Character 4	**Character 5**	**Character 6**	**Character 7**
0 Lumbar Vertebra **1** Sacrum **2** Pelvic Bone, Right **3** Pelvic Bone, Left **4** Acetabulum, Right **5** Acetabulum, Left **6** Upper Femur, Right **7** Upper Femur, Left **8** Femoral Shaft, Right **9** Femoral Shaft, Left **B** Lower Femur, Right **C** Lower Femur, Left **D** Patella, Right **F** Patella, Left **G** Tibia, Right **H** Tibia, Left **J** Fibula, Right **K** Fibula, Left **L** Tarsal, Right **M** Tarsal, Left **N** Metatarsal, Right **P** Metatarsal, Left **Q** Toe Phalanx, Right **R** Toe Phalanx, Left **S** Coccyx	**0** Open **3** Percutaneous **4** Percutaneous Endoscopic	**Z** No Device	**Z** No Qualifier

0 Medical and Surgical
Q Lower Bones
8 Division: Cutting into a body part, without draining fluids and/or gases from the body part, in order to separate or transect a body part

Body Part Character 4	Approach Character 5	Device Character 6	Qualifier Character 7
0 Lumbar Vertebra **1** Sacrum **2** Pelvic Bone, Right **3** Pelvic Bone, Left **4** Acetabulum, Right **5** Acetabulum, Left **6** Upper Femur, Right **7** Upper Femur, Left **8** Femoral Shaft, Right CC **9** Femoral Shaft, Left CC **B** Lower Femur, Right **C** Lower Femur, Left **D** Patella, Right **F** Patella, Left **G** Tibia, Right CC **H** Tibia, Left CC **J** Fibula, Right CC **K** Fibula, Left CC **L** Tarsal, Right CC **M** Tarsal, Left CC **N** Metatarsal, Right CC **P** Metatarsal, Left CC **Q** Toe Phalanx, Right CC **R** Toe Phalanx, Left CC **S** Coccyx	**0** Open **3** Percutaneous **4** Percutaneous Endoscopic	**Z** No Device	**Z** No Qualifier

CC 0Q880ZZ 0Q883ZZ 0Q884ZZ 0Q890ZZ 0Q893ZZ 0Q894ZZ 0Q8G0ZZ 0Q8G3ZZ 0Q8G4ZZ 0Q8H0ZZ 0Q8H3ZZ 0Q8H4ZZ 0Q8J0ZZ 0Q8J3ZZ 0Q8J4ZZ 0Q8K0ZZ 0Q8K3ZZ 0Q8K4ZZ 0Q8L0ZZ 0Q8L3ZZ 0Q8L4ZZ 0Q8M0ZZ 0Q8M3ZZ 0Q8M4ZZ 0Q8N0ZZ 0Q8N3ZZ 0Q8N4ZZ 0Q8P0ZZ 0Q8P3ZZ 0Q8P4ZZ 0Q8Q0ZZ 0Q8Q3ZZ 0Q8Q4ZZ 0Q8R0ZZ 0Q8R3ZZ 0Q8R4ZZ

0 Medical and Surgical
Q Lower Bones
9 Drainage: Taking or letting out fluids and/or gases from a body part

Body Part Character 4	Approach Character 5	Device Character 6	Qualifier Character 7
0 Lumbar Vertebra **1** Sacrum **2** Pelvic Bone, Right **3** Pelvic Bone, Left **4** Acetabulum, Right **5** Acetabulum, Left **6** Upper Femur, Right **7** Upper Femur, Left **8** Femoral Shaft, Right **9** Femoral Shaft, Left **B** Lower Femur, Right **C** Lower Femur, Left **D** Patella, Right **F** Patella, Left **G** Tibia, Right **H** Tibia, Left **J** Fibula, Right **K** Fibula, Left **L** Tarsal, Right **M** Tarsal, Left **N** Metatarsal, Right **P** Metatarsal, Left **Q** Toe Phalanx, Right **R** Toe Phalanx, Left **S** Coccyx	**0** Open **3** Percutaneous **4** Percutaneous Endoscopic	**0** Drainage Device	**Z** No Qualifier
0 Lumbar Vertebra **1** Sacrum **2** Pelvic Bone, Right **3** Pelvic Bone, Left **4** Acetabulum, Right **5** Acetabulum, Left **6** Upper Femur, Right **7** Upper Femur, Left **8** Femoral Shaft, Right **9** Femoral Shaft, Left **B** Lower Femur, Right **C** Lower Femur, Left **D** Patella, Right **F** Patella, Left **G** Tibia, Right **H** Tibia, Left **J** Fibula, Right **K** Fibula, Left **L** Tarsal, Right **M** Tarsal, Left **N** Metatarsal, Right **P** Metatarsal, Left **Q** Toe Phalanx, Right **R** Toe Phalanx, Left **S** Coccyx	**0** Open **3** Percutaneous **4** Percutaneous Endoscopic	**Z** No Device	**X** Diagnostic **Z** No Qualifier

0 Medical and Surgical
Q Lower Bones
B Excision: Cutting out or off, without replacement, a portion of a body part

Body Part Character 4	Approach Character 5	Device Character 6	Qualifier Character 7
0 Lumbar Vertebra **1** Sacrum **2** Pelvic Bone, Right **3** Pelvic Bone, Left **4** Acetabulum, Right **5** Acetabulum, Left **6** Upper Femur, Right **7** Upper Femur, Left **8** Femoral Shaft, Right **9** Femoral Shaft, Left **B** Lower Femur, Right **C** Lower Femur, Left **D** Patella, Right **F** Patella, Left **G** Tibia, Right **H** Tibia, Left **J** Fibula, Right **K** Fibula, Left **L** Tarsal, Right **M** Tarsal, Left **N** Metatarsal, Right CC **P** Metatarsal, Left CC **Q** Toe Phalanx, Right **R** Toe Phalanx, Left **S** Coccyx	**0** Open **3** Percutaneous **4** Percutaneous Endoscopic	**Z** No Device	**X** Diagnostic **Z** No Qualifier

CC 0QBN0ZZ 0QBN3ZZ 0QBN4ZZ 0QBP0ZZ 0QBP3ZZ 0QBP4ZZ

0 Medical and Surgical
Q Lower Bones
C Extirpation: Taking or cutting out solid matter from a body part

Body Part Character 4	Approach Character 5	Device Character 6	Qualifier Character 7
0 Lumbar Vertebra **1** Sacrum **2** Pelvic Bone, Right **3** Pelvic Bone, Left **4** Acetabulum, Right **5** Acetabulum, Left **6** Upper Femur, Right **7** Upper Femur, Left **8** Femoral Shaft, Right **9** Femoral Shaft, Left **B** Lower Femur, Right **C** Lower Femur, Left **D** Patella, Right **F** Patella, Left **G** Tibia, Right **H** Tibia, Left **J** Fibula, Right **K** Fibula, Left **L** Tarsal, Right **M** Tarsal, Left **N** Metatarsal, Right **P** Metatarsal, Left **Q** Toe Phalanx, Right **R** Toe Phalanx, Left **S** Coccyx	**0** Open **3** Percutaneous **4** Percutaneous Endoscopic	**Z** No Device	**Z** No Qualifier

0 Medical and Surgical
Q Lower Bones
D Extraction: Pulling or stripping out or off all or a portion of a body part by the use of force

Body Part Character 4	Approach Character 5	Device Character 6	Qualifier Character 7
0 Lumbar Vertebra **1** Sacrum **2** Pelvic Bone, Right **3** Pelvic Bone, Left **4** Acetabulum, Right **5** Acetabulum, Left **6** Upper Femur, Right **7** Upper Femur, Left **8** Femoral Shaft, Right **9** Femoral Shaft, Left **B** Lower Femur, Right **C** Lower Femur, Left **D** Patella, Right **F** Patella, Left **G** Tibia, Right **H** Tibia, Left **J** Fibula, Right **K** Fibula, Left **L** Tarsal, Right **M** Tarsal, Left **N** Metatarsal, Right **P** Metatarsal, Left **Q** Toe Phalanx, Right **R** Toe Phalanx, Left **S** Coccyx	**0** Open	**Z** No Device	**Z** No Qualifier

0 Medical and Surgical
Q Lower Bones
H Insertion: Putting in a nonbiological appliance that monitors, assists, performs, or prevents a physiological function but does not physically take the place of a body part

Body Part Character 4	Approach Character 5	Device Character 6	Qualifier Character 7
0 Lumbar Vertebra **1** Sacrum **2** Pelvic Bone, Right **3** Pelvic Bone, Left **4** Acetabulum, Right **5** Acetabulum, Left **D** Patella, Right **F** Patella, Left **L** Tarsal, Right **M** Tarsal, Left **N** Metatarsal, Right **P** Metatarsal, Left **Q** Toe Phalanx, Right **R** Toe Phalanx, Left **S** Coccyx	**0** Open **3** Percutaneous **4** Percutaneous Endoscopic	**4** Internal Fixation Device **5** External Fixation Device	**Z** No Qualifier
6 Upper Femur, Right **7** Upper Femur, Left **8** Femoral Shaft, Right **9** Femoral Shaft, Left **B** Lower Femur, Right **C** Lower Femur, Left **G** Tibia, Right **H** Tibia, Left **J** Fibula, Right **K** Fibula, Left	**0** Open **3** Percutaneous **4** Percutaneous Endoscopic	**4** Internal Fixation Device **5** External Fixation Device **6** Internal Fixation Device, Intramedullary **8** External Fixation Device, Limb Lengthening **B** External Fixation Device, Monoplanar **C** External Fixation Device, Ring **D** External Fixation Device, Hybrid	**Z** No Qualifier

0QH continued on next page

0QH continued from previous page

0 Medical and Surgical
Q Lower Bones
H Insertion: Putting in a nonbiological appliance that monitors, assists, performs, or prevents a physiological function but does not physically take the place of a body part

Body Part	Approach	Device	Qualifier
Character 4	**Character 5**	**Character 6**	**Character 7**
Y Lower Bone	**0** Open **3** Percutaneous **4** Percutaneous Endoscopic	**M** Bone Growth Stimulator	**Z** No Qualifier

0 Medical and Surgical
Q Lower Bones
J Inspection: Visually and/or manually exploring a body part

Body Part	Approach	Device	Qualifier
Character 4	**Character 5**	**Character 6**	**Character 7**
Y Lower Bone	**0** Open **3** Percutaneous **4** Percutaneous Endoscopic **X** External	**Z** No Device	**Z** No Qualifier

0 Medical and Surgical
Q Lower Bones
N Release: Freeing a body part from an abnormal physical constraint by cutting or by the use of force

Body Part	Approach	Device	Qualifier
Character 4	**Character 5**	**Character 6**	**Character 7**
0 Lumbar Vertebra **1** Sacrum **2** Pelvic Bone, Right **3** Pelvic Bone, Left **4** Acetabulum, Right **5** Acetabulum, Left **6** Upper Femur, Right **7** Upper Femur, Left **8** Femoral Shaft, Right **9** Femoral Shaft, Left **B** Lower Femur, Right **C** Lower Femur, Left **D** Patella, Right **F** Patella, Left **G** Tibia, Right **H** Tibia, Left **J** Fibula, Right **K** Fibula, Left **L** Tarsal, Right **M** Tarsal, Left **N** Metatarsal, Right **P** Metatarsal, Left **Q** Toe Phalanx, Right **R** Toe Phalanx, Left **S** Coccyx	**0** Open **3** Percutaneous **4** Percutaneous Endoscopic	**Z** No Device	**Z** No Qualifier

0 Medical and Surgical
Q Lower Bones
P Removal: Taking out or off a device from a body part

Body Part Character 4	Approach Character 5	Device Character 6	Qualifier Character 7
0 Lumbar Vertebra **1** Sacrum **4** Acetabulum, Right **5** Acetabulum, Left **S** Coccyx	**0** Open **3** Percutaneous **4** Percutaneous Endoscopic	**4** Internal Fixation Device **7** Autologous Tissue Substitute **J** Synthetic Substitute **K** Nonautologous Tissue Substitute	**Z** No Qualifier
0 Lumbar Vertebra **1** Sacrum **4** Acetabulum, Right **5** Acetabulum, Left **S** Coccyx	**X** External	**4** Internal Fixation Device	**Z** No Qualifier
2 Pelvic Bone, Right **3** Pelvic Bone, Left **6** Upper Femur, Right **7** Upper Femur, Left **8** Femoral Shaft, Right **9** Femoral Shaft, Left **B** Lower Femur, Right **C** Lower Femur, Left **D** Patella, Right CC **F** Patella, Left CC **G** Tibia, Right **H** Tibia, Left **J** Fibula, Right **K** Fibula, Left **L** Tarsal, Right **M** Tarsal, Left **N** Metatarsal, Right **P** Metatarsal, Left **Q** Toe Phalanx, Right **R** Toe Phalanx, Left	**0** Open **3** Percutaneous **4** Percutaneous Endoscopic	**4** Internal Fixation Device **5** External Fixation Device **7** Autologous Tissue Substitute **J** Synthetic Substitute **K** Nonautologous Tissue Substitute	**Z** No Qualifier
2 Pelvic Bone, Right **3** Pelvic Bone, Left **6** Upper Femur, Right **7** Upper Femur, Left **8** Femoral Shaft, Right **9** Femoral Shaft, Left **B** Lower Femur, Right **C** Lower Femur, Left **D** Patella, Right **F** Patella, Left **G** Tibia, Right **H** Tibia, Left **J** Fibula, Right **K** Fibula, Left **L** Tarsal, Right **M** Tarsal, Left **N** Metatarsal, Right **P** Metatarsal, Left **Q** Toe Phalanx, Right **R** Toe Phalanx, Left	**X** External	**4** Internal Fixation Device **5** External Fixation Device	**Z** No Qualifier
Y Lower Bone	**0** Open **3** Percutaneous **4** Percutaneous Endoscopic **X** External	**0** Drainage Device **M** Bone Growth Stimulator	**Z** No Qualifier

CC 0QPD0JZ 0QPD3JZ 0QPD4JZ 0QPF0JZ 0QPF3JZ 0QPF4JZ

0 Medical and Surgical
Q Lower Bones
Q Repair: Restoring, to the extent possible, a body part to its normal anatomic structure and function

Body Part Character 4	Approach Character 5	Device Character 6	Qualifier Character 7
0 Lumbar Vertebra	**0** Open	**Z** No Device	**Z** No Qualifier
1 Sacrum	**3** Percutaneous		
2 Pelvic Bone, Right	**4** Percutaneous Endoscopic		
3 Pelvic Bone, Left	**X** External		
4 Acetabulum, Right			
5 Acetabulum, Left			
6 Upper Femur, Right			
7 Upper Femur, Left			
8 Femoral Shaft, Right			
9 Femoral Shaft, Left			
B Lower Femur, Right			
C Lower Femur, Left			
D Patella, Right			
F Patella, Left			
G Tibia, Right			
H Tibia, Left			
J Fibula, Right			
K Fibula, Left			
L Tarsal, Right			
M Tarsal, Left			
N Metatarsal, Right			
P Metatarsal, Left			
Q Toe Phalanx, Right			
R Toe Phalanx, Left			
S Coccyx			

0 Medical and Surgical
Q Lower Bones
R Replacement: Putting in or on biological or synthetic material that physically takes the place and/or function of all or a portion of a body part

Body Part Character 4	Approach Character 5	Device Character 6	Qualifier Character 7
0 Lumbar Vertebra	**0** Open	**7** Autologous Tissue Substitute	**Z** No Qualifier
1 Sacrum	**3** Percutaneous	**J** Synthetic Substitute	
2 Pelvic Bone, Right	**4** Percutaneous Endoscopic	**K** Nonautologous Tissue Substitute	
3 Pelvic Bone, Left			
4 Acetabulum, Right			
5 Acetabulum, Left			
6 Upper Femur, Right			
7 Upper Femur, Left			
8 Femoral Shaft, Right CC			
9 Femoral Shaft, Left CC			
B Lower Femur, Right			
C Lower Femur, Left			
D Patella, Right CC			
F Patella, Left CC			
G Tibia, Right CC			
H Tibia, Left CC			
J Fibula, Right CC			
K Fibula, Left CC			
L Tarsal, Right CC			
M Tarsal, Left CC			
N Metatarsal, Right CC			
P Metatarsal, Left CC			
Q Toe Phalanx, Right CC			
R Toe Phalanx, Left CC			
S Coccyx			

CC 0QR807Z 0QR80KZ 0QR837Z 0QR83KZ 0QR847Z 0QR84KZ 0QR907Z 0QR90KZ 0QR937Z 0QR93KZ 0QR947Z 0QR94KZ 0QRD0JZ 0QRD3JZ 0QRD4JZ 0QRF0JZ 0QRF3JZ 0QRF4JZ 0QRG07Z 0QRG0KZ 0QRG37Z 0QRG3KZ 0QRG47Z 0QRG4KZ 0QRH07Z 0QRH0KZ 0QRH37Z 0QRH3KZ 0QRH47Z 0QRH4KZ 0QRJ07Z 0QRJ0KZ 0QRJ37Z 0QRJ3KZ 0QRJ47Z 0QRJ4KZ 0QRK07Z 0QRK0KZ 0QRK37Z 0QRK3KZ 0QRK47Z 0QRK4KZ 0QRL07Z 0QRL0KZ 0QRL37Z 0QRL3KZ 0QRL47Z 0QRL4KZ 0QRM07Z 0QRM0KZ 0QRM37Z 0QRM3KZ 0QRM47Z 0QRM4KZ 0QRN07Z 0QRN0KZ 0QRN37Z 0QRN3KZ 0QRN47Z 0QRN4KZ 0QRP07Z 0QRP0KZ 0QRP37Z 0QRP3KZ 0QRP47Z 0QRP4KZ 0QRQ07Z 0QRQ0KZ 0QRQ37Z 0QRQ3KZ 0QRQ47Z 0QRQ4KZ 0QRR07Z 0QRR0KZ 0QRR37Z 0QRR3KZ 0QRR47Z 0QRR4KZ

LC Limited Coverage NC Noncovered HAC HAC-associated Procedure CC Combination Cluster - See Appendix G for code lists
DRG Non-OR-Affecting MS-DRG Assignment New/Revised Text in **Orange** ♂ Male ♀ Female

0 Medical and Surgical
Q Lower Bones
S Reposition: Moving to its normal location, or other suitable location, all or a portion of a body part

Body Part Character 4	Approach Character 5	Device Character 6	Qualifier Character 7
0 Lumbar Vertebra CC **1** Sacrum CC **4** Acetabulum, Right **5** Acetabulum, Left **S** Coccyx CC	**0** Open **3** Percutaneous **4** Percutaneous Endoscopic	**4** Internal Fixation Device **Z** No Device	**Z** No Qualifier
0 Lumbar Vertebra **1** Sacrum **4** Acetabulum, Right **5** Acetabulum, Left **S** Coccyx	**X** External	**Z** No Device	**Z** No Qualifier
2 Pelvic Bone, Right **3** Pelvic Bone, Left **D** Patella, Right **F** Patella, Left **L** Tarsal, Right **M** Tarsal, Left **Q** Toe Phalanx, Right **R** Toe Phalanx, Left	**0** Open **3** Percutaneous **4** Percutaneous Endoscopic	**4** Internal Fixation Device **5** External Fixation Device **Z** No Device	**Z** No Qualifier
2 Pelvic Bone, Right **3** Pelvic Bone, Left **D** Patella, Right **F** Patella, Left **L** Tarsal, Right **M** Tarsal, Left **Q** Toe Phalanx, Right **R** Toe Phalanx, Left	**X** External	**Z** No Device	**Z** No Qualifier
6 Upper Femur, Right **7** Upper Femur, Left **8** Femoral Shaft, Right **9** Femoral Shaft, Left **B** Lower Femur, Right **C** Lower Femur, Left **G** Tibia, Right **H** Tibia, Left **J** Fibula, Right **K** Fibula, Left	**0** Open **3** Percutaneous **4** Percutaneous Endoscopic	**4** Internal Fixation Device **5** External Fixation Device **6** Internal Fixation Device, Intramedullary **B** External Fixation Device, Monoplanar **C** External Fixation Device, Ring **D** External Fixation Device, Hybrid **Z** No Device	**Z** No Qualifier
6 Upper Femur, Right **7** Upper Femur, Left **8** Femoral Shaft, Right **9** Femoral Shaft, Left **B** Lower Femur, Right **C** Lower Femur, Left **G** Tibia, Right **H** Tibia, Left **J** Fibula, Right **K** Fibula, Left	**X** External	**Z** No Device	**Z** No Qualifier
N Metatarsal, Right **P** Metatarsal, Left	**0** Open **3** Percutaneous **4** Percutaneous Endoscopic	**4** Internal Fixation Device **5** External Fixation Device **Z** No Device	**2** Sesamoid Bone(s) 1st Toe **Z** No Qualifier
N Metatarsal, Right **P** Metatarsal, Left	**X** External	**Z** No Device	**2** Sesamoid Bone(s) 1st Toe **Z** No Qualifier

CC 0QS03ZZ 0QS13ZZ 0QSS3ZZ

0 Medical and Surgical
Q Lower Bones
T Resection: Cutting out or off, without replacement, all of a body part

Body Part	Approach	Device	Qualifier
Character 4	Character 5	Character 6	Character 7
2 Pelvic Bone, Right 3 Pelvic Bone, Left 4 Acetabulum, Right 5 Acetabulum, Left 6 Upper Femur, Right CC 7 Upper Femur, Left CC 8 Femoral Shaft, Right CC 9 Femoral Shaft, Left CC B Lower Femur, Right CC C Lower Femur, Left CC D Patella, Right F Patella, Left G Tibia, Right H Tibia, Left J Fibula, Right K Fibula, Left L Tarsal, Right M Tarsal, Left N Metatarsal, Right P Metatarsal, Left Q Toe Phalanx, Right R Toe Phalanx, Left S Coccyx	0 Open	Z No Device	Z No Qualifier

CC 0QT60ZZ 0QT70ZZ 0QT80ZZ 0QT90ZZ 0QTB0ZZ 0QTC0ZZ

0 Medical and Surgical
Q Lower Bones
U Supplement: Putting in or on biological or synthetic material that physically reinforces and/or augments the function of a portion of a body part

Body Part	Approach	Device	Qualifier
Character 4	Character 5	Character 6	Character 7
0 Lumbar Vertebra CC 1 Sacrum CC 2 Pelvic Bone, Right 3 Pelvic Bone, Left 4 Acetabulum, Right 5 Acetabulum, Left 6 Upper Femur, Right 7 Upper Femur, Left 8 Femoral Shaft, Right CC 9 Femoral Shaft, Left CC B Lower Femur, Right C Lower Femur, Left D Patella, Right CC F Patella, Left CC G Tibia, Right CC H Tibia, Left CC J Fibula, Right CC K Fibula, Left CC L Tarsal, Right CC M Tarsal, Left CC N Metatarsal, Right CC P Metatarsal, Left CC Q Toe Phalanx, Right CC R Toe Phalanx, Left CC S Coccyx CC	0 Open 3 Percutaneous 4 Percutaneous Endoscopic	7 Autologous Tissue Substitute J Synthetic Substitute K Nonautologous Tissue Substitute	Z No Qualifier

CC 0QU03JZ 0QU13JZ 0QU807Z 0QU80KZ 0QU837Z 0QU83KZ 0QU847Z 0QU84KZ 0QU907Z 0QU90KZ 0QU937Z 0QU93KZ 0QU947Z 0QU94KZ 0QUD0JZ 0QUD3JZ 0QUD4JZ 0QUF0JZ 0QUF3JZ 0QUF4JZ 0QUG07Z 0QUG0KZ 0QUG37Z 0QUG3KZ 0QUG47Z 0QUG4KZ 0QUH07Z 0QUH0KZ 0QUH37Z 0QUH3KZ 0QUH47Z 0QUH4KZ 0QUJ07Z 0QUJ0KZ 0QUJ37Z 0QUJ3KZ 0QUJ47Z 0QUJ4KZ 0QUK07Z 0QUK0KZ 0QUK37Z 0QUK3KZ 0QUK47Z 0QUK4KZ 0QUL07Z 0QUL0KZ 0QUL37Z 0QUL3KZ 0QUL47Z 0QUL4KZ 0QUM07Z 0QUM0KZ 0QUM37Z 0QUM3KZ 0QUM47Z 0QUM4KZ 0QUN07Z 0QUN0KZ 0QUN37Z 0QUN3KZ 0QUN47Z 0QUN4KZ 0QUP07Z 0QUP0KZ 0QUP37Z 0QUP3KZ 0QUP47Z 0QUP4KZ 0QUQ07Z 0QUQ0KZ 0QUQ37Z 0QUQ3KZ 0QUQ47Z 0QUQ4KZ 0QUR07Z 0QUR0KZ 0QUR37Z 0QUR3KZ 0QUR47Z 0QUR4KZ 0QUS3JZ

LC Limited Coverage NC Noncovered HAC HAC-associated Procedure CC Combination Cluster - See Appendix G for code lists
DRG Non-OR-Affecting MS-DRG Assignment New/Revised Text in **Orange** ♂ Male ♀ Female

0 Medical and Surgical
Q Lower Bones
W Revision: Correcting, to the extent possible, a portion of a malfunctioning device or the position of a displaced device

Body Part Character 4	Approach Character 5	Device Character 6	Qualifier Character 7
0 Lumbar Vertebra **1** Sacrum **4** Acetabulum, Right **5** Acetabulum, Left **S** Coccyx	**0** Open **3** Percutaneous **4** Percutaneous Endoscopic **X** External	**4** Internal Fixation Device **7** Autologous Tissue Substitute **J** Synthetic Substitute **K** Nonautologous Tissue Substitute	**Z** No Qualifier
2 Pelvic Bone, Right **3** Pelvic Bone, Left **6** Upper Femur, Right **7** Upper Femur, Left **8** Femoral Shaft, Right **9** Femoral Shaft, Left **B** Lower Femur, Right **C** Lower Femur, Left **D** Patella, Right **F** Patella, Left **G** Tibia, Right **H** Tibia, Left **J** Fibula, Right **K** Fibula, Left **L** Tarsal, Right **M** Tarsal, Left **N** Metatarsal, Right **P** Metatarsal, Left **Q** Toe Phalanx, Right **R** Toe Phalanx, Left	**0** Open **3** Percutaneous **4** Percutaneous Endoscopic **X** External	**4** Internal Fixation Device **5** External Fixation Device **7** Autologous Tissue Substitute **J** Synthetic Substitute **K** Nonautologous Tissue Substitute	**Z** No Qualifier
Y Lower Bone	**0** Open **3** Percutaneous **4** Percutaneous Endoscopic **X** External	**0** Drainage Device **M** Bone Growth Stimulator	**Z** No Qualifier

NOTES

Upper Joints 0R2-0RW

0 Medical and Surgical
R Upper Joints
2 Change: Taking out or off a device from a body part and putting back an identical or similar device in or on the same body part without cutting or puncturing the skin or a mucous membrane

Body Part Character 4	Approach Character 5	Device Character 6	Qualifier Character 7
Y Upper Joint	**X** External	**0** Drainage Device **Y** Other Device	**Z** No Qualifier

0 Medical and Surgical
R Upper Joints
5 Destruction: Physical eradication of all or a portion of a body part by the direct use of energy, force, or a destructive agent

Body Part Character 4	Approach Character 5	Device Character 6	Qualifier Character 7
0 Occipital-cervical Joint **1** Cervical Vertebral Joint **3** Cervical Vertebral Disc **4** Cervicothoracic Vertebral Joint **5** Cervicothoracic Vertebral Disc **6** Thoracic Vertebral Joint **9** Thoracic Vertebral Disc **A** Thoracolumbar Vertebral Joint **B** Thoracolumbar Vertebral Disc **C** Temporomandibular Joint, Right **D** Temporomandibular Joint, Left **E** Sternoclavicular Joint, Right **F** Sternoclavicular Joint, Left **G** Acromioclavicular Joint, Right **H** Acromioclavicular Joint, Left **J** Shoulder Joint, Right **K** Shoulder Joint, Left **L** Elbow Joint, Right **M** Elbow Joint, Left **N** Wrist Joint, Right **P** Wrist Joint, Left **Q** Carpal Joint, Right **R** Carpal Joint, Left **S** Carpometacarpal Joint, Right **T** Carpometacarpal Joint, Left **U** Metacarpophalangeal Joint, Right **V** Metacarpophalangeal Joint, Left **W** Finger Phalangeal Joint, Right **X** Finger Phalangeal Joint, Left	**0** Open **3** Percutaneous **4** Percutaneous Endoscopic	**Z** No Device	**Z** No Qualifier

0 Medical and Surgical
R Upper Joints
9 Drainage: Taking or letting out fluids and/or gases from a body part

Body Part Character 4	Approach Character 5	Device Character 6	Qualifier Character 7
0 Occipital-cervical Joint **1** Cervical Vertebral Joint **3** Cervical Vertebral Disc **4** Cervicothoracic Vertebral Joint **5** Cervicothoracic Vertebral Disc **6** Thoracic Vertebral Joint **9** Thoracic Vertebral Disc **A** Thoracolumbar Vertebral Joint **B** Thoracolumbar Vertebral Disc **C** Temporomandibular Joint, Right **D** Temporomandibular Joint, Left **E** Sternoclavicular Joint, Right **F** Sternoclavicular Joint, Left **G** Acromioclavicular Joint, Right **H** Acromioclavicular Joint, Left **J** Shoulder Joint, Right **K** Shoulder Joint, Left **L** Elbow Joint, Right **M** Elbow Joint, Left **N** Wrist Joint, Right **P** Wrist Joint, Left **Q** Carpal Joint, Right **R** Carpal Joint, Left **S** Carpometacarpal Joint, Right **T** Carpometacarpal Joint, Left **U** Metacarpophalangeal Joint, Right **V** Metacarpophalangeal Joint, Left **W** Finger Phalangeal Joint, Right **X** Finger Phalangeal Joint, Left	**0** Open **3** Percutaneous **4** Percutaneous Endoscopic	**0** Drainage Device	**Z** No Qualifier
0 Occipital-cervical Joint **1** Cervical Vertebral Joint **3** Cervical Vertebral Disc **4** Cervicothoracic Vertebral Joint **5** Cervicothoracic Vertebral Disc **6** Thoracic Vertebral Joint **9** Thoracic Vertebral Disc **A** Thoracolumbar Vertebral Joint **B** Thoracolumbar Vertebral Disc **C** Temporomandibular Joint, Right **D** Temporomandibular Joint, Left **E** Sternoclavicular Joint, Right **F** Sternoclavicular Joint, Left **G** Acromioclavicular Joint, Right **H** Acromioclavicular Joint, Left **J** Shoulder Joint, Right **K** Shoulder Joint, Left **L** Elbow Joint, Right **M** Elbow Joint, Left **N** Wrist Joint, Right **P** Wrist Joint, Left **Q** Carpal Joint, Right **R** Carpal Joint, Left **S** Carpometacarpal Joint, Right **T** Carpometacarpal Joint, Left **U** Metacarpophalangeal Joint, Right **V** Metacarpophalangeal Joint, Left **W** Finger Phalangeal Joint, Right **X** Finger Phalangeal Joint, Left	**0** Open **3** Percutaneous **4** Percutaneous Endoscopic	**Z** No Device	**X** Diagnostic **Z** No Qualifier

0 Medical and Surgical
R Upper Joints
B Excision: Cutting out or off, without replacement, a portion of a body part

Body Part Character 4	Approach Character 5	Device Character 6	Qualifier Character 7
0 Occipital-cervical Joint **1** Cervical Vertebral Joint **3** Cervical Vertebral Disc **4** Cervicothoracic Vertebral Joint **5** Cervicothoracic Vertebral Disc **6** Thoracic Vertebral Joint **9** Thoracic Vertebral Disc **A** Thoracolumbar Vertebral Joint **B** Thoracolumbar Vertebral Disc **C** Temporomandibular Joint, Right **D** Temporomandibular Joint, Left **E** Sternoclavicular Joint, Right **F** Sternoclavicular Joint, Left **G** Acromioclavicular Joint, Right **H** Acromioclavicular Joint, Left **J** Shoulder Joint, Right **K** Shoulder Joint, Left **L** Elbow Joint, Right **M** Elbow Joint, Left **N** Wrist Joint, Right **P** Wrist Joint, Left **Q** Carpal Joint, Right **R** Carpal Joint, Left **S** Carpometacarpal Joint, Right **T** Carpometacarpal Joint, Left **U** Metacarpophalangeal Joint, Right **V** Metacarpophalangeal Joint, Left **W** Finger Phalangeal Joint, Right **X** Finger Phalangeal Joint, Left	**0** Open **3** Percutaneous **4** Percutaneous Endoscopic	**Z** No Device	**X** Diagnostic **Z** No Qualifier

0 Medical and Surgical
R Upper Joints
C Extirpation: Taking or cutting out solid matter from a body part

Body Part Character 4	Approach Character 5	Device Character 6	Qualifier Character 7
0 Occipital-cervical Joint **1** Cervical Vertebral Joint **3** Cervical Vertebral Disc **4** Cervicothoracic Vertebral Joint **5** Cervicothoracic Vertebral Disc **6** Thoracic Vertebral Joint **9** Thoracic Vertebral Disc **A** Thoracolumbar Vertebral Joint **B** Thoracolumbar Vertebral Disc **C** Temporomandibular Joint, Right **D** Temporomandibular Joint, Left **E** Sternoclavicular Joint, Right **F** Sternoclavicular Joint, Left **G** Acromioclavicular Joint, Right **H** Acromioclavicular Joint, Left **J** Shoulder Joint, Right **K** Shoulder Joint, Left **L** Elbow Joint, Right **M** Elbow Joint, Left **N** Wrist Joint, Right **P** Wrist Joint, Left **Q** Carpal Joint, Right **R** Carpal Joint, Left **S** Carpometacarpal Joint, Right **T** Carpometacarpal Joint, Left **U** Metacarpophalangeal Joint, Right **V** Metacarpophalangeal Joint, Left **W** Finger Phalangeal Joint, Right **X** Finger Phalangeal Joint, Left	**0** Open **3** Percutaneous **4** Percutaneous Endoscopic	**Z** No Device	**Z** No Qualifier

0 Medical and Surgical
R Upper Joints
G Fusion: Joining together portions of an articular body part rendering the articular body part immobile

Body Part Character 4	Approach Character 5	Device Character 6	Qualifier Character 7
0 Occipital-cervical Joint HAC **1** Cervical Vertebral Joint HAC **2** Cervical Vertebral Joints, 2 or more HAC **4** Cervicothoracic Vertebral Joint HAC **6** Thoracic Vertebral Joint HAC **7** Thoracic Vertebral Joints, 2 to 7 CC HAC **8** Thoracic Vertebral Joints, 8 or more HAC **A** Thoracolumbar Vertebral Joint HAC	**0** Open **3** Percutaneous **4** Percutaneous Endoscopic	**7** Autologous Tissue Substitute **J** Synthetic Substitute **K** Nonautologous Tissue Substitute	**0** Anterior Approach, Anterior Column **1** Posterior Approach, Posterior Column **J** Posterior Approach, Anterior Column
0 Occipital-cervical Joint HAC **1** Cervical Vertebral Joint HAC **2** Cervical Vertebral Joints, 2 or more HAC **4** Cervicothoracic Vertebral Joint HAC **6** Thoracic Vertebral Joint HAC **7** Thoracic Vertebral Joints, 2 to 7 CC HAC **8** Thoracic Vertebral Joints, 8 or more HAC **A** Thoracolumbar Vertebral Joint HAC	**0** Open **3** Percutaneous **4** Percutaneous Endoscopic	**A** Interbody Fusion Device	**0** Anterior Approach, Anterior Column **J** Posterior Approach, Anterior Column

0RG continued on next page

LC Limited Coverage NC Noncovered HAC HAC-associated Procedure CC Combination Cluster - See Appendix G for code lists
ORG Non-OR-Affecting MS-DRG Assignment New/Revised Text in **Orange** ♂ Male ♀ Female

0 Medical and Surgical
R Upper Joints
G Fusion: Joining together portions of an articular body part rendering the articular body part immobile

0RG continued from previous page

Body Part	Approach	Device	Qualifier
Character 4	**Character 5**	**Character 6**	**Character 7**
C Temporomandibular Joint, Right **D** Temporomandibular Joint, Left **E** Sternoclavicular Joint, Right HAC **F** Sternoclavicular Joint, Left HAC **G** Acromioclavicular Joint, Right HAC **H** Acromioclavicular Joint, Left HAC **J** Shoulder Joint, Right HAC **K** Shoulder Joint, Left HAC	**0** Open **3** Percutaneous **4** Percutaneous Endoscopic	**4** Internal Fixation Device **7** Autologous Tissue Substitute **J** Synthetic Substitute **K** Nonautologous Tissue Substitute	**Z** No Qualifier
L Elbow Joint, Right HAC **M** Elbow Joint, Left HAC **N** Wrist Joint, Right **P** Wrist Joint, Left **Q** Carpal Joint, Right **R** Carpal Joint, Left **S** Carpometacarpal Joint, Right **T** Carpometacarpal Joint, Left **U** Metacarpophalangeal Joint, Right **V** Metacarpophalangeal Joint, Left **W** Finger Phalangeal Joint, Right **X** Finger Phalangeal Joint, Left	**0** Open **3** Percutaneous **4** Percutaneous Endoscopic	**4** Internal Fixation Device **5** External Fixation Device **7** Autologous Tissue Substitute **J** Synthetic Substitute **K** Nonautologous Tissue Substitute	**Z** No Qualifier

CC 0RG7070 0RG7071 0RG707J 0RG70A0 0RG70A1 0RG70AJ 0RG70J0 0RG70J1 0RG70JJ 0RG70K0 0RG70K1 0RG70KJ 0RG7370 0RG7371 0RG737J 0RG73A0 0RG73A1 0RG73AJ 0RG73J0 0RG73J1 0RG73JJ 0RG73K0 0RG73K1 0RG73KJ 0RG7470 0RG7471 0RG747J 0RG74A0 0RG74A1 0RG74AJ 0RG74J0 0RG74J1 0RG74JJ 0RG74K0 0RG74K1 0RG74KJ

HAC 0RG0070 0RG0071 0RG007J 0RG00A0 0RG00AJ 0RG00J0 0RG00J1 0RG00JJ 0RG00K0 0RG00K1 0RG00KJ 0RG0370 0RG0371 0RG037J 0RG03A0 0RG03AJ 0RG03J0 0RG03J1 0RG03JJ 0RG03K0 0RG03K1 0RG03KJ 0RG0470 0RG0471 0RG047J 0RG04A0 0RG04AJ 0RG04J0 0RG04J1 0RG04JJ 0RG04K0 0RG04K1 0RG04KJ 0RG1070 0RG1071 0RG107J 0RG10A0 0RG10AJ 0RG10J0 0RG10J1 0RG10JJ 0RG10K0 0RG10K1 0RG10KJ 0RG1370 0RG1371 0RG137J 0RG13A0 0RG13AJ 0RG13J0 0RG13J1 0RG13JJ 0RG13K0 0RG13K1 0RG13KJ 0RG1470 0RG1471 0RG147J 0RG14A0 0RG14AJ 0RG14J0 0RG14J1 0RG14JJ 0RG14K0 0RG14K1 0RG14KJ 0RG2070 0RG2071 0RG207J 0RG20A0 0RG20AJ 0RG20J0 0RG20J1 0RG20JJ 0RG20K0 0RG20K1 0RG20KJ 0RG2370 0RG2371 0RG237J 0RG23A0 0RG23AJ 0RG23J0 0RG23J1 0RG23JJ 0RG23K0 0RG23K1 0RG23KJ 0RG2470 0RG2471 0RG247J 0RG24A0 0RG24AJ 0RG24J0 0RG24J1 0RG24JJ 0RG24K0 0RG24K1 0RG24KJ 0RG4070 0RG4071 0RG407J 0RG40A0 0RG40AJ 0RG40J0 0RG40J1 0RG40JJ 0RG40K0 0RG40K1 0RG40KJ 0RG4370 0RG4371 0RG437J 0RG43A0 0RG43AJ 0RG43J0 0RG43J1 0RG43JJ 0RG43K0 0RG43K1 0RG43KJ 0RG4470 0RG4471 0RG447J 0RG44A0 0RG44AJ 0RG44J0 0RG44J1 0RG44JJ 0RG44K0 0RG44K1 0RG44KJ 0RG6070 0RG6071 0RG607J 0RG60A0 0RG60AJ 0RG60J0 0RG60J1 0RG60JJ 0RG60K0 0RG60K1 0RG60KJ 0RG6370 0RG6371 0RG637J 0RG63A0 0RG63AJ 0RG63J0 0RG63J1 0RG63JJ 0RG63K0 0RG63K1 0RG63KJ 0RG6470 0RG6471 0RG647J 0RG64A0 0RG64AJ 0RG64J0 0RG64J1 0RG64JJ 0RG64K0 0RG64K1 0RG64KJ 0RG7070 0RG7071 0RG707J 0RG70A0 0RG70AJ 0RG70J0 0RG70J1 0RG70JJ 0RG70K0 0RG70K1 0RG70KJ 0RG7370 0RG7371 0RG737J 0RG73A0 0RG73AJ 0RG73J0 0RG73J1 0RG73JJ 0RG73K0 0RG73K1 0RG73KJ 0RG7470 0RG7471 0RG747J 0RG74A0 0RG74AJ 0RG74J0 0RG74J1 0RG74JJ 0RG74K0 0RG74K1 0RG74KJ 0RG8070 0RG8071 0RG807J 0RG80A0 0RG80AJ 0RG80J0 0RG80J1 0RG80JJ 0RG80K0 0RG80K1 0RG80KJ 0RG8370 0RG8371 0RG837J 0RG83A0 0RG83AJ 0RG83J0 0RG83J1 0RG83JJ 0RG83K0 0RG83K1 0RG83KJ 0RG8470 0RG8471 0RG847J 0RG84A0 0RG84AJ 0RG84J0 0RG84J1 0RG84JJ 0RG84K0 0RG84K1 0RG84KJ 0RGA070 0RGA071 0RGA07J 0RGA0A0 0RGA0AJ 0RGA0J0 0RGA0J1 0RGA0JJ 0RGA0K0 0RGA0K1 0RGA0KJ 0RGA370 0RGA371 0RGA37J 0RGA3A0 0RGA3AJ 0RGA3J0 0RGA3J1 0RGA3JJ 0RGA3K0 0RGA3K1 0RGA3KJ 0RGA470 0RGA471 0RGA47J 0RGA4A0 0RGA4AJ 0RGA4J0 0RGA4J1 0RGA4JJ 0RGA4K0 0RGA4K1 0RGA4KJ 0RGE04Z 0RGE07Z 0RGE0JZ 0RGE0KZ 0RGE34Z 0RGE37Z 0RGE3JZ 0RGE3KZ 0RGE44Z 0RGE47Z 0RGE4JZ 0RGE4KZ 0RGF04Z 0RGF07Z 0RGF0JZ 0RGF0KZ 0RGF34Z 0RGF37Z 0RGF3JZ 0RGF3KZ 0RGF44Z 0RGF47Z 0RGF4JZ 0RGF4KZ 0RGG04Z 0RGG07Z 0RGG0JZ 0RGG0KZ 0RGG34Z 0RGG37Z 0RGG3JZ 0RGG3KZ 0RGG44Z 0RGG47Z 0RGG4JZ 0RGG4KZ 0RGH04Z 0RGH07Z 0RGH0JZ 0RGH0KZ 0RGH34Z 0RGH37Z 0RGH3JZ 0RGH3KZ 0RGH44Z 0RGH47Z 0RGH4JZ 0RGH4KZ 0RGJ04Z 0RGJ07Z 0RGJ0JZ 0RGJ0KZ 0RGJ34Z 0RGJ37Z 0RGJ3JZ 0RGJ3KZ 0RGJ44Z 0RGJ47Z 0RGJ4JZ 0RGJ4KZ 0RGK04Z 0RGK07Z 0RGK0JZ 0RGK0KZ 0RGK34Z 0RGK37Z 0RGK3JZ 0RGK3KZ 0RGK44Z 0RGK47Z 0RGK4JZ 0RGK4KZ 0RGL04Z 0RGL05Z 0RGL07Z 0RGL0JZ 0RGL0KZ 0RGL34Z 0RGL35Z 0RGL37Z 0RGL3JZ 0RGL3KZ 0RGL44Z 0RGL45Z 0RGL47Z 0RGL4JZ 0RGL4KZ 0RGM04Z 0RGM05Z 0RGM07Z 0RGM0JZ 0RGM0KZ 0RGM34Z 0RGM35Z 0RGM37Z 0RGM3JZ 0RGM3KZ 0RGM44Z 0RGM45Z 0RGM47Z 0RGM4JZ 0RGM4KZ

Surgical site infection following certain orthopedic procedures of spine, shoulder or elbow procedures and secondary diagnosis K68.11, T84.60XA, T84.610A, T84.611A, T84.612A, T84.613A, T84.614A, T84.615A, T84.619A, T84.63XA, T84.69XA, T84.7XXA, T81.4XXA.

0 Medical and Surgical
R Upper Joints
H Insertion: Putting in a nonbiological appliance that monitors, assists, performs, or prevents a physiological function but does not physically take the place of a body part

Body Part Character 4	Approach Character 5	Device Character 6	Qualifier Character 7
0 Occipital-cervical Joint **1** Cervical Vertebral Joint **4** Cervicothoracic Vertebral Joint **6** Thoracic Vertebral Joint **A** Thoracolumbar Vertebral Joint	**0** Open **3** Percutaneous **4** Percutaneous Endoscopic	**3** Infusion Device **4** Internal Fixation Device **8** Spacer **B** Spinal Stabilization Device, Interspinous Process **C** Spinal Stabilization Device, Pedicle-Based **D** Spinal Stabilization Device, Facet Replacement	**Z** No Qualifier
3 Cervical Vertebral Disc **5** Cervicothoracic Vertebral Disc **9** Thoracic Vertebral Disc **B** Thoracolumbar Vertebral Disc	**0** Open **3** Percutaneous **4** Percutaneous Endoscopic	**3** Infusion Device	**Z** No Qualifier
C Temporomandibular Joint, Right **D** Temporomandibular Joint, Left **E** Sternoclavicular Joint, Right **F** Sternoclavicular Joint, Left **G** Acromioclavicular Joint, Right **H** Acromioclavicular Joint, Left **J** Shoulder Joint, Right **K** Shoulder Joint, Left	**0** Open **3** Percutaneous **4** Percutaneous Endoscopic	**3** Infusion Device **4** Internal Fixation Device **8** Spacer	**Z** No Qualifier
L Elbow Joint, Right **M** Elbow Joint, Left **N** Wrist Joint, Right **P** Wrist Joint, Left **Q** Carpal Joint, Right **R** Carpal Joint, Left **S** Carpometacarpal Joint, Right **T** Carpometacarpal Joint, Left **U** Metacarpophalangeal Joint, Right **V** Metacarpophalangeal Joint, Left **W** Finger Phalangeal Joint, Right **X** Finger Phalangeal Joint, Left	**0** Open **3** Percutaneous **4** Percutaneous Endoscopic	**3** Infusion Device **4** Internal Fixation Device **5** External Fixation Device **8** Spacer	**Z** No Qualifier

0RG continued on next page

0 Medical and Surgical
R Upper Joints
J Inspection: Visually and/or manually exploring a body part

Body Part Character 4	Approach Character 5	Device Character 6	Qualifier Character 7
0 Occipital-cervical Joint **1** Cervical Vertebral Joint **3** Cervical Vertebral Disc **4** Cervicothoracic Vertebral Joint **5** Cervicothoracic Vertebral Disc **6** Thoracic Vertebral Joint **9** Thoracic Vertebral Disc **A** Thoracolumbar Vertebral Joint **B** Thoracolumbar Vertebral Disc **C** Temporomandibular Joint, Right **D** Temporomandibular Joint, Left **E** Sternoclavicular Joint, Right **F** Sternoclavicular Joint, Left **G** Acromioclavicular Joint, Right **H** Acromioclavicular Joint, Left **J** Shoulder Joint, Right **K** Shoulder Joint, Left **L** Elbow Joint, Right **M** Elbow Joint, Left **N** Wrist Joint, Right **P** Wrist Joint, Left **Q** Carpal Joint, Right **R** Carpal Joint, Left **S** Carpometacarpal Joint, Right **T** Carpometacarpal Joint, Left **U** Metacarpophalangeal Joint, Right **V** Metacarpophalangeal Joint, Left **W** Finger Phalangeal Joint, Right **X** Finger Phalangeal Joint, Left	**0** Open **3** Percutaneous **4** Percutaneous Endoscopic **X** External	**Z** No Device	**Z** No Qualifier

0 Medical and Surgical
R Upper Joints
N Release: Freeing a body part from an abnormal physical constraint by cutting or by the use of force

Body Part Character 4	Approach Character 5	Device Character 6	Qualifier Character 7
0 Occipital-cervical Joint **1** Cervical Vertebral Joint **3** Cervical Vertebral Disc **4** Cervicothoracic Vertebral Joint **5** Cervicothoracic Vertebral Disc **6** Thoracic Vertebral Joint **9** Thoracic Vertebral Disc **A** Thoracolumbar Vertebral Joint **B** Thoracolumbar Vertebral Disc **C** Temporomandibular Joint, Right **D** Temporomandibular Joint, Left **E** Sternoclavicular Joint, Right **F** Sternoclavicular Joint, Left **G** Acromioclavicular Joint, Right **H** Acromioclavicular Joint, Left **J** Shoulder Joint, Right **K** Shoulder Joint, Left **L** Elbow Joint, Right **M** Elbow Joint, Left **N** Wrist Joint, Right **P** Wrist Joint, Left **Q** Carpal Joint, Right **R** Carpal Joint, Left **S** Carpometacarpal Joint, Right **T** Carpometacarpal Joint, Left **U** Metacarpophalangeal Joint, Right **V** Metacarpophalangeal Joint, Left **W** Finger Phalangeal Joint, Right **X** Finger Phalangeal Joint, Left	**0** Open **3** Percutaneous **4** Percutaneous Endoscopic **X** External	**Z** No Device	**Z** No Qualifier

0 Medical and Surgical
R Upper Joints
P Removal: Taking out or off a device from a body part

Body Part Character 4	Approach Character 5	Device Character 6	Qualifier Character 7
0 Occipital-cervical Joint **1** Cervical Vertebral Joint **4** Cervicothoracic Vertebral Joint **6** Thoracic Vertebral Joint **A** Thoracolumbar Vertebral Joint	**0** Open **3** Percutaneous **4** Percutaneous Endoscopic	**0** Drainage Device **3** Infusion Device **4** Internal Fixation Device **7** Autologous Tissue Substitute **8** Spacer **A** Interbody Fusion Device **J** Synthetic Substitute **K** Nonautologous Tissue Substitute	**Z** No Qualifier
0 Occipital-cervical Joint **1** Cervical Vertebral Joint **4** Cervicothoracic Vertebral Joint **6** Thoracic Vertebral Joint **A** Thoracolumbar Vertebral Joint	**X** External	**0** Drainage Device **3** Infusion Device **4** Internal Fixation Device	**Z** No Qualifier
3 Cervical Vertebral Disc **5** Cervicothoracic Vertebral Disc **9** Thoracic Vertebral Disc **B** Thoracolumbar Vertebral Disc	**0** Open **3** Percutaneous **4** Percutaneous Endoscopic	**0** Drainage Device **3** Infusion Device **7** Autologous Tissue Substitute **J** Synthetic Substitute **K** Nonautologous Tissue Substitute	**Z** No Qualifier

0RP continued on next page

0RP continued from previous page

0 Medical and Surgical
R Upper Joints
P Removal: Taking out or off a device from a body part

Body Part Character 4	Approach Character 5	Device Character 6	Qualifier Character 7
3 Cervical Vertebral Disc **5** Cervicothoracic Vertebral Disc **9** Thoracic Vertebral Disc **B** Thoracolumbar Vertebral Disc	**X** External	**0** Drainage Device **3** Infusion Device	**Z** No Qualifier
C Temporomandibular Joint, Right **D** Temporomandibular Joint, Left **E** Sternoclavicular Joint, Right **F** Sternoclavicular Joint, Left **G** Acromioclavicular Joint, Right **H** Acromioclavicular Joint, Left **J** Shoulder Joint, Right **K** Shoulder Joint, Left	**0** Open **3** Percutaneous **4** Percutaneous Endoscopic	**0** Drainage Device **3** Infusion Device **4** Internal Fixation Device **7** Autologous Tissue Substitute **8** Spacer **J** Synthetic Substitute **K** Nonautologous Tissue Substitute	**Z** No Qualifier
C Temporomandibular Joint, Right **D** Temporomandibular Joint, Left **E** Sternoclavicular Joint, Right **F** Sternoclavicular Joint, Left **G** Acromioclavicular Joint, Right **H** Acromioclavicular Joint, Left **J** Shoulder Joint, Right **K** Shoulder Joint, Left	**X** External	**0** Drainage Device **3** Infusion Device **4** Internal Fixation Device	**Z** No Qualifier
L Elbow Joint, Right **M** Elbow Joint, Left **N** Wrist Joint, Right **P** Wrist Joint, Left **Q** Carpal Joint, Right **R** Carpal Joint, Left **S** Carpometacarpal Joint, Right **T** Carpometacarpal Joint, Left **U** Metacarpophalangeal Joint, Right **V** Metacarpophalangeal Joint, Left **W** Finger Phalangeal Joint, Right **X** Finger Phalangeal Joint, Left	**0** Open **3** Percutaneous **4** Percutaneous Endoscopic	**0** Drainage Device **3** Infusion Device **4** Internal Fixation Device **5** External Fixation Device **7** Autologous Tissue Substitute **8** Spacer **J** Synthetic Substitute **K** Nonautologous Tissue Substitute	**Z** No Qualifier
L Elbow Joint, Right **M** Elbow Joint, Left **N** Wrist Joint, Right **P** Wrist Joint, Left **Q** Carpal Joint, Right **R** Carpal Joint, Left **S** Carpometacarpal Joint, Right **T** Carpometacarpal Joint, Left **U** Metacarpophalangeal Joint, Right **V** Metacarpophalangeal Joint, Left **W** Finger Phalangeal Joint, Right **X** Finger Phalangeal Joint, Left	**X** External	**0** Drainage Device **3** Infusion Device **4** Internal Fixation Device **5** External Fixation Device	**Z** No Qualifier

0 Medical and Surgical
R Upper Joints
Q Repair: Restoring, to the extent possible, a body part to its normal anatomic structure and function

Body Part Character 4	Approach Character 5	Device Character 6	Qualifier Character 7
0 Occipital-cervical Joint **1** Cervical Vertebral Joint **3** Cervical Vertebral Disc **4** Cervicothoracic Vertebral Joint **5** Cervicothoracic Vertebral Disc **6** Thoracic Vertebral Joint **9** Thoracic Vertebral Disc **A** Thoracolumbar Vertebral Joint **B** Thoracolumbar Vertebral Disc **C** Temporomandibular Joint, Right **D** Temporomandibular Joint, Left **E** Sternoclavicular Joint, Right HAC **F** Sternoclavicular Joint, Left HAC **G** Acromioclavicular Joint, Right HAC **H** Acromioclavicular Joint, Left HAC **J** Shoulder Joint, Right HAC **K** Shoulder Joint, Left HAC **L** Elbow Joint, Right HAC **M** Elbow Joint, Left HAC **N** Wrist Joint, Right **P** Wrist Joint, Left **Q** Carpal Joint, Right **R** Carpal Joint, Left **S** Carpometacarpal Joint, Right **T** Carpometacarpal Joint, Left **U** Metacarpophalangeal Joint, Right **V** Metacarpophalangeal Joint, Left **W** Finger Phalangeal Joint, Right **X** Finger Phalangeal Joint, Left	**0** Open **3** Percutaneous **4** Percutaneous Endoscopic **X** External	**Z** No Device	**Z** No Qualifier

HAC 0RQE0ZZ 0RQE3ZZ 0RQE4ZZ 0RQEXZZ 0RQF0ZZ 0RQF3ZZ 0RQF4ZZ 0RQFXZZ 0RQG0ZZ 0RQG3ZZ 0RQG4ZZ 0RQGXZZ 0RQH0ZZ 0RQH3ZZ 0RQH4ZZ 0RQHXZZ 0RQJ0ZZ 0RQJ3ZZ 0RQJ4ZZ 0RQJXZZ 0RQK0ZZ 0RQK3ZZ 0RQK4ZZ 0RQKXZZ 0RQL0ZZ 0RQL3ZZ 0RQL4ZZ 0RQLXZZ 0RQM0ZZ 0RQM3ZZ 0RQM4ZZ 0RQMXZZ
Surgical site infection following certain orthopedic procedures of spine, shoulder or elbow procedures and secondary diagnosis K68.11, T84.60XA, T84.610A, T84.611A, T84.612A, T84.613A, T84.614A, T84.615A, T84.619A, T84.63XA, T84.69XA, T84.7XXA, T81.4XXA.

0 Medical and Surgical
R Upper Joints
R Replacement: Putting in or on biological or synthetic material that physically takes the place and/or function of all or a portion of a body part

Body Part Character 4	Approach Character 5	Device Character 6	Qualifier Character 7
0 Occipital-cervical Joint **1** Cervical Vertebral Joint **3** Cervical Vertebral Disc **4** Cervicothoracic Vertebral Joint **5** Cervicothoracic Vertebral Disc **6** Thoracic Vertebral Joint **9** Thoracic Vertebral Disc **A** Thoracolumbar Vertebral Joint **B** Thoracolumbar Vertebral Disc **C** Temporomandibular Joint, Right **D** Temporomandibular Joint, Left **E** Sternoclavicular Joint, Right **F** Sternoclavicular Joint, Left **G** Acromioclavicular Joint, Right **H** Acromioclavicular Joint, Left **L** Elbow Joint, Right **M** Elbow Joint, Left **N** Wrist Joint, Right **P** Wrist Joint, Left **Q** Carpal Joint, Right **R** Carpal Joint, Left **S** Carpometacarpal Joint, Right **T** Carpometacarpal Joint, Left **U** Metacarpophalangeal Joint, Right **V** Metacarpophalangeal Joint, Left **W** Finger Phalangeal Joint, Right **X** Finger Phalangeal Joint, Left	**0** Open	**7** Autologous Tissue Substitute **J** Synthetic Substitute **K** Nonautologous Tissue Substitute	**Z** No Qualifier
J Shoulder Joint, Right **K** Shoulder Joint, Left	**0** Open	**0** Synthetic Substitute, Reverse Ball and Socket **7** Autologous Tissue Substitute **K** Nonautologous Tissue Substitute	**Z** No Qualifier
J Shoulder Joint, Right **K** Shoulder Joint, Left	**0** Open	**J** Synthetic Substitute	**6** Humeral Surface **7** Glenoid Surface **Z** No Qualifier

0 Medical and Surgical
R Upper Joints
S Reposition: Moving to its normal location, or other suitable location, all or a portion of a body part

Body Part Character 4	Approach Character 5	Device Character 6	Qualifier Character 7
0 Occipital-cervical Joint **1** Cervical Vertebral Joint **4** Cervicothoracic Vertebral Joint **6** Thoracic Vertebral Joint **A** Thoracolumbar Vertebral Joint **C** Temporomandibular Joint, Right **D** Temporomandibular Joint, Left **E** Sternoclavicular Joint, Right **F** Sternoclavicular Joint, Left **G** Acromioclavicular Joint, Right **H** Acromioclavicular Joint, Left **J** Shoulder Joint, Right **K** Shoulder Joint, Left	**0** Open **3** Percutaneous **4** Percutaneous Endoscopic **X** External	**4** Internal Fixation Device **Z** No Device	**Z** No Qualifier
L Elbow Joint, Right **M** Elbow Joint, Left **N** Wrist Joint, Right **P** Wrist Joint, Left **Q** Carpal Joint, Right **R** Carpal Joint, Left **S** Carpometacarpal Joint, Right **T** Carpometacarpal Joint, Left **U** Metacarpophalangeal Joint, Right **V** Metacarpophalangeal Joint, Left **W** Finger Phalangeal Joint, Right **X** Finger Phalangeal Joint, Left	**0** Open **3** Percutaneous **4** Percutaneous Endoscopic **X** External	**4** Internal Fixation Device **5** External Fixation Device **Z** No Device	**Z** No Qualifier

0 Medical and Surgical
R Upper Joints
T Resection: Cutting out or off, without replacement, all of a body part

Body Part Character 4	Approach Character 5	Device Character 6	Qualifier Character 7
3 Cervical Vertebral Disc **4** Cervicothoracic Vertebral Joint **5** Cervicothoracic Vertebral Disc **9** Thoracic Vertebral Disc **B** Thoracolumbar Vertebral Disc **C** Temporomandibular Joint, Right **D** Temporomandibular Joint, Left **E** Sternoclavicular Joint, Right **F** Sternoclavicular Joint, Left **G** Acromioclavicular Joint, Right **H** Acromioclavicular Joint, Left **J** Shoulder Joint, Right **K** Shoulder Joint, Left **L** Elbow Joint, Right **M** Elbow Joint, Left **N** Wrist Joint, Right **P** Wrist Joint, Left **Q** Carpal Joint, Right **R** Carpal Joint, Left **S** Carpometacarpal Joint, Right **T** Carpometacarpal Joint, Left **U** Metacarpophalangeal Joint, Right **V** Metacarpophalangeal Joint, Left **W** Finger Phalangeal Joint, Right **X** Finger Phalangeal Joint, Left	**0** Open	**Z** No Device	**Z** No Qualifier

0 Medical and Surgical
R Upper Joints
U Supplement: Putting in or on biological or synthetic material that physically reinforces and/or augments the function of a portion of a body part

Body Part Character 4	Approach Character 5	Device Character 6	Qualifier Character 7
0 Occipital-cervical Joint 1 Cervical Vertebral Joint 3 Cervical Vertebral Disc 4 Cervicothoracic Vertebral Joint 5 Cervicothoracic Vertebral Disc 6 Thoracic Vertebral Joint 9 Thoracic Vertebral Disc A Thoracolumbar Vertebral Joint B Thoracolumbar Vertebral Disc C Temporomandibular Joint, Right D Temporomandibular Joint, Left E Sternoclavicular Joint, Right HAC F Sternoclavicular Joint, Left HAC G Acromioclavicular Joint, Right HAC H Acromioclavicular Joint, Left HAC J Shoulder Joint, Right HAC K Shoulder Joint, Left HAC L Elbow Joint, Right HAC M Elbow Joint, Left HAC N Wrist Joint, Right P Wrist Joint, Left Q Carpal Joint, Right R Carpal Joint, Left S Carpometacarpal Joint, Right T Carpometacarpal Joint, Left U Metacarpophalangeal Joint, Right V Metacarpophalangeal Joint, Left W Finger Phalangeal Joint, Right X Finger Phalangeal Joint, Left	0 Open 3 Percutaneous 4 Percutaneous Endoscopic	7 Autologous Tissue Substitute J Synthetic Substitute K Nonautologous Tissue Substitute	Z No Qualifier

HAC 0RUE07Z 0RUE0JZ 0RUE0KZ 0RUE37Z 0RUE3JZ 0RUE3KZ 0RUE47Z 0RUE4JZ 0RUE4KZ 0RUF07Z 0RUF0JZ 0RUF0KZ 0RUF37Z 0RUF3JZ 0RUF3KZ 0RUF47Z 0RUF4JZ 0RUF4KZ 0RUG07Z 0RUG0JZ 0RUG0KZ 0RUG37Z 0RUG3JZ 0RUG3KZ 0RUG47Z 0RUG4JZ 0RUG4KZ 0RUH07Z 0RUH0JZ 0RUH0KZ 0RUH37Z 0RUH3JZ 0RUH3KZ 0RUH47Z 0RUH4JZ 0RUH4KZ 0RUJ07Z 0RUJ0JZ 0RUJ0KZ 0RUJ37Z 0RUJ3JZ 0RUJ3KZ 0RUJ47Z 0RUJ4JZ 0RUJ4KZ 0RUK07Z 0RUK0JZ 0RUK0KZ 0RUK37Z 0RUK3JZ 0RUK3KZ 0RUK47Z 0RUK4JZ 0RUK4KZ 0RUL07Z 0RUL0JZ 0RUL0KZ 0RUL37Z 0RUL3JZ 0RUL3KZ 0RUL47Z 0RUL4JZ 0RUL4KZ 0RUM07Z 0RUM0JZ 0RUM0KZ 0RUM37Z 0RUM3JZ 0RUM3KZ 0RUM47Z 0RUM4JZ 0RUM4KZ

Surgical site infection following certain orthopedic procedures of spine, shoulder or elbow procedures and secondary diagnosis K68.11, T84.60XA, T84.610A, T84.611A, T84.612A, T84.613A, T84.614A, T84.615A, T84.619A, T84.63XA, T84.69XA, T84.7XXA, T81.4XXA.

0 Medical and Surgical
R Upper Joints
W Revision: Correcting, to the extent possible, a portion of a malfunctioning device or the position of a displaced device

Body Part Character 4	Approach Character 5	Device Character 6	Qualifier Character 7
0 Occipital-cervical Joint **1** Cervical Vertebral Joint **4** Cervicothoracic Vertebral Joint **6** Thoracic Vertebral Joint **A** Thoracolumbar Vertebral Joint	**0** Open **3** Percutaneous **4** Percutaneous Endoscopic **X** External	**0** Drainage Device **3** Infusion Device **4** Internal Fixation Device **7** Autologous Tissue Substitute **8** Spacer **A** Interbody Fusion Device **J** Synthetic Substitute **K** Nonautologous Tissue Substitute	**Z** No Qualifier
3 Cervical Vertebral Disc **5** Cervicothoracic Vertebral Disc **9** Thoracic Vertebral Disc **B** Thoracolumbar Vertebral Disc	**0** Open **3** Percutaneous **4** Percutaneous Endoscopic **X** External	**0** Drainage Device **3** Infusion Device **7** Autologous Tissue Substitute **J** Synthetic Substitute **K** Nonautologous Tissue Substitute	**Z** No Qualifier
C Temporomandibular Joint, Right **D** Temporomandibular Joint, Left **E** Sternoclavicular Joint, Right **F** Sternoclavicular Joint, Left **G** Acromioclavicular Joint, Right **H** Acromioclavicular Joint, Left **J** Shoulder Joint, Right **K** Shoulder Joint, Left	**0** Open **3** Percutaneous **4** Percutaneous Endoscopic **X** External	**0** Drainage Device **3** Infusion Device **4** Internal Fixation Device **7** Autologous Tissue Substitute **8** Spacer **J** Synthetic Substitute **K** Nonautologous Tissue Substitute	**Z** No Qualifier
L Elbow Joint, Right **M** Elbow Joint, Left **N** Wrist Joint, Right **P** Wrist Joint, Left **Q** Carpal Joint, Right **R** Carpal Joint, Left **S** Carpometacarpal Joint, Right **T** Carpometacarpal Joint, Left **U** Metacarpophalangeal Joint, Right **V** Metacarpophalangeal Joint, Left **W** Finger Phalangeal Joint, Right **X** Finger Phalangeal Joint, Left	**0** Open **3** Percutaneous **4** Percutaneous Endoscopic **X** External	**0** Drainage Device **3** Infusion Device **4** Internal Fixation Device **5** External Fixation Device **7** Autologous Tissue Substitute **8** Spacer **J** Synthetic Substitute **K** Nonautologous Tissue Substitute	**Z** No Qualifier

NOTES

Lower Joints 0S2-0SW

0 Medical and Surgical
S Lower Joints
2 Change: Taking out or off a device from a body part and putting back an identical or similar device in or on the same body part without cutting or puncturing the skin or a mucous membrane

Body Part Character 4	Approach Character 5	Device Character 6	Qualifier Character 7
Y Lower Joint	**X** External	**0** Drainage Device **Y** Other Device	**Z** No Qualifier

0 Medical and Surgical
S Lower Joints
5 Destruction: Physical eradication of all or a portion of a body part by the direct use of energy, force, or a destructive agent

Body Part Character 4	Approach Character 5	Device Character 6	Qualifier Character 7
0 Lumbar Vertebral Joint **2** Lumbar Vertebral Disc **3** Lumbosacral Joint **4** Lumbosacral Disc **5** Sacrococcygeal Joint **6** Coccygeal Joint **7** Sacroiliac Joint, Right **8** Sacroiliac Joint, Left **9** Hip Joint, Right **B** Hip Joint, Left **C** Knee Joint, Right **D** Knee Joint, Left **F** Ankle Joint, Right **G** Ankle Joint, Left **H** Tarsal Joint, Right **J** Tarsal Joint, Left **K** Tarsometatarsal Joint, Right **L** Tarsometatarsal Joint, Left **M** Metatarsal-Phalangeal Joint, Right **N** Metatarsal-Phalangeal Joint, Left **P** Toe Phalangeal Joint, Right **Q** Toe Phalangeal Joint, Left	**0** Open **3** Percutaneous **4** Percutaneous Endoscopic	**Z** No Device	**Z** No Qualifier

0 Medical and Surgical
S Lower Joints
9 Drainage: Taking or letting out fluids and/or gases from a body part

Body Part Character 4	Approach Character 5	Device Character 6	Qualifier Character 7
0 Lumbar Vertebral Joint **2** Lumbar Vertebral Disc **3** Lumbosacral Joint **4** Lumbosacral Disc **5** Sacrococcygeal Joint **6** Coccygeal Joint **7** Sacroiliac Joint, Right **8** Sacroiliac Joint, Left **9** Hip Joint, Right **B** Hip Joint, Left **C** Knee Joint, Right **D** Knee Joint, Left **F** Ankle Joint, Right **G** Ankle Joint, Left **H** Tarsal Joint, Right **J** Tarsal Joint, Left **K** Tarsometatarsal Joint, Right **L** Tarsometatarsal Joint, Left **M** Metatarsal-Phalangeal Joint, Right **N** Metatarsal-Phalangeal Joint, Left **P** Toe Phalangeal Joint, Right **Q** Toe Phalangeal Joint, Left	**0** Open **3** Percutaneous **4** Percutaneous Endoscopic	**0** Drainage Device	**Z** No Qualifier
0 Lumbar Vertebral Joint **2** Lumbar Vertebral Disc **3** Lumbosacral Joint **4** Lumbosacral Disc **5** Sacrococcygeal Joint **6** Coccygeal Joint **7** Sacroiliac Joint, Right **8** Sacroiliac Joint, Left **9** Hip Joint, Right **B** Hip Joint, Left **C** Knee Joint, Right **D** Knee Joint, Left **F** Ankle Joint, Right **G** Ankle Joint, Left **H** Tarsal Joint, Right **J** Tarsal Joint, Left **K** Tarsometatarsal Joint, Right **L** Tarsometatarsal Joint, Left **M** Metatarsal-Phalangeal Joint, Right **N** Metatarsal-Phalangeal Joint, Left **P** Toe Phalangeal Joint, Right **Q** Toe Phalangeal Joint, Left	**0** Open **3** Percutaneous **4** Percutaneous Endoscopic	**Z** No Device	**X** Diagnostic **Z** No Qualifier

0 Medical and Surgical
S Lower Joints
B Excision: Cutting out or off, without replacement, a portion of a body part

Body Part Character 4	Approach Character 5	Device Character 6	Qualifier Character 7
0 Lumbar Vertebral Joint **2** Lumbar Vertebral Disc **3** Lumbosacral Joint **4** Lumbosacral Disc **5** Sacrococcygeal Joint **6** Coccygeal Joint **7** Sacroiliac Joint, Right **8** Sacroiliac Joint, Left **9** Hip Joint, Right **B** Hip Joint, Left **C** Knee Joint, Right CC **D** Knee Joint, Left CC **F** Ankle Joint, Right **G** Ankle Joint, Left **H** Tarsal Joint, Right **J** Tarsal Joint, Left **K** Tarsometatarsal Joint, Right **L** Tarsometatarsal Joint, Left **M** Metatarsal-Phalangeal Joint, Right **N** Metatarsal-Phalangeal Joint, Left **P** Toe Phalangeal Joint, Right **Q** Toe Phalangeal Joint, Left	**0** Open **3** Percutaneous **4** Percutaneous Endoscopic	**Z** No Device	**X** Diagnostic **Z** No Qualifier

CC 0SBC0ZZ 0SBC3ZZ 0SBC4ZZ 0SBD0ZZ 0SBD3ZZ 0SBD4ZZ

0 Medical and Surgical
S Lower Joints
C Extirpation: Taking or cutting out solid matter from a body part

Body Part Character 4	Approach Character 5	Device Character 6	Qualifier Character 7
0 Lumbar Vertebral Joint **2** Lumbar Vertebral Disc **3** Lumbosacral Joint **4** Lumbosacral Disc **5** Sacrococcygeal Joint **6** Coccygeal Joint **7** Sacroiliac Joint, Right **8** Sacroiliac Joint, Left **9** Hip Joint, Right **B** Hip Joint, Left **C** Knee Joint, Right **D** Knee Joint, Left **F** Ankle Joint, Right **G** Ankle Joint, Left **H** Tarsal Joint, Right **J** Tarsal Joint, Left **K** Tarsometatarsal Joint, Right **L** Tarsometatarsal Joint, Left **M** Metatarsal-Phalangeal Joint, Right **N** Metatarsal-Phalangeal Joint, Left **P** Toe Phalangeal Joint, Right **Q** Toe Phalangeal Joint, Left	**0** Open **3** Percutaneous **4** Percutaneous Endoscopic	**Z** No Device	**Z** No Qualifier

0 Medical and Surgical
S Lower Joints
G Fusion: Joining together portions of an articular body part rendering the articular body part immobile

Body Part Character 4	Approach Character 5	Device Character 6	Qualifier Character 7
0 Lumbar Vertebral Joint HAC **1** Lumbar Vertebral Joints, 2 or more CC HAC **3** Lumbosacral Joint HAC	**0** Open **3** Percutaneous **4** Percutaneous Endoscopic	**7** Autologous Tissue Substitute **J** Synthetic Substitute **K** Nonautologous Tissue Substitute	**0** Anterior Approach, Anterior Column **1** Posterior Approach, Posterior Column **J** Posterior Approach, Anterior Column
0 Lumbar Vertebral Joint HAC **1** Lumbar Vertebral Joints, 2 or more CC HAC **3** Lumbosacral Joint HAC	**0** Open **3** Percutaneous **4** Percutaneous Endoscopic	**A** Interbody Fusion Device	**0** Anterior Approach, Anterior Column **J** Posterior Approach, Anterior Column
5 Sacrococcygeal Joint **6** Coccygeal Joint **7** Sacroiliac Joint, Right HAC **8** Sacroiliac Joint, Left HAC	**0** Open **3** Percutaneous **4** Percutaneous Endoscopic	**4** Internal Fixation Device **7** Autologous Tissue Substitute **J** Synthetic Substitute **K** Nonautologous Tissue Substitute	**Z** No Qualifier
9 Hip Joint, Right **B** Hip Joint, Left **C** Knee Joint, Right **D** Knee Joint, Left **F** Ankle Joint, Right **G** Ankle Joint, Left **H** Tarsal Joint, Right **J** Tarsal Joint, Left **K** Tarsometatarsal Joint, Right **L** Tarsometatarsal Joint, Left **M** Metatarsal-Phalangeal Joint, Right CC **N** Metatarsal-Phalangeal Joint, Left CC **P** Toe Phalangeal Joint, Right **Q** Toe Phalangeal Joint, Left	**0** Open **3** Percutaneous **4** Percutaneous Endoscopic	**4** Internal Fixation Device **5** External Fixation Device **7** Autologous Tissue Substitute **J** Synthetic Substitute **K** Nonautologous Tissue Substitute	**Z** No Qualifier

0SG continued on next page

LC Limited Coverage NC Noncovered HAC HAC-associated Procedure CC Combination Cluster - See Appendix G for code lists
DRG Non-OR-Affecting MS-DRG Assignment New/Revised Text in **Orange** ♂ Male ♀ Female

0SG continued from previous page

CC 0SG1070 0SG1071 0SG107J 0SG10A0 0SG10A1 0SG10AJ 0SG10J0 0SG10J1 0SG10JJ 0SG10K0 0SG10K1 0SG10KJ 0SG1370 0SG1371 0SG137J 0SG13A0 0SG13A1 0SG13AJ 0SG13J0 0SG13J1 0SG13JJ 0SG13K0 0SG13K1 0SG13KJ 0SG1470 0SG1471 0SG147J 0SG14A0 0SG14A1 0SG14AJ 0SG14J0 0SG14J1 0SG14JJ 0SG14K0 0SG14K1 0SG14KJ

HAC 0SG0070 0SG0071 0SG007J 0SG00A0 0SG00AJ 0SG00J0 0SG00J1 0SG00JJ 0SG00K0 0SG00K1 0SG00KJ 0SG0370 0SG0371 0SG037J 0SG03A0 0SG03AJ 0SG03J0 0SG03J1 0SG03JJ 0SG03K0 0SG03K1 0SG03KJ 0SG0470 0SG0471 0SG047J 0SG04A0 0SG04AJ 0SG04J0 0SG04J1 0SG04JJ 0SG04K0 0SG04K1 0SG04KJ 0SG1070 0SG1071 0SG107J 0SG10A0 0SG10AJ 0SG10J0 0SG10J1 0SG10JJ 0SG10K0 0SG10K1 0SG10KJ 0SG1370 0SG1371 0SG137J 0SG13A0 0SG13AJ 0SG13J0 0SG13J1 0SG13JJ 0SG13K0 0SG13K1 0SG13KJ 0SG1470 0SG1471 0SG147J 0SG14A0 0SG14AJ 0SG14J0 0SG14J1 0SG14JJ 0SG14K0 0SG14K1 0SG14KJ 0SG3070 0SG3071 0SG307J 0SG30A0 0SG30AJ 0SG30J0 0SG30J1 0SG30JJ 0SG30K0 0SG30K1 0SG30KJ 0SG3370 0SG3371 0SG337J 0SG33A0 0SG33AJ 0SG33J0 0SG33J1 0SG33JJ 0SG33K0 0SG33K1 0SG33KJ 0SG3470 0SG3471 0SG347J 0SG34A0 0SG34AJ 0SG34J0 0SG34J1 0SG34JJ 0SG34K0 0SG34K1 0SG34KJ 0SG704Z 0SG707Z 0SG70JZ 0SG70KZ 0SG734Z 0SG737Z 0SG73JZ 0SG73KZ 0SG744Z 0SG747Z 0SG74JZ 0SG74KZ 0SG804Z 0SG807Z 0SG80JZ 0SG80KZ 0SG834Z 0SG837Z 0SG83JZ 0SG83KZ 0SG844Z 0SG847Z 0SG84JZ 0SG84KZ

Surgical site infection following certain orthopedic procedures of spine, shoulder or elbow procedures and secondary diagnosis K68.11, T84.60XA, T84.610A, T84.611A, T84.612A, T84.613A, T84.614A, T84.615A, T84.619A, T84.63XA, T84.69XA, T84.7XXA, T81.4XXA.

0 Medical and Surgical

S Lower Joints

H Insertion: Putting in a nonbiological appliance that monitors, assists, performs, or prevents a physiological function but does not physically take the place of a body part

Body Part Character 4	Approach Character 5	Device Character 6	Qualifier Character 7
0 Lumbar Vertebral Joint **3** Lumbosacral Joint	**0** Open **3** Percutaneous **4** Percutaneous Endoscopic	**3** Infusion Device **4** Internal Fixation Device **8** Spacer **B** Spinal Stabilization Device, Interspinous Process **C** Spinal Stabilization Device, Pedicle-Based **D** Spinal Stabilization Device, Facet Replacement	**Z** No Qualifier
2 Lumbar Vertebral Disc **4** Lumbosacral Disc	**0** Open **3** Percutaneous **4** Percutaneous Endoscopic	**3** Infusion Device **8** Spacer	**Z** No Qualifier
5 Sacrococcygeal Joint **6** Coccygeal Joint **7** Sacroiliac Joint, Right **8** Sacroiliac Joint, Left	**0** Open **3** Percutaneous **4** Percutaneous Endoscopic	**3** Infusion Device **4** Internal Fixation Device **8** Spacer	**Z** No Qualifier
9 Hip Joint, Right **B** Hip Joint, Left **C** Knee Joint, Right **D** Knee Joint, Left **F** Ankle Joint, Right **G** Ankle Joint, Left **H** Tarsal Joint, Right **J** Tarsal Joint, Left **K** Tarsometatarsal Joint, Right **L** Tarsometatarsal Joint, Left **M** Metatarsal-Phalangeal Joint, Right **N** Metatarsal-Phalangeal Joint, Left **P** Toe Phalangeal Joint, Right **Q** Toe Phalangeal Joint, Left	**0** Open **3** Percutaneous **4** Percutaneous Endoscopic	**3** Infusion Device **4** Internal Fixation Device **5** External Fixation Device **8** Spacer	**Z** No Qualifier

0 Medical and Surgical
S Lower Joints
J Inspection: Visually and/or manually exploring a body part

Body Part Character 4	Approach Character 5	Device Character 6	Qualifier Character 7
0 Lumbar Vertebral Joint **2** Lumbar Vertebral Disc **3** Lumbosacral Joint **4** Lumbosacral Disc **5** Sacrococcygeal Joint **6** Coccygeal Joint **7** Sacroiliac Joint, Right **8** Sacroiliac Joint, Left **9** Hip Joint, Right **B** Hip Joint, Left **C** Knee Joint, Right **D** Knee Joint, Left **F** Ankle Joint, Right **G** Ankle Joint, Left **H** Tarsal Joint, Right **J** Tarsal Joint, Left **K** Tarsometatarsal Joint, Right **L** Tarsometatarsal Joint, Left **M** Metatarsal-Phalangeal Joint, Right **N** Metatarsal-Phalangeal Joint, Left **P** Toe Phalangeal Joint, Right **Q** Toe Phalangeal Joint, Left	**0** Open **3** Percutaneous **4** Percutaneous Endoscopic **X** External	**Z** No Device	**Z** No Qualifier

0 Medical and Surgical
S Lower Joints
N Release: Freeing a body part from an abnormal physical constraint by cutting or by the use of force

Body Part Character 4	Approach Character 5	Device Character 6	Qualifier Character 7
0 Lumbar Vertebral Joint **2** Lumbar Vertebral Disc **3** Lumbosacral Joint **4** Lumbosacral Disc **5** Sacrococcygeal Joint **6** Coccygeal Joint **7** Sacroiliac Joint, Right **8** Sacroiliac Joint, Left **9** Hip Joint, Right **B** Hip Joint, Left **C** Knee Joint, Right **D** Knee Joint, Left **F** Ankle Joint, Right **G** Ankle Joint, Left **H** Tarsal Joint, Right **J** Tarsal Joint, Left **K** Tarsometatarsal Joint, Right **L** Tarsometatarsal Joint, Left **M** Metatarsal-Phalangeal Joint, Right **N** Metatarsal-Phalangeal Joint, Left **P** Toe Phalangeal Joint, Right **Q** Toe Phalangeal Joint, Left	**0** Open **3** Percutaneous **4** Percutaneous Endoscopic **X** External	**Z** No Device	**Z** No Qualifier

0 Medical and Surgical
S Lower Joints
P Removal: Taking out or off a device from a body part

Body Part Character 4	Approach Character 5	Device Character 6	Qualifier Character 7
0 Lumbar Vertebral Joint **3** Lumbosacral Joint	**0** Open **3** Percutaneous **4** Percutaneous Endoscopic	**0** Drainage Device **3** Infusion Device **4** Internal Fixation Device **7** Autologous Tissue Substitute **8** Spacer **A** Interbody Fusion Device **J** Synthetic Substitute **K** Nonautologous Tissue Substitute	**Z** No Qualifier
0 Lumbar Vertebral Joint **3** Lumbosacral Joint	**X** External	**0** Drainage Device **3** Infusion Device **4** Internal Fixation Device	**Z** No Qualifier
2 Lumbar Vertebral Disc **4** Lumbosacral Disc	**0** Open **3** Percutaneous **4** Percutaneous Endoscopic	**0** Drainage Device **3** Infusion Device **7** Autologous Tissue Substitute **J** Synthetic Substitute **K** Nonautologous Tissue Substitute	**Z** No Qualifier
2 Lumbar Vertebral Disc **4** Lumbosacral Disc	**X** External	**0** Drainage Device **3** Infusion Device	**Z** No Qualifier
5 Sacrococcygeal Joint **6** Coccygeal Joint **7** Sacroiliac Joint, Right **8** Sacroiliac Joint, Left	**0** Open **3** Percutaneous **4** Percutaneous Endoscopic	**0** Drainage Device **3** Infusion Device **4** Internal Fixation Device **7** Autologous Tissue Substitute **8** Spacer **J** Synthetic Substitute **K** Nonautologous Tissue Substitute	**Z** No Qualifier
5 Sacrococcygeal Joint **6** Coccygeal Joint **7** Sacroiliac Joint, Right **8** Sacroiliac Joint, Left	**X** External	**0** Drainage Device **3** Infusion Device **4** Internal Fixation Device	**Z** No Qualifier
9 Hip Joint, Right CC **B** Hip Joint, Left CC	**0** Open	**0** Drainage Device **3** Infusion Device **4** Internal Fixation Device **5** External Fixation Device **7** Autologous Tissue Substitute **8** Spacer **9** Liner **B** Resurfacing Device **E** Articulating Spacer **J** Synthetic Substitute **K** Nonautologous Tissue Substitute	**Z** No Qualifier
9 Hip Joint, Right CC **B** Hip Joint, Left CC	**3** Percutaneous **4** Percutaneous Endoscopic	**0** Drainage Device **3** Infusion Device **4** Internal Fixation Device **5** External Fixation Device **7** Autologous Tissue Substitute **8** Spacer **J** Synthetic Substitute **K** Nonautologous Tissue Substitute	**Z** No Qualifier
9 Hip Joint, Right **B** Hip Joint, Left	**X** External	**0** Drainage Device **3** Infusion Device **4** Internal Fixation Device **5** External Fixation Device	**Z** No Qualifier

0SP continued on next page

0SP continued from previous page

0 Medical and Surgical
S Lower Joints
P Removal: Taking out or off a device from a body part

Body Part Character 4	Approach Character 5	Device Character 6	Qualifier Character 7
A Hip Joint, Acetabular Surface, Right **E** Hip Joint, Acetabular Surface, Left **R** Hip Joint, Femoral Surface, Right **S** Hip Joint, Femoral Surface, Left **T** Knee Joint, Femoral Surface, Right **U** Knee Joint, Femoral Surface, Left **V** Knee Joint, Tibial Surface, Right **W** Knee Joint, Tibial Surface, Left	**0** Open **3** Percutaneous **4** Percutaneous Endoscopic	**J** Synthetic Substitute	**Z** No Qualifier
C Knee Joint, Right CC **D** Knee Joint, Left CC	**0** Open	**0** Drainage Device **3** Infusion Device **4** Internal Fixation Device **5** External Fixation Device **7** Autologous Tissue Substitute **8** Spacer **9** Liner **E** Articulating Spacer **K** Nonautologous Tissue Substitute **L** Synthetic Substitute, Unicondylar Medial **M** Synthetic Substitute, Unicondylar Lateral **N** Synthetic Substitute, Patellofemoral	**Z** No Qualifier
C Knee Joint, Right CC **D** Knee Joint, Left CC	**0** Open	**J** Synthetic Substitute	**C** Patellar Surface **Z** No Qualifier
C Knee Joint, Right CC **D** Knee Joint, Left CC	**3** Percutaneous **4** Percutaneous Endoscopic	**0** Drainage Device **3** Infusion Device **4** Internal Fixation Device **5** External Fixation Device **7** Autologous Tissue Substitute **8** Spacer **K** Nonautologous Tissue Substitute **L** Synthetic Substitute, Unicondylar Medial **M** Synthetic Substitute, Unicondylar Lateral **N** Synthetic Substitute, Patellofemoral	**Z** No Qualifier
C Knee Joint, Right CC **D** Knee Joint, Left CC	**3** Percutaneous **4** Percutaneous Endoscopic	**J** Synthetic Substitute	**C** Patellar Surface **Z** No Qualifier
C Knee Joint, Right **D** Knee Joint, Left	**X** External	**0** Drainage Device **3** Infusion Device **4** Internal Fixation Device **5** External Fixation Device	**Z** No Qualifier

0SP continued on next page

0SP continued from previous page

0 Medical and Surgical
S Lower Joints
P Removal: Taking out or off a device from a body part

Body Part	Approach	Device	Qualifier
Character 4	**Character 5**	**Character 6**	**Character 7**
F Ankle Joint, Right **G** Ankle Joint, Left **H** Tarsal Joint, Right **J** Tarsal Joint, Left **K** Tarsometatarsal Joint, Right **L** Tarsometatarsal Joint, Left **M** Metatarsal-Phalangeal Joint, Right **N** Metatarsal-Phalangeal Joint, Left **P** Toe Phalangeal Joint, Right **Q** Toe Phalangeal Joint, Left	**0** Open **3** Percutaneous **4** Percutaneous Endoscopic	**0** Drainage Device **3** Infusion Device **4** Internal Fixation Device **5** External Fixation Device **7** Autologous Tissue Substitute **8** Spacer **J** Synthetic Substitute **K** Nonautologous Tissue Substitute	**Z** No Qualifier
F Ankle Joint, Right **G** Ankle Joint, Left **H** Tarsal Joint, Right **J** Tarsal Joint, Left **K** Tarsometatarsal Joint, Right **L** Tarsometatarsal Joint, Left **M** Metatarsal-Phalangeal Joint, Right **N** Metatarsal-Phalangeal Joint, Left **P** Toe Phalangeal Joint, Right **Q** Toe Phalangeal Joint, Left	**X** External	**0** Drainage Device **3** Infusion Device **4** Internal Fixation Device **5** External Fixation Device	**Z** No Qualifier

CC 0SP908Z 0SP909Z 0SP90BZ 0SP90JZ 0SP948Z 0SP94JZ 0SPB08Z 0SPB09Z 0SPB0BZ 0SPB0JZ 0SPB48Z 0SPB4JZ 0SPC08Z 0SPC09Z 0SPC0JZ 0SPC38Z 0SPC48Z 0SPC4JZ 0SPD08Z 0SPD09Z 0SPD0JZ 0SPD38Z 0SPD48Z 0SPD4JZ

0 Medical and Surgical
S Lower Joints
Q Repair: Restoring, to the extent possible, a body part to its normal anatomic structure and function

Body Part	Approach	Device	Qualifier
Character 4	**Character 5**	**Character 6**	**Character 7**
0 Lumbar Vertebral Joint **2** Lumbar Vertebral Disc **3** Lumbosacral Joint **4** Lumbosacral Disc **5** Sacrococcygeal Joint **6** Coccygeal Joint **7** Sacroiliac Joint, Right **8** Sacroiliac Joint, Left **9** Hip Joint, Right **B** Hip Joint, Left **C** Knee Joint, Right **D** Knee Joint, Left **F** Ankle Joint, Right **G** Ankle Joint, Left **H** Tarsal Joint, Right **J** Tarsal Joint, Left **K** Tarsometatarsal Joint, Right **L** Tarsometatarsal Joint, Left **M** Metatarsal-Phalangeal Joint, Right **N** Metatarsal-Phalangeal Joint, Left **P** Toe Phalangeal Joint, Right **Q** Toe Phalangeal Joint, Left	**0** Open **3** Percutaneous **4** Percutaneous Endoscopic **X** External	**Z** No Device	**Z** No Qualifier

0 Medical and Surgical
S Lower Joints
R Replacement: Putting in or on biological or synthetic material that physically takes the place and/or function of all or a portion of a body part

Body Part Character 4	Approach Character 5	Device Character 6	Qualifier Character 7
0 Lumbar Vertebral Joint **2** Lumbar Vertebral Disc NC **3** Lumbosacral Joint **4** Lumbosacral Disc NC **5** Sacrococcygeal Joint **6** Coccygeal Joint **7** Sacroiliac Joint, Right **8** Sacroiliac Joint, Left **H** Tarsal Joint, Right **J** Tarsal Joint, Left **K** Tarsometatarsal Joint, Right **L** Tarsometatarsal Joint, Left **M** Metatarsal-Phalangeal Joint, Right **N** Metatarsal-Phalangeal Joint, Left **P** Toe Phalangeal Joint, Right **Q** Toe Phalangeal Joint, Left	**0** Open	**7** Autologous Tissue Substitute **J** Synthetic Substitute **K** Nonautologous Tissue Substitute	**Z** No Qualifier
9 Hip Joint, Right CC HAC **B** Hip Joint, Left CC HAC	**0** Open	**1** Synthetic Substitute, Metal **2** Synthetic Substitute, Metal on Polyethylene **3** Synthetic Substitute, Ceramic **4** Synthetic Substitute, Ceramic on Polyethylene **6** Synthetic Substitute, Oxidized Zirconium on Polyethylene **J** Synthetic Substitute	**9** Cemented **A** Uncemented **Z** No Qualifier
9 Hip Joint, Right HAC **B** Hip Joint, Left HAC	**0** Open	**7** Autologous Tissue Substitute **E** Articulating Spacer **K** Nonautologous Tissue Substitute	**Z** No Qualifier
A Hip Joint, Acetabular Surface, Right CC HAC **E** Hip Joint, Acetabular Surface, Left CC HAC	**0** Open	**0** Synthetic Substitute, Polyethylene **1** Synthetic Substitute, Metal **3** Synthetic Substitute, Ceramic **J** Synthetic Substitute	**9** Cemented **A** Uncemented **Z** No Qualifier
A Hip Joint, Acetabular Surface, Right HAC **E** Hip Joint, Acetabular Surface, Left HAC	**0** Open	**7** Autologous Tissue Substitute **K** Nonautologous Tissue Substitute	**Z** No Qualifier
C Knee Joint, Right CC HAC **D** Knee Joint, Left CC HAC	**0** Open	**6** Synthetic Substitute, Oxidized Zirconium on Polyethylene **J** Synthetic Substitute **L** Synthetic Substitute, Unicondylar Medial **M** Synthetic Substitute, Unicondylar Lateral **N** Synthetic Substitute, Patellofemoral	**9** Cemented **A** Uncemented **Z** No Qualifier
C Knee Joint, Right HAC **D** Knee Joint, Left HAC	**0** Open	**7** Autologous Tissue Substitute **E** Articulating Spacer **K** Nonautologous Tissue Substitute	**Z** No Qualifier

0SR continued on next page

0SR continued from previous page

0 Medical and Surgical
S Lower Joints
R Replacement: Putting in or on biological or synthetic material that physically takes the place and/or function of all or a portion of a body part

Body Part Character 4	Approach Character 5	Device Character 6	Qualifier Character 7
F Ankle Joint, Right **G** Ankle Joint, Left **T** Knee Joint, Femoral Surface, Right HAC **U** Knee Joint, Femoral Surface, Left HAC **V** Knee Joint, Tibial Surface, Right HAC **W** Knee Joint, Tibial Surface, Left HAC	**0** Open	**7** Autologous Tissue Substitute **K** Nonautologous Tissue Substitute	**Z** No Qualifier
F Ankle Joint, Right **G** Ankle Joint, Left **T** Knee Joint, Femoral Surface, Right CC HAC **U** Knee Joint, Femoral Surface, Left CC HAC **V** Knee Joint, Tibial Surface, Right CC HAC **W** Knee Joint, Tibial Surface, Left CC HAC	**0** Open	**J** Synthetic Substitute	**9** Cemented **A** Uncemented **Z** No Qualifier
R Hip Joint, Femoral Surface, Right CC HAC **S** Hip Joint, Femoral Surface, Left CC HAC	**0** Open	**1** Synthetic Substitute, Metal **3** Synthetic Substitute, Ceramic **J** Synthetic Substitute	**9** Cemented **A** Uncemented **Z** No Qualifier
R Hip Joint, Femoral Surface, Right HAC **S** Hip Joint, Femoral Surface, Left HAC	**0** Open	**7** Autologous Tissue Substitute **K** Nonautologous Tissue Substitute	**Z** No Qualifier

CC 0SR9019 0SR901A 0SR901Z 0SR9029 0SR902A 0SR902Z 0SR9039 0SR903A 0SR903Z 0SR9049 0SR904A 0SR904Z 0SR90J9 0SR90JA 0SR90JZ 0SRA009 0SRA00A 0SRA00Z 0SRA019 0SRA01A 0SRA01Z 0SRA039 0SRA03A 0SRA03Z 0SRA0J9 0SRA0JA 0SRA0JZ 0SRB019 0SRB01A 0SRB01Z 0SRB029 0SRB02A 0SRB02Z 0SRB039 0SRB03A 0SRB03Z 0SRB049 0SRB04A 0SRB04Z 0SRB0J9 0SRB0JA 0SRB0JZ 0SRC0J9 0SRC0JA 0SRC0JZ 0SRD0J9 0SRD0JA 0SRD0JZ 0SRE009 0SRE00A 0SRE00Z 0SRE019 0SRE01A 0SRE01Z 0SRE039 0SRE03A 0SRE03Z 0SRE0J9 0SRE0JA 0SRE0JZ 0SRR019 0SRR01A 0SRR01Z 0SRR039 0SRR03A 0SRR03Z 0SRR0J9 0SRR0JA 0SRR0JZ 0SRS019 0SRS01A 0SRS01Z 0SRS039 0SRS03A 0SRS03Z 0SRS0J9 0SRS0JA 0SRS0JZ 0SRT0J9 0SRT0JA 0SRT0JZ 0SRU0J9 0SRU0JA 0SRU0JZ 0SRV0J9 0SRV0JA 0SRV0JZ 0SRW0J9 0SRW0JA 0SRW0JZ

NC 0SR20JZ 0SR40JZ
When the beneficiary is over age 60.

HAC 0SR9019 0SR901A 0SR901Z 0SR9029 0SR902A 0SR902Z 0SR9039 0SR903A 0SR903Z 0SR9049 0SR904A 0SR904Z 0SR9069 0SR906A 0SR906Z 0SR907Z 0SR90J9 0SR90JA 0SR90JZ 0SR90KZ 0SRA009 0SRA00A 0SRA00Z 0SRA019 0SRA01A 0SRA01Z 0SRA039 0SRA03A 0SRA03Z 0SRA07Z 0SRA0J9 0SRA0JA 0SRA0JZ 0SRA0KZ 0SRB019 0SRB01A 0SRB01Z 0SRB029 0SRB02A 0SRB02Z 0SRB039 0SRB03A 0SRB03Z 0SRB049 0SRB04A 0SRB04Z 0SRB069 0SRB06A 0SRB06Z 0SRB07Z 0SRB0J9 0SRB0JA 0SRB0JZ 0SRB0KZ 0SRC069 0SRC06A 0SRC06Z 0SRC07Z 0SRC0J9 0SRC0JA 0SRC0JZ 0SRC0KZ 0SRC0L9 0SRC0LA 0SRC0LZ 0SRD069 0SRD06A 0SRD06Z 0SRD07Z 0SRD0J9 0SRD0JA 0SRD0JZ 0SRD0KZ 0SRD0L9 0SRD0LA 0SRD0LZ 0SRE009 0SRE00A 0SRE00Z 0SRE019 0SRE01A 0SRE01Z 0SRE039 0SRE03A 0SRE03Z 0SRE07Z 0SRE0J9 0SRE0JA 0SRE0JZ 0SRE0KZ 0SRR019 0SRR01A 0SRR01Z 0SRR039 0SRR03A 0SRR03Z 0SRR07Z 0SRR0J9 0SRR0JA 0SRR0JZ 0SRR0KZ 0SRS019 0SRS01A 0SRS01Z 0SRS039 0SRS03A 0SRS03Z 0SRS07Z 0SRS0J9 0SRS0JA 0SRS0JZ 0SRS0KZ 0SRT07Z 0SRT0J9 0SRT0JA 0SRT0JZ 0SRT0KZ 0SRU07Z 0SRU0J9 0SRU0JA 0SRU0JZ 0SRU0KZ 0SRV07Z 0SRV0J9 0SRV0JA 0SRV0JZ 0SRV0KZ 0SRW07Z 0SRW0J9 0SRW0JA 0SRW0JZ 0SRW0KZ
Surgical site infection, mediastinitis, following coronary artery bypass graft (CABG) and secondary diagnosis I26.02, I26.09, I26.92, I26.99, I82.401, I82.402, I82.403, I82.409, I82.411, I82.412, I82.413, I82.419, I82.421, I82.422, I82.423, I82.429, I82.431, I82.432, I82.433, I82.439, I82.441, I82.442, I82.443, I82.449, I82.491, I82.492, I82.493, I82.499, I82.4Y1, I82.4Y2, I82.4Y3, I82.4Y9, I82.4Z1, I82.4Z2, I82.4Z3, I82.4Z9.

LC Limited Coverage NC Noncovered HAC HAC-associated Procedure CC Combination Cluster - See Appendix G for code lists
DRG Non-OR-Affecting MS-DRG Assignment New/Revised Text in **Orange** ♂ Male ♀ Female

0 Medical and Surgical
S Lower Joints
S Reposition: Moving to its normal location, or other suitable location, all or a portion of a body part

Body Part Character 4	Approach Character 5	Device Character 6	Qualifier Character 7
0 Lumbar Vertebral Joint **3** Lumbosacral Joint **5** Sacrococcygeal Joint **6** Coccygeal Joint **7** Sacroiliac Joint, Right **8** Sacroiliac Joint, Left	**0** Open **3** Percutaneous **4** Percutaneous Endoscopic **X** External	**4** Internal Fixation Device **Z** No Device	**Z** No Qualifier
9 Hip Joint, Right **B** Hip Joint, Left **C** Knee Joint, Right **D** Knee Joint, Left **F** Ankle Joint, Right **G** Ankle Joint, Left **H** Tarsal Joint, Right **J** Tarsal Joint, Left **K** Tarsometatarsal Joint, Right **L** Tarsometatarsal Joint, Left **M** Metatarsal-Phalangeal Joint, Right **N** Metatarsal-Phalangeal Joint, Left **P** Toe Phalangeal Joint, Right **Q** Toe Phalangeal Joint, Left	**0** Open **3** Percutaneous **4** Percutaneous Endoscopic **X** External	**4** Internal Fixation Device **5** External Fixation Device **Z** No Device	**Z** No Qualifier

0 Medical and Surgical
S Lower Joints
T Resection: Cutting out or off, without replacement, all of a body part

Body Part Character 4	Approach Character 5	Device Character 6	Qualifier Character 7
2 Lumbar Vertebral Disc **4** Lumbosacral Disc **5** Sacrococcygeal Joint **6** Coccygeal Joint **7** Sacroiliac Joint, Right **8** Sacroiliac Joint, Left **9** Hip Joint, Right **B** Hip Joint, Left **C** Knee Joint, Right **D** Knee Joint, Left **F** Ankle Joint, Right **G** Ankle Joint, Left **H** Tarsal Joint, Right **J** Tarsal Joint, Left **K** Tarsometatarsal Joint, Right **L** Tarsometatarsal Joint, Left **M** Metatarsal-Phalangeal Joint, Right **N** Metatarsal-Phalangeal Joint, Left **P** Toe Phalangeal Joint, Right **Q** Toe Phalangeal Joint, Left	**0** Open	**Z** No Device	**Z** No Qualifier

0 Medical and Surgical
S Lower Joints
U Supplement: Putting in or on biological or synthetic material that physically reinforces and/or augments the function of a portion of a body part

Body Part Character 4	Approach Character 5	Device Character 6	Qualifier Character 7
0 Lumbar Vertebral Joint **2** Lumbar Vertebral Disc **3** Lumbosacral Joint **4** Lumbosacral Disc **5** Sacrococcygeal Joint **6** Coccygeal Joint **7** Sacroiliac Joint, Right **8** Sacroiliac Joint, Left **F** Ankle Joint, Right **G** Ankle Joint, Left **H** Tarsal Joint, Right **J** Tarsal Joint, Left **K** Tarsometatarsal Joint, Right **L** Tarsometatarsal Joint, Left **M** Metatarsal-Phalangeal Joint, Right **N** Metatarsal-Phalangeal Joint, Left **P** Toe Phalangeal Joint, Right **Q** Toe Phalangeal Joint, Left	**0** Open **3** Percutaneous **4** Percutaneous Endoscopic	**7** Autologous Tissue Substitute **J** Synthetic Substitute **K** Nonautologous Tissue Substitute	**Z** No Qualifier
9 Hip Joint, Right [CC] [HAC] **B** Hip Joint, Left [CC] [HAC]	**0** Open	**7** Autologous Tissue Substitute **9** Liner **B** Resurfacing Device **J** Synthetic Substitute **K** Nonautologous Tissue Substitute	**Z** No Qualifier
9 Hip Joint, Right **B** Hip Joint, Left	**3** Percutaneous **4** Percutaneous Endoscopic	**7** Autologous Tissue Substitute **J** Synthetic Substitute **K** Nonautologous Tissue Substitute	**Z** No Qualifier
A Hip Joint, Acetabular Surface, Right [CC] [HAC] **E** Hip Joint, Acetabular Surface, Left [CC] [HAC] **R** Hip Joint, Femoral Surface, Right [CC] [HAC] **S** Hip Joint, Femoral Surface, Left [CC] [HAC]	**0** Open	**9** Liner **B** Resurfacing Device	**Z** No Qualifier
C Knee Joint, Right [CC] **D** Knee Joint, Left [CC]	**0** Open	**7** Autologous Tissue Substitute **J** Synthetic Substitute **K** Nonautologous Tissue Substitute	**Z** No Qualifier
C Knee Joint, Right [CC] **D** Knee Joint, Left [CC]	**0** Open	**9** Liner	**C** Patellar Surface **Z** No Qualifier
C Knee Joint, Right [CC] **D** Knee Joint, Left [CC]	**3** Percutaneous **4** Percutaneous Endoscopic	**7** Autologous Tissue Substitute **J** Synthetic Substitute **K** Nonautologous Tissue Substitute	**Z** No Qualifier
T Knee Joint, Femoral Surface, Right [CC] **U** Knee Joint, Femoral Surface, Left [CC] **V** Knee Joint, Tibial Surface, Right [CC] **W** Knee Joint, Tibial Surface, Left [CC]	**0** Open	**9** Liner	**Z** No Qualifier

[CC] 0SU909Z 0SUA09Z 0SUB09Z 0SUC09C 0SUC0JZ 0SUC4JZ 0SUD09C 0SUD0JZ 0SUD4JZ 0SUE09Z 0SUR09Z 0SUS09Z 0SUT09Z 0SUU09Z 0SUV09Z 0SUW09Z

[HAC] 0SU90BZ 0SUA0BZ 0SUB0BZ 0SUE0BZ 0SUR0BZ 0SUS0BZ
Surgical site infection, mediastinitis, following coronary artery bypass graft (CABG) and secondary diagnosis I26.02, I26.09, I26.92, I26.99, I82.401, I82.402, I82.403, I82.409, I82.411, I82.412, I82.413, I82.419, I82.421, I82.422, I82.423, I82.429, I82.431, I82.432, I82.433, I82.439, I82.441, I82.442, I82.443, I82.449, I82.491, I82.492, I82.493, I82.499, I82.4Y1, I82.4Y2, I82.4Y3, I82.4Y9, I82.4Z1, I82.4Z2, I82.4Z3, I82.4Z9.

0 Medical and Surgical
S Lower Joints
W Revision: Correcting, to the extent possible, a portion of a malfunctioning device or the position of a displaced device

Body Part Character 4	Approach Character 5	Device Character 6	Qualifier Character 7
0 Lumbar Vertebral Joint **3** Lumbosacral Joint	**0** Open **3** Percutaneous **4** Percutaneous Endoscopic **X** External	**0** Drainage Device **3** Infusion Device **4** Internal Fixation Device **7** Autologous Tissue Substitute **8** Spacer **A** Interbody Fusion Device **J** Synthetic Substitute **K** Nonautologous Tissue Substitute	**Z** No Qualifier
2 Lumbar Vertebral Disc **4** Lumbosacral Disc	**0** Open **3** Percutaneous **4** Percutaneous Endoscopic **X** External	**0** Drainage Device **3** Infusion Device **7** Autologous Tissue Substitute **J** Synthetic Substitute **K** Nonautologous Tissue Substitute	**Z** No Qualifier
5 Sacrococcygeal Joint **6** Coccygeal Joint **7** Sacroiliac Joint, Right **8** Sacroiliac Joint, Left	**0** Open **3** Percutaneous **4** Percutaneous Endoscopic **X** External	**0** Drainage Device **3** Infusion Device **4** Internal Fixation Device **7** Autologous Tissue Substitute **8** Spacer **J** Synthetic Substitute **K** Nonautologous Tissue Substitute	**Z** No Qualifier
9 Hip Joint, Right **B** Hip Joint, Left	**0** Open	**0** Drainage Device **3** Infusion Device **4** Internal Fixation Device **5** External Fixation Device **7** Autologous Tissue Substitute **8** Spacer **9** Liner **B** Resurfacing Device **J** Synthetic Substitute **K** Nonautologous Tissue Substitute	**Z** No Qualifier
9 Hip Joint, Right **B** Hip Joint, Left	**3** Percutaneous **4** Percutaneous Endoscopic **X** External	**0** Drainage Device **3** Infusion Device **4** Internal Fixation Device **5** External Fixation Device **7** Autologous Tissue Substitute **8** Spacer **J** Synthetic Substitute **K** Nonautologous Tissue Substitute	**Z** No Qualifier
A Hip Joint, Acetabular Surface, Right **E** Hip Joint, Acetabular Surface, Left **R** Hip Joint, Femoral Surface, Right **S** Hip Joint, Femoral Surface, Left **T** Knee Joint, Femoral Surface, Right **U** Knee Joint, Femoral Surface, Left **V** Knee Joint, Tibial Surface, Right **W** Knee Joint, Tibial Surface, Left	**0** Open **3** Percutaneous **4** Percutaneous Endoscopic **X** External	**J** Synthetic Substitute	**Z** No Qualifier

0SW continued on next page

0SW continued from previous page

0 Medical and Surgical
S Lower Joints
W Revision: Correcting, to the extent possible, a portion of a malfunctioning device or the position of a displaced device

Body Part	Approach	Device	Qualifier
Character 4	**Character 5**	**Character 6**	**Character 7**
C Knee Joint, Right **D** Knee Joint, Left	**0** Open	**0** Drainage Device **3** Infusion Device **4** Internal Fixation Device **5** External Fixation Device **7** Autologous Tissue Substitute **8** Spacer **9** Liner **K** Nonautologous Tissue Substitute	**Z** No Qualifier
C Knee Joint, Right **D** Knee Joint, Left	**0** Open	**J** Synthetic Substitute	**C** Patellar Surface **Z** No Qualifier
C Knee Joint, Right **D** Knee Joint, Left	**3** Percutaneous **4** Percutaneous Endoscopic **X** External	**0** Drainage Device **3** Infusion Device **4** Internal Fixation Device **5** External Fixation Device **7** Autologous Tissue Substitute **8** Spacer **K** Nonautologous Tissue Substitute	**Z** No Qualifier
C Knee Joint, Right **D** Knee Joint, Left	**3** Percutaneous **4** Percutaneous Endoscopic **X** External	**J** Synthetic Substitute	**C** Patellar Surface **Z** No Qualifier
F Ankle Joint, Right **G** Ankle Joint, Left **H** Tarsal Joint, Right **J** Tarsal Joint, Left **K** Tarsometatarsal Joint, Right **L** Tarsometatarsal Joint, Left **M** Metatarsal-Phalangeal Joint, Right **N** Metatarsal-Phalangeal Joint, Left **P** Toe Phalangeal Joint, Right **Q** Toe Phalangeal Joint, Left	**0** Open **3** Percutaneous **4** Percutaneous Endoscopic **X** External	**0** Drainage Device **3** Infusion Device **4** Internal Fixation Device **5** External Fixation Device **7** Autologous Tissue Substitute **8** Spacer **J** Synthetic Substitute **K** Nonautologous Tissue Substitute	**Z** No Qualifier

NOTES

Urinary System 0T1-0TY

0 Medical and Surgical
T Urinary System
1 Bypass: Altering the route of passage of the contents of a tubular body part

Body Part	Approach	Device	Qualifier
Character 4	**Character 5**	**Character 6**	**Character 7**
3 Kidney Pelvis, Right **4** Kidney Pelvis, Left	**0** Open **4** Percutaneous Endoscopic	**7** Autologous Tissue Substitute **J** Synthetic Substitute **K** Nonautologous Tissue Substitute **Z** No Device	**3** Kidney Pelvis, Right **4** Kidney Pelvis, Left **6** Ureter, Right **7** Ureter, Left **8** Colon **9** Colocutaneous **A** Ileum **B** Bladder **C** Ileocutaneous **D** Cutaneous
3 Kidney Pelvis, Right **4** Kidney Pelvis, Left	**3** Percutaneous	**J** Synthetic Substitute	**D** Cutaneous
6 Ureter, Right **7** Ureter, Left **8** Ureters, Bilateral	**0** Open **4** Percutaneous Endoscopic	**7** Autologous Tissue Substitute **J** Synthetic Substitute **K** Nonautologous Tissue Substitute **Z** No Device	**6** Ureter, Right **7** Ureter, Left **8** Colon **9** Colocutaneous **A** Ileum **B** Bladder **C** Ileocutaneous **D** Cutaneous
6 Ureter, Right **7** Ureter, Left **8** Ureters, Bilateral	**3** Percutaneous	**J** Synthetic Substitute	**D** Cutaneous
B Bladder	**0** Open **4** Percutaneous Endoscopic	**7** Autologous Tissue Substitute **J** Synthetic Substitute **K** Nonautologous Tissue Substitute **Z** No Device	**9** Colocutaneous **C** Ileocutaneous **D** Cutaneous
B Bladder	**3** Percutaneous	**J** Synthetic Substitute	**D** Cutaneous

0 Medical and Surgical
T Urinary System
2 Change: Taking out or off a device from a body part and putting back an identical or similar device in or on the same body part without cutting or puncturing the skin or a mucous membrane

Body Part	Approach	Device	Qualifier
Character 4	**Character 5**	**Character 6**	**Character 7**
5 Kidney **9** Ureter **B** Bladder **D** Urethra	**X** External	**0** Drainage Device **Y** Other Device	**Z** No Qualifier

0 Medical and Surgical
T Urinary System
5 Destruction: Physical eradication of all or a portion of a body part by the direct use of energy, force, or a destructive agent

Body Part Character 4	Approach Character 5	Device Character 6	Qualifier Character 7
0 Kidney, Right **1** Kidney, Left **3** Kidney Pelvis, Right **4** Kidney Pelvis, Left **6** Ureter, Right **7** Ureter, Left **B** Bladder **C** Bladder Neck	**0** Open **3** Percutaneous **4** Percutaneous Endoscopic **7** Via Natural or Artificial Opening **8** Via Natural or Artificial Opening Endoscopic	**Z** No Device	**Z** No Qualifier
D Urethra	**0** Open **3** Percutaneous **4** Percutaneous Endoscopic **7** Via Natural or Artificial Opening **8** Via Natural or Artificial Opening Endoscopic **X** External	**Z** No Device	**Z** No Qualifier

0 Medical and Surgical
T Urinary System
7 Dilation: Expanding an orifice or the lumen of a tubular body part

Body Part Character 4	Approach Character 5	Device Character 6	Qualifier Character 7
3 Kidney Pelvis, Right **4** Kidney Pelvis, Left **6** Ureter, Right **7** Ureter, Left **8** Ureters, Bilateral **B** Bladder **C** Bladder Neck **D** Urethra	**0** Open **3** Percutaneous **4** Percutaneous Endoscopic **7** Via Natural or Artificial Opening **8** Via Natural or Artificial Opening Endoscopic	**D** Intraluminal Device **Z** No Device	**Z** No Qualifier

0 Medical and Surgical
T Urinary System
8 Division: Cutting into a body part, without draining fluids and/or gases from the body part, in order to separate or transect a body part

Body Part Character 4	Approach Character 5	Device Character 6	Qualifier Character 7
2 Kidneys, Bilateral **C** Bladder Neck	**0** Open **3** Percutaneous **4** Percutaneous Endoscopic	**Z** No Device	**Z** No Qualifier

0 Medical and Surgical
T Urinary System
9 Drainage: Taking or letting out fluids and/or gases from a body part

Body Part Character 4	Approach Character 5	Device Character 6	Qualifier Character 7
0 Kidney, Right **1** Kidney, Left **3** Kidney Pelvis, Right DRG **4** Kidney Pelvis, Left DRG **6** Ureter, Right **7** Ureter, Left **8** Ureters, Bilateral **B** Bladder **C** Bladder Neck	**0** Open **3** Percutaneous **4** Percutaneous Endoscopic **7** Via Natural or Artificial Opening **8** Via Natural or Artificial Opening Endoscopic	**0** Drainage Device	**Z** No Qualifier
0 Kidney, Right **1** Kidney, Left **3** Kidney Pelvis, Right **4** Kidney Pelvis, Left **6** Ureter, Right **7** Ureter, Left **8** Ureters, Bilateral **B** Bladder **C** Bladder Neck	**0** Open **3** Percutaneous **4** Percutaneous Endoscopic **7** Via Natural or Artificial Opening **8** Via Natural or Artificial Opening Endoscopic	**Z** No Device	**X** Diagnostic **Z** No Qualifier
D Urethra	**0** Open **3** Percutaneous **4** Percutaneous Endoscopic **7** Via Natural or Artificial Opening **8** Via Natural or Artificial Opening Endoscopic **X** External	**0** Drainage Device	**Z** No Qualifier
D Urethra	**0** Open **3** Percutaneous **4** Percutaneous Endoscopic **7** Via Natural or Artificial Opening **8** Via Natural or Artificial Opening Endoscopic **X** External	**Z** No Device	**X** Diagnostic **Z** No Qualifier

DRG 0T9330Z 0T9430Z

0 Medical and Surgical
T Urinary System
B Excision: Cutting out or off, without replacement, a portion of a body part

Body Part Character 4	Approach Character 5	Device Character 6	Qualifier Character 7
0 Kidney, Right **1** Kidney, Left **3** Kidney Pelvis, Right **4** Kidney Pelvis, Left **6** Ureter, Right **7** Ureter, Left **B** Bladder **C** Bladder Neck	**0** Open **3** Percutaneous **4** Percutaneous Endoscopic **7** Via Natural or Artificial Opening **8** Via Natural or Artificial Opening Endoscopic	**Z** No Device	**X** Diagnostic **Z** No Qualifier
D Urethra	**0** Open **3** Percutaneous **4** Percutaneous Endoscopic **7** Via Natural or Artificial Opening **8** Via Natural or Artificial Opening Endoscopic **X** External	**Z** No Device	**X** Diagnostic **Z** No Qualifier

0 Medical and Surgical
T Urinary System
C Extirpation: Taking or cutting out solid matter from a body part

Body Part	Approach	Device	Qualifier
Character 4	Character 5	Character 6	Character 7
0 Kidney, Right **1** Kidney, Left **3** Kidney Pelvis, Right **4** Kidney Pelvis, Left **6** Ureter, Right **7** Ureter, Left **B** Bladder **C** Bladder Neck	**0** Open **3** Percutaneous **4** Percutaneous Endoscopic **7** Via Natural or Artificial Opening **8** Via Natural or Artificial Opening Endoscopic	**Z** No Device	**Z** No Qualifier
D Urethra	**0** Open **3** Percutaneous **4** Percutaneous Endoscopic **7** Via Natural or Artificial Opening **8** Via Natural or Artificial Opening Endoscopic **X** External	**Z** No Device	**Z** No Qualifier

0 Medical and Surgical
T Urinary System
D Extraction: Pulling or stripping out or off all or a portion of a body part by the use of force

Body Part	Approach	Device	Qualifier
Character 4	Character 5	Character 6	Character 7
0 Kidney, Right **1** Kidney, Left	**0** Open **3** Percutaneous **4** Percutaneous Endoscopic	**Z** No Device	**Z** No Qualifier

0 Medical and Surgical
T Urinary System
F Fragmentation: Breaking solid matter in a body part into pieces

Body Part	Approach	Device	Qualifier
Character 4	Character 5	Character 6	Character 7
3 Kidney Pelvis, Right **4** Kidney Pelvis, Left **6** Ureter, Right **7** Ureter, Left **B** Bladder **C** Bladder Neck **D** Urethra NC	**0** Open **3** Percutaneous **4** Percutaneous Endoscopic **7** Via Natural or Artificial Opening **8** Via Natural or Artificial Opening Endoscopic **X** External	**Z** No Device	**Z** No Qualifier

NC 0TFDXZZ

0 Medical and Surgical
T Urinary System
H Insertion: Putting in a nonbiological appliance that monitors, assists, performs, or prevents a physiological function but does not physically take the place of a body part

Body Part	Approach	Device	Qualifier
Character 4	Character 5	Character 6	Character 7
5 Kidney	0 Open 3 Percutaneous 4 Percutaneous Endoscopic 7 Via Natural or Artificial Opening 8 Via Natural or Artificial Opening Endoscopic	2 Monitoring Device 3 Infusion Device Y Other Device	Z No Qualifier
9 Ureter CC	0 Open 3 Percutaneous 4 Percutaneous Endoscopic 7 Via Natural or Artificial Opening 8 Via Natural or Artificial Opening Endoscopic	2 Monitoring Device 3 Infusion Device M Stimulator Lead Y Other Device	Z No Qualifier
B Bladder NC CC	0 Open 3 Percutaneous 4 Percutaneous Endoscopic 7 Via Natural or Artificial Opening 8 Via Natural or Artificial Opening Endoscopic	2 Monitoring Device 3 Infusion Device L Artificial Sphincter M Stimulator Lead Y Other Device	Z No Qualifier
C Bladder Neck	0 Open 3 Percutaneous 4 Percutaneous Endoscopic 7 Via Natural or Artificial Opening 8 Via Natural or Artificial Opening Endoscopic	L Artificial Sphincter	Z No Qualifier
D Urethra	0 Open 3 Percutaneous 4 Percutaneous Endoscopic 7 Via Natural or Artificial Opening 8 Via Natural or Artificial Opening Endoscopic	2 Monitoring Device 3 Infusion Device L Artificial Sphincter Y Other Device	Z No Qualifier
D Urethra	X External	2 Monitoring Device 3 Infusion Device L Artificial Sphincter	Z No Qualifier

NC 0THB0MZ 0THB3MZ 0THB4MZ 0THB7MZ 0THB8MZ
CC 0TH90MZ 0TH93MZ 0TH94MZ 0TH97MZ 0TH98MZ 0THB0MZ 0THB3MZ 0THB4MZ 0THB7MZ 0THB8MZ

0 Medical and Surgical
T Urinary System
J Inspection: Visually and/or manually exploring a body part

Body Part	Approach	Device	Qualifier
Character 4	Character 5	Character 6	Character 7
5 Kidney 9 Ureter B Bladder D Urethra	0 Open 3 Percutaneous 4 Percutaneous Endoscopic 7 Via Natural or Artificial Opening 8 Via Natural or Artificial Opening Endoscopic X External	Z No Device	Z No Qualifier

0 Medical and Surgical
T Urinary System
L Occlusion: Completely closing an orifice or the lumen of a tubular body part

Body Part Character 4	Approach Character 5	Device Character 6	Qualifier Character 7
3 Kidney Pelvis, Right **4** Kidney Pelvis, Left **6** Ureter, Right **7** Ureter, Left **B** Bladder **C** Bladder Neck	**0** Open **3** Percutaneous **4** Percutaneous Endoscopic	**C** Extraluminal Device **D** Intraluminal Device **Z** No Device	**Z** No Qualifier
3 Kidney Pelvis, Right **4** Kidney Pelvis, Left **6** Ureter, Right **7** Ureter, Left **B** Bladder **C** Bladder Neck	**7** Via Natural or Artificial Opening **8** Via Natural or Artificial Opening Endoscopic	**D** Intraluminal Device **Z** No Device	**Z** No Qualifier
D Urethra	**0** Open **3** Percutaneous **4** Percutaneous Endoscopic **X** External	**C** Extraluminal Device **D** Intraluminal Device **Z** No Device	**Z** No Qualifier
D Urethra	**7** Via Natural or Artificial Opening **8** Via Natural or Artificial Opening Endoscopic	**D** Intraluminal Device **Z** No Device	**Z** No Qualifier

0 Medical and Surgical
T Urinary System
M Reattachment: Putting back in or on all or a portion of a separated body part to its normal location or other suitable location

Body Part Character 4	Approach Character 5	Device Character 6	Qualifier Character 7
0 Kidney, Right **1** Kidney, Left **2** Kidneys, Bilateral **3** Kidney Pelvis, Right **4** Kidney Pelvis, Left **6** Ureter, Right **7** Ureter, Left **8** Ureters, Bilateral **B** Bladder **C** Bladder Neck **D** Urethra	**0** Open **4** Percutaneous Endoscopic	**Z** No Device	**Z** No Qualifier

0 Medical and Surgical
T Urinary System
N Release: Freeing a body part from an abnormal physical constraint by cutting or by the use of force

Body Part Character 4	Approach Character 5	Device Character 6	Qualifier Character 7
0 Kidney, Right **1** Kidney, Left **3** Kidney Pelvis, Right **4** Kidney Pelvis, Left **6** Ureter, Right **7** Ureter, Left **B** Bladder **C** Bladder Neck	**0** Open **3** Percutaneous **4** Percutaneous Endoscopic **7** Via Natural or Artificial Opening **8** Via Natural or Artificial Opening Endoscopic	**Z** No Device	**Z** No Qualifier
D Urethra	**0** Open **3** Percutaneous **4** Percutaneous Endoscopic **7** Via Natural or Artificial Opening **8** Via Natural or Artificial Opening Endoscopic **X** External	**Z** No Device	**Z** No Qualifier

0 **Medical and Surgical**
T **Urinary System**
P **Removal:** Taking out or off a device from a body part

Body Part Character 4	Approach Character 5	Device Character 6	Qualifier Character 7
5 Kidney	0 Open 3 Percutaneous 4 Percutaneous Endoscopic 7 Via Natural or Artificial Opening 8 Via Natural or Artificial Opening Endoscopic	0 Drainage Device 2 Monitoring Device 3 Infusion Device 7 Autologous Tissue Substitute C Extraluminal Device D Intraluminal Device J Synthetic Substitute K Nonautologous Tissue Substitute Y Other Device	Z No Qualifier
5 Kidney	X External	0 Drainage Device 2 Monitoring Device 3 Infusion Device D Intraluminal Device	Z No Qualifier
9 Ureter CC	0 Open 3 Percutaneous 4 Percutaneous Endoscopic 7 Via Natural or Artificial Opening 8 Via Natural or Artificial Opening Endoscopic	0 Drainage Device 2 Monitoring Device 3 Infusion Device 7 Autologous Tissue Substitute C Extraluminal Device D Intraluminal Device J Synthetic Substitute K Nonautologous Tissue Substitute M Stimulator Lead Y Other Device	Z No Qualifier
9 Ureter	X External	0 Drainage Device 2 Monitoring Device 3 Infusion Device D Intraluminal Device M Stimulator Lead	Z No Qualifier
B Bladder NC CC	0 Open 3 Percutaneous 4 Percutaneous Endoscopic 7 Via Natural or Artificial Opening 8 Via Natural or Artificial Opening Endoscopic	0 Drainage Device 2 Monitoring Device 3 Infusion Device 7 Autologous Tissue Substitute C Extraluminal Device D Intraluminal Device J Synthetic Substitute K Nonautologous Tissue Substitute L Artificial Sphincter M Stimulator Lead Y Other Device	Z No Qualifier
B Bladder	X External	0 Drainage Device 2 Monitoring Device 3 Infusion Device D Intraluminal Device L Artificial Sphincter M Stimulator Lead	Z No Qualifier
D Urethra	0 Open 3 Percutaneous 4 Percutaneous Endoscopic 7 Via Natural or Artificial Opening 8 Via Natural or Artificial Opening Endoscopic	0 Drainage Device 2 Monitoring Device 3 Infusion Device 7 Autologous Tissue Substitute C Extraluminal Device D Intraluminal Device J Synthetic Substitute K Nonautologous Tissue Substitute L Artificial Sphincter Y Other Device	Z No Qualifier

0TP continued on next page

0TP continued from previous page

0 Medical and Surgical
T Urinary System
P Removal: Taking out or off a device from a body part

Body Part Character 4	Approach Character 5	Device Character 6	Qualifier Character 7
D Urethra	X External	0 Drainage Device 2 Monitoring Device 3 Infusion Device D Intraluminal Device L Artificial Sphincter	Z No Qualifier

NC 0TPB0MZ 0TPB3MZ 0TPB4MZ 0TPB7MZ 0TPB8MZ
CC 0TP90MZ 0TP93MZ 0TP94MZ 0TP97MZ 0TP98MZ 0TPB0MZ 0TPB3MZ 0TPB4MZ 0TPB7MZ 0TPB8MZ

0 Medical and Surgical
T Urinary System
Q Repair: Restoring, to the extent possible, a body part to its normal anatomic structure and function

Body Part Character 4	Approach Character 5	Device Character 6	Qualifier Character 7
0 Kidney, Right CC 1 Kidney, Left CC 3 Kidney Pelvis, Right CC 4 Kidney Pelvis, Left CC 6 Ureter, Right CC 7 Ureter, Left CC B Bladder CC C Bladder Neck	0 Open 3 Percutaneous 4 Percutaneous Endoscopic 7 Via Natural or Artificial Opening 8 Via Natural or Artificial Opening Endoscopic	Z No Device	Z No Qualifier
D Urethra CC	0 Open 3 Percutaneous 4 Percutaneous Endoscopic 7 Via Natural or Artificial Opening 8 Via Natural or Artificial Opening Endoscopic X External	Z No Device	Z No Qualifier

CC 0TQ00ZZ 0TQ03ZZ 0TQ04ZZ 0TQ10ZZ 0TQ13ZZ 0TQ14ZZ 0TQ30ZZ 0TQ33ZZ 0TQ34ZZ 0TQ40ZZ 0TQ43ZZ 0TQ44ZZ 0TQ60ZZ 0TQ63ZZ 0TQ64ZZ 0TQ70ZZ 0TQ73ZZ 0TQ74ZZ 0TQB0ZZ 0TQB3ZZ 0TQB4ZZ 0TQD0ZZ 0TQD3ZZ 0TQD4ZZ

0 Medical and Surgical
T Urinary System
R Replacement: Putting in or on biological or synthetic material that physically takes the place and/or function of all or a portion of a body part

Body Part Character 4	Approach Character 5	Device Character 6	Qualifier Character 7
3 Kidney Pelvis, Right 4 Kidney Pelvis, Left 6 Ureter, Right 7 Ureter, Left B Bladder CC C Bladder Neck	0 Open 4 Percutaneous Endoscopic 7 Via Natural or Artificial Opening 8 Via Natural or Artificial Opening Endoscopic	7 Autologous Tissue Substitute J Synthetic Substitute K Nonautologous Tissue Substitute	Z No Qualifier
D Urethra	0 Open 4 Percutaneous Endoscopic 7 Via Natural or Artificial Opening 8 Via Natural or Artificial Opening Endoscopic X External	7 Autologous Tissue Substitute J Synthetic Substitute K Nonautologous Tissue Substitute	Z No Qualifier

CC 0TRB07Z

0 Medical and Surgical
T Urinary System
S Reposition: Moving to its normal location, or other suitable location, all or a portion of a body part

Body Part Character 4	Approach Character 5	Device Character 6	Qualifier Character 7
0 Kidney, Right **1** Kidney, Left **2** Kidneys, Bilateral **3** Kidney Pelvis, Right **4** Kidney Pelvis, Left **6** Ureter, Right **7** Ureter, Left **8** Ureters, Bilateral **B** Bladder **C** Bladder Neck **D** Urethra	**0** Open **4** Percutaneous Endoscopic	**Z** No Device	**Z** No Qualifier

0 Medical and Surgical
T Urinary System
T Resection: Cutting out or off, without replacement, all of a body part

Body Part Character 4	Approach Character 5	Device Character 6	Qualifier Character 7
0 Kidney, Right **1** Kidney, Left **2** Kidneys, Bilateral	**0** Open **4** Percutaneous Endoscopic	**Z** No Device	**Z** No Qualifier
3 Kidney Pelvis, Right **4** Kidney Pelvis, Left **6** Ureter, Right **7** Ureter, Left **B** Bladder CC **C** Bladder Neck **D** Urethra CC	**0** Open **4** Percutaneous Endoscopic **7** Via Natural or Artificial Opening **8** Via Natural or Artificial Opening Endoscopic	**Z** No Device	**Z** No Qualifier

CC 0TTB0ZZ 0TTB4ZZ 0TTB7ZZ 0TTB8ZZ 0TTD0ZZ

0 Medical and Surgical
T Urinary System
U Supplement: Putting in or on biological or synthetic material that physically reinforces and/or augments the function of a portion of a body part

Body Part Character 4	Approach Character 5	Device Character 6	Qualifier Character 7
3 Kidney Pelvis, Right **4** Kidney Pelvis, Left **6** Ureter, Right **7** Ureter, Left **B** Bladder **C** Bladder Neck	**0** Open **4** Percutaneous Endoscopic **7** Via Natural or Artificial Opening **8** Via Natural or Artificial Opening Endoscopic	**7** Autologous Tissue Substitute **J** Synthetic Substitute **K** Nonautologous Tissue Substitute	**Z** No Qualifier
D Urethra	**0** Open **4** Percutaneous Endoscopic **7** Via Natural or Artificial Opening **8** Via Natural or Artificial Opening Endoscopic **X** External	**7** Autologous Tissue Substitute **J** Synthetic Substitute **K** Nonautologous Tissue Substitute	**Z** No Qualifier

LC Limited Coverage NC Noncovered HAC HAC-associated Procedure CC Combination Cluster - See Appendix G for code lists
DRG Non-OR-Affecting MS-DRG Assignment New/Revised Text in **Orange** ♂ Male ♀ Female

0 Medical and Surgical
T Urinary System
V Restriction: Partially closing an orifice or the lumen of a tubular body part

Body Part Character 4	Approach Character 5	Device Character 6	Qualifier Character 7
3 Kidney Pelvis, Right **4** Kidney Pelvis, Left **6** Ureter, Right **7** Ureter, Left **B** Bladder **C** Bladder Neck	**0** Open **3** Percutaneous **4** Percutaneous Endoscopic	**C** Extraluminal Device **D** Intraluminal Device **Z** No Device	**Z** No Qualifier
3 Kidney Pelvis, Right **4** Kidney Pelvis, Left **6** Ureter, Right **7** Ureter, Left **B** Bladder **C** Bladder Neck	**7** Via Natural or Artificial Opening **8** Via Natural or Artificial Opening Endoscopic	**D** Intraluminal Device **Z** No Device	**Z** No Qualifier
D Urethra	**0** Open **3** Percutaneous **4** Percutaneous Endoscopic	**C** Extraluminal Device **D** Intraluminal Device **Z** No Device	**Z** No Qualifier
D Urethra	**7** Via Natural or Artificial Opening **8** Via Natural or Artificial Opening Endoscopic	**D** Intraluminal Device **Z** No Device	**Z** No Qualifier
D Urethra	**X** External	**Z** No Device	**Z** No Qualifier

0 Medical and Surgical
T Urinary System
W Revision: Correcting, to the extent possible, a portion of a malfunctioning device or the position of a displaced device

Body Part Character 4	Approach Character 5	Device Character 6	Qualifier Character 7
5 Kidney	**0** Open **3** Percutaneous **4** Percutaneous Endoscopic **7** Via Natural or Artificial Opening **8** Via Natural or Artificial Opening Endoscopic	**0** Drainage Device **2** Monitoring Device **3** Infusion Device **7** Autologous Tissue Substitute **C** Extraluminal Device **D** Intraluminal Device **J** Synthetic Substitute **K** Nonautologous Tissue Substitute **Y** Other Device	**Z** No Qualifier
5 Kidney	**X** External	**0** Drainage Device **2** Monitoring Device **3** Infusion Device **7** Autologous Tissue Substitute **C** Extraluminal Device **D** Intraluminal Device **J** Synthetic Substitute **K** Nonautologous Tissue Substitute	**Z** No Qualifier
9 Ureter	**0** Open **3** Percutaneous **4** Percutaneous Endoscopic **7** Via Natural or Artificial Opening **8** Via Natural or Artificial Opening Endoscopic	**0** Drainage Device **2** Monitoring Device **3** Infusion Device **7** Autologous Tissue Substitute **C** Extraluminal Device **D** Intraluminal Device **J** Synthetic Substitute **K** Nonautologous Tissue Substitute **M** Stimulator Lead **Y** Other Device	**Z** No Qualifier
9 Ureter	**X** External	**0** Drainage Device **2** Monitoring Device **3** Infusion Device **7** Autologous Tissue Substitute **C** Extraluminal Device **D** Intraluminal Device **J** Synthetic Substitute **K** Nonautologous Tissue Substitute **M** Stimulator Lead	**Z** No Qualifier

0TW continued on next page

0TW continued from previous page

0 Medical and Surgical
T Urinary System
W Revision: Correcting, to the extent possible, a portion of a malfunctioning device or the position of a displaced device

Body Part Character 4	Approach Character 5	Device Character 6	Qualifier Character 7
B Bladder	**0** Open **3** Percutaneous **4** Percutaneous Endoscopic **7** Via Natural or Artificial Opening **8** Via Natural or Artificial Opening Endoscopic	**0** Drainage Device **2** Monitoring Device **3** Infusion Device **7** Autologous Tissue Substitute **C** Extraluminal Device **D** Intraluminal Device **J** Synthetic Substitute **K** Nonautologous Tissue Substitute **L** Artificial Sphincter **M** Stimulator Lead **Y** Other Device	**Z** No Qualifier
B Bladder	**X** External	**0** Drainage Device **2** Monitoring Device **3** Infusion Device **7** Autologous Tissue Substitute **C** Extraluminal Device **D** Intraluminal Device **J** Synthetic Substitute **K** Nonautologous Tissue Substitute **L** Artificial Sphincter **M** Stimulator Lead	**Z** No Qualifier
D Urethra	**0** Open **3** Percutaneous **4** Percutaneous Endoscopic **7** Via Natural or Artificial Opening **8** Via Natural or Artificial Opening Endoscopic	**0** Drainage Device **2** Monitoring Device **3** Infusion Device **7** Autologous Tissue Substitute **C** Extraluminal Device **D** Intraluminal Device **J** Synthetic Substitute **K** Nonautologous Tissue Substitute **L** Artificial Sphincter **Y** Other Device	**Z** No Qualifier
D Urethra	**X** External	**0** Drainage Device **2** Monitoring Device **3** Infusion Device **7** Autologous Tissue Substitute **C** Extraluminal Device **D** Intraluminal Device **J** Synthetic Substitute **K** Nonautologous Tissue Substitute **L** Artificial Sphincter	**Z** No Qualifier

0 Medical and Surgical
T Urinary System
Y Transplantation: Putting in or on all or a portion of a living body part taken from another individual or animal to physically take the place and/or function of all or a portion of a similar body part

Body Part Character 4	Approach Character 5	Device Character 6	Qualifier Character 7
0 Kidney, Right LC CC NC **1** Kidney, Left LC CC NC	**0** Open	**Z** No Device	**0** Allogeneic **1** Syngeneic **2** Zooplastic

LC 0TY00Z0 0TY00Z1 0TY00Z2 0TY10Z0 0TY10Z1 0TY10Z2
CC 0TY00Z0 0TY00Z1 0TY00Z2 0TY10Z0 0TY10Z1 0TY10Z2
NC 0TY00Z0 0TY00Z1 0TY00Z2 0TY10Z0 0TY10Z1 0TY10Z2

NOTES

Female Reproductive System 0U1-0UY

0 Medical and Surgical
U Female Reproductive System
1 Bypass: Altering the route of passage of the contents of a tubular body part

Body Part Character 4	Approach Character 5	Device Character 6	Qualifier Character 7
5 Fallopian Tube, Right ♀ **6** Fallopian Tube, Left ♀	**0** Open **4** Percutaneous Endoscopic	**7** Autologous Tissue Substitute **J** Synthetic Substitute **K** Nonautologous Tissue Substitute **Z** No Device	**5** Fallopian Tube, Right **6** Fallopian Tube, Left **9** Uterus

♀ 0U15075 0U15076 0U15079 0U150J5 0U150J6 0U150J9 0U150K5 0U150K6 0U150K9 0U150Z5 0U150Z6 0U150Z9 0U15475 0U15476 0U15479 0U154J5 0U154J6 0U154J9 0U154K5 0U154K6 0U154K9 0U154Z5 0U154Z6 0U154Z9 0U16075 0U16076 0U16079 0U160J5 0U160J6 0U160J9 0U160K5 0U160K6 0U160K9 0U160Z5 0U160Z6 0U160Z9 0U16475 0U16476 0U16479 0U164J5 0U164J6 0U164J9 0U164K5 0U164K6 0U164K9 0U164Z5 0U164Z6 0U164Z9

0 Medical and Surgical
U Female Reproductive System
2 Change: Taking out or off a device from a body part and putting back an identical or similar device in or on the same body part without cutting or puncturing the skin or a mucous membrane

Body Part Character 4	Approach Character 5	Device Character 6	Qualifier Character 7
3 Ovary ♀ **8** Fallopian Tube ♀ **M** Vulva ♀	**X** External	**0** Drainage Device **Y** Other Device	**Z** No Qualifier
D Uterus and Cervix ♀	**X** External	**0** Drainage Device **H** Contraceptive Device **Y** Other Device	**Z** No Qualifier
H Vagina and Cul-de-sac ♀	**X** External	**0** Drainage Device **G** Intraluminal Device, Pessary **Y** Other Device	**Z** No Qualifier

♀ 0U23X0Z 0U23XYZ 0U28X0Z 0U28XYZ 0U2DX0Z 0U2DXHZ 0U2DXYZ 0U2HX0Z 0U2HXGZ 0U2HXYZ 0U2MX0Z 0U2MXYZ

0 Medical and Surgical
U Female Reproductive System
5 Destruction: Physical eradication of all or a portion of a body part by the direct use of energy, force, or a destructive agent

Body Part Character 4	Approach Character 5	Device Character 6	Qualifier Character 7
0 Ovary, Right ♀ **1** Ovary, Left ♀ **2** Ovaries, Bilateral ♀ **4** Uterine Supporting Structure ♀	**0** Open **3** Percutaneous **4** Percutaneous Endoscopic **8** Via Natural or Artificial Opening Endoscopic	**Z** No Device	**Z** No Qualifier
5 Fallopian Tube, Right ♀ **6** Fallopian Tube, Left ♀ **7** Fallopian Tubes, Bilateral ♀ NC **9** Uterus ♀ **B** Endometrium ♀ **C** Cervix ♀ **F** Cul-de-sac ♀	**0** Open **3** Percutaneous **4** Percutaneous Endoscopic **7** Via Natural or Artificial Opening **8** Via Natural or Artificial Opening Endoscopic	**Z** No Device	**Z** No Qualifier
G Vagina ♀ **K** Hymen ♀	**0** Open **3** Percutaneous **4** Percutaneous Endoscopic **7** Via Natural or Artificial Opening **8** Via Natural or Artificial Opening Endoscopic **X** External	**Z** No Device	**Z** No Qualifier

0U5 continued on next page

0U5 continued from previous page

0 Medical and Surgical
U Female Reproductive System
5 Destruction: Physical eradication of all or a portion of a body part by the direct use of energy, force, or a destructive agent

Body Part Character 4	Approach Character 5	Device Character 6	Qualifier Character 7
J Clitoris ♀ **L** Vestibular Gland ♀ **M** Vulva ♀	**0** Open **X** External	**Z** No Device	**Z** No Qualifier

♀ 0U500ZZ 0U503ZZ 0U504ZZ 0U508ZZ 0U510ZZ 0U513ZZ 0U514ZZ 0U518ZZ 0U520ZZ 0U523ZZ 0U524ZZ 0U528ZZ 0U540ZZ 0U543ZZ 0U544ZZ 0U548ZZ 0U550ZZ 0U553ZZ 0U554ZZ 0U557ZZ 0U558ZZ 0U560ZZ 0U563ZZ 0U564ZZ 0U567ZZ 0U568ZZ 0U570ZZ 0U573ZZ 0U574ZZ 0U577ZZ 0U578ZZ 0U590ZZ 0U593ZZ 0U594ZZ 0U597ZZ 0U598ZZ 0U5B0ZZ 0U5B3ZZ 0U5B4ZZ 0U5B7ZZ 0U5B8ZZ 0U5C0ZZ 0U5C3ZZ 0U5C4ZZ 0U5C7ZZ 0U5C8ZZ 0U5F0ZZ 0U5F3ZZ 0U5F4ZZ 0U5F7ZZ 0U5F8ZZ 0U5G0ZZ 0U5G3ZZ 0U5G4ZZ 0U5G7ZZ 0U5G8ZZ 0U5GXZZ 0U5J0ZZ 0U5JXZZ 0U5K0ZZ 0U5K3ZZ 0U5K4ZZ 0U5K7ZZ 0U5K8ZZ 0U5KXZZ 0U5L0ZZ 0U5LXZZ 0U5M0ZZ 0U5MXZZ

NC 0U570ZZ 0U573ZZ 0U574ZZ 0U577ZZ 0U578ZZ Codes in this list are noncovered procedures only when reported with Z30.2 as either a principal or secondary diagnosis.

0 Medical and Surgical
U Female Reproductive System
7 Dilation: Expanding an orifice or the lumen of a tubular body part

Body Part Character 4	Approach Character 5	Device Character 6	Qualifier Character 7
5 Fallopian Tube, Right ♀ **6** Fallopian Tube, Left ♀ **7** Fallopian Tubes, Bilateral ♀ **9** Uterus ♀ **C** Cervix ♀ **G** Vagina ♀	**0** Open **3** Percutaneous **4** Percutaneous Endoscopic **7** Via Natural or Artificial Opening **8** Via Natural or Artificial Opening Endoscopic	**D** Intraluminal Device **Z** No Device	**Z** No Qualifier
K Hymen ♀	**0** Open **3** Percutaneous **4** Percutaneous Endoscopic **7** Via Natural or Artificial Opening **8** Via Natural or Artificial Opening Endoscopic **X** External	**D** Intraluminal Device **Z** No Device	**Z** No Qualifier

♀ 0U750DZ 0U750ZZ 0U753DZ 0U753ZZ 0U754DZ 0U754ZZ 0U757DZ 0U757ZZ 0U758DZ 0U758ZZ 0U760DZ 0U760ZZ 0U763DZ 0U763ZZ 0U764DZ 0U764ZZ 0U767DZ 0U767ZZ 0U768DZ 0U768ZZ 0U770DZ 0U770ZZ 0U773DZ 0U773ZZ 0U774DZ 0U774ZZ 0U777DZ 0U777ZZ 0U778DZ 0U778ZZ 0U790DZ 0U790ZZ 0U793DZ 0U793ZZ 0U794DZ 0U794ZZ 0U797DZ 0U797ZZ 0U798DZ 0U798ZZ 0U7C0DZ 0U7C0ZZ 0U7C3DZ 0U7C3ZZ 0U7C4DZ 0U7C4ZZ 0U7C7DZ 0U7C7ZZ 0U7C8DZ 0U7C8ZZ 0U7G0DZ 0U7G0ZZ 0U7G3DZ 0U7G3ZZ 0U7G4DZ 0U7G4ZZ 0U7G7DZ 0U7G7ZZ 0U7G8DZ 0U7G8ZZ 0U7K0DZ 0U7K0ZZ 0U7K3DZ 0U7K3ZZ 0U7K4DZ 0U7K4ZZ 0U7K7DZ 0U7K7ZZ 0U7K8DZ 0U7K8ZZ 0U7KXDZ 0U7KXZZ

0 Medical and Surgical
U Female Reproductive System
8 Division: Cutting into a body part, without draining fluids and/or gases from the body part, in order to separate or transect a body part

Body Part Character 4	Approach Character 5	Device Character 6	Qualifier Character 7
0 Ovary, Right ♀ **1** Ovary, Left ♀ **2** Ovaries, Bilateral ♀ **4** Uterine Supporting Structure ♀	**0** Open **3** Percutaneous **4** Percutaneous Endoscopic	**Z** No Device	**Z** No Qualifier
K Hymen ♀	**7** Via Natural or Artificial Opening **8** Via Natural or Artificial Opening Endoscopic **X** External	**Z** No Device	**Z** No Qualifier

♀ 0U800ZZ 0U803ZZ 0U804ZZ 0U810ZZ 0U813ZZ 0U814ZZ 0U820ZZ 0U823ZZ 0U824ZZ 0U840ZZ 0U843ZZ 0U844ZZ 0U8K7ZZ 0U8K8ZZ 0U8KXZZ

0 Medical and Surgical
U Female Reproductive System
9 Drainage: Taking or letting out fluids and/or gases from a body part

Body Part Character 4	Approach Character 5	Device Character 6	Qualifier Character 7
0 Ovary, Right ♀ **1** Ovary, Left ♀ **2** Ovaries, Bilateral ♀	**0** Open **3** Percutaneous **4** Percutaneous Endoscopic **8** Via Natural or Artificial Opening Endoscopic	**0** Drainage Device	**Z** No Qualifier
0 Ovary, Right ♀ **1** Ovary, Left ♀ **2** Ovaries, Bilateral ♀	**0** Open **3** Percutaneous **4** Percutaneous Endoscopic **8** Via Natural or Artificial Opening Endoscopic	**Z** No Device	**X** Diagnostic **Z** No Qualifier
0 Ovary, Right ♀ **1** Ovary, Left ♀ **2** Ovaries, Bilateral ♀	**X** External	**Z** No Device	**Z** No Qualifier
4 Uterine Supporting Structure ♀	**0** Open **3** Percutaneous **4** Percutaneous Endoscopic **8** Via Natural or Artificial Opening Endoscopic	**0** Drainage Device	**Z** No Qualifier
4 Uterine Supporting Structure ♀	**0** Open **3** Percutaneous **4** Percutaneous Endoscopic **8** Via Natural or Artificial Opening Endoscopic	**Z** No Device	**X** Diagnostic **Z** No Qualifier
5 Fallopian Tube, Right ♀ **6** Fallopian Tube, Left ♀ **7** Fallopian Tubes, Bilateral ♀ **9** Uterus ♀ **C** Cervix ♀ **F** Cul-de-sac ♀	**0** Open **3** Percutaneous **4** Percutaneous Endoscopic **7** Via Natural or Artificial Opening **8** Via Natural or Artificial Opening Endoscopic	**0** Drainage Device	**Z** No Qualifier
5 Fallopian Tube, Right ♀ **6** Fallopian Tube, Left ♀ **7** Fallopian Tubes, Bilateral ♀ **9** Uterus ♀ **C** Cervix ♀ **F** Cul-de-sac ♀	**0** Open **3** Percutaneous **4** Percutaneous Endoscopic **7** Via Natural or Artificial Opening **8** Via Natural or Artificial Opening Endoscopic	**Z** No Device	**X** Diagnostic **Z** No Qualifier
G Vagina ♀ **K** Hymen ♀	**0** Open **3** Percutaneous **4** Percutaneous Endoscopic **7** Via Natural or Artificial Opening **8** Via Natural or Artificial Opening Endoscopic **X** External	**0** Drainage Device	**Z** No Qualifier
G Vagina ♀ **K** Hymen ♀	**0** Open **3** Percutaneous **4** Percutaneous Endoscopic **7** Via Natural or Artificial Opening **8** Via Natural or Artificial Opening Endoscopic **X** External	**Z** No Device	**X** Diagnostic **Z** No Qualifier
J Clitoris ♀ **L** Vestibular Gland ♀ **M** Vulva ♀	**0** Open **X** External	**0** Drainage Device	**Z** No Qualifier
J Clitoris ♀ **L** Vestibular Gland ♀ **M** Vulva ♀	**0** Open **X** External	**Z** No Device	**X** Diagnostic **Z** No Qualifier

0U9 continued on next page

0U9 continued from previous page

♀ 0U9000Z 0U900ZX 0U900ZZ 0U9030Z 0U903ZX 0U903ZZ 0U9040Z 0U904ZX 0U904ZZ 0U9080Z 0U908ZX 0U908ZZ 0U90XZZ
0U9100Z 0U910ZX 0U910ZZ 0U9130Z 0U913ZX 0U913ZZ 0U9140Z 0U914ZX 0U914ZZ 0U9180Z 0U918ZX 0U918ZZ 0U91XZZ
0U9200Z 0U920ZX 0U920ZZ 0U9230Z 0U923ZX 0U923ZZ 0U9240Z 0U924ZX 0U924ZZ 0U9280Z 0U928ZX 0U928ZZ 0U92XZZ
0U9400Z 0U940ZX 0U940ZZ 0U9430Z 0U943ZX 0U943ZZ 0U9440Z 0U944ZX 0U944ZZ 0U9480Z 0U948ZX 0U948ZZ 0U9500Z
0U950ZX 0U950ZZ 0U9530Z 0U953ZX 0U953ZZ 0U9540Z 0U954ZX 0U954ZZ 0U9570Z 0U957ZX 0U957ZZ 0U9580Z 0U958ZX
0U958ZZ 0U9600Z 0U960ZX 0U960ZZ 0U9630Z 0U963ZX 0U963ZZ 0U9640Z 0U964ZX 0U964ZZ 0U9670Z 0U967ZX 0U967ZZ
0U9680Z 0U968ZX 0U968ZZ 0U9700Z 0U970ZX 0U970ZZ 0U9730Z 0U973ZX 0U973ZZ 0U9740Z 0U974ZX 0U974ZZ 0U9770Z
0U977ZX 0U977ZZ 0U9780Z 0U978ZX 0U978ZZ 0U9900Z 0U990ZX 0U990ZZ 0U9930Z 0U993ZX 0U993ZZ 0U9940Z 0U994ZX
0U994ZZ 0U9970Z 0U997ZX 0U997ZZ 0U9980Z 0U998ZX 0U998ZZ 0U9C00Z 0U9C0ZX 0U9C0ZZ 0U9C30Z 0U9C3ZX 0U9C3ZZ
0U9C40Z 0U9C4ZX 0U9C4ZZ 0U9C70Z 0U9C7ZX 0U9C7ZZ 0U9C80Z 0U9C8ZX 0U9C8ZZ 0U9F00Z 0U9F0ZX 0U9F0ZZ 0U9F30Z
0U9F3ZX 0U9F3ZZ 0U9F40Z 0U9F4ZX 0U9F4ZZ 0U9F70Z 0U9F7ZX 0U9F7ZZ 0U9F80Z 0U9F8ZX 0U9F8ZZ 0U9G00Z 0U9G0ZX
0U9G0ZZ 0U9G30Z 0U9G3ZX 0U9G3ZZ 0U9G40Z 0U9G4ZX 0U9G4ZZ 0U9G70Z 0U9G7ZX 0U9G7ZZ 0U9G80Z 0U9G8ZX 0U9G8ZZ
0U9GX0Z 0U9GXZX 0U9GXZZ 0U9J00Z 0U9J0ZX 0U9J0ZZ 0U9JX0Z 0U9JXZX 0U9JXZZ 0U9K00Z 0U9K0ZX 0U9K0ZZ 0U9K30Z
0U9K3ZX 0U9K3ZZ 0U9K40Z 0U9K4ZX 0U9K4ZZ 0U9K70Z 0U9K7ZX 0U9K7ZZ 0U9K80Z 0U9K8ZX 0U9K8ZZ 0U9KX0Z 0U9KXZX
0U9KXZZ 0U9L00Z 0U9L0ZX 0U9L0ZZ 0U9LX0Z 0U9LXZX 0U9LXZZ 0U9M00Z 0U9M0ZX 0U9M0ZZ 0U9MX0Z 0U9MXZX 0U9MXZZ

0 Medical and Surgical
U Female Reproductive System
B Excision: Cutting out or off, without replacement, a portion of a body part

Body Part Character 4	Approach Character 5	Device Character 6	Qualifier Character 7
0 Ovary, Right ♀ **1** Ovary, Left ♀ **2** Ovaries, Bilateral ♀ **4** Uterine Supporting Structure ♀ **5** Fallopian Tube, Right ♀ **6** Fallopian Tube, Left ♀ **7** Fallopian Tubes, Bilateral ♀ **9** Uterus ♀ **C** Cervix ♀ **F** Cul-de-sac ♀	**0** Open **3** Percutaneous **4** Percutaneous Endoscopic **7** Via Natural or Artificial Opening **8** Via Natural or Artificial Opening Endoscopic	**Z** No Device	**X** Diagnostic **Z** No Qualifier
G Vagina ♀ **K** Hymen ♀	**0** Open **3** Percutaneous **4** Percutaneous Endoscopic **7** Via Natural or Artificial Opening **8** Via Natural or Artificial Opening Endoscopic **X** External	**Z** No Device	**X** Diagnostic **Z** No Qualifier
J Clitoris ♀ **L** Vestibular Gland ♀ **M** Vulva ♀	**0** Open **X** External	**Z** No Device	**X** Diagnostic **Z** No Qualifier

♀ 0UB00ZX 0UB00ZZ 0UB03ZX 0UB03ZZ 0UB04ZX 0UB04ZZ 0UB07ZX 0UB07ZZ 0UB08ZX 0UB08ZZ 0UB10ZX 0UB10ZZ 0UB13ZX
0UB13ZZ 0UB14ZX 0UB14ZZ 0UB17ZX 0UB17ZZ 0UB18ZX 0UB18ZZ 0UB20ZX 0UB20ZZ 0UB23ZX 0UB23ZZ 0UB24ZX 0UB24ZZ
0UB27ZX 0UB27ZZ 0UB28ZX 0UB28ZZ 0UB40ZX 0UB40ZZ 0UB43ZX 0UB43ZZ 0UB44ZX 0UB44ZZ 0UB47ZX 0UB47ZZ 0UB48ZX
0UB48ZZ 0UB50ZX 0UB50ZZ 0UB53ZX 0UB53ZZ 0UB54ZX 0UB54ZZ 0UB57ZX 0UB57ZZ 0UB58ZX 0UB58ZZ 0UB60ZX 0UB60ZZ
0UB63ZX 0UB63ZZ 0UB64ZX 0UB64ZZ 0UB67ZX 0UB67ZZ 0UB68ZX 0UB68ZZ 0UB70ZX 0UB70ZZ 0UB73ZX 0UB73ZZ 0UB74ZX
0UB74ZZ 0UB77ZX 0UB77ZZ 0UB78ZX 0UB78ZZ 0UB90ZX 0UB90ZZ 0UB93ZX 0UB93ZZ 0UB94ZX 0UB94ZZ 0UB97ZX 0UB97ZZ
0UB98ZX 0UB98ZZ 0UBC0ZX 0UBC0ZZ 0UBC3ZX 0UBC3ZZ 0UBC4ZX 0UBC4ZZ 0UBC7ZX 0UBC7ZZ 0UBC8ZX 0UBC8ZZ 0UBF0ZX
0UBF0ZZ 0UBF3ZX 0UBF3ZZ 0UBF4ZX 0UBF4ZZ 0UBF7ZX 0UBF7ZZ 0UBF8ZX 0UBF8ZZ 0UBG0ZX 0UBG0ZZ 0UBG3ZX 0UBG3ZZ
0UBG4ZX 0UBG4ZZ 0UBG7ZX 0UBG7ZZ 0UBG8ZX 0UBG8ZZ 0UBGXZX 0UBGXZZ 0UBJ0ZX 0UBJ0ZZ 0UBJXZX 0UBJXZZ 0UBK0ZX
0UBK0ZZ 0UBK3ZX 0UBK3ZZ 0UBK4ZX 0UBK4ZZ 0UBK7ZX 0UBK7ZZ 0UBK8ZX 0UBK8ZZ 0UBKXZX 0UBKXZZ 0UBL0ZX 0UBL0ZZ
0UBLXZX 0UBLXZZ 0UBM0ZX 0UBM0ZZ 0UBMXZX 0UBMXZZ

0 Medical and Surgical
U Female Reproductive System
C Extirpation: Taking or cutting out solid matter from a body part

Body Part Character 4	Approach Character 5	Device Character 6	Qualifier Character 7
0 Ovary, Right ♀ **1** Ovary, Left ♀ **2** Ovaries, Bilateral ♀ **4** Uterine Supporting Structure ♀	**0** Open **3** Percutaneous **4** Percutaneous Endoscopic **8** Via Natural or Artificial Opening Endoscopic	**Z** No Device	**Z** No Qualifier
5 Fallopian Tube, Right ♀ **6** Fallopian Tube, Left ♀ **7** Fallopian Tubes, Bilateral ♀ **9** Uterus ♀ **B** Endometrium ♀ **C** Cervix ♀ **F** Cul-de-sac ♀	**0** Open **3** Percutaneous **4** Percutaneous Endoscopic **7** Via Natural or Artificial Opening **8** Via Natural or Artificial Opening Endoscopic	**Z** No Device	**Z** No Qualifier
G Vagina ♀ **K** Hymen ♀	**0** Open **3** Percutaneous **4** Percutaneous Endoscopic **7** Via Natural or Artificial Opening **8** Via Natural or Artificial Opening Endoscopic **X** External	**Z** No Device	**Z** No Qualifier
J Clitoris ♀ **L** Vestibular Gland ♀ **M** Vulva ♀	**0** Open **X** External	**Z** No Device	**Z** No Qualifier

♀ 0UC00ZZ 0UC03ZZ 0UC04ZZ 0UC08ZZ 0UC10ZZ 0UC13ZZ 0UC14ZZ 0UC18ZZ 0UC20ZZ 0UC23ZZ 0UC24ZZ 0UC28ZZ 0UC40ZZ 0UC43ZZ 0UC44ZZ 0UC48ZZ 0UC50ZZ 0UC53ZZ 0UC54ZZ 0UC57ZZ 0UC58ZZ 0UC60ZZ 0UC63ZZ 0UC64ZZ 0UC67ZZ 0UC68ZZ 0UC70ZZ 0UC73ZZ 0UC74ZZ 0UC77ZZ 0UC78ZZ 0UC90ZZ 0UC93ZZ 0UC94ZZ 0UC97ZZ 0UC98ZZ 0UCB0ZZ 0UCB3ZZ 0UCB4ZZ 0UCB7ZZ 0UCB8ZZ 0UCC0ZZ 0UCC3ZZ 0UCC4ZZ 0UCC7ZZ 0UCC8ZZ 0UCF0ZZ 0UCF3ZZ 0UCF4ZZ 0UCF7ZZ 0UCF8ZZ 0UCG0ZZ 0UCG3ZZ 0UCG4ZZ 0UCG7ZZ 0UCG8ZZ 0UCGXZZ 0UCJ0ZZ 0UCJXZZ 0UCK0ZZ 0UCK3ZZ 0UCK4ZZ 0UCK7ZZ 0UCK8ZZ 0UCKXZZ 0UCL0ZZ 0UCLXZZ 0UCM0ZZ 0UCMXZZ

0 Medical and Surgical
U Female Reproductive System
D Extraction: Pulling or stripping out or off all or a portion of a body part by the use of force

Body Part Character 4	Approach Character 5	Device Character 6	Qualifier Character 7
B Endometrium ♀	**7** Via Natural or Artificial Opening **8** Via Natural or Artificial Opening Endoscopic	**Z** No Device	**X** Diagnostic **Z** No Qualifier
N Ova ♀	**0** Open **3** Percutaneous **4** Percutaneous Endoscopic	**Z** No Device	**Z** No Qualifier

♀ 0UDB7ZX 0UDB7ZZ 0UDB8ZX 0UDB8ZZ 0UDN0ZZ 0UDN3ZZ 0UDN4ZZ

0 Medical and Surgical
U Female Reproductive System
F Fragmentation: Breaking solid matter in a body part into pieces

Body Part Character 4	Approach Character 5	Device Character 6	Qualifier Character 7
5 Fallopian Tube, Right NC ♀ **6** Fallopian Tube, Left NC ♀ **7** Fallopian Tubes, Bilateral NC ♀ **9** Uterus NC ♀	**0** Open **3** Percutaneous **4** Percutaneous Endoscopic **7** Via Natural or Artificial Opening **8** Via Natural or Artificial Opening Endoscopic **X** External	**Z** No Device	**Z** No Qualifier

♀ 0UF50ZZ 0UF53ZZ 0UF54ZZ 0UF57ZZ 0UF58ZZ 0UF5XZZ 0UF60ZZ 0UF63ZZ 0UF64ZZ 0UF67ZZ 0UF68ZZ 0UF6XZZ 0UF70ZZ 0UF73ZZ 0UF74ZZ 0UF77ZZ 0UF78ZZ 0UF7XZZ 0UF90ZZ 0UF93ZZ 0UF94ZZ 0UF97ZZ 0UF98ZZ 0UF9XZZ

NC 0UF5XZZ 0UF6XZZ 0UF7XZZ 0UF9XZZ

0 Medical and Surgical
U Female Reproductive System
H Insertion: Putting in a nonbiological appliance that monitors, assists, performs, or prevents a physiological function but does not physically take the place of a body part

Body Part	Approach	Device	Qualifier
Character 4	Character 5	Character 6	Character 7
3 Ovary ♀	**0** Open **3** Percutaneous **4** Percutaneous Endoscopic	**3** Infusion Device **Y** Other Device	**Z** No Qualifier
3 Ovary ♀	**7** Via Natural or Artificial Opening **8** Via Natural or Artificial Opening Endoscopic	**Y** Other Device	**Z** No Qualifier
8 Fallopian Tube ♀ **D** Uterus and Cervix ♀ **H** Vagina and Cul-de-sac ♀	**0** Open **3** Percutaneous **4** Percutaneous Endoscopic **7** Via Natural or Artificial Opening **8** Via Natural or Artificial Opening Endoscopic	**3** Infusion Device **Y** Other Device	**Z** No Qualifier
9 Uterus ♀	**0** Open **7** Via Natural or Artificial Opening **8** Via Natural or Artificial Opening Endoscopic	**H** Contraceptive Device	**Z** No Qualifier
C Cervix ♀	**0** Open **3** Percutaneous **4** Percutaneous Endoscopic	**1** Radioactive Element	**Z** No Qualifier
C Cervix ♀	**7** Via Natural or Artificial Opening **8** Via Natural or Artificial Opening Endoscopic	**1** Radioactive Element **H** Contraceptive Device	**Z** No Qualifier
F Cul-de-sac ♀	**7** Via Natural or Artificial Opening **8** Via Natural or Artificial Opening Endoscopic	**G** Intraluminal Device, Pessary	**Z** No Qualifier
G Vagina ♀	**0** Open **3** Percutaneous **4** Percutaneous Endoscopic **X** External	**1** Radioactive Element	**Z** No Qualifier
G Vagina ♀	**7** Via Natural or Artificial Opening **8** Via Natural or Artificial Opening Endoscopic	**1** Radioactive Element **G** Intraluminal Device, Pessary	**Z** No Qualifier

♀ 0UH303Z 0UH30YZ 0UH333Z 0UH33YZ 0UH343Z 0UH34YZ 0UH37YZ 0UH38YZ 0UH803Z 0UH80YZ 0UH833Z 0UH83YZ 0UH843Z 0UH84YZ 0UH873Z 0UH87YZ 0UH883Z 0UH88YZ 0UH90HZ 0UH97HZ 0UH98HZ 0UHC01Z 0UHC31Z 0UHC41Z 0UHC71Z 0UHC7HZ 0UHC81Z 0UHC8HZ 0UHD03Z 0UHD0YZ 0UHD33Z 0UHD3YZ 0UHD43Z 0UHD4YZ 0UHD73Z 0UHD7YZ 0UHD83Z 0UHD8YZ 0UHF7GZ 0UHF8GZ 0UHG01Z 0UHG31Z 0UHG41Z 0UHG71Z 0UHG7GZ 0UHG81Z 0UHG8GZ 0UHGX1Z 0UHH03Z 0UHH0YZ 0UHH33Z 0UHH3YZ 0UHH43Z 0UHH4YZ 0UHH73Z 0UHH7YZ 0UHH83Z 0UHH8YZ

0 Medical and Surgical
U Female Reproductive System
J Inspection: Visually and/or manually exploring a body part

Body Part	Approach	Device	Qualifier
Character 4	Character 5	Character 6	Character 7
3 Ovary ♀	**0** Open **3** Percutaneous **4** Percutaneous Endoscopic **8** Via Natural or Artificial Opening Endoscopic **X** External	**Z** No Device	**Z** No Qualifier

0UJ continued on next page

0UJ continued from previous page

0 Medical and Surgical
U Female Reproductive System
J Inspection: Visually and/or manually exploring a body part

Body Part Character 4	Approach Character 5	Device Character 6	Qualifier Character 7
8 Fallopian Tube ♀ **D** Uterus and Cervix ♀ **H** Vagina and Cul-de-sac ♀	**0** Open **3** Percutaneous **4** Percutaneous Endoscopic **7** Via Natural or Artificial Opening **8** Via Natural or Artificial Opening Endoscopic **X** External	**Z** No Device	**Z** No Qualifier
M Vulva ♀	**0** Open **X** External	**Z** No Device	**Z** No Qualifier

♀ 0UJ30ZZ 0UJ33ZZ 0UJ34ZZ 0UJ38ZZ 0UJ3XZZ 0UJ80ZZ 0UJ83ZZ 0UJ84ZZ 0UJ87ZZ 0UJ88ZZ 0UJ8XZZ 0UJD0ZZ 0UJD3ZZ 0UJD4ZZ 0UJD7ZZ 0UJD8ZZ 0UJDXZZ 0UJH0ZZ 0UJH3ZZ 0UJH4ZZ 0UJH7ZZ 0UJH8ZZ 0UJHXZZ 0UJM0ZZ 0UJMXZZ

0 Medical and Surgical
U Female Reproductive System
L Occlusion: Completely closing an orifice or the lumen of a tubular body part

Body Part Character 4	Approach Character 5	Device Character 6	Qualifier Character 7
5 Fallopian Tube, Right ♀ **6** Fallopian Tube, Left ♀ **7** Fallopian Tubes, Bilateral ♀ NC	**0** Open **3** Percutaneous **4** Percutaneous Endoscopic	**C** Extraluminal Device **D** Intraluminal Device **Z** No Device	**Z** No Qualifier
5 Fallopian Tube, Right ♀ **6** Fallopian Tube, Left ♀ **7** Fallopian Tubes, Bilateral ♀ NC	**7** Via Natural or Artificial Opening **8** Via Natural or Artificial Opening Endoscopic	**D** Intraluminal Device **Z** No Device	**Z** No Qualifier
F Cul-de-sac ♀ **G** Vagina ♀	**7** Via Natural or Artificial Opening **8** Via Natural or Artificial Opening Endoscopic	**D** Intraluminal Device **Z** No Device	**Z** No Qualifier

♀ 0UL50CZ 0UL50DZ 0UL50ZZ 0UL53CZ 0UL53DZ 0UL53ZZ 0UL54CZ 0UL54DZ 0UL54ZZ 0UL57DZ 0UL57ZZ 0UL58DZ 0UL58ZZ 0UL60CZ 0UL60DZ 0UL60ZZ 0UL63CZ 0UL63DZ 0UL63ZZ 0UL64CZ 0UL64DZ 0UL64ZZ 0UL67DZ 0UL67ZZ 0UL68DZ 0UL68ZZ 0UL70CZ 0UL70DZ 0UL70ZZ 0UL73CZ 0UL73DZ 0UL73ZZ 0UL74CZ 0UL74DZ 0UL74ZZ 0UL77DZ 0UL77ZZ 0UL78DZ 0UL78ZZ 0ULF7DZ 0ULF7ZZ 0ULF8DZ 0ULF8ZZ 0ULG7DZ 0ULG7ZZ 0ULG8DZ 0ULG8ZZ

NC 0UL70CZ 0UL70DZ 0UL70ZZ 0UL73CZ 0UL73DZ 0UL73ZZ 0UL74CZ 0UL74DZ 0UL74ZZ 0UL77DZ 0UL77ZZ 0UL78DZ 0UL78ZZ
Codes in this list are noncovered procedures only when reported with Z30.2 as either a principal or secondary diagnosis.

0 Medical and Surgical
U Female Reproductive System
M Reattachment: Putting back in or on all or a portion of a separated body part to its normal location or other suitable location

Body Part Character 4	Approach Character 5	Device Character 6	Qualifier Character 7
0 Ovary, Right ♀ **1** Ovary, Left ♀ **2** Ovaries, Bilateral ♀ **4** Uterine Supporting Structure ♀ **5** Fallopian Tube, Right ♀ **6** Fallopian Tube, Left ♀ **7** Fallopian Tubes, Bilateral ♀ **9** Uterus ♀ **C** Cervix ♀ **F** Cul-de-sac ♀ **G** Vagina ♀	**0** Open **4** Percutaneous Endoscopic	**Z** No Device	**Z** No Qualifier
J Clitoris ♀ **M** Vulva ♀	**X** External	**Z** No Device	**Z** No Qualifier
K Hymen ♀	**0** Open **4** Percutaneous Endoscopic **X** External	**Z** No Device	**Z** No Qualifier

♀ 0UM00ZZ 0UM04ZZ 0UM10ZZ 0UM14ZZ 0UM20ZZ 0UM24ZZ 0UM40ZZ 0UM44ZZ 0UM50ZZ 0UM54ZZ 0UM60ZZ 0UM64ZZ 0UM70ZZ 0UM74ZZ 0UM90ZZ 0UM94ZZ 0UMC0ZZ 0UMC4ZZ 0UMF0ZZ 0UMF4ZZ 0UMG0ZZ 0UMG4ZZ 0UMJXZZ 0UMK0ZZ 0UMK4ZZ 0UMKXZZ 0UMMXZZ

LC Limited Coverage NC Noncovered HAC HAC-associated Procedure CC Combination Cluster - See Appendix G for code lists
DRG Non-OR-Affecting MS-DRG Assignment New/Revised Text in **Orange** ♂ Male ♀ Female

0 Medical and Surgical
U Female Reproductive System
N Release: Freeing a body part from an abnormal physical constraint by cutting or by the use of force

Body Part Character 4	Approach Character 5	Device Character 6	Qualifier Character 7
0 Ovary, Right ♀ **1** Ovary, Left ♀ **2** Ovaries, Bilateral ♀ **4** Uterine Supporting Structure ♀	**0** Open **3** Percutaneous **4** Percutaneous Endoscopic **8** Via Natural or Artificial Opening Endoscopic	**Z** No Device	**Z** No Qualifier
5 Fallopian Tube, Right ♀ **6** Fallopian Tube, Left ♀ **7** Fallopian Tubes, Bilateral ♀ **9** Uterus ♀ **C** Cervix ♀ **F** Cul-de-sac ♀	**0** Open **3** Percutaneous **4** Percutaneous Endoscopic **7** Via Natural or Artificial Opening **8** Via Natural or Artificial Opening Endoscopic	**Z** No Device	**Z** No Qualifier
G Vagina ♀ **K** Hymen ♀	**0** Open **3** Percutaneous **4** Percutaneous Endoscopic **7** Via Natural or Artificial Opening **8** Via Natural or Artificial Opening Endoscopic **X** External	**Z** No Device	**Z** No Qualifier
J Clitoris ♀ **L** Vestibular Gland ♀ **M** Vulva ♀	**0** Open **X** External	**Z** No Device	**Z** No Qualifier

♀ 0UN00ZZ 0UN03ZZ 0UN04ZZ 0UN08ZZ 0UN10ZZ 0UN13ZZ 0UN14ZZ 0UN18ZZ 0UN20ZZ 0UN23ZZ 0UN24ZZ 0UN28ZZ 0UN40ZZ 0UN43ZZ 0UN44ZZ 0UN48ZZ 0UN50ZZ 0UN53ZZ 0UN54ZZ 0UN57ZZ 0UN58ZZ 0UN60ZZ 0UN63ZZ 0UN64ZZ 0UN67ZZ 0UN68ZZ 0UN70ZZ 0UN73ZZ 0UN74ZZ 0UN77ZZ 0UN78ZZ 0UN90ZZ 0UN93ZZ 0UN94ZZ 0UN97ZZ 0UN98ZZ 0UNC0ZZ 0UNC3ZZ 0UNC4ZZ 0UNC7ZZ 0UNC8ZZ 0UNF0ZZ 0UNF3ZZ 0UNF4ZZ 0UNF7ZZ 0UNF8ZZ 0UNG0ZZ 0UNG3ZZ 0UNG4ZZ 0UNG7ZZ 0UNG8ZZ 0UNGXZZ 0UNJ0ZZ 0UNJXZZ 0UNK0ZZ 0UNK3ZZ 0UNK4ZZ 0UNK7ZZ 0UNK8ZZ 0UNKXZZ 0UNL0ZZ 0UNLXZZ 0UNM0ZZ 0UNMXZZ

0 Medical and Surgical
U Female Reproductive System
P Removal: Taking out or off a device from a body part

Body Part Character 4	Approach Character 5	Device Character 6	Qualifier Character 7
3 Ovary ♀	**0** Open **3** Percutaneous **4** Percutaneous Endoscopic	**0** Drainage Device **3** Infusion Device **Y** Other Device	**Z** No Qualifier
3 Ovary ♀	**7** Via Natural or Artificial Opening **8** Via Natural or Artificial Opening Endoscopic	**Y** Other Device	**Z** No Qualifier
3 Ovary ♀	**X** External	**0** Drainage Device **3** Infusion Device	**Z** No Qualifier
8 Fallopian Tube ♀	**0** Open **3** Percutaneous **4** Percutaneous Endoscopic **7** Via Natural or Artificial Opening **8** Via Natural or Artificial Opening Endoscopic	**0** Drainage Device **3** Infusion Device **7** Autologous Tissue Substitute **C** Extraluminal Device **D** Intraluminal Device **J** Synthetic Substitute **K** Nonautologous Tissue Substitute **Y** Other Device	**Z** No Qualifier
8 Fallopian Tube ♀	**X** External	**0** Drainage Device **3** Infusion Device **D** Intraluminal Device	**Z** No Qualifier

0UP continued on next page

0 Medical and Surgical
U Female Reproductive System
P Removal: Taking out or off a device from a body part

0UP continued from previous page

Body Part Character 4	Approach Character 5	Device Character 6	Qualifier Character 7
D Uterus and Cervix ♀	**0** Open **3** Percutaneous **4** Percutaneous Endoscopic **7** Via Natural or Artificial Opening **8** Via Natural or Artificial Opening Endoscopic	**0** Drainage Device **1** Radioactive Element **3** Infusion Device **7** Autologous Tissue Substitute **C** Extraluminal Device **D** Intraluminal Device **H** Contraceptive Device **J** Synthetic Substitute **K** Nonautologous Tissue Substitute **Y** Other Device	**Z** No Qualifier
D Uterus and Cervix ♀	**X** External	**0** Drainage Device **3** Infusion Device **D** Intraluminal Device **H** Contraceptive Device	**Z** No Qualifier
H Vagina and Cul-de-sac ♀	**0** Open **3** Percutaneous **4** Percutaneous Endoscopic **7** Via Natural or Artificial Opening **8** Via Natural or Artificial Opening Endoscopic	**0** Drainage Device **1** Radioactive Element **3** Infusion Device **7** Autologous Tissue Substitute **D** Intraluminal Device **J** Synthetic Substitute **K** Nonautologous Tissue Substitute **Y** Other Device	**Z** No Qualifier
H Vagina and Cul-de-sac ♀	**X** External	**0** Drainage Device **1** Radioactive Element **3** Infusion Device **D** Intraluminal Device	**Z** No Qualifier
M Vulva ♀	**0** Open	**0** Drainage Device **7** Autologous Tissue Substitute **J** Synthetic Substitute **K** Nonautologous Tissue Substitute	**Z** No Qualifier
M Vulva ♀	**X** External	**0** Drainage Device	**Z** No Qualifier

♀ 0UP300Z 0UP303Z 0UP30YZ 0UP330Z 0UP333Z 0UP33YZ 0UP340Z 0UP343Z 0UP34YZ 0UP37YZ 0UP38YZ 0UP3X0Z 0UP3X3Z 0UP800Z 0UP803Z 0UP807Z 0UP80CZ 0UP80DZ 0UP80JZ 0UP80KZ 0UP80YZ 0UP830Z 0UP833Z 0UP837Z 0UP83CZ 0UP83DZ 0UP83JZ 0UP83KZ 0UP83YZ 0UP840Z 0UP843Z 0UP847Z 0UP84CZ 0UP84DZ 0UP84JZ 0UP84KZ 0UP84YZ 0UP870Z 0UP873Z 0UP877Z 0UP87CZ 0UP87DZ 0UP87JZ 0UP87KZ 0UP87YZ 0UP880Z 0UP883Z 0UP887Z 0UP88CZ 0UP88DZ 0UP88JZ 0UP88KZ 0UP88YZ 0UP8X0Z 0UP8X3Z 0UP8XDZ 0UPD00Z 0UPD01Z 0UPD03Z 0UPD07Z 0UPD0CZ 0UPD0DZ 0UPD0HZ 0UPD0JZ 0UPD0KZ 0UPD0YZ 0UPD30Z 0UPD31Z 0UPD33Z 0UPD37Z 0UPD3CZ 0UPD3DZ 0UPD3HZ 0UPD3JZ 0UPD3KZ 0UPD3YZ 0UPD40Z 0UPD41Z 0UPD43Z 0UPD47Z 0UPD4CZ 0UPD4DZ 0UPD4HZ 0UPD4JZ 0UPD4KZ 0UPD4YZ 0UPD70Z 0UPD71Z 0UPD73Z 0UPD77Z 0UPD7CZ 0UPD7DZ 0UPD7HZ 0UPD7JZ 0UPD7KZ 0UPD7YZ 0UPD80Z 0UPD81Z 0UPD83Z 0UPD87Z 0UPD8CZ 0UPD8DZ 0UPD8HZ 0UPD8JZ 0UPD8KZ 0UPD8YZ 0UPDX0Z 0UPDX3Z 0UPDXDZ 0UPDXHZ 0UPH00Z 0UPH01Z 0UPH03Z 0UPH07Z 0UPH0DZ 0UPH0JZ 0UPH0KZ 0UPH0YZ 0UPH30Z 0UPH31Z 0UPH33Z 0UPH37Z 0UPH3DZ 0UPH3JZ 0UPH3KZ 0UPH3YZ 0UPH40Z 0UPH41Z 0UPH43Z 0UPH47Z 0UPH4DZ 0UPH4JZ 0UPH4KZ 0UPH4YZ 0UPH70Z 0UPH71Z 0UPH73Z 0UPH77Z 0UPH7DZ 0UPH7JZ 0UPH7KZ 0UPH7YZ 0UPH80Z 0UPH81Z 0UPH83Z 0UPH87Z 0UPH8DZ 0UPH8JZ 0UPH8KZ 0UPH8YZ 0UPHX0Z 0UPHX1Z 0UPHX3Z 0UPHXDZ 0UPM00Z 0UPM07Z 0UPM0JZ 0UPM0KZ 0UPMX0Z

0 Medical and Surgical
U Female Reproductive System
Q Repair: Restoring, to the extent possible, a body part to its normal anatomic structure and function

Body Part Character 4	Approach Character 5	Device Character 6	Qualifier Character 7
0 Ovary, Right ♀ CC **1** Ovary, Left ♀ CC **2** Ovaries, Bilateral ♀ CC **4** Uterine Supporting Structure ♀	**0** Open **3** Percutaneous **4** Percutaneous Endoscopic **8** Via Natural or Artificial Opening Endoscopic	**Z** No Device	**Z** No Qualifier
5 Fallopian Tube, Right ♀ CC **6** Fallopian Tube, Left ♀ CC **7** Fallopian Tubes, Bilateral ♀ CC **9** Uterus ♀ **C** Cervix ♀ **F** Cul-de-sac ♀	**0** Open **3** Percutaneous **4** Percutaneous Endoscopic **7** Via Natural or Artificial Opening **8** Via Natural or Artificial Opening Endoscopic	**Z** No Device	**Z** No Qualifier
G Vagina ♀ **K** Hymen ♀	**0** Open **3** Percutaneous **4** Percutaneous Endoscopic **7** Via Natural or Artificial Opening **8** Via Natural or Artificial Opening Endoscopic **X** External	**Z** No Device	**Z** No Qualifier
J Clitoris ♀ **L** Vestibular Gland ♀ **M** Vulva ♀ CC	**0** Open **X** External	**Z** No Device	**Z** No Qualifier

♀ 0UQ00ZZ 0UQ03ZZ 0UQ04ZZ 0UQ08ZZ 0UQ10ZZ 0UQ13ZZ 0UQ14ZZ 0UQ18ZZ 0UQ20ZZ 0UQ23ZZ 0UQ24ZZ 0UQ28ZZ 0UQ40ZZ 0UQ43ZZ 0UQ44ZZ 0UQ48ZZ 0UQ50ZZ 0UQ53ZZ 0UQ54ZZ 0UQ57ZZ 0UQ58ZZ 0UQ60ZZ 0UQ63ZZ 0UQ64ZZ 0UQ67ZZ 0UQ68ZZ 0UQ70ZZ 0UQ73ZZ 0UQ74ZZ 0UQ77ZZ 0UQ78ZZ 0UQ90ZZ 0UQ93ZZ 0UQ94ZZ 0UQ97ZZ 0UQ98ZZ 0UQC0ZZ 0UQC3ZZ 0UQC4ZZ 0UQC7ZZ 0UQC8ZZ 0UQF0ZZ 0UQF3ZZ 0UQF4ZZ 0UQF7ZZ 0UQF8ZZ 0UQG0ZZ 0UQG3ZZ 0UQG4ZZ 0UQG7ZZ 0UQG8ZZ 0UQGXZZ 0UQJ0ZZ 0UQJXZZ 0UQK0ZZ 0UQK3ZZ 0UQK4ZZ 0UQK7ZZ 0UQK8ZZ 0UQKXZZ 0UQL0ZZ 0UQLXZZ 0UQM0ZZ 0UQMXZZ

CC 0UQ00ZZ 0UQ03ZZ 0UQ04ZZ 0UQ10ZZ 0UQ13ZZ 0UQ14ZZ 0UQ20ZZ 0UQ23ZZ 0UQ24ZZ 0UQ50ZZ 0UQ53ZZ 0UQ54ZZ 0UQ60ZZ 0UQ63ZZ 0UQ64ZZ 0UQ70ZZ 0UQ73ZZ 0UQ74ZZ 0UQM0ZZ 0UQMXZZ

0 Medical and Surgical
U Female Reproductive System
S Reposition: Moving to its normal location, or other suitable location, all or a portion of a body part

Body Part Character 4	Approach Character 5	Device Character 6	Qualifier Character 7
0 Ovary, Right ♀ **1** Ovary, Left ♀ **2** Ovaries, Bilateral ♀ **4** Uterine Supporting Structure ♀ **5** Fallopian Tube, Right ♀ **6** Fallopian Tube, Left ♀ **7** Fallopian Tubes, Bilateral ♀ **C** Cervix ♀ **F** Cul-de-sac ♀	**0** Open **4** Percutaneous Endoscopic **8** Via Natural or Artificial Opening Endoscopic	**Z** No Device	**Z** No Qualifier
9 Uterus ♀ **G** Vagina ♀	**0** Open **4** Percutaneous Endoscopic **7** Via Natural or Artificial Opening **8** Via Natural or Artificial Opening Endoscopic **X** External	**Z** No Device	**Z** No Qualifier

♀ 0US00ZZ 0US04ZZ 0US08ZZ 0US10ZZ 0US14ZZ 0US18ZZ 0US20ZZ 0US24ZZ 0US28ZZ 0US40ZZ 0US44ZZ 0US48ZZ 0US50ZZ 0US54ZZ 0US58ZZ 0US60ZZ 0US64ZZ 0US68ZZ 0US70ZZ 0US74ZZ 0US78ZZ 0US90ZZ 0US94ZZ 0US97ZZ 0US98ZZ 0US9XZZ 0USC0ZZ 0USC4ZZ 0USC8ZZ 0USF0ZZ 0USF4ZZ 0USF8ZZ 0USG0ZZ 0USG4ZZ 0USG7ZZ 0USG8ZZ 0USGXZZ

0 Medical and Surgical
U Female Reproductive System
T Resection: Cutting out or off, without replacement, all of a body part

Body Part	Approach	Device	Qualifier
Character 4	Character 5	Character 6	Character 7
0 Ovary, Right CC ♀ **1** Ovary, Left CC ♀ **2** Ovaries, Bilateral CC ♀ **5** Fallopian Tube, Right CC ♀ **6** Fallopian Tube, Left CC ♀ **7** Fallopian Tubes, Bilateral CC ♀	**0** Open **4** Percutaneous Endoscopic **7** Via Natural or Artificial Opening **8** Via Natural or Artificial Opening Endoscopic **F** Via Natural or Artificial Opening With Percutaneous Endoscopic Assistance	**Z** No Device	**Z** No Qualifier
4 Uterine Supporting Structure CC ♀ **C** Cervix CC ♀ **F** Cul-de-sac ♀ **G** Vagina CC ♀	**0** Open **4** Percutaneous Endoscopic **7** Via Natural or Artificial Opening **8** Via Natural or Artificial Opening Endoscopic	**Z** No Device	**Z** No Qualifier
9 Uterus CC ♀	**0** Open **4** Percutaneous Endoscopic **7** Via Natural or Artificial Opening **8** Via Natural or Artificial Opening Endoscopic **F** Via Natural or Artificial Opening With Percutaneous Endoscopic Assistance	**Z** No Device	**L** Supracervical **Z** No Qualifier
J Clitoris ♀ **L** Vestibular Gland ♀ **M** Vulva CC ♀	**0** Open **X** External	**Z** No Device	**Z** No Qualifier
K Hymen ♀	**0** Open **4** Percutaneous Endoscopic **7** Via Natural or Artificial Opening **8** Via Natural or Artificial Opening Endoscopic **X** External	**Z** No Device	**Z** No Qualifier

♀ 0UT00ZZ 0UT04ZZ 0UT07ZZ 0UT08ZZ 0UT0FZZ 0UT10ZZ 0UT14ZZ 0UT17ZZ 0UT18ZZ 0UT1FZZ 0UT20ZZ 0UT24ZZ 0UT27ZZ 0UT28ZZ 0UT2FZZ 0UT40ZZ 0UT44ZZ 0UT47ZZ 0UT48ZZ 0UT50ZZ 0UT54ZZ 0UT57ZZ 0UT58ZZ 0UT5FZZ 0UT60ZZ 0UT64ZZ 0UT67ZZ 0UT68ZZ 0UT6FZZ 0UT70ZZ 0UT74ZZ 0UT77ZZ 0UT78ZZ 0UT7FZZ 0UT90ZL 0UT90ZZ 0UT94ZL 0UT94ZZ 0UT97ZL 0UT97ZZ 0UT98ZL 0UT98ZZ 0UT9FZL 0UT9FZZ 0UTC0ZZ 0UTC4ZZ 0UTC7ZZ 0UTC8ZZ 0UTF0ZZ 0UTF4ZZ 0UTF7ZZ 0UTF8ZZ 0UTG0ZZ 0UTG4ZZ 0UTG7ZZ 0UTG8ZZ 0UTJ0ZZ 0UTJXZZ 0UTK0ZZ 0UTK4ZZ 0UTK7ZZ 0UTK8ZZ 0UTKXZZ 0UTL0ZZ 0UTLXZZ 0UTM0ZZ 0UTMXZZ

CC 0UT00ZZ 0UT04ZZ 0UT10ZZ 0UT14ZZ 0UT20ZZ 0UT24ZZ 0UT40ZZ 0UT44ZZ 0UT47ZZ 0UT48ZZ 0UT50ZZ 0UT54ZZ 0UT60ZZ 0UT64ZZ 0UT70ZZ 0UT74ZZ 0UT90ZZ 0UT94ZZ 0UT97ZZ 0UT98ZZ 0UT9FZZ 0UTC0ZZ 0UTC4ZZ 0UTC7ZZ 0UTC8ZZ 0UTG0ZZ 0UTM0ZZ 0UTMXZZ

0 Medical and Surgical
U Female Reproductive System
U Supplement: Putting in or on biological or synthetic material that physically reinforces and/or augments the function of a portion of a body part

Body Part	Approach	Device	Qualifier
Character 4	Character 5	Character 6	Character 7
4 Uterine Supporting Structure ♀	**0** Open **4** Percutaneous Endoscopic	**7** Autologous Tissue Substitute **J** Synthetic Substitute **K** Nonautologous Tissue Substitute	**Z** No Qualifier
5 Fallopian Tube, Right ♀ **6** Fallopian Tube, Left ♀ **7** Fallopian Tubes, Bilateral ♀ **F** Cul-de-sac ♀	**0** Open **4** Percutaneous Endoscopic **7** Via Natural or Artificial Opening **8** Via Natural or Artificial Opening Endoscopic	**7** Autologous Tissue Substitute **J** Synthetic Substitute **K** Nonautologous Tissue Substitute	**Z** No Qualifier
G Vagina ♀ **K** Hymen ♀	**0** Open **4** Percutaneous Endoscopic **7** Via Natural or Artificial Opening **8** Via Natural or Artificial Opening Endoscopic **X** External	**7** Autologous Tissue Substitute **J** Synthetic Substitute **K** Nonautologous Tissue Substitute	**Z** No Qualifier

0UU continued on next page

LC Limited Coverage NC Noncovered HAC HAC-associated Procedure CC Combination Cluster - See Appendix G for code lists
DRG Non-OR-Affecting MS-DRG Assignment New/Revised Text in **Orange** ♂ Male ♀ Female

0UU continued from previous page

0 Medical and Surgical
U Female Reproductive System
U Supplement: Putting in or on biological or synthetic material that physically reinforces and/or augments the function of a portion of a body part

Body Part Character 4	Approach Character 5	Device Character 6	Qualifier Character 7
J Clitoris ♀ **M** Vulva ♀	**0** Open **X** External	**7** Autologous Tissue Substitute **J** Synthetic Substitute **K** Nonautologous Tissue Substitute	**Z** No Qualifier

♀ 0UU407Z 0UU40JZ 0UU40KZ 0UU447Z 0UU44JZ 0UU44KZ 0UU507Z 0UU50JZ 0UU50KZ 0UU547Z 0UU54JZ 0UU54KZ 0UU577Z 0UU57JZ 0UU57KZ 0UU587Z 0UU58JZ 0UU58KZ 0UU607Z 0UU60JZ 0UU60KZ 0UU647Z 0UU64JZ 0UU64KZ 0UU677Z 0UU67JZ 0UU67KZ 0UU687Z 0UU68JZ 0UU68KZ 0UU707Z 0UU70JZ 0UU70KZ 0UU747Z 0UU74JZ 0UU74KZ 0UU777Z 0UU77JZ 0UU77KZ 0UU787Z 0UU78JZ 0UU78KZ 0UUF07Z 0UUF0JZ 0UUF0KZ 0UUF47Z 0UUF4JZ 0UUF4KZ 0UUF77Z 0UUF7JZ 0UUF7KZ 0UUF87Z 0UUF8JZ 0UUF8KZ 0UUG07Z 0UUG0JZ 0UUG0KZ 0UUG47Z 0UUG4JZ 0UUG4KZ 0UUG77Z 0UUG7JZ 0UUG7KZ 0UUG87Z 0UUG8JZ 0UUG8KZ 0UUGX7Z 0UUGXJZ 0UUGXKZ 0UUJ07Z 0UUJ0JZ 0UUJ0KZ 0UUJX7Z 0UUJXJZ 0UUJXKZ 0UUK07Z 0UUK0JZ 0UUK0KZ 0UUK47Z 0UUK4JZ 0UUK4KZ 0UUK77Z 0UUK7JZ 0UUK7KZ 0UUK87Z 0UUK8JZ 0UUK8KZ 0UUKX7Z 0UUKXJZ 0UUKXKZ 0UUM07Z 0UUM0JZ 0UUM0KZ 0UUMX7Z 0UUMXJZ 0UUMXKZ

0 Medical and Surgical
U Female Reproductive System
V Restriction: Partially closing an orifice or the lumen of a tubular body part

Body Part Character 4	Approach Character 5	Device Character 6	Qualifier Character 7
C Cervix ♀	**0** Open **3** Percutaneous **4** Percutaneous Endoscopic	**C** Extraluminal Device **D** Intraluminal Device **Z** No Device	**Z** No Qualifier
C Cervix ♀	**7** Via Natural or Artificial Opening **8** Via Natural or Artificial Opening Endoscopic	**D** Intraluminal Device **Z** No Device	**Z** No Qualifier

♀ 0UVC0CZ 0UVC0DZ 0UVC0ZZ 0UVC3CZ 0UVC3DZ 0UVC3ZZ 0UVC4CZ 0UVC4DZ 0UVC4ZZ 0UVC7DZ 0UVC7ZZ 0UVC8DZ 0UVC8ZZ

0 Medical and Surgical
U Female Reproductive System
W Revision: Correcting, to the extent possible, a portion of a malfunctioning device or the position of a displaced device

Body Part Character 4	Approach Character 5	Device Character 6	Qualifier Character 7
3 Ovary ♀	**0** Open **3** Percutaneous **4** Percutaneous Endoscopic	**0** Drainage Device **3** Infusion Device **Y** Other Device	**Z** No Qualifier
3 Ovary ♀	**7** Via Natural or Artificial Opening **8** Via Natural or Artificial Opening Endoscopic	**Y** Other Device	**Z** No Qualifier
3 Ovary ♀	**X** External	**0** Drainage Device **3** Infusion Device	**Z** No Qualifier
8 Fallopian Tube ♀	**0** Open **3** Percutaneous **4** Percutaneous Endoscopic **7** Via Natural or Artificial Opening **8** Via Natural or Artificial Opening Endoscopic	**0** Drainage Device **3** Infusion Device **7** Autologous Tissue Substitute **C** Extraluminal Device **D** Intraluminal Device **J** Synthetic Substitute **K** Nonautologous Tissue Substitute **Y** Other Device	**Z** No Qualifier
8 Fallopian Tube ♀	**X** External	**0** Drainage Device **3** Infusion Device **7** Autologous Tissue Substitute **C** Extraluminal Device **D** Intraluminal Device **J** Synthetic Substitute **K** Nonautologous Tissue Substitute	**Z** No Qualifier

0UW continued on next page

0 Medical and Surgical
U Female Reproductive System
W Revision: Correcting, to the extent possible, a portion of a malfunctioning device or the position of a displaced device

0UW continued from previous page

Body Part Character 4	Approach Character 5	Device Character 6	Qualifier Character 7
D Uterus and Cervix ♀	**0** Open **3** Percutaneous **4** Percutaneous Endoscopic **7** Via Natural or Artificial Opening **8** Via Natural or Artificial Opening Endoscopic	**0** Drainage Device **1** Radioactive Element **3** Infusion Device **7** Autologous Tissue Substitute **C** Extraluminal Device **D** Intraluminal Device **H** Contraceptive Device **J** Synthetic Substitute **K** Nonautologous Tissue Substitute **Y** Other Device	**Z** No Qualifier
D Uterus and Cervix ♀	**X** External	**0** Drainage Device **3** Infusion Device **7** Autologous Tissue Substitute **C** Extraluminal Device **D** Intraluminal Device **H** Contraceptive Device **J** Synthetic Substitute **K** Nonautologous Tissue Substitute	**Z** No Qualifier
H Vagina and Cul-de-sac ♀	**0** Open **3** Percutaneous **4** Percutaneous Endoscopic **7** Via Natural or Artificial Opening **8** Via Natural or Artificial Opening Endoscopic	**0** Drainage Device **1** Radioactive Element **3** Infusion Device **7** Autologous Tissue Substitute **D** Intraluminal Device **J** Synthetic Substitute **K** Nonautologous Tissue Substitute **Y** Other Device	**Z** No Qualifier
H Vagina and Cul-de-sac ♀	**X** External	**0** Drainage Device **3** Infusion Device **7** Autologous Tissue Substitute **D** Intraluminal Device **J** Synthetic Substitute **K** Nonautologous Tissue Substitute	**Z** No Qualifier
M Vulva ♀	**0** Open **X** External	**0** Drainage Device **7** Autologous Tissue Substitute **J** Synthetic Substitute **K** Nonautologous Tissue Substitute	**Z** No Qualifier

♀ 0UW300Z 0UW303Z 0UW30YZ 0UW330Z 0UW333Z 0UW33YZ 0UW340Z 0UW343Z 0UW34YZ 0UW37YZ 0UW38YZ 0UW3X0Z 0UW3X3Z 0UW800Z 0UW803Z 0UW807Z 0UW80CZ 0UW80DZ 0UW80JZ 0UW80KZ 0UW80YZ 0UW830Z 0UW833Z 0UW837Z 0UW83CZ 0UW83DZ 0UW83JZ 0UW83KZ 0UW83YZ 0UW840Z 0UW843Z 0UW847Z 0UW84CZ 0UW84DZ 0UW84JZ 0UW84KZ 0UW84YZ 0UW870Z 0UW873Z 0UW877Z 0UW87CZ 0UW87DZ 0UW87JZ 0UW87KZ 0UW87YZ 0UW880Z 0UW883Z 0UW887Z 0UW88CZ 0UW88DZ 0UW88JZ 0UW88KZ 0UW88YZ 0UW8X0Z 0UW8X3Z 0UW8X7Z 0UW8XCZ 0UW8XDZ 0UW8XJZ 0UW8XKZ 0UWD00Z 0UWD01Z 0UWD03Z 0UWD07Z 0UWD0CZ 0UWD0DZ 0UWD0HZ 0UWD0JZ 0UWD0KZ 0UWD0YZ 0UWD30Z 0UWD31Z 0UWD33Z 0UWD37Z 0UWD3CZ 0UWD3DZ 0UWD3HZ 0UWD3JZ 0UWD3KZ 0UWD3YZ 0UWD40Z 0UWD41Z 0UWD43Z 0UWD47Z 0UWD4CZ 0UWD4DZ 0UWD4HZ 0UWD4JZ 0UWD4KZ 0UWD4YZ 0UWD70Z 0UWD71Z 0UWD73Z 0UWD77Z 0UWD7CZ 0UWD7DZ 0UWD7HZ 0UWD7JZ 0UWD7KZ 0UWD7YZ 0UWD80Z 0UWD81Z 0UWD83Z 0UWD87Z 0UWD8CZ 0UWD8DZ 0UWD8HZ 0UWD8JZ 0UWD8KZ 0UWD8YZ 0UWDX0Z 0UWDX3Z 0UWDX7Z 0UWDXCZ 0UWDXDZ 0UWDXHZ 0UWDXJZ 0UWDXKZ 0UWH00Z 0UWH01Z 0UWH03Z 0UWH07Z 0UWH0DZ 0UWH0JZ 0UWH0KZ 0UWH0YZ 0UWH30Z 0UWH31Z 0UWH33Z 0UWH37Z 0UWH3DZ 0UWH3JZ 0UWH3KZ 0UWH3YZ 0UWH40Z 0UWH41Z 0UWH43Z 0UWH47Z 0UWH4DZ 0UWH4JZ 0UWH4KZ 0UWH4YZ 0UWH70Z 0UWH71Z 0UWH73Z 0UWH77Z 0UWH7DZ 0UWH7JZ 0UWH7KZ 0UWH7YZ 0UWH80Z 0UWH81Z 0UWH83Z 0UWH87Z 0UWH8DZ 0UWH8JZ 0UWH8KZ 0UWH8YZ 0UWHX0Z 0UWHX3Z 0UWHX7Z 0UWHXDZ 0UWHXJZ 0UWHXKZ 0UWM00Z 0UWM07Z 0UWM0JZ 0UWM0KZ 0UWMX0Z 0UWMX7Z 0UWMXJZ 0UWMXKZ

LC Limited Coverage NC Noncovered HAC HAC-associated Procedure CC Combination Cluster - See Appendix G for code lists
DRG Non-OR-Affecting MS-DRG Assignment New/Revised Text in Orange ♂ Male ♀ Female

0 Medical and Surgical
U Female Reproductive System
Y Transplantation: Putting in or on all or a portion of a living body part taken from another individual or animal to physically take the place and/or function of all or a portion of a similar body part

Body Part Character 4	Approach Character 5	Device Character 6	Qualifier Character 7
0 Ovary, Right ♀ **1** Ovary, Left ♀ **9** Uterus ♀	**0** Open	**Z** No Device	**0** Allogeneic **1** Syngeneic **2** Zooplastic

♀ 0UY00Z0 0UY00Z1 0UY00Z2 0UY10Z0 0UY10Z1 0UY10Z2 0UY90Z0 0UY90Z1 0UY90Z2

NOTES

NOTES

Male Reproductive System 0V1-0VX

0 Medical and Surgical
V Male Reproductive System
1 Bypass: Altering the route of passage of the contents of a tubular body part

Body Part Character 4	Approach Character 5	Device Character 6	Qualifier Character 7
N Vas Deferens, Right ♂ **P** Vas Deferens, Left ♂ **Q** Vas Deferens, Bilateral ♂	**0** Open **4** Percutaneous Endoscopic	**7** Autologous Tissue Substitute **J** Synthetic Substitute **K** Nonautologous Tissue Substitute **Z** No Device	**J** Epididymis, Right **K** Epididymis, Left **N** Vas Deferens, Right **P** Vas Deferens, Left

♂ 0V1N07J 0V1N07K 0V1N07N 0V1N07P 0V1N0JJ 0V1N0JK 0V1N0JN 0V1N0JP 0V1N0KJ 0V1N0KK 0V1N0KN 0V1N0KP 0V1N0ZJ 0V1N0ZK 0V1N0ZN 0V1N0ZP 0V1N47J 0V1N47K 0V1N47N 0V1N47P 0V1N4JJ 0V1N4JK 0V1N4JN 0V1N4JP 0V1N4KJ 0V1N4KK 0V1N4KN 0V1N4KP 0V1N4ZJ 0V1N4ZK 0V1N4ZN 0V1N4ZP 0V1P07J 0V1P07K 0V1P07N 0V1P07P 0V1P0JJ 0V1P0JK 0V1P0JN 0V1P0JP 0V1P0KJ 0V1P0KK 0V1P0KN 0V1P0KP 0V1P0ZJ 0V1P0ZK 0V1P0ZN 0V1P0ZP 0V1P47J 0V1P47K 0V1P47N 0V1P47P 0V1P4JJ 0V1P4JK 0V1P4JN 0V1P4JP 0V1P4KJ 0V1P4KK 0V1P4KN 0V1P4KP 0V1P4ZJ 0V1P4ZK 0V1P4ZN 0V1P4ZP 0V1Q07J 0V1Q07K 0V1Q07N 0V1Q07P 0V1Q0JJ 0V1Q0JK 0V1Q0JN 0V1Q0JP 0V1Q0KJ 0V1Q0KK 0V1Q0KN 0V1Q0KP 0V1Q0ZJ 0V1Q0ZK 0V1Q0ZN 0V1Q0ZP 0V1Q47J 0V1Q47K 0V1Q47N 0V1Q47P 0V1Q4JJ 0V1Q4JK 0V1Q4JN 0V1Q4JP 0V1Q4KJ 0V1Q4KK 0V1Q4KN 0V1Q4KP 0V1Q4ZJ 0V1Q4ZK 0V1Q4ZN 0V1Q4ZP

0 Medical and Surgical
V Male Reproductive System
2 Change: Taking out or off a device from a body part and putting back an identical or similar device in or on the same body part without cutting or puncturing the skin or a mucous membrane

Body Part Character 4	Approach Character 5	Device Character 6	Qualifier Character 7
4 Prostate and Seminal Vesicles ♂ **8** Scrotum and Tunica Vaginalis ♂ **D** Testis ♂ **M** Epididymis and Spermatic Cord ♂ **R** Vas Deferens ♂ **S** Penis ♂	**X** External	**0** Drainage Device **Y** Other Device	**Z** No Qualifier

♂ 0V24X0Z 0V24XYZ 0V28X0Z 0V28XYZ 0V2DX0Z 0V2DXYZ 0V2MX0Z 0V2MXYZ 0V2RX0Z 0V2RXYZ 0V2SX0Z 0V2SXYZ

LC Limited Coverage NC Noncovered HAC HAC-associated Procedure CC Combination Cluster - See Appendix G for code lists
DRG Non-OR-Affecting MS-DRG Assignment New/Revised Text in **Orange** ♂ Male ♀ Female

0 Medical and Surgical
V Male Reproductive System
5 Destruction: Physical eradication of all or a portion of a body part by the direct use of energy, force, or a destructive agent

Body Part	Approach	Device	Qualifier
Character 4	Character 5	Character 6	Character 7
0 Prostate ♂	0 Open 3 Percutaneous 4 Percutaneous Endoscopic 7 Via Natural or Artificial Opening 8 Via Natural or Artificial Opening Endoscopic	Z No Device	Z No Qualifier
1 Seminal Vesicle, Right ♂ 2 Seminal Vesicle, Left ♂ 3 Seminal Vesicles, Bilateral ♂ 6 Tunica Vaginalis, Right ♂ 7 Tunica Vaginalis, Left ♂ 9 Testis, Right ♂ B Testis, Left ♂ C Testes, Bilateral ♂	0 Open 3 Percutaneous 4 Percutaneous Endoscopic	Z No Device	Z No Qualifier
5 Scrotum ♂ S Penis ♂ T Prepuce ♂	0 Open 3 Percutaneous 4 Percutaneous Endoscopic X External	Z No Device	Z No Qualifier
F Spermatic Cord, Right ♂ G Spermatic Cord, Left ♂ H Spermatic Cords, Bilateral ♂ J Epididymis, Right ♂ K Epididymis, Left ♂ L Epididymis, Bilateral ♂ N Vas Deferens, Right ♂ NC P Vas Deferens, Left ♂ NC Q Vas Deferens, Bilateral ♂ NC	0 Open 3 Percutaneous 4 Percutaneous Endoscopic 8 Via Natural or Artificial Opening Endoscopic	Z No Device	Z No Qualifier

♂ 0V500ZZ 0V503ZZ 0V504ZZ 0V507ZZ 0V508ZZ 0V510ZZ 0V513ZZ 0V514ZZ 0V520ZZ 0V523ZZ 0V524ZZ 0V530ZZ 0V533ZZ 0V534ZZ 0V550ZZ 0V553ZZ 0V554ZZ 0V55XZZ 0V560ZZ 0V563ZZ 0V564ZZ 0V570ZZ 0V573ZZ 0V574ZZ 0V590ZZ 0V593ZZ 0V594ZZ 0V5B0ZZ 0V5B3ZZ 0V5B4ZZ 0V5C0ZZ 0V5C3ZZ 0V5C4ZZ 0V5F0ZZ 0V5F3ZZ 0V5F4ZZ 0V5F8ZZ 0V5G0ZZ 0V5G3ZZ 0V5G4ZZ 0V5G8ZZ 0V5H0ZZ 0V5H3ZZ 0V5H4ZZ 0V5H8ZZ 0V5J0ZZ 0V5J3ZZ 0V5J4ZZ 0V5J8ZZ 0V5K0ZZ 0V5K3ZZ 0V5K4ZZ 0V5K8ZZ 0V5L0ZZ 0V5L3ZZ 0V5L4ZZ 0V5L8ZZ 0V5N0ZZ 0V5N3ZZ 0V5N4ZZ 0V5N8ZZ 0V5P0ZZ 0V5P3ZZ 0V5P4ZZ 0V5P8ZZ 0V5Q0ZZ 0V5Q3ZZ 0V5Q4ZZ 0V5Q8ZZ 0V5S0ZZ 0V5S3ZZ 0V5S4ZZ 0V5SXZZ 0V5T0ZZ 0V5T3ZZ 0V5T4ZZ 0V5TXZZ

NC 0V5N0ZZ 0V5N3ZZ 0V5N4ZZ 0V5P0ZZ 0V5P3ZZ 0V5P4ZZ 0V5Q0ZZ 0V5Q3ZZ 0V5Q4ZZ Codes in this list are noncovered procedures only when reported with Z30.2 as either a principal or secondary diagnosis.

0 Medical and Surgical
V Male Reproductive System
7 Dilation: Expanding an orifice or the lumen of a tubular body part

Body Part	Approach	Device	Qualifier
Character 4	Character 5	Character 6	Character 7
N Vas Deferens, Right ♂ P Vas Deferens, Left ♂ Q Vas Deferens, Bilateral ♂	0 Open 3 Percutaneous 4 Percutaneous Endoscopic	D Intraluminal Device Z No Device	Z No Qualifier

♂ 0V7N0DZ 0V7N0ZZ 0V7N3DZ 0V7N3ZZ 0V7N4DZ 0V7N4ZZ 0V7P0DZ 0V7P0ZZ 0V7P3DZ 0V7P3ZZ 0V7P4DZ 0V7P4ZZ 0V7Q0DZ 0V7Q0ZZ 0V7Q3DZ 0V7Q3ZZ 0V7Q4DZ 0V7Q4ZZ

LC Limited Coverage NC Noncovered HAC HAC-associated Procedure CC Combination Cluster - See Appendix G for code lists
DRG Non-OR-Affecting MS-DRG Assignment New/Revised Text in **Orange** ♂ Male ♀ Female

0 Medical and Surgical
V Male Reproductive System
9 Drainage: Taking or letting out fluids and/or gases from a body part

Body Part Character 4	Approach Character 5	Device Character 6	Qualifier Character 7
0 Prostate ♂	**0** Open **3** Percutaneous **4** Percutaneous Endoscopic **7** Via Natural or Artificial Opening **8** Via Natural or Artificial Opening Endoscopic	**0** Drainage Device	**Z** No Qualifier
0 Prostate ♂	**0** Open **3** Percutaneous **4** Percutaneous Endoscopic **7** Via Natural or Artificial Opening **8** Via Natural or Artificial Opening Endoscopic	**Z** No Device	**X** Diagnostic **Z** No Qualifier
1 Seminal Vesicle, Right ♂ **2** Seminal Vesicle, Left ♂ **3** Seminal Vesicles, Bilateral ♂ **6** Tunica Vaginalis, Right ♂ **7** Tunica Vaginalis, Left ♂ **9** Testis, Right ♂ **B** Testis, Left ♂ **C** Testes, Bilateral ♂ **F** Spermatic Cord, Right ♂ **G** Spermatic Cord, Left ♂ **H** Spermatic Cords, Bilateral ♂ **J** Epididymis, Right ♂ **K** Epididymis, Left ♂ **L** Epididymis, Bilateral ♂ **N** Vas Deferens, Right ♂ **P** Vas Deferens, Left ♂ **Q** Vas Deferens, Bilateral ♂	**0** Open **3** Percutaneous **4** Percutaneous Endoscopic	**0** Drainage Device	**Z** No Qualifier
1 Seminal Vesicle, Right ♂ **2** Seminal Vesicle, Left ♂ **3** Seminal Vesicles, Bilateral ♂ **6** Tunica Vaginalis, Right ♂ **7** Tunica Vaginalis, Left ♂ **9** Testis, Right ♂ **B** Testis, Left ♂ **C** Testes, Bilateral ♂ **F** Spermatic Cord, Right ♂ **G** Spermatic Cord, Left ♂ **H** Spermatic Cords, Bilateral ♂ **J** Epididymis, Right ♂ **K** Epididymis, Left ♂ **L** Epididymis, Bilateral ♂ **N** Vas Deferens, Right ♂ **P** Vas Deferens, Left ♂ **Q** Vas Deferens, Bilateral ♂	**0** Open **3** Percutaneous **4** Percutaneous Endoscopic	**Z** No Device	**X** Diagnostic **Z** No Qualifier
5 Scrotum ♂ **S** Penis ♂ **T** Prepuce ♂	**0** Open **3** Percutaneous **4** Percutaneous Endoscopic **X** External	**0** Drainage Device	**Z** No Qualifier
5 Scrotum ♂ **S** Penis ♂ **T** Prepuce ♂	**0** Open **3** Percutaneous **4** Percutaneous Endoscopic **X** External	**Z** No Device	**X** Diagnostic **Z** No Qualifier

♂ 0V9000Z 0V900ZX 0V900ZZ 0V9030Z 0V903ZX 0V903ZZ 0V9040Z 0V904ZX 0V904ZZ 0V9070Z 0V907ZX 0V907ZZ 0V9080Z 0V908ZX 0V908ZZ 0V9100Z 0V910ZX 0V910ZZ 0V9130Z 0V913ZX 0V913ZZ 0V9140Z 0V914ZX 0V914ZZ 0V9200Z 0V920ZX 0V920ZZ 0V9230Z 0V923ZX 0V923ZZ 0V9240Z 0V924ZX 0V924ZZ 0V9300Z 0V930ZX 0V930ZZ 0V9330Z 0V933ZX 0V933ZZ 0V9340Z 0V934ZX 0V934ZZ 0V9500Z 0V950ZX 0V950ZZ 0V9530Z 0V953ZX 0V953ZZ 0V9540Z 0V954ZX 0V954ZZ 0V95X0Z

0V9 continued on next page

0V9 continued from previous page

0V95XZX 0V95XZZ 0V9600Z 0V960ZX 0V960ZZ 0V9630Z 0V963ZX 0V963ZZ 0V9640Z 0V964ZX 0V964ZZ 0V9700Z 0V970ZX
0V970ZZ 0V9730Z 0V973ZX 0V973ZZ 0V9740Z 0V974ZX 0V974ZZ 0V9900Z 0V990ZX 0V990ZZ 0V9930Z 0V993ZX 0V993ZZ
0V9940Z 0V994ZX 0V994ZZ 0V9B00Z 0V9B0ZX 0V9B0ZZ 0V9B30Z 0V9B3ZX 0V9B3ZZ 0V9B40Z 0V9B4ZX 0V9B4ZZ 0V9C00Z
0V9C0ZX 0V9C0ZZ 0V9C30Z 0V9C3ZX 0V9C3ZZ 0V9C40Z 0V9C4ZX 0V9C4ZZ 0V9F00Z 0V9F0ZX 0V9F0ZZ 0V9F30Z 0V9F3ZX
0V9F3ZZ 0V9F40Z 0V9F4ZX 0V9F4ZZ 0V9G00Z 0V9G0ZX 0V9G0ZZ 0V9G30Z 0V9G3ZX 0V9G3ZZ 0V9G40Z 0V9G4ZX 0V9G4ZZ
0V9H00Z 0V9H0ZX 0V9H0ZZ 0V9H30Z 0V9H3ZX 0V9H3ZZ 0V9H40Z 0V9H4ZX 0V9H4ZZ 0V9J00Z 0V9J0ZX 0V9J0ZZ 0V9J30Z
0V9J3ZX 0V9J3ZZ 0V9J40Z 0V9J4ZX 0V9J4ZZ 0V9K00Z 0V9K0ZX 0V9K0ZZ 0V9K30Z 0V9K3ZX 0V9K3ZZ 0V9K40Z 0V9K4ZX
0V9K4ZZ 0V9L00Z 0V9L0ZX 0V9L0ZZ 0V9L30Z 0V9L3ZX 0V9L3ZZ 0V9L40Z 0V9L4ZX 0V9L4ZZ 0V9N00Z 0V9N0ZX 0V9N0ZZ
0V9N30Z 0V9N3ZX 0V9N3ZZ 0V9N40Z 0V9N4ZX 0V9N4ZZ 0V9P00Z 0V9P0ZX 0V9P0ZZ 0V9P30Z 0V9P3ZX 0V9P3ZZ 0V9P40Z
0V9P4ZX 0V9P4ZZ 0V9Q00Z 0V9Q0ZX 0V9Q0ZZ 0V9Q30Z 0V9Q3ZX 0V9Q3ZZ 0V9Q40Z 0V9Q4ZX 0V9Q4ZZ 0V9S00Z 0V9S0ZX
0V9S0ZZ 0V9S30Z 0V9S3ZX 0V9S3ZZ 0V9S40Z 0V9S4ZX 0V9S4ZZ 0V9SX0Z 0V9SXZX 0V9SXZZ 0V9T00Z 0V9T0ZX 0V9T0ZZ
0V9T30Z 0V9T3ZX 0V9T3ZZ 0V9T40Z 0V9T4ZX 0V9T4ZZ 0V9TX0Z 0V9TXZX 0V9TXZZ

0 Medical and Surgical
V Male Reproductive System
B Excision: Cutting out or off, without replacement, a portion of a body part

Body Part Character 4	Approach Character 5	Device Character 6	Qualifier Character 7
0 Prostate ♂	**0** Open **3** Percutaneous **4** Percutaneous Endoscopic **7** Via Natural or Artificial Opening **8** Via Natural or Artificial Opening Endoscopic	**Z** No Device	**X** Diagnostic **Z** No Qualifier
1 Seminal Vesicle, Right ♂ **2** Seminal Vesicle, Left ♂ **3** Seminal Vesicles, Bilateral ♂ **6** Tunica Vaginalis, Right ♂ **7** Tunica Vaginalis, Left ♂ **9** Testis, Right ♂ **B** Testis, Left ♂ **C** Testes, Bilateral ♂	**0** Open **3** Percutaneous **4** Percutaneous Endoscopic	**Z** No Device	**X** Diagnostic **Z** No Qualifier
5 Scrotum ♂ **S** Penis ♂ **T** Prepuce ♂	**0** Open **3** Percutaneous **4** Percutaneous Endoscopic **X** External	**Z** No Device	**X** Diagnostic **Z** No Qualifier
F Spermatic Cord, Right ♂ **G** Spermatic Cord, Left ♂ **H** Spermatic Cords, Bilateral ♂ **J** Epididymis, Right ♂ **K** Epididymis, Left ♂ **L** Epididymis, Bilateral ♂ **N** Vas Deferens, Right ♂ NC **P** Vas Deferens, Left ♂ NC **Q** Vas Deferens, Bilateral ♂ NC	**0** Open **3** Percutaneous **4** Percutaneous Endoscopic **8** Via Natural or Artificial Opening Endoscopic	**Z** No Device	**X** Diagnostic **Z** No Qualifier

♂ 0VB00ZX 0VB00ZZ 0VB03ZX 0VB03ZZ 0VB04ZX 0VB04ZZ 0VB07ZX 0VB07ZZ 0VB08ZX 0VB08ZZ 0VB10ZX 0VB10ZZ 0VB13ZX
0VB13ZZ 0VB14ZX 0VB14ZZ 0VB20ZX 0VB20ZZ 0VB23ZX 0VB23ZZ 0VB24ZX 0VB24ZZ 0VB30ZX 0VB30ZZ 0VB33ZX 0VB33ZZ
0VB34ZX 0VB34ZZ 0VB50ZX 0VB50ZZ 0VB53ZX 0VB53ZZ 0VB54ZX 0VB54ZZ 0VB5XZX 0VB5XZZ 0VB60ZX 0VB60ZZ 0VB63ZX
0VB63ZZ 0VB64ZX 0VB64ZZ 0VB70ZX 0VB70ZZ 0VB73ZX 0VB73ZZ 0VB74ZX 0VB74ZZ 0VB90ZX 0VB90ZZ 0VB93ZX 0VB93ZZ
0VB94ZX 0VB94ZZ 0VBB0ZX 0VBB0ZZ 0VBB3ZX 0VBB3ZZ 0VBB4ZX 0VBB4ZZ 0VBC0ZX 0VBC0ZZ 0VBC3ZX 0VBC3ZZ 0VBC4ZX
0VBC4ZZ 0VBF0ZX 0VBF0ZZ 0VBF3ZX 0VBF3ZZ 0VBF4ZX 0VBF4ZZ 0VBF8ZX 0VBF8ZZ 0VBG0ZX 0VBG0ZZ 0VBG3ZX 0VBG3ZZ
0VBG4ZX 0VBG4ZZ 0VBG8ZX 0VBG8ZZ 0VBH0ZX 0VBH0ZZ 0VBH3ZX 0VBH3ZZ 0VBH4ZX 0VBH4ZZ 0VBH8ZX 0VBH8ZZ 0VBJ0ZX
0VBJ0ZZ 0VBJ3ZX 0VBJ3ZZ 0VBJ4ZX 0VBJ4ZZ 0VBJ8ZX 0VBJ8ZZ 0VBK0ZX 0VBK0ZZ 0VBK3ZX 0VBK3ZZ 0VBK4ZX 0VBK4ZZ
0VBK8ZX 0VBK8ZZ 0VBL0ZX 0VBL0ZZ 0VBL3ZX 0VBL3ZZ 0VBL4ZX 0VBL4ZZ 0VBL8ZX 0VBL8ZZ 0VBN0ZX 0VBN0ZZ 0VBN3ZX
0VBN3ZZ 0VBN4ZX 0VBN4ZZ 0VBN8ZX 0VBN8ZZ 0VBP0ZX 0VBP0ZZ 0VBP3ZX 0VBP3ZZ 0VBP4ZX 0VBP4ZZ 0VBP8ZX 0VBP8ZZ
0VBQ0ZX 0VBQ0ZZ 0VBQ3ZX 0VBQ3ZZ 0VBQ4ZX 0VBQ4ZZ 0VBQ8ZX 0VBQ8ZZ 0VBS0ZX 0VBS0ZZ 0VBS3ZX 0VBS3ZZ 0VBS4ZX
0VBS4ZZ 0VBSXZX 0VBSXZZ 0VBT0ZX 0VBT0ZZ 0VBT3ZX 0VBT3ZZ 0VBT4ZX 0VBT4ZZ 0VBTXZX 0VBTXZZ

NC 0VBN0ZZ 0VBN3ZZ 0VBN4ZZ 0VBP0ZZ 0VBP3ZZ 0VBP4ZZ 0VBQ0ZZ 0VBQ3ZZ 0VBQ4ZZ Codes in this list are noncovered procedures only when reported with Z30.2 as either a principal or secondary diagnosis.

0 Medical and Surgical
V Male Reproductive System
C Extirpation: Taking or cutting out solid matter from a body part

Body Part Character 4	Approach Character 5	Device Character 6	Qualifier Character 7
0 Prostate ♂	**0** Open **3** Percutaneous **4** Percutaneous Endoscopic **7** Via Natural or Artificial Opening **8** Via Natural or Artificial Opening Endoscopic	**Z** No Device	**Z** No Qualifier
1 Seminal Vesicle, Right ♂ **2** Seminal Vesicle, Left ♂ **3** Seminal Vesicles, Bilateral ♂ **6** Tunica Vaginalis, Right ♂ **7** Tunica Vaginalis, Left ♂ **9** Testis, Right ♂ **B** Testis, Left ♂ **C** Testes, Bilateral ♂ **F** Spermatic Cord, Right ♂ **G** Spermatic Cord, Left ♂ **H** Spermatic Cords, Bilateral ♂ **J** Epididymis, Right ♂ **K** Epididymis, Left ♂ **L** Epididymis, Bilateral ♂ **N** Vas Deferens, Right ♂ **P** Vas Deferens, Left ♂ **Q** Vas Deferens, Bilateral ♂	**0** Open **3** Percutaneous **4** Percutaneous Endoscopic	**Z** No Device	**Z** No Qualifier
5 Scrotum ♂ **S** Penis ♂ **T** Prepuce ♂	**0** Open **3** Percutaneous **4** Percutaneous Endoscopic **X** External	**Z** No Device	**Z** No Qualifier

♂ 0VC00ZZ 0VC03ZZ 0VC04ZZ 0VC07ZZ 0VC08ZZ 0VC10ZZ 0VC13ZZ 0VC14ZZ 0VC20ZZ 0VC23ZZ 0VC24ZZ 0VC30ZZ 0VC33ZZ 0VC34ZZ 0VC50ZZ 0VC53ZZ 0VC54ZZ 0VC5XZZ 0VC60ZZ 0VC63ZZ 0VC64ZZ 0VC70ZZ 0VC73ZZ 0VC74ZZ 0VC90ZZ 0VC93ZZ 0VC94ZZ 0VCB0ZZ 0VCB3ZZ 0VCB4ZZ 0VCC0ZZ 0VCC3ZZ 0VCC4ZZ 0VCF0ZZ 0VCF3ZZ 0VCF4ZZ 0VCG0ZZ 0VCG3ZZ 0VCG4ZZ 0VCH0ZZ 0VCH3ZZ 0VCH4ZZ 0VCJ0ZZ 0VCJ3ZZ 0VCJ4ZZ 0VCK0ZZ 0VCK3ZZ 0VCK4ZZ 0VCL0ZZ 0VCL3ZZ 0VCL4ZZ 0VCN0ZZ 0VCN3ZZ 0VCN4ZZ 0VCP0ZZ 0VCP3ZZ 0VCP4ZZ 0VCQ0ZZ 0VCQ3ZZ 0VCQ4ZZ 0VCS0ZZ 0VCS3ZZ 0VCS4ZZ 0VCSXZZ 0VCT0ZZ 0VCT3ZZ 0VCT4ZZ 0VCTXZZ

0 Medical and Surgical
V Male Reproductive System
H Insertion: Putting in a nonbiological appliance that monitors, assists, performs, or prevents a physiological function but does not physically take the place of a body part

Body Part	Approach	Device	Qualifier
Character 4	Character 5	Character 6	Character 7
0 Prostate ♂	0 Open 3 Percutaneous 4 Percutaneous Endoscopic 7 Via Natural or Artificial Opening 8 Via Natural or Artificial Opening Endoscopic	1 Radioactive Element	Z No Qualifier
4 Prostate and Seminal Vesicles ♂ 8 Scrotum and Tunica Vaginalis ♂ D Testis ♂ M Epididymis and Spermatic Cord ♂ R Vas Deferens ♂	0 Open 3 Percutaneous 4 Percutaneous Endoscopic 7 Via Natural or Artificial Opening 8 Via Natural or Artificial Opening Endoscopic	3 Infusion Device Y Other Device	Z No Qualifier
S Penis ♂	0 Open 3 Percutaneous 4 Percutaneous Endoscopic	3 Infusion Device Y Other Device	Z No Qualifier
S Penis ♂	7 Via Natural or Artificial Opening 8 Via Natural or Artificial Opening Endoscopic	Y Other Device	Z No Qualifier
S Penis ♂	X External	3 Infusion Device	Z No Qualifier

♂ 0VH001Z 0VH031Z 0VH041Z 0VH071Z 0VH081Z 0VH403Z 0VH40YZ 0VH433Z 0VH43YZ 0VH443Z 0VH44YZ 0VH473Z 0VH47YZ 0VH483Z 0VH48YZ 0VH803Z 0VH80YZ 0VH833Z 0VH83YZ 0VH843Z 0VH84YZ 0VH873Z 0VH87YZ 0VH883Z 0VH88YZ 0VHD03Z 0VHD0YZ 0VHD33Z 0VHD3YZ 0VHD43Z 0VHD4YZ 0VHD73Z 0VHD7YZ 0VHD83Z 0VHD8YZ 0VHM03Z 0VHM0YZ 0VHM33Z 0VHM3YZ 0VHM43Z 0VHM4YZ 0VHM73Z 0VHM7YZ 0VHM83Z 0VHM8YZ 0VHR03Z 0VHR0YZ 0VHR33Z 0VHR3YZ 0VHR43Z 0VHR4YZ 0VHR73Z 0VHR7YZ 0VHR83Z 0VHR8YZ 0VHS03Z 0VHS0YZ 0VHS33Z 0VHS3YZ 0VHS43Z 0VHS4YZ 0VHS7YZ 0VHS8YZ 0VHSX3Z

0 Medical and Surgical
V Male Reproductive System
J Inspection: Visually and/or manually exploring a body part

Body Part	Approach	Device	Qualifier
Character 4	Character 5	Character 6	Character 7
4 Prostate and Seminal Vesicles ♂ 8 Scrotum and Tunica Vaginalis ♂ D Testis ♂ M Epididymis and Spermatic Cord ♂ R Vas Deferens ♂ S Penis ♂	0 Open 3 Percutaneous 4 Percutaneous Endoscopic X External	Z No Device	Z No Qualifier

♂ 0VJ40ZZ 0VJ43ZZ 0VJ44ZZ 0VJ4XZZ 0VJ80ZZ 0VJ83ZZ 0VJ84ZZ 0VJ8XZZ 0VJD0ZZ 0VJD3ZZ 0VJD4ZZ 0VJDXZZ 0VJM0ZZ 0VJM3ZZ 0VJM4ZZ 0VJMXZZ 0VJR0ZZ 0VJR3ZZ 0VJR4ZZ 0VJRXZZ 0VJS0ZZ 0VJS3ZZ 0VJS4ZZ 0VJSXZZ

0 Medical and Surgical
V Male Reproductive System
L Occlusion: Completely closing an orifice or the lumen of a tubular body part

Body Part Character 4	Approach Character 5	Device Character 6	Qualifier Character 7
F Spermatic Cord, Right ♂ NC **G** Spermatic Cord, Left ♂ NC **H** Spermatic Cords, Bilateral ♂ NC **N** Vas Deferens, Right ♂ NC **P** Vas Deferens, Left ♂ NC **Q** Vas Deferens, Bilateral ♂ NC	**0** Open **3** Percutaneous **4** Percutaneous Endoscopic **8** Via Natural or Artificial Opening Endoscopic	**C** Extraluminal Device **D** Intraluminal Device **Z** No Device	**Z** No Qualifier

♂ 0VLF0CZ 0VLF0DZ 0VLF0ZZ 0VLF3CZ 0VLF3DZ 0VLF3ZZ 0VLF4CZ 0VLF4DZ 0VLF4ZZ 0VLF8CZ 0VLF8DZ 0VLF8ZZ 0VLG0CZ 0VLG0DZ 0VLG0ZZ 0VLG3CZ 0VLG3DZ 0VLG3ZZ 0VLG4CZ 0VLG4DZ 0VLG4ZZ 0VLG8CZ 0VLG8DZ 0VLG8ZZ 0VLH0CZ 0VLH0DZ 0VLH0ZZ 0VLH3CZ 0VLH3DZ 0VLH3ZZ 0VLH4CZ 0VLH4DZ 0VLH4ZZ 0VLH8CZ 0VLH8DZ 0VLH8ZZ 0VLN0CZ 0VLN0DZ 0VLN0ZZ 0VLN3CZ 0VLN3DZ 0VLN3ZZ 0VLN4CZ 0VLN4DZ 0VLN4ZZ 0VLN8CZ 0VLN8DZ 0VLN8ZZ 0VLP0CZ 0VLP0DZ 0VLP0ZZ 0VLP3CZ 0VLP3DZ 0VLP3ZZ 0VLP4CZ 0VLP4DZ 0VLP4ZZ 0VLP8CZ 0VLP8DZ 0VLP8ZZ 0VLQ0CZ 0VLQ0DZ 0VLQ0ZZ 0VLQ3CZ 0VLQ3DZ 0VLQ3ZZ 0VLQ4CZ 0VLQ4DZ 0VLQ4ZZ 0VLQ8CZ 0VLQ8DZ 0VLQ8ZZ

NC 0VLF0CZ 0VLF0DZ 0VLF0ZZ 0VLF3CZ 0VLF3DZ 0VLF3ZZ 0VLF4CZ 0VLF4DZ 0VLF4ZZ 0VLG0CZ 0VLG0DZ 0VLG0ZZ 0VLG3CZ 0VLG3DZ 0VLG3ZZ 0VLG4CZ 0VLG4DZ 0VLG4ZZ 0VLH0CZ 0VLH0DZ 0VLH0ZZ 0VLH3CZ 0VLH3DZ 0VLH3ZZ 0VLH4CZ 0VLH4DZ 0VLH4ZZ 0VLN0CZ 0VLN0ZZ 0VLN3CZ 0VLN3ZZ 0VLN4CZ 0VLN4ZZ 0VLP0CZ 0VLP0ZZ 0VLP3CZ 0VLP3ZZ 0VLP4CZ 0VLP4ZZ 0VLQ0CZ 0VLQ0ZZ 0VLQ3CZ 0VLQ3ZZ 0VLQ4CZ 0VLQ4ZZ Codes in this list are noncovered procedures only when reported with Z30.2 as either a principal or secondary diagnosis.

0 Medical and Surgical
V Male Reproductive System
M Reattachment: Putting back in or on all or a portion of a separated body part to its normal location or other suitable location

Body Part Character 4	Approach Character 5	Device Character 6	Qualifier Character 7
5 Scrotum ♂ **S** Penis ♂	**X** External	**Z** No Device	**Z** No Qualifier
6 Tunica Vaginalis, Right ♂ **7** Tunica Vaginalis, Left ♂ **9** Testis, Right ♂ **B** Testis, Left ♂ **C** Testes, Bilateral ♂ **F** Spermatic Cord, Right ♂ **G** Spermatic Cord, Left ♂ **H** Spermatic Cords, Bilateral ♂	**0** Open **4** Percutaneous Endoscopic	**Z** No Device	**Z** No Qualifier

♂ 0VM5XZZ 0VM60ZZ 0VM64ZZ 0VM70ZZ 0VM74ZZ 0VM90ZZ 0VM94ZZ 0VMB0ZZ 0VMB4ZZ 0VMC0ZZ 0VMC4ZZ 0VMF0ZZ 0VMF4ZZ 0VMG0ZZ 0VMG4ZZ 0VMH0ZZ 0VMH4ZZ 0VMSXZZ

0 Medical and Surgical
V Male Reproductive System
N Release: Freeing a body part from an abnormal physical constraint by cutting or by the use of force

Body Part Character 4	Approach Character 5	Device Character 6	Qualifier Character 7
0 Prostate ♂	**0** Open **3** Percutaneous **4** Percutaneous Endoscopic **7** Via Natural or Artificial Opening **8** Via Natural or Artificial Opening Endoscopic	**Z** No Device	**Z** No Qualifier
1 Seminal Vesicle, Right ♂ **2** Seminal Vesicle, Left ♂ **3** Seminal Vesicles, Bilateral ♂ **6** Tunica Vaginalis, Right ♂ **7** Tunica Vaginalis, Left ♂ **9** Testis, Right ♂ **B** Testis, Left ♂ **C** Testes, Bilateral ♂	**0** Open **3** Percutaneous **4** Percutaneous Endoscopic	**Z** No Device	**Z** No Qualifier
5 Scrotum ♂ **S** Penis ♂ **T** Prepuce ♂	**0** Open **3** Percutaneous **4** Percutaneous Endoscopic **X** External	**Z** No Device	**Z** No Qualifier
F Spermatic Cord, Right ♂ **G** Spermatic Cord, Left ♂ **H** Spermatic Cords, Bilateral ♂ **J** Epididymis, Right ♂ **K** Epididymis, Left ♂ **L** Epididymis, Bilateral ♂ **N** Vas Deferens, Right ♂ **P** Vas Deferens, Left ♂ **Q** Vas Deferens, Bilateral ♂	**0** Open **3** Percutaneous **4** Percutaneous Endoscopic **8** Via Natural or Artificial Opening Endoscopic	**Z** No Device	**Z** No Qualifier

♂ 0VN00ZZ 0VN03ZZ 0VN04ZZ 0VN07ZZ 0VN08ZZ 0VN10ZZ 0VN13ZZ 0VN14ZZ 0VN20ZZ 0VN23ZZ 0VN24ZZ 0VN30ZZ 0VN33ZZ
0VN34ZZ 0VN50ZZ 0VN53ZZ 0VN54ZZ 0VN5XZZ 0VN60ZZ 0VN63ZZ 0VN64ZZ 0VN70ZZ 0VN73ZZ 0VN74ZZ 0VN90ZZ 0VN93ZZ
0VN94ZZ 0VNB0ZZ 0VNB3ZZ 0VNB4ZZ 0VNC0ZZ 0VNC3ZZ 0VNC4ZZ 0VNF0ZZ 0VNF3ZZ 0VNF4ZZ 0VNF8ZZ 0VNG0ZZ 0VNG3ZZ
0VNG4ZZ 0VNG8ZZ 0VNH0ZZ 0VNH3ZZ 0VNH4ZZ 0VNH8ZZ 0VNJ0ZZ 0VNJ3ZZ 0VNJ4ZZ 0VNJ8ZZ 0VNK0ZZ 0VNK3ZZ 0VNK4ZZ
0VNK8ZZ 0VNL0ZZ 0VNL3ZZ 0VNL4ZZ 0VNL8ZZ 0VNN0ZZ 0VNN3ZZ 0VNN4ZZ 0VNN8ZZ 0VNP0ZZ 0VNP3ZZ 0VNP4ZZ 0VNP8ZZ
0VNQ0ZZ 0VNQ3ZZ 0VNQ4ZZ 0VNQ8ZZ 0VNS0ZZ 0VNS3ZZ 0VNS4ZZ 0VNSXZZ 0VNT0ZZ 0VNT3ZZ 0VNT4ZZ 0VNTXZZ

0 Medical and Surgical
V Male Reproductive System
P Removal: Taking out or off a device from a body part

Body Part Character 4	Approach Character 5	Device Character 6	Qualifier Character 7
4 Prostate and Seminal Vesicles ♂	**0** Open **3** Percutaneous **4** Percutaneous Endoscopic **7** Via Natural or Artificial Opening **8** Via Natural or Artificial Opening Endoscopic	**0** Drainage Device **1** Radioactive Element **3** Infusion Device **7** Autologous Tissue Substitute **J** Synthetic Substitute **K** Nonautologous Tissue Substitute **Y** Other Device	**Z** No Qualifier
4 Prostate and Seminal Vesicles ♂	**X** External	**0** Drainage Device **1** Radioactive Element **3** Infusion Device	**Z** No Qualifier
8 Scrotum and Tunica Vaginalis ♂ **D** Testis ♂ **S** Penis ♂	**0** Open **3** Percutaneous **4** Percutaneous Endoscopic **7** Via Natural or Artificial Opening **8** Via Natural or Artificial Opening Endoscopic	**0** Drainage Device **3** Infusion Device **7** Autologous Tissue Substitute **J** Synthetic Substitute **K** Nonautologous Tissue Substitute **Y** Other Device	**Z** No Qualifier
8 Scrotum and Tunica Vaginalis ♂ **D** Testis ♂ **S** Penis ♂	**X** External	**0** Drainage Device **3** Infusion Device	**Z** No Qualifier
M Epididymis and Spermatic Cord ♂	**0** Open **3** Percutaneous **4** Percutaneous Endoscopic **7** Via Natural or Artificial Opening **8** Via Natural or Artificial Opening Endoscopic	**0** Drainage Device **3** Infusion Device **7** Autologous Tissue Substitute **C** Extraluminal Device **J** Synthetic Substitute **K** Nonautologous Tissue Substitute **Y** Other Device	**Z** No Qualifier
M Epididymis and Spermatic Cord ♂	**X** External	**0** Drainage Device **3** Infusion Device	**Z** No Qualifier
R Vas Deferens ♂	**0** Open **3** Percutaneous **4** Percutaneous Endoscopic **7** Via Natural or Artificial Opening **8** Via Natural or Artificial Opening Endoscopic	**0** Drainage Device **3** Infusion Device **7** Autologous Tissue Substitute **C** Extraluminal Device **D** Intraluminal Device **J** Synthetic Substitute **K** Nonautologous Tissue Substitute **Y** Other Device	**Z** No Qualifier
R Vas Deferens ♂	**X** External	**0** Drainage Device **3** Infusion Device **D** Intraluminal Device	**Z** No Qualifier

♂ 0VP400Z 0VP401Z 0VP403Z 0VP407Z 0VP40JZ 0VP40KZ 0VP40YZ 0VP430Z 0VP431Z 0VP433Z 0VP437Z 0VP43JZ 0VP43KZ
0VP43YZ 0VP440Z 0VP441Z 0VP443Z 0VP447Z 0VP44JZ 0VP44KZ 0VP44YZ 0VP470Z 0VP471Z 0VP473Z 0VP477Z 0VP47JZ
0VP47KZ 0VP47YZ 0VP480Z 0VP481Z 0VP483Z 0VP487Z 0VP48JZ 0VP48KZ 0VP48YZ 0VP4X0Z 0VP4X1Z 0VP4X3Z 0VP800Z
0VP803Z 0VP807Z 0VP80JZ 0VP80KZ 0VP80YZ 0VP830Z 0VP833Z 0VP837Z 0VP83JZ 0VP83KZ 0VP83YZ 0VP840Z 0VP843Z
0VP847Z 0VP84JZ 0VP84KZ 0VP84YZ 0VP870Z 0VP873Z 0VP877Z 0VP87JZ 0VP87KZ 0VP87YZ 0VP880Z 0VP883Z 0VP887Z
0VP88JZ 0VP88KZ 0VP88YZ 0VP8X0Z 0VP8X3Z 0VPD00Z 0VPD03Z 0VPD07Z 0VPD0JZ 0VPD0KZ 0VPD0YZ 0VPD30Z 0VPD33Z
0VPD37Z 0VPD3JZ 0VPD3KZ 0VPD3YZ 0VPD40Z 0VPD43Z 0VPD47Z 0VPD4JZ 0VPD4KZ 0VPD4YZ 0VPD70Z 0VPD73Z 0VPD77Z
0VPD7JZ 0VPD7KZ 0VPD7YZ 0VPD80Z 0VPD83Z 0VPD87Z 0VPD8JZ 0VPD8KZ 0VPD8YZ 0VPDX0Z 0VPDX3Z 0VPM00Z 0VPM03Z
0VPM07Z 0VPM0CZ 0VPM0JZ 0VPM0KZ 0VPM0YZ 0VPM30Z 0VPM33Z 0VPM37Z 0VPM3CZ 0VPM3JZ 0VPM3KZ 0VPM3YZ 0VPM40Z
0VPM43Z 0VPM47Z 0VPM4CZ 0VPM4JZ 0VPM4KZ 0VPM4YZ 0VPM70Z 0VPM73Z 0VPM77Z 0VPM7CZ 0VPM7JZ 0VPM7KZ 0VPM7YZ
0VPM80Z 0VPM83Z 0VPM87Z 0VPM8CZ 0VPM8JZ 0VPM8KZ 0VPM8YZ 0VPMX0Z 0VPMX3Z 0VPR00Z 0VPR03Z 0VPR07Z 0VPR0CZ
0VPR0DZ 0VPR0JZ 0VPR0KZ 0VPR0YZ 0VPR30Z 0VPR33Z 0VPR37Z 0VPR3CZ 0VPR3DZ 0VPR3JZ 0VPR3KZ 0VPR3YZ 0VPR40Z
0VPR43Z 0VPR47Z 0VPR4CZ 0VPR4DZ 0VPR4JZ 0VPR4KZ 0VPR4YZ 0VPR70Z 0VPR73Z 0VPR77Z 0VPR7CZ 0VPR7DZ 0VPR7JZ
0VPR7KZ 0VPR7YZ 0VPR80Z 0VPR83Z 0VPR87Z 0VPR8CZ 0VPR8DZ 0VPR8JZ 0VPR8KZ 0VPR8YZ 0VPRX0Z 0VPRX3Z 0VPRXDZ
0VPS00Z 0VPS03Z 0VPS07Z 0VPS0JZ 0VPS0KZ 0VPS0YZ 0VPS30Z 0VPS33Z 0VPS37Z 0VPS3JZ 0VPS3KZ 0VPS3YZ 0VPS40Z
0VPS43Z 0VPS47Z 0VPS4JZ 0VPS4KZ 0VPS4YZ 0VPS70Z 0VPS73Z 0VPS77Z 0VPS7JZ 0VPS7KZ 0VPS7YZ 0VPS80Z 0VPS83Z
0VPS87Z 0VPS8JZ 0VPS8KZ 0VPS8YZ 0VPSX0Z 0VPSX3Z

0 Medical and Surgical
V Male Reproductive System
Q Repair: Restoring, to the extent possible, a body part to its normal anatomic structure and function

Body Part Character 4	Approach Character 5	Device Character 6	Qualifier Character 7
0 Prostate ♂	**0** Open **3** Percutaneous **4** Percutaneous Endoscopic **7** Via Natural or Artificial Opening **8** Via Natural or Artificial Opening Endoscopic	**Z** No Device	**Z** No Qualifier
1 Seminal Vesicle, Right ♂ **2** Seminal Vesicle, Left ♂ **3** Seminal Vesicles, Bilateral ♂ **6** Tunica Vaginalis, Right ♂ **7** Tunica Vaginalis, Left ♂ **9** Testis, Right ♂ **B** Testis, Left ♂ **C** Testes, Bilateral ♂	**0** Open **3** Percutaneous **4** Percutaneous Endoscopic	**Z** No Device	**Z** No Qualifier
5 Scrotum ♂ **S** Penis ♂ **T** Prepuce ♂	**0** Open **3** Percutaneous **4** Percutaneous Endoscopic **X** External	**Z** No Device	**Z** No Qualifier
F Spermatic Cord, Right ♂ **G** Spermatic Cord, Left ♂ **H** Spermatic Cords, Bilateral ♂ **J** Epididymis, Right ♂ **K** Epididymis, Left ♂ **L** Epididymis, Bilateral ♂ **N** Vas Deferens, Right ♂ **P** Vas Deferens, Left ♂ **Q** Vas Deferens, Bilateral ♂	**0** Open **3** Percutaneous **4** Percutaneous Endoscopic **8** Via Natural or Artificial Opening Endoscopic	**Z** No Device	**Z** No Qualifier

♂ 0VQ00ZZ 0VQ03ZZ 0VQ04ZZ 0VQ07ZZ 0VQ08ZZ 0VQ10ZZ 0VQ13ZZ 0VQ14ZZ 0VQ20ZZ 0VQ23ZZ 0VQ24ZZ 0VQ30ZZ 0VQ33ZZ 0VQ34ZZ 0VQ50ZZ 0VQ53ZZ 0VQ54ZZ 0VQ5XZZ 0VQ60ZZ 0VQ63ZZ 0VQ64ZZ 0VQ70ZZ 0VQ73ZZ 0VQ74ZZ 0VQ90ZZ 0VQ93ZZ 0VQ94ZZ 0VQB0ZZ 0VQB3ZZ 0VQB4ZZ 0VQC0ZZ 0VQC3ZZ 0VQC4ZZ 0VQF0ZZ 0VQF3ZZ 0VQF4ZZ 0VQF8ZZ 0VQG0ZZ 0VQG3ZZ 0VQG4ZZ 0VQG8ZZ 0VQH0ZZ 0VQH3ZZ 0VQH4ZZ 0VQH8ZZ 0VQJ0ZZ 0VQJ3ZZ 0VQJ4ZZ 0VQJ8ZZ 0VQK0ZZ 0VQK3ZZ 0VQK4ZZ 0VQK8ZZ 0VQL0ZZ 0VQL3ZZ 0VQL4ZZ 0VQL8ZZ 0VQN0ZZ 0VQN3ZZ 0VQN4ZZ 0VQN8ZZ 0VQP0ZZ 0VQP3ZZ 0VQP4ZZ 0VQP8ZZ 0VQQ0ZZ 0VQQ3ZZ 0VQQ4ZZ 0VQQ8ZZ 0VQS0ZZ 0VQS3ZZ 0VQS4ZZ 0VQSXZZ 0VQT0ZZ 0VQT3ZZ 0VQT4ZZ 0VQTXZZ

0 Medical and Surgical
V Male Reproductive System
R Replacement: Putting in or on biological or synthetic material that physically takes the place and/or function of all or a portion of a body part

Body Part Character 4	Approach Character 5	Device Character 6	Qualifier Character 7
9 Testis, Right ♂ **B** Testis, Left ♂ **C** Testes, Bilateral ♂	**0** Open	**J** Synthetic Substitute	**Z** No Qualifier

♂ 0VR90JZ 0VRB0JZ 0VRC0JZ

0 Medical and Surgical
V Male Reproductive System
S Reposition: Moving to its normal location, or other suitable location, all or a portion of a body part

Body Part Character 4	Approach Character 5	Device Character 6	Qualifier Character 7
9 Testis, Right ♂ B Testis, Left ♂ C Testes, Bilateral ♂ F Spermatic Cord, Right ♂ G Spermatic Cord, Left ♂ H Spermatic Cords, Bilateral ♂	0 Open 3 Percutaneous 4 Percutaneous Endoscopic 8 Via Natural or Artificial Opening Endoscopic	Z No Device	Z No Qualifier

♂ 0VS90ZZ 0VS93ZZ 0VS94ZZ 0VS98ZZ 0VSB0ZZ 0VSB3ZZ 0VSB4ZZ 0VSB8ZZ 0VSC0ZZ 0VSC3ZZ 0VSC4ZZ 0VSC8ZZ 0VSF0ZZ 0VSF3ZZ 0VSF4ZZ 0VSF8ZZ 0VSG0ZZ 0VSG3ZZ 0VSG4ZZ 0VSG8ZZ 0VSH0ZZ 0VSH3ZZ 0VSH4ZZ 0VSH8ZZ

0 Medical and Surgical
V Male Reproductive System
T Resection: Cutting out or off, without replacement, all of a body part

Body Part Character 4	Approach Character 5	Device Character 6	Qualifier Character 7
0 Prostate CC ♂	0 Open 4 Percutaneous Endoscopic 7 Via Natural or Artificial Opening 8 Via Natural or Artificial Opening Endoscopic	Z No Device	Z No Qualifier
1 Seminal Vesicle, Right ♂ 2 Seminal Vesicle, Left ♂ 3 Seminal Vesicles, Bilateral CC ♂ 6 Tunica Vaginalis, Right ♂ 7 Tunica Vaginalis, Left ♂ 9 Testis, Right ♂ B Testis, Left ♂ C Testes, Bilateral ♂ F Spermatic Cord, Right ♂ G Spermatic Cord, Left ♂ H Spermatic Cords, Bilateral ♂ J Epididymis, Right ♂ K Epididymis, Left ♂ L Epididymis, Bilateral ♂ N Vas Deferens, Right ♂ NC P Vas Deferens, Left ♂ NC Q Vas Deferens, Bilateral ♂ NC	0 Open 4 Percutaneous Endoscopic	Z No Device	Z No Qualifier
5 Scrotum ♂ S Penis ♂ T Prepuce ♂	0 Open 4 Percutaneous Endoscopic X External	Z No Device	Z No Qualifier

♂ 0VT00ZZ 0VT04ZZ 0VT07ZZ 0VT08ZZ 0VT10ZZ 0VT14ZZ 0VT20ZZ 0VT24ZZ 0VT30ZZ 0VT34ZZ 0VT50ZZ 0VT54ZZ 0VT5XZZ 0VT60ZZ 0VT64ZZ 0VT70ZZ 0VT74ZZ 0VT90ZZ 0VT94ZZ 0VTB0ZZ 0VTB4ZZ 0VTC0ZZ 0VTC4ZZ 0VTF0ZZ 0VTF4ZZ 0VTG0ZZ 0VTG4ZZ 0VTH0ZZ 0VTH4ZZ 0VTJ0ZZ 0VTJ4ZZ 0VTK0ZZ 0VTK4ZZ 0VTL0ZZ 0VTL4ZZ 0VTN0ZZ 0VTN4ZZ 0VTP0ZZ 0VTP4ZZ 0VTQ0ZZ 0VTQ4ZZ 0VTS0ZZ 0VTS4ZZ 0VTSXZZ 0VTT0ZZ 0VTT4ZZ 0VTTXZZ
CC 0VT00ZZ 0VT04ZZ 0VT07ZZ 0VT08ZZ 0VT30ZZ 0VT34ZZ
NC 0VTN0ZZ 0VTN4ZZ 0VTP0ZZ 0VTP4ZZ 0VTQ0ZZ 0VTQ4ZZ Codes in this list are noncovered procedures only when reported with Z30.2 as either a principal or secondary diagnosis.

0 Medical and Surgical
V Male Reproductive System
U Supplement: Putting in or on biological or synthetic material that physically reinforces and/or augments the function of a portion of a body part

Body Part Character 4	Approach Character 5	Device Character 6	Qualifier Character 7
1 Seminal Vesicle, Right ♂ **2** Seminal Vesicle, Left ♂ **3** Seminal Vesicles, Bilateral ♂ **6** Tunica Vaginalis, Right ♂ **7** Tunica Vaginalis, Left ♂ **F** Spermatic Cord, Right ♂ **G** Spermatic Cord, Left ♂ **H** Spermatic Cords, Bilateral ♂ **J** Epididymis, Right ♂ **K** Epididymis, Left ♂ **L** Epididymis, Bilateral ♂ **N** Vas Deferens, Right ♂ **P** Vas Deferens, Left ♂ **Q** Vas Deferens, Bilateral ♂	**0** Open **4** Percutaneous Endoscopic **8** Via Natural or Artificial Opening Endoscopic	**7** Autologous Tissue Substitute **J** Synthetic Substitute **K** Nonautologous Tissue Substitute	**Z** No Qualifier
5 Scrotum ♂ **S** Penis ♂ **T** Prepuce ♂	**0** Open **4** Percutaneous Endoscopic **X** External	**7** Autologous Tissue Substitute **J** Synthetic Substitute **K** Nonautologous Tissue Substitute	**Z** No Qualifier
9 Testis, Right ♂ **B** Testis, Left ♂ **C** Testes, Bilateral ♂	**0** Open	**7** Autologous Tissue Substitute **J** Synthetic Substitute **K** Nonautologous Tissue Substitute	**Z** No Qualifier

♂ 0VU107Z 0VU10JZ 0VU10KZ 0VU147Z 0VU14JZ 0VU14KZ 0VU187Z 0VU18JZ 0VU18KZ 0VU207Z 0VU20JZ 0VU20KZ 0VU247Z 0VU24JZ 0VU24KZ 0VU287Z 0VU28JZ 0VU28KZ 0VU307Z 0VU30JZ 0VU30KZ 0VU347Z 0VU34JZ 0VU34KZ 0VU387Z 0VU38JZ 0VU38KZ 0VU507Z 0VU50JZ 0VU50KZ 0VU547Z 0VU54JZ 0VU54KZ 0VU5X7Z 0VU5XJZ 0VU5XKZ 0VU607Z 0VU60JZ 0VU60KZ 0VU647Z 0VU64JZ 0VU64KZ 0VU687Z 0VU68JZ 0VU68KZ 0VU707Z 0VU70JZ 0VU70KZ 0VU747Z 0VU74JZ 0VU74KZ 0VU787Z 0VU78JZ 0VU78KZ 0VU907Z 0VU90JZ 0VU90KZ 0VUB07Z 0VUB0JZ 0VUB0KZ 0VUC07Z 0VUC0JZ 0VUC0KZ 0VUF07Z 0VUF0JZ 0VUF0KZ 0VUF47Z 0VUF4JZ 0VUF4KZ 0VUF87Z 0VUF8JZ 0VUF8KZ 0VUG07Z 0VUG0JZ 0VUG0KZ 0VUG47Z 0VUG4JZ 0VUG4KZ 0VUG87Z 0VUG8JZ 0VUG8KZ 0VUH07Z 0VUH0JZ 0VUH0KZ 0VUH47Z 0VUH4JZ 0VUH4KZ 0VUH87Z 0VUH8JZ 0VUH8KZ 0VUJ07Z 0VUJ0JZ 0VUJ0KZ 0VUJ47Z 0VUJ4JZ 0VUJ4KZ 0VUJ87Z 0VUJ8JZ 0VUJ8KZ 0VUK07Z 0VUK0JZ 0VUK0KZ 0VUK47Z 0VUK4JZ 0VUK4KZ 0VUK87Z 0VUK8JZ 0VUK8KZ 0VUL07Z 0VUL0JZ 0VUL0KZ 0VUL47Z 0VUL4JZ 0VUL4KZ 0VUL87Z 0VUL8JZ 0VUL8KZ 0VUN07Z 0VUN0JZ 0VUN0KZ 0VUN47Z 0VUN4JZ 0VUN4KZ 0VUN87Z 0VUN8JZ 0VUN8KZ 0VUP07Z 0VUP0JZ 0VUP0KZ 0VUP47Z 0VUP4JZ 0VUP4KZ 0VUP87Z 0VUP8JZ 0VUP8KZ 0VUQ07Z 0VUQ0JZ 0VUQ0KZ 0VUQ47Z 0VUQ4JZ 0VUQ4KZ 0VUQ87Z 0VUQ8JZ 0VUQ8KZ 0VUS07Z 0VUS0JZ 0VUS0KZ 0VUS47Z 0VUS4JZ 0VUS4KZ 0VUSX7Z 0VUSXJZ 0VUSXKZ 0VUT07Z 0VUT0JZ 0VUT0KZ 0VUT47Z 0VUT4JZ 0VUT4KZ 0VUTX7Z 0VUTXJZ 0VUTXKZ

0 Medical and Surgical
V Male Reproductive System
W Revision: Correcting, to the extent possible, a portion of a malfunctioning device or the position of a displaced device

Body Part Character 4	Approach Character 5	Device Character 6	Qualifier Character 7
4 Prostate and Seminal Vesicles ♂ **8** Scrotum and Tunica Vaginalis ♂ **D** Testis ♂ **S** Penis ♂	**0** Open **3** Percutaneous **4** Percutaneous Endoscopic **7** Via Natural or Artificial Opening **8** Via Natural or Artificial Opening Endoscopic	**0** Drainage Device **3** Infusion Device **7** Autologous Tissue Substitute **J** Synthetic Substitute **K** Nonautologous Tissue Substitute **Y** Other Device	**Z** No Qualifier
4 Prostate and Seminal Vesicles ♂ **8** Scrotum and Tunica Vaginalis ♂ **D** Testis ♂ **S** Penis ♂	**X** External	**0** Drainage Device **3** Infusion Device **7** Autologous Tissue Substitute **J** Synthetic Substitute **K** Nonautologous Tissue Substitute	**Z** No Qualifier
M Epididymis and Spermatic Cord ♂	**0** Open **3** Percutaneous **4** Percutaneous Endoscopic **7** Via Natural or Artificial Opening **8** Via Natural or Artificial Opening Endoscopic	**0** Drainage Device **3** Infusion Device **7** Autologous Tissue Substitute **C** Extraluminal Device **J** Synthetic Substitute **K** Nonautologous Tissue Substitute **Y** Other Device	**Z** No Qualifier
M Epididymis and Spermatic Cord ♂	**X** External	**0** Drainage Device **3** Infusion Device **7** Autologous Tissue Substitute **C** Extraluminal Device **J** Synthetic Substitute **K** Nonautologous Tissue Substitute	**Z** No Qualifier
R Vas Deferens ♂	**0** Open **3** Percutaneous **4** Percutaneous Endoscopic **7** Via Natural or Artificial Opening **8** Via Natural or Artificial Opening Endoscopic	**0** Drainage Device **3** Infusion Device **7** Autologous Tissue Substitute **C** Extraluminal Device **D** Intraluminal Device **J** Synthetic Substitute **K** Nonautologous Tissue Substitute **Y** Other Device	**Z** No Qualifier
R Vas Deferens ♂	**X** External	**0** Drainage Device **3** Infusion Device **7** Autologous Tissue Substitute **C** Extraluminal Device **D** Intraluminal Device **J** Synthetic Substitute **K** Nonautologous Tissue Substitute	**Z** No Qualifier

♂ 0VW400Z 0VW403Z 0VW407Z 0VW40JZ 0VW40KZ 0VW40YZ 0VW430Z 0VW433Z 0VW437Z 0VW43JZ 0VW43KZ 0VW43YZ 0VW440Z 0VW443Z 0VW447Z 0VW44JZ 0VW44KZ 0VW44YZ 0VW470Z 0VW473Z 0VW477Z 0VW47JZ 0VW47KZ 0VW47YZ 0VW480Z 0VW483Z 0VW487Z 0VW48JZ 0VW48KZ 0VW48YZ 0VW4X0Z 0VW4X3Z 0VW4X7Z 0VW4XJZ 0VW4XKZ 0VW800Z 0VW803Z 0VW807Z 0VW80JZ 0VW80KZ 0VW80YZ 0VW830Z 0VW833Z 0VW837Z 0VW83JZ 0VW83KZ 0VW83YZ 0VW840Z 0VW843Z 0VW847Z 0VW84JZ 0VW84KZ 0VW84YZ 0VW870Z 0VW873Z 0VW877Z 0VW87JZ 0VW87KZ 0VW87YZ 0VW880Z 0VW883Z 0VW887Z 0VW88JZ 0VW88KZ 0VW88YZ 0VW8X0Z 0VW8X3Z 0VW8X7Z 0VW8XJZ 0VW8XKZ 0VWD00Z 0VWD03Z 0VWD07Z 0VWD0JZ 0VWD0KZ 0VWD0YZ 0VWD30Z 0VWD33Z 0VWD37Z 0VWD3JZ 0VWD3KZ 0VWD3YZ 0VWD40Z 0VWD43Z 0VWD47Z 0VWD4JZ 0VWD4KZ 0VWD4YZ 0VWD70Z 0VWD73Z 0VWD77Z 0VWD7JZ 0VWD7KZ 0VWD7YZ 0VWD80Z 0VWD83Z 0VWD87Z 0VWD8JZ 0VWD8KZ 0VWD8YZ 0VWDX0Z 0VWDX3Z 0VWDX7Z 0VWDXJZ 0VWDXKZ 0VWM00Z 0VWM03Z 0VWM07Z 0VWM0CZ 0VWM0JZ 0VWM0KZ 0VWM0YZ 0VWM30Z 0VWM33Z 0VWM37Z 0VWM3CZ 0VWM3JZ 0VWM3KZ 0VWM3YZ 0VWM40Z 0VWM43Z 0VWM47Z 0VWM4CZ 0VWM4JZ 0VWM4KZ 0VWM4YZ 0VWM70Z 0VWM73Z 0VWM77Z 0VWM7CZ 0VWM7JZ 0VWM7KZ 0VWM7YZ 0VWM80Z 0VWM83Z 0VWM87Z 0VWM8CZ 0VWM8JZ 0VWM8KZ 0VWM8YZ 0VWMX0Z 0VWMX3Z 0VWMX7Z 0VWMXCZ 0VWMXJZ 0VWMXKZ 0VWR00Z 0VWR03Z 0VWR07Z 0VWR0CZ 0VWR0DZ 0VWR0JZ 0VWR0KZ 0VWR0YZ 0VWR30Z 0VWR33Z 0VWR37Z 0VWR3CZ 0VWR3DZ 0VWR3JZ 0VWR3KZ 0VWR3YZ 0VWR40Z 0VWR43Z 0VWR47Z 0VWR4CZ 0VWR4DZ 0VWR4JZ 0VWR4KZ 0VWR4YZ 0VWR70Z 0VWR73Z 0VWR77Z 0VWR7CZ 0VWR7DZ 0VWR7JZ 0VWR7KZ 0VWR7YZ 0VWR80Z 0VWR83Z 0VWR87Z 0VWR8CZ 0VWR8DZ 0VWR8JZ 0VWR8KZ 0VWR8YZ 0VWRX0Z 0VWRX3Z 0VWRX7Z 0VWRXCZ 0VWRXDZ 0VWRXJZ 0VWRXKZ 0VWS00Z 0VWS03Z 0VWS07Z 0VWS0JZ 0VWS0KZ 0VWS0YZ 0VWS30Z 0VWS33Z 0VWS37Z 0VWS3JZ 0VWS3KZ 0VWS3YZ 0VWS40Z 0VWS43Z 0VWS47Z 0VWS4JZ 0VWS4KZ 0VWS4YZ 0VWS70Z 0VWS73Z 0VWS77Z 0VWS7JZ 0VWS7KZ 0VWS7YZ 0VWS80Z 0VWS83Z 0VWS87Z 0VWS8JZ 0VWS8KZ 0VWS8YZ 0VWSX0Z 0VWSX3Z 0VWSX7Z 0VWSXJZ 0VWSXKZ

0 Medical and Surgical
V Male Reproductive System
X Transfer: Moving, without taking out, all or a portion of a body part to another locationto take over the function of all or a portion of a body part

Body Part Character 4	Approach Character 5	Device Character 6	Qualifier Character 7
T Prepuce ♂	0 Open X External	Z No Device	D Urethra S Penis

♂ 0VXT0ZD 0VXT0ZS 0VXTXZD 0VXTXZS

NOTES

NOTES

Anatomical Regions, General 0W0-0WY

0 Medical and Surgical
W Anatomical Regions, General
0 Alteration: Modifying the anatomic structure of a body part without affecting the function of the body part

Body Part Character 4	Approach Character 5	Device Character 6	Qualifier Character 7
0 Head **2** Face **4** Upper Jaw **5** Lower Jaw **6** Neck **8** Chest Wall **F** Abdominal Wall **K** Upper Back **L** Lower Back **M** Perineum, Male ♂ **N** Perineum, Female ♀	**0** Open **3** Percutaneous **4** Percutaneous Endoscopic	**7** Autologous Tissue Substitute **J** Synthetic Substitute **K** Nonautologous Tissue Substitute **Z** No Device	**Z** No Qualifier

♂ 0W0M07Z 0W0M0JZ 0W0M0KZ 0W0M0ZZ 0W0M37Z 0W0M3JZ 0W0M3KZ 0W0M3ZZ 0W0M47Z 0W0M4JZ 0W0M4KZ 0W0M4ZZ
♀ 0W0N07Z 0W0N0JZ 0W0N0KZ 0W0N0ZZ 0W0N37Z 0W0N3JZ 0W0N3KZ 0W0N3ZZ 0W0N47Z 0W0N4JZ 0W0N4KZ 0W0N4ZZ

0 Medical and Surgical
W Anatomical Regions, General
1 Bypass: Altering the route of passage of the contents of a tubular body part

Body Part Character 4	Approach Character 5	Device Character 6	Qualifier Character 7
1 Cranial Cavity	**0** Open	**J** Synthetic Substitute	**9** Pleural Cavity, Right **B** Pleural Cavity, Left **G** Peritoneal Cavity **J** Pelvic Cavity
9 Pleural Cavity, Right **B** Pleural Cavity, Left **G** Peritoneal Cavity **J** Pelvic Cavity	**0** Open **3** Percutaneous **4** Percutaneous Endoscopic	**J** Synthetic Substitute	**4** Cutaneous **9** Pleural Cavity, Right **B** Pleural Cavity, Left **G** Peritoneal Cavity **J** Pelvic Cavity **W** Upper Vein **Y** Lower Vein

0 Medical and Surgical
W Anatomical Regions, General
2 Change: Taking out or off a device from a body part and putting back an identical or similar device in or on the same body part without cutting or puncturing the skin or a mucous membrane

Body Part Character 4	Approach Character 5	Device Character 6	Qualifier Character 7
0 Head **1** Cranial Cavity **2** Face **4** Upper Jaw **5** Lower Jaw **6** Neck **8** Chest Wall **9** Pleural Cavity, Right **B** Pleural Cavity, Left **C** Mediastinum **D** Pericardial Cavity **F** Abdominal Wall **G** Peritoneal Cavity **H** Retroperitoneum **J** Pelvic Cavity **K** Upper Back **L** Lower Back **M** Perineum, Male ♂ **N** Perineum, Female ♀	**X** External	**0** Drainage Device **Y** Other Device	**Z** No Qualifier

♂ 0W2MX0Z 0W2MXYZ
♀ 0W2NX0Z 0W2NXYZ

0 Medical and Surgical
W Anatomical Regions, General
3 Control: Stopping, or attempting to stop, postprocedural or other acute bleeding

Body Part Character 4	Approach Character 5	Device Character 6	Qualifier Character 7
0 Head **1** Cranial Cavity **2** Face **4** Upper Jaw **5** Lower Jaw **6** Neck **8** Chest Wall **9** Pleural Cavity, Right **B** Pleural Cavity, Left **C** Mediastinum **D** Pericardial Cavity **F** Abdominal Wall **G** Peritoneal Cavity **H** Retroperitoneum **J** Pelvic Cavity **K** Upper Back **L** Lower Back **M** Perineum, Male ♂ **N** Perineum, Female ♀	**0** Open **3** Percutaneous **4** Percutaneous Endoscopic	**Z** No Device	**Z** No Qualifier
3 Oral Cavity and Throat	**0** Open **3** Percutaneous **4** Percutaneous Endoscopic **7** Via Natural or Artificial Opening **8** Via Natural or Artificial Opening Endoscopic **X** External	**Z** No Device	**Z** No Qualifier
P Gastrointestinal Tract **Q** Respiratory Tract **R** Genitourinary Tract	**0** Open **3** Percutaneous **4** Percutaneous Endoscopic **7** Via Natural or Artificial Opening **8** Via Natural or Artificial Opening Endoscopic	**Z** No Device	**Z** No Qualifier

♂ 0W3M0ZZ 0W3M3ZZ 0W3M4ZZ
♀ 0W3N0ZZ 0W3N3ZZ 0W3N4ZZ

0 Medical and Surgical
W Anatomical Regions, General
4 Creation: Putting in or on biological or synthetic material to form a new body part that to the extent possible replicates the anatomic structure or function of an absent body part

Body Part	Approach	Device	Qualifier
Character 4	**Character 5**	**Character 6**	**Character 7**
M Perineum, Male ♂	**0** Open	**7** Autologous Tissue Substitute **J** Synthetic Substitute **K** Nonautologous Tissue Substitute	**0** Vagina
N Perineum, Female ♀	**0** Open	**7** Autologous Tissue Substitute **J** Synthetic Substitute **K** Nonautologous Tissue Substitute	**1** Penis

♂ 0W4M070 0W4M0J0 0W4M0K0
♀ 0W4N071 0W4N0J1 0W4N0K1

0 Medical and Surgical
W Anatomical Regions, General
8 Division: Cutting into a body part, without draining fluids and/or gases from the body part, in order to separate or transect a body part

Body Part	Approach	Device	Qualifier
Character 4	**Character 5**	**Character 6**	**Character 7**
N Perineum, Female ♀	**X** External	**Z** No Device	**Z** No Qualifier

♀ 0W8NXZZ

0 Medical and Surgical
W Anatomical Regions, General
9 Drainage: Taking or letting out fluids and/or gases from a body part

Body Part	Approach	Device	Qualifier
Character 4	**Character 5**	**Character 6**	**Character 7**
0 Head **1** Cranial Cavity **2** Face **3** Oral Cavity and Throat **4** Upper Jaw **5** Lower Jaw **6** Neck **8** Chest Wall **9** Pleural Cavity, Right **B** Pleural Cavity, Left **C** Mediastinum **D** Pericardial Cavity **F** Abdominal Wall **G** Peritoneal Cavity **H** Retroperitoneum **J** Pelvic Cavity **K** Upper Back **L** Lower Back **M** Perineum, Male ♂ **N** Perineum, Female ♀	**0** Open **3** Percutaneous **4** Percutaneous Endoscopic	**0** Drainage Device	**Z** No Qualifier

0W9 continued on next page

0W9 continued from previous page

0 Medical and Surgical
W Anatomical Regions, General
9 Drainage: Taking or letting out fluids and/or gases from a body part

Body Part Character 4	Approach Character 5	Device Character 6	Qualifier Character 7
0 Head **1** Cranial Cavity **2** Face **3** Oral Cavity and Throat **4** Upper Jaw **5** Lower Jaw **6** Neck **8** Chest Wall **9** Pleural Cavity, Right **B** Pleural Cavity, Left **C** Mediastinum **D** Pericardial Cavity **F** Abdominal Wall **G** Peritoneal Cavity **H** Retroperitoneum **J** Pelvic Cavity **K** Upper Back **L** Lower Back **M** Perineum, Male ♂ **N** Perineum, Female ♀	**0** Open **3** Percutaneous **4** Percutaneous Endoscopic	**Z** No Device	**X** Diagnostic **Z** No Qualifier

♂ 0W9M00Z 0W9M0ZX 0W9M0ZZ 0W9M30Z 0W9M3ZX 0W9M3ZZ 0W9M40Z 0W9M4ZX 0W9M4ZZ
♀ 0W9N00Z 0W9N0ZX 0W9N0ZZ 0W9N30Z 0W9N3ZX 0W9N3ZZ 0W9N40Z 0W9N4ZZ

0 Medical and Surgical
W Anatomical Regions, General
B Excision: Cutting out or off, without replacement, a portion of a body part

Body Part Character 4	Approach Character 5	Device Character 6	Qualifier Character 7
0 Head **2** Face **3** Oral Cavity and Throat **4** Upper Jaw **5** Lower Jaw **8** Chest Wall **K** Upper Back **L** Lower Back **M** Perineum, Male ♂ **N** Perineum, Female ♀	**0** Open **3** Percutaneous **4** Percutaneous Endoscopic **X** External	**Z** No Device	**X** Diagnostic **Z** No Qualifier
6 Neck **F** Abdominal Wall	**0** Open **3** Percutaneous **4** Percutaneous Endoscopic	**Z** No Device	**X** Diagnostic **Z** No Qualifier
6 Neck **F** Abdominal Wall	**X** External	**Z** No Device	**2** Stoma **X** Diagnostic **Z** No Qualifier
C Mediastinum **H** Retroperitoneum	**0** Open **3** Percutaneous **4** Percutaneous Endoscopic	**Z** No Device	**X** Diagnostic **Z** No Qualifier

♂ 0WBM0ZX 0WBM0ZZ 0WBM3ZX 0WBM3ZZ 0WBM4ZX 0WBM4ZZ 0WBMXZX 0WBMXZZ
♀ 0WBN0ZX 0WBN0ZZ 0WBN3ZX 0WBN3ZZ 0WBN4ZX 0WBN4ZZ 0WBNXZX 0WBNXZZ

0 Medical and Surgical
W Anatomical Regions, General
C Extirpation: Taking or cutting out solid matter from a body part

Body Part Character 4	Approach Character 5	Device Character 6	Qualifier Character 7
1 Cranial Cavity **3** Oral Cavity and Throat **9** Pleural Cavity, Right **B** Pleural Cavity, Left **C** Mediastinum **D** Pericardial Cavity **G** Peritoneal Cavity **H** Retroperitoneum **J** Pelvic Cavity	**0** Open **3** Percutaneous **4** Percutaneous Endoscopic **X** External	**Z** No Device	**Z** No Qualifier
P Gastrointestinal Tract **Q** Respiratory Tract **R** Genitourinary Tract	**0** Open **3** Percutaneous **4** Percutaneous Endoscopic **7** Via Natural or Artificial Opening **8** Via Natural or Artificial Opening Endoscopic **X** External	**Z** No Device	**Z** No Qualifier

0 Medical and Surgical
W Anatomical Regions, General
F Fragmentation: Breaking solid matter in a body part into pieces

Body Part Character 4	Approach Character 5	Device Character 6	Qualifier Character 7
1 Cranial Cavity NC **3** Oral Cavity and Throat NC **9** Pleural Cavity, Right NC **B** Pleural Cavity, Left NC **C** Mediastinum NC **D** Pericardial Cavity **G** Peritoneal Cavity NC **J** Pelvic Cavity NC	**0** Open **3** Percutaneous **4** Percutaneous Endoscopic **X** External	**Z** No Device	**Z** No Qualifier
P Gastrointestinal Tract NC **Q** Respiratory Tract NC **R** Genitourinary Tract	**0** Open **3** Percutaneous **4** Percutaneous Endoscopic **7** Via Natural or Artificial Opening **8** Via Natural or Artificial Opening Endoscopic **X** External	**Z** No Device	**Z** No Qualifier

NC 0WF1XZZ 0WF3XZZ 0WF9XZZ 0WFBXZZ 0WFCXZZ 0WFGXZZ 0WFJXZZ 0WFPXZZ 0WFQXZZ

0 Medical and Surgical
W Anatomical Regions, General
H Insertion: Putting in a nonbiological appliance that monitors, assists, performs, or prevents a physiological function but does not physically take the place of a body part

Body Part Character 4	Approach Character 5	Device Character 6	Qualifier Character 7
0 Head **1** Cranial Cavity **2** Face **3** Oral Cavity and Throat **4** Upper Jaw **5** Lower Jaw **6** Neck **8** Chest Wall **9** Pleural Cavity, Right **B** Pleural Cavity, Left **C** Mediastinum **D** Pericardial Cavity **F** Abdominal Wall **G** Peritoneal Cavity **H** Retroperitoneum **J** Pelvic Cavity **K** Upper Back **L** Lower Back **M** Perineum, Male **N** Perineum, Female ♀	**0** Open **3** Percutaneous **4** Percutaneous Endoscopic	**1** Radioactive Element **3** Infusion Device **Y** Other Device	**Z** No Qualifier
P Gastrointestinal Tract **Q** Respiratory Tract **R** Genitourinary Tract	**0** Open **3** Percutaneous **4** Percutaneous Endoscopic **7** Via Natural or Artificial Opening **8** Via Natural or Artificial Opening Endoscopic	**1** Radioactive Element **3** Infusion Device **Y** Other Device	**Z** No Qualifier

♀ 0WHN03Z 0WHN0YZ 0WHN33Z 0WHN3YZ 0WHN43Z 0WHN4YZ

0 Medical and Surgical
W Anatomical Regions, General
J Inspection: Visually and/or manually exploring a body part

Body Part Character 4	Approach Character 5	Device Character 6	Qualifier Character 7
0 Head **2** Face **3** Oral Cavity and Throat **4** Upper Jaw **5** Lower Jaw **6** Neck **8** Chest Wall **F** Abdominal Wall **K** Upper Back DRG **L** Lower Back DRG **M** Perineum, Male ♂ DRG **N** Perineum, Female ♀	**0** Open **3** Percutaneous **4** Percutaneous Endoscopic **X** External	**Z** No Device	**Z** No Qualifier
1 Cranial Cavity **9** Pleural Cavity, Right **B** Pleural Cavity, Left **C** Mediastinum **D** Pericardial Cavity **G** Peritoneal Cavity **H** Retroperitoneum **J** Pelvic Cavity	**0** Open **3** Percutaneous **4** Percutaneous Endoscopic	**Z** No Device	**Z** No Qualifier
P Gastrointestinal Tract **Q** Respiratory Tract **R** Genitourinary Tract	**0** Open **3** Percutaneous **4** Percutaneous Endoscopic **7** Via Natural or Artificial Opening **8** Via Natural or Artificial Opening Endoscopic	**Z** No Device	**Z** No Qualifier

♂ 0WJM0ZZ 0WJM3ZZ 0WJM4ZZ 0WJMXZZ
♀ 0WJN0ZZ 0WJN3ZZ 0WJN4ZZ 0WJNXZZ
DRG 0WJK0ZZ 0WJL0ZZ 0WJM0ZZ 0WJM4ZZ

0 Medical and Surgical
W Anatomical Regions, General
M Reattachment: Putting back in or on all or a portion of a separated body part to its normal location or other suitable location

Body Part Character 4	Approach Character 5	Device Character 6	Qualifier Character 7
2 Face **4** Upper Jaw **5** Lower Jaw **6** Neck **8** Chest Wall **F** Abdominal Wall **K** Upper Back **L** Lower Back **M** Perineum, Male ♂ **N** Perineum, Female ♀	**0** Open	**Z** No Device	**Z** No Qualifier

♂ 0WMM0ZZ
♀ 0WMN0ZZ

0 Medical and Surgical
W Anatomical Regions, General
P Removal: Taking out or off a device from a body part

Body Part Character 4	Approach Character 5	Device Character 6	Qualifier Character 7
0 Head **2** Face **4** Upper Jaw **5** Lower Jaw **6** Neck **8** Chest Wall **C** Mediastinum **F** Abdominal Wall **K** Upper Back **L** Lower Back **M** Perineum, Male ♂ **N** Perineum, Female ♀	**0** Open **3** Percutaneous **4** Percutaneous Endoscopic **X** External	**0** Drainage Device **1** Radioactive Element **3** Infusion Device **7** Autologous Tissue Substitute **J** Synthetic Substitute **K** Nonautologous Tissue Substitute **Y** Other Device	**Z** No Qualifier
1 Cranial Cavity **9** Pleural Cavity, Right **B** Pleural Cavity, Left **G** Peritoneal Cavity **J** Pelvic Cavity	**0** Open **3** Percutaneous **4** Percutaneous Endoscopic	**0** Drainage Device **1** Radioactive Element **3** Infusion Device **J** Synthetic Substitute **Y** Other Device	**Z** No Qualifier
1 Cranial Cavity **9** Pleural Cavity, Right **B** Pleural Cavity, Left **G** Peritoneal Cavity **J** Pelvic Cavity	**X** External	**0** Drainage Device **1** Radioactive Element **3** Infusion Device	**Z** No Qualifier
D Pericardial Cavity **H** Retroperitoneum	**0** Open **3** Percutaneous **4** Percutaneous Endoscopic	**0** Drainage Device **1** Radioactive Element **3** Infusion Device **Y** Other Device	**Z** No Qualifier
D Pericardial Cavity **H** Retroperitoneum	**X** External	**0** Drainage Device **1** Radioactive Element **3** Infusion Device	**Z** No Qualifier
P Gastrointestinal Tract **Q** Respiratory Tract **R** Genitourinary Tract	**0** Open **3** Percutaneous **4** Percutaneous Endoscopic **7** Via Natural or Artificial Opening **8** Via Natural or Artificial Opening Endoscopic **X** External	**1** Radioactive Element **3** Infusion Device **Y** Other Device	**Z** No Qualifier

♂ 0WPM00Z 0WPM01Z 0WPM03Z 0WPM07Z 0WPM0JZ 0WPM0KZ 0WPM0YZ 0WPM30Z 0WPM31Z 0WPM33Z 0WPM37Z 0WPM3JZ 0WPM3KZ 0WPM3YZ 0WPM40Z 0WPM41Z 0WPM43Z 0WPM47Z 0WPM4JZ 0WPM4KZ 0WPM4YZ 0WPMX0Z 0WPMX1Z 0WPMX3Z 0WPMX7Z 0WPMXJZ 0WPMXKZ 0WPMXYZ

♀ 0WPN00Z 0WPN01Z 0WPN03Z 0WPN07Z 0WPN0JZ 0WPN0KZ 0WPN0YZ 0WPN30Z 0WPN31Z 0WPN33Z 0WPN37Z 0WPN3JZ 0WPN3KZ 0WPN3YZ 0WPN40Z 0WPN41Z 0WPN43Z 0WPN47Z 0WPN4JZ 0WPN4KZ 0WPN4YZ 0WPNX0Z 0WPNX1Z 0WPNX3Z 0WPNX7Z 0WPNXJZ 0WPNXKZ 0WPNXYZ

0 Medical and Surgical
W Anatomical Regions, General
Q Repair: Restoring, to the extent possible, a body part to its normal anatomic structure and function

Body Part Character 4	Approach Character 5	Device Character 6	Qualifier Character 7
0 Head **2** Face **3** Oral Cavity and Throat **4** Upper Jaw **5** Lower Jaw **8** Chest Wall CC **K** Upper Back **L** Lower Back **M** Perineum, Male ♂ **N** Perineum, Female CC ♀	**0** Open **3** Percutaneous **4** Percutaneous Endoscopic **X** External	**Z** No Device	**Z** No Qualifier
6 Neck **F** Abdominal Wall	**0** Open **3** Percutaneous **4** Percutaneous Endoscopic	**Z** No Device	**Z** No Qualifier
6 Neck **F** Abdominal Wall CC	**X** External	**Z** No Device	**2** Stoma **Z** No Qualifier
C Mediastinum CC	**0** Open **3** Percutaneous **4** Percutaneous Endoscopic	**Z** No Device	**Z** No Qualifier

♂ 0WQM0ZZ 0WQM3ZZ 0WQM4ZZ 0WQMXZZ
♀ 0WQN0ZZ 0WQN3ZZ 0WQN4ZZ 0WQNXZZ
CC 0WQ80ZZ 0WQ83ZZ 0WQ84ZZ 0WQC0ZZ 0WQC3ZZ 0WQC4ZZ 0WQFXZ2 0WQFXZZ 0WQN0ZZ 0WQN3ZZ 0WQN4ZZ

0 Medical and Surgical
W Anatomical Regions, General
U Supplement: Putting in or on biological or synthetic material that physically reinforces and/or augments the function of a portion of a body part

Body Part Character 4	Approach Character 5	Device Character 6	Qualifier Character 7
0 Head **2** Face **4** Upper Jaw **5** Lower Jaw **6** Neck **8** Chest Wall **C** Mediastinum **F** Abdominal Wall **K** Upper Back **L** Lower Back **M** Perineum, Male ♂ **N** Perineum, Female ♀	**0** Open **4** Percutaneous Endoscopic	**7** Autologous Tissue Substitute **J** Synthetic Substitute **K** Nonautologous Tissue Substitute	**Z** No Qualifier

♂ 0WUM07Z 0WUM0JZ 0WUM0KZ 0WUM47Z 0WUM4JZ 0WUM4KZ
♀ 0WUN07Z 0WUN0JZ 0WUN0KZ 0WUN47Z 0WUN4JZ 0WUN4KZ

0 Medical and Surgical
W Anatomical Regions, General
W Revision: Correcting, to the extent possible, a portion of a malfunctioning device or the position of a displaced device

Body Part Character 4	Approach Character 5	Device Character 6	Qualifier Character 7
0 Head **2** Face **4** Upper Jaw **5** Lower Jaw **6** Neck **8** Chest Wall **C** Mediastinum **F** Abdominal Wall **K** Upper Back DRG **L** Lower Back DRG **M** Perineum, Male ♂ DRG **N** Perineum, Female ♀	**0** Open **3** Percutaneous **4** Percutaneous Endoscopic **X** External	**0** Drainage Device **1** Radioactive Element **3** Infusion Device **7** Autologous Tissue Substitute **J** Synthetic Substitute **K** Nonautologous Tissue Substitute **Y** Other Device	**Z** No Qualifier
1 Cranial Cavity **9** Pleural Cavity, Right **B** Pleural Cavity, Left **G** Peritoneal Cavity **J** Pelvic Cavity	**0** Open **3** Percutaneous **4** Percutaneous Endoscopic **X** External	**0** Drainage Device **1** Radioactive Element **3** Infusion Device **J** Synthetic Substitute **Y** Other Device	**Z** No Qualifier
D Pericardial Cavity **H** Retroperitoneum	**0** Open **3** Percutaneous **4** Percutaneous Endoscopic **X** External	**0** Drainage Device **1** Radioactive Element **3** Infusion Device **Y** Other Device	**Z** No Qualifier
P Gastrointestinal Tract **Q** Respiratory Tract **R** Genitourinary Tract	**0** Open **3** Percutaneous **4** Percutaneous Endoscopic **7** Via Natural or Artificial Opening **8** Via Natural or Artificial Opening Endoscopic **X** External	**1** Radioactive Element **3** Infusion Device **Y** Other Device	**Z** No Qualifier

♂ 0WWM00Z 0WWM01Z 0WWM03Z 0WWM07Z 0WWM0JZ 0WWM0KZ 0WWM0YZ 0WWM30Z 0WWM31Z 0WWM33Z 0WWM37Z 0WWM3JZ 0WWM3KZ 0WWM3YZ 0WWM40Z 0WWM41Z 0WWM43Z 0WWM47Z 0WWM4JZ 0WWM4KZ 0WWM4YZ 0WWMX0Z 0WWMX1Z 0WWMX3Z 0WWMX7Z 0WWMXJZ 0WWMXKZ 0WWMXYZ

♀ 0WWN00Z 0WWN01Z 0WWN03Z 0WWN07Z 0WWN0JZ 0WWN0KZ 0WWN0YZ 0WWN30Z 0WWN31Z 0WWN33Z 0WWN37Z 0WWN3JZ 0WWN3KZ 0WWN3YZ 0WWN40Z 0WWN41Z 0WWN43Z 0WWN47Z 0WWN4JZ 0WWN4KZ 0WWN4YZ 0WWNX0Z 0WWNX1Z 0WWNX3Z 0WWNX7Z 0WWNXJZ 0WWNXKZ 0WWNXYZ

DRG 0WWK00Z 0WWK01Z 0WWK03Z 0WWK07Z 0WWK0JZ 0WWK0KZ 0WWK0YZ 0WWK30Z 0WWK31Z 0WWK33Z 0WWK37Z 0WWK3JZ 0WWK3KZ 0WWK3YZ 0WWK40Z 0WWK41Z 0WWK43Z 0WWK47Z 0WWK4JZ 0WWK4KZ 0WWK4YZ 0WWL00Z 0WWL01Z 0WWL03Z 0WWL07Z 0WWL0JZ 0WWL0KZ 0WWL0YZ 0WWL30Z 0WWL31Z 0WWL33Z 0WWL37Z 0WWL3JZ 0WWL3KZ 0WWL3YZ 0WWL40Z 0WWL41Z 0WWL43Z 0WWL47Z 0WWL4JZ 0WWL4KZ 0WWL4YZ 0WWM00Z 0WWM01Z 0WWM03Z 0WWM0JZ 0WWM0YZ 0WWM30Z 0WWM31Z 0WWM33Z 0WWM3JZ 0WWM3YZ 0WWM40Z 0WWM41Z 0WWM43Z 0WWM4JZ 0WWM4YZ

0 Medical and Surgical
W Anatomical Regions, General
Y Transplantation: Putting in or on all or a portion of a living body part taken from another individual or animal to physically take the place and/or function of all or a portion of a similar body part

Body Part Character 4	Approach Character 5	Device Character 6	Qualifier Character 7
2 Face	**0** Open	**Z** No Device	**0** Allogeneic **1** Syngeneic

NOTES

NOTES

Anatomical Regions, Upper Extremities 0X0-0XY

0 Medical and Surgical
X Anatomical Regions, Upper Extremities
0 Alteration: Modifying the anatomic structure of a body part without affecting the function of the body part

Body Part	Approach	Device	Qualifier
Character 4	**Character 5**	**Character 6**	**Character 7**
2 Shoulder Region, Right **3** Shoulder Region, Left **4** Axilla, Right **5** Axilla, Left **6** Upper Extremity, Right **7** Upper Extremity, Left **8** Upper Arm, Right **9** Upper Arm, Left **B** Elbow Region, Right **C** Elbow Region, Left **D** Lower Arm, Right **F** Lower Arm, Left **G** Wrist Region, Right **H** Wrist Region, Left	**0** Open **3** Percutaneous **4** Percutaneous Endoscopic	**7** Autologous Tissue Substitute **J** Synthetic Substitute **K** Nonautologous Tissue Substitute **Z** No Device	**Z** No Qualifier

0 Medical and Surgical
X Anatomical Regions, Upper Extremities
2 Change: Taking out or off a device from a body part and putting back an identical or similar device in or on the same body part without cutting or puncturing the skin or a mucous membrane

Body Part	Approach	Device	Qualifier
Character 4	**Character 5**	**Character 6**	**Character 7**
6 Upper Extremity, Right **7** Upper Extremity, Left	**X** External	**0** Drainage Device **Y** Other Device	**Z** No Qualifier

0 Medical and Surgical
X Anatomical Regions, Upper Extremities
3 Control: Stopping, or attempting to stop, postprocedural or other acute bleeding

Body Part	Approach	Device	Qualifier
Character 4	**Character 5**	**Character 6**	**Character 7**
2 Shoulder Region, Right **3** Shoulder Region, Left **4** Axilla, Right **5** Axilla, Left **6** Upper Extremity, Right **7** Upper Extremity, Left **8** Upper Arm, Right **9** Upper Arm, Left **B** Elbow Region, Right **C** Elbow Region, Left **D** Lower Arm, Right **F** Lower Arm, Left **G** Wrist Region, Right **H** Wrist Region, Left **J** Hand, Right **K** Hand, Left	**0** Open **3** Percutaneous **4** Percutaneous Endoscopic	**Z** No Device	**Z** No Qualifier

0 Medical and Surgical
X Anatomical Regions, Upper Extremities
6 Detachment: Cutting off all or a portion of the upper or lower extremities

Body Part Character 4	Approach Character 5	Device Character 6	Qualifier Character 7
0 Forequarter, Right **1** Forequarter, Left **2** Shoulder Region, Right **3** Shoulder Region, Left **B** Elbow Region, Right **C** Elbow Region, Left	**0** Open	**Z** No Device	**Z** No Qualifier
8 Upper Arm, Right **9** Upper Arm, Left **D** Lower Arm, Right **F** Lower Arm, Left	**0** Open	**Z** No Device	**1** High **2** Mid **3** Low
J Hand, Right **K** Hand, Left	**0** Open	**Z** No Device	**0** Complete **4** Complete 1st Ray **5** Complete 2nd Ray **6** Complete 3rd Ray **7** Complete 4th Ray **8** Complete 5th Ray **9** Partial 1st Ray **B** Partial 2nd Ray **C** Partial 3rd Ray **D** Partial 4th Ray **F** Partial 5th Ray
L Thumb, Right **M** Thumb, Left **N** Index Finger, Right **P** Index Finger, Left **Q** Middle Finger, Right **R** Middle Finger, Left **S** Ring Finger, Right **T** Ring Finger, Left **V** Little Finger, Right **W** Little Finger, Left	**0** Open	**Z** No Device	**0** Complete **1** High **2** Mid **3** Low

0 Medical and Surgical
X Anatomical Regions, Upper Extremities
9 Drainage: Taking or letting out fluids and/or gases from a body part

Body Part	Approach	Device	Qualifier
Character 4	**Character 5**	**Character 6**	**Character 7**
2 Shoulder Region, Right **3** Shoulder Region, Left **4** Axilla, Right **5** Axilla, Left **6** Upper Extremity, Right **7** Upper Extremity, Left **8** Upper Arm, Right **9** Upper Arm, Left **B** Elbow Region, Right **C** Elbow Region, Left **D** Lower Arm, Right **F** Lower Arm, Left **G** Wrist Region, Right **H** Wrist Region, Left **J** Hand, Right **K** Hand, Left	**0** Open **3** Percutaneous **4** Percutaneous Endoscopic	**0** Drainage Device	**Z** No Qualifier
2 Shoulder Region, Right **3** Shoulder Region, Left **4** Axilla, Right **5** Axilla, Left **6** Upper Extremity, Right **7** Upper Extremity, Left **8** Upper Arm, Right **9** Upper Arm, Left **B** Elbow Region, Right **C** Elbow Region, Left **D** Lower Arm, Right **F** Lower Arm, Left **G** Wrist Region, Right **H** Wrist Region, Left **J** Hand, Right **K** Hand, Left	**0** Open **3** Percutaneous **4** Percutaneous Endoscopic	**Z** No Device	**X** Diagnostic **Z** No Qualifier

0 Medical and Surgical
X Anatomical Regions, Upper Extremities
B Excision: Cutting out or off, without replacement, a portion of a body part

Body Part Character 4	Approach Character 5	Device Character 6	Qualifier Character 7
2 Shoulder Region, Right 3 Shoulder Region, Left 4 Axilla, Right 5 Axilla, Left 6 Upper Extremity, Right 7 Upper Extremity, Left 8 Upper Arm, Right 9 Upper Arm, Left B Elbow Region, Right C Elbow Region, Left D Lower Arm, Right F Lower Arm, Left G Wrist Region, Right H Wrist Region, Left J Hand, Right K Hand, Left	0 Open 3 Percutaneous 4 Percutaneous Endoscopic	Z No Device	X Diagnostic Z No Qualifier

0 Medical and Surgical
X Anatomical Regions, Upper Extremities
H Insertion: Putting in a nonbiological appliance that monitors, assists, performs, or prevents a physiological function but does not physically take the place of a body part

Body Part Character 4	Approach Character 5	Device Character 6	Qualifier Character 7
2 Shoulder Region, Right DRG 3 Shoulder Region, Left DRG 4 Axilla, Right DRG 5 Axilla, Left DRG 6 Upper Extremity, Right 7 Upper Extremity, Left 8 Upper Arm, Right 9 Upper Arm, Left B Elbow Region, Right C Elbow Region, Left D Lower Arm, Right F Lower Arm, Left G Wrist Region, Right H Wrist Region, Left J Hand, Right K Hand, Left	0 Open 3 Percutaneous 4 Percutaneous Endoscopic	1 Radioactive Element 3 Infusion Device Y Other Device	Z No Qualifier

DRG 0XH203Z 0XH20YZ 0XH233Z 0XH23YZ 0XH243Z 0XH24YZ 0XH303Z 0XH30YZ 0XH333Z 0XH33YZ 0XH343Z 0XH34YZ 0XH403Z 0XH40YZ 0XH433Z 0XH43YZ 0XH443Z 0XH44YZ 0XH503Z 0XH50YZ 0XH533Z 0XH53YZ

0 Medical and Surgical
X Anatomical Regions, Upper Extremities
J Inspection: Visually and/or manually exploring a body part

Body Part Character 4	Approach Character 5	Device Character 6	Qualifier Character 7
2 Shoulder Region, Right **3** Shoulder Region, Left **4** Axilla, Right **5** Axilla, Left **6** Upper Extremity, Right **7** Upper Extremity, Left **8** Upper Arm, Right **9** Upper Arm, Left **B** Elbow Region, Right **C** Elbow Region, Left **D** Lower Arm, Right **F** Lower Arm, Left **G** Wrist Region, Right **H** Wrist Region, Left **J** Hand, Right **K** Hand, Left	**0** Open **3** Percutaneous **4** Percutaneous Endoscopic **X** External	**Z** No Device	**Z** No Qualifier

0 Medical and Surgical
X Anatomical Regions, Upper Extremities
M Reattachment: Putting back in or on all or a portion of a separated body part to its normal location or other suitable location

Body Part Character 4	Approach Character 5	Device Character 6	Qualifier Character 7
0 Forequarter, Right **1** Forequarter, Left **2** Shoulder Region, Right **3** Shoulder Region, Left **4** Axilla, Right **5** Axilla, Left **6** Upper Extremity, Right **7** Upper Extremity, Left **8** Upper Arm, Right **9** Upper Arm, Left **B** Elbow Region, Right **C** Elbow Region, Left **D** Lower Arm, Right **F** Lower Arm, Left **G** Wrist Region, Right **H** Wrist Region, Left **J** Hand, Right **K** Hand, Left **L** Thumb, Right **M** Thumb, Left **N** Index Finger, Right **P** Index Finger, Left **Q** Middle Finger, Right **R** Middle Finger, Left **S** Ring Finger, Right **T** Ring Finger, Left **V** Little Finger, Right **W** Little Finger, Left	**0** Open	**Z** No Device	**Z** No Qualifier

0 Medical and Surgical
X Anatomical Regions, Upper Extremities
P Removal: Taking out or off a device from a body part

Body Part Character 4	Approach Character 5	Device Character 6	Qualifier Character 7
6 Upper Extremity, Right **7** Upper Extremity, Left	**0** Open **3** Percutaneous **4** Percutaneous Endoscopic **X** External	**0** Drainage Device **1** Radioactive Element **3** Infusion Device **7** Autologous Tissue Substitute **J** Synthetic Substitute **K** Nonautologous Tissue Substitute **Y** Other Device	**Z** No Qualifier

0 Medical and Surgical
X Anatomical Regions, Upper Extremities
Q Repair: Restoring, to the extent possible, a body part to its normal anatomic structure and function

Body Part Character 4	Approach Character 5	Device Character 6	Qualifier Character 7
2 Shoulder Region, Right **3** Shoulder Region, Left **4** Axilla, Right **5** Axilla, Left **6** Upper Extremity, Right **7** Upper Extremity, Left **8** Upper Arm, Right **9** Upper Arm, Left **B** Elbow Region, Right **C** Elbow Region, Left **D** Lower Arm, Right **F** Lower Arm, Left **G** Wrist Region, Right **H** Wrist Region, Left **J** Hand, Right **K** Hand, Left **L** Thumb, Right **M** Thumb, Left **N** Index Finger, Right **P** Index Finger, Left **Q** Middle Finger, Right **R** Middle Finger, Left **S** Ring Finger, Right **T** Ring Finger, Left **V** Little Finger, Right **W** Little Finger, Left	**0** Open **3** Percutaneous **4** Percutaneous Endoscopic **X** External	**Z** No Device	**Z** No Qualifier

0 Medical and Surgical
X Anatomical Regions, Upper Extremities
R Replacement: Putting in or on biological or synthetic material that physically takes the place and/or function of all or a portion of a body part

Body Part Character 4	Approach Character 5	Device Character 6	Qualifier Character 7
L Thumb, Right **M** Thumb, Left	**0** Open **4** Percutaneous Endoscopic	**7** Autologous Tissue Substitute	**N** Toe, Right **P** Toe, Left

0 Medical and Surgical
X Anatomical Regions, Upper Extremities
U Supplement: Putting in or on biological or synthetic material that physically reinforces and/or augments the function of a portion of a body part

Body Part	Approach	Device	Qualifier
Character 4	Character 5	Character 6	Character 7
2 Shoulder Region, Right **3** Shoulder Region, Left **4** Axilla, Right **5** Axilla, Left **6** Upper Extremity, Right **7** Upper Extremity, Left **8** Upper Arm, Right **9** Upper Arm, Left **B** Elbow Region, Right **C** Elbow Region, Left **D** Lower Arm, Right **F** Lower Arm, Left **G** Wrist Region, Right **H** Wrist Region, Left **J** Hand, Right **K** Hand, Left **L** Thumb, Right **M** Thumb, Left **N** Index Finger, Right **P** Index Finger, Left **Q** Middle Finger, Right **R** Middle Finger, Left **S** Ring Finger, Right **T** Ring Finger, Left **V** Little Finger, Right **W** Little Finger, Left	**0** Open **4** Percutaneous Endoscopic	**7** Autologous Tissue Substitute **J** Synthetic Substitute **K** Nonautologous Tissue Substitute	**Z** No Qualifier

0 Medical and Surgical
X Anatomical Regions, Upper Extremities
W Revision: Correcting, to the extent possible, a portion of a malfunctioning device or the position of a displaced device

Body Part	Approach	Device	Qualifier
Character 4	Character 5	Character 6	Character 7
6 Upper Extremity, Right DRG **7** Upper Extremity, Left DRG	**0** Open **3** Percutaneous **4** Percutaneous Endoscopic **X** External	**0** Drainage Device **3** Infusion Device **7** Autologous Tissue Substitute **J** Synthetic Substitute **K** Nonautologous Tissue Substitute **Y** Other Device	**Z** No Qualifier

DRG 0XW600Z 0XW603Z 0XW607Z 0XW60JZ 0XW60KZ 0XW60YZ 0XW630Z 0XW633Z 0XW637Z 0XW63JZ 0XW63KZ 0XW63YZ 0XW640Z 0XW643Z 0XW647Z 0XW64JZ 0XW64KZ 0XW64YZ 0XW700Z 0XW703Z 0XW707Z 0XW70JZ 0XW70KZ 0XW70YZ 0XW730Z 0XW733Z 0XW737Z 0XW73JZ 0XW73KZ 0XW73YZ 0XW740Z 0XW743Z 0XW747Z 0XW74JZ 0XW74KZ 0XW74YZ

0 Medical and Surgical
X Anatomical Regions, Upper Extremities
X Transfer: Moving, without taking out, all or a portion of a body part to another location to take over the function of all or a portion of a body part

Body Part	Approach	Device	Qualifier
Character 4	Character 5	Character 6	Character 7
N Index Finger, Right	**0** Open	**Z** No Device	**L** Thumb, Right
P Index Finger, Left	**0** Open	**Z** No Device	**M** Thumb, Left

0 Medical and Surgical
X Anatomical Regions, Upper Extremities
Y Transplantation: Putting in or on all or a portion of a living body part taken from another individual or animal to physically take the place and/or function of all or a portion of a similar body part

Body Part	Approach	Device	Qualifier
Character 4	Character 5	Character 6	Character 7
J Hand, Right **K** Hand, Left	**0** Open	**Z** No Device	**0** Allogeneic **1** Syngeneic

LC Limited Coverage NC Noncovered HAC HAC-associated Procedure CC Combination Cluster - See Appendix G for code lists
DRG Non-OR-Affecting MS-DRG Assignment New/Revised Text in **Orange** ♂ Male ♀ Female

NOTES

Anatomical Regions, Lower Extremities 0Y0-0YW

0 Medical and Surgical
Y Anatomical Regions, Lower Extremities
0 Alteration: Modifying the anatomic structure of a body part without affecting the function of the body part

Body Part Character 4	Approach Character 5	Device Character 6	Qualifier Character 7
0 Buttock, Right **1** Buttock, Left **9** Lower Extremity, Right **B** Lower Extremity, Left **C** Upper Leg, Right **D** Upper Leg, Left **F** Knee Region, Right **G** Knee Region, Left **H** Lower Leg, Right **J** Lower Leg, Left **K** Ankle Region, Right **L** Ankle Region, Left	**0** Open **3** Percutaneous **4** Percutaneous Endoscopic	**7** Autologous Tissue Substitute **J** Synthetic Substitute **K** Nonautologous Tissue Substitute **Z** No Device	**Z** No Qualifier

0 Medical and Surgical
Y Anatomical Regions, Lower Extremities
2 Change: Taking out or off a device from a body part and putting back an identical or similar device in or on the same body part without cutting or puncturing the skin or a mucous membrane

Body Part Character 4	Approach Character 5	Device Character 6	Qualifier Character 7
9 Lower Extremity, Right **B** Lower Extremity, Left	**X** External	**0** Drainage Device **Y** Other Device	**Z** No Qualifier

0 Medical and Surgical
Y Anatomical Regions, Lower Extremities
3 Control: Stopping, or attempting to stop, postprocedural or other acute bleeding

Body Part Character 4	Approach Character 5	Device Character 6	Qualifier Character 7
0 Buttock, Right **1** Buttock, Left **5** Inguinal Region, Right **6** Inguinal Region, Left **7** Femoral Region, Right **8** Femoral Region, Left **9** Lower Extremity, Right **B** Lower Extremity, Left **C** Upper Leg, Right **D** Upper Leg, Left **F** Knee Region, Right **G** Knee Region, Left **H** Lower Leg, Right **J** Lower Leg, Left **K** Ankle Region, Right **L** Ankle Region, Left **M** Foot, Right **N** Foot, Left	**0** Open **3** Percutaneous **4** Percutaneous Endoscopic	**Z** No Device	**Z** No Qualifier

0 Medical and Surgical
Y Anatomical Regions, Lower Extremities
6 Detachment: Cutting off all or a portion of the upper or lower extremities

Body Part Character 4	Approach Character 5	Device Character 6	Qualifier Character 7
2 Hindquarter, Right **3** Hindquarter, Left **4** Hindquarter, Bilateral **7** Femoral Region, Right **8** Femoral Region, Left **F** Knee Region, Right **G** Knee Region, Left	**0** Open	**Z** No Device	**Z** No Qualifier
C Upper Leg, Right **D** Upper Leg, Left **H** Lower Leg, Right **J** Lower Leg, Left	**0** Open	**Z** No Device	**1** High **2** Mid **3** Low
M Foot, Right **N** Foot, Left	**0** Open	**Z** No Device	**0** Complete **4** Complete 1st Ray **5** Complete 2nd Ray **6** Complete 3rd Ray **7** Complete 4th Ray **8** Complete 5th Ray **9** Partial 1st Ray **B** Partial 2nd Ray **C** Partial 3rd Ray **D** Partial 4th Ray **F** Partial 5th Ray
P 1st Toe, Right **Q** 1st Toe, Left **R** 2nd Toe, Right **S** 2nd Toe, Left **T** 3rd Toe, Right **U** 3rd Toe, Left **V** 4th Toe, Right **W** 4th Toe, Left **X** 5th Toe, Right **Y** 5th Toe, Left	**0** Open	**Z** No Device	**0** Complete **1** High **2** Mid **3** Low

0 Medical and Surgical
Y Anatomical Regions, Lower Extremities
9 Drainage: Taking or letting out fluids and/or gases from a body part

Body Part Character 4	Approach Character 5	Device Character 6	Qualifier Character 7
0 Buttock, Right **1** Buttock, Left **5** Inguinal Region, Right **6** Inguinal Region, Left **7** Femoral Region, Right **8** Femoral Region, Left **9** Lower Extremity, Right **B** Lower Extremity, Left **C** Upper Leg, Right **D** Upper Leg, Left **F** Knee Region, Right **G** Knee Region, Left **H** Lower Leg, Right **J** Lower Leg, Left **K** Ankle Region, Right **L** Ankle Region, Left **M** Foot, Right **N** Foot, Left	**0** Open **3** Percutaneous **4** Percutaneous Endoscopic	**0** Drainage Device	**Z** No Qualifier
0 Buttock, Right **1** Buttock, Left **5** Inguinal Region, Right **6** Inguinal Region, Left **7** Femoral Region, Right **8** Femoral Region, Left **9** Lower Extremity, Right **B** Lower Extremity, Left **C** Upper Leg, Right **D** Upper Leg, Left **F** Knee Region, Right **G** Knee Region, Left **H** Lower Leg, Right **J** Lower Leg, Left **K** Ankle Region, Right **L** Ankle Region, Left **M** Foot, Right **N** Foot, Left	**0** Open **3** Percutaneous **4** Percutaneous Endoscopic	**Z** No Device	**X** Diagnostic **Z** No Qualifier

0 Medical and Surgical
Y Anatomical Regions, Lower Extremities
B Excision: Cutting out or off, without replacement, a portion of a body part

Body Part Character 4	Approach Character 5	Device Character 6	Qualifier Character 7
0 Buttock, Right **1** Buttock, Left **5** Inguinal Region, Right **6** Inguinal Region, Left **7** Femoral Region, Right **8** Femoral Region, Left **9** Lower Extremity, Right **B** Lower Extremity, Left **C** Upper Leg, Right **D** Upper Leg, Left **F** Knee Region, Right **G** Knee Region, Left **H** Lower Leg, Right **J** Lower Leg, Left **K** Ankle Region, Right **L** Ankle Region, Left **M** Foot, Right **N** Foot, Left	**0** Open **3** Percutaneous **4** Percutaneous Endoscopic	**Z** No Device	**X** Diagnostic **Z** No Qualifier

0 Medical and Surgical
Y Anatomical Regions, Lower Extremities
H Insertion: Putting in a nonbiological appliance that monitors, assists, performs, or prevents a physiological function but does not physically take the place of a body part

Body Part Character 4	Approach Character 5	Device Character 6	Qualifier Character 7
0 Buttock, Right **1** Buttock, Left **5** Inguinal Region, Right **6** Inguinal Region, Left **7** Femoral Region, Right **8** Femoral Region, Left **9** Lower Extremity, Right **B** Lower Extremity, Left **C** Upper Leg, Right **D** Upper Leg, Left **F** Knee Region, Right **G** Knee Region, Left **H** Lower Leg, Right **J** Lower Leg, Left **K** Ankle Region, Right **L** Ankle Region, Left **M** Foot, Right **N** Foot, Left	**0** Open **3** Percutaneous **4** Percutaneous Endoscopic	**1** Radioactive Element **3** Infusion Device **Y** Other Device	**Z** No Qualifier

0 Medical and Surgical
Y Anatomical Regions, Lower Extremities
J Inspection: Visually and/or manually exploring a body part

Body Part Character 4	Approach Character 5	Device Character 6	Qualifier Character 7
0 Buttock, Right **1** Buttock, Left **5** Inguinal Region, Right **6** Inguinal Region, Left **7** Femoral Region, Right **8** Femoral Region, Left **9** Lower Extremity, Right **A** Inguinal Region, Bilateral **B** Lower Extremity, Left **C** Upper Leg, Right **D** Upper Leg, Left **E** Femoral Region, Bilateral **F** Knee Region, Right **G** Knee Region, Left **H** Lower Leg, Right **J** Lower Leg, Left **K** Ankle Region, Right **L** Ankle Region, Left **M** Foot, Right **N** Foot, Left	**0** Open **3** Percutaneous **4** Percutaneous Endoscopic **X** External	**Z** No Device	**Z** No Qualifier

0 Medical and Surgical
Y Anatomical Regions, Lower Extremities
M Reattachment: Putting back in or on all or a portion of a separated body part to its normal location or other suitable location

Body Part Character 4	Approach Character 5	Device Character 6	Qualifier Character 7
0 Buttock, Right **1** Buttock, Left **2** Hindquarter, Right **3** Hindquarter, Left **4** Hindquarter, Bilateral **5** Inguinal Region, Right **6** Inguinal Region, Left **7** Femoral Region, Right **8** Femoral Region, Left **9** Lower Extremity, Right **B** Lower Extremity, Left **C** Upper Leg, Right **D** Upper Leg, Left **F** Knee Region, Right **G** Knee Region, Left **H** Lower Leg, Right **J** Lower Leg, Left **K** Ankle Region, Right **L** Ankle Region, Left **M** Foot, Right **N** Foot, Left **P** 1st Toe, Right **Q** 1st Toe, Left **R** 2nd Toe, Right **S** 2nd Toe, Left **T** 3rd Toe, Right **U** 3rd Toe, Left **V** 4th Toe, Right **W** 4th Toe, Left **X** 5th Toe, Right **Y** 5th Toe, Left	**0** Open	**Z** No Device	**Z** No Qualifier

0 Medical and Surgical
Y Anatomical Regions, Lower Extremities
P Removal: Taking out or off a device from a body part

Body Part Character 4	Approach Character 5	Device Character 6	Qualifier Character 7
9 Lower Extremity, Right **B** Lower Extremity, Left	**0** Open **3** Percutaneous **4** Percutaneous Endoscopic **X** External	**0** Drainage Device **1** Radioactive Element **3** Infusion Device **7** Autologous Tissue Substitute **J** Synthetic Substitute **K** Nonautologous Tissue Substitute **Y** Other Device	**Z** No Qualifier

0 Medical and Surgical
Y Anatomical Regions, Lower Extremities
Q Repair: Restoring, to the extent possible, a body part to its normal anatomic structure and function

Body Part Character 4	Approach Character 5	Device Character 6	Qualifier Character 7
0 Buttock, Right **1** Buttock, Left **5** Inguinal Region, Right **6** Inguinal Region, Left **7** Femoral Region, Right **8** Femoral Region, Left **9** Lower Extremity, Right **A** Inguinal Region, Bilateral **B** Lower Extremity, Left **C** Upper Leg, Right **D** Upper Leg, Left **E** Femoral Region, Bilateral **F** Knee Region, Right **G** Knee Region, Left **H** Lower Leg, Right **J** Lower Leg, Left **K** Ankle Region, Right **L** Ankle Region, Left **M** Foot, Right **N** Foot, Left **P** 1st Toe, Right **Q** 1st Toe, Left **R** 2nd Toe, Right **S** 2nd Toe, Left **T** 3rd Toe, Right **U** 3rd Toe, Left **V** 4th Toe, Right **W** 4th Toe, Left **X** 5th Toe, Right **Y** 5th Toe, Left	**0** Open **3** Percutaneous **4** Percutaneous Endoscopic **X** External	**Z** No Device	**Z** No Qualifier

0 Medical and Surgical
Y Anatomical Regions, Lower Extremities
U Supplement: Putting in or on biological or synthetic material that physically reinforces and/or augments the function of a portion of a body part

Body Part	Approach	Device	Qualifier
Character 4	**Character 5**	**Character 6**	**Character 7**
0 Buttock, Right **1** Buttock, Left **5** Inguinal Region, Right **6** Inguinal Region, Left **7** Femoral Region, Right **8** Femoral Region, Left **9** Lower Extremity, Right **A** Inguinal Region, Bilateral **B** Lower Extremity, Left **C** Upper Leg, Right **D** Upper Leg, Left **E** Femoral Region, Bilateral **F** Knee Region, Right **G** Knee Region, Left **H** Lower Leg, Right **J** Lower Leg, Left **K** Ankle Region, Right **L** Ankle Region, Left **M** Foot, Right **N** Foot, Left **P** 1st Toe, Right **Q** 1st Toe, Left **R** 2nd Toe, Right **S** 2nd Toe, Left **T** 3rd Toe, Right **U** 3rd Toe, Left **V** 4th Toe, Right **W** 4th Toe, Left **X** 5th Toe, Right **Y** 5th Toe, Left	**0** Open **4** Percutaneous Endoscopic	**7** Autologous Tissue Substitute **J** Synthetic Substitute **K** Nonautologous Tissue Substitute	**Z** No Qualifier

0 Medical and Surgical
Y Anatomical Regions, Lower Extremities
W Revision: Correcting, to the extent possible, a portion of a malfunctioning device or the position of a displaced device

Body Part	Approach	Device	Qualifier
Character 4	**Character 5**	**Character 6**	**Character 7**
9 Lower Extremity, Right **B** Lower Extremity, Left	**0** Open **3** Percutaneous **4** Percutaneous Endoscopic **X** External	**0** Drainage Device **3** Infusion Device **7** Autologous Tissue Substitute **J** Synthetic Substitute **K** Nonautologous Tissue Substitute **Y** Other Device	**Z** No Qualifier

NOTES

Obstetrics 102-10Y

1 Obstetrics
0 Pregnancy
2 Change: Taking out or off a device from a body part and putting back an identical or similar device in or on the same body part without cutting or puncturing the skin or a mucous membrane

Body Part	Approach	Device	Qualifier
Character 4	**Character 5**	**Character 6**	**Character 7**
0 Products of Conception ♀	**7** Via Natural or Artificial Opening	**3** Monitoring Electrode **Y** Other Device	**Z** No Qualifier

♀ 102073Z 10207YZ

1 Obstetrics
0 Pregnancy
9 Drainage: Taking or letting out fluids and/or gases from a body part

Body Part	Approach	Device	Qualifier
Character 4	**Character 5**	**Character 6**	**Character 7**
0 Products of Conception ♀	**0** Open **3** Percutaneous **4** Percutaneous Endoscopic **7** Via Natural or Artificial Opening **8** Via Natural or Artificial Opening Endoscopic	**Z** No Device	**9** Fetal Blood **A** Fetal Cerebrospinal Fluid **B** Fetal Fluid, Other **C** Amniotic Fluid, Therapeutic **D** Fluid, Other **U** Amniotic Fluid, Diagnostic

♀ 10900Z9 10900ZA 10900ZB 10900ZC 10900ZD 10900ZU 10903Z9 10903ZA 10903ZB 10903ZC 10903ZD 10903ZU 10904Z9 10904ZA 10904ZB 10904ZC 10904ZD 10904ZU 10907Z9 10907ZA 10907ZB 10907ZC 10907ZD 10907ZU 10908Z9 10908ZA 10908ZB 10908ZC 10908ZD 10908ZU

1 Obstetrics
0 Pregnancy
A Abortion: Artificially terminating a pregnancy

Body Part	Approach	Device	Qualifier
Character 4	**Character 5**	**Character 6**	**Character 7**
0 Products of Conception ♀	**0** Open **3** Percutaneous **4** Percutaneous Endoscopic **8** Via Natural or Artificial Opening Endoscopic	**Z** No Device	**Z** No Qualifier
0 Products of Conception ♀	**7** Via Natural or Artificial Opening	**Z** No Device	**6** Vacuum **W** Laminaria **X** Abortifacient **Z** No Qualifier

♀ 10A00ZZ 10A03ZZ 10A04ZZ 10A07Z6 10A07ZW 10A07ZX 10A07ZZ 10A08ZZ

1 Obstetrics
0 Pregnancy
D Extraction: Pulling or stripping out or off all or a portion of a body part by the use of force

Body Part Character 4	Approach Character 5	Device Character 6	Qualifier Character 7
0 Products of Conception ♀	0 Open	Z No Device	0 High 1 Low 2 Extraperitoneal
0 Products of Conception ♀ CC	7 Via Natural or Artificial Opening	Z No Device	3 Low Forceps 4 Mid Forceps 5 High Forceps 6 Vacuum 7 Internal Version 8 Other
1 Products of Conception, Retained ♀	7 Via Natural or Artificial Opening 8 Via Natural or Artificial Opening Endoscopic	Z No Device	9 Manual Z No Qualifier
2 Products of Conception, Ectopic ♀	7 Via Natural or Artificial Opening 8 Via Natural or Artificial Opening Endoscopic	Z No Device	Z No Qualifier

♀ 10D00Z0 10D00Z1 10D00Z2 10D07Z3 10D07Z4 10D07Z5 10D07Z6 10D07Z7 10D07Z8 10D17Z9 10D17ZZ 10D18Z9 10D18ZZ 10D27ZZ 10D28ZZ

CC 10D07Z3 10D07Z4 10D07Z5 10D07Z6

1 Obstetrics
0 Pregnancy
E Delivery: Assisting the passage of the products of conception from the genital canal

Body Part Character 4	Approach Character 5	Device Character 6	Qualifier Character 7
0 Products of Conception ♀ CC	X External	Z No Device	Z No Qualifier

♀ 10E0XZZ

CC 10E0XZZ

1 Obstetrics
0 Pregnancy
H Insertion: Putting in a nonbiological appliance that monitors, assists, performs, or prevents a physiological function but does not physically take the place of a body part

Body Part Character 4	Approach Character 5	Device Character 6	Qualifier Character 7
0 Products of Conception ♀	0 Open 7 Via Natural or Artificial Opening	3 Monitoring Electrode Y Other Device	Z No Qualifier

♀ 10H003Z 10H00YZ 10H073Z 10H07YZ

1 Obstetrics
0 Pregnancy
J Inspection: Visually and/or manually exploring a body part

Body Part Character 4	Approach Character 5	Device Character 6	Qualifier Character 7
0 Products of Conception ♀ 1 Products of Conception, Retained ♀ 2 Products of Conception, Ectopic ♀	0 Open 3 Percutaneous 4 Percutaneous Endoscopic 7 Via Natural or Artificial Opening 8 Via Natural or Artificial Opening Endoscopic X External	Z No Device	Z No Qualifier

♀ 10J00ZZ 10J03ZZ 10J04ZZ 10J07ZZ 10J08ZZ 10J0XZZ 10J10ZZ 10J13ZZ 10J14ZZ 10J17ZZ 10J18ZZ 10J1XZZ 10J20ZZ 10J23ZZ 10J24ZZ 10J27ZZ 10J28ZZ 10J2XZZ

1 Obstetrics
0 Pregnancy
P Removal: Taking out or off a device from a body part, region, or orifice

Body Part Character 4	Approach Character 5	Device Character 6	Qualifier Character 7
0 Products of Conception ♀	**0** Open **7** Via Natural or Artificial Opening	**3** Monitoring Electrode **Y** Other Device	**Z** No Qualifier

♀ 10P003Z 10P00YZ 10P073Z 10P07YZ

1 Obstetrics
0 Pregnancy
Q Repair: Restoring, to the extent possible, a body part to its normal anatomic structure and function

Body Part Character 4	Approach Character 5	Device Character 6	Qualifier Character 7
0 Products of Conception ♀	**0** Open **3** Percutaneous **4** Percutaneous Endoscopic **7** Via Natural or Artificial Opening **8** Via Natural or Artificial Opening Endoscopic	**Y** Other Device **Z** No Device	**E** Nervous System **F** Cardiovascular System **G** Lymphatics and Hemic **H** Eye **J** Ear, Nose and Sinus **K** Respiratory System **L** Mouth and Throat **M** Gastrointestinal System **N** Hepatobiliary and Pancreas **P** Endocrine System **Q** Skin **R** Musculoskeletal System **S** Urinary System **T** Female Reproductive System **V** Male Reproductive System **Y** Other Body System

♀ 10Q00YE 10Q00YF 10Q00YG 10Q00YH 10Q00YJ 10Q00YK 10Q00YL 10Q00YM 10Q00YN 10Q00YP 10Q00YQ 10Q00YR 10Q00YS
10Q00YT 10Q00YV 10Q00YY 10Q00ZE 10Q00ZF 10Q00ZG 10Q00ZH 10Q00ZJ 10Q00ZK 10Q00ZL 10Q00ZM 10Q00ZN 10Q00ZP
10Q00ZQ 10Q00ZR 10Q00ZS 10Q00ZT 10Q00ZV 10Q00ZY 10Q03YE 10Q03YF 10Q03YG 10Q03YH 10Q03YJ 10Q03YK 10Q03YL
10Q03YM 10Q03YN 10Q03YP 10Q03YQ 10Q03YR 10Q03YS 10Q03YT 10Q03YV 10Q03YY 10Q03ZE 10Q03ZF 10Q03ZG 10Q03ZH
10Q03ZJ 10Q03ZK 10Q03ZL 10Q03ZM 10Q03ZN 10Q03ZP 10Q03ZQ 10Q03ZR 10Q03ZS 10Q03ZT 10Q03ZV 10Q03ZY 10Q04YE
10Q04YF 10Q04YG 10Q04YH 10Q04YJ 10Q04YK 10Q04YL 10Q04YM 10Q04YN 10Q04YP 10Q04YQ 10Q04YR 10Q04YS 10Q04YT
10Q04YV 10Q04YY 10Q04ZE 10Q04ZF 10Q04ZG 10Q04ZH 10Q04ZJ 10Q04ZK 10Q04ZL 10Q04ZM 10Q04ZN 10Q04ZP 10Q04ZQ
10Q04ZR 10Q04ZS 10Q04ZT 10Q04ZV 10Q04ZY 10Q07YE 10Q07YF 10Q07YG 10Q07YH 10Q07YJ 10Q07YK 10Q07YL 10Q07YM
10Q07YN 10Q07YP 10Q07YQ 10Q07YR 10Q07YS 10Q07YT 10Q07YV 10Q07YY 10Q07ZE 10Q07ZF 10Q07ZG 10Q07ZH 10Q07ZJ
10Q07ZK 10Q07ZL 10Q07ZM 10Q07ZN 10Q07ZP 10Q07ZQ 10Q07ZR 10Q07ZS 10Q07ZT 10Q07ZV 10Q07ZY 10Q08YE 10Q08YF
10Q08YG 10Q08YH 10Q08YJ 10Q08YK 10Q08YL 10Q08YM 10Q08YN 10Q08YP 10Q08YQ 10Q08YR 10Q08YS 10Q08YT 10Q08YV
10Q08YY 10Q08ZE 10Q08ZF 10Q08ZG 10Q08ZH 10Q08ZJ 10Q08ZK 10Q08ZL 10Q08ZM 10Q08ZN 10Q08ZP 10Q08ZQ 10Q08ZR
10Q08ZS 10Q08ZT 10Q08ZV 10Q08ZY

1 Obstetrics
0 Pregnancy
S Reposition: Moving to its normal location, or other suitable location, all or a portion of a body part

Body Part Character 4	Approach Character 5	Device Character 6	Qualifier Character 7
0 Products of Conception ♀	**7** Via Natural or Artificial Opening **X** External	**Z** No Device	**Z** No Qualifier
2 Products of Conception, Ectopic ♀	**0** Open **3** Percutaneous **4** Percutaneous Endoscopic **7** Via Natural or Artificial Opening **8** Via Natural or Artificial Opening Endoscopic	**Z** No Device	**Z** No Qualifier

♀ 10S07ZZ 10S0XZZ 10S20ZZ 10S23ZZ 10S24ZZ 10S27ZZ 10S28ZZ

1 Obstetrics
0 Pregnancy
T Resection: Cutting out or off, without replacement, all of a body part

Body Part Character 4	Approach Character 5	Device Character 6	Qualifier Character 7
2 Products of Conception, Ectopic ♀	**0** Open **3** Percutaneous **4** Percutaneous Endoscopic **7** Via Natural or Artificial Opening **8** Via Natural or Artificial Opening Endoscopic	**Z** No Device	**Z** No Qualifier

♀ 10T20ZZ 10T23ZZ 10T24ZZ 10T27ZZ 10T28ZZ

1 Obstetrics
0 Pregnancy
Y Transplantation: Putting in or on all or a portion of a living body part taken from another individual or animal to physically take the place and/or function of all or a portion of a similar body part

Body Part Character 4	Approach Character 5	Device Character 6	Qualifier Character 7
0 Products of Conception ♀	**3** Percutaneous **4** Percutaneous Endoscopic **7** Via Natural or Artificial Opening	**Z** No Device	**E** Nervous System **F** Cardiovascular System **G** Lymphatics and Hemic **H** Eye **J** Ear, Nose and Sinus **K** Respiratory System **L** Mouth and Throat **M** Gastrointestinal System **N** Hepatobiliary and Pancreas **P** Endocrine System **Q** Skin **R** Musculoskeletal System **S** Urinary System **T** Female Reproductive System **V** Male Reproductive System **Y** Other Body System

♀ 10Y03ZE 10Y03ZF 10Y03ZG 10Y03ZH 10Y03ZJ 10Y03ZK 10Y03ZL 10Y03ZM 10Y03ZN 10Y03ZP 10Y03ZQ 10Y03ZR 10Y03ZS 10Y03ZT 10Y03ZV 10Y03ZY 10Y04ZE 10Y04ZF 10Y04ZG 10Y04ZH 10Y04ZJ 10Y04ZK 10Y04ZL 10Y04ZM 10Y04ZN 10Y04ZP 10Y04ZQ 10Y04ZR 10Y04ZS 10Y04ZT 10Y04ZV 10Y04ZY 10Y07ZE 10Y07ZF 10Y07ZG 10Y07ZH 10Y07ZJ 10Y07ZK 10Y07ZL 10Y07ZM 10Y07ZN 10Y07ZP 10Y07ZQ 10Y07ZR 10Y07ZS 10Y07ZT 10Y07ZV 10Y07ZY

NOTES

NOTES

Placement-Anatomical Regions 2W0-2W6

2 Placement
W Anatomical Regions
0 Change: Taking out or off a device from a body part and putting back an identical or similar device in or on the same body part without cutting or puncturing the skin or a mucous membrane

Body Region Character 4	Approach Character 5	Device Character 6	Qualifier Character 7
0 Head **2** Neck **3** Abdominal Wall **4** Chest Wall **5** Back **6** Inguinal Region, Right **7** Inguinal Region, Left **8** Upper Extremity, Right **9** Upper Extremity, Left **A** Upper Arm, Right **B** Upper Arm, Left **C** Lower Arm, Right **D** Lower Arm, Left **E** Hand, Right **F** Hand, Left **G** Thumb, Right **H** Thumb, Left **J** Finger, Right **K** Finger, Left **L** Lower Extremity, Right **M** Lower Extremity, Left **N** Upper Leg, Right **P** Upper Leg, Left **Q** Lower Leg, Right **R** Lower Leg, Left **S** Foot, Right **T** Foot, Left **U** Toe, Right **V** Toe, Left	**X** External	**0** Traction Apparatus **1** Splint **2** Cast **3** Brace **4** Bandage **5** Packing Material **6** Pressure Dressing **7** Intermittent Pressure Device **Y** Other Device	**Z** No Qualifier
1 Face	**X** External	**0** Traction Apparatus **1** Splint **2** Cast **3** Brace **4** Bandage **5** Packing Material **6** Pressure Dressing **7** Intermittent Pressure Device **9** Wire **Y** Other Device	**Z** No Qualifier

2 Placement
W Anatomical Regions
1 Compression: Putting pressure on a body region

Body Region Character 4	Approach Character 5	Device Character 6	Qualifier Character 7
0 Head **1** Face **2** Neck **3** Abdominal Wall **4** Chest Wall **5** Back **6** Inguinal Region, Right **7** Inguinal Region, Left **8** Upper Extremity, Right **9** Upper Extremity, Left **A** Upper Arm, Right **B** Upper Arm, Left **C** Lower Arm, Right **D** Lower Arm, Left **E** Hand, Right **F** Hand, Left **G** Thumb, Right **H** Thumb, Left **J** Finger, Right **K** Finger, Left **L** Lower Extremity, Right **M** Lower Extremity, Left **N** Upper Leg, Right **P** Upper Leg, Left **Q** Lower Leg, Right **R** Lower Leg, Left **S** Foot, Right **T** Foot, Left **U** Toe, Right **V** Toe, Left	**X** External	**6** Pressure Dressing **7** Intermittent Pressure Device	**Z** No Qualifier

2 Placement
W Anatomical Regions
2 Dressing: Putting material on a body region for protection

Body Region Character 4	Approach Character 5	Device Character 6	Qualifier Character 7
0 Head **1** Face **2** Neck **3** Abdominal Wall **4** Chest Wall **5** Back **6** Inguinal Region, Right **7** Inguinal Region, Left **8** Upper Extremity, Right **9** Upper Extremity, Left **A** Upper Arm, Right **B** Upper Arm, Left **C** Lower Arm, Right **D** Lower Arm, Left **E** Hand, Right **F** Hand, Left **G** Thumb, Right **H** Thumb, Left **J** Finger, Right **K** Finger, Left **L** Lower Extremity, Right **M** Lower Extremity, Left **N** Upper Leg, Right **P** Upper Leg, Left **Q** Lower Leg, Right **R** Lower Leg, Left **S** Foot, Right **T** Foot, Left **U** Toe, Right **V** Toe, Left	**X** External	**4** Bandage	**Z** No Qualifier

2 Placement
W Anatomical Regions
3 Immobilization: Limiting or preventing motion of a body region

Body Region Character 4	Approach Character 5	Device Character 6	Qualifier Character 7
0 Head **2** Neck **3** Abdominal Wall **4** Chest Wall **5** Back **6** Inguinal Region, Right **7** Inguinal Region, Left **8** Upper Extremity, Right **9** Upper Extremity, Left **A** Upper Arm, Right **B** Upper Arm, Left **C** Lower Arm, Right **D** Lower Arm, Left **E** Hand, Right **F** Hand, Left **G** Thumb, Right **H** Thumb, Left **J** Finger, Right **K** Finger, Left **L** Lower Extremity, Right **M** Lower Extremity, Left **N** Upper Leg, Right **P** Upper Leg, Left **Q** Lower Leg, Right **R** Lower Leg, Left **S** Foot, Right **T** Foot, Left **U** Toe, Right **V** Toe, Left	**X** External	**1** Splint **2** Cast **3** Brace **Y** Other Device	**Z** No Qualifier
1 Face	**X** External	**1** Splint **2** Cast **3** Brace **9** Wire **Y** Other Device	**Z** No Qualifier

2 Placement
W Anatomical Regions
4 Packing: Putting material in a body region or orifice

Body Region Character 4	Approach Character 5	Device Character 6	Qualifier Character 7
0 Head **1** Face **2** Neck **3** Abdominal Wall **4** Chest Wall **5** Back **6** Inguinal Region, Right **7** Inguinal Region, Left **8** Upper Extremity, Right **9** Upper Extremity, Left **A** Upper Arm, Right **B** Upper Arm, Left **C** Lower Arm, Right **D** Lower Arm, Left **E** Hand, Right **F** Hand, Left **G** Thumb, Right **H** Thumb, Left **J** Finger, Right **K** Finger, Left **L** Lower Extremity, Right **M** Lower Extremity, Left **N** Upper Leg, Right **P** Upper Leg, Left **Q** Lower Leg, Right **R** Lower Leg, Left **S** Foot, Right **T** Foot, Left **U** Toe, Right **V** Toe, Left	**X** External	**5** Packing Material	**Z** No Qualifier

2 Placement
W Anatomical Regions
5 Removal: Taking out or off a device from a body part

Body Region Character 4	Approach Character 5	Device Character 6	Qualifier Character 7
0 Head **2** Neck **3** Abdominal Wall **4** Chest Wall **5** Back **6** Inguinal Region, Right **7** Inguinal Region, Left **8** Upper Extremity, Right **9** Upper Extremity, Left **A** Upper Arm, Right **B** Upper Arm, Left **C** Lower Arm, Right **D** Lower Arm, Left **E** Hand, Right **F** Hand, Left **G** Thumb, Right **H** Thumb, Left **J** Finger, Right **K** Finger, Left **L** Lower Extremity, Right **M** Lower Extremity, Left **N** Upper Leg, Right **P** Upper Leg, Left **Q** Lower Leg, Right **R** Lower Leg, Left **S** Foot, Right **T** Foot, Left **U** Toe, Right **V** Toe, Left	**X** External	**0** Traction Apparatus **1** Splint **2** Cast **3** Brace **4** Bandage **5** Packing Material **6** Pressure Dressing **7** Intermittent Pressure Device **Y** Other Device	**Z** No Qualifier
1 Face	**X** External	**0** Traction Apparatus **1** Splint **2** Cast **3** Brace **4** Bandage **5** Packing Material **6** Pressure Dressing **7** Intermittent Pressure Device **9** Wire **Y** Other Device	**Z** No Qualifier

2 Placement
W Anatomical Regions
6 Traction: Exerting a pulling force on a body region in a distal direction

Body Region Character 4	Approach Character 5	Device Character 6	Qualifier Character 7
0 Head **1** Face **2** Neck **3** Abdominal Wall **4** Chest Wall **5** Back **6** Inguinal Region, Right **7** Inguinal Region, Left **8** Upper Extremity, Right **9** Upper Extremity, Left **A** Upper Arm, Right **B** Upper Arm, Left **C** Lower Arm, Right **D** Lower Arm, Left **E** Hand, Right **F** Hand, Left **G** Thumb, Right **H** Thumb, Left **J** Finger, Right **K** Finger, Left **L** Lower Extremity, Right **M** Lower Extremity, Left **N** Upper Leg, Right **P** Upper Leg, Left **Q** Lower Leg, Right **R** Lower Leg, Left **S** Foot, Right **T** Foot, Left **U** Toe, Right **V** Toe, Left	**X** External	**0** Traction Apparatus **Z** No Device	**Z** No Qualifier

NOTES

Placement-Anatomical Orifices 2Y0-2Y5

2 Placement
Y Anatomical Orifices
0 Change: Taking out or off a device from a body part and putting back an identical or similar device in or on the same body part without cutting or puncturing the skin or a mucous membrane

Body Region	Approach	Device	Qualifier
Character 4	Character 5	Character 6	Character 7
0 Mouth and Pharynx **1** Nasal **2** Ear **3** Anorectal **4** Female Genital Tract ♀ **5** Urethra	**X** External	**5** Packing Material	**Z** No Qualifier

♀ 2Y04X5Z

2 Placement
Y Anatomical Orifices
4 Packing: Putting material in a body region or orifice

Body Region	Approach	Device	Qualifier
Character 4	Character 5	Character 6	Character 7
0 Mouth and Pharynx **1** Nasal **2** Ear **3** Anorectal **4** Female Genital Tract ♀ **5** Urethra	**X** External	**5** Packing Material	**Z** No Qualifier

♀ 2Y44X5Z

2 Placement
Y Anatomical Orifices
5 Removal: Taking out or off a device from a body part

Body Region	Approach	Device	Qualifier
Character 4	Character 5	Character 6	Character 7
0 Mouth and Pharynx **1** Nasal **2** Ear **3** Anorectal **4** Female Genital Tract ♀ **5** Urethra	**X** External	**5** Packing Material	**Z** No Qualifier

♀ 2Y54X5Z

NOTES

Administration 302-3E1

3 Administration
0 Circulatory
2 Transfusion: Putting in blood or blood products

Body System / Region	Approach	Substance	Qualifier
Character 4	Character 5	Character 6	Character 7
3 Peripheral Vein NC **4** Central Vein NC	**0** Open **3** Percutaneous	**A** Stem Cells, Embryonic	**Z** No Qualifier
3 Peripheral Vein NC **4** Central Vein NC	**0** Open **3** Percutaneous	**G** Bone Marrow **X** Stem Cells, Cord Blood **Y** Stem Cells, Hematopoietic	**0** Autologous **2** Allogeneic, Related **3** Allogeneic, Unrelated **4** Allogeneic, Unspecified
3 Peripheral Vein **4** Central Vein	**0** Open **3** Percutaneous	**H** Whole Blood **J** Serum Albumin **K** Frozen Plasma **L** Fresh Plasma **M** Plasma Cryoprecipitate **N** Red Blood Cells **P** Frozen Red Cells **Q** White Cells **R** Platelets **S** Globulin **T** Fibrinogen **V** Antihemophilic Factors **W** Factor IX	**0** Autologous **1** Nonautologous
5 Peripheral Artery NC **6** Central Artery NC	**0** Open **3** Percutaneous	**G** Bone Marrow **H** Whole Blood **J** Serum Albumin **K** Frozen Plasma **L** Fresh Plasma **M** Plasma Cryoprecipitate **N** Red Blood Cells **P** Frozen Red Cells **Q** White Cells **R** Platelets **S** Globulin **T** Fibrinogen **V** Antihemophilic Factors **W** Factor IX **X** Stem Cells, Cord Blood **Y** Stem Cells, Hematopoietic	**0** Autologous **1** Nonautologous
7 Products of Conception, Circulatory ♀	**3** Percutaneous **7** Via Natural or Artificial Opening	**H** Whole Blood **J** Serum Albumin **K** Frozen Plasma **L** Fresh Plasma **M** Plasma Cryoprecipitate **N** Red Blood Cells **P** Frozen Red Cells **Q** White Cells **R** Platelets **S** Globulin **T** Fibrinogen **V** Antihemophilic Factors **W** Factor IX	**1** Nonautologous
8 Vein	**0** Open **3** Percutaneous	**B** 4-Factor Prothrombin Complex Concentrate	**1** Nonautologous

♀ 30273H1 30273J1 30273K1 30273L1 30273M1 30273N1 30273P1 30273Q1 30273R1 30273S1 30273T1 30273V1 30273W1 30277H1 30277J1 30277K1 30277L1 30277M1 30277N1 30277P1 30277Q1 30277R1 30277S1 30277T1 30277V1 30277W1

NC 30230G2 30230G3 30230G4 30230Y2 30230Y3 30230Y4 30233G2 30233G3 30233G4 30233Y2 30233Y3 30233Y4 30240G2 30240G3 30240G4 30240Y2 30240Y3 30240Y4 30243G2 30243G3 30243G4 30243Y2 30243Y3 30243Y4 30250G1 30250Y1 30253G1 30253Y1 30260G1 30260Y1 30263G1 30263Y1 Codes in this list are noncovered procedures only when reported with C90.00 or C90.01 as either a principal or secondary diagnosis.

302 continued on next page

302 continued from previous page

NC 30230AZ 30230G0 30230Y0 30233AZ 30233G0 30233Y0 30240AZ 30240G0 30240Y0 30243AZ 30243G0 30243Y0 30250G0 30250Y0 30253G0 30253Y0 30260G0 30260Y0 30263G0 30263Y0 Codes in this list are noncovered procedures only when reported with C91.00, C92.00, C92.10, C92.11, C92.40, C92.50, C92.60, C92.A0, C93.00, C94.00, or C95.00 as either a principal or secondary diagnosis.

3 Administration
C Indwelling Device
1 Irrigation: Putting in or on a cleansing substance

Body System / Region	Approach	Substance	Qualifier
Character 4	**Character 5**	**Character 6**	**Character 7**
Z None	**X** External	**8** Irrigating Substance	**Z** No Qualifier

3 Administration
E Physiological Systems and Anatomical Regions
0 Introduction: Putting in or on a therapeutic, diagnostic, nutritional, physiological, or prophylactic substance except blood or blood products

Body System / Region	Approach	Substance	Qualifier
Character 4	**Character 5**	**Character 6**	**Character 7**
0 Skin and Mucous Membranes	**X** External	**0** Antineoplastic	**5** Other Antineoplastic **M** Monoclonal Antibody
0 Skin and Mucous Membranes	**X** External	**2** Anti-infective	**8** Oxazolidinones **9** Other Anti-infective
0 Skin and Mucous Membranes	**X** External	**3** Anti-inflammatory **4** Serum, Toxoid and Vaccine **B** Anesthetic Agent **K** Other Diagnostic Substance **M** Pigment **N** Analgesics, Hypnotics, Sedatives **T** Destructive Agent	**Z** No Qualifier
0 Skin and Mucous Membranes	**X** External	**G** Other Therapeutic Substance	**C** Other Substance
1 Subcutaneous Tissue	**0** Open	**2** Anti-infective	**A** Anti-Infective Envelope
1 Subcutaneous Tissue	**3** Percutaneous	**0** Antineoplastic	**5** Other Antineoplastic **M** Monoclonal Antibody
1 Subcutaneous Tissue	**3** Percutaneous	**2** Anti-infective	**8** Oxazolidinones **9** Other Anti-infective **A** Anti-Infective Envelope
1 Subcutaneous Tissue	**3** Percutaneous	**3** Anti-inflammatory **6** Nutritional Substance **7** Electrolytic and Water Balance Substance **B** Anesthetic Agent **H** Radioactive Substance **K** Other Diagnostic Substance **N** Analgesics, Hypnotics, Sedatives **T** Destructive Agent	**Z** No Qualifier
1 Subcutaneous Tissue	**3** Percutaneous	**4** Serum, Toxoid and Vaccine	**0** Influenza Vaccine **Z** No Qualifier
1 Subcutaneous Tissue	**3** Percutaneous	**G** Other Therapeutic Substance	**C** Other Substance
1 Subcutaneous Tissue	**3** Percutaneous	**V** Hormone	**G** Insulin **J** Other Hormone
2 Muscle	**3** Percutaneous	**0** Antineoplastic	**5** Other Antineoplastic **M** Monoclonal Antibody
2 Muscle	**3** Percutaneous	**2** Anti-infective	**8** Oxazolidinones **9** Other Anti-infective

3E0 continued on next page

3E0 continued from previous page

3 Administration
E Physiological Systems and Anatomical Regions
0 Introduction: Putting in or on a therapeutic, diagnostic, nutritional, physiological, or prophylactic substance except blood or blood products

Body System / Region Character 4	Approach Character 5	Substance Character 6	Qualifier Character 7
2 Muscle	**3** Percutaneous	**3** Anti-inflammatory **6** Nutritional Substance **7** Electrolytic and Water Balance Substance **B** Anesthetic Agent **H** Radioactive Substance **K** Other Diagnostic Substance **N** Analgesics, Hypnotics, Sedatives **T** Destructive Agent	**Z** No Qualifier
2 Muscle	3 Percutaneous	4 Serum, Toxoid and Vaccine	0 Influenza Vaccine Z No Qualifier
2 Muscle	**3** Percutaneous	**G** Other Therapeutic Substance	**C** Other Substance
3 Peripheral Vein	**0** Open	**0** Antineoplastic	**2** High-dose Interleukin-2 **3** Low-dose Interleukin-2 **5** Other Antineoplastic **M** Monoclonal Antibody **P** Clofarabine
3 Peripheral Vein	**0** Open	**1** Thrombolytic	**6** Recombinant Human-activated Protein C **7** Other Thrombolytic
3 Peripheral Vein	**0** Open	**2** Anti-infective	**8** Oxazolidinones **9** Other Anti-infective
3 Peripheral Vein	**0** Open	**3** Anti-inflammatory **4** Serum, Toxoid and Vaccine **6** Nutritional Substance **7** Electrolytic and Water Balance Substance **F** Intracirculatory Anesthetic **H** Radioactive Substance **K** Other Diagnostic Substance **N** Analgesics, Hypnotics, Sedatives **P** Platelet Inhibitor **R** Antiarrhythmic **T** Destructive Agent **X** Vasopressor	**Z** No Qualifier
3 Peripheral Vein	**0** Open	**G** Other Therapeutic Substance	**C** Other Substance **N** Blood Brain Barrier Disruption
3 Peripheral Vein	**0** Open	**U** Pancreatic Islet Cells	**0** Autologous **1** Nonautologous
3 Peripheral Vein	**0** Open	**V** Hormone	**G** Insulin **H** Human B -type Natriuretic Peptide **J** Other Hormone
3 Peripheral Vein	**0** Open	**W** Immunotherapeutic	**K** Immunostimulator **L** Immunosuppressive
3 Peripheral Vein	**3** Percutaneous	**0** Antineoplastic	**2** High-dose Interleukin-2 **3** Low-dose Interleukin-2 **5** Other Antineoplastic **M** Monoclonal Antibody **P** Clofarabine

3E0 continued on next page

3E0 continued from previous page

3 Administration
E Physiological Systems and Anatomical Regions
0 Introduction: Putting in or on a therapeutic, diagnostic, nutritional, physiological, or prophylactic substance except blood or blood products

Body System / Region Character 4	Approach Character 5	Substance Character 6	Qualifier Character 7
3 Peripheral Vein	**3** Percutaneous	**1** Thrombolytic	**6** Recombinant Human-activated Protein C **7** Other Thrombolytic
3 Peripheral Vein	**3** Percutaneous	**2** Anti-infective	**8** Oxazolidinones **9** Other Anti-infective
3 Peripheral Vein	**3** Percutaneous	**3** Anti-inflammatory **4** Serum, Toxoid and Vaccine **6** Nutritional Substance **7** Electrolytic and Water Balance Substance **F** Intracirculatory Anesthetic **H** Radioactive Substance **K** Other Diagnostic Substance **N** Analgesics, Hypnotics, Sedatives **P** Platelet Inhibitor **R** Antiarrhythmic **T** Destructive Agent **X** Vasopressor	**Z** No Qualifier
3 Peripheral Vein	**3** Percutaneous	**G** Other Therapeutic Substance	**C** Other Substance **N** Blood Brain Barrier Disruption **Q** Glucarpidase
3 Peripheral Vein	**3** Percutaneous	**U** Pancreatic Islet Cells	**0** Autologous **1** Nonautologous
3 Peripheral Vein	**3** Percutaneous	**V** Hormone	**G** Insulin **H** Human B-type Natriuretic Peptide **J** Other Hormone
3 Peripheral Vein	**3** Percutaneous	**W** Immunotherapeutic	**K** Immunostimulator **L** Immunosuppressive
4 Central Vein	**0** Open	**0** Antineoplastic	**2** High-dose Interleukin-2 **3** Low-dose Interleukin-2 **5** Other Antineoplastic **M** Monoclonal Antibody **P** Clofarabine
4 Central Vein	**0** Open	**1** Thrombolytic	**6** Recombinant Human-activated Protein C **7** Other Thrombolytic
4 Central Vein	**0** Open	**2** Anti-infective	**8** Oxazolidinones **9** Other Anti-infective
4 Central Vein	**0** Open	**3** Anti-inflammatory **4** Serum, Toxoid and Vaccine **6** Nutritional Substance **7** Electrolytic and Water Balance Substance **F** Intracirculatory Anesthetic **H** Radioactive Substance **K** Other Diagnostic Substance **N** Analgesics, Hypnotics, Sedatives **P** Platelet Inhibitor **R** Antiarrhythmic **T** Destructive Agent **X** Vasopressor	**Z** No Qualifier
4 Central Vein	**0** Open	**G** Other Therapeutic Substance	**C** Other Substance **N** Blood Brain Barrier Disruption

3E0 continued on next page

3E0 continued from previous page

3 **Administration**
E **Physiological Systems and Anatomical Regions**
0 **Introduction:** Putting in or on a therapeutic, diagnostic, nutritional, physiological, or prophylactic substance except blood or blood products

Body System / Region Character 4	Approach Character 5	Substance Character 6	Qualifier Character 7
4 Central Vein	**0** Open	**V** Hormone	**G** Insulin **H** Human B-type Natriuretic Peptide **J** Other Hormone
4 Central Vein	**0** Open	**W** Immunotherapeutic	**K** Immunostimulator **L** Immunosuppressive
4 Central Vein	**3** Percutaneous	**0** Antineoplastic	**2** High-dose Interleukin-2 **3** Low-dose Interleukin-2 **5** Other Antineoplastic **M** Monoclonal Antibody **P** Clofarabine
4 Central Vein	**3** Percutaneous	**1** Thrombolytic	**6** Recombinant Human-activated Protein C **7** Other Thrombolytic
4 Central Vein	**3** Percutaneous	**2** Anti-infective	**8** Oxazolidinones **9** Other Anti-infective
4 Central Vein	**3** Percutaneous	**3** Anti-inflammatory **4** Serum, Toxoid and Vaccine **6** Nutritional Substance **7** Electrolytic and Water Balance Substance **F** Intracirculatory Anesthetic **H** Radioactive Substance **K** Other Diagnostic Substance **N** Analgesics, Hypnotics, Sedatives **P** Platelet Inhibitor **R** Antiarrhythmic **T** Destructive Agent **X** Vasopressor	**Z** No Qualifier
4 Central Vein	**3** Percutaneous	**G** Other Therapeutic Substance	**C** Other Substance **N** Blood Brain Barrier Disruption **Q** Glucarpidase
4 Central Vein	**3** Percutaneous	**V** Hormone	**G** Insulin **H** Human B-type Natriuretic Peptide **J** Other Hormone
4 Central Vein	**3** Percutaneous	**W** Immunotherapeutic	**K** Immunostimulator **L** Immunosuppressive
5 Peripheral Artery **6** Central Artery	**0** Open **3** Percutaneous	**0** Antineoplastic	**2** High-dose Interleukin-2 **3** Low-dose Interleukin-2 **5** Other Antineoplastic **M** Monoclonal Antibody **P** Clofarabine
5 Peripheral Artery **6** Central Artery	**0** Open **3** Percutaneous	**1** Thrombolytic	**6** Recombinant Human-activated Protein C **7** Other Thrombolytic
5 Peripheral Artery **6** Central Artery	**0** Open **3** Percutaneous	**2** Anti-infective	**8** Oxazolidinones **9** Other Anti-infective

3E0 continued on next page

3E0 continued from previous page

3 Administration
E Physiological Systems and Anatomical Regions
0 Introduction: Putting in or on a therapeutic, diagnostic, nutritional, physiological, or prophylactic substance except blood or blood products

Body System / Region Character 4	Approach Character 5	Substance Character 6	Qualifier Character 7
5 Peripheral Artery **6** Central Artery	**0** Open **3** Percutaneous	**3** Anti-inflammatory **4** Serum, Toxoid and Vaccine **6** Nutritional Substance **7** Electrolytic and Water Balance Substance **F** Intracirculatory Anesthetic **H** Radioactive Substance **K** Other Diagnostic Substance **N** Analgesics, Hypnotics, Sedatives **P** Platelet Inhibitor **R** Antiarrhythmic **T** Destructive Agent **X** Vasopressor	**Z** No Qualifier
5 Peripheral Artery **6** Central Artery	**0** Open **3** Percutaneous	**G** Other Therapeutic Substance	**C** Other Substance **N** Blood Brain Barrier Disruption
5 Peripheral Artery **6** Central Artery	**0** Open **3** Percutaneous	**V** Hormone	**G** Insulin **H** Human B-type Natriuretic Peptide **J** Other Hormone
5 Peripheral Artery **6** Central Artery	**0** Open **3** Percutaneous	**W** Immunotherapeutic	**K** Immunostimulator **L** Immunosuppressive
7 Coronary Artery **8** Heart	**0** Open **3** Percutaneous	**1** Thrombolytic	**6** Recombinant Human-activated Protein C **7** Other Thrombolytic
7 Coronary Artery **8** Heart	**0** Open **3** Percutaneous	**G** Other Therapeutic Substance	**C** Other Substance
7 Coronary Artery **8** Heart	**0** Open **3** Percutaneous	**K** Other Diagnostic Substance **P** Platelet Inhibitor	**Z** No Qualifier
7 Coronary Artery **8** Heart	**4** Percutaneous Endoscopic	**G** Other Therapeutic Substance	**C** Other Substance
9 Nose	**3** Percutaneous **7** Via Natural or Artificial Opening **X** External	**0** Antineoplastic	**5** Other Antineoplastic **M** Monoclonal Antibody
9 Nose	**3** Percutaneous **7** Via Natural or Artificial Opening **X** External	**2** Anti-infective	**8** Oxazolidinones **9** Other Anti-infective
9 Nose	**3** Percutaneous **7** Via Natural or Artificial Opening **X** External	**3** Anti-inflammatory **4** Serum, Toxoid and Vaccine **B** Anesthetic Agent **H** Radioactive Substance **K** Other Diagnostic Substance **N** Analgesics, Hypnotics, Sedatives **T** Destructive Agent	**Z** No Qualifier
9 Nose	**3** Percutaneous **7** Via Natural or Artificial Opening **X** External	**G** Other Therapeutic Substance	**C** Other Substance
A Bone Marrow	**3** Percutaneous	**0** Antineoplastic	**5** Other Antineoplastic **M** Monoclonal Antibody
A Bone Marrow	**3** Percutaneous	**G** Other Therapeutic Substance	**C** Other Substance
B Ear	**3** Percutaneous **7** Via Natural or Artificial Opening **X** External	**0** Antineoplastic	**4** Liquid Brachytherapy Radioisotope **5** Other Antineoplastic **M** Monoclonal Antibody

3E0 continued on next page

3E0 continued from previous page

3 Administration
E Physiological Systems and Anatomical Regions
0 Introduction: Putting in or on a therapeutic, diagnostic, nutritional, physiological, or prophylactic substance except blood or blood products

Body System / Region Character 4	Approach Character 5	Substance Character 6	Qualifier Character 7
B Ear	**3** Percutaneous **7** Via Natural or Artificial Opening **X** External	**2** Anti-infective	**8** Oxazolidinones **9** Other Anti-infective
B Ear	**3** Percutaneous **7** Via Natural or Artificial Opening **X** External	**3** Anti-inflammatory **B** Anesthetic Agent **H** Radioactive Substance **K** Other Diagnostic Substance **N** Analgesics, Hypnotics, Sedatives **T** Destructive Agent	**Z** No Qualifier
B Ear	**3** Percutaneous **7** Via Natural or Artificial Opening **X** External	**G** Other Therapeutic Substance	**C** Other Substance
C Eye	**3** Percutaneous **7** Via Natural or Artificial Opening **X** External	**0** Antineoplastic	**4** Liquid Brachytherapy Radioisotope **5** Other Antineoplastic **M** Monoclonal Antibody
C Eye	**3** Percutaneous **7** Via Natural or Artificial Opening **X** External	**2** Anti-infective	**8** Oxazolidinones **9** Other Anti-infective
C Eye	**3** Percutaneous **7** Via Natural or Artificial Opening **X** External	**3** Anti-inflammatory **B** Anesthetic Agent **H** Radioactive Substance **K** Other Diagnostic Substance **M** Pigment **N** Analgesics, Hypnotics, Sedatives **T** Destructive Agent	**Z** No Qualifier
C Eye	**3** Percutaneous **7** Via Natural or Artificial Opening **X** External	**G** Other Therapeutic Substance	**C** Other Substance
C Eye	**3** Percutaneous **7** Via Natural or Artificial Opening **X** External	**S** Gas	**F** Other Gas
D Mouth and Pharynx	**3** Percutaneous **7** Via Natural or Artificial Opening **X** External	**0** Antineoplastic	**4** Liquid Brachytherapy Radioisotope **5** Other Antineoplastic **M** Monoclonal Antibody
D Mouth and Pharynx	**3** Percutaneous **7** Via Natural or Artificial Opening **X** External	**2** Anti-infective	**8** Oxazolidinones **9** Other Anti-infective
D Mouth and Pharynx	**3** Percutaneous **7** Via Natural or Artificial Opening **X** External	**3** Anti-inflammatory **4** Serum, Toxoid and Vaccine **6** Nutritional Substance **7** Electrolytic and Water Balance Substance **B** Anesthetic Agent **H** Radioactive Substance **K** Other Diagnostic Substance **N** Analgesics, Hypnotics, Sedatives **R** Antiarrhythmic **T** Destructive Agent	**Z** No Qualifier
D Mouth and Pharynx	**3** Percutaneous **7** Via Natural or Artificial Opening **X** External	**G** Other Therapeutic Substance	**C** Other Substance

3E0 continued on next page

3E0 continued from previous page

3 Administration
E Physiological Systems and Anatomical Regions
0 Introduction: Putting in or on a therapeutic, diagnostic, nutritional, physiological, or prophylactic substance except blood or blood products

Body System / Region Character 4	Approach Character 5	Substance Character 6	Qualifier Character 7
E Products of Conception ♀ **G** Upper GI **H** Lower GI **K** Genitourinary Tract **N** Male Reproductive ♂	**3** Percutaneous **7** Via Natural or Artificial Opening **8** Via Natural or Artificial Opening Endoscopic	**0** Antineoplastic	**4** Liquid Brachytherapy Radioisotope **5** Other Antineoplastic **M** Monoclonal Antibody
E Products of Conception ♀ **G** Upper GI **H** Lower GI **K** Genitourinary Tract **N** Male Reproductive ♂	**3** Percutaneous **7** Via Natural or Artificial Opening **8** Via Natural or Artificial Opening Endoscopic	**2** Anti-infective	**8** Oxazolidinones **9** Other Anti-infective
E Products of Conception ♀ **G** Upper GI **H** Lower GI **K** Genitourinary Tract **N** Male Reproductive ♂	**3** Percutaneous **7** Via Natural or Artificial Opening **8** Via Natural or Artificial Opening Endoscopic	**3** Anti-inflammatory **6** Nutritional Substance **7** Electrolytic and Water Balance Substance **B** Anesthetic Agent **H** Radioactive Substance **K** Other Diagnostic Substance **N** Analgesics, Hypnotics, Sedatives **T** Destructive Agent	**Z** No Qualifier
E Products of Conception ♀ **G** Upper GI **H** Lower GI **K** Genitourinary Tract **N** Male Reproductive ♂	**3** Percutaneous **7** Via Natural or Artificial Opening **8** Via Natural or Artificial Opening Endoscopic	**G** Other Therapeutic Substance	**C** Other Substance
E Products of Conception ♀ **G** Upper GI **H** Lower GI **K** Genitourinary Tract **N** Male Reproductive ♂	**3** Percutaneous **7** Via Natural or Artificial Opening **8** Via Natural or Artificial Opening Endoscopic	**S** Gas	**F** Other Gas
E Products of Conception ♀ **G** Upper GI **H** Lower GI **K** Genitourinary Tract **N** Male Reproductive ♂	**4** Percutaneous Endoscopic	**G** Other Therapeutic Substance	**C** Other Substance
F Respiratory Tract	**3** Percutaneous **7** Via Natural or Artificial Opening **8** Via Natural or Artificial Opening Endoscopic	**0** Antineoplastic	**4** Liquid Brachytherapy Radioisotope **5** Other Antineoplastic **M** Monoclonal Antibody
F Respiratory Tract	**3** Percutaneous **7** Via Natural or Artificial Opening **8** Via Natural or Artificial Opening Endoscopic	**2** Anti-infective	**8** Oxazolidinones **9** Other Anti-infective
F Respiratory Tract	**3** Percutaneous **7** Via Natural or Artificial Opening **8** Via Natural or Artificial Opening Endoscopic	**3** Anti-inflammatory **6** Nutritional Substance **7** Electrolytic and Water Balance Substance **B** Anesthetic Agent **H** Radioactive Substance **K** Other Diagnostic Substance **N** Analgesics, Hypnotics, Sedatives **T** Destructive Agent	**Z** No Qualifier
F Respiratory Tract	**3** Percutaneous **7** Via Natural or Artificial Opening **8** Via Natural or Artificial Opening Endoscopic	**G** Other Therapeutic Substance	**C** Other Substance

3E0 continued on next page

3 **Administration**
E **Physiological Systems and Anatomical Regions**
0 **Introduction:** Putting in or on a therapeutic, diagnostic, nutritional, physiological, or prophylactic substance except blood or blood products

3E0 continued from previous page

Body System / Region Character 4	Approach Character 5	Substance Character 6	Qualifier Character 7
F Respiratory Tract	**3** Percutaneous **7** Via Natural or Artificial Opening **8** Via Natural or Artificial Opening Endoscopic	**S** Gas	**D** Nitric Oxide **F** Other Gas
F Respiratory Tract	**4** Percutaneous Endoscopic	**G** Other Therapeutic Substance	**C** Other Substance
J Biliary and Pancreatic Tract	**3** Percutaneous **7** Via Natural or Artificial Opening **8** Via Natural or Artificial Opening Endoscopic	**0** Antineoplastic	**4** Liquid Brachytherapy Radioisotope **5** Other Antineoplastic **M** Monoclonal Antibody
J Biliary and Pancreatic Tract	**3** Percutaneous **7** Via Natural or Artificial Opening **8** Via Natural or Artificial Opening Endoscopic	**2** Anti-infective	**8** Oxazolidinones **9** Other Anti-infective
J Biliary and Pancreatic Tract	**3** Percutaneous **7** Via Natural or Artificial Opening **8** Via Natural or Artificial Opening Endoscopic	**3** Anti-inflammatory **6** Nutritional Substance **7** Electrolytic and Water Balance Substance **B** Anesthetic Agent **H** Radioactive Substance **K** Other Diagnostic Substance **N** Analgesics, Hypnotics, Sedatives **T** Destructive Agent	**Z** No Qualifier
J Biliary and Pancreatic Tract	**3** Percutaneous **7** Via Natural or Artificial Opening **8** Via Natural or Artificial Opening Endoscopic	**G** Other Therapeutic Substance	**C** Other Substance
J Biliary and Pancreatic Tract	**3** Percutaneous **7** Via Natural or Artificial Opening **8** Via Natural or Artificial Opening Endoscopic	**S** Gas	**F** Other Gas
J Biliary and Pancreatic Tract	**3** Percutaneous **7** Via Natural or Artificial Opening **8** Via Natural or Artificial Opening Endoscopic	**U** Pancreatic Islet Cells	**0** Autologous **1** Nonautologous
J Biliary and Pancreatic Tract	**4** Percutaneous Endoscopic	**G** Other Therapeutic Substance	**C** Other Substance
L Pleural Cavity **M** Peritoneal Cavity	**0** Open	**5** Adhesion Barrier	**Z** No Qualifier
L Pleural Cavity **M** Peritoneal Cavity	**3** Percutaneous	**0** Antineoplastic	**4** Liquid Brachytherapy Radioisotope **5** Other Antineoplastic **M** Monoclonal Antibody
L Pleural Cavity **M** Peritoneal Cavity	**3** Percutaneous	**2** Anti-infective	**8** Oxazolidinones **9** Other Anti-infective
L Pleural Cavity **M** Peritoneal Cavity	**3** Percutaneous	**3** Anti-inflammatory **5** Adhesion Barrier **6** Nutritional Substance **7** Electrolytic and Water Balance Substance **B** Anesthetic Agent **H** Radioactive Substance **K** Other Diagnostic Substance **N** Analgesics, Hypnotics, Sedatives **T** Destructive Agent	**Z** No Qualifier
L Pleural Cavity **M** Peritoneal Cavity	**3** Percutaneous	**G** Other Therapeutic Substance	**C** Other Substance

3E0 continued on next page

3 Administration

E Physiological Systems and Anatomical Regions

0 Introduction: Putting in or on a therapeutic, diagnostic, nutritional, physiological, or prophylactic substance except blood or blood products

3E0 continued from previous page

Body System / Region Character 4	Approach Character 5	Substance Character 6	Qualifier Character 7
L Pleural Cavity **M** Peritoneal Cavity	**3** Percutaneous	**S** Gas	**F** Other Gas
L Pleural Cavity **M** Peritoneal Cavity	**4** Percutaneous Endoscopic	**5** Adhesion Barrier	**Z** No Qualifier
L Pleural Cavity **M** Peritoneal Cavity	**4** Percutaneous Endoscopic	**G** Other Therapeutic Substance	**C** Other Substance
L Pleural Cavity **M** Peritoneal Cavity	**7** Via Natural or Artificial Opening	**0** Antineoplastic	**4** Liquid Brachytherapy Radioisotope **5** Other Antineoplastic **M** Monoclonal Antibody
L Pleural Cavity **M** Peritoneal Cavity	**7** Via Natural or Artificial Opening	**S** Gas	**F** Other Gas
P Female Reproductive ♀	**0** Open	**5** Adhesion Barrier	**Z** No Qualifier
P Female Reproductive ♀	**3** Percutaneous	**0** Antineoplastic	**4** Liquid Brachytherapy Radioisotope **5** Other Antineoplastic **M** Monoclonal Antibody
P Female Reproductive ♀	**3** Percutaneous	**2** Anti-infective	**8** Oxazolidinones **9** Other Anti-infective
P Female Reproductive ♀	**3** Percutaneous	**3** Anti-inflammatory **5** Adhesion Barrier **6** Nutritional Substance **7** Electrolytic and Water Balance Substance **B** Anesthetic Agent **H** Radioactive Substance **K** Other Diagnostic Substance **L** Sperm **N** Analgesics, Hypnotics, Sedatives **T** Destructive Agent **V** Hormone	**Z** No Qualifier
P Female Reproductive ♀	**3** Percutaneous	**G** Other Therapeutic Substance	**C** Other Substance
P Female Reproductive ♀	**3** Percutaneous	**Q** Fertilized Ovum	**0** Autologous **1** Nonautologous
P Female Reproductive ♀	**3** Percutaneous	**S** Gas	**F** Other Gas
P Female Reproductive ♀	**4** Percutaneous Endoscopic	**5** Adhesion Barrier	**Z** No Qualifier
P Female Reproductive ♀	**4** Percutaneous Endoscopic	**G** Other Therapeutic Substance	**C** Other Substance
P Female Reproductive ♀	**7** Via Natural or Artificial Opening	**0** Antineoplastic	**4** Liquid Brachytherapy Radioisotope **5** Other Antineoplastic **M** Monoclonal Antibody
P Female Reproductive ♀	**7** Via Natural or Artificial Opening	**2** Anti-infective	**8** Oxazolidinones **9** Other Anti-infective
P Female Reproductive ♀	**7** Via Natural or Artificial Opening	**3** Anti-inflammatory **6** Nutritional Substance **7** Electrolytic and Water Balance Substance **B** Anesthetic Agent **H** Radioactive Substance **K** Other Diagnostic Substance **L** Sperm **N** Analgesics, Hypnotics, Sedatives **T** Destructive Agent **V** Hormone	**Z** No Qualifier

3E0 continued on next page

3E0 continued from previous page

3 Administration
E Physiological Systems and Anatomical Regions
0 Introduction: Putting in or on a therapeutic, diagnostic, nutritional, physiological, or prophylactic substance except blood or blood products

Body System / Region	Approach	Substance	Qualifier
Character 4	**Character 5**	**Character 6**	**Character 7**
P Female Reproductive ♀	**7** Via Natural or Artificial Opening	**G** Other Therapeutic Substance	**C** Other Substance
P Female Reproductive ♀	**7** Via Natural or Artificial Opening	**Q** Fertilized Ovum	**0** Autologous **1** Nonautologous
P Female Reproductive ♀	**7** Via Natural or Artificial Opening	**S** Gas	**F** Other Gas
P Female Reproductive ♀	**8** Via Natural or Artificial Opening Endoscopic	**0** Antineoplastic	**4** Liquid Brachytherapy Radioisotope **5** Other Antineoplastic **M** Monoclonal Antibody
P Female Reproductive ♀	**8** Via Natural or Artificial Opening Endoscopic	**2** Anti-infective	**8** Oxazolidinones **9** Other Anti-infective
P Female Reproductive ♀	**8** Via Natural or Artificial Opening Endoscopic	**3** Anti-inflammatory **6** Nutritional Substance **7** Electrolytic and Water Balance Substance **B** Anesthetic Agent **H** Radioactive Substance **K** Other Diagnostic Substance **N** Analgesics, Hypnotics, Sedatives **T** Destructive Agent	**Z** No Qualifier
P Female Reproductive ♀	**8** Via Natural or Artificial Opening Endoscopic	**G** Other Therapeutic Substance	**C** Other Substance
P Female Reproductive ♀	**8** Via Natural or Artificial Opening Endoscopic	**S** Gas	**F** Other Gas
Q Cranial Cavity and Brain	**0** Open **3** Percutaneous	**0** Antineoplastic	**4** Liquid Brachytherapy Radioisotope **5** Other Antineoplastic **M** Monoclonal Antibody
Q Cranial Cavity and Brain	**0** Open **3** Percutaneous	**2** Anti-infective	**8** Oxazolidinones **9** Other Anti-infective
Q Cranial Cavity and Brain	**0** Open **3** Percutaneous	**3** Anti-inflammatory **6** Nutritional Substance **7** Electrolytic and Water Balance Substance **A** Stem Cells, Embryonic **B** Anesthetic Agent **H** Radioactive Substance **K** Other Diagnostic Substance **N** Analgesics, Hypnotics, Sedatives **T** Destructive Agent	**Z** No Qualifier
Q Cranial Cavity and Brain	**0** Open **3** Percutaneous	**E** Stem Cells, Somatic	**0** Autologous **1** Nonautologous
Q Cranial Cavity and Brain	**0** Open **3** Percutaneous	**G** Other Therapeutic Substance	**C** Other Substance
Q Cranial Cavity and Brain	**0** Open **3** Percutaneous	**S** Gas	**F** Other Gas
Q Cranial Cavity and Brain	**7** Via Natural or Artificial Opening	**0** Antineoplastic	**4** Liquid Brachytherapy Radioisotope **5** Other Antineoplastic **M** Monoclonal Antibody
Q Cranial Cavity and Brain	**7** Via Natural or Artificial Opening	**S** Gas	**F** Other Gas
R Spinal Canal	**0** Open	**A** Stem Cells, Embryonic	**Z** No Qualifier
R Spinal Canal	**0** Open	**E** Stem Cells, Somatic	**0** Autologous **1** Nonautologous

3E0 continued on next page

3 Administration

3E0 continued from previous page

E Physiological Systems and Anatomical Regions

0 Introduction: Putting in or on a therapeutic, diagnostic, nutritional, physiological, or prophylactic substance except blood or blood products

Body System / Region Character 4	Approach Character 5	Substance Character 6	Qualifier Character 7
R Spinal Canal	**3** Percutaneous	**0** Antineoplastic	**2** High-dose Interleukin-2 **3** Low-dose Interleukin-2 **4** Liquid Brachytherapy Radioisotope **5** Other Antineoplastic **M** Monoclonal Antibody
R Spinal Canal	**3** Percutaneous	**2** Anti-infective	**8** Oxazolidinones **9** Other Anti-infective
R Spinal Canal	**3** Percutaneous	**3** Anti-inflammatory **6** Nutritional Substance **7** Electrolytic and Water Balance Substance **A** Stem Cells, Embryonic **B** Anesthetic Agent **H** Radioactive Substance **K** Other Diagnostic Substance **N** Analgesics, Hypnotics, Sedatives **T** Destructive Agent	**Z** No Qualifier
R Spinal Canal	**3** Percutaneous	**E** Stem Cells, Somatic	**0** Autologous **1** Nonautologous
R Spinal Canal	**3** Percutaneous	**G** Other Therapeutic Substance	**C** Other Substance
R Spinal Canal	**3** Percutaneous	**S** Gas	**F** Other Gas
R Spinal Canal	**7** Via Natural or Artificial Opening	**S** Gas	**F** Other Gas
S Epidural Space	**3** Percutaneous	**0** Antineoplastic	**2** High-dose Interleukin-2 **3** Low-dose Interleukin-2 **4** Liquid Brachytherapy Radioisotope **5** Other Antineoplastic **M** Monoclonal Antibody
S Epidural Space	**3** Percutaneous	**2** Anti-infective	**8** Oxazolidinones **9** Other Anti-infective
S Epidural Space	**3** Percutaneous	**3** Anti-inflammatory **6** Nutritional Substance **7** Electrolytic and Water Balance Substance **B** Anesthetic Agent **H** Radioactive Substance **K** Other Diagnostic Substance **N** Analgesics, Hypnotics, Sedatives **T** Destructive Agent	**Z** No Qualifier
S Epidural Space	**3** Percutaneous	**G** Other Therapeutic Substance	**C** Other Substance
S Epidural Space	**3** Percutaneous	**S** Gas	**F** Other Gas
S Epidural Space	**7** Via Natural or Artificial Opening	**S** Gas	**F** Other Gas
T Peripheral Nerves and Plexi **X** Cranial Nerves	**3** Percutaneous	**3** Anti-inflammatory **B** Anesthetic Agent **T** Destructive Agent	**Z** No Qualifier
T Peripheral Nerves and Plexi **X** Cranial Nerves	**3** Percutaneous	**G** Other Therapeutic Substance	**C** Other Substance
U Joints	**0** Open	**2** Anti-infective	**8** Oxazolidinones **9** Other Anti-infective
U Joints	**0** Open	**G** Other Therapeutic Substance	**B** Recombinant Bone Morphogenetic Protein

3E0 continued on next page

3E0 continued from previous page

3 **Administration**
E **Physiological Systems and Anatomical Regions**
0 **Introduction:** Putting in or on a therapeutic, diagnostic, nutritional, physiological, or prophylactic substance except blood or blood products

Body System / Region Character 4	Approach Character 5	Substance Character 6	Qualifier Character 7
U Joints	**3** Percutaneous	**0** Antineoplastic	**4** Liquid Brachytherapy Radioisotope **5** Other Antineoplastic **M** Monoclonal Antibody
U Joints	**3** Percutaneous	**2** Anti-infective	**8** Oxazolidinones **9** Other Anti-infective
U Joints	**3** Percutaneous	**3** Anti-inflammatory **6** Nutritional Substance **7** Electrolytic and Water Balance Substance **B** Anesthetic Agent **H** Radioactive Substance **K** Other Diagnostic Substance **N** Analgesics, Hypnotics, Sedatives **T** Destructive Agent	**Z** No Qualifier
U Joints	**3** Percutaneous	**G** Other Therapeutic Substance	**B** Recombinant Bone Morphogenetic Protein **C** Other Substance
U Joints	**3** Percutaneous	**S** Gas	**F** Other Gas
U Joints	**4** Percutaneous Endoscopic	**G** Other Therapeutic Substance	**C** Other Substance
V Bones	**0** Open	**G** Other Therapeutic Substance	**B** Recombinant Bone Morphogenetic Protein
V Bones	**3** Percutaneous	**0** Antineoplastic	**5** Other Antineoplastic **M** Monoclonal Antibody
V Bones	**3** Percutaneous	**2** Anti-infective	**8** Oxazolidinones **9** Other Anti-infective
V Bones	**3** Percutaneous	**3** Anti-inflammatory **6** Nutritional Substance **7** Electrolytic and Water Balance Substance **B** Anesthetic Agent **H** Radioactive Substance **K** Other Diagnostic Substance **N** Analgesics, Hypnotics, Sedatives **T** Destructive Agent	**Z** No Qualifier
V Bones	**3** Percutaneous	**G** Other Therapeutic Substance	**B** Recombinant Bone Morphogenetic Protein **C** Other Substance
W Lymphatics	**3** Percutaneous	**0** Antineoplastic	**5** Other Antineoplastic **M** Monoclonal Antibody
W Lymphatics	**3** Percutaneous	**2** Anti-infective	**8** Oxazolidinones **9** Other Anti-infective
W Lymphatics	**3** Percutaneous	**3** Anti-inflammatory **6** Nutritional Substance **7** Electrolytic and Water Balance Substance **B** Anesthetic Agent **H** Radioactive Substance **K** Other Diagnostic Substance **N** Analgesics, Hypnotics, Sedatives **T** Destructive Agent	**Z** No Qualifier
W Lymphatics	**3** Percutaneous	**G** Other Therapeutic Substance	**C** Other Substance

3E0 continued on next page

3 Administration

3E0 continued from previous page

E Physiological Systems and Anatomical Regions

0 Introduction: Putting in or on a therapeutic, diagnostic, nutritional, physiological, or prophylactic substance except blood or blood products

Body System / Region Character 4	Approach Character 5	Substance Character 6	Qualifier Character 7
Y Pericardial Cavity	**3** Percutaneous	**0** Antineoplastic	**4** Liquid Brachytherapy Radioisotope **5** Other Antineoplastic **M** Monoclonal Antibody
Y Pericardial Cavity	**3** Percutaneous	**2** Anti-infective	**8** Oxazolidinones **9** Other Anti-infective
Y Pericardial Cavity	**3** Percutaneous	**3** Anti-inflammatory **6** Nutritional Substance **7** Electrolytic and Water Balance Substance **B** Anesthetic Agent **H** Radioactive Substance **K** Other Diagnostic Substance **N** Analgesics, Hypnotics, Sedatives **T** Destructive Agent	**Z** No Qualifier
Y Pericardial Cavity	**3** Percutaneous	**G** Other Therapeutic Substance	**C** Other Substance
Y Pericardial Cavity	**3** Percutaneous	**S** Gas	**F** Other Gas
Y Pericardial Cavity	**4** Percutaneous Endoscopic	**G** Other Therapeutic Substance	**C** Other Substance
Y Pericardial Cavity	**7** Via Natural or Artificial Opening	**0** Antineoplastic	**4** Liquid Brachytherapy Radioisotope **5** Other Antineoplastic **M** Monoclonal Antibody
Y Pericardial Cavity	**7** Via Natural or Artificial Opening	**S** Gas	**F** Other Gas

♂ 3E0N304 3E0N305 3E0N30M 3E0N328 3E0N329 3E0N33Z 3E0N36Z 3E0N37Z 3E0N3BZ 3E0N3GC 3E0N3HZ 3E0N3KZ 3E0N3NZ 3E0N3SF 3E0N3TZ 3E0N704 3E0N705 3E0N70M 3E0N728 3E0N729 3E0N73Z 3E0N76Z 3E0N77Z 3E0N7BZ 3E0N7GC 3E0N7HZ 3E0N7KZ 3E0N7NZ 3E0N7SF 3E0N7TZ 3E0N804 3E0N805 3E0N80M 3E0N828 3E0N829 3E0N83Z 3E0N86Z 3E0N87Z 3E0N8BZ 3E0N8GC 3E0N8HZ 3E0N8KZ 3E0N8NZ 3E0N8SF 3E0N8TZ

♀ 3E0E304 3E0E305 3E0E30M 3E0E328 3E0E329 3E0E33Z 3E0E36Z 3E0E37Z 3E0E3BZ 3E0E3GC 3E0E3HZ 3E0E3KZ 3E0E3NZ 3E0E3SF 3E0E3TZ 3E0E4GC 3E0E704 3E0E705 3E0E70M 3E0E728 3E0E729 3E0E73Z 3E0E76Z 3E0E77Z 3E0E7BZ 3E0E7GC 3E0E7HZ 3E0E7KZ 3E0E7NZ 3E0E7SF 3E0E7TZ 3E0E804 3E0E805 3E0E80M 3E0E828 3E0E829 3E0E83Z 3E0E86Z 3E0E87Z 3E0E8BZ 3E0E8GC 3E0E8HZ 3E0E8KZ 3E0E8NZ 3E0E8SF 3E0E8TZ 3E0P05Z 3E0P304 3E0P305 3E0P30M 3E0P328 3E0P329 3E0P33Z 3E0P35Z 3E0P36Z 3E0P37Z 3E0P3BZ 3E0P3GC 3E0P3HZ 3E0P3KZ 3E0P3LZ 3E0P3NZ 3E0P3Q0 3E0P3Q1 3E0P3SF 3E0P3TZ 3E0P3VZ 3E0P45Z 3E0P4GC 3E0P704 3E0P705 3E0P70M 3E0P728 3E0P729 3E0P73Z 3E0P76Z 3E0P77Z 3E0P7BZ 3E0P7GC 3E0P7HZ 3E0P7KZ 3E0P7LZ 3E0P7NZ 3E0P7Q0 3E0P7Q1 3E0P7SF 3E0P7TZ 3E0P7VZ 3E0P804 3E0P805 3E0P80M 3E0P828 3E0P829 3E0P83Z 3E0P86Z 3E0P87Z 3E0P8BZ 3E0P8GC 3E0P8HZ 3E0P8KZ 3E0P8NZ 3E0P8SF 3E0P8TZ

3 **Administration**
E **Physiological Systems and Anatomical Regions**
1 **Irrigation:** Putting in or on a cleansing substance

Body System / Region Character 4	Approach Character 5	Substance Character 6	Qualifier Character 7
0 Skin and Mucous Membranes **C** Eye	**3** Percutaneous **X** External	**8** Irrigating Substance	**X** Diagnostic **Z** No Qualifier
9 Nose **B** Ear **F** Respiratory Tract **G** Upper GI **H** Lower GI **J** Biliary and Pancreatic Tract **K** Genitourinary Tract **N** Male Reproductive ♂ **P** Female Reproductive ♀	**3** Percutaneous **7** Via Natural or Artificial Opening **8** Via Natural or Artificial Opening Endoscopic	**8** Irrigating Substance	**X** Diagnostic **Z** No Qualifier
L Pleural Cavity **Q** Cranial Cavity and Brain **R** Spinal Canal **S** Epidural Space **U** Joints **Y** Pericardial Cavity	**3** Percutaneous	**8** Irrigating Substance	**X** Diagnostic **Z** No Qualifier
M Peritoneal Cavity	**3** Percutaneous	**8** Irrigating Substance	**X** Diagnostic **Z** No Qualifier
M Peritoneal Cavity	**3** Percutaneous	**9** Dialysate	**Z** No Qualifier

♂ 3E1N38X 3E1N38Z 3E1N78X 3E1N78Z 3E1N88X 3E1N88Z
♀ 3E1P38X 3E1P38Z 3E1P78X 3E1P78Z 3E1P88X 3E1P88Z

NOTES

Measurement and Monitoring 4A0-4B0

4 Measurement and Monitoring
A Physiological Systems
0 Measurement: Determining the level of a physiological or physical function at a point in time

Body System	Approach	Function/Device	Qualifier
Character 4	Character 5	Character 6	Character 7
0 Central Nervous	**0** Open	**2** Conductivity **4** Electrical Activity **B** Pressure	**Z** No Qualifier
0 Central Nervous	**3** Percutaneous **7** Via Natural or Artificial Opening **8** Via Natural or Artificial Opening Endoscopic	**4** Electrical Activity	**Z** No Qualifier
0 Central Nervous	**3** Percutaneous **7** Via Natural or Artificial Opening **8** Via Natural or Artificial Opening Endoscopic	**B** Pressure **K** Temperature **R** Saturation	**D** Intracranial
0 Central Nervous	**X** External	**2** Conductivity **4** Electrical Activity	**Z** No Qualifier
1 Peripheral Nervous	**0** Open **3** Percutaneous **7** Via Natural or Artificial Opening **8** Via Natural or Artificial Opening Endoscopic **X** External	**2** Conductivity	**9** Sensory **B** Motor
1 Peripheral Nervous	**0** Open **3** Percutaneous **7** Via Natural or Artificial Opening **8** Via Natural or Artificial Opening Endoscopic **X** External	**4** Electrical Activity	**Z** No Qualifier
2 Cardiac	**0** Open **3** Percutaneous **7** Via Natural or Artificial Opening **8** Via Natural or Artificial Opening Endoscopic	**4** Electrical Activity **9** Output **C** Rate **F** Rhythm **H** Sound **P** Action Currents	**Z** No Qualifier
2 Cardiac	**0** Open **3** Percutaneous **7** Via Natural or Artificial Opening **8** Via Natural or Artificial Opening Endoscopic	**N** Sampling and Pressure	**6** Right Heart **7** Left Heart **8** Bilateral
2 Cardiac	**X** External	**4** Electrical Activity	**A** Guidance **Z** No Qualifier
2 Cardiac	**X** External	**9** Output **C** Rate **F** Rhythm **H** Sound **P** Action Currents	**Z** No Qualifier
2 Cardiac	**X** External	**M** Total Activity	**4** Stress
3 Arterial	**0** Open **3** Percutaneous	**5** Flow **J** Pulse	**1** Peripheral **3** Pulmonary **C** Coronary
3 Arterial	**0** Open **3** Percutaneous	**B** Pressure	**1** Peripheral **3** Pulmonary **C** Coronary **F** Other Thoracic

4A0 continued on next page

4A0 continued from previous page

4 Measurement and Monitoring
A Physiological Systems
0 Measurement: Determining the level of a physiological or physical function at a point in time

Body System	Approach	Function/Device	Qualifier
Character 4	**Character 5**	**Character 6**	**Character 7**
3 Arterial	**0** Open **3** Percutaneous	**H** Sound **R** Saturation	**1** Peripheral
3 Arterial	**X** External	**5** Flow **B** Pressure **H** Sound **J** Pulse **R** Saturation	**1** Peripheral
4 Venous	**0** Open **3** Percutaneous	**5** Flow **B** Pressure **J** Pulse	**0** Central **1** Peripheral **2** Portal **3** Pulmonary
4 Venous	**0** Open **3** Percutaneous	**R** Saturation	**1** Peripheral
4 Venous	**X** External	**5** Flow **B** Pressure **J** Pulse **R** Saturation	**1** Peripheral
5 Circulatory	**X** External	**L** Volume	**Z** No Qualifier
6 Lymphatic	**0** Open **3** Percutaneous **7** Via Natural or Artificial Opening **8** Via Natural or Artificial Opening Endoscopic	**5** Flow **B** Pressure	**Z** No Qualifier
7 Visual	**X** External	**0** Acuity **7** Mobility **B** Pressure	**Z** No Qualifier
8 Olfactory	**X** External	**0** Acuity	**Z** No Qualifier
9 Respiratory	**7** Via Natural or Artificial Opening **8** Via Natural or Artificial Opening Endoscopic **X** External	**1** Capacity **5** Flow **C** Rate **D** Resistance **L** Volume **M** Total Activity	**Z** No Qualifier
B Gastrointestinal	**7** Via Natural or Artificial Opening **8** Via Natural or Artificial Opening Endoscopic	**8** Motility **B** Pressure **G** Secretion	**Z** No Qualifier
C Biliary	**3** Percutaneous **4** Percutaneous Endoscopic **7** Via Natural or Artificial Opening **8** Via Natural or Artificial Opening Endoscopic	**5** Flow **B** Pressure	**Z** No Qualifier
D Urinary	**7** Via Natural or Artificial Opening **8** Via Natural or Artificial Opening Endoscopic	**3** Contractility **5** Flow **B** Pressure **D** Resistance **L** Volume	**Z** No Qualifier
F Musculoskeletal	**3** Percutaneous **X** External	**3** Contractility	**Z** No Qualifier
H Products of Conception, Cardiac ♀	**7** Via Natural or Artificial Opening **8** Via Natural or Artificial Opening Endoscopic **X** External	**4** Electrical Activity **C** Rate **F** Rhythm **H** Sound	**Z** No Qualifier

4A0 continued on next page

4A0 continued from previous page

4 Measurement and Monitoring
A Physiological Systems
0 Measurement: Determining the level of a physiological or physical function at a point in time

Body System Character 4	Approach Character 5	Function/Device Character 6	Qualifier Character 7
J Products of Conception, Nervous ♀	**7** Via Natural or Artificial Opening **8** Via Natural or Artificial Opening Endoscopic **X** External	**2** Conductivity **4** Electrical Activity **B** Pressure	**Z** No Qualifier
Z None	**7** Via Natural or Artificial Opening	**6** Metabolism **K** Temperature	**Z** No Qualifier
Z None	**X** External	**6** Metabolism **K** Temperature **Q** Sleep	**Z** No Qualifier

♀ 4A0H74Z 4A0H7CZ 4A0H7FZ 4A0H7HZ 4A0H84Z 4A0H8CZ 4A0H8FZ 4A0H8HZ 4A0HX4Z 4A0HXCZ 4A0HXFZ 4A0HXHZ 4A0J72Z 4A0J74Z 4A0J7BZ 4A0J82Z 4A0J84Z 4A0J8BZ 4A0JX2Z 4A0JX4Z 4A0JXBZ

4 Measurement and Monitoring
A Physiological Systems
1 Monitoring: Determining the level of a physiological or physical function repetitively over a period of time

Body System Character 4	Approach Character 5	Function/Device Character 6	Qualifier Character 7
0 Central Nervous	**0** Open	**2** Conductivity **B** Pressure	**Z** No Qualifier
0 Central Nervous	**0** Open	**4** Electrical Activity	**G** Intraoperative **Z** No Qualifier
0 Central Nervous	**3** Percutaneous **7** Via Natural or Artificial Opening **8** Via Natural or Artificial Opening Endoscopic	**4** Electrical Activity	**G** Intraoperative **Z** No Qualifier
0 Central Nervous	**3** Percutaneous **7** Via Natural or Artificial Opening **8** Via Natural or Artificial Opening Endoscopic	**B** Pressure **K** Temperature **R** Saturation	**D** Intracranial
0 Central Nervous	**X** External	**2** Conductivity	**Z** No Qualifier
0 Central Nervous	**X** External	**4** Electrical Activity	**G** Intraoperative **Z** No Qualifier
1 Peripheral Nervous	**0** Open **3** Percutaneous **7** Via Natural or Artificial Opening **8** Via Natural or Artificial Opening Endoscopic **X** External	**2** Conductivity	**9** Sensory **B** Motor
1 Peripheral Nervous	**0** Open **3** Percutaneous **7** Via Natural or Artificial Opening **8** Via Natural or Artificial Opening Endoscopic **X** External	**4** Electrical Activity	**G** Intraoperative **Z** No Qualifier
2 Cardiac	**0** Open **3** Percutaneous **7** Via Natural or Artificial Opening **8** Via Natural or Artificial Opening Endoscopic	**4** Electrical Activity **9** Output **C** Rate **F** Rhythm **H** Sound	**Z** No Qualifier
2 Cardiac	**X** External	**4** Electrical Activity	**5** Ambulatory **Z** No Qualifier

4A1 continued on next page

4 **Measurement and Monitoring**
A **Physiological Systems**
1 **Monitoring:** Determining the level of a physiological or physical function repetitively over a period of time

4A1 continued from previous page

Body System	Approach	Function/Device	Qualifier
Character 4	Character 5	Character 6	Character 7
2 Cardiac	X External	9 Output C Rate F Rhythm H Sound	Z No Qualifier
2 Cardiac	X External	M Total Activity	4 Stress
2 Cardiac	X External	S Vascular Perfusion	H Indocyanine Green Dye
3 Arterial	0 Open 3 Percutaneous	5 Flow B Pressure J Pulse	1 Peripheral 3 Pulmonary C Coronary
3 Arterial	0 Open 3 Percutaneous	H Sound R Saturation	1 Peripheral
3 Arterial	X External	5 Flow B Pressure H Sound J Pulse R Saturation	1 Peripheral
4 Venous	0 Open 3 Percutaneous	5 Flow B Pressure J Pulse	0 Central 1 Peripheral 2 Portal 3 Pulmonary
4 Venous	0 Open 3 Percutaneous	R Saturation	0 Central 2 Portal 3 Pulmonary
4 Venous	X External	5 Flow B Pressure J Pulse	1 Peripheral
6 Lymphatic	0 Open 3 Percutaneous 7 Via Natural or Artificial Opening 8 Via Natural or Artificial Opening Endoscopic	5 Flow B Pressure	Z No Qualifier
9 Respiratory	7 Via Natural or Artificial Opening X External	1 Capacity 5 Flow C Rate D Resistance L Volume	Z No Qualifier
B Gastrointestinal	7 Via Natural or Artificial Opening 8 Via Natural or Artificial Opening Endoscopic	8 Motility B Pressure G Secretion	Z No Qualifier
B Gastrointestinal	X External	S Vascular Perfusion	H Indocyanine Green Dye
D Urinary	7 Via Natural or Artificial Opening 8 Via Natural or Artificial Opening Endoscopic	3 Contractility 5 Flow B Pressure D Resistance L Volume	Z No Qualifier
G Skin and Breast	X External	S Vascular Perfusion	H Indocyanine Green Dye
H Products of Conception, Cardiac ♀	7 Via Natural or Artificial Opening 8 Via Natural or Artificial Opening Endoscopic X External	4 Electrical Activity C Rate F Rhythm H Sound	Z No Qualifier

4A1 continued on next page

4A1 continued from previous page

4 Measurement and Monitoring
A Physiological Systems
1 Monitoring: Determining the level of a physiological or physical function repetitively over a period of time

Body System	Approach	Function/Device	Qualifier
Character 4	**Character 5**	**Character 6**	**Character 7**
J Products of Conception, Nervous ♀	**7** Via Natural or Artificial Opening **8** Via Natural or Artificial Opening Endoscopic **X** External	**2** Conductivity **4** Electrical Activity **B** Pressure	**Z** No Qualifier
Z None	**7** Via Natural or Artificial Opening	**K** Temperature	**Z** No Qualifier
Z None	**X** External	**K** Temperature **Q** Sleep	**Z** No Qualifier

♀ 4A1H74Z 4A1H7CZ 4A1H7FZ 4A1H7HZ 4A1H84Z 4A1H8CZ 4A1H8FZ 4A1H8HZ 4A1HX4Z 4A1HXCZ 4A1HXFZ 4A1HXHZ 4A1J72Z 4A1J74Z 4A1J7BZ 4A1J82Z 4A1J84Z 4A1J8BZ 4A1JX2Z 4A1JX4Z 4A1JXBZ

4 Measurement and Monitoring
B Physiological Devices
0 Measurement: Determining the level of a physiological or physical function at a point in time

Body System	Approach	Function/Device	Qualifier
Character 4	**Character 5**	**Character 6**	**Character 7**
0 Central Nervous **1** Peripheral Nervous **F** Musculoskeletal	**X** External	**V** Stimulator	**Z** No Qualifier
2 Cardiac	**X** External	**S** Pacemaker **T** Defibrillator	**Z** No Qualifier
9 Respiratory	**X** External	**S** Pacemaker	**Z** No Qualifier

NOTES

Extracorporeal or Systemic Assistance and Performance 5A0-5A2

5 Extracorporeal or Systemic Assistance and Performance
A Physiological Systems
0 Assistance: Taking over a portion of a physiological function by extracorporeal means

Body System	Approach	Function/Device	Qualifier
Character 4	**Character 5**	**Character 6**	**Character 7**
2 Cardiac	**1** Intermittent **2** Continuous	**1** Output	**0** Balloon Pump **5** Pulsatile Compression **6** Other Pump **D** Impeller Pump
5 Circulatory	**1** Intermittent **2** Continuous	**2** Oxygenation	**1** Hyperbaric **C** Supersaturated
9 Respiratory	**2** Continuous	**0** Filtration	**Z** No Qualifier
9 Respiratory	**3** Less than 24 Consecutive Hours **4** 24-96 Consecutive Hours **5** Greater than 96 Consecutive Hours	**5** Ventilation	**7** Continuous Positive Airway Pressure **8** Intermittent Positive Airway Pressure **9** Continuous Negative Airway Pressure **B** Intermittent Negative Airway Pressure **Z** No Qualifier

5 Extracorporeal or Systemic Assistance and Performance
A Physiological Systems
1 Performance: Completely taking over a physiological function by extracorporeal means

Body System	Approach	Function/Device	Qualifier
Character 4	**Character 5**	**Character 6**	**Character 7**
2 Cardiac	**0** Single	**1** Output	**2** Manual
2 Cardiac	**1** Intermittent	**3** Pacing	**Z** No Qualifier
2 Cardiac	**2** Continuous	**1** Output **3** Pacing	**Z** No Qualifier
5 Circulatory	**2** Continuous	**2** Oxygenation	**F** Membrane, Central **G** Membrane, Peripheral Veno-arterial **H** Membrane, Peripheral Veno-venous
9 Respiratory	**0** Single	**5** Ventilation	**4** Nonmechanical
9 Respiratory	**3** Less than 24 Consecutive Hours **4** 24-96 Consecutive Hours **5** Greater than 96 Consecutive Hours	**5** Ventilation	**Z** No Qualifier
C Biliary	**0** Single **6** Multiple	**0** Filtration	**Z** No Qualifier
D Urinary	**7** Intermittent, Less than 6 Hours Per Day **8** Prolonged Intermittent, 6-18 hours Per Day **9** Continuous, Greater than 18 hours Per Day	**0** Filtration	**Z** No Qualifier

5 Extracorporeal or Systemic Assistance and Performance
A Physiological Systems
2 Restoration: Returning, or attempting to return, a physiological function to its original state by extracorporeal means.

Body System	Approach	Function/Device	Qualifier
Character 4	**Character 5**	**Character 6**	**Character 7**
2 Cardiac	**0** Single	**4** Rhythm	**Z** No Qualifier

NOTES

Extracorporeal or Systemic Therapies 6A0-6AB

6 Extracorporeal or Systemic Therapies
A Physiological Systems
0 Atmospheric Control: Extracorporeal control of atmospheric pressure and composition

Body System	Duration	Qualifier	Qualifier
Character 4	**Character 5**	**Character 6**	**Character 7**
Z None	0 Single 1 Multiple	Z No Qualifier	Z No Qualifier

6 Extracorporeal or Systemic Therapies
A Physiological Systems
1 Decompression: Extracorporeal elimination of undissolved gas from body fluids

Body System	Duration	Qualifier	Qualifier
Character 4	**Character 5**	**Character 6**	**Character 7**
5 Circulatory	0 Single 1 Multiple	Z No Qualifier	Z No Qualifier

6 Extracorporeal or Systemic Therapies
A Physiological Systems
2 Electromagnetic Therapy: Extracorporeal treatment by electromagnetic rays

Body System	Duration	Qualifier	Qualifier
Character 4	**Character 5**	**Character 6**	**Character 7**
1 Urinary 2 Central Nervous	0 Single 1 Multiple	Z No Qualifier	Z No Qualifier

6 Extracorporeal or Systemic Therapies
A Physiological Systems
3 Hyperthermia: Extracorporeal raising of body temperature

Body System	Duration	Qualifier	Qualifier
Character 4	**Character 5**	**Character 6**	**Character 7**
Z None	0 Single 1 Multiple	Z No Qualifier	Z No Qualifier

6 Extracorporeal or Systemic Therapies
A Physiological Systems
4 Hypothermia: Extracorporeal lowering of body temperature

Body System	Duration	Qualifier	Qualifier
Character 4	**Character 5**	**Character 6**	**Character 7**
Z None	0 Single 1 Multiple	Z No Qualifier	Z No Qualifier

6 Extracorporeal or Systemic Therapies
A Physiological Systems
5 Pheresis: Extracorporeal separation of blood products

Body System	Duration	Qualifier	Qualifier
Character 4	**Character 5**	**Character 6**	**Character 7**
5 Circulatory	0 Single 1 Multiple	Z No Qualifier	0 Erythrocytes 1 Leukocytes 2 Platelets 3 Plasma T Stem Cells, Cord Blood V Stem Cells, Hematopoietic

6 Extracorporeal or Systemic Therapies
A Physiological Systems
6 Phototherapy: Extracorporeal treatment by light rays

Body System	Duration	Qualifier	Qualifier
Character 4	**Character 5**	**Character 6**	**Character 7**
0 Skin **5** Circulatory	**0** Single **1** Multiple	**Z** No Qualifier	**Z** No Qualifier

6 Extracorporeal or Systemic Therapies
A Physiological Systems
7 Ultrasound Therapy: Extracorporeal treatment by ultrasound

Body System Character 4	Duration Character 5	Qualifier Character 6	Qualifier Character 7
5 Circulatory	**0** Single **1** Multiple	**Z** No Qualifier	**4** Head and Neck Vessels **5** Heart **6** Peripheral Vessels **7** Other Vessels **Z** No Qualifier

6 Extracorporeal or Systemic Therapies
A Physiological Systems
8 Ultraviolet Light Therapy: Extracorporeal treatment by ultraviolet light

Body System	Duration	Qualifier	Qualifier
Character 4	**Character 5**	**Character 6**	**Character 7**
0 Skin	**0** Single **1** Multiple	**Z** No Qualifier	**Z** No Qualifier

6 Extracorporeal or Systemic Therapies
A Physiological Systems
9 Shock Wave Therapy: Extracorporeal treatment by shock waves

Body System	Duration	Qualifier	Qualifier
Character 4	**Character 5**	**Character 6**	**Character 7**
3 Musculoskeletal	**0** Single **1** Multiple	**Z** No Qualifier	**Z** No Qualifier

6 Extracorporeal or Systemic Therapies
A Physiological Systems
B Perfusion: Extracorporeal treatment by diffusion of therapeutic fluid

Body System	Duration	Qualifier	Qualifier
Character 4	**Character 5**	**Character 6**	**Character 7**
5 Circulatory **B** Respiratory System **F** Hepatobiliary System and Pancreas **T** Urinary System	**0** Single	**B** Donor Organ	**Z** No Qualifier

NOTES

NOTES

Osteopathic 7W0

7 Osteopathic
W Anatomical Regions
0 Treatment: Manual treatment to eliminate or alleviate somatic dysfunction and related disorders

Body Region Character 4	Approach Character 5	Method Character 6	Qualifier Character 7
0 Head **1** Cervical **2** Thoracic **3** Lumbar **4** Sacrum **5** Pelvis **6** Lower Extremities **7** Upper Extremities **8** Rib Cage **9** Abdomen	**X** External	**0** Articulatory-Raising **1** Fascial Release **2** General Mobilization **3** High Velocity-Low Amplitude **4** Indirect **5** Low Velocity-High Amplitude **6** Lymphatic Pump **7** Muscle Energy-Isometric **8** Muscle Energy-Isotonic **9** Other Method	**Z** None

NOTES

Other Procedures 8C0-8E0

8 Other Procedures
C Indwelling Device
0 Other Procedures: Methodologies which attempt to remediate or cure a disorder or disease

Body Region Character 4	Approach Character 5	Method Character 6	Qualifier Character 7
1 Nervous System	**X** External	**6** Collection	**J** Cerebrospinal Fluid **L** Other Fluid
2 Circulatory System	**X** External	**6** Collection	**K** Blood **L** Other Fluid

8 Other Procedures
E Physiological Systems and Anatomical Regions
0 Other Procedures: Methodologies which attempt to remediate or cure a disorder or disease

Body Region Character 4	Approach Character 5	Method Character 6	Qualifier Character 7
1 Nervous System **U** Female Reproductive System ♀	**X** External	**Y** Other Method	**7** Examination
2 Circulatory System	**3** Percutaneous	**D** Near Infrared Spectroscopy	**Z** No Qualifier
9 Head and Neck Region **W** Trunk Region	**0** Open **3** Percutaneous **4** Percutaneous Endoscopic **7** Via Natural or Artificial Opening **8** Via Natural or Artificial Opening Endoscopic	**C** Robotic Assisted Procedure	**Z** No Qualifier
9 Head and Neck Region **W** Trunk Region	**X** External	**B** Computer Assisted Procedure	**F** With Fluoroscopy **G** With Computerized Tomography **H** With Magnetic Resonance Imaging **Z** No Qualifier
9 Head and Neck Region **W** Trunk Region	**X** External	**C** Robotic Assisted Procedure	**Z** No Qualifier
9 Head and Neck Region **W** Trunk Region	**X** External	**Y** Other Method	**8** Suture Removal
H Integumentary System and Breast	**3** Percutaneous	**0** Acupuncture	**0** Anesthesia **Z** No Qualifier
H Integumentary System and Breast ♀	**X** External	**6** Collection	**2** Breast Milk
H Integumentary System and Breast	**X** External	**Y** Other Method	**9** Piercing
K Musculoskeletal System	**X** External	**1** Therapeutic Massage	**Z** No Qualifier
K Musculoskeletal System	**X** External	**Y** Other Method	**7** Examination
V Male Reproductive System ♂	**X** External	**1** Therapeutic Massage	**C** Prostate **D** Rectum
V Male Reproductive System ♂	**X** External	**6** Collection	**3** Sperm
X Upper Extremity **Y** Lower Extremity	**0** Open **3** Percutaneous **4** Percutaneous Endoscopic	**C** Robotic Assisted Procedure	**Z** No Qualifier
X Upper Extremity **Y** Lower Extremity	**X** External	**B** Computer Assisted Procedure	**F** With Fluoroscopy **G** With Computerized Tomography **H** With Magnetic Resonance Imaging **Z** No Qualifier

8E0 continued on next page

8E0 continued from previous page

8 **Other Procedures**
E **Physiological Systems and Anatomical Regions**
0 **Other Procedures:** Methodologies which attempt to remediate or cure a disorder or disease

Body Region	Approach	Method	Qualifier
Character 4	**Character 5**	**Character 6**	**Character 7**
X Upper Extremity **Y** Lower Extremity	**X** External	**C** Robotic Assisted Procedure	**Z** No Qualifier
X Upper Extremity **Y** Lower Extremity	**X** External	**Y** Other Method	**8** Suture Removal
Z None	**X** External	**Y** Other Method	**1** In Vitro Fertilization **4** Yoga Therapy **5** Meditation **6** Isolation

♂ 8E0VX1C 8E0VX63
♀ 8E0HX62 8E0UXY7

NOTES

NOTES

Chiropractic 9WB

9 Chiropractic
W Anatomical Regions
B Manipulation: Manual procedure that involves a directed thrust to move a joint past the physiological range of motion, without exceeding the anatomical limit

Body Region	Approach	Method	Qualifier
Character 4	**Character 5**	**Character 6**	**Character 7**
0 Head **1** Cervical **2** Thoracic **3** Lumbar **4** Sacrum **5** Pelvis **6** Lower Extremities **7** Upper Extremities **8** Rib Cage **9** Abdomen	**X** External	**B** Non-Manual **C** Indirect Visceral **D** Extra-Articular **F** Direct Visceral **G** Long Lever Specific Contact **H** Short Lever Specific Contact **J** Long and Short Lever Specific Contact **K** Mechanically Assisted **L** Other Method	**Z** None

NOTES

Imaging B00-BY4

B Imaging
0 Central Nervous System
0 Plain Radiography: Planar display of an image developed from the capture of external ionizing radiation on photographic or photoconductive plate

Body Part	Contrast	Qualifier	Qualifier
Character 4	Character 5	Character 6	Character 7
B Spinal Cord	**0** High Osmolar **1** Low Osmolar **Y** Other Contrast **Z** None	**Z** None	**Z** None

B Imaging
0 Central Nervous System
1 Fluoroscopy: Single plane or bi-plane real time display of an image developed from the capture of external ionizing radiation on a fluorescent screen. The image may also be stored by either digital or analog means

Body Part	Contrast	Qualifier	Qualifier
Character 4	Character 5	Character 6	Character 7
B Spinal Cord	**0** High Osmolar **1** Low Osmolar **Y** Other Contrast **Z** None	**Z** None	**Z** None

B Imaging
0 Central Nervous System
2 Computerized Tomography (CT Scan): Computer reformatted digital display of multiplanar images developed from the capture of multiple exposures of external ionizing radiation

Body Part	Contrast	Qualifier	Qualifier
Character 4	Character 5	Character 6	Character 7
0 Brain **7** Cisterna **8** Cerebral Ventricle(s) **9** Sella Turcica/Pituitary Gland **B** Spinal Cord	**0** High Osmolar **1** Low Osmolar **Y** Other Contrast	**0** Unenhanced and Enhanced **Z** None	**Z** None
0 Brain **7** Cisterna **8** Cerebral Ventricle(s) **9** Sella Turcica/Pituitary Gland **B** Spinal Cord	**Z** None	**Z** None	**Z** None

B Imaging
0 Central Nervous System
3 Magnetic Resonance Imaging (MRI): Computer reformatted digital display of multiplanar images developed from the capture of radiofrequency signals emitted by nuclei in a body site excited within a magnetic field

Body Part	Contrast	Qualifier	Qualifier
Character 4	Character 5	Character 6	Character 7
0 Brain **9** Sella Turcica/Pituitary Gland **B** Spinal Cord **C** Acoustic Nerves	**Y** Other Contrast	**0** Unenhanced and Enhanced **Z** None	**Z** None
0 Brain **9** Sella Turcica/Pituitary Gland **B** Spinal Cord **C** Acoustic Nerves	**Z** None	**Z** None	**Z** None

B Imaging
0 Central Nervous System
4 Ultrasonography: Real time display of images of anatomy or flow information developed from the capture of reflected and attenuated high frequency sound waves

Body Part	Contrast	Qualifier	Qualifier
Character 4	Character 5	Character 6	Character 7
0 Brain **B** Spinal Cord	**Z** None	**Z** None	**Z** None

B Imaging
2 Heart
0 Plain Radiography: Planar display of an image developed from the capture of external ionizing radiation on photographic or photoconductive plate

Body Part	Contrast	Qualifier	Qualifier
Character 4	Character 5	Character 6	Character 7
0 Coronary Artery, Single **1** Coronary Arteries, Multiple **2** Coronary Artery Bypass Graft, Single **3** Coronary Artery Bypass Grafts, Multiple **4** Heart, Right **5** Heart, Left **6** Heart, Right and Left **7** Internal Mammary Bypass Graft, Right **8** Internal Mammary Bypass Graft, Left **F** Bypass Graft, Other	**0** High Osmolar **1** Low Osmolar **Y** Other Contrast	**Z** None	**Z** None

B Imaging
2 Heart
1 Fluoroscopy: Single plane or bi-plane real time display of an image developed from the capture of external ionizing radiation on a fluorescent screen. The image may also be stored by either digital or analog means

Body Part	Contrast	Qualifier	Qualifier
Character 4	Character 5	Character 6	Character 7
0 Coronary Artery, Single **1** Coronary Arteries, Multiple **2** Coronary Artery Bypass Graft, Single **3** Coronary Artery Bypass Grafts, Multiple	**0** High Osmolar **1** Low Osmolar **Y** Other Contrast	**1** Laser	**0** Intraoperative
0 Coronary Artery, Single **1** Coronary Arteries, Multiple **2** Coronary Artery Bypass Graft, Single **3** Coronary Artery Bypass Grafts, Multiple	**0** High Osmolar **1** Low Osmolar **Y** Other Contrast	**Z** None	**Z** None
4 Heart, Right **5** Heart, Left **6** Heart, Right and Left **7** Internal Mammary Bypass Graft, Right **8** Internal Mammary Bypass Graft, Left **F** Bypass Graft, Other	**0** High Osmolar **1** Low Osmolar **Y** Other Contrast	**Z** None	**Z** None

B Imaging
2 Heart
2 Computerized Tomography (CT Scan): Computer reformatted digital display of multiplanar images developed from the capture of multiple exposures of external ionizing radiation

Body Part	Contrast	Qualifier	Qualifier
Character 4	**Character 5**	**Character 6**	**Character 7**
1 Coronary Arteries, Multiple **3** Coronary Artery Bypass Grafts, Multiple **6** Heart, Right and Left	**0** High Osmolar **1** Low Osmolar **Y** Other Contrast	**0** Unenhanced and Enhanced **Z** None	**Z** None
1 Coronary Arteries, Multiple **3** Coronary Artery Bypass Grafts, Multiple **6** Heart, Right and Left	**Z** None	**2** Intravascular Optical Coherence **Z** None	**Z** None

B Imaging
2 Heart
3 Magnetic Resonance Imaging (MRI): Computer reformatted digital display of multiplanar images developed from the capture of radiofrequency signals emitted by nuclei in a body site excited within a magnetic field

Body Part	Contrast	Qualifier	Qualifier
Character 4	**Character 5**	**Character 6**	**Character 7**
1 Coronary Arteries, Multiple **3** Coronary Artery Bypass Grafts, Multiple **6** Heart, Right and Left	**Y** Other Contrast	**0** Unenhanced and Enhanced **Z** None	**Z** None
1 Coronary Arteries, Multiple **3** Coronary Artery Bypass Grafts, Multiple **6** Heart, Right and Left	**Z** None	**Z** None	**Z** None

B Imaging
2 Heart
4 Ultrasonography: Real time display of images of anatomy or flow information developed from the capture of reflected and attenuated high frequency sound waves

Body Part	Contrast	Qualifier	Qualifier
Character 4	**Character 5**	**Character 6**	**Character 7**
0 Coronary Artery, Single **1** Coronary Arteries, Multiple **4** Heart, Right **5** Heart, Left **6** Heart, Right and Left **B** Heart with Aorta **C** Pericardium **D** Pediatric Heart	**Y** Other Contrast	**Z** None	**Z** None
0 Coronary Artery, Single **1** Coronary Arteries, Multiple **4** Heart, Right **5** Heart, Left **6** Heart, Right and Left **B** Heart with Aorta **C** Pericardium **D** Pediatric Heart	**Z** None	**Z** None	**3** Intravascular **4** Transesophageal **Z** None

B Imaging
3 Upper Arteries
0 Plain Radiography: Planar display of an image developed from the capture of external ionizing radiation on photographic or photoconductive plate

Body Part	Contrast	Qualifier	Qualifier
Character 4	**Character 5**	**Character 6**	**Character 7**
0 Thoracic Aorta **1** Brachiocephalic-Subclavian Artery, Right **2** Subclavian Artery, Left **3** Common Carotid Artery, Right **4** Common Carotid Artery, Left **5** Common Carotid Arteries, Bilateral **6** Internal Carotid Artery, Right **7** Internal Carotid Artery, Left **8** Internal Carotid Arteries, Bilateral **9** External Carotid Artery, Right **B** External Carotid Artery, Left **C** External Carotid Arteries, Bilateral **D** Vertebral Artery, Right **F** Vertebral Artery, Left **G** Vertebral Arteries, Bilateral **H** Upper Extremity Arteries, Right **J** Upper Extremity Arteries, Left **K** Upper Extremity Arteries, Bilateral **L** Intercostal and Bronchial Arteries **M** Spinal Arteries **N** Upper Arteries, Other **P** Thoraco-Abdominal Aorta **Q** Cervico-Cerebral Arch **R** Intracranial Arteries **S** Pulmonary Artery, Right **T** Pulmonary Artery, Left	**0** High Osmolar **1** Low Osmolar **Y** Other Contrast **Z** None	**Z** None	**Z** None

B Imaging
3 Upper Arteries
1 Fluoroscopy: Single plane or bi-plane real time display of an image developed from the capture of external ionizing radiation on a fluorescent screen. The image may also be stored by either digital or analog means

Body Part Character 4	Contrast Character 5	Qualifier Character 6	Qualifier Character 7
0 Thoracic Aorta **1** Brachiocephalic-Subclavian Artery, Right **2** Subclavian Artery, Left **3** Common Carotid Artery, Right **4** Common Carotid Artery, Left **5** Common Carotid Arteries, Bilateral **6** Internal Carotid Artery, Right **7** Internal Carotid Artery, Left **8** Internal Carotid Arteries, Bilateral **9** External Carotid Artery, Right **B** External Carotid Artery, Left **C** External Carotid Arteries, Bilateral **D** Vertebral Artery, Right **F** Vertebral Artery, Left **G** Vertebral Arteries, Bilateral **H** Upper Extremity Arteries, Right **J** Upper Extremity Arteries, Left **K** Upper Extremity Arteries, Bilateral **L** Intercostal and Bronchial Arteries **M** Spinal Arteries **N** Upper Arteries, Other **P** Thoraco-Abdominal Aorta **Q** Cervico-Cerebral Arch **R** Intracranial Arteries **S** Pulmonary Artery, Right **T** Pulmonary Artery, Left **U** Pulmonary Trunk	**0** High Osmolar **1** Low Osmolar **Y** Other Contrast	**1** Laser	**0** Intraoperative

B31 continued on next page

B Imaging
3 Upper Arteries
1 Fluoroscopy: Single plane or bi-plane real time display of an image developed from the capture of external ionizing radiation on a fluorescent screen. The image may also be stored by either digital or analog means

B31 continued from previous page

Body Part Character 4	Contrast Character 5	Qualifier Character 6	Qualifier Character 7
0 Thoracic Aorta **1** Brachiocephalic-Subclavian Artery, Right **2** Subclavian Artery, Left **3** Common Carotid Artery, Right **4** Common Carotid Artery, Left **5** Common Carotid Arteries, Bilateral **6** Internal Carotid Artery, Right **7** Internal Carotid Artery, Left **8** Internal Carotid Arteries, Bilateral **9** External Carotid Artery, Right **B** External Carotid Artery, Left **C** External Carotid Arteries, Bilateral **D** Vertebral Artery, Right **F** Vertebral Artery, Left **G** Vertebral Arteries, Bilateral **H** Upper Extremity Arteries, Right **J** Upper Extremity Arteries, Left **K** Upper Extremity Arteries, Bilateral **L** Intercostal and Bronchial Arteries **M** Spinal Arteries **N** Upper Arteries, Other **P** Thoraco-Abdominal Aorta **Q** Cervico-Cerebral Arch **R** Intracranial Arteries **S** Pulmonary Artery, Right **T** Pulmonary Artery, Left **U** Pulmonary Trunk	**0** High Osmolar **1** Low Osmolar **Y** Other Contrast	**Z** None	**Z** None

B31 continued on next page

B31 continued from previous page

B Imaging
3 Upper Arteries
1 Fluoroscopy: Single plane or bi-plane real time display of an image developed from the capture of external ionizing radiation on a fluorescent screen. The image may also be stored by either digital or analog means

Body Part Character 4	Contrast Character 5	Qualifier Character 6	Qualifier Character 7
0 Thoracic Aorta **1** Brachiocephalic-Subclavian Artery, Right **2** Subclavian Artery, Left **3** Common Carotid Artery, Right **4** Common Carotid Artery, Left **5** Common Carotid Arteries, Bilateral **6** Internal Carotid Artery, Right **7** Internal Carotid Artery, Left **8** Internal Carotid Arteries, Bilateral **9** External Carotid Artery, Right **B** External Carotid Artery, Left **C** External Carotid Arteries, Bilateral **D** Vertebral Artery, Right **F** Vertebral Artery, Left **G** Vertebral Arteries, Bilateral **H** Upper Extremity Arteries, Right **J** Upper Extremity Arteries, Left **K** Upper Extremity Arteries, Bilateral **L** Intercostal and Bronchial Arteries **M** Spinal Arteries **N** Upper Arteries, Other **P** Thoraco-Abdominal Aorta **Q** Cervico-Cerebral Arch **R** Intracranial Arteries **S** Pulmonary Artery, Right **T** Pulmonary Artery, Left **U** Pulmonary Trunk	**Z** None	**Z** None	**Z** None

B Imaging
3 Upper Arteries
2 Computerized Tomography (CT Scan): Computer reformatted digital display of multiplanar images developed from the capture of multiple exposures of external ionizing radiation

Body Part Character 4	Contrast Character 5	Qualifier Character 6	Qualifier Character 7
0 Thoracic Aorta **5** Common Carotid Arteries, Bilateral **8** Internal Carotid Arteries, Bilateral **G** Vertebral Arteries, Bilateral **R** Intracranial Arteries **S** Pulmonary Artery, Right **T** Pulmonary Artery, Left	**0** High Osmolar **1** Low Osmolar **Y** Other Contrast	**Z** None	**Z** None
0 Thoracic Aorta **5** Common Carotid Arteries, Bilateral **8** Internal Carotid Arteries, Bilateral **G** Vertebral Arteries, Bilateral **R** Intracranial Arteries **S** Pulmonary Artery, Right **T** Pulmonary Artery, Left	**Z** None	**2** Intravascular Optical Coherence **Z** None	**Z** None

B Imaging
3 Upper Arteries
3 Magnetic Resonance Imaging (MRI): Computer reformatted digital display of multiplanar images developed from the capture of radiofrequency signals emitted by nuclei in a body site excited within a magnetic field

Body Part Character 4	Contrast Character 5	Qualifier Character 6	Qualifier Character 7
0 Thoracic Aorta **5** Common Carotid Arteries, Bilateral **8** Internal Carotid Arteries, Bilateral **G** Vertebral Arteries, Bilateral **H** Upper Extremity Arteries, Right **J** Upper Extremity Arteries, Left **K** Upper Extremity Arteries, Bilateral **M** Spinal Arteries **Q** Cervico-Cerebral Arch **R** Intracranial Arteries	**Y** Other Contrast	**0** Unenhanced and Enhanced **Z** None	**Z** None
0 Thoracic Aorta **5** Common Carotid Arteries, Bilateral **8** Internal Carotid Arteries, Bilateral **G** Vertebral Arteries, Bilateral **H** Upper Extremity Arteries, Right **J** Upper Extremity Arteries, Left **K** Upper Extremity Arteries, Bilateral **M** Spinal Arteries **Q** Cervico-Cerebral Arch **R** Intracranial Arteries	**Z** None	**Z** None	**Z** None

B Imaging
3 Upper Arteries
4 Ultrasonography: Real time display of images of anatomy or flow information developed from the capture of reflected and attenuated high frequency sound waves

Body Part Character 4	Contrast Character 5	Qualifier Character 6	Qualifier Character 7
0 Thoracic Aorta **1** Brachiocephalic-Subclavian Artery, Right **2** Subclavian Artery, Left **3** Common Carotid Artery, Right **4** Common Carotid Artery, Left **5** Common Carotid Arteries, Bilateral **6** Internal Carotid Artery, Right **7** Internal Carotid Artery, Left **8** Internal Carotid Arteries, Bilateral **H** Upper Extremity Arteries, Right **J** Upper Extremity Arteries, Left **K** Upper Extremity Arteries, Bilateral **R** Intracranial Arteries **S** Pulmonary Artery, Right **T** Pulmonary Artery, Left **V** Ophthalmic Arteries	**Z** None	**Z** None	**3** Intravascular **Z** None

B Imaging
4 Lower Arteries
0 Plain Radiography: Planar display of an image developed from the capture of external ionizing radiation on photographic or photoconductive plate

Body Part Character 4	Contrast Character 5	Qualifier Character 6	Qualifier Character 7
0 Abdominal Aorta **2** Hepatic Artery **3** Splenic Arteries **4** Superior Mesenteric Artery **5** Inferior Mesenteric Artery **6** Renal Artery, Right **7** Renal Artery, Left **8** Renal Arteries, Bilateral **9** Lumbar Arteries **B** Intra-Abdominal Arteries, Other **C** Pelvic Arteries **D** Aorta and Bilateral Lower Extremity Arteries **F** Lower Extremity Arteries, Right **G** Lower Extremity Arteries, Left **J** Lower Arteries, Other **M** Renal Artery Transplant	**0** High Osmolar **1** Low Osmolar **Y** Other Contrast	**Z** None	**Z** None

B Imaging
4 Lower Arteries
1 Fluoroscopy: Single plane or bi-plane real time display of an image developed from the capture of external ionizing radiation on a fluorescent screen. The image may also be stored by either digital or analog means

Body Part Character 4	Contrast Character 5	Qualifier Character 6	Qualifier Character 7
0 Abdominal Aorta **2** Hepatic Artery **3** Splenic Arteries **4** Superior Mesenteric Artery **5** Inferior Mesenteric Artery **6** Renal Artery, Right **7** Renal Artery, Left **8** Renal Arteries, Bilateral **9** Lumbar Arteries **B** Intra-Abdominal Arteries, Other **C** Pelvic Arteries **D** Aorta and Bilateral Lower Extremity Arteries **F** Lower Extremity Arteries, Right **G** Lower Extremity Arteries, Left **J** Lower Arteries, Other	**0** High Osmolar **1** Low Osmolar **Y** Other Contrast	**1** Laser	**0** Intraoperative
0 Abdominal Aorta **2** Hepatic Artery **3** Splenic Arteries **4** Superior Mesenteric Artery **5** Inferior Mesenteric Artery **6** Renal Artery, Right **7** Renal Artery, Left **8** Renal Arteries, Bilateral **9** Lumbar Arteries **B** Intra-Abdominal Arteries, Other **C** Pelvic Arteries **D** Aorta and Bilateral Lower Extremity Arteries **F** Lower Extremity Arteries, Right **G** Lower Extremity Arteries, Left **J** Lower Arteries, Other	**0** High Osmolar **1** Low Osmolar **Y** Other Contrast	**Z** None	**Z** None
0 Abdominal Aorta **2** Hepatic Artery **3** Splenic Arteries **4** Superior Mesenteric Artery **5** Inferior Mesenteric Artery **6** Renal Artery, Right **7** Renal Artery, Left **8** Renal Arteries, Bilateral **9** Lumbar Arteries **B** Intra-Abdominal Arteries, Other **C** Pelvic Arteries **D** Aorta and Bilateral Lower Extremity Arteries **F** Lower Extremity Arteries, Right **G** Lower Extremity Arteries, Left **J** Lower Arteries, Other	**Z** None	**Z** None	**Z** None

B Imaging
4 Lower Arteries
2 Computerized Tomography (CT Scan): Computer reformatted digital display of multiplanar images developed from the capture of multiple exposures of external ionizing radiation

Body Part Character 4	Contrast Character 5	Qualifier Character 6	Qualifier Character 7
0 Abdominal Aorta **1** Celiac Artery **4** Superior Mesenteric Artery **8** Renal Arteries, Bilateral **C** Pelvic Arteries **F** Lower Extremity Arteries, Right **G** Lower Extremity Arteries, Left **H** Lower Extremity Arteries, Bilateral **M** Renal Artery Transplant	**0** High Osmolar **1** Low Osmolar **Y** Other Contrast	**Z** None	**Z** None
0 Abdominal Aorta **1** Celiac Artery **4** Superior Mesenteric Artery **8** Renal Arteries, Bilateral **C** Pelvic Arteries **F** Lower Extremity Arteries, Right **G** Lower Extremity Arteries, Left **H** Lower Extremity Arteries, Bilateral **M** Renal Artery Transplant	**Z** None	**2** Intravascular Optical Coherence **Z** None	**Z** None

B Imaging
4 Lower Arteries
3 Magnetic Resonance Imaging (MRI): Computer reformatted digital display of multiplanar images developed from the capture of radiofrequency signals emitted by nuclei in a body site excited within a magnetic field

Body Part Character 4	Contrast Character 5	Qualifier Character 6	Qualifier Character 7
0 Abdominal Aorta **1** Celiac Artery **4** Superior Mesenteric Artery **8** Renal Arteries, Bilateral **C** Pelvic Arteries **F** Lower Extremity Arteries, Right **G** Lower Extremity Arteries, Left **H** Lower Extremity Arteries, Bilateral	**Y** Other Contrast	**0** Unenhanced and Enhanced **Z** None	**Z** None
0 Abdominal Aorta **1** Celiac Artery **4** Superior Mesenteric Artery **8** Renal Arteries, Bilateral **C** Pelvic Arteries **F** Lower Extremity Arteries, Right **G** Lower Extremity Arteries, Left **H** Lower Extremity Arteries, Bilateral	**Z** None	**Z** None	**Z** None

B Imaging
4 Lower Arteries
4 Ultrasonography: Real time display of images of anatomy or flow information developed from the capture of reflected and attenuated high frequency sound waves

Body Part	Contrast	Qualifier	Qualifier
Character 4	Character 5	Character 6	Character 7
0 Abdominal Aorta **4** Superior Mesenteric Artery **5** Inferior Mesenteric Artery **6** Renal Artery, Right **7** Renal Artery, Left **8** Renal Arteries, Bilateral **B** Intra-Abdominal Arteries, Other **F** Lower Extremity Arteries, Right **G** Lower Extremity Arteries, Left **H** Lower Extremity Arteries, Bilateral **K** Celiac and Mesenteric Arteries **L** Femoral Artery **N** Penile Arteries	**Z** None	**Z** None	**3** Intravascular **Z** None

B Imaging
5 Veins
0 Plain Radiography: Planar display of an image developed from the capture of external ionizing radiation on photographic or photoconductive plate

Body Part	Contrast	Qualifier	Qualifier
Character 4	Character 5	Character 6	Character 7
0 Epidural Veins **1** Cerebral and Cerebellar Veins **2** Intracranial Sinuses **3** Jugular Veins, Right **4** Jugular Veins, Left **5** Jugular Veins, Bilateral **6** Subclavian Vein, Right **7** Subclavian Vein, Left **8** Superior Vena Cava **9** Inferior Vena Cava **B** Lower Extremity Veins, Right **C** Lower Extremity Veins, Left **D** Lower Extremity Veins, Bilateral **F** Pelvic (Iliac) Veins, Right **G** Pelvic (Iliac) Veins, Left **H** Pelvic (Iliac) Veins, Bilateral **J** Renal Vein, Right **K** Renal Vein, Left **L** Renal Veins, Bilateral **M** Upper Extremity Veins, Right **N** Upper Extremity Veins, Left **P** Upper Extremity Veins, Bilateral **Q** Pulmonary Vein, Right **R** Pulmonary Vein, Left **S** Pulmonary Veins, Bilateral **T** Portal and Splanchnic Veins **V** Veins, Other **W** Dialysis Shunt/Fistula	**0** High Osmolar **1** Low Osmolar **Y** Other Contrast	**Z** None	**Z** None

B Imaging
5 Veins
1 Fluoroscopy: Single plane or bi-plane real time display of an image developed from the capture of external ionizing radiation on a fluorescent screen. The image may also be stored by either digital or analog means

Body Part Character 4	Contrast Character 5	Qualifier Character 6	Qualifier Character 7
0 Epidural Veins **1** Cerebral and Cerebellar Veins **2** Intracranial Sinuses **3** Jugular Veins, Right **4** Jugular Veins, Left **5** Jugular Veins, Bilateral **6** Subclavian Vein, Right **7** Subclavian Vein, Left **8** Superior Vena Cava **9** Inferior Vena Cava **B** Lower Extremity Veins, Right **C** Lower Extremity Veins, Left **D** Lower Extremity Veins, Bilateral **F** Pelvic (Iliac) Veins, Right **G** Pelvic (Iliac) Veins, Left **H** Pelvic (Iliac) Veins, Bilateral **J** Renal Vein, Right **K** Renal Vein, Left **L** Renal Veins, Bilateral **M** Upper Extremity Veins, Right **N** Upper Extremity Veins, Left **P** Upper Extremity Veins, Bilateral **Q** Pulmonary Vein, Right **R** Pulmonary Vein, Left **S** Pulmonary Veins, Bilateral **T** Portal and Splanchnic Veins **V** Veins, Other **W** Dialysis Shunt/Fistula	**0** High Osmolar **1** Low Osmolar **Y** Other Contrast **Z** None	**Z** None	**A** Guidance **Z** None

B Imaging
5 Veins
2 Computerized Tomography (CT Scan): Computer reformatted digital display of multiplanar images developed from the capture of multiple exposures of external ionizing radiation

Body Part Character 4	Contrast Character 5	Qualifier Character 6	Qualifier Character 7
2 Intracranial Sinuses **8** Superior Vena Cava **9** Inferior Vena Cava **F** Pelvic (Iliac) Veins, Right **G** Pelvic (Iliac) Veins, Left **H** Pelvic (Iliac) Veins, Bilateral **J** Renal Vein, Right **K** Renal Vein, Left **L** Renal Veins, Bilateral **Q** Pulmonary Vein, Right **R** Pulmonary Vein, Left **S** Pulmonary Veins, Bilateral **T** Portal and Splanchnic Veins	**0** High Osmolar **1** Low Osmolar **Y** Other Contrast	**0** Unenhanced and Enhanced **Z** None	**Z** None
2 Intracranial Sinuses **8** Superior Vena Cava **9** Inferior Vena Cava **F** Pelvic (Iliac) Veins, Right **G** Pelvic (Iliac) Veins, Left **H** Pelvic (Iliac) Veins, Bilateral **J** Renal Vein, Right **K** Renal Vein, Left **L** Renal Veins, Bilateral **Q** Pulmonary Vein, Right **R** Pulmonary Vein, Left **S** Pulmonary Veins, Bilateral **T** Portal and Splanchnic Veins	**Z** None	**2** Intravascular Optical Coherence **Z** None	**Z** None

B Imaging
5 Veins
3 Magnetic Resonance Imaging (MRI): Computer reformatted digital display of multiplanar images developed from the capture of radiofrequency signals emitted by nuclei in a body site excited within a magnetic field

Body Part Character 4	Contrast Character 5	Qualifier Character 6	Qualifier Character 7
1 Cerebral and Cerebellar Veins **2** Intracranial Sinuses **5** Jugular Veins, Bilateral **8** Superior Vena Cava **9** Inferior Vena Cava **B** Lower Extremity Veins, Right **C** Lower Extremity Veins, Left **D** Lower Extremity Veins, Bilateral **H** Pelvic (Iliac) Veins, Bilateral **L** Renal Veins, Bilateral **M** Upper Extremity Veins, Right **N** Upper Extremity Veins, Left **P** Upper Extremity Veins, Bilateral **S** Pulmonary Veins, Bilateral **T** Portal and Splanchnic Veins **V** Veins, Other	**Y** Other Contrast	**0** Unenhanced and Enhanced **Z** None	**Z** None
1 Cerebral and Cerebellar Veins **2** Intracranial Sinuses **5** Jugular Veins, Bilateral **8** Superior Vena Cava **9** Inferior Vena Cava **B** Lower Extremity Veins, Right **C** Lower Extremity Veins, Left **D** Lower Extremity Veins, Bilateral **H** Pelvic (Iliac) Veins, Bilateral **L** Renal Veins, Bilateral **M** Upper Extremity Veins, Right **N** Upper Extremity Veins, Left **P** Upper Extremity Veins, Bilateral **S** Pulmonary Veins, Bilateral **T** Portal and Splanchnic Veins **V** Veins, Other	**Z** None	**Z** None	**Z** None

B Imaging
5 Veins
4 Ultrasonography: Real time display of images of anatomy or flow information developed from the capture of reflected and attenuated high frequency sound waves

Body Part Character 4	Contrast Character 5	Qualifier Character 6	Qualifier Character 7
3 Jugular Veins, Right **4** Jugular Veins, Left **6** Subclavian Vein, Right **7** Subclavian Vein, Left **8** Superior Vena Cava **9** Inferior Vena Cava **B** Lower Extremity Veins, Right **C** Lower Extremity Veins, Left **D** Lower Extremity Veins, Bilateral **J** Renal Vein, Right **K** Renal Vein, Left **L** Renal Veins, Bilateral **M** Upper Extremity Veins, Right **N** Upper Extremity Veins, Left **P** Upper Extremity Veins, Bilateral **T** Portal and Splanchnic Veins	**Z** None	**Z** None	**3** Intravascular **A** Guidance **Z** None

B Imaging
7 Lymphatic System
0 Plain Radiography: Planar display of an image developed from the capture of external ionizing radiation on photographic or photoconductive plate

Body Part Character 4	Contrast Character 5	Qualifier Character 6	Qualifier Character 7
0 Abdominal/Retroperitoneal Lymphatics, Unilateral **1** Abdominal/Retroperitoneal Lymphatics, Bilateral **4** Lymphatics, Head and Neck **5** Upper Extremity Lymphatics, Right **6** Upper Extremity Lymphatics, Left **7** Upper Extremity Lymphatics, Bilateral **8** Lower Extremity Lymphatics, Right **9** Lower Extremity Lymphatics, Left **B** Lower Extremity Lymphatics, Bilateral **C** Lymphatics, Pelvic	**0** High Osmolar **1** Low Osmolar **Y** Other Contrast	**Z** None	**Z** None

B Imaging
8 Eye
0 Plain Radiography: Planar display of an image developed from the capture of external ionizing radiation on photographic or photoconductive plate

Body Part Character 4	Contrast Character 5	Qualifier Character 6	Qualifier Character 7
0 Lacrimal Duct, Right **1** Lacrimal Duct, Left **2** Lacrimal Ducts, Bilateral	**0** High Osmolar **1** Low Osmolar **Y** Other Contrast	**Z** None	**Z** None
3 Optic Foramina, Right **4** Optic Foramina, Left **5** Eye, Right **6** Eye, Left **7** Eyes, Bilateral	**Z** None	**Z** None	**Z** None

B Imaging
8 Eye
2 Computerized Tomography (CT Scan): Computer reformatted digital display of multiplanar images developed from the capture of multiple exposures of external ionizing radiation

Body Part Character 4	Contrast Character 5	Qualifier Character 6	Qualifier Character 7
5 Eye, Right **6** Eye, Left **7** Eyes, Bilateral	**0** High Osmolar **1** Low Osmolar **Y** Other Contrast	**0** Unenhanced and Enhanced **Z** None	**Z** None
5 Eye, Right **6** Eye, Left **7** Eyes, Bilateral	**Z** None	**Z** None	**Z** None

B Imaging
8 Eye
3 Magnetic Resonance Imaging (MRI): Computer reformatted digital display of multiplanar images developed from the capture of radiofrequency signals emitted by nuclei in a body site excited within a magnetic field

Body Part Character 4	Contrast Character 5	Qualifier Character 6	Qualifier Character 7
5 Eye, Right **6** Eye, Left **7** Eyes, Bilateral	**Y** Other Contrast	**0** Unenhanced and Enhanced **Z** None	**Z** None
5 Eye, Right **6** Eye, Left **7** Eyes, Bilateral	**Z** None	**Z** None	**Z** None

B Imaging
8 Eye
4 Ultrasonography: Real time display of images of anatomy or flow information developed from the capture of reflected and attenuated high frequency sound waves

Body Part Character 4	Contrast Character 5	Qualifier Character 6	Qualifier Character 7
5 Eye, Right **6** Eye, Left **7** Eyes, Bilateral	**Z** None	**Z** None	**Z** None

B Imaging
9 Ear, Nose, Mouth and Throat
0 Plain Radiography: Planar display of an image developed from the capture of external ionizing radiation on photographic or photoconductive plate

Body Part Character 4	Contrast Character 5	Qualifier Character 6	Qualifier Character 7
2 Paranasal Sinuses **F** Nasopharynx/Oropharynx **H** Mastoids	**Z** None	**Z** None	**Z** None
4 Parotid Gland, Right **5** Parotid Gland, Left **6** Parotid Glands, Bilateral **7** Submandibular Gland, Right **8** Submandibular Gland, Left **9** Submandibular Glands, Bilateral **B** Salivary Gland, Right **C** Salivary Gland, Left **D** Salivary Glands, Bilateral	**0** High Osmolar **1** Low Osmolar **Y** Other Contrast	**Z** None	**Z** None

B Imaging
9 Ear, Nose, Mouth and Throat
1 Fluoroscopy: Single plane or bi-plane real time display of an image developed from the capture of external ionizing radiation on a fluorescent screen. The image may also be stored by either digital or analog means

Body Part Character 4	Contrast Character 5	Qualifier Character 6	Qualifier Character 7
G Pharynx and Epiglottis **J** Larynx	**Y** Other Contrast **Z** None	**Z** None	**Z** None

B Imaging
9 Ear, Nose, Mouth and Throat
2 Computerized Tomography (CT Scan): Computer reformatted digital display of multiplanar images developed from the capture of multiple exposures of external ionizing radiation

Body Part Character 4	Contrast Character 5	Qualifier Character 6	Qualifier Character 7
0 Ear **2** Paranasal Sinuses **6** Parotid Glands, Bilateral **9** Submandibular Glands, Bilateral **D** Salivary Glands, Bilateral **F** Nasopharynx/Oropharynx **J** Larynx	**0** High Osmolar **1** Low Osmolar **Y** Other Contrast	**0** Unenhanced and Enhanced **Z** None	**Z** None
0 Ear **2** Paranasal Sinuses **6** Parotid Glands, Bilateral **9** Submandibular Glands, Bilateral **D** Salivary Glands, Bilateral **F** Nasopharynx/Oropharynx **J** Larynx	**Z** None	**Z** None	**Z** None

B Imaging
9 Ear, Nose, Mouth and Throat
3 Magnetic Resonance Imaging (MRI): Computer reformatted digital display of multiplanar images developed from the capture of radiofrequency signals emitted by nuclei in a body site excited within a magnetic field

Body Part Character 4	Contrast Character 5	Qualifier Character 6	Qualifier Character 7
0 Ear **2** Paranasal Sinuses **6** Parotid Glands, Bilateral **9** Submandibular Glands, Bilateral **D** Salivary Glands, Bilateral **F** Nasopharynx/Oropharynx **J** Larynx	**Y** Other Contrast	**0** Unenhanced and Enhanced **Z** None	**Z** None
0 Ear **2** Paranasal Sinuses **6** Parotid Glands, Bilateral **9** Submandibular Glands, Bilateral **D** Salivary Glands, Bilateral **F** Nasopharynx/Oropharynx **J** Larynx	**Z** None	**Z** None	**Z** None

B Imaging
B Respiratory System
0 Plain Radiography: Planar display of an image developed from the capture of external ionizing radiation on photographic or photoconductive plate

Body Part Character 4	Contrast Character 5	Qualifier Character 6	Qualifier Character 7
7 Tracheobronchial Tree, Right **8** Tracheobronchial Tree, Left **9** Tracheobronchial Trees, Bilateral	**Y** Other Contrast	**Z** None	**Z** None
D Upper Airways	**Z** None	**Z** None	**Z** None

B Imaging
B Respiratory System
1 Fluoroscopy: Single plane or bi-plane real time display of an image developed from the capture of external ionizing radiation on a fluorescent screen. The image may also be stored by either digital or analog means

Body Part Character 4	Contrast Character 5	Qualifier Character 6	Qualifier Character 7
2 Lung, Right **3** Lung, Left **4** Lungs, Bilateral **6** Diaphragm **C** Mediastinum **D** Upper Airways	**Z** None	**Z** None	**Z** None
7 Tracheobronchial Tree, Right **8** Tracheobronchial Tree, Left **9** Tracheobronchial Trees, Bilateral	**Y** Other Contrast	**Z** None	**Z** None

B Imaging
B Respiratory System
2 Computerized Tomography (CT Scan): Computer reformatted digital display of multiplanar images developed from the capture of multiple exposures of external ionizing radiation

Body Part	Contrast	Qualifier	Qualifier
Character 4	**Character 5**	**Character 6**	**Character 7**
4 Lungs, Bilateral **7** Tracheobronchial Tree, Right **8** Tracheobronchial Tree, Left **9** Tracheobronchial Trees, Bilateral **F** Trachea/Airways	**0** High Osmolar **1** Low Osmolar **Y** Other Contrast	**0** Unenhanced and Enhanced **Z** None	**Z** None
4 Lungs, Bilateral **7** Tracheobronchial Tree, Right **8** Tracheobronchial Tree, Left **9** Tracheobronchial Trees, Bilateral **F** Trachea/Airways	**Z** None	**Z** None	**Z** None

B Imaging
B Respiratory System
3 Magnetic Resonance Imaging (MRI): Computer reformatted digital display of multiplanar images developed from the capture of radiofrequency signals emitted by nuclei in a body site excited within a magnetic field

Body Part	Contrast	Qualifier	Qualifier
Character 4	**Character 5**	**Character 6**	**Character 7**
G Lung Apices	**Y** Other Contrast	**0** Unenhanced and Enhanced **Z** None	**Z** None
G Lung Apices	**Z** None	**Z** None	**Z** None

B Imaging
B Respiratory System
4 Ultrasonography: Real time display of images of anatomy or flow information developed from the capture of reflected and attenuated high frequency sound waves

Body Part	Contrast	Qualifier	Qualifier
Character 4	**Character 5**	**Character 6**	**Character 7**
B Pleura **C** Mediastinum	**Z** None	**Z** None	**Z** None

B Imaging
D Gastrointestinal System
1 Fluoroscopy: Single plane or bi-plane real time display of an image developed from the capture of external ionizing radiation on a fluorescent screen. The image may also be stored by either digital or analog means

Body Part	Contrast	Qualifier	Qualifier
Character 4	**Character 5**	**Character 6**	**Character 7**
1 Esophagus **2** Stomach **3** Small Bowel **4** Colon **5** Upper GI **6** Upper GI and Small Bowel **9** Duodenum **B** Mouth/Oropharynx	**Y** Other Contrast **Z** None	**Z** None	**Z** None

B Imaging
D Gastrointestinal System
2 Computerized Tomography (CT Scan): Computer reformatted digital display of multiplanar images developed from the capture of multiple exposures of external ionizing radiation

Body Part Character 4	Contrast Character 5	Qualifier Character 6	Qualifier Character 7
4 Colon	0 High Osmolar 1 Low Osmolar Y Other Contrast	0 Unenhanced and Enhanced Z None	Z None
4 Colon	Z None	Z None	Z None

B Imaging
D Gastrointestinal System
4 Ultrasonography: Real time display of images of anatomy or flow information developed from the capture of reflected and attenuated high frequency sound waves

Body Part Character 4	Contrast Character 5	Qualifier Character 6	Qualifier Character 7
1 Esophagus 2 Stomach 7 Gastrointestinal Tract 8 Appendix 9 Duodenum C Rectum	Z None	Z None	Z None

B Imaging
F Hepatobiliary System and Pancreas
0 Plain Radiography: Planar display of an image developed from the capture of external ionizing radiation on photographic or photoconductive plate

Body Part Character 4	Contrast Character 5	Qualifier Character 6	Qualifier Character 7
0 Bile Ducts 3 Gallbladder and Bile Ducts C Hepatobiliary System, All	0 High Osmolar 1 Low Osmolar Y Other Contrast	Z None	Z None

B Imaging
F Hepatobiliary System and Pancreas
1 Fluoroscopy: Single plane or bi-plane real time display of an image developed from the capture of external ionizing radiation on a fluorescent screen. The image may also be stored by either digital or analog means

Body Part Character 4	Contrast Character 5	Qualifier Character 6	Qualifier Character 7
0 Bile Ducts 1 Biliary and Pancreatic Ducts 2 Gallbladder 3 Gallbladder and Bile Ducts 4 Gallbladder, Bile Ducts and Pancreatic Ducts 8 Pancreatic Ducts	0 High Osmolar 1 Low Osmolar Y Other Contrast	Z None	Z None

B Imaging
F Hepatobiliary System and Pancreas
2 Computerized Tomography (CT Scan): Computer reformatted digital display of multiplanar images developed from the capture of multiple exposures of external ionizing radiation

Body Part Character 4	Contrast Character 5	Qualifier Character 6	Qualifier Character 7
5 Liver **6** Liver and Spleen **7** Pancreas **C** Hepatobiliary System, All	**0** High Osmolar **1** Low Osmolar **Y** Other Contrast	**0** Unenhanced and Enhanced **Z** None	**Z** None
5 Liver **6** Liver and Spleen **7** Pancreas **C** Hepatobiliary System, All	**Z** None	**Z** None	**Z** None

B Imaging
F Hepatobiliary System and Pancreas
3 Magnetic Resonance Imaging (MRI): Computer reformatted digital display of multiplanar images developed from the capture of radiofrequency signals emitted by nuclei in a body site excited within a magnetic field

Body Part Character 4	Contrast Character 5	Qualifier Character 6	Qualifier Character 7
5 Liver **6** Liver and Spleen **7** Pancreas	**Y** Other Contrast	**0** Unenhanced and Enhanced **Z** None	**Z** None
5 Liver **6** Liver and Spleen **7** Pancreas	**Z** None	**Z** None	**Z** None

B Imaging
F Hepatobiliary System and Pancreas
4 Ultrasonography: Real time display of images of anatomy or flow information developed from the capture of reflected and attenuated high frequency sound waves

Body Part Character 4	Contrast Character 5	Qualifier Character 6	Qualifier Character 7
0 Bile Ducts **2** Gallbladder **3** Gallbladder and Bile Ducts **5** Liver **6** Liver and Spleen **7** Pancreas **C** Hepatobiliary System, All	**Z** None	**Z** None	**Z** None

B Imaging
G Endocrine System
2 Computerized Tomography (CT Scan): Computer reformatted digital display of multiplanar images developed from the capture of multiple exposures of external ionizing radiation

Body Part Character 4	Contrast Character 5	Qualifier Character 6	Qualifier Character 7
2 Adrenal Glands, Bilateral **3** Parathyroid Glands **4** Thyroid Gland	**0** High Osmolar **1** Low Osmolar **Y** Other Contrast	**0** Unenhanced and Enhanced **Z** None	**Z** None
2 Adrenal Glands, Bilateral **3** Parathyroid Glands **4** Thyroid Gland	**Z** None	**Z** None	**Z** None

B Imaging
G Endocrine System
3 Magnetic Resonance Imaging (MRI): Computer reformatted digital display of multiplanar images developed from the capture of radiofrequency signals emitted by nuclei in a body site excited within a magnetic field

Body Part	Contrast	Qualifier	Qualifier
Character 4	**Character 5**	**Character 6**	**Character 7**
2 Adrenal Glands, Bilateral **3** Parathyroid Glands **4** Thyroid Gland	**Y** Other Contrast	**0** Unenhanced and Enhanced **Z** None	**Z** None
2 Adrenal Glands, Bilateral **3** Parathyroid Glands **4** Thyroid Gland	**Z** None	**Z** None	**Z** None

B Imaging
G Endocrine System
4 Ultrasonography: Real time display of images of anatomy or flow information developed from the capture of reflected and attenuated high frequency sound waves

Body Part	Contrast	Qualifier	Qualifier
Character 4	**Character 5**	**Character 6**	**Character 7**
0 Adrenal Gland, Right **1** Adrenal Gland, Left **2** Adrenal Glands, Bilateral **3** Parathyroid Glands **4** Thyroid Gland	**Z** None	**Z** None	**Z** None

B Imaging
H Skin, Subcutaneous Tissue and Breast
0 Plain Radiography: Planar display of an image developed from the capture of external ionizing radiation on photographic or photoconductive plate

Body Part	Contrast	Qualifier	Qualifier
Character 4	**Character 5**	**Character 6**	**Character 7**
0 Breast, Right **1** Breast, Left **2** Breasts, Bilateral	**Z** None	**Z** None	**Z** None
3 Single Mammary Duct, Right **4** Single Mammary Duct, Left **5** Multiple Mammary Ducts, Right **6** Multiple Mammary Ducts, Left	**0** High Osmolar **1** Low Osmolar **Y** Other Contrast **Z** None	**Z** None	**Z** None

B Imaging
H Skin, Subcutaneous Tissue and Breast
3 Magnetic Resonance Imaging (MRI): Computer reformatted digital display of multiplanar images developed from the capture of radiofrequency signals emitted by nuclei in a body site excited within a magnetic field

Body Part Character 4	Contrast Character 5	Qualifier Character 6	Qualifier Character 7
0 Breast, Right **1** Breast, Left **2** Breasts, Bilateral **D** Subcutaneous Tissue, Head/ Neck **F** Subcutaneous Tissue, Upper Extremity **G** Subcutaneous Tissue, Thorax **H** Subcutaneous Tissue, Abdomen and Pelvis **J** Subcutaneous Tissue, Lower Extremity	**Y** Other Contrast	**0** Unenhanced and Enhanced **Z** None	**Z** None
0 Breast, Right **1** Breast, Left **2** Breasts, Bilateral **D** Subcutaneous Tissue, Head/ Neck **F** Subcutaneous Tissue, Upper Extremity **G** Subcutaneous Tissue, Thorax **H** Subcutaneous Tissue, Abdomen and Pelvis **J** Subcutaneous Tissue, Lower Extremity	**Z** None	**Z** None	**Z** None

B Imaging
H Skin, Subcutaneous Tissue and Breast
4 Ultrasonography: Real time display of images of anatomy or flow information developed from the capture of reflected and attenuated high frequency sound waves

Body Part Character 4	Contrast Character 5	Qualifier Character 6	Qualifier Character 7
0 Breast, Right **1** Breast, Left **2** Breasts, Bilateral **7** Extremity, Upper **8** Extremity, Lower **9** Abdominal Wall **B** Chest Wall **C** Head and Neck	**Z** None	**Z** None	**Z** None

B Imaging
L Connective Tissue
3 Magnetic Resonance Imaging (MRI): Computer reformatted digital display of multiplanar images developed from the capture of radiofrequency signals emitted by nuclei in a body site excited within a magnetic field

Body Part	Contrast	Qualifier	Qualifier
Character 4	**Character 5**	**Character 6**	**Character 7**
0 Connective Tissue, Upper Extremity **1** Connective Tissue, Lower Extremity **2** Tendons, Upper Extremity **3** Tendons, Lower Extremity	**Y** Other Contrast	**0** Unenhanced and Enhanced **Z** None	**Z** None
0 Connective Tissue, Upper Extremity **1** Connective Tissue, Lower Extremity **2** Tendons, Upper Extremity **3** Tendons, Lower Extremity	**Z** None	**Z** None	**Z** None

B Imaging
L Connective Tissue
4 Ultrasonography: Real time display of images of anatomy or flow information developed from the capture of reflected and attenuated high frequency sound waves

Body Part	Contrast	Qualifier	Qualifier
Character 4	**Character 5**	**Character 6**	**Character 7**
0 Connective Tissue, Upper Extremity **1** Connective Tissue, Lower Extremity **2** Tendons, Upper Extremity **3** Tendons, Lower Extremity	**Z** None	**Z** None	**Z** None

B Imaging
N Skull and Facial Bones
0 Plain Radiography: Planar display of an image developed from the capture of external ionizing radiation on photographic or photoconductive plate

Body Part	Contrast	Qualifier	Qualifier
Character 4	**Character 5**	**Character 6**	**Character 7**
0 Skull **1** Orbit, Right **2** Orbit, Left **3** Orbits, Bilateral **4** Nasal Bones **5** Facial Bones **6** Mandible **B** Zygomatic Arch, Right **C** Zygomatic Arch, Left **D** Zygomatic Arches, Bilateral **G** Tooth, Single **H** Teeth, Multiple **J** Teeth, All	**Z** None	**Z** None	**Z** None
7 Temporomandibular Joint, Right **8** Temporomandibular Joint, Left **9** Temporomandibular Joints, Bilateral	**0** High Osmolar **1** Low Osmolar **Y** Other Contrast **Z** None	**Z** None	**Z** None

B Imaging
N Skull and Facial Bones
1 Fluoroscopy: Single plane or bi-plane real time display of an image developed from the capture of external ionizing radiation on a fluorescent screen. The image may also be stored by either digital or analog means

Body Part	Contrast	Qualifier	Qualifier
Character 4	Character 5	Character 6	Character 7
7 Temporomandibular Joint, Right 8 Temporomandibular Joint, Left 9 Temporomandibular Joints, Bilateral	0 High Osmolar 1 Low Osmolar Y Other Contrast Z None	Z None	Z None

B Imaging
N Skull and Facial Bones
2 Computerized Tomography (CT Scan): Computer reformatted digital display of multiplanar images developed from the capture of multiple exposures of external ionizing radiation

Body Part	Contrast	Qualifier	Qualifier
Character 4	Character 5	Character 6	Character 7
0 Skull 3 Orbits, Bilateral 5 Facial Bones 6 Mandible 9 Temporomandibular Joints, Bilateral F Temporal Bones	0 High Osmolar 1 Low Osmolar Y Other Contrast Z None	Z None	Z None

B Imaging
N Skull and Facial Bones
3 Magnetic Resonance Imaging (MRI): Computer reformatted digital display of multiplanar images developed from the capture of radiofrequency signals emitted by nuclei in a body site excited within a magnetic field

Body Part	Contrast	Qualifier	Qualifier
Character 4	Character 5	Character 6	Character 7
9 Temporomandibular Joints, Bilateral	Y Other Contrast Z None	Z None	Z None

B Imaging
P Non-Axial Upper Bones
0 Plain Radiography: Planar display of an image developed from the capture of external ionizing radiation on photographic or photoconductive plate

Body Part	Contrast	Qualifier	Qualifier
Character 4	Character 5	Character 6	Character 7
0 Sternoclavicular Joint, Right 1 Sternoclavicular Joint, Left 2 Sternoclavicular Joints, Bilateral 3 Acromioclavicular Joints, Bilateral 4 Clavicle, Right 5 Clavicle, Left 6 Scapula, Right 7 Scapula, Left A Humerus, Right B Humerus, Left E Upper Arm, Right F Upper Arm, Left J Forearm, Right K Forearm, Left N Hand, Right P Hand, Left R Finger(s), Right S Finger(s), Left X Ribs, Right Y Ribs, Left	Z None	Z None	Z None

BP0 continued on next page

B Imaging
P Non-Axial Upper Bones
0 Plain Radiography: Planar display of an image developed from the capture of external ionizing radiation on photographic or photoconductive plate

BP0 continued from previous page

Body Part	Contrast	Qualifier	Qualifier
Character 4	Character 5	Character 6	Character 7
8 Shoulder, Right **9** Shoulder, Left **C** Hand/Finger Joint, Right **D** Hand/Finger Joint, Left **G** Elbow, Right **H** Elbow, Left **L** Wrist, Right **M** Wrist, Left	**0** High Osmolar **1** Low Osmolar **Y** Other Contrast **Z** None	**Z** None	**Z** None

B Imaging
P Non-Axial Upper Bones
1 Fluoroscopy: Single plane or bi-plane real time display of an image developed from the capture of external ionizing radiation on a fluorescent screen. The image may also be stored by either digital or analog means

Body Part	Contrast	Qualifier	Qualifier
Character 4	Character 5	Character 6	Character 7
0 Sternoclavicular Joint, Right **1** Sternoclavicular Joint, Left **2** Sternoclavicular Joints, Bilateral **3** Acromioclavicular Joints, Bilateral **4** Clavicle, Right **5** Clavicle, Left **6** Scapula, Right **7** Scapula, Left **A** Humerus, Right **B** Humerus, Left **E** Upper Arm, Right **F** Upper Arm, Left **J** Forearm, Right **K** Forearm, Left **N** Hand, Right **P** Hand, Left **R** Finger(s), Right **S** Finger(s), Left **X** Ribs, Right **Y** Ribs, Left	**Z** None	**Z** None	**Z** None
8 Shoulder, Right **9** Shoulder, Left **L** Wrist, Right **M** Wrist, Left	**0** High Osmolar **1** Low Osmolar **Y** Other Contrast **Z** None	**Z** None	**Z** None
C Hand/Finger Joint, Right **D** Hand/Finger Joint, Left **G** Elbow, Right **H** Elbow, Left	**0** High Osmolar **1** Low Osmolar **Y** Other Contrast	**Z** None	**Z** None

B Imaging
P Non-Axial Upper Bones
2 Computerized Tomography (CT Scan): Computer reformatted digital display of multiplanar images developed from the capture of multiple exposures of external ionizing radiation

Body Part	Contrast	Qualifier	Qualifier
Character 4	**Character 5**	**Character 6**	**Character 7**
0 Sternoclavicular Joint, Right **1** Sternoclavicular Joint, Left **W** Thorax	**0** High Osmolar **1** Low Osmolar **Y** Other Contrast	**Z** None	**Z** None
2 Sternoclavicular Joints, Bilateral **3** Acromioclavicular Joints, Bilateral **4** Clavicle, Right **5** Clavicle, Left **6** Scapula, Right **7** Scapula, Left **8** Shoulder, Right **9** Shoulder, Left **A** Humerus, Right **B** Humerus, Left **E** Upper Arm, Right **F** Upper Arm, Left **G** Elbow, Right **H** Elbow, Left **J** Forearm, Right **K** Forearm, Left **L** Wrist, Right **M** Wrist, Left **N** Hand, Right **P** Hand, Left **Q** Hands and Wrists, Bilateral **R** Finger(s), Right **S** Finger(s), Left **T** Upper Extremity, Right **U** Upper Extremity, Left **V** Upper Extremities, Bilateral **X** Ribs, Right **Y** Ribs, Left	**0** High Osmolar **1** Low Osmolar **Y** Other Contrast **Z** None	**Z** None	**Z** None
C Hand/Finger Joint, Right **D** Hand/Finger Joint, Left	**Z** None	**Z** None	**Z** None

B Imaging
P Non-Axial Upper Bones
3 Magnetic Resonance Imaging (MRI): Computer reformatted digital display of multiplanar images developed from the capture of radiofrequency signals emitted by nuclei in a body site excited within a magnetic field

Body Part	Contrast	Qualifier	Qualifier
Character 4	**Character 5**	**Character 6**	**Character 7**
8 Shoulder, Right **9** Shoulder, Left **C** Hand/Finger Joint, Right **D** Hand/Finger Joint, Left **E** Upper Arm, Right **F** Upper Arm, Left **G** Elbow, Right **H** Elbow, Left **J** Forearm, Right **K** Forearm, Left **L** Wrist, Right **M** Wrist, Left	**Y** Other Contrast	**0** Unenhanced and Enhanced **Z** None	**Z** None

BP3 continued on next page

B Imaging
P Non-Axial Upper Bones
3 Magnetic Resonance Imaging (MRI): Computer reformatted digital display of multiplanar images developed from the capture of radiofrequency signals emitted by nuclei in a body site excited within a magnetic field

BP3 continued from previous page

Body Part	Contrast	Qualifier	Qualifier
Character 4	Character 5	Character 6	Character 7
8 Shoulder, Right 9 Shoulder, Left C Hand/Finger Joint, Right D Hand/Finger Joint, Left E Upper Arm, Right F Upper Arm, Left G Elbow, Right H Elbow, Left J Forearm, Right K Forearm, Left L Wrist, Right M Wrist, Left	Z None	Z None	Z None

B Imaging
P Non-Axial Upper Bones
4 Ultrasonography: Real time display of images of anatomy or flow information developed from the capture of reflected and attenuated high frequency sound waves

Body Part	Contrast	Qualifier	Qualifier
Character 4	Character 5	Character 6	Character 7
8 Shoulder, Right 9 Shoulder, Left G Elbow, Right H Elbow, Left L Wrist, Right M Wrist, Left N Hand, Right P Hand, Left	Z None	Z None	1 Densitometry Z None

B Imaging
Q Non-Axial Lower Bones
0 Plain Radiography: Planar display of an image developed from the capture of external ionizing radiation on photographic or photoconductive plate

Body Part	Contrast	Qualifier	Qualifier
Character 4	Character 5	Character 6	Character 7
0 Hip, Right 1 Hip, Left	0 High Osmolar 1 Low Osmolar Y Other Contrast	Z None	Z None
0 Hip, Right 1 Hip, Left	Z None	Z None	1 Densitometry Z None
3 Femur, Right 4 Femur, Left	Z None	Z None	1 Densitometry Z None
7 Knee, Right 8 Knee, Left G Ankle, Right H Ankle, Left	0 High Osmolar 1 Low Osmolar Y Other Contrast Z None	Z None	Z None
D Lower Leg, Right F Lower Leg, Left J Calcaneus, Right K Calcaneus, Left L Foot, Right M Foot, Left P Toe(s), Right Q Toe(s), Left V Patella, Right W Patella, Left	Z None	Z None	Z None
X Foot/Toe Joint, Right Y Foot/Toe Joint, Left	0 High Osmolar 1 Low Osmolar Y Other Contrast	Z None	Z None

LC Limited Coverage NC Noncovered HAC HAC-associated Procedure CC Combination Cluster - See Appendix G for code lists
DRG Non-OR-Affecting MS-DRG Assignment New/Revised Text in **Orange** ♂ Male ♀ Female

B Imaging
Q Non-Axial Lower Bones
1 Fluoroscopy: Single plane or bi-plane real time display of an image developed from the capture of external ionizing radiation on a fluorescent screen. The image may also be stored by either digital or analog means

Body Part Character 4	Contrast Character 5	Qualifier Character 6	Qualifier Character 7
0 Hip, Right **1** Hip, Left **7** Knee, Right **8** Knee, Left **G** Ankle, Right **H** Ankle, Left **X** Foot/Toe Joint, Right **Y** Foot/Toe Joint, Left	**0** High Osmolar **1** Low Osmolar **Y** Other Contrast **Z** None	**Z** None	**Z** None
3 Femur, Right **4** Femur, Left **D** Lower Leg, Right **F** Lower Leg, Left **J** Calcaneus, Right **K** Calcaneus, Left **L** Foot, Right **M** Foot, Left **P** Toe(s), Right **Q** Toe(s), Left **V** Patella, Right **W** Patella, Left	**Z** None	**Z** None	**Z** None

B Imaging
Q Non-Axial Lower Bones
2 Computerized Tomography (CT Scan): Computer reformatted digital display of multiplanar images developed from the capture of multiple exposures of external ionizing radiation

Body Part Character 4	Contrast Character 5	Qualifier Character 6	Qualifier Character 7
0 Hip, Right **1** Hip, Left **3** Femur, Right **4** Femur, Left **7** Knee, Right **8** Knee, Left **D** Lower Leg, Right **F** Lower Leg, Left **G** Ankle, Right **H** Ankle, Left **J** Calcaneus, Right **K** Calcaneus, Left **L** Foot, Right **M** Foot, Left **P** Toe(s), Right **Q** Toe(s), Left **R** Lower Extremity, Right **S** Lower Extremity, Left **V** Patella, Right **W** Patella, Left **X** Foot/Toe Joint, Right **Y** Foot/Toe Joint, Left	**0** High Osmolar **1** Low Osmolar **Y** Other Contrast **Z** None	**Z** None	**Z** None
B Tibia/Fibula, Right **C** Tibia/Fibula, Left	**0** High Osmolar **1** Low Osmolar **Y** Other Contrast	**Z** None	**Z** None

B Imaging
Q Non-Axial Lower Bones
3 Magnetic Resonance Imaging (MRI): Computer reformatted digital display of multiplanar images developed from the capture of radiofrequency signals emitted by nuclei in a body site excited within a magnetic field

Body Part Character 4	Contrast Character 5	Qualifier Character 6	Qualifier Character 7
0 Hip, Right **1** Hip, Left **3** Femur, Right **4** Femur, Left **7** Knee, Right **8** Knee, Left **D** Lower Leg, Right **F** Lower Leg, Left **G** Ankle, Right **H** Ankle, Left **J** Calcaneus, Right **K** Calcaneus, Left **L** Foot, Right **M** Foot, Left **P** Toe(s), Right **Q** Toe(s), Left **V** Patella, Right **W** Patella, Left	**Y** Other Contrast	**0** Unenhanced and Enhanced **Z** None	**Z** None
0 Hip, Right **1** Hip, Left **3** Femur, Right **4** Femur, Left **7** Knee, Right **8** Knee, Left **D** Lower Leg, Right **F** Lower Leg, Left **G** Ankle, Right **H** Ankle, Left **J** Calcaneus, Right **K** Calcaneus, Left **L** Foot, Right **M** Foot, Left **P** Toe(s), Right **Q** Toe(s), Left **V** Patella, Right **W** Patella, Left	**Z** None	**Z** None	**Z** None

B Imaging
Q Non-Axial Lower Bones
4 Ultrasonography: Real time display of images of anatomy or flow information developed from the capture of reflected and attenuated high frequency sound waves

Body Part Character 4	Contrast Character 5	Qualifier Character 6	Qualifier Character 7
0 Hip, Right **1** Hip, Left **2** Hips, Bilateral **7** Knee, Right **8** Knee, Left **9** Knees, Bilateral	**Z** None	**Z** None	**Z** None

B Imaging
R Axial Skeleton, Except Skull and Facial Bones
0 Plain Radiography: Planar display of an image developed from the capture of external ionizing radiation on photographic or photoconductive plate

Body Part Character 4	Contrast Character 5	Qualifier Character 6	Qualifier Character 7
0 Cervical Spine **7** Thoracic Spine **9** Lumbar Spine **G** Whole Spine	**Z** None	**Z** None	**1** Densitometry **Z** None
1 Cervical Disc(s) **2** Thoracic Disc(s) **3** Lumbar Disc(s) **4** Cervical Facet Joint(s) **5** Thoracic Facet Joint(s) **6** Lumbar Facet Joint(s) **D** Sacroiliac Joints	**0** High Osmolar **1** Low Osmolar **Y** Other Contrast **Z** None	**Z** None	**Z** None
8 Thoracolumbar Joint **B** Lumbosacral Joint **C** Pelvis **F** Sacrum and Coccyx **H** Sternum	**Z** None	**Z** None	**Z** None

B Imaging
R Axial Skeleton, Except Skull and Facial Bones
1 Fluoroscopy: Single plane or bi-plane real time display of an image developed from the capture of external ionizing radiation on a fluorescent screen. The image may also be stored by either digital or analog means

Body Part Character 4	Contrast Character 5	Qualifier Character 6	Qualifier Character 7
0 Cervical Spine **1** Cervical Disc(s) **2** Thoracic Disc(s) **3** Lumbar Disc(s) **4** Cervical Facet Joint(s) **5** Thoracic Facet Joint(s) **6** Lumbar Facet Joint(s) **7** Thoracic Spine **8** Thoracolumbar Joint **9** Lumbar Spine **B** Lumbosacral Joint **C** Pelvis **D** Sacroiliac Joints **F** Sacrum and Coccyx **G** Whole Spine **H** Sternum	**0** High Osmolar **1** Low Osmolar **Y** Other Contrast **Z** None	**Z** None	**Z** None

B Imaging
R Axial Skeleton, Except Skull and Facial Bones
2 Computerized Tomography (CT Scan): Computer reformatted digital display of multiplanar images developed from the capture of multiple exposures of external ionizing radiation

Body Part Character 4	Contrast Character 5	Qualifier Character 6	Qualifier Character 7
0 Cervical Spine **7** Thoracic Spine **9** Lumbar Spine **C** Pelvis **D** Sacroiliac Joints **F** Sacrum and Coccyx	**0** High Osmolar **1** Low Osmolar **Y** Other Contrast **Z** None	**Z** None	**Z** None

B Imaging
R Axial Skeleton, Except Skull and Facial Bones
3 Magnetic Resonance Imaging (MRI): Computer reformatted digital display of multiplanar images developed from the capture of radiofrequency signals emitted by nuclei in a body site excited within a magnetic field

Body Part Character 4	Contrast Character 5	Qualifier Character 6	Qualifier Character 7
0 Cervical Spine **1** Cervical Disc(s) **2** Thoracic Disc(s) **3** Lumbar Disc(s) **7** Thoracic Spine **9** Lumbar Spine **C** Pelvis **F** Sacrum and Coccyx	**Y** Other Contrast	**0** Unenhanced and Enhanced **Z** None	**Z** None
0 Cervical Spine **1** Cervical Disc(s) **2** Thoracic Disc(s) **3** Lumbar Disc(s) **7** Thoracic Spine **9** Lumbar Spine **C** Pelvis **F** Sacrum and Coccyx	**Z** None	**Z** None	**Z** None

B Imaging
R Axial Skeleton, Except Skull and Facial Bones
4 Ultrasonography: Real time display of images of anatomy or flow information developed from the capture of reflected and attenuated high frequency sound waves

Body Part Character 4	Contrast Character 5	Qualifier Character 6	Qualifier Character 7
0 Cervical Spine **7** Thoracic Spine **9** Lumbar Spine **F** Sacrum and Coccyx	**Z** None	**Z** None	**Z** None

B Imaging
T Urinary System
0 Plain Radiography: Planar display of an image developed from the capture of external ionizing radiation on photographic or photoconductive plate

Body Part Character 4	Contrast Character 5	Qualifier Character 6	Qualifier Character 7
0 Bladder **1** Kidney, Right **2** Kidney, Left **3** Kidneys, Bilateral **4** Kidneys, Ureters and Bladder **5** Urethra **6** Ureter, Right **7** Ureter, Left **8** Ureters, Bilateral **B** Bladder and Urethra **C** Ileal Diversion Loop	**0** High Osmolar **1** Low Osmolar **Y** Other Contrast **Z** None	**Z** None	**Z** None

LC Limited Coverage NC Noncovered HAC HAC-associated Procedure CC Combination Cluster - See Appendix G for code lists
DRG Non-OR-Affecting MS-DRG Assignment New/Revised Text in **Orange** ♂ Male ♀ Female

B Imaging
T Urinary System
1 Fluoroscopy: Single plane or bi-plane real time display of an image developed from the capture of external ionizing radiation on a fluorescent screen. The image may also be stored by either digital or analog means

Body Part	Contrast	Qualifier	Qualifier
Character 4	**Character 5**	**Character 6**	**Character 7**
0 Bladder **1** Kidney, Right **2** Kidney, Left **3** Kidneys, Bilateral **4** Kidneys, Ureters and Bladder **5** Urethra **6** Ureter, Right **7** Ureter, Left **B** Bladder and Urethra **C** Ileal Diversion Loop **D** Kidney, Ureter and Bladder, Right **F** Kidney, Ureter and Bladder, Left **G** Ileal Loop, Ureters and Kidneys	**0** High Osmolar **1** Low Osmolar **Y** Other Contrast **Z** None	**Z** None	**Z** None

B Imaging
T Urinary System
2 Computerized Tomography (CT Scan): Computer reformatted digital display of multiplanar images developed from the capture of multiple exposures of external ionizing radiation

Body Part	Contrast	Qualifier	Qualifier
Character 4	**Character 5**	**Character 6**	**Character 7**
0 Bladder **1** Kidney, Right **2** Kidney, Left **3** Kidneys, Bilateral **9** Kidney Transplant	**0** High Osmolar **1** Low Osmolar **Y** Other Contrast	**0** Unenhanced and Enhanced **Z** None	**Z** None
0 Bladder **1** Kidney, Right **2** Kidney, Left **3** Kidneys, Bilateral **9** Kidney Transplant	**Z** None	**Z** None	**Z** None

B Imaging
T Urinary System
3 Magnetic Resonance Imaging (MRI): Computer reformatted digital display of multiplanar images developed from the capture of radiofrequency signals emitted by nuclei in a body site excited within a magnetic field

Body Part	Contrast	Qualifier	Qualifier
Character 4	**Character 5**	**Character 6**	**Character 7**
0 Bladder **1** Kidney, Right **2** Kidney, Left **3** Kidneys, Bilateral **9** Kidney Transplant	**Y** Other Contrast	**0** Unenhanced and Enhanced **Z** None	**Z** None
0 Bladder **1** Kidney, Right **2** Kidney, Left **3** Kidneys, Bilateral **9** Kidney Transplant	**Z** None	**Z** None	**Z** None

B Imaging
T Urinary System
4 Ultrasonography: Real time display of images of anatomy or flow information developed from the capture of reflected and attenuated high frequency sound waves

Body Part	Contrast	Qualifier	Qualifier
Character 4	Character 5	Character 6	Character 7
0 Bladder 1 Kidney, Right 2 Kidney, Left 3 Kidneys, Bilateral 5 Urethra 6 Ureter, Right 7 Ureter, Left 8 Ureters, Bilateral 9 Kidney Transplant J Kidneys and Bladder	Z None	Z None	Z None

B Imaging
U Female Reproductive System
0 Plain Radiography: Planar display of an image developed from the capture of external ionizing radiation on photographic or photoconductive plate

Body Part	Contrast	Qualifier	Qualifier
Character 4	Character 5	Character 6	Character 7
0 Fallopian Tube, Right ♀ 1 Fallopian Tube, Left ♀ 2 Fallopian Tubes, Bilateral ♀ 6 Uterus ♀ 8 Uterus and Fallopian Tubes ♀ 9 Vagina ♀	0 High Osmolar 1 Low Osmolar Y Other Contrast	Z None	Z None

♀ BU000ZZ BU001ZZ BU00YZZ BU010ZZ BU011ZZ BU01YZZ BU020ZZ BU021ZZ BU02YZZ BU060ZZ BU061ZZ BU06YZZ BU080ZZ BU081ZZ BU08YZZ BU090ZZ BU091ZZ BU09YZZ

B Imaging
U Female Reproductive System
1 Fluoroscopy: Single plane or bi-plane real time display of an image developed from the capture of external ionizing radiation on a fluorescent screen. The image may also be stored by either digital or analog means

Body Part	Contrast	Qualifier	Qualifier
Character 4	Character 5	Character 6	Character 7
0 Fallopian Tube, Right ♀ 1 Fallopian Tube, Left ♀ 2 Fallopian Tubes, Bilateral ♀ 6 Uterus ♀ 8 Uterus and Fallopian Tubes ♀ 9 Vagina ♀	0 High Osmolar 1 Low Osmolar Y Other Contrast Z None	Z None	Z None

♀ BU100ZZ BU101ZZ BU10YZZ BU10ZZZ BU110ZZ BU111ZZ BU11YZZ BU11ZZZ BU120ZZ BU121ZZ BU12YZZ BU12ZZZ BU160ZZ BU161ZZ BU16YZZ BU16ZZZ BU180ZZ BU181ZZ BU18YZZ BU18ZZZ BU190ZZ BU191ZZ BU19YZZ BU19ZZZ

B Imaging
U Female Reproductive System
3 Magnetic Resonance Imaging (MRI): Computer reformatted digital display of multiplanar images developed from the capture of radiofrequency signals emitted by nuclei in a body site excited within a magnetic field

Body Part	Contrast	Qualifier	Qualifier
Character 4	Character 5	Character 6	Character 7
3 Ovary, Right ♀ 4 Ovary, Left ♀ 5 Ovaries, Bilateral ♀ 6 Uterus ♀ 9 Vagina ♀ B Pregnant Uterus ♀ C Uterus and Ovaries ♀	Y Other Contrast	0 Unenhanced and Enhanced Z None	Z None
3 Ovary, Right ♀ 4 Ovary, Left ♀ 5 Ovaries, Bilateral ♀ 6 Uterus ♀ 9 Vagina ♀ B Pregnant Uterus ♀ C Uterus and Ovaries ♀	Z None	Z None	Z None

♀ BU33Y0Z BU33YZZ BU33ZZZ BU34Y0Z BU34YZZ BU34ZZZ BU35Y0Z BU35YZZ BU35ZZZ BU36Y0Z BU36YZZ BU36ZZZ BU39Y0Z BU39YZZ BU39ZZZ BU3BY0Z BU3BYZZ BU3BZZZ BU3CY0Z BU3CYZZ BU3CZZZ

B Imaging
U Female Reproductive System
4 Ultrasonography: Real time display of images of anatomy or flow information developed from the capture of reflected and attenuated high frequency sound waves

Body Part	Contrast	Qualifier	Qualifier
Character 4	Character 5	Character 6	Character 7
0 Fallopian Tube, Right ♀ 1 Fallopian Tube, Left ♀ 2 Fallopian Tubes, Bilateral ♀ 3 Ovary, Right ♀ 4 Ovary, Left ♀ 5 Ovaries, Bilateral ♀ 6 Uterus ♀ C Uterus and Ovaries ♀	Y Other Contrast Z None	Z None	Z None

♀ BU40YZZ BU40ZZZ BU41YZZ BU41ZZZ BU42YZZ BU42ZZZ BU43YZZ BU43ZZZ BU44YZZ BU44ZZZ BU45YZZ BU45ZZZ BU46YZZ BU46ZZZ BU4CYZZ BU4CZZZ

B Imaging
V Male Reproductive System
0 Plain Radiography: Planar display of an image developed from the capture of external ionizing radiation on photographic or photoconductive plate

Body Part	Contrast	Qualifier	Qualifier
Character 4	Character 5	Character 6	Character 7
0 Corpora Cavernosa ♂ 1 Epididymis, Right ♂ 2 Epididymis, Left ♂ 3 Prostate ♂ 5 Testicle, Right ♂ 6 Testicle, Left ♂ 8 Vasa Vasorum ♂	0 High Osmolar 1 Low Osmolar Y Other Contrast	Z None	Z None

♂ BV000ZZ BV001ZZ BV00YZZ BV010ZZ BV011ZZ BV01YZZ BV020ZZ BV021ZZ BV02YZZ BV030ZZ BV031ZZ BV03YZZ BV050ZZ BV051ZZ BV05YZZ BV060ZZ BV061ZZ BV06YZZ BV080ZZ BV081ZZ BV08YZZ

B Imaging
V Male Reproductive System
1 Fluoroscopy: Single plane or bi-plane real time display of an image developed from the capture of external ionizing radiation on a fluorescent screen. The image may also be stored by either digital or analog means

Body Part	Contrast	Qualifier	Qualifier
Character 4	Character 5	Character 6	Character 7
0 Corpora Cavernosa ♂ 8 Vasa Vasorum ♂	0 High Osmolar 1 Low Osmolar Y Other Contrast Z None	Z None	Z None

♂ BV100ZZ BV101ZZ BV10YZZ BV10ZZZ BV180ZZ BV181ZZ BV18YZZ BV18ZZZ

B Imaging
V Male Reproductive System
2 Computerized Tomography (CT Scan): Computer reformatted digital display of multiplanar images developed from the capture of multiple exposures of external ionizing radiation

Body Part	Contrast	Qualifier	Qualifier
Character 4	Character 5	Character 6	Character 7
3 Prostate ♂	0 High Osmolar 1 Low Osmolar Y Other Contrast	0 Unenhanced and Enhanced Z None	Z None
3 Prostate ♂	Z None	Z None	Z None

♂ BV2300Z BV230ZZ BV2310Z BV23Y0Z BV23YZZ BV23ZZZ

B Imaging
V Male Reproductive System
3 Magnetic Resonance Imaging (MRI): Computer reformatted digital display of multiplanar images developed from the capture of radiofrequency signals emitted by nuclei in a body site excited within a magnetic field

Body Part	Contrast	Qualifier	Qualifier
Character 4	Character 5	Character 6	Character 7
0 Corpora Cavernosa ♂ 3 Prostate ♂ 4 Scrotum ♂ 5 Testicle, Right ♂ 6 Testicle, Left ♂ 7 Testicles, Bilateral ♂	Y Other Contrast	0 Unenhanced and Enhanced Z None	Z None
0 Corpora Cavernosa ♂ 3 Prostate ♂ 4 Scrotum ♂ 5 Testicle, Right ♂ 6 Testicle, Left ♂ 7 Testicles, Bilateral ♂	Z None	Z None	Z None

♂ BV30Y0Z BV30YZZ BV30ZZZ BV33Y0Z BV33YZZ BV33ZZZ BV34Y0Z BV34YZZ BV34ZZZ BV35Y0Z BV35YZZ BV35ZZZ BV36Y0Z BV36YZZ BV36ZZZ BV37Y0Z BV37YZZ BV37ZZZ

B Imaging
V Male Reproductive System
4 Ultrasonography: Real time display of images of anatomy or flow information developed from the capture of reflected and attenuated high frequency sound waves

Body Part	Contrast	Qualifier	Qualifier
Character 4	Character 5	Character 6	Character 7
4 Scrotum ♂ 9 Prostate and Seminal Vesicles ♂ B Penis ♂	Z None	Z None	Z None

♂ BV44ZZZ BV49ZZZ BV4BZZZ

B Imaging
W Anatomical Regions
0 Plain Radiography: Planar display of an image developed from the capture of external ionizing radiation on photographic or photoconductive plate

Body Part	Contrast	Qualifier	Qualifier
Character 4	Character 5	Character 6	Character 7
0 Abdomen 1 Abdomen and Pelvis 3 Chest B Long Bones, All C Lower Extremity J Upper Extremity K Whole Body L Whole Skeleton M Whole Body, Infant	Z None	Z None	Z None

B Imaging
W Anatomical Regions
1 Fluoroscopy: Single plane or bi-plane real time display of an image developed from the capture of external ionizing radiation on a fluorescent screen. The image may also be stored by either digital or analog means

Body Part	Contrast	Qualifier	Qualifier
Character 4	Character 5	Character 6	Character 7
1 Abdomen and Pelvis 9 Head and Neck C Lower Extremity J Upper Extremity	0 High Osmolar 1 Low Osmolar Y Other Contrast Z None	Z None	Z None

B Imaging
W Anatomical Regions
2 Computerized Tomography (CT Scan): Computer reformatted digital display of multiplanar images developed from the capture of multiple exposures of external ionizing radiation

Body Part	Contrast	Qualifier	Qualifier
Character 4	Character 5	Character 6	Character 7
0 Abdomen 1 Abdomen and Pelvis 4 Chest and Abdomen 5 Chest, Abdomen and Pelvis 8 Head 9 Head and Neck F Neck G Pelvic Region	0 High Osmolar 1 Low Osmolar Y Other Contrast	0 Unenhanced and Enhanced Z None	Z None
0 Abdomen 1 Abdomen and Pelvis 4 Chest and Abdomen 5 Chest, Abdomen and Pelvis 8 Head 9 Head and Neck F Neck G Pelvic Region	Z None	Z None	Z None

B Imaging
W Anatomical Regions
3 Magnetic Resonance Imaging (MRI): Computer reformatted digital display of multiplanar images developed from the capture of radiofrequency signals emitted by nuclei in a body site excited within a magnetic field

Body Part	Contrast	Qualifier	Qualifier
Character 4	Character 5	Character 6	Character 7
0 Abdomen **8** Head **F** Neck **G** Pelvic Region **H** Retroperitoneum **P** Brachial Plexus	**Y** Other Contrast	**0** Unenhanced and Enhanced **Z** None	**Z** None
0 Abdomen **8** Head **F** Neck **G** Pelvic Region **H** Retroperitoneum **P** Brachial Plexus	**Z** None	**Z** None	**Z** None
3 Chest	**Y** Other Contrast	**0** Unenhanced and Enhanced **Z** None	**Z** None

B Imaging
W Anatomical Regions
4 Ultrasonography: Real time display of images of anatomy or flow information developed from the capture of reflected and attenuated high frequency sound waves

Body Part	Contrast	Qualifier	Qualifier
Character 4	Character 5	Character 6	Character 7
0 Abdomen **1** Abdomen and Pelvis **F** Neck **G** Pelvic Region	**Z** None	**Z** None	**Z** None

B Imaging
Y Fetus and Obstetrical
3 Magnetic Resonance Imaging (MRI): Computer reformatted digital display of multiplanar images developed from the capture of radiofrequency signals emitted by nuclei in a body site excited within a magnetic field

Body Part	Contrast	Qualifier	Qualifier
Character 4	Character 5	Character 6	Character 7
0 Fetal Head ♀ **1** Fetal Heart ♀ **2** Fetal Thorax ♀ **3** Fetal Abdomen ♀ **4** Fetal Spine ♀ **5** Fetal Extremities ♀ **6** Whole Fetus ♀	**Y** Other Contrast	**0** Unenhanced and Enhanced **Z** None	**Z** None
0 Fetal Head ♀ **1** Fetal Heart ♀ **2** Fetal Thorax ♀ **3** Fetal Abdomen ♀ **4** Fetal Spine ♀ **5** Fetal Extremities ♀ **6** Whole Fetus ♀	**Z** None	**Z** None	**Z** None

♀ BY30Y0Z BY30YZZ BY30ZZZ BY31Y0Z BY31YZZ BY31ZZZ BY32Y0Z BY32YZZ BY32ZZZ BY33Y0Z BY33YZZ BY33ZZZ BY34YZZ BY34ZZZ BY35Y0Z BY35YZZ BY35ZZZ BY36Y0Z BY36YZZ BY36ZZZ

LC Limited Coverage NC Noncovered HAC HAC-associated Procedure CC Combination Cluster - See Appendix G for code lists
DRG Non-OR-Affecting MS-DRG Assignment New/Revised Text in **Orange** ♂ Male ♀ Female

B Imaging
Y Fetus and Obstetrical
4 Ultrasonography: Real time display of images of anatomy or flow information developed from the capture of reflected and attenuated high frequency sound waves

Body Part Character 4	Contrast Character 5	Qualifier Character 6	Qualifier Character 7
7 Fetal Umbilical Cord ♀ **8** Placenta ♀ **9** First Trimester, Single Fetus ♀ **B** First Trimester, Multiple Gestation ♀ **C** Second Trimester, Single Fetus ♀ **D** Second Trimester, Multiple Gestation ♀ **F** Third Trimester, Single Fetus ♀ **G** Third Trimester, Multiple Gestation ♀	**Z** None	**Z** None	**Z** None

♀ BY47ZZZ BY48ZZZ BY49ZZZ BY4BZZZ BY4CZZZ BY4DZZZ BY4FZZZ BY4GZZZ

NOTES

NOTES

Nuclear Medicine C01-CW7

C Nuclear Medicine
0 Central Nervous System
1 Planar Nuclear Medicine Imaging: Introduction of radioactive materials into the body for single plane display of images developed from the capture of radioactive emissions

Body Part	Radionuclide	Qualifier	Qualifier
Character 4	Character 5	Character 6	Character 7
0 Brain	1 Technetium 99m (Tc-99m) Y Other Radionuclide	Z None	Z None
5 Cerebrospinal Fluid	D Indium 111 (In-111) Y Other Radionuclide	Z None	Z None
Y Central Nervous System	Y Other Radionuclide	Z None	Z None

C Nuclear Medicine
0 Central Nervous System
2 Tomographic (Tomo) Nuclear Medicine Imaging: Introduction of radioactive materials into the body for three dimensional display of images developed from the capture of radioactive emissions

Body Part	Radionuclide	Qualifier	Qualifier
Character 4	Character 5	Character 6	Character 7
0 Brain	1 Technetium 99m (Tc-99m) F Iodine 123 (I-123) S Thallium 201 (Tl-201) Y Other Radionuclide	Z None	Z None
5 Cerebrospinal Fluid	D Indium 111 (In-111) Y Other Radionuclide	Z None	Z None
Y Central Nervous System	Y Other Radionuclide	Z None	Z None

C Nuclear Medicine
0 Central Nervous System
3 Positron Emission Tomographic (PET) Imaging: Introduction of radioactive materials into the body for three dimensional display of images developed from the simultaneous capture, 180 degrees apart, of radioactive emissions

Body Part	Radionuclide	Qualifier	Qualifier
Character 4	Character 5	Character 6	Character 7
0 Brain	B Carbon 11 (C-11) K Fluorine 18 (F-18) M Oxygen 15 (O-15) Y Other Radionuclide	Z None	Z None
Y Central Nervous System	Y Other Radionuclide	Z None	Z None

C Nuclear Medicine
0 Central Nervous System
5 Nonimaging Nuclear Medicine Probe: Introduction of radioactive materials into the body for the study of distribution and fate of certain substances by the detection of radioactive emissions; or, alternatively, measurement of absorption of radioactive emissions from an external source

Body Part	Radionuclide	Qualifier	Qualifier
Character 4	Character 5	Character 6	Character 7
0 Brain	V Xenon 133 (Xe-133) Y Other Radionuclide	Z None	Z None
Y Central Nervous System	Y Other Radionuclide	Z None	Z None

C Nuclear Medicine
2 Heart
1 Planar Nuclear Medicine Imaging: Introduction of radioactive materials into the body for single plane display of images developed from the capture of radioactive emissions

Body Part Character 4	Radionuclide Character 5	Qualifier Character 6	Qualifier Character 7
6 Heart, Right and Left	**1** Technetium 99m (Tc-99m) **Y** Other Radionuclide	**Z** None	**Z** None
G Myocardium	**1** Technetium 99m (Tc-99m) **D** Indium 111 (In-111) **S** Thallium 201 (Tl-201) **Y** Other Radionuclide **Z** None	**Z** None	**Z** None
Y Heart	**Y** Other Radionuclide	**Z** None	**Z** None

C Nuclear Medicine
2 Heart
2 Tomographic (Tomo) Nuclear Medicine Imaging: Introduction of radioactive materials into the body for three dimensional display of images developed from the capture of radioactive emissions

Body Part Character 4	Radionuclide Character 5	Qualifier Character 6	Qualifier Character 7
6 Heart, Right and Left	**1** Technetium 99m (Tc-99m) **Y** Other Radionuclide	**Z** None	**Z** None
G Myocardium	**1** Technetium 99m (Tc-99m) **D** Indium 111 (In-111) **K** Fluorine 18 (F-18) **S** Thallium 201 (Tl-201) **Y** Other Radionuclide **Z** None	**Z** None	**Z** None
Y Heart	**Y** Other Radionuclide	**Z** None	**Z** None

C Nuclear Medicine
2 Heart
3 Positron Emission Tomographic (PET) Imaging: Introduction of radioactive materials into the body for three dimensional display of images developed from the simultaneous capture, 180 degrees apart, of radioactive emissions

Body Part Character 4	Radionuclide Character 5	Qualifier Character 6	Qualifier Character 7
G Myocardium	**K** Fluorine 18 (F-18) **M** Oxygen 15 (O-15) **Q** Rubidium 82 (Rb-82) **R** Nitrogen 13 (N-13) **Y** Other Radionuclide	**Z** None	**Z** None
Y Heart	**Y** Other Radionuclide	**Z** None	**Z** None

C Nuclear Medicine
2 Heart
5 Nonimaging Nuclear Medicine Probe: Introduction of radioactive materials into the body for the study of distribution and fate of certain substances by the detection of radioactive emissions; or, alternatively, measurement of absorption of radioactive emissions from an external source

Body Part Character 4	Radionuclide Character 5	Qualifier Character 6	Qualifier Character 7
6 Heart, Right and Left	**1** Technetium 99m (Tc-99m) **Y** Other Radionuclide	**Z** None	**Z** None
Y Heart	**Y** Other Radionuclide	**Z** None	**Z** None

C Nuclear Medicine
5 Veins
1 Planar Nuclear Medicine Imaging: Introduction of radioactive materials into the body for single plane display of images developed from the capture of radioactive emissions

Body Part	Radionuclide	Qualifier	Qualifier
Character 4	**Character 5**	**Character 6**	**Character 7**
B Lower Extremity Veins, Right **C** Lower Extremity Veins, Left **D** Lower Extremity Veins, Bilateral **N** Upper Extremity Veins, Right **P** Upper Extremity Veins, Left **Q** Upper Extremity Veins, Bilateral **R** Central Veins	**1** Technetium 99m (Tc-99m) **Y** Other Radionuclide	**Z** None	**Z** None
Y Veins	**Y** Other Radionuclide	**Z** None	**Z** None

C Nuclear Medicine
7 Lymphatic and Hematologic System
1 Planar Nuclear Medicine Imaging: Introduction of radioactive materials into the body for single plane display of images developed from the capture of radioactive emissions

Body Part	Radionuclide	Qualifier	Qualifier
Character 4	**Character 5**	**Character 6**	**Character 7**
0 Bone Marrow	**1** Technetium 99m (Tc-99m) **D** Indium 111 (In-111) **Y** Other Radionuclide	**Z** None	**Z** None
2 Spleen **5** Lymphatics, Head and Neck **D** Lymphatics, Pelvic **J** Lymphatics, Head **K** Lymphatics, Neck **L** Lymphatics, Upper Chest **M** Lymphatics, Trunk **N** Lymphatics, Upper Extremity **P** Lymphatics, Lower Extremity	**1** Technetium 99m (Tc-99m) **Y** Other Radionuclide	**Z** None	**Z** None
3 Blood	**D** Indium 111 (In-111) **Y** Other Radionuclide	**Z** None	**Z** None
Y Lymphatic and Hematologic System	**Y** Other Radionuclide	**Z** None	**Z** None

C Nuclear Medicine
7 Lymphatic and Hematologic System
2 Tomographic (Tomo) Nuclear Medicine Imaging: Introduction of radioactive materials into the body for three dimensional display of images developed from the capture of radioactive emissions

Body Part	Radionuclide	Qualifier	Qualifier
Character 4	**Character 5**	**Character 6**	**Character 7**
2 Spleen	**1** Technetium 99m (Tc-99m) **Y** Other Radionuclide	**Z** None	**Z** None
Y Lymphatic and Hematologic System	**Y** Other Radionuclide	**Z** None	**Z** None

LC Limited Coverage NC Noncovered HAC HAC-associated Procedure CC Combination Cluster - See Appendix G for code lists
DRG Non-OR-Affecting MS-DRG Assignment New/Revised Text in **Orange** ♂ Male ♀ Female

C Nuclear Medicine
7 Lymphatic and Hematologic System
5 Nonimaging Nuclear Medicine Probe: Introduction of radioactive materials into the body for the study of distribution and fate of certain substances by the detection of radioactive emissions; or, alternatively, measurement of absorption of radioactive emissions from an external source

Body Part	Radionuclide	Qualifier	Qualifier
Character 4	**Character 5**	**Character 6**	**Character 7**
5 Lymphatics, Head and Neck **D** Lymphatics, Pelvic **J** Lymphatics, Head **K** Lymphatics, Neck **L** Lymphatics, Upper Chest **M** Lymphatics, Trunk **N** Lymphatics, Upper Extremity **P** Lymphatics, Lower Extremity	**1** Technetium 99m (Tc-99m) **Y** Other Radionuclide	**Z** None	**Z** None
Y Lymphatic and Hematologic System	**Y** Other Radionuclide	**Z** None	**Z** None

C Nuclear Medicine
7 Lymphatic and Hematologic System
6 Nonimaging Nuclear Medicine Assay: Introduction of radioactive materials into the body for the study of body fluids and blood elements, by the detection of radioactive emissions

Body Part	Radionuclide	Qualifier	Qualifier
Character 4	**Character 5**	**Character 6**	**Character 7**
3 Blood	**1** Technetium 99m (Tc-99m) **7** Cobalt 58 (Co-58) **C** Cobalt 57 (Co-57) **D** Indium 111 (In-111) **H** Iodine 125 (I-125) **W** Chromium (Cr-51) **Y** Other Radionuclide	**Z** None	**Z** None
Y Lymphatic and Hematologic System	**Y** Other Radionuclide	**Z** None	**Z** None

C Nuclear Medicine
8 Eye
1 Planar Nuclear Medicine Imaging: Introduction of radioactive materials into the body for single plane display of images developed from the capture of radioactive emissions

Body Part	Radionuclide	Qualifier	Qualifier
Character 4	**Character 5**	**Character 6**	**Character 7**
9 Lacrimal Ducts, Bilateral	**1** Technetium 99m (Tc-99m) **Y** Other Radionuclide	**Z** None	**Z** None
Y Eye	**Y** Other Radionuclide	**Z** None	**Z** None

C Nuclear Medicine
9 Ear, Nose, Mouth and Throat
1 Planar Nuclear Medicine Imaging: Introduction of radioactive materials into the body for single plane display of images developed from the capture of radioactive emissions

Body Part	Radionuclide	Qualifier	Qualifier
Character 4	**Character 5**	**Character 6**	**Character 7**
B Salivary Glands, Bilateral	**1** Technetium 99m (Tc-99m) **Y** Other Radionuclide	**Z** None	**Z** None
Y Ear, Nose, Mouth and Throat	**Y** Other Radionuclide	**Z** None	**Z** None

C Nuclear Medicine
B Respiratory System
1 Planar Nuclear Medicine Imaging: Introduction of radioactive materials into the body for single plane display of images developed from the capture of radioactive emissions

Body Part Character 4	Radionuclide Character 5	Qualifier Character 6	Qualifier Character 7
2 Lungs and Bronchi	**1** Technetium 99m (Tc-99m) **9** Krypton (Kr-81m) **T** Xenon 127 (Xe-127) **V** Xenon 133 (Xe-133) **Y** Other Radionuclide	**Z** None	**Z** None
Y Respiratory System	**Y** Other Radionuclide	**Z** None	**Z** None

C Nuclear Medicine
B Respiratory System
2 Tomographic (Tomo) Nuclear Medicine Imaging: Introduction of radioactive materials into the body for three dimensional display of images developed from the capture of radioactive emissions

Body Part Character 4	Radionuclide Character 5	Qualifier Character 6	Qualifier Character 7
2 Lungs and Bronchi	**1** Technetium 99m (Tc-99m) **9** Krypton (Kr-81m) **Y** Other Radionuclide	**Z** None	**Z** None
Y Respiratory System	**Y** Other Radionuclide	**Z** None	**Z** None

C Nuclear Medicine
B Respiratory System
3 Positron Emission Tomographic (PET) Imaging: Introduction of radioactive materials into the body for three dimensional display of images developed from the simultaneous capture, 180 degrees apart, of radioactive emissions

Body Part Character 4	Radionuclide Character 5	Qualifier Character 6	Qualifier Character 7
2 Lungs and Bronchi	**K** Fluorine 18 (F-18) **Y** Other Radionuclide	**Z** None	**Z** None
Y Respiratory System	**Y** Other Radionuclide	**Z** None	**Z** None

C Nuclear Medicine
D Gastrointestinal System
1 Planar Nuclear Medicine Imaging: Introduction of radioactive materials into the body for single plane display of images developed from the capture of radioactive emissions

Body Part Character 4	Radionuclide Character 5	Qualifier Character 6	Qualifier Character 7
5 Upper Gastrointestinal Tract **7** Gastrointestinal Tract	**1** Technetium 99m (Tc-99m) **D** Indium 111 (In-111) **Y** Other Radionuclide	**Z** None	**Z** None
Y Digestive System	**Y** Other Radionuclide	**Z** None	**Z** None

C Nuclear Medicine
D Gastrointestinal System
2 Tomographic (Tomo) Nuclear Medicine Imaging: Introduction of radioactive materials into the body for three dimensional display of images developed from the capture of radioactive emissions

Body Part Character 4	Radionuclide Character 5	Qualifier Character 6	Qualifier Character 7
7 Gastrointestinal Tract	**1** Technetium 99m (Tc-99m) **D** Indium 111 (In-111) **Y** Other Radionuclide	**Z** None	**Z** None
Y Digestive System	**Y** Other Radionuclide	**Z** None	**Z** None

C Nuclear Medicine
F Hepatobiliary System and Pancreas
1 Planar Nuclear Medicine Imaging: Introduction of radioactive materials into the body for single plane display of images developed from the capture of radioactive emissions

Body Part	Radionuclide	Qualifier	Qualifier
Character 4	Character 5	Character 6	Character 7
4 Gallbladder 5 Liver 6 Liver and Spleen C Hepatobiliary System, All	1 Technetium 99m (Tc-99m) Y Other Radionuclide	Z None	Z None
Y Hepatobiliary System and Pancreas	Y Other Radionuclide	Z None	Z None

C Nuclear Medicine
F Hepatobiliary System and Pancreas
2 Tomographic (Tomo) Nuclear Medicine Imaging: Introduction of radioactive materials into the body for three dimensional display of images developed from the capture of radioactive emissions

Body Part	Radionuclide	Qualifier	Qualifier
Character 4	Character 5	Character 6	Character 7
4 Gallbladder 5 Liver 6 Liver and Spleen	1 Technetium 99m (Tc-99m) Y Other Radionuclide	Z None	Z None
Y Hepatobiliary System and Pancreas	Y Other Radionuclide	Z None	Z None

C Nuclear Medicine
G Endocrine System
1 Planar Nuclear Medicine Imaging: Introduction of radioactive materials into the body for single plane display of images developed from the capture of radioactive emissions

Body Part	Radionuclide	Qualifier	Qualifier
Character 4	Character 5	Character 6	Character 7
1 Parathyroid Glands	1 Technetium 99m (Tc-99m) S Thallium 201 (Tl-201) Y Other Radionuclide	Z None	Z None
2 Thyroid Gland	1 Technetium 99m (Tc-99m) F Iodine 123 (I-123) G Iodine 131 (I-131) Y Other Radionuclide	Z None	Z None
4 Adrenal Glands, Bilateral	G Iodine 131 (I-131) Y Other Radionuclide	Z None	Z None
Y Endocrine System	Y Other Radionuclide	Z None	Z None

C Nuclear Medicine
G Endocrine System
2 Tomographic (Tomo) Nuclear Medicine Imaging: Introduction of radioactive materials into the body for three dimensional display of images developed from the capture of radioactive emissions

Body Part	Radionuclide	Qualifier	Qualifier
Character 4	Character 5	Character 6	Character 7
1 Parathyroid Glands	1 Technetium 99m (Tc-99m) S Thallium 201 (Tl-201) Y Other Radionuclide	Z None	Z None
Y Endocrine System	Y Other Radionuclide	Z None	Z None

C Nuclear Medicine
G Endocrine System
4 Nonimaging Nuclear Medicine Uptake: Introduction of radioactive materials into the body for measurements of organ function, from the detection of radioactive emissions

Body Part Character 4	Radionuclide Character 5	Qualifier Character 6	Qualifier Character 7
2 Thyroid Gland	1 Technetium 99m (Tc-99m) F Iodine 123 (I-123) G Iodine 131 (I-131) Y Other Radionuclide	Z None	Z None
Y Endocrine System	Y Other Radionuclide	Z None	Z None

C Nuclear Medicine
H Skin, Subcutaneous Tissue and Breast
1 Planar Nuclear Medicine Imaging: Introduction of radioactive materials into the body for single plane display of images developed from the capture of radioactive emissions

Body Part Character 4	Radionuclide Character 5	Qualifier Character 6	Qualifier Character 7
0 Breast, Right 1 Breast, Left 2 Breasts, Bilateral	1 Technetium 99m (Tc-99m) S Thallium 201 (Tl-201) Y Other Radionuclide	Z None	Z None
Y Skin, Subcutaneous Tissue and Breast	Y Other Radionuclide	Z None	Z None

C Nuclear Medicine
H Skin, Subcutaneous Tissue and Breast
2 Tomographic (Tomo) Nuclear Medicine Imaging: Introduction of radioactive materials into the body for three dimensional display of images developed from the capture of radioactive emissions

Body Part Character 4	Radionuclide Character 5	Qualifier Character 6	Qualifier Character 7
0 Breast, Right 1 Breast, Left 2 Breasts, Bilateral	1 Technetium 99m (Tc-99m) S Thallium 201 (Tl-201) Y Other Radionuclide	Z None	Z None
Y Skin, Subcutaneous Tissue and Breast	Y Other Radionuclide	Z None	Z None

C Nuclear Medicine
P Musculoskeletal System
1 Planar Nuclear Medicine Imaging: Introduction of radioactive materials into the body for single plane display of images developed from the capture of radioactive emissions

Body Part Character 4	Radionuclide Character 5	Qualifier Character 6	Qualifier Character 7
1 Skull 4 Thorax 5 Spine 6 Pelvis 7 Spine and Pelvis 8 Upper Extremity, Right 9 Upper Extremity, Left B Upper Extremities, Bilateral C Lower Extremity, Right D Lower Extremity, Left F Lower Extremities, Bilateral Z Musculoskeletal System, All	1 Technetium 99m (Tc-99m) Y Other Radionuclide	Z None	Z None
Y Musculoskeletal System, Other	Y Other Radionuclide	Z None	Z None

C Nuclear Medicine
P Musculoskeletal System
2 Tomographic (Tomo) Nuclear Medicine Imaging: Introduction of radioactive materials into the body for three dimensional display of images developed from the capture of radioactive emissions

Body Part Character 4	Radionuclide Character 5	Qualifier Character 6	Qualifier Character 7
1 Skull **2** Cervical Spine **3** Skull and Cervical Spine **4** Thorax **6** Pelvis **7** Spine and Pelvis **8** Upper Extremity, Right **9** Upper Extremity, Left **B** Upper Extremities, Bilateral **C** Lower Extremity, Right **D** Lower Extremity, Left **F** Lower Extremities, Bilateral **G** Thoracic Spine **H** Lumbar Spine **J** Thoracolumbar Spine	**1** Technetium 99m (Tc-99m) **Y** Other Radionuclide	**Z** None	**Z** None
Y Musculoskeletal System, Other	**Y** Other Radionuclide	**Z** None	**Z** None

C Nuclear Medicine
P Musculoskeletal System
5 Nonimaging Nuclear Medicine Probe: Introduction of radioactive materials into the body for the study of distribution and fate of certain substances by the detection of radioactive emissions; or, alternatively, measurement of absorption of radioactive emissions from an external source

Body Part Character 4	Radionuclide Character 5	Qualifier Character 6	Qualifier Character 7
5 Spine **N** Upper Extremities **P** Lower Extremities	**Z** None	**Z** None	**Z** None
Y Musculoskeletal System, Other	**Y** Other Radionuclide	**Z** None	**Z** None

C Nuclear Medicine
T Urinary System
1 Planar Nuclear Medicine Imaging: Introduction of radioactive materials into the body for single plane display of images developed from the capture of radioactive emissions

Body Part Character 4	Radionuclide Character 5	Qualifier Character 6	Qualifier Character 7
3 Kidneys, Ureters and Bladder	**1** Technetium 99m (Tc-99m) **F** Iodine 123 (I-123) **G** Iodine 131 (I-131) **Y** Other Radionuclide	**Z** None	**Z** None
H Bladder and Ureters	**1** Technetium 99m (Tc-99m) **Y** Other Radionuclide	**Z** None	**Z** None
Y Urinary System	**Y** Other Radionuclide	**Z** None	**Z** None

C Nuclear Medicine
T Urinary System
2 Tomographic (Tomo) Nuclear Medicine Imaging: Introduction of radioactive materials into the body for three dimensional display of images developed from the capture of radioactive emissions

Body Part Character 4	Radionuclide Character 5	Qualifier Character 6	Qualifier Character 7
3 Kidneys, Ureters and Bladder	**1** Technetium 99m (Tc-99m) **Y** Other Radionuclide	**Z** None	**Z** None
Y Urinary System	**Y** Other Radionuclide	**Z** None	**Z** None

C Nuclear Medicine
T Urinary System
6 Nonimaging Nuclear Medicine Assay: Introduction of radioactive materials into the body for the study of body fluids and blood elements, by the detection of radioactive emissions

Body Part Character 4	Radionuclide Character 5	Qualifier Character 6	Qualifier Character 7
3 Kidneys, Ureters and Bladder	**1** Technetium 99m (Tc-99m) **F** Iodine 123 (I-123) **G** Iodine 131 (I-131) **H** Iodine 125 (I-125) **Y** Other Radionuclide	**Z** None	**Z** None
Y Urinary System	**Y** Other Radionuclide	**Z** None	**Z** None

C Nuclear Medicine
V Male Reproductive System
1 Planar Nuclear Medicine Imaging: Introduction of radioactive materials into the body for single plane display of images developed from the capture of radioactive emissions

Body Part Character 4	Radionuclide Character 5	Qualifier Character 6	Qualifier Character 7
9 Testicles, Bilateral ♂	**1** Technetium 99m (Tc-99m) **Y** Other Radionuclide	**Z** None	**Z** None
Y Male Reproductive System ♂	**Y** Other Radionuclide	**Z** None	**Z** None

♂ CV191ZZ CV19YZZ CV1YYZZ

C Nuclear Medicine
W Anatomical Regions
1 Planar Nuclear Medicine Imaging: Introduction of radioactive materials into the body for single plane display of images developed from the capture of radioactive emissions

Body Part Character 4	Radionuclide Character 5	Qualifier Character 6	Qualifier Character 7
0 Abdomen **1** Abdomen and Pelvis **4** Chest and Abdomen **6** Chest and Neck **B** Head and Neck **D** Lower Extremity **J** Pelvic Region **M** Upper Extremity **N** Whole Body	**1** Technetium 99m (Tc-99m) **D** Indium 111 (In-111) **F** Iodine 123 (I-123) **G** Iodine 131 (I-131) **L** Gallium 67 (Ga-67) **S** Thallium 201 (Tl-201) **Y** Other Radionuclide	**Z** None	**Z** None
3 Chest	**1** Technetium 99m (Tc-99m) **D** Indium 111 (In-111) **F** Iodine 123 (I-123) **G** Iodine 131 (I-131) **K** Fluorine 18 (F-18) **L** Gallium 67 (Ga-67) **S** Thallium 201 (Tl-201) **Y** Other Radionuclide	**Z** None	**Z** None
Y Anatomical Regions, Multiple	**Y** Other Radionuclide	**Z** None	**Z** None
Z Anatomical Region, Other	**Z** None	**Z** None	**Z** None

C Nuclear Medicine
W Anatomical Regions
2 Tomographic (Tomo) Nuclear Medicine Imaging: Introduction of radioactive materials into the body for three dimensional display of images developed from the capture of radioactive emissions

Body Part Character 4	Radionuclide Character 5	Qualifier Character 6	Qualifier Character 7
0 Abdomen **1** Abdomen and Pelvis **3** Chest **4** Chest and Abdomen **6** Chest and Neck **B** Head and Neck **D** Lower Extremity **J** Pelvic Region **M** Upper Extremity	**1** Technetium 99m (Tc-99m) **D** Indium 111 (In-111) **F** Iodine 123 (I-123) **G** Iodine 131 (I-131) **K** Fluorine 18 (F-18) **L** Gallium 67 (Ga-67) **S** Thallium 201 (Tl-201) **Y** Other Radionuclide	**Z** None	**Z** None
Y Anatomical Regions, Multiple	**Y** Other Radionuclide	**Z** None	**Z** None

C Nuclear Medicine
W Anatomical Regions
3 Positron Emission Tomographic (PET) Imaging: Introduction of radioactive materials into the body for three dimensional display of images developed from the simultaneous capture, 180 degrees apart, of radioactive emissions

Body Part Character 4	Radionuclide Character 5	Qualifier Character 6	Qualifier Character 7
N Whole Body	**Y** Other Radionuclide	**Z** None	**Z** None

C Nuclear Medicine
W Anatomical Regions
5 Nonimaging Nuclear Medicine Probe: Introduction of radioactive materials into the body for the study of distribution and fate of certain substances by the detection of radioactive emissions; or, alternatively, measurement of absorption of radioactive emissions from an external source

Body Part Character 4	Radionuclide Character 5	Qualifier Character 6	Qualifier Character 7
0 Abdomen **1** Abdomen and Pelvis **3** Chest **4** Chest and Abdomen **6** Chest and Neck **B** Head and Neck **D** Lower Extremity **J** Pelvic Region **M** Upper Extremity	**1** Technetium 99m (Tc-99m) **D** Indium 111 (In-111) **Y** Other Radionuclide	**Z** None	**Z** None

C Nuclear Medicine
W Anatomical Regions
7 Systemic Nuclear Medicine Therapy: Introduction of unsealed radioactive materials into the body for treatment

Body Part Character 4	Radionuclide Character 5	Qualifier Character 6	Qualifier Character 7
0 Abdomen **3** Chest	**N** Phosphorus 32 (P-32) **Y** Other Radionuclide	**Z** None	**Z** None
G Thyroid	**G** Iodine 131 (I-131) **Y** Other Radionuclide	**Z** None	**Z** None
N Whole Body	**8** Samarium 153 (Sm-153) **G** Iodine 131 (I-131) **N** Phosphorus 32 (P-32) **P** Strontium 89 (Sr-89) **Y** Other Radionuclide	**Z** None	**Z** None
Y Anatomical Regions, Multiple	**Y** Other Radionuclide	**Z** None	**Z** None

NOTES

NOTES

Radiation Therapy D00-DWY

D Radiation Therapy
0 Central and Peripheral Nervous System
0 Beam Radiation

Treatment Site Character 4	Modality Qualifier Character 5	Isotope Character 6	Qualifier Character 7
0 Brain **1** Brain Stem **6** Spinal Cord **7** Peripheral Nerve	**0** Photons <1 MeV **1** Photons 1 - 10 MeV **2** Photons >10 MeV **4** Heavy Particles (Protons, Ions) **5** Neutrons **6** Neutron Capture	**Z** None	**Z** None
0 Brain **1** Brain Stem **6** Spinal Cord **7** Peripheral Nerve	**3** Electrons	**Z** None	**0** Intraoperative **Z** None

D Radiation Therapy
0 Central and Peripheral Nervous System
1 Brachytherapy

Treatment Site Character 4	Modality Qualifier Character 5	Isotope Character 6	Qualifier Character 7
0 Brain **1** Brain Stem **6** Spinal Cord **7** Peripheral Nerve	**9** High Dose Rate (HDR) **B** Low Dose Rate (LDR)	**7** Cesium 137 (Cs-137) **8** Iridium 192 (Ir-192) **9** Iodine 125 (I-125) **B** Palladium 103 (Pd-103) **C** Californium 252 (Cf-252) **Y** Other Isotope	**Z** None

D Radiation Therapy
0 Central and Peripheral Nervous System
2 Stereotactic Radiosurgery

Treatment Site Character 4	Modality Qualifier Character 5	Isotope Character 6	Qualifier Character 7
0 Brain DRG **1** Brain Stem DRG **6** Spinal Cord DRG **7** Peripheral Nerve DRG	**D** Stereotactic Other Photon Radiosurgery **H** Stereotactic Particulate Radiosurgery **J** Stereotactic Gamma Beam Radiosurgery	**Z** None	**Z** None

DRG D020DZZ D020HZZ D020JZZ D021DZZ D021HZZ D021JZZ D026DZZ D026HZZ D026JZZ D027DZZ D027HZZ D027JZZ

D Radiation Therapy
0 Central and Peripheral Nervous System
Y Other Radiation

Treatment Site Character 4	Modality Qualifier Character 5	Isotope Character 6	Qualifier Character 7
0 Brain **1** Brain Stem **6** Spinal Cord **7** Peripheral Nerve	**7** Contact Radiation **8** Hyperthermia **F** Plaque Radiation **K** Laser Interstitial Thermal Therapy	**Z** None	**Z** None

LC Limited Coverage NC Noncovered HAC HAC-associated Procedure CC Combination Cluster - See Appendix G for code lists
DRG Non-OR-Affecting MS-DRG Assignment New/Revised Text in **Orange** ♂ Male ♀ Female

D Radiation Therapy
7 Lymphatic and Hematologic System
0 Beam Radiation

Treatment Site Character 4	Modality Qualifier Character 5	Isotope Character 6	Qualifier Character 7
0 Bone Marrow 1 Thymus 2 Spleen 3 Lymphatics, Neck 4 Lymphatics, Axillary 5 Lymphatics, Thorax 6 Lymphatics, Abdomen 7 Lymphatics, Pelvis 8 Lymphatics, Inguinal	0 Photons <1 MeV 1 Photons 1 - 10 MeV 2 Photons >10 MeV 4 Heavy Particles (Protons, Ions) 5 Neutrons 6 Neutron Capture	Z None	Z None
0 Bone Marrow 1 Thymus 2 Spleen 3 Lymphatics, Neck 4 Lymphatics, Axillary 5 Lymphatics, Thorax 6 Lymphatics, Abdomen 7 Lymphatics, Pelvis 8 Lymphatics, Inguinal	3 Electrons	Z None	0 Intraoperative Z None

D Radiation Therapy
7 Lymphatic and Hematologic System
1 Brachytherapy

Treatment Site Character 4	Modality Qualifier Character 5	Isotope Character 6	Qualifier Character 7
0 Bone Marrow 1 Thymus 2 Spleen 3 Lymphatics, Neck 4 Lymphatics, Axillary 5 Lymphatics, Thorax 6 Lymphatics, Abdomen 7 Lymphatics, Pelvis 8 Lymphatics, Inguinal	9 High Dose Rate (HDR) B Low Dose Rate (LDR)	7 Cesium 137 (Cs-137) 8 Iridium 192 (Ir-192) 9 Iodine 125 (I-125) B Palladium 103 (Pd-103) C Californium 252 (Cf-252) Y Other Isotope	Z None

D Radiation Therapy
7 Lymphatic and Hematologic System
2 Stereotactic Radiosurgery

Treatment Site Character 4	Modality Qualifier Character 5	Isotope Character 6	Qualifier Character 7
0 Bone Marrow DRG 1 Thymus DRG 2 Spleen DRG 3 Lymphatics, Neck DRG 4 Lymphatics, Axillary DRG 5 Lymphatics, Thorax DRG 6 Lymphatics, Abdomen DRG 7 Lymphatics, Pelvis DRG 8 Lymphatics, Inguinal DRG	D Stereotactic Other Photon Radiosurgery H Stereotactic Particulate Radiosurgery J Stereotactic Gamma Beam Radiosurgery	Z None	Z None

DRG D720DZZ D720HZZ D720JZZ D721DZZ D721HZZ D721JZZ D722DZZ D722HZZ D722JZZ D723DZZ D723HZZ D723JZZ D724DZZ D724HZZ D724JZZ D725DZZ D725HZZ D725JZZ D726DZZ D726HZZ D726JZZ D727DZZ D727HZZ D727JZZ D728DZZ D728HZZ D728JZZ

LC Limited Coverage NC Noncovered HAC HAC-associated Procedure CC Combination Cluster - See Appendix G for code lists
DRG Non-OR-Affecting MS-DRG Assignment New/Revised Text in Orange ♂ Male ♀ Female

D Radiation Therapy
7 Lymphatic and Hematologic System
Y Other Radiation

Treatment Site	Modality Qualifier	Isotope	Qualifier
Character 4	**Character 5**	**Character 6**	**Character 7**
0 Bone Marrow **1** Thymus **2** Spleen **3** Lymphatics, Neck **4** Lymphatics, Axillary **5** Lymphatics, Thorax **6** Lymphatics, Abdomen **7** Lymphatics, Pelvis **8** Lymphatics, Inguinal	**8** Hyperthermia **F** Plaque Radiation	**Z** None	**Z** None

D Radiation Therapy
8 Eye
0 Beam Radiation

Treatment Site	Modality Qualifier	Isotope	Qualifier
Character 4	**Character 5**	**Character 6**	**Character 7**
0 Eye	**0** Photons <1 MeV **1** Photons 1 - 10 MeV **2** Photons >10 MeV **4** Heavy Particles (Protons, Ions) **5** Neutrons **6** Neutron Capture	**Z** None	**Z** None
0 Eye	**3** Electrons	**Z** None	**0** Intraoperative **Z** None

D Radiation Therapy
8 Eye
1 Brachytherapy

Treatment Site	Modality Qualifier	Isotope	Qualifier
Character 4	**Character 5**	**Character 6**	**Character 7**
0 Eye	**9** High Dose Rate (HDR) **B** Low Dose Rate (LDR)	**7** Cesium 137 (Cs-137) **8** Iridium 192 (Ir-192) **9** Iodine 125 (I-125) **B** Palladium 103 (Pd-103) **C** Californium 252 (Cf-252) **Y** Other Isotope	**Z** None

D Radiation Therapy
8 Eye
2 Stereotactic Radiosurgery

Treatment Site	Modality Qualifier	Isotope	Qualifier
Character 4	**Character 5**	**Character 6**	**Character 7**
0 Eye DRG	**D** Stereotactic Other Photon Radiosurgery **H** Stereotactic Particulate Radiosurgery **J** Stereotactic Gamma Beam Radiosurgery	**Z** None	**Z** None

DRG D820DZZ D820HZZ D820JZZ

D Radiation Therapy
8 Eye
Y Other Radiation

Treatment Site Character 4	Modality Qualifier Character 5	Isotope Character 6	Qualifier Character 7
0 Eye	**7** Contact Radiation **8** Hyperthermia **F** Plaque Radiation	**Z** None	**Z** None

D Radiation Therapy
9 Ear, Nose, Mouth and Throat
0 Beam Radiation

Treatment Site Character 4	Modality Qualifier Character 5	Isotope Character 6	Qualifier Character 7
0 Ear **1** Nose **3** Hypopharynx **4** Mouth **5** Tongue **6** Salivary Glands **7** Sinuses **8** Hard Palate **9** Soft Palate **B** Larynx **D** Nasopharynx **F** Oropharynx	**0** Photons <1 MeV **1** Photons 1 - 10 MeV **2** Photons >10 MeV **4** Heavy Particles (Protons, Ions) **5** Neutrons **6** Neutron Capture	**Z** None	**Z** None
0 Ear **1** Nose **3** Hypopharynx **4** Mouth **5** Tongue **6** Salivary Glands **7** Sinuses **8** Hard Palate **9** Soft Palate **B** Larynx **D** Nasopharynx **F** Oropharynx	**3** Electrons	**Z** None	**0** Intraoperative **Z** None

D Radiation Therapy
9 Ear, Nose, Mouth and Throat
1 Brachytherapy

Treatment Site Character 4	Modality Qualifier Character 5	Isotope Character 6	Qualifier Character 7
0 Ear **1** Nose **3** Hypopharynx **4** Mouth **5** Tongue **6** Salivary Glands **7** Sinuses **8** Hard Palate **9** Soft Palate **B** Larynx **D** Nasopharynx **F** Oropharynx	**9** High Dose Rate (HDR) **B** Low Dose Rate (LDR)	**7** Cesium 137 (Cs-137) **8** Iridium 192 (Ir-192) **9** Iodine 125 (I-125) **B** Palladium 103 (Pd-103) **C** Californium 252 (Cf-252) **Y** Other Isotope	**Z** None

D Radiation Therapy
9 Ear, Nose, Mouth and Throat
2 Stereotactic Radiosurgery

Treatment Site Character 4	Modality Qualifier Character 5	Isotope Character 6	Qualifier Character 7
0 Ear DRG 1 Nose DRG 4 Mouth DRG 5 Tongue DRG 6 Salivary Glands DRG 7 Sinuses DRG 8 Hard Palate DRG 9 Soft Palate DRG B Larynx DRG C Pharynx DRG D Nasopharynx DRG	D Stereotactic Other Photon Radiosurgery H Stereotactic Particulate Radiosurgery J Stereotactic Gamma Beam Radiosurgery	Z None	Z None

DRG D920DZZ D920HZZ D920JZZ D921DZZ D921HZZ D921JZZ D924DZZ D924HZZ D924JZZ D925DZZ D925HZZ D925JZZ D926DZZ D926HZZ D926JZZ D927DZZ D927HZZ D927JZZ D928DZZ D928HZZ D928JZZ D929DZZ D929HZZ D929JZZ D92BDZZ D92BHZZ D92BJZZ D92CDZZ D92CHZZ D92CJZZ D92DDZZ D92DHZZ D92DJZZ

D Radiation Therapy
9 Ear, Nose, Mouth and Throat
Y Other Radiation

Treatment Site Character 4	Modality Qualifier Character 5	Isotope Character 6	Qualifier Character 7
0 Ear 1 Nose 5 Tongue 6 Salivary Glands 7 Sinuses 8 Hard Palate 9 Soft Palate	7 Contact Radiation 8 Hyperthermia F Plaque Radiation	Z None	Z None
3 Hypopharynx F Oropharynx	7 Contact Radiation 8 Hyperthermia	Z None	Z None
4 Mouth B Larynx D Nasopharynx	7 Contact Radiation 8 Hyperthermia C Intraoperative Radiation Therapy (IORT) F Plaque Radiation	Z None	Z None
C Pharynx	C Intraoperative Radiation Therapy (IORT) F Plaque Radiation	Z None	Z None

D Radiation Therapy
B Respiratory System
0 Beam Radiation

Treatment Site Character 4	Modality Qualifier Character 5	Isotope Character 6	Qualifier Character 7
0 Trachea 1 Bronchus 2 Lung 5 Pleura 6 Mediastinum 7 Chest Wall 8 Diaphragm	0 Photons <1 MeV 1 Photons 1 - 10 MeV 2 Photons >10 MeV 4 Heavy Particles (Protons, Ions) 5 Neutrons 6 Neutron Capture	Z None	Z None
0 Trachea 1 Bronchus 2 Lung 5 Pleura 6 Mediastinum 7 Chest Wall 8 Diaphragm	3 Electrons	Z None	0 Intraoperative Z None

D Radiation Therapy
B Respiratory System
1 Brachytherapy

Treatment Site	Modality Qualifier	Isotope	Qualifier
Character 4	Character 5	Character 6	Character 7
0 Trachea 1 Bronchus 2 Lung 5 Pleura 6 Mediastinum 7 Chest Wall 8 Diaphragm	9 High Dose Rate (HDR) B Low Dose Rate (LDR)	7 Cesium 137 (Cs-137) 8 Iridium 192 (Ir-192) 9 Iodine 125 (I-125) B Palladium 103 (Pd-103) C Californium 252 (Cf-252) Y Other Isotope	Z None

D Radiation Therapy
B Respiratory System
2 Stereotactic Radiosurgery

Treatment Site	Modality Qualifier	Isotope	Qualifier
Character 4	Character 5	Character 6	Character 7
0 Trachea DRG 1 Bronchus DRG 2 Lung DRG 5 Pleura DRG 6 Mediastinum DRG 7 Chest Wall DRG 8 Diaphragm	D Stereotactic Other Photon Radiosurgery H Stereotactic Particulate Radiosurgery J Stereotactic Gamma Beam Radiosurgery	Z None	Z None

DRG DB20DZZ DB20HZZ DB20JZZ DB21DZZ DB21HZZ DB21JZZ DB22DZZ DB22HZZ DB22JZZ DB25DZZ DB25HZZ DB25JZZ DB26DZZ DB26HZZ DB26JZZ DB27DZZ

D Radiation Therapy
B Respiratory System
Y Other Radiation

Treatment Site	Modality Qualifier	Isotope	Qualifier
Character 4	Character 5	Character 6	Character 7
0 Trachea 1 Bronchus 2 Lung 5 Pleura 6 Mediastinum 7 Chest Wall 8 Diaphragm	7 Contact Radiation 8 Hyperthermia F Plaque Radiation K Laser Interstitial Thermal Therapy	Z None	Z None

D Radiation Therapy
D Gastrointestinal System
0 Beam Radiation

Treatment Site	Modality Qualifier	Isotope	Qualifier
Character 4	Character 5	Character 6	Character 7
0 Esophagus 1 Stomach 2 Duodenum 3 Jejunum 4 Ileum 5 Colon 7 Rectum	0 Photons <1 MeV 1 Photons 1 - 10 MeV 2 Photons >10 MeV 4 Heavy Particles (Protons, Ions) 5 Neutrons 6 Neutron Capture	Z None	Z None
0 Esophagus 1 Stomach 2 Duodenum 3 Jejunum 4 Ileum 5 Colon 7 Rectum	3 Electrons	Z None	0 Intraoperative Z None

D Radiation Therapy
D Gastrointestinal System
1 Brachytherapy

Treatment Site Character 4	Modality Qualifier Character 5	Isotope Character 6	Qualifier Character 7
0 Esophagus **1** Stomach **2** Duodenum **3** Jejunum **4** Ileum **5** Colon **7** Rectum	**9** High Dose Rate (HDR) **B** Low Dose Rate (LDR)	**7** Cesium 137 (Cs-137) **8** Iridium 192 (Ir-192) **9** Iodine 125 (I-125) **B** Palladium 103 (Pd-103) **C** Californium 252 (Cf-252) **Y** Other Isotope	**Z** None

D Radiation Therapy
D Gastrointestinal System
2 Stereotactic Radiosurgery

Treatment Site Character 4	Modality Qualifier Character 5	Isotope Character 6	Qualifier Character 7
0 Esophagus **1** Stomach **2** Duodenum **3** Jejunum **4** Ileum **5** Colon **7** Rectum	**D** Stereotactic Other Photon Radiosurgery **H** Stereotactic Particulate Radiosurgery **J** Stereotactic Gamma Beam Radiosurgery	**Z** None	**Z** None

D Radiation Therapy
D Gastrointestinal System
Y Other Radiation

Treatment Site Character 4	Modality Qualifier Character 5	Isotope Character 6	Qualifier Character 7
0 Esophagus	**7** Contact Radiation **8** Hyperthermia **F** Plaque Radiation **K** Laser Interstitial Thermal Therapy	**Z** None	**Z** None
1 Stomach **2** Duodenum **3** Jejunum **4** Ileum **5** Colon **7** Rectum	**7** Contact Radiation **8** Hyperthermia **C** Intraoperative Radiation Therapy (IORT) **F** Plaque Radiation **K** Laser Interstitial Thermal Therapy	**Z** None	**Z** None
8 Anus	**C** Intraoperative Radiation Therapy (IORT) **F** Plaque Radiation **K** Laser Interstitial Thermal Therapy	**Z** None	**Z** None

D Radiation Therapy
F Hepatobiliary System and Pancreas
0 Beam Radiation

Treatment Site	Modality Qualifier	Isotope	Qualifier
Character 4	**Character 5**	**Character 6**	**Character 7**
0 Liver **1** Gallbladder **2** Bile Ducts **3** Pancreas	**0** Photons <1 MeV **1** Photons 1 - 10 MeV **2** Photons >10 MeV **4** Heavy Particles (Protons, Ions) **5** Neutrons **6** Neutron Capture	**Z** None	**Z** None
0 Liver **1** Gallbladder **2** Bile Ducts **3** Pancreas	**3** Electrons	**Z** None	**0** Intraoperative **Z** None

D Radiation Therapy
F Hepatobiliary System and Pancreas
1 Brachytherapy

Treatment Site	Modality Qualifier	Isotope	Qualifier
Character 4	**Character 5**	**Character 6**	**Character 7**
0 Liver **1** Gallbladder **2** Bile Ducts **3** Pancreas	**9** High Dose Rate (HDR) **B** Low Dose Rate (LDR)	**7** Cesium 137 (Cs-137) **8** Iridium 192 (Ir-192) **9** Iodine 125 (I-125) **B** Palladium 103 (Pd-103) **C** Californium 252 (Cf-252) **Y** Other Isotope	**Z** None

D Radiation Therapy
F Hepatobiliary System and Pancreas
2 Stereotactic Radiosurgery

Treatment Site	Modality Qualifier	Isotope	Qualifier
Character 4	**Character 5**	**Character 6**	**Character 7**
0 Liver **1** Gallbladder **2** Bile Ducts **3** Pancreas	**D** Stereotactic Other Photon Radiosurgery **H** Stereotactic Particulate Radiosurgery **J** Stereotactic Gamma Beam Radiosurgery	**Z** None	**Z** None

D Radiation Therapy
F Hepatobiliary System and Pancreas
Y Other Radiation

Treatment Site	Modality Qualifier	Isotope	Qualifier
Character 4	**Character 5**	**Character 6**	**Character 7**
0 Liver **1** Gallbladder **2** Bile Ducts **3** Pancreas	**7** Contact Radiation **8** Hyperthermia **C** Intraoperative Radiation Therapy (IORT) **F** Plaque Radiation **K** Laser Interstitial Thermal Therapy	**Z** None	**Z** None

D Radiation Therapy
G Endocrine System
0 Beam Radiation

Treatment Site Character 4	Modality Qualifier Character 5	Isotope Character 6	Qualifier Character 7
0 Pituitary Gland 1 Pineal Body 2 Adrenal Glands 4 Parathyroid Glands 5 Thyroid	0 Photons <1 MeV 1 Photons 1 - 10 MeV 2 Photons >10 MeV 5 Neutrons 6 Neutron Capture	Z None	Z None
0 Pituitary Gland 1 Pineal Body 2 Adrenal Glands 4 Parathyroid Glands 5 Thyroid	3 Electrons	Z None	0 Intraoperative Z None

D Radiation Therapy
G Endocrine System
1 Brachytherapy

Treatment Site Character 4	Modality Qualifier Character 5	Isotope Character 6	Qualifier Character 7
0 Pituitary Gland 1 Pineal Body 2 Adrenal Glands 4 Parathyroid Glands 5 Thyroid	9 High Dose Rate (HDR) B Low Dose Rate (LDR)	7 Cesium 137 (Cs-137) 8 Iridium 192 (Ir-192) 9 Iodine 125 (I-125) B Palladium 103 (Pd-103) C Californium 252 (Cf-252) Y Other Isotope	Z None

D Radiation Therapy
G Endocrine System
2 Stereotactic Radiosurgery

Treatment Site Character 4	Modality Qualifier Character 5	Isotope Character 6	Qualifier Character 7
0 Pituitary Gland 1 Pineal Body 2 Adrenal Glands 4 Parathyroid Glands 5 Thyroid	D Stereotactic Other Photon Radiosurgery H Stereotactic Particulate Radiosurgery J Stereotactic Gamma Beam Radiosurgery	Z None	Z None

D Radiation Therapy
G Endocrine System
Y Other Radiation

Treatment Site Character 4	Modality Qualifier Character 5	Isotope Character 6	Qualifier Character 7
0 Pituitary Gland 1 Pineal Body 2 Adrenal Glands 4 Parathyroid Glands 5 Thyroid	7 Contact Radiation 8 Hyperthermia F Plaque Radiation K Laser Interstitial Thermal Therapy	Z None	Z None

D Radiation Therapy
H Skin
0 Beam Radiation

Treatment Site Character 4	Modality Qualifier Character 5	Isotope Character 6	Qualifier Character 7
2 Skin, Face **3** Skin, Neck **4** Skin, Arm **6** Skin, Chest **7** Skin, Back **8** Skin, Abdomen **9** Skin, Buttock **B** Skin, Leg	**0** Photons <1 MeV **1** Photons 1 - 10 MeV **2** Photons >10 MeV **4** Heavy Particles (Protons, Ions) **5** Neutrons **6** Neutron Capture	**Z** None	**Z** None
2 Skin, Face **3** Skin, Neck **4** Skin, Arm **6** Skin, Chest **7** Skin, Back **8** Skin, Abdomen **9** Skin, Buttock **B** Skin, Leg	**3** Electrons	**Z** None	**0** Intraoperative **Z** None

D Radiation Therapy
H Skin
Y Other Radiation

Treatment Site Character 4	Modality Qualifier Character 5	Isotope Character 6	Qualifier Character 7
2 Skin, Face **3** Skin, Neck **4** Skin, Arm **6** Skin, Chest **7** Skin, Back **8** Skin, Abdomen **9** Skin, Buttock **B** Skin, Leg	**7** Contact Radiation **8** Hyperthermia **F** Plaque Radiation	**Z** None	**Z** None
5 Skin, Hand **C** Skin, Foot	**F** Plaque Radiation	**Z** None	**Z** None

D Radiation Therapy
M Breast
0 Beam Radiation

Treatment Site Character 4	Modality Qualifier Character 5	Isotope Character 6	Qualifier Character 7
0 Breast, Left **1** Breast, Right	**0** Photons <1 MeV **1** Photons 1 - 10 MeV **2** Photons >10 MeV **4** Heavy Particles (Protons, Ions) **5** Neutrons **6** Neutron Capture	**Z** None	**Z** None
0 Breast, Left **1** Breast, Right	**3** Electrons	**Z** None	**0** Intraoperative **Z** None

D Radiation Therapy
M Breast
1 Brachytherapy

Treatment Site	Modality Qualifier	Isotope	Qualifier
Character 4	**Character 5**	**Character 6**	**Character 7**
0 Breast, Left **1** Breast, Right	**9** High Dose Rate (HDR) **B** Low Dose Rate (LDR)	**7** Cesium 137 (Cs-137) **8** Iridium 192 (Ir-192) **9** Iodine 125 (I-125) **B** Palladium 103 (Pd-103) **C** Californium 252 (Cf-252) **Y** Other Isotope	**Z** None

D Radiation Therapy
M Breast
2 Stereotactic Radiosurgery

Treatment Site	Modality Qualifier	Isotope	Qualifier
Character 4	**Character 5**	**Character 6**	**Character 7**
0 Breast, Left **1** Breast, Right	**D** Stereotactic Other Photon Radiosurgery **H** Stereotactic Particulate Radiosurgery **J** Stereotactic Gamma Beam Radiosurgery	**Z** None	**Z** None

D Radiation Therapy
M Breast
Y Other Radiation

Treatment Site	Modality Qualifier	Isotope	Qualifier
Character 4	**Character 5**	**Character 6**	**Character 7**
0 Breast, Left **1** Breast, Right	**7** Contact Radiation **8** Hyperthermia **F** Plaque Radiation **K** Laser Interstitial Thermal Therapy	**Z** None	**Z** None

D Radiation Therapy
P Musculoskeletal System
0 Beam Radiation

Treatment Site Character 4	Modality Qualifier Character 5	Isotope Character 6	Qualifier Character 7
0 Skull **2** Maxilla **3** Mandible **4** Sternum **5** Rib(s) **6** Humerus **7** Radius/Ulna **8** Pelvic Bones **9** Femur **B** Tibia/Fibula **C** Other Bone	**0** Photons <1 MeV **1** Photons 1 - 10 MeV **2** Photons >10 MeV **4** Heavy Particles (Protons, Ions) **5** Neutrons **6** Neutron Capture	**Z** None	**Z** None
0 Skull **2** Maxilla **3** Mandible **4** Sternum **5** Rib(s) **6** Humerus **7** Radius/Ulna **8** Pelvic Bones **9** Femur **B** Tibia/Fibula **C** Other Bone	**3** Electrons	**Z** None	**0** Intraoperative **Z** None

D Radiation Therapy
P Musculoskeletal System
Y Other Radiation

Treatment Site Character 4	Modality Qualifier Character 5	Isotope Character 6	Qualifier Character 7
0 Skull **2** Maxilla **3** Mandible **4** Sternum **5** Rib(s) **6** Humerus **7** Radius/Ulna **8** Pelvic Bones **9** Femur **B** Tibia/Fibula **C** Other Bone	**7** Contact Radiation **8** Hyperthermia **F** Plaque Radiation	**Z** None	**Z** None

D Radiation Therapy
T Urinary System
0 Beam Radiation

Treatment Site Character 4	Modality Qualifier Character 5	Isotope Character 6	Qualifier Character 7
0 Kidney **1** Ureter **2** Bladder **3** Urethra	**0** Photons <1 MeV **1** Photons 1 - 10 MeV **2** Photons >10 MeV **4** Heavy Particles (Protons, Ions) **5** Neutrons **6** Neutron Capture	**Z** None	**Z** None
0 Kidney **1** Ureter **2** Bladder **3** Urethra	**3** Electrons	**Z** None	**0** Intraoperative **Z** None

D Radiation Therapy
T Urinary System
1 Brachytherapy

Treatment Site Character 4	Modality Qualifier Character 5	Isotope Character 6	Qualifier Character 7
0 Kidney **1** Ureter **2** Bladder **3** Urethra	**9** High Dose Rate (HDR) **B** Low Dose Rate (LDR)	**7** Cesium 137 (Cs-137) **8** Iridium 192 (Ir-192) **9** Iodine 125 (I-125) **B** Palladium 103 (Pd-103) **C** Californium 252 (Cf-252) **Y** Other Isotope	**Z** None

D Radiation Therapy
T Urinary System
2 Stereotactic Radiosurgery

Treatment Site Character 4	Modality Qualifier Character 5	Isotope Character 6	Qualifier Character 7
0 Kidney **1** Ureter **2** Bladder **3** Urethra	**D** Stereotactic Other Photon Radiosurgery **H** Stereotactic Particulate Radiosurgery **J** Stereotactic Gamma Beam Radiosurgery	**Z** None	**Z** None

D Radiation Therapy
T Urinary System
Y Other Radiation

Treatment Site Character 4	Modality Qualifier Character 5	Isotope Character 6	Qualifier Character 7
0 Kidney **1** Ureter **2** Bladder **3** Urethra	**7** Contact Radiation **8** Hyperthermia **C** Intraoperative Radiation Therapy (IORT) **F** Plaque Radiation	**Z** None	**Z** None

D Radiation Therapy
U Female Reproductive System
0 Beam Radiation

Treatment Site	Modality Qualifier	Isotope	Qualifier
Character 4	**Character 5**	**Character 6**	**Character 7**
0 Ovary ♀ **1** Cervix ♀ **2** Uterus ♀	**0** Photons <1 MeV **1** Photons 1 - 10 MeV **2** Photons >10 MeV **4** Heavy Particles (Protons, Ions) **5** Neutrons **6** Neutron Capture	**Z** None	**Z** None
0 Ovary ♀ **1** Cervix ♀ **2** Uterus ♀	**3** Electrons	**Z** None	**0** Intraoperative **Z** None

♀ DU000ZZ DU001ZZ DU002ZZ DU003Z0 DU003ZZ DU004ZZ DU005ZZ DU006ZZ DU010ZZ DU011ZZ DU012ZZ DU013Z0 DU013ZZ DU014ZZ DU015ZZ DU016ZZ DU020ZZ DU021ZZ DU022ZZ DU023Z0 DU023ZZ DU024ZZ DU025ZZ DU026ZZ

D Radiation Therapy
U Female Reproductive System
1 Brachytherapy

Treatment Site	Modality Qualifier	Isotope	Qualifier
Character 4	**Character 5**	**Character 6**	**Character 7**
0 Ovary ♀ **1** Cervix ♀ **2** Uterus ♀	**9** High Dose Rate (HDR) **B** Low Dose Rate (LDR)	**7** Cesium 137 (Cs-137) **8** Iridium 192 (Ir-192) **9** Iodine 125 (I-125) **B** Palladium 103 (Pd-103) **C** Californium 252 (Cf-252) **Y** Other Isotope	**Z** None

♀ DU1097Z DU1098Z DU1099Z DU109BZ DU109CZ DU109YZ DU10B7Z DU10B8Z DU10B9Z DU10BBZ DU10BCZ DU10BYZ DU1197Z DU1198Z DU1199Z DU119BZ DU119CZ DU119YZ DU11B7Z DU11B8Z DU11B9Z DU11BBZ DU11BCZ DU11BYZ DU1297Z DU1298Z DU1299Z DU129BZ DU129CZ DU129YZ DU12B7Z DU12B8Z DU12B9Z DU12BBZ DU12BCZ DU12BYZ

D Radiation Therapy
U Female Reproductive System
2 Stereotactic Radiosurgery

Treatment Site	Modality Qualifier	Isotope	Qualifier
Character 4	**Character 5**	**Character 6**	**Character 7**
0 Ovary ♀ **1** Cervix ♀ **2** Uterus ♀	**D** Stereotactic Other Photon Radiosurgery **H** Stereotactic Particulate Radiosurgery **J** Stereotactic Gamma Beam Radiosurgery	**Z** None	**Z** None

♀ DU20DZZ DU20HZZ DU20JZZ DU21DZZ DU21HZZ DU21JZZ DU22DZZ DU22HZZ DU22JZZ

D Radiation Therapy
U Female Reproductive System
Y Other Radiation

Treatment Site	Modality Qualifier	Isotope	Qualifier
Character 4	**Character 5**	**Character 6**	**Character 7**
0 Ovary ♀ **1** Cervix ♀ **2** Uterus ♀	**7** Contact Radiation **8** Hyperthermia **C** Intraoperative Radiation Therapy (IORT) **F** Plaque Radiation	**Z** None	**Z** None

♀ DUY07ZZ DUY08ZZ DUY0CZZ DUY0FZZ DUY17ZZ DUY18ZZ DUY1CZZ DUY1FZZ DUY27ZZ DUY28ZZ DUY2CZZ DUY2FZZ

D Radiation Therapy
V Male Reproductive System
0 Beam Radiation

Treatment Site Character 4	Modality Qualifier Character 5	Isotope Character 6	Qualifier Character 7
0 Prostate ♂ **1** Testis ♂	**0** Photons <1 MeV **1** Photons 1 - 10 MeV **2** Photons >10 MeV **4** Heavy Particles (Protons, Ions) **5** Neutrons **6** Neutron Capture	**Z** None	**Z** None
0 Prostate ♂ **1** Testis ♂	**3** Electrons	**Z** None	**0** Intraoperative **Z** None

♂ DV000ZZ DV001ZZ DV002ZZ DV003Z0 DV003ZZ DV004ZZ DV005ZZ DV006ZZ DV010ZZ DV011ZZ DV012ZZ DV013Z0 DV013ZZ DV014ZZ DV015ZZ DV016ZZ

D Radiation Therapy
V Male Reproductive System
1 Brachytherapy

Treatment Site Character 4	Modality Qualifier Character 5	Isotope Character 6	Qualifier Character 7
0 Prostate ♂ **1** Testis ♂	**9** High Dose Rate (HDR) **B** Low Dose Rate (LDR)	**7** Cesium 137 (Cs-137) **8** Iridium 192 (Ir-192) **9** Iodine 125 (I-125) **B** Palladium 103 (Pd-103) **C** Californium 252 (Cf-252) **Y** Other Isotope	**Z** None

♂ DV1097Z DV1098Z DV1099Z DV109BZ DV109CZ DV109YZ DV10B7Z DV10B8Z DV10B9Z DV10BBZ DV10BCZ DV10BYZ DV1197Z DV1198Z DV1199Z DV119BZ DV119CZ DV119YZ DV11B7Z DV11B8Z DV11B9Z DV11BBZ DV11BCZ DV11BYZ

D Radiation Therapy
V Male Reproductive System
2 Stereotactic Radiosurgery

Treatment Site Character 4	Modality Qualifier Character 5	Isotope Character 6	Qualifier Character 7
0 Prostate ♂ **1** Testis ♂	**D** Stereotactic Other Photon Radiosurgery **H** Stereotactic Particulate Radiosurgery **J** Stereotactic Gamma Beam Radiosurgery	**Z** None	**Z** None

♂ DV20DZZ DV20HZZ DV20JZZ DV21DZZ DV21HZZ DV21JZZ

D Radiation Therapy
V Male Reproductive System
Y Other Radiation

Treatment Site Character 4	Modality Qualifier Character 5	Isotope Character 6	Qualifier Character 7
0 Prostate ♂	**7** Contact Radiation **8** Hyperthermia **C** Intraoperative Radiation Therapy (IORT) **F** Plaque Radiation **K** Laser Interstitial Thermal Therapy	**Z** None	**Z** None
1 Testis ♂	**7** Contact Radiation **8** Hyperthermia **F** Plaque Radiation	**Z** None	**Z** None

♂ DVY07ZZ DVY08ZZ DVY0CZZ DVY0FZZ DVY0KZZ DVY17ZZ DVY18ZZ DVY1FZZ

D Radiation Therapy
W Anatomical Regions
0 Beam Radiation

Treatment Site Character 4	Modality Qualifier Character 5	Isotope Character 6	Qualifier Character 7
1 Head and Neck 2 Chest 3 Abdomen 4 Hemibody 5 Whole Body 6 Pelvic Region	0 Photons <1 MeV 1 Photons 1 - 10 MeV 2 Photons >10 MeV 4 Heavy Particles (Protons, Ions) 5 Neutrons 6 Neutron Capture	Z None	Z None
1 Head and Neck 2 Chest 3 Abdomen 4 Hemibody 5 Whole Body 6 Pelvic Region	3 Electrons	Z None	0 Intraoperative Z None

D Radiation Therapy
W Anatomical Regions
1 Brachytherapy

Treatment Site Character 4	Modality Qualifier Character 5	Isotope Character 6	Qualifier Character 7
1 Head and Neck 2 Chest 3 Abdomen 6 Pelvic Region	9 High Dose Rate (HDR) B Low Dose Rate (LDR)	7 Cesium 137 (Cs-137) 8 Iridium 192 (Ir-192) 9 Iodine 125 (I-125) B Palladium 103 (Pd-103) C Californium 252 (Cf-252) Y Other Isotope	Z None

D Radiation Therapy
W Anatomical Regions
2 Stereotactic Radiosurgery

Treatment Site Character 4	Modality Qualifier Character 5	Isotope Character 6	Qualifier Character 7
1 Head and Neck 2 Chest 3 Abdomen 6 Pelvic Region	D Stereotactic Other Photon Radiosurgery H Stereotactic Particulate Radiosurgery J Stereotactic Gamma Beam Radiosurgery	Z None	Z None

D Radiation Therapy
W Anatomical Regions
Y Other Radiation

Treatment Site Character 4	Modality Qualifier Character 5	Isotope Character 6	Qualifier Character 7
1 Head and Neck 2 Chest 3 Abdomen 4 Hemibody 6 Pelvic Region	7 Contact Radiation 8 Hyperthermia F Plaque Radiation	Z None	Z None
5 Whole Body	7 Contact Radiation 8 Hyperthermia F Plaque Radiation	Z None	Z None
5 Whole Body	G Isotope Administration	D Iodine 131 (I-131) F Phosphorus 32 (P-32) G Strontium 89 (Sr-89) H Strontium 90 (Sr-90) Y Other Isotope	Z None

NOTES

NOTES

Physical Rehabilitation and Diagnostic Audiology F00-F15

F Physical Rehabilitation and Diagnostic Audiology
0 Rehabilitation
0 Speech Assessment: Measurement of speech and related functions

Body system/ Region	Type Qualifier	Equipment	Qualifier
Character 4	**Character 5**	**Character 6**	**Character 7**
3 Neurological System - Whole Body	**G** Communicative/Cognitive Integration Skills	**K** Audiovisual **M** Augmentative / Alternative Communication **P** Computer **Y** Other Equipment **Z** None	**Z** None
Z None	**0** Filtered Speech **3** Staggered Spondaic Word **Q** Performance Intensity Phonetically Balanced Speech Discrimination **R** Brief Tone Stimuli **S** Distorted Speech **T** Dichotic Stimuli **V** Temporal Ordering of Stimuli **W** Masking Patterns	**1** Audiometer **2** Sound Field / Booth **K** Audiovisual **Z** None	**Z** None
Z None	**1** Speech Threshold **2** Speech/Word Recognition	**1** Audiometer **2** Sound Field / Booth **9** Cochlear Implant **K** Audiovisual **Z** None	**Z** None
Z None	**4** Sensorineural Acuity Level	**1** Audiometer **2** Sound Field / Booth **Z** None	**Z** None
Z None	**5** Synthetic Sentence Identification	**1** Audiometer **2** Sound Field / Booth **9** Cochlear Implant **K** Audiovisual	**Z** None
Z None	**6** Speech and/or Language Screening **7** Nonspoken Language **8** Receptive/Expressive Language **C** Aphasia **G** Communicative/Cognitive Integration Skills **L** Augmentative/Alternative Communication System	**K** Audiovisual **M** Augmentative / Alternative Communication **P** Computer **Y** Other Equipment **Z** None	**Z** None
Z None	**9** Articulation/Phonology	**K** Audiovisual **P** Computer **Q** Speech Analysis **Y** Other Equipment **Z** None	**Z** None
Z None	**B** Motor Speech	**K** Audiovisual **N** Biosensory Feedback **P** Computer **Q** Speech Analysis **T** Aerodynamic Function **Y** Other Equipment **Z** None	**Z** None

F00 continued on next page

F Physical Rehabilitation and Diagnostic Audiology
0 Rehabilitation
0 Speech Assessment: Measurement of speech and related functions

F00 continued from previous page

Body system/ Region	Type Qualifier	Equipment	Qualifier
Character 4	**Character 5**	**Character 6**	**Character 7**
Z None	**D** Fluency	**K** Audiovisual **N** Biosensory Feedback **P** Computer **Q** Speech Analysis **S** Voice Analysis **T** Aerodynamic Function **Y** Other Equipment **Z** None	**Z** None
Z None	**F** Voice	**K** Audiovisual **N** Biosensory Feedback **P** Computer **S** Voice Analysis **T** Aerodynamic Function **Y** Other Equipment **Z** None	**Z** None
Z None	**H** Bedside Swallowing and Oral Function **P** Oral Peripheral Mechanism	**Y** Other Equipment **Z** None	**Z** None
Z None	**J** Instrumental Swallowing and Oral Function	**T** Aerodynamic Function **W** Swallowing **Y** Other Equipment	**Z** None
Z None	**K** Orofacial Myofunctional	**K** Audiovisual **P** Computer **Y** Other Equipment **Z** None	**Z** None
Z None	**M** Voice Prosthetic	**K** Audiovisual **P** Computer **S** Voice Analysis **V** Speech Prosthesis **Y** Other Equipment **Z** None	**Z** None
Z None	**N** Non-invasive Instrumental Status	**N** Biosensory Feedback **P** Computer **Q** Speech Analysis **S** Voice Analysis **T** Aerodynamic Function **Y** Other Equipment	**Z** None
Z None	**X** Other Specified Central Auditory Processing	**Z** None	**Z** None

F Physical Rehabilitation and Diagnostic Audiology
0 Rehabilitation
1 Motor and/or Nerve Function Assessment: Measurement of motor, nerve, and related functions

Body system/ Region Character 4	Type Qualifier Character 5	Equipment Character 6	Qualifier Character 7
0 Neurological System - Head and Neck **1** Neurological System - Upper Back / Upper Extremity **2** Neurological System - Lower Back / Lower Extremity **3** Neurological System - Whole Body	**0** Muscle Performance	**E** Orthosis **F** Assistive, Adaptive, Supportive or Protective **U** Prosthesis **Y** Other Equipment **Z** None	**Z** None
0 Neurological System - Head and Neck **1** Neurological System - Upper Back / Upper Extremity **2** Neurological System - Lower Back / Lower Extremity **3** Neurological System - Whole Body	**1** Integumentary Integrity **3** Coordination/Dexterity **4** Motor Function **G** Reflex Integrity	**Z** None	**Z** None
0 Neurological System - Head and Neck **1** Neurological System - Upper Back / Upper Extremity **2** Neurological System - Lower Back / Lower Extremity **3** Neurological System - Whole Body	**5** Range of Motion and Joint Integrity **6** Sensory Awareness/Processing/ Integrity	**Y** Other Equipment **Z** None	**Z** None
D Integumentary System - Head and Neck **F** Integumentary System - Upper Back / Upper Extremity **G** Integumentary System - Lower Back / Lower Extremity **H** Integumentary System - Whole Body **J** Musculoskeletal System - Head and Neck **K** Musculoskeletal System - Upper Back / Upper Extremity **L** Musculoskeletal System - Lower Back / Lower Extremity **M** Musculoskeletal System - Whole Body	**0** Muscle Performance	**E** Orthosis **F** Assistive, Adaptive, Supportive or Protective **U** Prosthesis **Y** Other Equipment **Z** None	**Z** None
D Integumentary System - Head and Neck **F** Integumentary System - Upper Back / Upper Extremity **G** Integumentary System - Lower Back / Lower Extremity **H** Integumentary System - Whole Body **J** Musculoskeletal System - Head and Neck **K** Musculoskeletal System - Upper Back / Upper Extremity **L** Musculoskeletal System - Lower Back / Lower Extremity **M** Musculoskeletal System - Whole Body	**1** Integumentary Integrity	**Z** None	**Z** None

F01 continued on next page

F01 continued from previous page

F Physical Rehabilitation and Diagnostic Audiology
0 Rehabilitation
1 Motor and/or Nerve Function Assessment: Measurement of motor, nerve, and related functions

Body system/ Region Character 4	Type Qualifier Character 5	Equipment Character 6	Qualifier Character 7
D Integumentary System - Head and Neck **F** Integumentary System - Upper Back / Upper Extremity **G** Integumentary System - Lower Back / Lower Extremity **H** Integumentary System - Whole Body **J** Musculoskeletal System - Head and Neck **K** Musculoskeletal System - Upper Back / Upper Extremity **L** Musculoskeletal System - Lower Back / Lower Extremity **M** Musculoskeletal System - Whole Body	**5** Range of Motion and Joint Integrity **6** Sensory Awareness/Processing/ Integrity	**Y** Other Equipment **Z** None	**Z** None
N Genitourinary System	**0** Muscle Performance	**E** Orthosis **F** Assistive, Adaptive, Supportive or Protective **U** Prosthesis **Y** Other Equipment **Z** None	**Z** None
Z None	**2** Visual Motor Integration	**K** Audiovisual **M** Augmentative / Alternative Communication **N** Biosensory Feedback **P** Computer **Q** Speech Analysis **S** Voice Analysis **Y** Other Equipment **Z** None	**Z** None
Z None	**7** Facial Nerve Function	**7** Electrophysiologic	**Z** None
Z None	**9** Somatosensory Evoked Potentials	**J** Somatosensory	**Z** None
Z None	**B** Bed Mobility **C** Transfer **F** Wheelchair Mobility	**E** Orthosis **F** Assistive, Adaptive, Supportive or Protective **U** Prosthesis **Z** None	**Z** None
Z None	**D** Gait and/or Balance	**E** Orthosis **F** Assistive, Adaptive, Supportive or Protective **U** Prosthesis **Y** Other Equipment **Z** None	**Z** None

F Physical Rehabilitation and Diagnostic Audiology
0 Rehabilitation
2 Activities of Daily Living Assessment: Measurement of functional level for activities of daily living

Body system/ Region	Type Qualifier	Equipment	Qualifier
Character 4	**Character 5**	**Character 6**	**Character 7**
0 Neurological System - Head and Neck DRG	**9** Cranial Nerve Integrity **D** Neuromotor Development	**Y** Other Equipment **Z** None	**Z** None
1 Neurological System - Upper Back / Upper Extremity DRG **2** Neurological System - Lower Back / Lower Extremity DRG **3** Neurological System - Whole Body DRG	**D** Neuromotor Development	**Y** Other Equipment **Z** None	**Z** None
4 Circulatory System - Head and Neck DRG **5** Circulatory System - Upper Back / Upper Extremity DRG **6** Circulatory System - Lower Back / Lower Extremity DRG **8** Respiratory System - Head and Neck DRG **9** Respiratory System - Upper Back / Upper Extremity DRG **B** Respiratory System - Lower Back / Lower Extremity DRG	**G** Ventilation, Respiration and Circulation	**C** Mechanical **G** Aerobic Endurance and Conditioning **Y** Other Equipment **Z** None	**Z** None
7 Circulatory System - Whole Body DRG **C** Respiratory System - Whole Body DRG	**7** Aerobic Capacity and Endurance	**E** Orthosis **G** Aerobic Endurance and Conditioning **U** Prosthesis **Y** Other Equipment **Z** None	**Z** None
7 Circulatory System - Whole Body DRG **C** Respiratory System - Whole Body DRG	**G** Ventilation, Respiration and Circulation	**C** Mechanical **G** Aerobic Endurance and Conditioning **Y** Other Equipment **Z** None	**Z** None
Z None DRG	**0** Bathing/Showering **1** Dressing **3** Grooming/Personal Hygiene **4** Home Management	**E** Orthosis **F** Assistive, Adaptive, Supportive or Protective **U** Prosthesis **Z** None	**Z** None
Z None DRG	**2** Feeding/Eating **8** Anthropometric Characteristics **F** Pain	**Y** Other Equipment **Z** None	**Z** None
Z None DRG	**5** Perceptual Processing	**K** Audiovisual **M** Augmentative / Alternative Communication **N** Biosensory Feedback **P** Computer **Q** Speech Analysis **S** Voice Analysis **Y** Other Equipment **Z** None	**Z** None
Z None DRG	**6** Psychosocial Skills	**Z** None	**Z** None
Z None DRG	**B** Environmental, Home and Work Barriers **C** Ergonomics and Body Mechanics	**E** Orthosis **F** Assistive, Adaptive, Supportive or Protective **U** Prosthesis **Y** Other Equipment **Z** None	**Z** None

F02 continued on next page

F Physical Rehabilitation and Diagnostic Audiology
0 Rehabilitation
2 Activities of Daily Living Assessment: Measurement of functional level for activities of daily living

F02 continued from previous page

Body system/ Region Character 4	Type Qualifier Character 5	Equipment Character 6	Qualifier Character 7
Z None DRG	**H** Vocational Activities and Functional Community or Work Reintegration Skills	**E** Orthosis **F** Assistive, Adaptive, Supportive or Protective **G** Aerobic Endurance and Conditioning **U** Prosthesis **Y** Other Equipment **Z** None	**Z** None

DRG F0209ZZ F020DYZ F020DZZ F021DYZ F021DZZ F022DYZ F022DZZ F023DYZ F023DZZ F024GCZ F024GGZ F024GYZ F024GZZ F025GCZ F025GGZ F025GYZ F025GZZ F026GCZ F026GGZ F026GYZ F026GZZ F0277EZ F0277GZ F0277UZ F0277YZ F0277ZZ F027GCZ F027GGZ F027GYZ F027GZZ F028GCZ F028GGZ F028GYZ F028GZZ F029GCZ F029GGZ F029GYZ F029GZZ F02BGCZ F02BGGZ F02BGYZ F02BGZZ F02C7EZ F02C7GZ F02C7UZ F02C7YZ F02C7ZZ F02CGCZ F02CGGZ F02CGYZ F02CGZZ F02Z0EZ F02Z0FZ F02Z0UZ F02Z0ZZ F02Z1EZ F02Z1FZ F02Z1UZ F02Z1ZZ F02Z2YZ F02Z2ZZ F02Z3EZ F02Z3FZ F02Z3UZ F02Z3ZZ F02Z4EZ F02Z4FZ F02Z4UZ F02Z4ZZ F02Z5KZ F02Z5MZ F02Z5NZ F02Z5PZ F02Z5QZ F02Z5SZ F02Z5YZ F02Z5ZZ F02Z6ZZ F02Z8YZ F02Z8ZZ F02ZBEZ F02ZBFZ F02ZBUZ F02ZBYZ F02ZBZZ F02ZCEZ F02ZCFZ F02ZCUZ F02ZCYZ F02ZCZZ F02ZFYZ F02ZFZZ F02ZHEZ F02ZHFZ F02ZHGZ F02ZHUZ F02ZHYZ F02ZHZZ

F Physical Rehabilitation and Diagnostic Audiology
0 Rehabilitation
6 Speech Treatment: Application of techniques to improve, augment, or compensate for speech and related functional impairment

Body system/ Region Character 4	Type Qualifier Character 5	Equipment Character 6	Qualifier Character 7
3 Neurological System - Whole Body DRG	**6** Communicative/Cognitive Integration Skills	**K** Audiovisual **M** Augmentative / Alternative Communication **P** Computer **Y** Other Equipment **Z** None	**Z** None
Z None DRG	**0** Nonspoken Language **3** Aphasia **6** Communicative/Cognitive Integration Skills	**K** Audiovisual **M** Augmentative / Alternative Communication **P** Computer **Y** Other Equipment **Z** None	**Z** None
Z None DRG	**1** Speech-Language Pathology and Related Disorders Counseling **2** Speech-Language Pathology and Related Disorders Prevention	**K** Audiovisual **Z** None	**Z** None
Z None DRG	**4** Articulation/Phonology	**K** Audiovisual **P** Computer **Q** Speech Analysis **T** Aerodynamic Function **Y** Other Equipment **Z** None	**Z** None
Z None DRG	**5** Aural Rehabilitation	**K** Audiovisual **L** Assistive Listening **M** Augmentative / Alternative Communication **N** Biosensory Feedback **P** Computer **Q** Speech Analysis **S** Voice Analysis **Y** Other Equipment **Z** None	**Z** None

F06 continued on next page

F06 continued from previous page

F Physical Rehabilitation and Diagnostic Audiology
0 Rehabilitation
6 Speech Treatment: Application of techniques to improve, augment, or compensate for speech and related functional impairment

Body system/ Region	Type Qualifier	Equipment	Qualifier
Character 4	**Character 5**	**Character 6**	**Character 7**
Z None DRG	**7** Fluency	**4** Electroacoustic Immittance / Acoustic Reflex **K** Audiovisual **N** Biosensory Feedback **Q** Speech Analysis **S** Voice Analysis **T** Aerodynamic Function **Y** Other Equipment **Z** None	**Z** None
Z None DRG	**8** Motor Speech	**K** Audiovisual **N** Biosensory Feedback **P** Computer **Q** Speech Analysis **S** Voice Analysis **T** Aerodynamic Function **Y** Other Equipment **Z** None	**Z** None
Z None DRG	**9** Orofacial Myofunctional	**K** Audiovisual **P** Computer **Y** Other Equipment **Z** None	**Z** None
Z None DRG	**B** Receptive/Expressive Language	**K** Audiovisual **L** Assistive Listening **M** Augmentative / Alternative Communication **P** Computer **Y** Other Equipment **Z** None	**Z** None
Z None DRG	**C** Voice	**K** Audiovisual **N** Biosensory Feedback **P** Computer **S** Voice Analysis **T** Aerodynamic Function **V** Speech Prosthesis **Y** Other Equipment **Z** None	**Z** None
Z None DRG	**D** Swallowing Dysfunction	**M** Augmentative / Alternative Communication **T** Aerodynamic Function **V** Speech Prosthesis **Y** Other Equipment **Z** None	**Z** None

DRG F0636KZ F0636MZ F0636PZ F0636YZ F0636ZZ F06Z0KZ F06Z0MZ F06Z0PZ F06Z0YZ F06Z0ZZ F06Z1KZ F06Z1ZZ F06Z2KZ F06Z2ZZ F06Z3KZ F06Z3MZ F06Z3PZ F06Z3YZ F06Z3ZZ F06Z4KZ F06Z4PZ F06Z4QZ F06Z4TZ F06Z4YZ F06Z4ZZ F06Z5KZ F06Z5LZ F06Z5MZ F06Z5NZ F06Z5PZ F06Z5QZ F06Z5SZ F06Z5YZ F06Z5ZZ F06Z6KZ F06Z6MZ F06Z6PZ F06Z6YZ F06Z6ZZ F06Z74Z F06Z7KZ F06Z7NZ F06Z7QZ F06Z7SZ F06Z7TZ F06Z7YZ F06Z7ZZ F06Z8KZ F06Z8NZ F06Z8PZ F06Z8QZ F06Z8SZ F06Z8TZ F06Z8YZ F06Z8ZZ F06Z9KZ F06Z9PZ F06Z9YZ F06Z9ZZ F06ZBKZ F06ZBLZ F06ZBMZ F06ZBPZ F06ZBYZ F06ZBZZ F06ZCKZ F06ZCNZ F06ZCPZ F06ZCSZ F06ZCTZ F06ZCVZ F06ZCYZ F06ZCZZ F06ZDMZ F06ZDTZ F06ZDVZ F06ZDYZ F06ZDZZ

F Physical Rehabilitation and Diagnostic Audiology
0 Rehabilitation
7 Motor Treatment: Exercise or activities to increase or facilitate motor function

Body system/ Region	Type Qualifier	Equipment	Qualifier
Character 4	Character 5	Character 6	Character 7
0 Neurological System - Head and Neck DRG 1 Neurological System - Upper Back / Upper Extremity DRG 2 Neurological System - Lower Back / Lower Extremity DRG 3 Neurological System - Whole Body DRG D Integumentary System - Head and Neck DRG F Integumentary System - Upper Back / Upper Extremity DRG G Integumentary System - Lower Back / Lower Extremity DRG H Integumentary System - Whole Body DRG J Musculoskeletal System - Head and Neck DRG K Musculoskeletal System - Upper Back / Upper Extremity DRG L Musculoskeletal System - Lower Back / Lower Extremity DRG M Musculoskeletal System - Whole Body DRG	0 Range of Motion and Joint Mobility 1 Muscle Performance 2 Coordination/Dexterity 3 Motor Function	E Orthosis F Assistive, Adaptive, Supportive or Protective U Prosthesis Y Other Equipment Z None	Z None
0 Neurological System - Head and Neck DRG 1 Neurological System - Upper Back / Upper Extremity DRG 2 Neurological System - Lower Back / Lower Extremity DRG 3 Neurological System - Whole Body DRG D Integumentary System - Head and Neck DRG F Integumentary System - Upper Back / Upper Extremity DRG G Integumentary System - Lower Back / Lower Extremity DRG H Integumentary System - Whole Body DRG J Musculoskeletal System - Head and Neck DRG K Musculoskeletal System - Upper Back / Upper Extremity DRG L Musculoskeletal System - Lower Back / Lower Extremity DRG M Musculoskeletal System - Whole Body DRG	6 Therapeutic Exercise	B Physical Agents C Mechanical D Electrotherapeutic E Orthosis F Assistive, Adaptive, Supportive or Protective G Aerobic Endurance and Conditioning H Mechanical or Electromechanical U Prosthesis Y Other Equipment Z None	Z None

F07 continued on next page

F07 continued from previous page

F Physical Rehabilitation and Diagnostic Audiology
0 Rehabilitation
7 Motor Treatment: Exercise or activities to increase or facilitate motor function

Body system/ Region Character 4	Type Qualifier Character 5	Equipment Character 6	Qualifier Character 7
0 Neurological System - Head and Neck DRG **1** Neurological System - Upper Back / Upper Extremity DRG **2** Neurological System - Lower Back / Lower Extremity DRG **3** Neurological System - Whole Body DRG **D** Integumentary System - Head and Neck DRG **F** Integumentary System - Upper Back / Upper Extremity DRG **G** Integumentary System - Lower Back / Lower Extremity DRG **H** Integumentary System - Whole Body DRG **J** Musculoskeletal System - Head and Neck DRG **K** Musculoskeletal System - Upper Back / Upper Extremity DRG **L** Musculoskeletal System - Lower Back / Lower Extremity DRG **M** Musculoskeletal System - Whole Body DRG	**7** Manual Therapy Techniques	**Z** None	**Z** None
4 Circulatory System - Head and Neck DRG **5** Circulatory System - Upper Back / Upper Extremity DRG **6** Circulatory System - Lower Back / Lower Extremity DRG **7** Circulatory System - Whole Body DRG **8** Respiratory System - Head and Neck DRG **9** Respiratory System - Upper Back / Upper Extremity DRG **B** Respiratory System - Lower Back / Lower Extremity DRG **C** Respiratory System - Whole Body DRG	**6** Therapeutic Exercise	**B** Physical Agents **C** Mechanical **D** Electrotherapeutic **E** Orthosis **F** Assistive, Adaptive, Supportive or Protective **G** Aerobic Endurance and Conditioning **H** Mechanical or Electromechanical **U** Prosthesis **Y** Other Equipment **Z** None	**Z** None
N Genitourinary System DRG	**1** Muscle Performance	**E** Orthosis **F** Assistive, Adaptive, Supportive or Protective **U** Prosthesis **Y** Other Equipment **Z** None	**Z** None
N Genitourinary System DRG	**6** Therapeutic Exercise	**B** Physical Agents **C** Mechanical **D** Electrotherapeutic **E** Orthosis **F** Assistive, Adaptive, Supportive or Protective **G** Aerobic Endurance and Conditioning **H** Mechanical or Electromechanical **U** Prosthesis **Y** Other Equipment **Z** None	**Z** None

F07 continued on next page

LC Limited Coverage NC Noncovered HAC HAC-associated Procedure CC Combination Cluster - See Appendix G for code lists
DRG Non-OR-Affecting MS-DRG Assignment New/Revised Text in **Orange** ♂ Male ♀ Female

F Physical Rehabilitation and Diagnostic Audiology
0 Rehabilitation
7 Motor Treatment: Exercise or activities to increase or facilitate motor function

F07 continued from previous page

Body system/ Region Character 4	Type Qualifier Character 5	Equipment Character 6	Qualifier Character 7
Z None DRG	**4** Wheelchair Mobility	**D** Electrotherapeutic **E** Orthosis **F** Assistive, Adaptive, Supportive or Protective **U** Prosthesis **Y** Other Equipment **Z** None	**Z** None
Z None DRG	**5** Bed Mobility	**C** Mechanical **E** Orthosis **F** Assistive, Adaptive, Supportive or Protective **U** Prosthesis **Y** Other Equipment **Z** None	**Z** None
Z None DRG	**8** Transfer Training	**C** Mechanical **D** Electrotherapeutic **E** Orthosis **F** Assistive, Adaptive, Supportive or Protective **U** Prosthesis **Y** Other Equipment **Z** None	**Z** None
Z None DRG	**9** Gait Training/Functional Ambulation	**C** Mechanical **D** Electrotherapeutic **E** Orthosis **F** Assistive, Adaptive, Supportive or Protective **G** Aerobic Endurance and Conditioning **U** Prosthesis **Y** Other Equipment **Z** None	**Z** None

DRG F0700EZ F0700FZ F0700UZ F0700YZ F0700ZZ F0701EZ F0701FZ F0701UZ F0701YZ F0701ZZ F0702EZ F0702FZ F0702UZ F0702YZ F0702ZZ F0703EZ F0703FZ F0703UZ F0703YZ F0703ZZ F0706BZ F0706CZ F0706DZ F0706EZ F0706FZ F0706GZ F0706HZ F0706UZ F0706YZ F0706ZZ F0707ZZ F0710EZ F0710FZ F0710UZ F0710YZ F0710ZZ F0711EZ F0711FZ F0711UZ F0711YZ F0711ZZ F0712EZ F0712FZ F0712UZ F0712YZ F0712ZZ F0713EZ F0713FZ F0713UZ F0713YZ F0713ZZ F0716BZ F0716CZ F0716DZ F0716EZ F0716FZ F0716GZ F0716HZ F0716UZ F0716YZ F0716ZZ F0717ZZ F0720EZ F0720FZ F0720UZ F0720YZ F0720ZZ F0721EZ F0721FZ F0721UZ F0721YZ F0721ZZ F0722EZ F0722FZ F0722UZ F0722YZ F0722ZZ F0723EZ F0723FZ F0723UZ F0723YZ F0723ZZ F0726BZ F0726CZ F0726DZ F0726EZ F0726FZ F0726GZ F0726HZ F0726UZ F0726YZ F0726ZZ F0727ZZ F0730EZ F0730FZ F0730UZ F0730YZ F0730ZZ F0731EZ F0731FZ F0731UZ F0731YZ F0731ZZ F0732EZ F0732FZ F0732UZ F0732YZ F0732ZZ F0733EZ F0733FZ F0733UZ F0733YZ F0733ZZ F0736BZ F0736CZ F0736DZ F0736EZ F0736FZ F0736GZ F0736HZ F0736UZ F0736YZ F0736ZZ F0737ZZ F0746BZ F0746CZ F0746DZ F0746EZ F0746FZ F0746GZ F0746HZ F0746UZ F0746YZ F0746ZZ F0756BZ F0756CZ F0756DZ F0756EZ F0756FZ F0756GZ F0756HZ F0756UZ F0756YZ F0756ZZ F0766BZ F0766CZ F0766DZ F0766EZ F0766FZ F0766GZ F0766HZ F0766UZ F0766YZ F0766ZZ F0776BZ F0776CZ F0776DZ F0776EZ F0776FZ F0776GZ F0776HZ F0776UZ F0776YZ F0776ZZ F0786BZ F0786CZ F0786DZ F0786EZ F0786FZ F0786GZ F0786HZ F0786UZ F0786YZ F0786ZZ F0796BZ F0796CZ F0796DZ F0796EZ F0796FZ F0796GZ F0796HZ F0796UZ F0796YZ F0796ZZ F07B6BZ F07B6CZ F07B6DZ F07B6EZ F07B6FZ F07B6GZ F07B6HZ F07B6UZ F07B6YZ F07B6ZZ F07C6BZ F07C6CZ F07C6DZ F07C6EZ F07C6FZ F07C6GZ F07C6HZ F07C6UZ F07C6YZ F07C6ZZ F07D0EZ F07D0FZ F07D0UZ F07D0YZ F07D0ZZ F07D1EZ F07D1FZ F07D1UZ F07D1YZ F07D1ZZ F07D2EZ F07D2FZ F07D2UZ F07D2YZ F07D2ZZ F07D3EZ F07D3FZ F07D3UZ F07D3YZ F07D3ZZ F07D6BZ

F Physical Rehabilitation and Diagnostic Audiology
0 Rehabilitation
8 Activities of Daily Living Treatment: Exercise or activities to facilitate functional competence for activities of daily living

Body system/ Region Character 4	Type Qualifier Character 5	Equipment Character 6	Qualifier Character 7
D Integumentary System - Head and Neck **F** Integumentary System - Upper Back / Upper Extremity **G** Integumentary System - Lower Back / Lower Extremity **H** Integumentary System - Whole Body **J** Musculoskeletal System - Head and Neck **K** Musculoskeletal System - Upper Back / Upper Extremity **L** Musculoskeletal System - Lower Back / Lower Extremity **M** Musculoskeletal System - Whole Body	**5** Wound Management	**B** Physical Agents **C** Mechanical **D** Electrotherapeutic **E** Orthosis **F** Assistive, Adaptive, Supportive or Protective **U** Prosthesis **Y** Other Equipment **Z** None	**Z** None
Z None	**0** Bathing/Showering Techniques **1** Dressing Techniques **2** Grooming/Personal Hygiene	**E** Orthosis **F** Assistive, Adaptive, Supportive or Protective **U** Prosthesis **Y** Other Equipment **Z** None	**Z** None
Z None	**3** Feeding/Eating	**C** Mechanical **D** Electrotherapeutic **E** Orthosis **F** Assistive, Adaptive, Supportive or Protective **U** Prosthesis **Y** Other Equipment **Z** None	**Z** None
Z None	**4** Home Management	**D** Electrotherapeutic **E** Orthosis **F** Assistive, Adaptive, Supportive or Protective **U** Prosthesis **Y** Other Equipment **Z** None	**Z** None
Z None	**6** Psychosocial Skills	**Z** None	**Z** None
Z None	**7** Vocational Activities and Functional Community or Work Reintegration Skills	**B** Physical Agents **C** Mechanical **D** Electrotherapeutic **E** Orthosis **F** Assistive, Adaptive, Supportive or Protective **G** Aerobic Endurance and Conditioning **U** Prosthesis **Y** Other Equipment **Z** None	**Z** None

F Physical Rehabilitation and Diagnostic Audiology
0 Rehabilitation
9 Hearing Treatment: Application of techniques to improve, augment, or compensate for hearing and related functional impairment

Body system/ Region	Type Qualifier	Equipment	Qualifier
Character 4	**Character 5**	**Character 6**	**Character 7**
Z None	**0** Hearing and Related Disorders Counseling **1** Hearing and Related Disorders Prevention	**K** Audiovisual **Z** None	**Z** None
Z None	**2** Auditory Processing	**K** Audiovisual **L** Assistive Listening **P** Computer **Y** Other Equipment **Z** None	**Z** None
Z None	**3** Cerumen Management	**X** Cerumen Management **Z** None	**Z** None

F Physical Rehabilitation and Diagnostic Audiology
0 Rehabilitation
B Cochlear Implant Treatment: Application of techniques to improve the communication abilities of individuals with cochlear implant

Body system/ Region	Type Qualifier	Equipment	Qualifier
Character 4	**Character 5**	**Character 6**	**Character 7**
Z None	**0** Cochlear Implant Rehabilitation	**1** Audiometer **2** Sound Field / Booth **9** Cochlear Implant **K** Audiovisual **P** Computer **Y** Other Equipment	**Z** None

F Physical Rehabilitation and Diagnostic Audiology
0 Rehabilitation
C Vestibular Treatment: Application of techniques to improve, augment, or compensate for vestibular and related functional impairment

Body system/ Region	Type Qualifier	Equipment	Qualifier
Character 4	**Character 5**	**Character 6**	**Character 7**
3 Neurological System - Whole Body **H** Integumentary System - Whole Body **M** Musculoskeletal System - Whole Body	**3** Postural Control	**E** Orthosis **F** Assistive, Adaptive, Supportive or Protective **U** Prosthesis **Y** Other Equipment **Z** None	**Z** None
Z None	**0** Vestibular	**8** Vestibular / Balance **Z** None	**Z** None
Z None	**1** Perceptual Processing **2** Visual Motor Integration	**K** Audiovisual **L** Assistive Listening **N** Biosensory Feedback **P** Computer **Q** Speech Analysis **S** Voice Analysis **T** Aerodynamic Function **Y** Other Equipment **Z** None	**Z** None

F Physical Rehabilitation and Diagnostic Audiology
0 Rehabilitation
D Device Fitting: Fitting of a device designed to facilitate or support achievement of a higher level of function

Body system/ Region	Type Qualifier	Equipment	Qualifier
Character 4	**Character 5**	**Character 6**	**Character 7**
Z None	**0** Tinnitus Masker	**5** Hearing Aid Selection / Fitting / Test **Z** None	**Z** None

F0D continued on next page

F Physical Rehabilitation and Diagnostic Audiology
0 Rehabilitation
D Device Fitting: Fitting of a device designed to facilitate or support achievement of a higher level of function

F0D continued from previous page

Body system/ Region	Type Qualifier	Equipment	Qualifier
Character 4	**Character 5**	**Character 6**	**Character 7**
Z None	**1** Monaural Hearing Aid **2** Binaural Hearing Aid **5** Assistive Listening Device	**1** Audiometer **2** Sound Field / Booth **5** Hearing Aid Selection / Fitting / Test **K** Audiovisual **L** Assistive Listening **Z** None	**Z** None
Z None	**3** Augmentative/Alternative Communication System	**M** Augmentative / Alternative Communication	**Z** None
Z None	**4** Voice Prosthetic	**S** Voice Analysis **V** Speech Prosthesis	**Z** None
Z None	**6** Dynamic Orthosis **7** Static Orthosis **8** Prosthesis **9** Assistive, Adaptive, Supportive or Protective Devices	**E** Orthosis **F** Assistive, Adaptive, Supportive or Protective **U** Prosthesis **Z** None	**Z** None

F Physical Rehabilitation and Diagnostic Audiology
0 Rehabilitation
F Caregiver Training: Training in activities to support patient's optimal level of function

Body system/ Region	Type Qualifier	Equipment	Qualifier
Character 4	**Character 5**	**Character 6**	**Character 7**
Z None	**0** Bathing/Showering Technique **1** Dressing **2** Feeding and Eating **3** Grooming/Personal Hygiene **4** Bed Mobility **5** Transfer **6** Wheelchair Mobility **7** Therapeutic Exercise **8** Airway Clearance Techniques **9** Wound Management **B** Vocational Activities and Functional Community or Work Reintegration Skills **C** Gait Training/Functional Ambulation **D** Application, Proper Use and Care of Devices **F** Application, Proper Use and Care of Orthoses **G** Application, Proper Use and Care of Prosthesis **H** Home Management	**E** Orthosis **F** Assistive, Adaptive, Supportive or Protective **U** Prosthesis **Z** None	**Z** None
Z None	**J** Communication Skills	**K** Audiovisual **L** Assistive Listening **M** Augmentative / Alternative Communication **P** Computer **Z** None	**Z** None

F Physical Rehabilitation and Diagnostic Audiology
1 Diagnostic Audiology
3 Hearing Assessment: Measurement of hearing and related functions

Body system/ Region Character 4	Type Qualifier Character 5	Equipment Character 6	Qualifier Character 7
Z None	**0** Hearing Screening	**0** Occupational Hearing **1** Audiometer **2** Sound Field / Booth **3** Tympanometer **8** Vestibular / Balance **9** Cochlear Implant **Z** None	**Z** None
Z None	**1** Pure Tone Audiometry, Air **2** Pure Tone Audiometry, Air and Bone	**0** Occupational Hearing **1** Audiometer **2** Sound Field / Booth **Z** None	**Z** None
Z None	**3** Bekesy Audiometry **6** Visual Reinforcement Audiometry **9** Short Increment Sensitivity Index **B** Stenger **C** Pure Tone Stenger	**1** Audiometer **2** Sound Field / Booth **Z** None	**Z** None
Z None	**4** Conditioned Play Audiometry **5** Select Picture Audiometry	**1** Audiometer **2** Sound Field / Booth **K** Audiovisual **Z** None	**Z** None
Z None	**7** Alternate Binaural or Monaural Loudness Balance	**1** Audiometer **K** Audiovisual **Z** None	**Z** None
Z None	**8** Tone Decay **D** Tympanometry **F** Eustachian Tube Function **G** Acoustic Reflex Patterns **H** Acoustic Reflex Threshold **J** Acoustic Reflex Decay	**3** Tympanometer **4** Electroacoustic Immittance / Acoustic Reflex **Z** None	**Z** None
Z None	**K** Electrocochleography **L** Auditory Evoked Potentials	**7** Electrophysiologic **Z** None	**Z** None
Z None	**M** Evoked Otoacoustic Emissions, Screening **N** Evoked Otoacoustic Emissions, Diagnostic	**6** Otoacoustic Emission (OAE) **Z** None	**Z** None
Z None	**P** Aural Rehabilitation Status	**1** Audiometer **2** Sound Field / Booth **4** Electroacoustic Immittance / Acoustic Reflex **9** Cochlear Implant **K** Audiovisual **L** Assistive Listening **P** Computer **Z** None	**Z** None
Z None	**Q** Auditory Processing	**K** Audiovisual **P** Computer **Y** Other Equipment **Z** None	**Z** None

F Physical Rehabilitation and Diagnostic Audiology
1 Diagnostic Audiology
4 Hearing Aid Assessment: Measurement of the appropriateness and/or effectiveness of a hearing device

Body system/ Region Character 4	Type Qualifier Character 5	Equipment Character 6	Qualifier Character 7
Z None	**0** Cochlear Implant	**1** Audiometer **2** Sound Field / Booth **3** Tympanometer **4** Electroacoustic Immittance / Acoustic Reflex **5** Hearing Aid Selection / Fitting / Test **7** Electrophysiologic **9** Cochlear Implant **K** Audiovisual **L** Assistive Listening **P** Computer **Y** Other Equipment **Z** None	**Z** None
Z None	**1** Ear Canal Probe Microphone **6** Binaural Electroacoustic Hearing Aid Check **8** Monaural Electroacoustic Hearing Aid Check	**5** Hearing Aid Selection / Fitting / Test **Z** None	**Z** None
Z None	**2** Monaural Hearing Aid **3** Binaural Hearing Aid	**1** Audiometer **2** Sound Field / Booth **3** Tympanometer **4** Electroacoustic Immittance / Acoustic Reflex **5** Hearing Aid Selection / Fitting / Test **K** Audiovisual **L** Assistive Listening **P** Computer **Z** None	**Z** None
Z None	**4** Assistive Listening System/ Device Selection	**1** Audiometer **2** Sound Field / Booth **3** Tympanometer **4** Electroacoustic Immittance / Acoustic Reflex **K** Audiovisual **L** Assistive Listening **Z** None	**Z** None
Z None	**5** Sensory Aids	**1** Audiometer **2** Sound Field / Booth **3** Tympanometer **4** Electroacoustic Immittance / Acoustic Reflex **5** Hearing Aid Selection / Fitting / Test **K** Audiovisual **L** Assistive Listening **Z** None	**Z** None
Z None	**7** Ear Protector Attenuation	**0** Occupational Hearing **Z** None	**Z** None

F Physical Rehabilitation and Diagnostic Audiology
1 Diagnostic Audiology
5 Vestibular Assessment: Measurement of the vestibular system and related functions

Body system/ Region	Type Qualifier	Equipment	Qualifier
Character 4	**Character 5**	**Character 6**	**Character 7**
Z None	**0** Bithermal, Binaural Caloric Irrigation **1** Bithermal, Monaural Caloric Irrigation **2** Unithermal Binaural Screen **3** Oscillating Tracking **4** Sinusoidal Vertical Axis Rotational **5** Dix-Hallpike Dynamic **6** Computerized Dynamic Posturography	**8** Vestibular / Balance **Z** None	**Z** None
Z None	**7** Tinnitus Masker	**5** Hearing Aid Selection / Fitting / Test **Z** None	**Z** None

NOTES

NOTES

Mental Health GZ1-GZJ

G Mental Health
Z None
1 Psychological Tests: The administration and interpretation of standardized psychological tests and measurement instruments for the assessment of psychological function

Qualifier	Qualifier	Qualifier	Qualifier
Character 4	**Character 5**	**Character 6**	**Character 7**
0 Developmental **1** Personality and Behavioral **2** Intellectual and Psychoeducational **3** Neuropsychological **4** Neurobehavioral and Cognitive Status	**Z** None	**Z** None	**Z** None

G Mental Health
Z None
2 Crisis Intervention: Treatment of a traumatized, acutely disturbed or distressed individual for the purpose of short-term stabilization

Qualifier	Qualifier	Qualifier	Qualifier
Character 4	**Character 5**	**Character 6**	**Character 7**
Z None	**Z** None	**Z** None	**Z** None

G Mental Health
Z None
3 Medication Management: Monitoring and adjusting the use of medications for the treatment of a mental health disorder

Qualifier	Qualifier	Qualifier	Qualifier
Character 4	**Character 5**	**Character 6**	**Character 7**
Z None	**Z** None	**Z** None	**Z** None

G Mental Health
Z None
5 Individual Psychotherapy: Treatment of an individual with a mental health disorder by behavioral, cognitive, psychoanalytic, psychodynamic or psychophysiological means to improve functioning or well-being

Qualifier	Qualifier	Qualifier	Qualifier
Character 4	**Character 5**	**Character 6**	**Character 7**
0 Interactive **1** Behavioral **2** Cognitive **3** Interpersonal **4** Psychoanalysis **5** Psychodynamic **6** Supportive **8** Cognitive-Behavioral **9** Psychophysiological	**Z** None	**Z** None	**Z** None

G Mental Health
Z None
6 Counseling: The application of psychological methods to treat an individual with normal developmental issues and psychological problems in order to increase function, improve well-being, alleviate distress, maladjustment or resolve crises

Qualifier	Qualifier	Qualifier	Qualifier
Character 4	**Character 5**	**Character 6**	**Character 7**
0 Educational **1** Vocational **3** Other Counseling	**Z** None	**Z** None	**Z** None

G Mental Health
Z None
7 Family Psychotherapy: Treatment that includes one or more family members of an individual with a mental health disorder by behavioral, cognitive, psychoanalytic, psychodynamic or psychophysiological means to improve functioning or well-being

Qualifier Character 4	Qualifier Character 5	Qualifier Character 6	Qualifier Character 7
2 Other Family Psychotherapy	**Z** None	**Z** None	**Z** None

G Mental Health
Z None
B Electroconvulsive Therapy: The application of controlled electrical voltages to treat a mental health disorder

Qualifier Character 4	Qualifier Character 5	Qualifier Character 6	Qualifier Character 7
0 Unilateral-Single Seizure **1** Unilateral-Multiple Seizure **2** Bilateral-Single Seizure **3** Bilateral-Multiple Seizure **4** Other Electroconvulsive Therapy	**Z** None	**Z** None	**Z** None

G Mental Health
Z None
C Biofeedback: Provision of information from the monitoring and regulating of physiological processes in conjunction with cognitive-behavioral techniques to improve patient functioning or well-being

Qualifier Character 4	Qualifier Character 5	Qualifier Character 6	Qualifier Character 7
9 Other Biofeedback	**Z** None	**Z** None	**Z** None

G Mental Health
Z None
F Hypnosis: Induction of a state of heightened suggestibility by auditory, visual and tactile techniques to elicit an emotional or behavioral response

Qualifier Character 4	Qualifier Character 5	Qualifier Character 6	Qualifier Character 7
Z None	**Z** None	**Z** None	**Z** None

G Mental Health
Z None
G Narcosynthesis: Administration of intravenous barbiturates in order to release suppressed or repressed thoughts

Qualifier Character 4	Qualifier Character 5	Qualifier Character 6	Qualifier Character 7
Z None	**Z** None	**Z** None	**Z** None

G Mental Health
Z None
H Group Psychotherapy: Treatment of two or more individuals with a mental health disorder by behavioral, cognitive, psychoanalytic, psychodynamic or psychophysiological means to improve functioning or well-being

Qualifier Character 4	Qualifier Character 5	Qualifier Character 6	Qualifier Character 7
Z None	**Z** None	**Z** None	**Z** None

G Mental Health
Z None
J Light Therapy: Application of specialized light treatments to improve functioning or well-being

Qualifier Character 4	Qualifier Character 5	Qualifier Character 6	Qualifier Character 7
Z None	**Z** None	**Z** None	**Z** None

NOTES

NOTES

Substance Abuse Treatment HZ2-HZ9

H Substance Abuse Treatment
Z None
2 Detoxification Services: Detoxification from alcohol and/or drugs

Qualifier Character 4	Qualifier Character 5	Qualifier Character 6	Qualifier Character 7
Z None	**Z** None	**Z** None	**Z** None

H Substance Abuse Treatment
Z None
3 Individual Counseling: The application of psychological methods to treat an individual with addictive behavior

Qualifier Character 4	Qualifier Character 5	Qualifier Character 6	Qualifier Character 7
0 Cognitive **1** Behavioral **2** Cognitive-Behavioral **3** 12-Step **4** Interpersonal **5** Vocational **6** Psychoeducation **7** Motivational Enhancement **8** Confrontational **9** Continuing Care **B** Spiritual **C** Pre/Post-Test Infectious Disease	**Z** None	**Z** None	**Z** None

H Substance Abuse Treatment
Z None
4 Group Counseling: The application of psychological methods to treat two or more individuals with addictive behavior

Qualifier Character 4	Qualifier Character 5	Qualifier Character 6	Qualifier Character 7
0 Cognitive **1** Behavioral **2** Cognitive-Behavioral **3** 12-Step **4** Interpersonal **5** Vocational **6** Psychoeducation **7** Motivational Enhancement **8** Confrontational **9** Continuing Care **B** Spiritual **C** Pre/Post-Test Infectious Disease	**Z** None	**Z** None	**Z** None

H Substance Abuse Treatment
Z None
5 Individual Psychotherapy: Treatment of an individual with addictive behavior by behavioral, cognitive, psychoanalytic, psychodynamic or psychophysiological means

Qualifier	Qualifier	Qualifier	Qualifier
Character 4	**Character 5**	**Character 6**	**Character 7**
0 Cognitive **1** Behavioral **2** Cognitive-Behavioral **3** 12-Step **4** Interpersonal **5** Interactive **6** Psychoeducation **7** Motivational Enhancement **8** Confrontational **9** Supportive **B** Psychoanalysis **C** Psychodynamic **D** Psychophysiological	**Z** None	**Z** None	**Z** None

H Substance Abuse Treatment
Z None
6 Family Counseling: The application of psychological methods that includes one or more family members to treat an individual with addictive behavior

Qualifier	Qualifier	Qualifier	Qualifier
Character 4	**Character 5**	**Character 6**	**Character 7**
3 Other Family Counseling	**Z** None	**Z** None	**Z** None

H Substance Abuse Treatment
Z None
8 Medication Management: Monitoring and adjusting the use of replacement medications for the treatment of addiction

Qualifier	Qualifier	Qualifier	Qualifier
Character 4	**Character 5**	**Character 6**	**Character 7**
0 Nicotine Replacement **1** Methadone Maintenance **2** Levo-alpha-acetyl-methadol (LAAM) **3** Antabuse **4** Naltrexone **5** Naloxone **6** Clonidine **7** Bupropion **8** Psychiatric Medication **9** Other Replacement Medication	**Z** None	**Z** None	**Z** None

H Substance Abuse Treatment
Z None
9 Pharmacotherapy: The use of replacement medications for the treatment of addiction

Qualifier Character 4	Qualifier Character 5	Qualifier Character 6	Qualifier Character 7
0 Nicotine Replacement **1** Methadone Maintenance **2** Levo-alpha-acetyl-methadol (LAAM) **3** Antabuse **4** Naltrexone **5** Naloxone **6** Clonidine **7** Bupropion **8** Psychiatric Medication **9** Other Replacement Medication	**Z** None	**Z** None	**Z** None

NOTES

New Technology X2A-XY0

Cardiovascular System X2A-X2R

X New Technology
2 Cardiovascular System
A Assistance: Taking over a portion of a physiological function by extracorporeal means

Body Part Character 4	Approach Character 5	Device/Substance/Technology Character 6	Qualifier Character 7
5 Innominate Artery and Left Common Carotid Artery	**3** Percutaneous	**1** Cerebral Embolic Filtration, Dual Filter	**2** New Technology Group 2

X New Technology
2 Cardiovascular System
C Extirpation: Taking or cutting out solid matter from a body part

Body Part Character 4	Approach Character 5	Device/Substance/Technology Character 6	Qualifier Character 7
0 Coronary Artery, One Artery **1** Coronary Artery, Two Arteries **2** Coronary Artery, Three Arteries **3** Coronary Artery, Four or More Arteries	**3** Percutaneous	**6** Orbital Atherectomy Technology	**1** New Technology Group 1

X New Technology
2 Cardiovascular System
R Replacement: Putting in or on biological or synthetic material that physically takes the place and/or function of all or a portion of a body part

Body Part Character 4	Approach Character 5	Device/Substance/Technology Character 6	Qualifier Character 7
F Aortic Valve	**0** Open **3** Percutaneous **4** Percutaneous Endoscopic	**3** Zooplastic Tissue, Rapid Deployment Technique	**2** New Technology Group 2

NOTES

Skin, Subcutaneous Tissue, Fascia, and Breast XHR

X New Technology
H Skin, Subcutaneous Tissue, Fascia and Breast
R Replacement: Putting in or on biological or synthetic material that physically takes the place and/or function of all or a portion of a body part

Body Part	Approach	Device/Substance/Technology	Qualifier
Character 4	**Character 5**	**Character 6**	**Character 7**
P Skin	**X** External	**L** Skin Substitute, Porcine Liver Derived	**2** New Technology Group 2

NOTES

Muscles, Tendons, Bursae, and Ligaments XK0

X New Technology
K Muscles, Tendons, Bursae and Ligaments
0 Introduction: Putting in or on a therapeutic, diagnostic, nutritional, physiological, or prophylactic substance except blood or blood products

Body Part	Approach	Device/Substance/Technology	Qualifier
Character 4	**Character 5**	**Character 6**	**Character 7**
2 Muscle	**3** Percutaneous	**0** Concentrated Bone Marrow Aspirate	**3** New Technology Group 3

NOTES

Bones XNS

X New Technology
N Bones
S Reposition: Moving to its normal location, or other suitable location, all or a portion of a body part

Body Part Character 4	Approach Character 5	Device/Substance/Technology Character 6	Qualifier Character 7
0 Lumbar Vertebra **3** Cervical Vertebra **4** Thoracic Vertebra	**0** Open **3** Percutaneous	**3** Magnetically Controlled Growth Rod(s)	**2** New Technology Group 2

NOTES

Joints XR2-XRG

X New Technology
R Joints
2 Monitoring: Determining the level of a physiological or physical function repetitively over a period of time

Body Part Character 4	Approach Character 5	Device/Substance/Technology Character 6	Qualifier Character 7
G Knee Joint, Right **H** Knee Joint, Left	**0** Open	**2** Intraoperative Knee Replacement Sensor	**1** New Technology Group 1

X New Technology
R Joints
G Fusion: Joining together portions of an articular body part rendering the articular body part immobile

Body Part Character 4	Approach Character 5	Device/Substance/Technology Character 6	Qualifier Character 7
0 Occipital-cervical Joint HAC	**0** Open	**9** Interbody Fusion Device, Nanotextured Surface	**2** New Technology Group 2
0 Occipital-cervical Joint HAC	**0** Open	**F** Interbody Fusion Device, Radiolucent Porous	**3** New Technology Group 3
1 Cervical Vertebral Joint HAC	**0** Open	**9** Interbody Fusion Device, Nanotextured Surface	**2** New Technology Group 2
1 Cervical Vertebral Joint HAC	**0** Open	**F** Interbody Fusion Device, Radiolucent Porous	**3** New Technology Group 3
2 Cervical Vertebral Joints, 2 or more HAC	**0** Open	**9** Interbody Fusion Device, Nanotextured Surface	**2** New Technology Group 2
2 Cervical Vertebral Joints, 2 or more HAC	**0** Open	**F** Interbody Fusion Device, Radiolucent Porous	**3** New Technology Group 3
4 Cervicothoracic Vertebral Joint HAC	**0** Open	**9** Interbody Fusion Device, Nanotextured Surface	**2** New Technology Group 2
4 Cervicothoracic Vertebral Joint HAC	**0** Open	**F** Interbody Fusion Device, Radiolucent Porous	**3** New Technology Group 3
6 Thoracic Vertebral Joint HAC	**0** Open	**9** Interbody Fusion Device, Nanotextured Surface	**2** New Technology Group 2
6 Thoracic Vertebral Joint HAC	**0** Open	**F** Interbody Fusion Device, Radiolucent Porous	**3** New Technology Group 3
7 Thoracic Vertebral Joints, 2 to 7 HAC	**0** Open	**9** Interbody Fusion Device, Nanotextured Surface	**2** New Technology Group 2
7 Thoracic Vertebral Joints, 2 to 7 HAC	**0** Open	**F** Interbody Fusion Device, Radiolucent Porous	**3** New Technology Group 3
8 Thoracic Vertebral Joints, 8 or more HAC	**0** Open	**9** Interbody Fusion Device, Nanotextured Surface	**2** New Technology Group 2
8 Thoracic Vertebral Joints, 8 or more HAC	**0** Open	**F** Interbody Fusion Device, Radiolucent Porous	**3** New Technology Group 3
A Thoracolumbar Vertebral Joint HAC	**0** Open	**9** Interbody Fusion Device, Nanotextured Surface	**2** New Technology Group 2
A Thoracolumbar Vertebral Joint HAC	**0** Open	**F** Interbody Fusion Device, Radiolucent Porous	**3** New Technology Group 3
B Lumbar Vertebral Joint HAC	**0** Open	**9** Interbody Fusion Device, Nanotextured Surface	**2** New Technology Group 2
B Lumbar Vertebral Joint HAC	**0** Open	**F** Interbody Fusion Device, Radiolucent Porous	**3** New Technology Group 3
C Lumbar Vertebral Joints, 2 or more HAC	**0** Open	**9** Interbody Fusion Device, Nanotextured Surface	**2** New Technology Group 2
C Lumbar Vertebral Joints, 2 or more HAC	**0** Open	**F** Interbody Fusion Device, Radiolucent Porous	**3** New Technology Group 3

XRG continued on next page

X New Technology
R Joints
G Fusion: Joining together portions of an articular body part rendering the articular body part immobile

XRG continued from previous page

Body Part Character 4	Approach Character 5	Device/Substance/Technology Character 6	Qualifier Character 7
D Lumbosacral Joint HAC	**0** Open	**9** Interbody Fusion Device, Nanotextured Surface	**2** New Technology Group 2
D Lumbosacral Joint HAC	**0** Open	**F** Interbody Fusion Device, Radiolucent Porous	**3** New Technology Group 3

HAC XRG0092 XRG00F3 XRG1092 XRG10F3 XRG2092 XRG20F3 XRG4092 XRG40F3 XRG6092 XRG60F3 XRG7092 XRG70F3 XRG8092 XRG80F3 XRGA092 XRGA0F3 XRGB092 XRGB0F3 XRGC092 XRGC0F3 XRGD092 XRGD0F3
Surgical site infection following certain orthopedic procedures of spine, shoulder or elbow procedures and secondary diagnosis K68.11, T84.60XA, T84.610A, T84.611A, T84.612A, T84.613A, T84.614A, T84.615A, T84.619A, T84.63XA, T84.69XA, T84.7XXA, T81.4XXA.

NOTES

NOTES

Male Reproductive System XV5

X New Technology
V Male Reproductive System
5 Destruction: Physical eradication of all or a portion of a body part by the direct use of energy, force, or a destructive agent

Body Part	Approach	Device/Substance/Technology	Qualifier
Character 4	**Character 5**	**Character 6**	**Character 7**
0 Prostate ♂	**8** Via Natural or Artificial Opening Endoscopic	**A** Robotic Waterjet Ablation	**4** New Technology Group 4

♂ XV508A4

NOTES

Anatomical Regions XW0

X New Technology
W Anatomical Regions
0 Introduction: Putting in or on a therapeutic, diagnostic, nutritional, physiological, or prophylactic substance except blood or blood products

Body Part Character 4	Approach Character 5	Device/Substance/Technology Character 6	Qualifier Character 7
3 Peripheral Vein	**3** Percutaneous	**2** Ceftazidime-Avibactam Anti-infective **3** Idarucizumab, Dabigatran Reversal Agent **4** Isavuconazole Anti-infective **5** Blinatumomab Antineoplastic Immunotherapy	**1** New Technology Group 1
3 Peripheral Vein	**3** Percutaneous	**7** Andexanet Alfa, Factor Xa Inhibitor Reversal Agent **9** Defibrotide Sodium Anticoagulant	**2** New Technology Group 2
3 Peripheral Vein	**3** Percutaneous	**A** Bezlotoxumab Monoclonal Antibody **B** Cytarabine and Daunorubicin Liposome Antineoplastic **C** Engineered Autologous Chimeric Antigen Receptor T-cell Immunotherapy **F** Other New Technology Therapeutic Substance	**3** New Technology Group 3
3 Peripheral Vein	**3** Percutaneous	**G** Plazomicin Anti-infective **H** Synthetic Human Angiotensin II	**4** New Technology Group 4
4 Central Vein	**3** Percutaneous	**2** Ceftazidime-Avibactam Anti-infective **3** Idarucizumab, Dabigatran Reversal Agent **4** Isavuconazole Antiinfective **5** Blinatumomab Antineoplastic Immunotherapy	**1** New Technology Group 1
4 Central Vein	**3** Percutaneous	**7** Andexanet Alfa, Factor Xa Inhibitor Reversal Agent **9** Defibrotide Sodium Anticoagulant	**2** New Technology Group 2
4 Central Vein	**3** Percutaneous	**A** Bezlotoxumab Monoclonal Antibody **B** Cytarabine and Daunorubicin Liposome Antineoplastic **C** Engineered Autologous Chimeric Antigen Receptor T-cell Immunotherapy **F** Other New Technology Therapeutic Substance	**3** New Technology Group 3
4 Central Vein	**3** Percutaneous	**G** Plazomicin Anti-infective **H** Synthetic Human Angiotensin II	**4** New Technology Group 4
D Mouth and Pharynx	**X** External	**8** Uridine Triacetate	**2** New Technology Group 2

NOTES

Extracorporeal XY0

X New Technology
Y Extracorporeal
0 Introduction: Putting in or on a therapeutic, diagnostic, nutritional, physiological, or prophylactic substance except blood or blood products

Body Part	Approach	Device/Substance/Technology	Qualifier
Character 4	**Character 5**	**Character 6**	**Character 7**
V Vein Graft	**X** External	**8** Endothelial Damage Inhibitor	**3** New Technology Group 3

NOTES

Appendix A: Root Operations Definitions

0 - Medical and Surgical		
Value	**Root Operation**	**Definition/Explanation**
0	Alteration	**Definition:** Modifying the anatomic structure of a body part without affecting the function of the body part **Explanation:** Principal purpose is to improve appearance **Includes/Examples:** Face lift, breast augmentation
1	Bypass	**Definition:** Altering the route of passage of the contents of a tubular body part **Explanation:** Rerouting contents of a body part to a downstream area of the normal route, to a similar route and body part, or to an abnormal route and dissimilar body part. Includes one or more anastomoses, with or without the use of a device. **Includes/Examples:** Coronary artery bypass, colostomy formation
2	Change	**Definition:** Taking out or off a device from a body part and putting back an identical or similar device in or on the same body part without cutting or puncturing the skin or a mucous membrane **Explanation:** All CHANGE procedures are coded using the approach EXTERNAL **Includes/Examples:** Urinary catheter change, gastrostomy tube change
3	Control	**Definition:** Stopping, or attempting to stop, postprocedural or other acute bleeding **Explanation:** The site of the bleeding is coded as an anatomical region and not to a specific body part **Includes/Examples:** Control of post-prostatectomy hemorrhage, control of intracranial subdural hemorrhage, control of bleeding duodenal ulcer, control of retroperitoneal hemorrhage
4	Creation	**Definition:** Putting in or on biological or synthetic material to form a new body part that to the extent possible replicates the anatomic structure or function of an absent body part **Explanation:** Used for gender reassignment surgery and corrective procedures in individuals with congenital anomalies **Includes/Examples:** Creation of vagina in a male, creation of right and left atrioventricular valve from common atrioventricular valve
5	Destruction	**Definition:** Physical eradication of all or a portion of a body part by the direct use of energy, force, or a destructive agent **Explanation:** None of the body part is physically taken out **Includes/Examples:** Fulguration of rectal polyp, cautery of skin lesion
6	Detachment	**Definition:** Cutting off all or a portion of the upper or lower extremities **Explanation:** The body part value is the site of the detachment, with a qualifier if applicable to further specify the level where the extremity was detached **Includes/Examples:** Below knee amputation, disarticulation of shoulder
7	Dilation	**Definition:** Expanding an orifice or the lumen of a tubular body part **Explanation:** The orifice can be a natural orifice or an artificially created orifice. Accomplished by stretching a tubular body part using intraluminal pressure or by cutting part of the orifice or wall of the tubular body part. **Includes/Examples:** Percutaneous transluminal angioplasty, internal urethrotomy
8	Division	**Definition:** Cutting into a body part, without draining fluids and/or gases from the body part, in order to separate or transect a body part **Explanation:** All or a portion of the body part is separated into two or more portions **Includes/Examples:** Spinal cordotomy, osteotomy
9	Drainage	**Definition:** Taking or letting out fluids and/or gases from a body part **Explanation:** The qualifier DIAGNOSTIC is used to identify drainage procedures that are biopsies **Includes/Examples:** Thoracentesis, incision and drainage
B	Excision	**Definition:** Cutting out or off, without replacement, a portion of a body part **Explanation:** The qualifier DIAGNOSTIC is used to identify excision procedures that are biopsies **Includes/Examples:** Partial nephrectomy, liver biopsy

0 - Medical and Surgical		
Value	**Root Operation**	**Definition/Explanation**
C	Extirpation	**Definition:** Taking or cutting out solid matter from a body part **Explanation:** The solid matter may be an abnormal byproduct of a biological function or a foreign body; it may be imbedded in a body part or in the lumen of a tubular body part. The solid matter may or may not have been previously broken into pieces. **Includes/Examples:** Thrombectomy, choledocholithotomy
D	Extraction	**Definition:** Pulling or stripping out or off all or a portion of a body part by the use of force **Explanation:** The qualifier DIAGNOSTIC is used to identify extraction procedures that are biopsies **Includes/Examples:** Dilation and curettage, vein stripping
F	Fragmentation	**Definition:** Breaking solid matter in a body part into pieces **Explanation:** Physical force (e.g., manual, ultrasonic) applied directly or indirectly is used to break the solid matter into pieces. The solid matter may be an abnormal byproduct of a biological function or a foreign body. The pieces of solid matter are not taken out. **Includes/Examples:** Extracorporeal shockwave lithotripsy, transurethral lithotripsy
G	Fusion	**Definition:** Joining together portions of an articular body part rendering the articular body part immobile **Explanation:** The body part is joined together by fixation device, bone graft, or other means **Includes/Examples:** Spinal fusion, ankle arthrodesis
H	Insertion	**Definition:** Putting in a nonbiological appliance that monitors, assists, performs, or prevents a physiological function but does not physically take the place of a body part **Includes/Examples:** Insertion of radioactive implant, insertion of central venous catheter
J	Inspection	**Definition:** Visually and/or manually exploring a body part **Explanation:** Visual exploration may be performed with or without optical instrumentation. Manual exploration may be performed directly or through intervening body layers. **Includes/Examples:** Diagnostic arthroscopy, exploratory laparotomy
K	Map	**Definition:** Locating the route of passage of electrical impulses and/or locating functional areas in a body part **Explanation:** Applicable only to the cardiac conduction mechanism and the central nervous system **Includes/Examples:** Cardiac mapping, cortical mapping
L	Occlusion	**Definition:** Completely closing an orifice or the lumen of a tubular body part **Explanation:** The orifice can be a natural orifice or an artificially created orifice **Includes/Examples:** Fallopian tube ligation, ligation of inferior vena cava
M	Reattachment	**Definition:** Putting back in or on all or a portion of a separated body part to its normal location or other suitable location **Explanation:** Vascular circulation and nervous pathways may or may not be reestablished **Includes/Examples:** Reattachment of hand, reattachment of avulsed kidney
N	Release	**Definition:** Freeing a body part from an abnormal physical constraint by cutting or by the use of force **Explanation:** Some of the restraining tissue may be taken out but none of the body part is taken out **Includes/Examples:** Adhesiolysis, carpal tunnel release
P	Removal	**Definition:** Taking out or off a device from a body part **Explanation:** If a device is taken out and a similar device put in without cutting or puncturing the skin or mucous membrane, the procedure is coded to the root operation CHANGE. Otherwise, the procedure for taking out a device is coded to the root operation REMOVAL. **Includes/Examples:** Drainage tube removal, cardiac pacemaker removal
Q	Repair	**Definition:** Restoring, to the extent possible, a body part to its normal anatomic structure and function **Explanation:** Used only when the method to accomplish the repair is not one of the other root operations **Includes/Examples:** Colostomy takedown, suture of laceration

0 - Medical and Surgical		
Value	**Root Operation**	**Definition/Explanation**
R	Replacement	**Definition:** Putting in or on biological or synthetic material that physically takes the place and/or function of all or a portion of a body part **Explanation:** The body part may have been taken out or replaced, or may be taken out, physically eradicated, or rendered nonfunctional during the Replacement procedure. A Removal procedure is coded for taking out the device used in a previous replacement procedure. **Includes/Examples:** Total hip replacement, bone graft, free skin graft
S	Reposition	**Definition:** Moving to its normal location, or other suitable location, all or a portion of a body part **Explanation:** The body part is moved to a new location from an abnormal location, or from a normal location where it is not functioning correctly. The body part may or may not be cut out or off to be moved to the new location. **Includes/Examples:** Reposition of undescended testicle, fracture reduction
T	Resection	**Definition:** Cutting out or off, without replacement, all of a body part **Includes/Examples:** Total nephrectomy, total lobectomy of lung
V	Restriction	**Definition:** Partially closing an orifice or the lumen of a tubular body part **Explanation:** The orifice can be a natural orifice or an artificially created orifice **Includes/Examples:** Esophagogastric fundoplication, cervical cerclage
W	Revision	**Definition:** Correcting, to the extent possible, a portion of a malfunctioning device or the position of a displaced device **Explanation:** Revision can include correcting a malfunctioning or displaced device by taking out or putting in components of the device such as a screw or pin **Includes/Examples:** Adjustment of position of pacemaker lead, recementing of hip prosthesis
U	Supplement	**Definition:** Putting in or on biological or synthetic material that physically reinforces and/or augments the function of a portion of a body part **Explanation:** The biological material is non-living, or is living and from the same individual. The body part may have been previously replaced, and the Supplement procedure is performed to physically reinforce and/or augment the function of the replaced body part. **Includes/Examples:** Herniorrhaphy using mesh, free nerve graft, mitral valve ring annuloplasty, put a new acetabular liner in a previous hip replacement
X	Transfer	**Definition:** Moving, without taking out, all or a portion of a body part to another location to take over the function of all or a portion of a body part **Explanation:** The body part transferred remains connected to its vascular and nervous supply **Includes/Examples:** Tendon transfer, skin pedicle flap transfer
Y	Transplantation	**Definition:** Putting in or on all or a portion of a living body part taken from another individual or animal to physically take the place and/or function of all or a portion of a similar body part **Explanation:** The native body part may or may not be taken out, and the transplanted body part may take over all or a portion of its function **Includes/Examples:** Kidney transplant, heart transplant

1 - Obstetrics		
Value	**Root Operation**	**Definition/Explanation**
A	Abortion	**Definition:** Artificially terminating a pregnancy
2	Change	**Definition:** Taking out or off a device from a body part and putting back an identical or similar device in or on the same body part without cutting or puncturing the skin or a mucous membrane
E	Delivery	**Definition:** Assisting the passage of the products of conception from the genital canal
9	Drainage	**Definition:** Taking or letting out fluids and/or gases from a body part
D	Extraction	**Definition:** Pulling or stripping out or off all or a portion of a body part by the use of force

1-Obstetrics continued on next page

1-Obstetrics continued from previous page

1 - Obstetrics		
Value	**Root Operation**	**Definition/Explanation**
H	Insertion	**Definition:** Putting in a nonbiological appliance that monitors, assists, performs, or prevents a physiological function but does not physically take the place of a body part
J	Inspection	**Definition:** Visually and/or manually exploring a body part **Explanation:** Visual exploration may be performed with or without optical instrumentation. Manual exploration may be performed directly or through intervening body layers
P	Removal	**Definition:** Taking out or off a device from a body part, region or orifice **Explanation:** If a device is taken out and a similar device put in without cutting or puncturing the skin or mucous membrane, the procedure is coded to the root operation CHANGE. Otherwise, the procedure for taking out a device is coded to the root operation REMOVAL.
Q	Repair	**Definition:** Restoring, to the extent possible, a body part to its normal anatomic structure and function **Explanation:** Used only when the method to accomplish the repair is not one of the other root operations
S	Reposition	**Definition:** Moving to its normal location, or other suitable location, all or a portion of a body part **Explanation:** The body part is moved to a new location from an abnormal location, or from a normal location where it is not functioning correctly. The body part may or may not be cut out or off to be moved to the new location.
T	Resection	**Definition:** Cutting out or off, without replacement, all of a body part
Y	Transplantation	**Definition:** Putting in or on all or a portion of a living body part taken from another individual or animal to physically take the place and/or function of all or a portion of a similar body part **Explanation:** The native body part may or may not be taken out, and the transplanted body part may take over all or a portion of its function

2 - Placement		
Value	**Root Operation**	**Definition/Explanation**
0	Change	**Definition:** Taking out or off a device from a body part and putting back an identical or similar device in or on the same body part without cutting or puncturing the skin or a mucous membrane
1	Compression	**Definition:** Putting pressure on a body region
2	Dressing	**Definition:** Putting material on a body region for protection
3	Immobilization	**Definition:** Limiting or preventing motion of a body region
4	Packing	**Definition:** Putting material in a body region or orifice
5	Removal	**Definition:** Taking out or off a device from a body part
6	Traction	**Definition:** Exerting a pulling force on a body region in a distal direction

3 - Administration		
Value	**Root Operation**	**Definition/Explanation**
0	Introduction	**Definition:** Putting in or on a therapeutic, diagnostic, nutritional, physiological, or prophylactic substance except blood or blood products
1	Irrigation	**Definition:** Putting in or on a cleansing substance
2	Transfusion	**Definition:** Putting in blood or blood products

4 - Measurement and Monitoring		
Value	**Root Operation**	**Definition/Explanation**
0	Measurement	**Definition:** Determining the level of a physiological or physical function at a point in time
1	Monitoring	**Definition:** Determining the level of a physiological or physical function repetitively over a period of time

5 - Extracorporeal or Systemic Assistance and Performance		
Value	**Root Operation**	**Definition/Explanation**
0	Assistance	**Definition:** Taking over a portion of a physiological function by extracorporeal means
1	Performance	**Definition:** Completely taking over a physiological function by extracorporeal means
2	Restoration	**Definition:** Returning, or attempting to return, a physiological function to its original state by extracorporeal means.

6 - Extracorporeal or Systemic Therapies		
Value	**Root Operation**	**Definition/Explanation**
0	Atmospheric Control	**Definition:** Extracorporeal control of atmospheric pressure and composition
1	Decompression	**Definition:** Extracorporeal elimination of undissolved gas from body fluids
2	Electromagnetic Therapy	**Definition:** Extracorporeal treatment by electromagnetic rays
3	Hyperthermia	**Definition:** Extracorporeal raising of body temperature
4	Hypothermia	**Definition:** Extracorporeal lowering of body temperature
B	Perfusion	**Definition:** Extracorporeal treatment by diffusion of therapeutic fluid
5	Pheresis	**Definition:** Extracorporeal separation of blood products
6	Phototherapy	**Definition:** Extracorporeal treatment by light rays
9	Shock Wave Therapy	**Definition:** Extracorporeal treatment by shock waves
7	Ultrasound Therapy	**Definition:** Extracorporeal treatment by ultrasound
8	Ultraviolet Light Therapy	**Definition:** Extracorporeal treatment by ultraviolet light

7 - Osteopathic		
Value	**Root Operation**	**Definition/Explanation**
0	Treatment	**Definition:** Manual treatment to eliminate or alleviate somatic dysfunction and related disorders

8 - Other Procedures		
Value	**Root Operation**	**Definition/Explanation**
0	Other Procedures	**Definition:** Methodologies which attempt to remediate or cure a disorder or disease

9 - Chiropractic		
Value	**Root Operation**	**Definition/Explanation**
B	Manipulation	**Definition:** Manual procedure that involves a directed thrust to move a joint past the physiological range of motion, without exceeding the anatomical limit

X - New Technology		
Value	**Root Operation**	**Definition/Explanation**
A	Assistance	**Definition:** Taking over a portion of a physiological function by extracorporeal means
5	Destruction	**Definition:** Physical eradication of all or a portion of a body part by the direct use of energy, force, or a destructive agent **Explanation:** None of the body part is physically taken out **Includes/Examples:** Fulguration of rectal polyp, cautery of skin lesion
C	Extirpation	**Definition:** Taking or cutting out solid matter from a body part **Explanation:** The solid matter may be an abnormal byproduct of a biological function or a foreign body; it may be imbedded in a body part or in the lumen of a tubular body part. The solid matter may or may not have been previously broken into pieces. **Includes/Examples:** Thrombectomy, choledocholithotomy
G	Fusion	**Definition:** Joining together portions of an articular body part rendering the articular body part immobile **Explanation:** The body part is joined together by fixation device, bone graft, or other means **Includes/Examples:** Spinal fusion, ankle arthrodesis
0	Introduction	**Definition:** Putting in or on a therapeutic, diagnostic, nutritional, physiological, or prophylactic substance except blood or blood products
2	Monitoring	**Definition:** Determining the level of a physiological or physical function repetitively over a period of time
R	Replacement	**Definition:** Putting in or on biological or synthetic material that physically takes the place and/or function of all or a portion of a body part **Explanation:** The body part may have been taken out or replaced, or may be taken out, physically eradicated, or rendered nonfunctional during the Replacement procedure. A Removal procedure is coded for taking out the device used in a previous replacement procedure. **Includes/Examples:** Total hip replacement, bone graft, free skin graft
S	Reposition	**Definition:** Moving to its normal location, or other suitable location, all or a portion of a body part **Explanation:** The body part is moved to a new location from an abnormal location, or from a normal location where it is not functioning correctly. The body part may or may not be cut out or off to be moved to the new location. **Includes/Examples:** Reposition of undescended testicle, fracture reduction

Appendix B: Body Part Key

Anatomical Term	ICD-10-PCS Value
Abdominal aortic plexus	Abdominal Sympathetic Nerve
Abdominal esophagus	Esophagus, Lower
Abductor hallucis muscle	Foot Muscle, Right
	Foot Muscle, Left
Accessory cephalic vein	Cephalic Vein, Right
	Cephalic Vein, Left
Accessory obturator nerve	Lumbar Plexus
Accessory phrenic nerve	Phrenic Nerve
Accessory spleen	Spleen
Acetabulofemoral joint	Hip Joint, Right
	Hip Joint, Left
Achilles tendon	Lower Leg Tendon, Right
	Lower Leg Tendon, Left
Acromioclavicular ligament	Shoulder Bursa and Ligament, Right
	Shoulder Bursa and Ligament, Left
Acromion (process)	Scapula, Right
	Scapula, Left
Adductor brevis muscle	Upper Leg Muscle, Right
	Upper Leg Muscle, Left
Adductor hallucis muscle	Foot Muscle, Right
	Foot Muscle, Left
Adductor longus muscle	Upper Leg Muscle, Right
	Upper Leg Muscle, Left
Adductor magnus muscle	Upper Leg Muscle, Right
	Upper Leg Muscle, Left
Adenohypophysis	Pituitary Gland
Alar ligament of axis	Head and Neck Bursa and Ligament
Alveolar process of mandible	Mandible, Right
	Mandible, Left
Alveolar process of maxilla	Maxilla
Anal orifice	Anus
Anatomical snuffbox	Lower Arm and Wrist Muscle, Right
	Lower Arm and Wrist Muscle, Left
Angular artery	Face Artery
Angular vein	Face Vein, Right
	Face Vein, Left
Annular ligament	Elbow Bursa and Ligament, Right
	Elbow Bursa and Ligament, Left
Anorectal junction	Rectum
Ansa cervicalis	Cervical Plexus
Antebrachial fascia	Subcutaneous Tissue and Fascia, Right Lower Arm
	Subcutaneous Tissue and Fascia, Left Lower Arm

Anatomical Term	ICD-10-PCS Value
Anterior (pectoral) lymph node	Lymphatic, Right Axillary
	Lymphatic, Left Axillary
Anterior cerebral artery	Intracranial Artery
Anterior cerebral vein	Intracranial Vein
Anterior choroidal artery	Intracranial Artery
Anterior circumflex humeral artery	Axillary Artery, Right
	Axillary Artery, Left
Anterior communicating artery	Intracranial Artery
Anterior cruciate ligament (ACL)	Knee Bursa and Ligament, Right
	Knee Bursa and Ligament, Left
Anterior crural nerve	Femoral Nerve
Anterior facial vein	Face Vein, Right
	Face Vein, Left
Anterior intercostal artery	Internal Mammary Artery, Right
	Internal Mammary Artery, Left
Anterior interosseous nerve	Median Nerve
Anterior lateral malleolar artery	Anterior Tibial Artery, Right
	Anterior Tibial Artery, Left
Anterior lingual gland	Minor Salivary Gland
Anterior medial malleolar artery	Anterior Tibial Artery, Right
	Anterior Tibial Artery, Left
Anterior spinal artery	Vertebral Artery, Right
	Vertebral Artery, Left
Anterior tibial recurrent artery	Anterior Tibial Artery, Right
	Anterior Tibial Artery, Left
Anterior ulnar recurrent artery	Ulnar Artery, Right
	Ulnar Artery, Left
Anterior vagal trunk	Vagus Nerve
Anterior vertebral muscle	Neck Muscle, Right
	Neck Muscle, Left
Antihelix	External Ear, Right
	External Ear, Left
	External Ear, Bilateral
Antitragus	External Ear, Right
	External Ear, Left
	External Ear, Bilateral
Antrum of Highmore	Maxillary Sinus, Right
	Maxillary Sinus, Left
Aortic annulus	Aortic Valve
Aortic arch	Thoracic Aorta, Ascending/Arch
Aortic intercostal artery	Upper Artery
Apical (subclavicular) lymph node	Lymphatic, Right Axillary
	Lymphatic, Left Axillary
Apneustic center	Pons
Aqueduct of Sylvius	Cerebral Ventricle

Anatomical Term	ICD-10-PCS Value
Aqueous humour	Anterior Chamber, Right
	Anterior Chamber, Left
Arachnoid mater, intracranial	Cerebral Meninges
Arachnoid mater, spinal	Spinal Meninges
Arcuate artery	Foot Artery, Right
	Foot Artery, Left
Areola	Nipple, Right
	Nipple, Left
Arterial canal (duct)	Pulmonary Artery, Left
Aryepiglottic fold	Larynx
Arytenoid cartilage	Larynx
Arytenoid muscle	Neck Muscle, Right
	Neck Muscle, Left
Ascending aorta	Thoracic Aorta, Ascending/Arch
Ascending palatine artery	Face Artery
Ascending pharyngeal artery	External Carotid Artery, Right
	External Carotid Artery, Left
Atlantoaxial joint	Cervical Vertebral Joint
Atrioventricular node	Conduction Mechanism
Atrium dextrum cordis	Atrium, Right
Atrium pulmonale	Atrium, Left
Auditory tube	Eustachian Tube, Right
	Eustachian Tube, Left
Auerbach's (myenteric) plexus	Abdominal Sympathetic Nerve
Auricle	External Ear, Right
	External Ear, Left
	External Ear, Bilateral
Auricularis muscle	Head Muscle
Axillary fascia	Subcutaneous Tissue and Fascia, Right Upper Arm
	Subcutaneous Tissue and Fascia, Left Upper Arm
Axillary nerve	Brachial Plexus
Bartholin's (greater vestibular) gland	Vestibular Gland
Basal (internal) cerebral vein	Intracranial Vein
Basal nuclei	Basal Ganglia
Base of Tongue	Pharynx
Basilar artery	Intracranial Artery
Basis pontis	Pons
Biceps brachii muscle	Upper Arm Muscle, Right
	Upper Arm Muscle, Left
Biceps femoris muscle	Upper Leg Muscle, Right
	Upper Leg Muscle, Left
Bicipital aponeurosis	Subcutaneous Tissue and Fascia, Right Lower Arm
	Subcutaneous Tissue and Fascia, Left Lower Arm

Anatomical Term	ICD-10-PCS Value
Bicuspid valve	Mitral Valve
Body of femur	Femoral Shaft, Right
	Femoral Shaft, Left
Body of fibula	Fibula, Right
	Fibula, Left
Bony labyrinth	Inner Ear, Right
	Inner Ear, Left
Bony orbit	Orbit, Right
	Orbit, Left
Bony vestibule	Inner Ear, Right
	Inner Ear, Left
Botallo's duct	Pulmonary Artery, Left
Brachial (lateral) lymph node	Lymphatic, Right Axillary
	Lymphatic, Left Axillary
Brachialis muscle	Upper Arm Muscle, Right
	Upper Arm Muscle, Left
Brachiocephalic artery	Innominate Artery
Brachiocephalic trunk	Innominate Artery
Brachiocephalic vein	Innominate Vein, Right
	Innominate Vein, Left
Brachioradialis muscle	Lower Arm and Wrist Muscle, Right
	Lower Arm and Wrist Muscle, Left
Broad ligament	Uterine Supporting Structure
Bronchial artery	Upper Artery
Bronchus intermedius	Main Bronchus, Right
Buccal gland	Buccal Mucosa
Buccinator lymph node	Lymphatic, Head
Buccinator muscle	Facial Muscle
Bulbospongiosus muscle	Perineum Muscle
Bulbourethral (Cowper's) gland	Urethra
Bundle of His	Conduction Mechanism
Bundle of Kent	Conduction Mechanism
Calcaneocuboid joint	Tarsal Joint, Right
	Tarsal Joint, Left
Calcaneocuboid ligament	Foot Bursa and Ligament, Right
	Foot Bursa and Ligament, Left
Calcaneofibular ligament	Ankle Bursa and Ligament, Right
	Ankle Bursa and Ligament, Left
Calcaneus	Tarsal, Right
	Tarsal, Left
Capitate bone	Carpal, Right
	Carpal, Left
Cardia	Esophagogastric Junction
Cardiac plexus	Thoracic Sympathetic Nerve
Cardioesophageal junction	Esophagogastric Junction
Caroticotympanic artery	Internal Carotid Artery, Right
	Internal Carotid Artery, Left

Anatomical Term	ICD-10-PCS Value
Carotid glomus	Carotid Body, Left
	Carotid Body, Right
	Carotid Bodies, Bilateral
Carotid sinus	Internal Carotid Artery, Right
	Internal Carotid Artery, Left
Carotid sinus nerve	Glossopharyngeal Nerve
Carpometacarpal ligament	Hand Bursa and Ligament, Right
	Hand Bursa and Ligament, Left
Cauda equina	Lumbar Spinal Cord
Cavernous plexus	Head and Neck Sympathetic Nerve
Celiac (solar) plexus	Abdominal Sympathetic Nerve
Celiac ganglion	Abdominal Sympathetic Nerve
Celiac lymph node	Lymphatic, Aortic
Celiac trunk	Celiac Artery
Central axillary lymph node	Lymphatic, Right Axillary
	Lymphatic, Left Axillary
Cerebral aqueduct (Sylvius)	Cerebral Ventricle
Cerebrum	Brain
Cervical esophagus	Esophagus, Upper
Cervical facet joint	Cervical Vertebral Joint
	Cervical Vertebral Joints, 2 or more
Cervical ganglion	Head and Neck Sympathetic Nerve
Cervical interspinous ligament	Head and Neck Bursa and Ligament
Cervical intertransverse ligament	Head and Neck Bursa and Ligament
Cervical ligamentum flavum	Head and Neck Bursa and Ligament
Cervical lymph node	Lymphatic, Right Neck
	Lymphatic, Left Neck
Cervicothoracic facet joint	Cervicothoracic Vertebral Joint
Choana	Nasopharynx
Chondroglossus muscle	Tongue, Palate, Pharynx Muscle
Chorda tympani	Facial Nerve
Choroid plexus	Cerebral Ventricle
Ciliary body	Eye, Right
	Eye, Left
Ciliary ganglion	Head and Neck Sympathetic Nerve
Circle of Willis	Intracranial Artery
Circumflex iliac artery	Femoral Artery, Right
	Femoral Artery, Left
Claustrum	Basal Ganglia
Coccygeal body	Coccygeal Glomus
Coccygeus muscle	Trunk Muscle, Right
	Trunk Muscle, Left
Cochlea	Inner Ear, Right
	Inner Ear, Left
Cochlear nerve	Acoustic Nerve

Anatomical Term	ICD-10-PCS Value
Columella	Nasal Mucosa and Soft Tissue
Common digital vein	Foot Vein, Right
	Foot Vein, Left
Common facial vein	Face Vein, Right
	Face Vein, Left
Common fibular nerve	Peroneal Nerve
Common hepatic artery	Hepatic Artery
Common iliac (subaortic) lymph node	Lymphatic, Pelvis
Common interosseous artery	Ulnar Artery, Right
	Ulnar Artery, Left
Common peroneal nerve	Peroneal Nerve
Condyloid process	Mandible, Right
	Mandible, Left
Conus arteriosus	Ventricle, Right
Conus medullaris	Lumbar Spinal Cord
Coracoacromial ligament	Shoulder Bursa and Ligament, Right
	Shoulder Bursa and Ligament, Left
Coracobrachialis muscle	Upper Arm Muscle, Right
	Upper Arm Muscle, Left
Coracoclavicular ligament	Shoulder Bursa and Ligament, Right
	Shoulder Bursa and Ligament, Left
Coracohumeral ligament	Shoulder Bursa and Ligament, Right
	Shoulder Bursa and Ligament, Left
Coracoid process	Scapula, Right
	Scapula, Left
Corniculate cartilage	Larynx
Corpus callosum	Brain
Corpus cavernosum	Penis
Corpus spongiosum	Penis
Corpus striatum	Basal Ganglia
Corrugator supercilii muscle	Facial Muscle
Costocervical trunk	Subclavian Artery, Right
	Subclavian Artery, Left
Costoclavicular ligament	Shoulder Bursa and Ligament, Right
	Shoulder Bursa and Ligament, Left
Costotransverse joint	Thoracic Vertebral Joint
Costotransverse ligament	Rib(s) Bursa and Ligament
Costovertebral joint	Thoracic Vertebral Joint
Costoxiphoid ligament	Sternum Bursa and Ligament
Cowper's (bulbourethral) gland	Urethra
Cremaster muscle	Perineum Muscle
Cribriform plate	Ethmoid Bone, Right
	Ethmoid Bone, Left

Anatomical Term	ICD-10-PCS Value
Cricoid cartilage	Trachea
Cricothyroid artery	Thyroid Artery, Right
	Thyroid Artery, Left
Cricothyroid muscle	Neck Muscle, Right
	Neck Muscle, Left
Crural fascia	Subcutaneous Tissue and Fascia, Right Upper Leg
	Subcutaneous Tissue and Fascia, Left Upper Leg
Cubital lymph node	Lymphatic, Right Upper Extremity
	Lymphatic, Left Upper Extremity
Cubital nerve	Ulnar Nerve
Cuboid bone	Tarsal, Right
	Tarsal, Left
Cuboideonavicular joint	Tarsal Joint, Right
	Tarsal Joint, Left
Culmen	Cerebellum
Cuneiform cartilage	Larynx
Cuneonavicular joint	Tarsal Joint, Right
	Tarsal Joint, Left
Cuneonavicular ligament	Foot Bursa and Ligament, Right
	Foot Bursa and Ligament, Left
Cutaneous (transverse) cervical nerve	Cervical Plexus
Deep cervical fascia	Subcutaneous Tissue and Fascia, Right Neck
	Subcutaneous Tissue and Fascia, Left Neck
Deep cervical vein	Vertebral Vein, Right
	Vertebral Vein, Left
Deep circumflex iliac artery	External Iliac Artery, Right
	External Iliac Artery, Left
Deep facial vein	Face Vein, Right
	Face Vein, Left
Deep femoral (profunda femoris) vein	Femoral Vein, Right
	Femoral Vein, Left
Deep femoral artery	Femoral Artery, Right
	Femoral Artery, Left
Deep palmar arch	Hand Artery, Right
	Hand Artery, Left
Deep transverse perineal muscle	Perineum Muscle
Deferential artery	Internal Iliac Artery, Right
	Internal Iliac Artery, Left
Deltoid fascia	Subcutaneous Tissue and Fascia, Right Upper Arm
	Subcutaneous Tissue and Fascia, Left Upper Arm
Deltoid ligament	Ankle Bursa and Ligament, Right
	Ankle Bursa and Ligament, Left

Anatomical Term	ICD-10-PCS Value
Deltoid muscle	Shoulder Muscle, Right
	Shoulder Muscle, Left
Deltopectoral (infraclavicular) lymph node	Lymphatic, Right Upper Extremity
	Lymphatic, Left Upper Extremity
Dens	Cervical Vertebra
Denticulate (dentate) ligament	Spinal Meninges
Depressor anguli oris muscle	Facial Muscle
Depressor labii inferioris muscle	Facial Muscle
Depressor septi nasi muscle	Facial Muscle
Depressor supercilii muscle	Facial Muscle
Dermis	Skin
Descending genicular artery	Femoral Artery, Right
	Femoral Artery, Left
Diaphragma sellae	Dura Mater
Distal humerus	Humeral Shaft, Right
	Humeral Shaft, Left
Distal humerus, involving joint	Elbow Joint, Right
	Elbow Joint, Left
Distal radioulnar joint	Wrist Joint, Right
	Wrist Joint, Left
Dorsal digital nerve	Radial Nerve
Dorsal metacarpal vein	Hand Vein, Right
	Hand Vein, Left
Dorsal metatarsal artery	Foot Artery, Right
	Foot Artery, Left
Dorsal metatarsal vein	Foot Vein, Right
	Foot Vein, Left
Dorsal scapular artery	Subclavian Artery, Right
	Subclavian Artery, Left
Dorsal scapular nerve	Brachial Plexus
Dorsal venous arch	Foot Vein, Right
	Foot Vein, Left
Dorsalis pedis artery	Anterior Tibial Artery, Right
	Anterior Tibial Artery, Left
Duct of Santorini	Pancreatic Duct, Accessory
Duct of Wirsung	Pancreatic Duct
Ductus deferens	Vas Deferens, Right
	Vas Deferens, Left
	Vas Deferens, Bilateral
	Vas Deferens
Duodenal ampulla	Ampulla of Vater
Duodenojejunal flexure	Jejunum
Dura mater, intracranial	Dura Mater
Dura mater, spinal	Spinal Meninges
Dural venous sinus	Intracranial Vein

Anatomical Term	ICD-10-PCS Value
Earlobe	External Ear, Right
	External Ear, Left
	External Ear, Bilateral
Eighth cranial nerve	Acoustic Nerve
Ejaculatory duct	Vas Deferens, Right
	Vas Deferens, Left
	Vas Deferens, Bilateral
	Vas Deferens
Eleventh cranial nerve	Accessory Nerve
Encephalon	Brain
Ependyma	Cerebral Ventricle
Epidermis	Skin
Epidural space, spinal	Spinal Canal
Epiploic foramen	Peritoneum
Epithalamus	Thalamus
Epitrochlear lymph node	Lymphatic, Right Upper Extremity
	Lymphatic, Left Upper Extremity
Erector spinae muscle	Trunk Muscle, Right
	Trunk Muscle, Left
Esophageal artery	Upper Artery
Esophageal plexus	Thoracic Sympathetic Nerve
Ethmoidal air cell	Ethmoid Sinus, Right
	Ethmoid Sinus, Left
Extensor carpi radialis muscle	Lower Arm and Wrist Muscle, Right
	Lower Arm and Wrist Muscle, Left
Extensor carpi ulnaris muscle	Lower Arm and Wrist Muscle, Right
	Lower Arm and Wrist Muscle, Left
Extensor digitorum brevis muscle	Foot Muscle, Right
	Foot Muscle, Left
Extensor digitorum longus muscle	Lower Leg Muscle, Right
	Lower Leg Muscle, Left
Extensor hallucis brevis muscle	Foot Muscle, Right
	Foot Muscle, Left
Extensor hallucis longus muscle	Lower Leg Muscle, Right
	Lower Leg Muscle, Left
External anal sphincter	Anal Sphincter
External auditory meatus	External Auditory Canal, Right
	External Auditory Canal, Left
External maxillary artery	Face Artery
External naris	Nasal Mucosa and Soft Tissue
External oblique aponeurosis	Subcutaneous Tissue and Fascia, Trunk
External oblique muscle	Abdomen Muscle, Right
	Abdomen Muscle, Left
External popliteal nerve	Peroneal Nerve
External pudendal artery	Femoral Artery, Right
	Femoral Artery, Left

Anatomical Term	ICD-10-PCS Value
External pudendal vein	Saphenous Vein, Right
	Saphenous Vein, Left
External urethral sphincter	Urethra
Extradural space, intracranial	Epidural Space, Intracranial
Extradural space, spinal	Spinal Canal
Facial artery	Face Artery
False vocal cord	Larynx
Falx cerebri	Dura Mater
Fascia lata	Subcutaneous Tissue and Fascia, Right Upper Leg
	Subcutaneous Tissue and Fascia, Left Upper Leg
Femoral head	Upper Femur, Right
	Upper Femur, Left
Femoral lymph node	Lymphatic, Right Lower Extremity
	Lymphatic, Left Lower Extremity
Femoropatellar joint	Knee Joint, Right
	Knee Joint, Left
	Knee Joint, Femoral Surface, Right
	Knee Joint, Femoral Surface, Left
Femorotibial joint	Knee Joint, Right
	Knee Joint, Left
	Knee Joint, Tibial Surface, Right
	Knee Joint, Tibial Surface, Left
Fibular artery	Peroneal Artery, Right
	Peroneal Artery, Left
Fibularis brevis muscle	Lower Leg Muscle, Right
	Lower Leg Muscle, Left
Fibularis longus muscle	Lower Leg Muscle, Right
	Lower Leg Muscle, Left
Fifth cranial nerve	Trigeminal Nerve
Filum terminale	Spinal Meninges
First cranial nerve	Olfactory Nerve
First intercostal nerve	Brachial Plexus
Flexor carpi radialis muscle	Lower Arm and Wrist Muscle, Right
	Lower Arm and Wrist Muscle, Left
Flexor carpi ulnaris muscle	Lower Arm and Wrist Muscle, Right
	Lower Arm and Wrist Muscle, Left
Flexor digitorum brevis muscle	Foot Muscle, Right
	Foot Muscle, Left
Flexor digitorum longus muscle	Lower Leg Muscle, Right
	Lower Leg Muscle, Left
Flexor hallucis brevis muscle	Foot Muscle, Right
	Foot Muscle, Left
Flexor hallucis longus muscle	Lower Leg Muscle, Right
	Lower Leg Muscle, Left
Flexor pollicis longus muscle	Lower Arm and Wrist Muscle, Right
	Lower Arm and Wrist Muscle, Left

Anatomical Term	ICD-10-PCS Value
Foramen magnum	Occipital Bone
Foramen of Monro (intraventricular)	Cerebral Ventricle
Foreskin	Prepuce
Fossa of Rosenmuller	Nasopharynx
Fourth cranial nerve	Trochlear Nerve
Fourth ventricle	Cerebral Ventricle
Fovea	Retina, Right
	Retina, Left
Frenulum labii inferioris	Lower Lip
Frenulum labii superioris	Upper Lip
Frenulum linguae	Tongue
Frontal lobe	Cerebral Hemisphere
Frontal vein	Face Vein, Right
	Face Vein, Left
Fundus uteri	Uterus
Galea aponeurotica	Subcutaneous Tissue and Fascia, Scalp
Ganglion impar (ganglion of Walther)	Sacral Sympathetic Nerve
Gasserian ganglion	Trigeminal Nerve
Gastric lymph node	Lymphatic, Aortic
Gastric plexus	Abdominal Sympathetic Nerve
Gastrocnemius muscle	Lower Leg Muscle, Right
	Lower Leg Muscle, Left
Gastrocolic ligament	Omentum
Gastrocolic omentum	Omentum
Gastroduodenal artery	Hepatic Artery
Gastroesophageal (GE) junction	Esophagogastric Junction
Gastrohepatic omentum	Omentum
Gastrophrenic ligament	Omentum
Gastrosplenic ligament	Omentum
Gemellus muscle	Hip Muscle, Right
	Hip Muscle, Left
Geniculate ganglion	Facial Nerve
Geniculate nucleus	Thalamus
Genioglossus muscle	Tongue, Palate, Pharynx Muscle
Genitofemoral nerve	Lumbar Plexus
Glans penis	Prepuce
Glenohumeral joint	Shoulder Joint, Right
	Shoulder Joint, Left
Glenohumeral ligament	Shoulder Bursa and Ligament, Right
	Shoulder Bursa and Ligament, Left
Glenoid fossa (of scapula)	Glenoid Cavity, Right
	Glenoid Cavity, Left
Glenoid ligament (labrum)	Shoulder Joint, Right
	Shoulder Joint, Left

Anatomical Term	ICD-10-PCS Value
Globus pallidus	Basal Ganglia
Glossoepiglottic fold	Epiglottis
Glottis	Larynx
Gluteal lymph node	Lymphatic, Pelvis
Gluteal vein	Hypogastric Vein, Right
	Hypogastric Vein, Left
Gluteus maximus muscle	Hip Muscle, Right
	Hip Muscle, Left
Gluteus medius muscle	Hip Muscle, Right
	Hip Muscle, Left
Gluteus minimus muscle	Hip Muscle, Right
	Hip Muscle, Left
Gracilis muscle	Upper Leg Muscle, Right
	Upper Leg Muscle, Left
Great auricular nerve	Cervical Plexus
Great cerebral vein	Intracranial Vein
Great(er) saphenous vein	Saphenous Vein, Right
	Saphenous Vein, Left
Greater alar cartilage	Nasal Mucosa and Soft Tissue
Greater occipital nerve	Cervical Nerve
Greater Omentum	Omentum
Greater splanchnic nerve	Thoracic Sympathetic Nerve
Greater superficial petrosal nerve	Facial Nerve
Greater trochanter	Upper Femur, Right
	Upper Femur, Left
Greater tuberosity	Humeral Head, Right
	Humeral Head, Left
Greater vestibular (Bartholin's) gland	Vestibular Gland
Greater wing	Sphenoid Bone
Hallux	1st Toe, Right
	1st Toe, Left
Hamate bone	Carpal, Right
	Carpal, Left
Head of fibula	Fibula, Right
	Fibula, Left
Helix	External Ear, Right
	External Ear, Left
	External Ear, Bilateral
Hepatic artery proper	Hepatic Artery
Hepatic flexure	Transverse Colon
Hepatic lymph node	Lymphatic, Aortic
Hepatic plexus	Abdominal Sympathetic Nerve
Hepatic portal vein	Portal Vein
Hepatogastric ligament	Omentum
Hepatopancreatic ampulla	Ampulla of Vater

Anatomical Term	ICD-10-PCS Value
Humeroradial joint	Elbow Joint, Right
	Elbow Joint, Left
Humeroulnar joint	Elbow Joint, Right
	Elbow Joint, Left
Humerus, distal	Humeral Shaft, Right
	Humeral Shaft, Left
Hyoglossus muscle	Tongue, Palate, Pharynx Muscle
Hyoid artery	Thyroid Artery, Right
	Thyroid Artery, Left
Hypogastric artery	Internal Iliac Artery, Right
	Internal Iliac Artery, Left
Hypopharynx	Pharynx
Hypophysis	Pituitary Gland
Hypothenar muscle	Hand Muscle, Right
	Hand Muscle, Left
Ileal artery	Superior Mesenteric Artery
Ileocolic artery	Superior Mesenteric Artery
Ileocolic vein	Colic Vein
Iliac crest	Pelvic Bone, Right
	Pelvic Bone, Left
Iliac fascia	Subcutaneous Tissue and Fascia, Right Upper Leg
	Subcutaneous Tissue and Fascia, Left Upper Leg
Iliac lymph node	Lymphatic, Pelvis
Iliacus muscle	Hip Muscle, Right
	Hip Muscle, Left
Iliofemoral ligament	Hip Bursa and Ligament, Right
	Hip Bursa and Ligament, Left
Iliohypogastric nerve	Lumbar Plexus
Ilioinguinal nerve	Lumbar Plexus
Iliolumbar artery	Internal Iliac Artery, Right
	Internal Iliac Artery, Left
Iliolumbar ligament	Lower Spine Bursa and Ligament
Iliotibial tract (band)	Subcutaneous Tissue and Fascia, Right Upper Leg
	Subcutaneous Tissue and Fascia, Left Upper Leg
Ilium	Pelvic Bone, Right
	Pelvic Bone, Left
Incus	Auditory Ossicle, Right
	Auditory Ossicle, Left
Inferior cardiac nerve	Thoracic Sympathetic Nerve
Inferior cerebellar vein	Intracranial Vein
Inferior cerebral vein	Intracranial Vein
Inferior epigastric artery	External Iliac Artery, Right
	External Iliac Artery, Left
Inferior epigastric lymph node	Lymphatic, Pelvis

Anatomical Term	ICD-10-PCS Value
Inferior genicular artery	Popliteal Artery, Right
	Popliteal Artery, Left
Inferior gluteal artery	Internal Iliac Artery, Right
	Internal Iliac Artery, Left
Inferior gluteal nerve	Sacral Plexus
Inferior hypogastric plexus	Abdominal Sympathetic Nerve
Inferior labial artery	Face Artery
Inferior longitudinal muscle	Tongue, Palate, Pharynx Muscle
Inferior mesenteric ganglion	Abdominal Sympathetic Nerve
Inferior mesenteric lymph node	Lymphatic, Mesenteric
Inferior mesenteric plexus	Abdominal Sympathetic Nerve
Inferior oblique muscle	Extraocular Muscle, Right
	Extraocular Muscle, Left
Inferior pancreaticoduodenal artery	Superior Mesenteric Artery
Inferior phrenic artery	Abdominal Aorta
Inferior rectus muscle	Extraocular Muscle, Right
	Extraocular Muscle, Left
Inferior suprarenal artery	Renal Artery, Right
	Renal Artery, Left
Inferior tarsal plate	Lower Eyelid, Right
	Lower Eyelid, Left
Inferior thyroid vein	Innominate Vein, Right
	Innominate Vein, Left
Inferior tibiofibular joint	Ankle Joint, Right
	Ankle Joint, Left
Inferior turbinate	Nasal Turbinate
Inferior ulnar collateral artery	Brachial Artery, Right
	Brachial Artery, Left
Inferior vesical artery	Internal Iliac Artery, Right
	Internal Iliac Artery, Left
Infraauricular lymph node	Lymphatic, Head
Infraclavicular (deltopectoral) lymphnode	Lymphatic, Right Upper Extremity
	Lymphatic, Left Upper Extremity
Infrahyoid muscle	Neck Muscle, Right
	Neck Muscle, Left
Infraparotid lymph node	Lymphatic, Head
Infraspinatus fascia	Subcutaneous Tissue and Fascia, Right Upper Arm
	Subcutaneous Tissue and Fascia, Left Upper Arm
Infraspinatus muscle	Shoulder Muscle, Right
	Shoulder Muscle, Left
Infundibulopelvic ligament	Uterine Supporting Structure
Inguinal canal	Inguinal Region, Right
	Inguinal Region, Left
	Inguinal Region, Bilateral

Anatomical Term	ICD-10-PCS Value
Inguinal triangle	Inguinal Region, Right
	Inguinal Region, Left
	Inguinal Region, Bilateral
Interatrial septum	Atrial Septum
Intercarpal joint	Carpal Joint, Right
	Carpal Joint, Left
Intercarpal ligament	Hand Bursa and Ligament, Right
	Hand Bursa and Ligament, Left
Interclavicular ligament	Shoulder Bursa and Ligament, Right
	Shoulder Bursa and Ligament, Left
Intercostal lymph node	Lymphatic, Thorax
Intercostal muscle	Thorax Muscle, Right
	Thorax Muscle, Left
Intercostal nerve	Thoracic Nerve
Intercostobrachial nerve	Thoracic Nerve
Intercuneiform joint	Tarsal Joint, Right
	Tarsal Joint, Left
Intercuneiform ligament	Foot Bursa and Ligament, Right
	Foot Bursa and Ligament, Left
Intermediate bronchus	Main Bronchus, Right
Intermediate cuneiform bone	Tarsal, Right
	Tarsal, Left
Internal (basal) cerebral vein	Intracranial Vein
Internal anal sphincter	Anal Sphincter
Internal carotid artery, intracranial portion	Intracranial Artery
Internal carotid plexus	Head and Neck Sympathetic Nerve
Internal iliac vein	Hypogastric Vein, Right
	Hypogastric Vein, Left
Internal maxillary artery	External Carotid Artery, Right
	External Carotid Artery, Left
Internal naris	Nasal Mucosa and Soft Tissue
Internal oblique muscle	Abdomen Muscle, Right
	Abdomen Muscle, Left
Internal pudendal artery	Internal Iliac Artery, Right
	Internal Iliac Artery, Left
Internal pudendal vein	Hypogastric Vein, Right
	Hypogastric Vein, Left
Internal thoracic artery	Internal Mammary Artery, Right
	Internal Mammary Artery, Left
	Subclavian Artery, Right
	Subclavian Artery, Left
Internal urethral sphincter	Urethra
Interphalangeal (IP) joint	Finger Phalangeal Joint, Right
	Finger Phalangeal Joint, Left
	Toe Phalangeal Joint, Right
	Toe Phalangeal Joint, Left

Anatomical Term	ICD-10-PCS Value
Interphalangeal ligament	Hand Bursa and Ligament, Right
	Hand Bursa and Ligament, Left
	Foot Bursa and Ligament, Right
	Foot Bursa and Ligament, Left
Interspinalis muscle	Trunk Muscle, Right
	Trunk Muscle, Left
Interspinous ligament, cervical	Head and Neck Bursa and Ligament
Interspinous ligament, lumbar	Lower Spine Bursa and Ligament
Interspinous ligament, thoracic	Upper Spine Bursa and Ligament
Intertransversarius muscle	Trunk Muscle, Right
	Trunk Muscle, Left
Intertransverse ligament, cervical	Head and Neck Bursa and Ligament
Intertransverse ligament, lumbar	Lower Spine Bursa and Ligament
Intertransverse ligament, thoracic	Upper Spine Bursa and Ligament
Interventricular foramen (Monro)	Cerebral Ventricle
Interventricular septum	Ventricular Septum
Intestinal lymphatic trunk	Cisterna Chyli
Ischiatic nerve	Sciatic Nerve
Ischiocavernosus muscle	Perineum Muscle
Ischiofemoral ligament	Hip Bursa and Ligament, Right
	Hip Bursa and Ligament, Left
Ischium	Pelvic Bone, Right
	Pelvic Bone, Left
Jejunal artery	Superior Mesenteric Artery
Jugular body	Glomus Jugulare
Jugular lymph node	Lymphatic, Right Neck
	Lymphatic, Left Neck
Labia majora	Vulva
Labia minora	Vulva
Labial gland	Upper Lip
	Lower Lip
Lacrimal canaliculus	Lacrimal Duct, Right
	Lacrimal Duct, Left
Lacrimal punctum	Lacrimal Duct, Right
	Lacrimal Duct, Left
Lacrimal sac	Lacrimal Duct, Right
	Lacrimal Duct, Left
Laryngopharynx	Pharynx
Lateral (brachial) lymph node	Lymphatic, Right Axillary
	Lymphatic, Left Axillary
Lateral canthus	Upper Eyelid, Right
	Upper Eyelid, Left

Anatomical Term	ICD-10-PCS Value
Lateral collateral ligament (LCL)	Knee Bursa and Ligament, Right
	Knee Bursa and Ligament, Left
Lateral condyle of femur	Lower Femur, Right
	Lower Femur, Left
Lateral condyle of tibia	Tibia, Right
	Tibia, Left
Lateral cuneiform bone	Tarsal, Right
	Tarsal, Left
Lateral epicondyle of femur	Lower Femur, Right
	Lower Femur, Left
Lateral epicondyle of humerus	Humeral Shaft, Right
	Humeral Shaft, Left
Lateral femoral cutaneous nerve	Lumbar Plexus
Lateral malleolus	Fibula, Right
	Fibula, Left
Lateral meniscus	Knee Joint, Right
	Knee Joint, Left
Lateral nasal cartilage	Nasal Mucosa and Soft Tissue
Lateral plantar artery	Foot Artery, Right
	Foot Artery, Left
Lateral plantar nerve	Tibial Nerve
Lateral rectus muscle	Extraocular Muscle, Right
	Extraocular Muscle, Left
Lateral sacral artery	Internal Iliac Artery, Right
	Internal Iliac Artery, Left
Lateral sacral vein	Hypogastric Vein, Right
	Hypogastric Vein, Left
Lateral sural cutaneous nerve	Peroneal Nerve
Lateral tarsal artery	Foot Artery, Right
	Foot Artery, Left
Lateral temporomandibular ligament	Head and Neck Bursa and Ligament
Lateral thoracic artery	Axillary Artery, Right
	Axillary Artery, Left
Latissimus dorsi muscle	Trunk Muscle, Right
	Trunk Muscle, Left
Least splanchnic nerve	Thoracic Sympathetic Nerve
Left ascending lumbar vein	Hemiazygos Vein
Left atrioventricular valve	Mitral Valve
Left auricular appendix	Atrium, Left
Left colic vein	Colic Vein
Left coronary sulcus	Heart, Left
Left gastric artery	Gastric Artery
Left gastroepiploic artery	Splenic Artery
Left gastroepiploic vein	Splenic Vein
Left inferior phrenic vein	Renal Vein, Left

Anatomical Term	ICD-10-PCS Value
Left inferior pulmonary vein	Pulmonary Vein, Left
Left jugular trunk	Thoracic Duct
Left lateral ventricle	Cerebral Ventricle
Left ovarian vein	Renal Vein, Left
Left second lumbar vein	Renal Vein, Left
Left subclavian trunk	Thoracic Duct
Left subcostal vein	Hemiazygos Vein
Left superior pulmonary vein	Pulmonary Vein, Left
Left suprarenal vein	Renal Vein, Left
Left testicular vein	Renal Vein, Left
Leptomeninges, intracranial	Cerebral Meninges
Leptomeninges, spinal	Spinal Meninges
Lesser alar cartilage	Nasal Mucosa and Soft Tissue
Lesser occipital nerve	Cervical Plexus
Lesser omentum	Omentum
Lesser saphenous vein	Saphenous Vein, Right
	Saphenous Vein, Left
Lesser splanchnic nerve	Thoracic Sympathetic Nerve
Lesser trochanter	Upper Femur, Right
	Upper Femur, Left
Lesser tuberosity	Humeral Head, Right
	Humeral Head, Left
Lesser wing	Sphenoid Bone
Levator anguli oris muscle	Facial Muscle
Levator ani muscle	Perineum Muscle
Levator labii superioris alaeque nasi muscle	Facial Muscle
Levator labii superioris muscle	Facial Muscle
Levator palpebrae superioris muscle	Upper Eyelid, Right
	Upper Eyelid, Left
Levator scapulae muscle	Neck Muscle, Right
	Neck Muscle, Left
Levator veli palatini muscle	Tongue, Palate, Pharynx Muscle
Levatores costarum muscle	Thorax Muscle, Right
	Thorax Muscle, Left
Ligament of head of fibula	Knee Bursa and Ligament, Right
	Knee Bursa and Ligament, Left
Ligament of the lateral malleolus	Ankle Bursa and Ligament, Right
	Ankle Bursa and Ligament, Left
Ligamentum flavum, cervical	Head and Neck Bursa and Ligament
Ligamentum flavum, lumbar	Lower Spine Bursa and Ligament
Ligamentum flavum, thoracic	Upper Spine Bursa and Ligament
Lingual artery	External Carotid Artery, Right
	External Carotid Artery, Left
Lingual tonsil	Pharynx
Locus ceruleus	Pons
Long thoracic nerve	Brachial Plexus

Anatomical Term	ICD-10-PCS Value
Lumbar artery	Abdominal Aorta
Lumbar facet joint	Lumbar Vertebral Joint
Lumbar ganglion	Lumbar Sympathetic Nerve
Lumbar lymph node	Lymphatic, Aortic
Lumbar lymphatic trunk	Cisterna Chyli
Lumbar splanchnic nerve	Lumbar Sympathetic Nerve
Lumbosacral facet joint	Lumbosacral Joint
Lumbosacral trunk	Lumbar Nerve
Lunate bone	Carpal, Right
	Carpal, Left
Lunotriquetral ligament	Hand Bursa and Ligament, Right
	Hand Bursa and Ligament, Left
Macula	Retina, Right
	Retina, Left
Malleus	Auditory Ossicle, Right
	Auditory Ossicle, Left
Mammary duct	Breast, Right
	Breast, Left
	Breast, Bilateral
Mammary gland	Breast, Right
	Breast, Left
	Breast, Bilateral
Mammillary body	Hypothalamus
Mandibular nerve	Trigeminal Nerve
Mandibular notch	Mandible, Right
	Mandible, Left
Manubrium	Sternum
Masseter muscle	Head Muscle
Masseteric fascia	Subcutaneous Tissue and Fascia, Face
Mastoid (postauricular) lymph node	Lymphatic, Right Neck
	Lymphatic, Left Neck
Mastoid air cells	Mastoid Sinus, Right
	Mastoid Sinus, Left
Mastoid process	Temporal Bone, Right
	Temporal Bone, Left
Maxillary artery	External Carotid Artery, Right
	External Carotid Artery, Left
Maxillary nerve	Trigeminal Nerve
Medial canthus	Lower Eyelid, Right
	Lower Eyelid, Left
Medial collateral ligament (MCL)	Knee Bursa and Ligament, Right
	Knee Bursa and Ligament, Left
Medial condyle of femur	Lower Femur, Right
	Lower Femur, Left
Medial condyle of tibia	Tibia, Right
	Tibia, Left

Anatomical Term	ICD-10-PCS Value
Medial cuneiform bone	Tarsal, Right
	Tarsal, Left
Medial epicondyle of femur	Lower Femur, Right
	Lower Femur, Left
Medial epicondyle of humerus	Humeral Shaft, Right
	Humeral Shaft, Left
Medial malleolus	Tibia, Right
	Tibia, Left
Medial meniscus	Knee Joint, Right
	Knee Joint, Left
Medial plantar artery	Foot Artery, Right
	Foot Artery, Left
Medial plantar nerve	Tibial Nerve
Medial popliteal nerve	Tibial Nerve
Medial rectus muscle	Extraocular Muscle, Right
	Extraocular Muscle, Left
Medial sural cutaneous nerve	Tibial Nerve
Median antebrachial vein	Basilic Vein, Right
	Basilic Vein, Left
Median cubital vein	Basilic Vein, Right
	Basilic Vein, Left
Median sacral artery	Abdominal Aorta
Mediastinal cavity	Mediastinum
Mediastinal lymph node	Lymphatic, Thorax
Mediastinal space	Mediastinum
Meissner's (submucous) plexus	Abdominal Sympathetic Nerve
Membranous urethra	Urethra
Mental foramen	Mandible, Right
	Mandible, Left
Mentalis muscle	Facial Muscle
Mesoappendix	Mesentery
Mesocolon	Mesentery
Metacarpal ligament	Hand Bursa and Ligament, Right
	Hand Bursa and Ligament, Left
Metacarpophalangeal ligament	Hand Bursa and Ligament, Right
	Hand Bursa and Ligament, Left
Metatarsal ligament	Foot Bursa and Ligament, Right
	Foot Bursa and Ligament, Left
Metatarsophalangeal (MTP) joint	Metatarsal-Phalangeal Joint, Right
	Metatarsal-Phalangeal Joint, Left
Metatarsophalangeal ligament	Foot Bursa and Ligament, Right
	Foot Bursa and Ligament, Left
Metathalamus	Thalamus
Midcarpal joint	Carpal Joint, Right
	Carpal Joint, Left
Middle cardiac nerve	Thoracic Sympathetic Nerve
Middle cerebral artery	Intracranial Artery

Anatomical Term	ICD-10-PCS Value
Middle cerebral vein	Intracranial Vein
Middle colic vein	Colic Vein
Middle genicular artery	Popliteal Artery, Right
	Popliteal Artery, Left
Middle hemorrhoidal vein	Hypogastric Vein, Right
	Hypogastric Vein, Left
Middle rectal artery	Internal Iliac Artery, Right
	Internal Iliac Artery, Left
Middle suprarenal artery	Abdominal Aorta
Middle temporal artery	Temporal Artery, Right
	Temporal Artery, Left
Middle turbinate	Nasal Turbinate
Mitral annulus	Mitral Valve
Molar gland	Buccal Mucosa
Musculocutaneous nerve	Brachial Plexus
Musculophrenic artery	Internal Mammary Artery, Right
	Internal Mammary Artery, Left
Musculospiral nerve	Radial Nerve
Myelencephalon	Medulla Oblongata
Myenteric (Auerbach's) plexus	Abdominal Sympathetic Nerve
Myometrium	Uterus
Nail bed	Finger Nail
	Toe Nail
Nail plate	Finger Nail
	Toe Nail
Nasal cavity	Nasal Mucosa and Soft Tissue
Nasal concha	Nasal Turbinate
Nasalis muscle	Facial Muscle
Nasolacrimal duct	Lacrimal Duct, Right
	Lacrimal Duct, Left
Navicular bone	Tarsal, Right
	Tarsal, Left
Neck of femur	Upper Femur, Right
	Upper Femur, Left
Neck of humerus (anatomical) (surgical)	Humeral Head, Right
	Humeral Head, Left
Nerve to the stapedius	Facial Nerve
Neurohypophysis	Pituitary Gland
Ninth cranial nerve	Glossopharyngeal Nerve
Nostril	Nasal Mucosa and Soft Tissue
Obturator artery	Internal Iliac Artery, Right
	Internal Iliac Artery, Left
Obturator lymph node	Lymphatic, Pelvis
Obturator muscle	Hip Muscle, Right
	Hip Muscle, Left
Obturator nerve	Lumbar Plexus

Anatomical Term	ICD-10-PCS Value
Obturator vein	Hypogastric Vein, Right
	Hypogastric Vein, Left
Obtuse margin	Heart, Left
Occipital artery	External Carotid Artery, Right
	External Carotid Artery, Left
Occipital lobe	Cerebral Hemisphere
Occipital lymph node	Lymphatic, Right Neck
	Lymphatic, Left Neck
Occipitofrontalis muscle	Facial Muscle
Odontoid process	Cervical Vertebra
Olecranon bursa	Elbow Bursa and Ligament, Right
	Elbow Bursa and Ligament, Left
Olecranon process	Ulna, Right
	Ulna, Left
Olfactory bulb	Olfactory Nerve
Ophthalmic artery	Intracranial Artery
Ophthalmic nerve	Trigeminal Nerve
Ophthalmic vein	Intracranial Vein
Optic chiasma	Optic Nerve
Optic disc	Retina, Right
	Retina, Left
Optic foramen	Sphenoid Bone
Orbicularis oculi muscle	Upper Eyelid, Right
	Upper Eyelid, Left
Orbicularis oris muscle	Facial Muscle
Orbital fascia	Subcutaneous Tissue and Fascia, Face
Orbital portion of ethmoid bone	Orbit, Right
	Orbit, Left
Orbital portion of frontal bone	Orbit, Right
	Orbit, Left
Orbital portion of lacrimal bone	Orbit, Right
	Orbit, Left
Orbital portion of maxilla	Orbit, Right
	Orbit, Left
Orbital portion of palatine bone	Orbit, Right
	Orbit, Left
Orbital portion of sphenoid bone	Orbit, Right
	Orbit, Left
Orbital portion of zygomatic bone	Orbit, Right
	Orbit, Left
Oropharynx	Pharynx
Otic ganglion	Head and Neck Sympathetic Nerve
Oval window	Middle Ear, Right
	Middle Ear, Left
Ovarian artery	Abdominal Aorta
Ovarian ligament	Uterine Supporting Structure

Anatomical Term	ICD-10-PCS Value
Oviduct	Fallopian Tube, Right
	Fallopian Tube, Left
Palatine gland	Buccal Mucosa
Palatine tonsil	Tonsils
Palatine uvula	Uvula
Palatoglossal muscle	Tongue, Palate, Pharynx Muscle
Palatopharyngeal muscle	Tongue, Palate, Pharynx Muscle
Palmar (volar) digital vein	Hand Vein, Right
	Hand Vein, Left
Palmar (volar) metacarpal vein	Hand Vein, Right
	Hand Vein, Left
Palmar cutaneous nerve	Median Nerve
	Radial Nerve
Palmar fascia (aponeurosis)	Subcutaneous Tissue and Fascia, Right Hand
	Subcutaneous Tissue and Fascia, Left Hand
Palmar interosseous muscle	Hand Muscle, Right
	Hand Muscle, Left
Palmar ulnocarpal ligament	Wrist Bursa and Ligament, Right
	Wrist Bursa and Ligament, Left
Palmaris longus muscle	Lower Arm and Wrist Muscle, Right
	Lower Arm and Wrist Muscle, Left
Pancreatic artery	Splenic Artery
Pancreatic plexus	Abdominal Sympathetic Nerve
Pancreatic vein	Splenic Vein
Pancreaticosplenic lymph node	Lymphatic, Aortic
Paraaortic lymph node	Lymphatic, Aortic
Pararectal lymph node	Lymphatic, Mesenteric
Parasternal lymph node	Lymphatic, Thorax
Paratracheal lymph node	Lymphatic, Thorax
Paraurethral (Skene's) gland	Vestibular Gland
Parietal lobe	Cerebral Hemisphere
Parotid lymph node	Lymphatic, Head
Parotid plexus	Facial Nerve
Pars flaccida	Tympanic Membrane, Right
	Tympanic Membrane, Left
Patellar ligament	Knee Bursa and Ligament, Right
	Knee Bursa and Ligament, Left
Patellar tendon	Knee Tendon, Right
	Knee Tendon, Left
Patellofemoral joint	Knee Joint, Right
	Knee Joint, Left
	Knee Joint, Femoral Surface, Right
	Knee Joint, Femoral Surface, Left
Pectineus muscle	Upper Leg Muscle, Right
	Upper Leg Muscle, Left

Anatomical Term	ICD-10-PCS Value
Pectoral (anterior) lymph node	Lymphatic, Right Axillary
	Lymphatic, Left Axillary
Pectoral fascia	Subcutaneous Tissue and Fascia, Chest
Pectoralis major muscle	Thorax Muscle, Right
	Thorax Muscle, Left
Pectoralis minor muscle	Thorax Muscle, Right
	Thorax Muscle, Left
Pelvic splanchnic nerve	Abdominal Sympathetic Nerve
	Sacral Sympathetic Nerve
Penile urethra	Urethra
Pericardiophrenic artery	Internal Mammary Artery, Right
	Internal Mammary Artery, Left
Perimetrium	Uterus
Peroneus brevis muscle	Lower Leg Muscle, Right
	Lower Leg Muscle, Left
Peroneus longus muscle	Lower Leg Muscle, Right
	Lower Leg Muscle, Left
Petrous part of temporal bone	Temporal Bone, Right
	Temporal Bone, Left
Pharyngeal constrictor muscle	Tongue, Palate, Pharynx Muscle
Pharyngeal plexus	Vagus Nerve
Pharyngeal recess	Nasopharynx
Pharyngeal tonsil	Adenoids
Pharyngotympanic tube	Eustachian Tube, Right
	Eustachian Tube, Left
Pia mater, intracranial	Cerebral Meninges
Pia mater, spinal	Spinal Meninges
Pinna	External Ear, Right
	External Ear, Left
	External Ear, Bilateral
Piriform recess (sinus)	Pharynx
Piriformis muscle	Hip Muscle, Right
	Hip Muscle, Left
Pisiform bone	Carpal, Right
	Carpal, Left
Pisohamate ligament	Hand Bursa and Ligament, Right
	Hand Bursa and Ligament, Left
Pisometacarpal ligament	Hand Bursa and Ligament, Right
	Hand Bursa and Ligament, Left
Plantar digital vein	Foot Vein, Right
	Foot Vein, Left
Plantar fascia (aponeurosis)	Subcutaneous Tissue and Fascia, Right Foot
	Subcutaneous Tissue and Fascia, Left Foot

Anatomical Term	ICD-10-PCS Value
Plantar metatarsal vein	Foot Vein, Right
	Foot Vein, Left
Plantar venous arch	Foot Vein, Right
	Foot Vein, Left
Platysma muscle	Neck Muscle, Right
	Neck Muscle, Left
Plica semilunaris	Conjunctiva, Right
	Conjunctiva, Left
Pneumogastric nerve	Vagus Nerve
Pneumotaxic center	Pons
Pontine tegmentum	Pons
Popliteal ligament	Knee Bursa and Ligament, Right
	Knee Bursa and Ligament, Left
Popliteal lymph node	Lymphatic, Right Lower Extremity
	Lymphatic, Left Lower Extremity
Popliteal vein	Femoral Vein, Right
	Femoral Vein, Left
Popliteus muscle	Lower Leg Muscle, Right
	Lower Leg Muscle, Left
Postauricular (mastoid) lymph node	Lymphatic, Right Neck
	Lymphatic, Left Neck
Postcava	Inferior Vena Cava
Posterior (subscapular) lymph node	Lymphatic, Right Axillary
	Lymphatic, Left Axillary
Posterior auricular artery	External Carotid Artery, Right
	External Carotid Artery, Left
Posterior auricular nerve	Facial Nerve
Posterior auricular vein	External Jugular Vein, Right
	External Jugular Vein, Left
Posterior cerebral artery	Intracranial Artery
Posterior chamber	Eye, Right
	Eye, Left
Posterior circumflex humeral artery	Axillary Artery, Right
	Axillary Artery, Left
Posterior communicating artery	Intracranial Artery
Posterior cruciate ligament (PCL)	Knee Bursa and Ligament, Right
	Knee Bursa and Ligament, Left
Posterior facial (retromandibular) vein	Face Vein, Right
	Face Vein, Left
Posterior femoral cutaneous nerve	Sacral Plexus
Posterior inferior cerebellar artery(PICA)	Intracranial Artery
Posterior interosseous nerve	Radial Nerve
Posterior labial nerve	Pudendal Nerve
Posterior scrotal nerve	Pudendal Nerve

Anatomical Term	ICD-10-PCS Value
Posterior spinal artery	Vertebral Artery, Right
	Vertebral Artery, Left
Posterior tibial recurrent artery	Anterior Tibial Artery, Right
	Anterior Tibial Artery, Left
Posterior ulnar recurrent artery	Ulnar Artery, Right
	Ulnar Artery, Left
Posterior vagal trunk	Vagus Nerve
Preauricular lymph node	Lymphatic, Head
Precava	Superior Vena Cava
Prepatellar bursa	Knee Bursa and Ligament, Right
	Knee Bursa and Ligament, Left
Pretracheal fascia	Subcutaneous Tissue and Fascia, Right Neck
	Subcutaneous Tissue and Fascia, Left Neck
Prevertebral fascia	Subcutaneous Tissue and Fascia, Right Neck
	Subcutaneous Tissue and Fascia, Left Neck
Princeps pollicis artery	Hand Artery, Right
	Hand Artery, Left
Procerus muscle	Facial Muscle
Profunda brachii	Brachial Artery, Right
	Brachial Artery, Left
Profunda femoris (deep femoral) vein	Femoral Vein, Right
	Femoral Vein, Left
Pronator quadratus muscle	Lower Arm and Wrist Muscle, Right
	Lower Arm and Wrist Muscle, Left
Pronator teres muscle	Lower Arm and Wrist Muscle, Right
	Lower Arm and Wrist Muscle, Left
Prostatic urethra	Urethra
Proximal radioulnar joint	Elbow Joint, Right
	Elbow Joint, Left
Psoas muscle	Hip Muscle, Right
	Hip Muscle, Left
Pterygoid muscle	Head Muscle
Pterygoid process	Sphenoid Bone
Pterygopalatine (sphenopalatine) ganglion	Head and Neck Sympathetic Nerve
Pubis	Pelvic Bone, Right
	Pelvic Bone, Left
Pubofemoral ligament	Hip Bursa and Ligament, Right
	Hip Bursa and Ligament, Left
Pudendal nerve	Sacral Plexus
Pulmoaortic canal	Pulmonary Artery, Left
Pulmonary annulus	Pulmonary Valve
Pulmonary plexus	Vagus Nerve
	Thoracic Sympathetic Nerve

Anatomical Term	ICD-10-PCS Value
Pulmonic valve	Pulmonary Valve
Pulvinar	Thalamus
Pyloric antrum	Stomach, Pylorus
Pyloric canal	Stomach, Pylorus
Pyloric sphincter	Stomach, Pylorus
Pyramidalis muscle	Abdomen Muscle, Right
	Abdomen Muscle, Left
Quadrangular cartilage	Nasal Septum
Quadrate lobe	Liver
Quadratus femoris muscle	Hip Muscle, Right
	Hip Muscle, Left
Quadratus lumborum muscle	Trunk Muscle, Right
	Trunk Muscle, Left
Quadratus plantae muscle	Foot Muscle, Right
	Foot Muscle, Left
Quadriceps (femoris)	Upper Leg Muscle, Right
	Upper Leg Muscle, Left
Radial collateral carpal ligament	Wrist Bursa and Ligament, Right
	Wrist Bursa and Ligament, Left
Radial collateral ligament	Elbow Bursa and Ligament, Right
	Elbow Bursa and Ligament, Left
Radial notch	Ulna, Right
	Ulna, Left
Radial recurrent artery	Radial Artery, Right
	Radial Artery, Left
Radial vein	Brachial Vein, Right
	Brachial Vein, Left
Radialis indicis	Hand Artery, Right
	Hand Artery, Left
Radiocarpal joint	Wrist Joint, Right
	Wrist Joint, Left
Radiocarpal ligament	Wrist Bursa and Ligament, Right
	Wrist Bursa and Ligament, Left
Radioulnar ligament	Wrist Bursa and Ligament, Right
	Wrist Bursa and Ligament, Left
Rectosigmoid junction	Sigmoid Colon
Rectus abdominis muscle	Abdomen Muscle, Right
	Abdomen Muscle, Left
Rectus femoris muscle	Upper Leg Muscle, Right
	Upper Leg Muscle, Left
Recurrent laryngeal nerve	Vagus Nerve
Renal calyx	Kidney, Right
	Kidney, Left
	Kidneys, Bilateral
	Kidney

Anatomical Term	ICD-10-PCS Value
Renal capsule	Kidney, Right
	Kidney, Left
	Kidneys, Bilateral
	Kidney
Renal cortex	Kidney, Right
	Kidney, Left
	Kidneys, Bilateral
	Kidney
Renal plexus	Abdominal Sympathetic Nerve
Renal segment	Kidney, Right
	Kidney, Left
	Kidneys, Bilateral
	Kidney
Renal segmental artery	Renal Artery, Right
	Renal Artery, Left
Retroperitoneal cavity	Retroperitoneum
Retroperitoneal lymph node	Lymphatic, Aortic
Retroperitoneal space	Retroperitoneum
Retropharyngeal lymph node	Lymphatic, Right Neck
	Lymphatic, Left Neck
Retropubic space	Pelvic Cavity
Rhinopharynx	Nasopharynx
Rhomboid major muscle	Trunk Muscle, Right
	Trunk Muscle, Left
Rhomboid minor muscle	Trunk Muscle, Right
	Trunk Muscle, Left
Right ascending lumbar vein	Azygos Vein
Right atrioventricular valve	Tricuspid Valve
Right auricular appendix	Atrium, Right
Right colic vein	Colic Vein
Right coronary sulcus	Heart, Right
Right gastric artery	Gastric Artery
Right gastroepiploic vein	Superior Mesenteric Vein
Right inferior phrenic vein	Inferior Vena Cava
Right inferior pulmonary vein	Pulmonary Vein, Right
Right jugular trunk	Lymphatic, Right Neck
Right lateral ventricle	Cerebral Ventricle
Right lymphatic duct	Lymphatic, Right Neck
Right ovarian vein	Inferior Vena Cava
Right second lumbar vein	Inferior Vena Cava
Right subclavian trunk	Lymphatic, Right Neck
Right subcostal vein	Azygos Vein
Right superior pulmonary vein	Pulmonary Vein, Right
Right suprarenal vein	Inferior Vena Cava
Right testicular vein	Inferior Vena Cava
Rima glottidis	Larynx
Risorius muscle	Facial Muscle

Anatomical Term	ICD-10-PCS Value
Round ligament of uterus	Uterine Supporting Structure
Round window	Inner Ear, Right
	Inner Ear, Left
Sacral ganglion	Sacral Sympathetic Nerve
Sacral lymph node	Lymphatic, Pelvis
Sacral splanchnic nerve	Sacral Sympathetic Nerve
Sacrococcygeal ligament	Lower Spine Bursa and Ligament
Sacrococcygeal symphysis	Sacrococcygeal Joint
Sacroiliac ligament	Lower Spine Bursa and Ligament
Sacrospinous ligament	Lower Spine Bursa and Ligament
Sacrotuberous ligament	Lower Spine Bursa and Ligament
Salpingopharyngeus muscle	Tongue, Palate, Pharynx Muscle
Salpinx	Fallopian Tube, Right
	Fallopian Tube, Left
Saphenous nerve	Femoral Nerve
Sartorius muscle	Upper Leg Muscle, Right
	Upper Leg Muscle, Left
Scalene muscle	Neck Muscle, Right
	Neck Muscle, Left
Scaphoid bone	Carpal, Right
	Carpal, Left
Scapholunate ligament	Hand Bursa and Ligament, Right
	Hand Bursa and Ligament, Left
Scaphotrapezium ligament	Hand Bursa and Ligament, Right
	Hand Bursa and Ligament, Left
Scarpa's (vestibular) ganglion	Acoustic Nerve
Sebaceous gland	Skin
Second cranial nerve	Optic Nerve
Sella turcica	Sphenoid Bone
Semicircular canal	Inner Ear, Right
	Inner Ear, Left
Semimembranosus muscle	Upper Leg Muscle, Right
	Upper Leg Muscle, Left
Semitendinosus muscle	Upper Leg Muscle, Right
	Upper Leg Muscle, Left
Septal cartilage	Nasal Septum
Serratus anterior muscle	Thorax Muscle, Right
	Thorax Muscle, Left
Serratus posterior muscle	Trunk Muscle, Right
	Trunk Muscle, Left
Seventh cranial nerve	Facial Nerve
Short gastric artery	Splenic Artery
Sigmoid artery	Inferior Mesenteric Artery
Sigmoid flexure	Sigmoid Colon
Sigmoid vein	Inferior Mesenteric Vein
Sinoatrial node	Conduction Mechanism
Sinus venosus	Atrium, Right
Sixth cranial nerve	Abducens Nerve

Anatomical Term	ICD-10-PCS Value
Skene's (paraurethral) gland	Vestibular Gland
Small saphenous vein	Saphenous Vein, Right
	Saphenous Vein, Left
Solar (celiac) plexus	Abdominal Sympathetic Nerve
Soleus muscle	Lower Leg Muscle, Right
	Lower Leg Muscle, Left
Sphenomandibular ligament	Head and Neck Bursa and Ligament
Sphenopalatine (pterygopalatine) ganglion	Head and Neck Sympathetic Nerve
Spinal nerve, cervical	Cervical Nerve
Spinal nerve, lumbar	Lumbar Nerve
Spinal nerve, sacral	Sacral Nerve
Spinal nerve, thoracic	Thoracic Nerve
Spinous process	Cervical Vertebra
	Thoracic Vertebra
	Lumbar Vertebra
Spiral ganglion	Acoustic Nerve
Splenic flexure	Transverse Colon
Splenic plexus	Abdominal Sympathetic Nerve
Splenius capitis muscle	Head Muscle
Splenius cervicis muscle	Neck Muscle, Right
	Neck Muscle, Left
Stapes	Auditory Ossicle, Right
	Auditory Ossicle, Left
Stellate ganglion	Head and Neck Sympathetic Nerve
Stensen's duct	Parotid Duct, Right
	Parotid Duct, Left
Sternoclavicular ligament	Shoulder Bursa and Ligament, Right
	Shoulder Bursa and Ligament, Left
Sternocleidomastoid artery	Thyroid Artery, Right
	Thyroid Artery, Left
Sternocleidomastoid muscle	Neck Muscle, Right
	Neck Muscle, Left
Sternocostal ligament	Sternum Bursa and Ligament
Styloglossus muscle	Tongue, Palate, Pharynx Muscle
Stylomandibular ligament	Head and Neck Bursa and Ligament
Stylopharyngeus muscle	Tongue, Palate, Pharynx Muscle
Subacromial bursa	Shoulder Bursa and Ligament, Right
	Shoulder Bursa and Ligament, Left
Subaortic (common iliac) lymph node	Lymphatic, Pelvis
Subarachnoid space, spinal	Spinal Canal
Subclavicular (apical) lymph node	Lymphatic, Right Axillary
	Lymphatic, Left Axillary
Subclavius muscle	Thorax Muscle, Right
	Thorax Muscle, Left

Anatomical Term	ICD-10-PCS Value
Subclavius nerve	Brachial Plexus
Subcostal artery	Upper Artery
Subcostal muscle	Thorax Muscle, Right
	Thorax Muscle, Left
Subcostal nerve	Thoracic Nerve
Subdural space, spinal	Spinal Canal
Submandibular ganglion	Facial Nerve
	Head and Neck Sympathetic Nerve
Submandibular gland	Submaxillary Gland, Right
	Submaxillary Gland, Left
Submandibular lymph node	Lymphatic, Head
Submaxillary ganglion	Head and Neck Sympathetic Nerve
Submaxillary lymph node	Lymphatic, Head
Submental artery	Face Artery
Submental lymph node	Lymphatic, Head
Submucous (Meissner's) plexus	Abdominal Sympathetic Nerve
Suboccipital nerve	Cervical Nerve
Suboccipital venous plexus	Vertebral Vein, Right
	Vertebral Vein, Left
Subparotid lymph node	Lymphatic, Head
Subscapular (posterior) lymph node	Lymphatic, Right Axillary
	Lymphatic, Left Axillary
Subscapular aponeurosis	Subcutaneous Tissue and Fascia, Right Upper Arm
	Subcutaneous Tissue and Fascia, Left Upper Arm
Subscapular artery	Axillary Artery, Right
	Axillary Artery, Left
Subscapularis muscle	Shoulder Muscle, Right
	Shoulder Muscle, Left
Substantia nigra	Basal Ganglia
Subtalar (talocalcaneal) joint	Tarsal Joint, Right
	Tarsal Joint, Left
Subtalar ligament	Foot Bursa and Ligament, Right
	Foot Bursa and Ligament, Left
Subthalamic nucleus	Basal Ganglia
Superficial circumflex iliac vein	Saphenous Vein, Right
	Saphenous Vein, Left
Superficial epigastric artery	Femoral Artery, Right
	Femoral Artery, Left
Superficial epigastric vein	Saphenous Vein, Right
	Saphenous Vein, Left
Superficial palmar arch	Hand Artery, Right
	Hand Artery, Left
Superficial palmar venous arch	Hand Vein, Right
	Hand Vein, Left

Anatomical Term	ICD-10-PCS Value
Superficial temporal artery	Temporal Artery, Right
	Temporal Artery, Left
Superficial transverse perineal muscle	Perineum Muscle
Superior cardiac nerve	Thoracic Sympathetic Nerve
Superior cerebellar vein	Intracranial Vein
Superior cerebral vein	Intracranial Vein
Superior clunic (cluneal) nerve	Lumbar Nerve
Superior epigastric artery	Internal Mammary Artery, Right
	Internal Mammary Artery, Left
Superior genicular artery	Popliteal Artery, Right
	Popliteal Artery, Left
Superior gluteal artery	Internal Iliac Artery, Right
	Internal Iliac Artery, Left
Superior gluteal nerve	Lumbar Plexus
Superior hypogastric plexus	Abdominal Sympathetic Nerve
Superior labial artery	Face Artery
Superior laryngeal artery	Thyroid Artery, Right
	Thyroid Artery, Left
Superior laryngeal nerve	Vagus Nerve
Superior longitudinal muscle	Tongue, Palate, Pharynx Muscle
Superior mesenteric ganglion	Abdominal Sympathetic Nerve
Superior mesenteric lymph node	Lymphatic, Mesenteric
Superior mesenteric plexus	Abdominal Sympathetic Nerve
Superior oblique muscle	Extraocular Muscle, Right
	Extraocular Muscle, Left
Superior olivary nucleus	Pons
Superior rectal artery	Inferior Mesenteric Artery
Superior rectal vein	Inferior Mesenteric Vein
Superior rectus muscle	Extraocular Muscle, Right
	Extraocular Muscle, Left
Superior tarsal plate	Upper Eyelid, Right
	Upper Eyelid, Left
Superior thoracic artery	Axillary Artery, Right
	Axillary Artery, Left
Superior thyroid artery	External Carotid Artery, Right
	External Carotid Artery, Left
	Thyroid Artery, Right
	Thyroid Artery, Left
Superior turbinate	Nasal Turbinate
Superior ulnar collateral artery	Brachial Artery, Right
	Brachial Artery, Left
Supraclavicular (Virchow's) lymph node	Lymphatic, Right Neck
	Lymphatic, Left Neck
Supraclavicular nerve	Cervical Plexus
Suprahyoid lymph node	Lymphatic, Head

Anatomical Term	ICD-10-PCS Value
Suprahyoid muscle	Neck Muscle, Right
	Neck Muscle, Left
Suprainguinal lymph node	Lymphatic, Pelvis
Supraorbital vein	Face Vein, Right
	Face Vein, Left
Suprarenal gland	Adrenal Gland, Left
	Adrenal Gland, Right
	Adrenal Glands, Bilateral
	Adrenal Gland
Suprarenal plexus	Abdominal Sympathetic Nerve
Suprascapular nerve	Brachial Plexus
Supraspinatus fascia	Subcutaneous Tissue and Fascia, Right Upper Arm
	Subcutaneous Tissue and Fascia, Left Upper Arm
Supraspinatus muscle	Shoulder Muscle, Right
	Shoulder Muscle, Left
Supraspinous ligament	Upper Spine Bursa and Ligament
	Lower Spine Bursa and Ligament
Suprasternal notch	Sternum
Supratrochlear lymph node	Lymphatic, Right Upper Extremity
	Lymphatic, Left Upper Extremity
Sural artery	Popliteal Artery, Right
	Popliteal Artery, Left
Sweat gland	Skin
Talocalcaneal (subtalar) joint	Tarsal Joint, Right
	Tarsal Joint, Left
Talocalcaneal ligament	Foot Bursa and Ligament, Right
	Foot Bursa and Ligament, Left
Talocalcaneonavicular joint	Tarsal Joint, Right
	Tarsal Joint, Left
Talocalcaneonavicular ligament	Foot Bursa and Ligament, Right
	Foot Bursa and Ligament, Left
Talocrural joint	Ankle Joint, Right
	Ankle Joint, Left
Talofibular ligament	Ankle Bursa and Ligament, Right
	Ankle Bursa and Ligament, Left
Talus bone	Tarsal, Right
	Tarsal, Left
Tarsometatarsal ligament	Foot Bursa and Ligament, Right
	Foot Bursa and Ligament, Left
Temporal lobe	Cerebral Hemisphere
Temporalis muscle	Head Muscle
Temporoparietalis muscle	Head Muscle
Tensor fasciae latae muscle	Hip Muscle, Right
	Hip Muscle, Left
Tensor veli palatini muscle	Tongue, Palate, Pharynx Muscle
Tenth cranial nerve	Vagus Nerve
Tentorium cerebelli	Dura Mater
Teres major muscle	Shoulder Muscle, Right
	Shoulder Muscle, Left
Teres minor muscle	Shoulder Muscle, Right
	Shoulder Muscle, Left
Testicular artery	Abdominal Aorta
Thenar muscle	Hand Muscle, Right
	Hand Muscle, Left
Third cranial nerve	Oculomotor Nerve
Third occipital nerve	Cervical Nerve
Third ventricle	Cerebral Ventricle
Thoracic aortic plexus	Thoracic Sympathetic Nerve
Thoracic esophagus	Esophagus, Middle
Thoracic facet joint	Thoracic Vertebral Joint
Thoracic ganglion	Thoracic Sympathetic Nerve
Thoracoacromial artery	Axillary Artery, Right
	Axillary Artery, Left
Thoracolumbar facet joint	Thoracolumbar Vertebral Joint
Thymus gland	Thymus
Thyroarytenoid muscle	Neck Muscle, Right
	Neck Muscle, Left
Thyrocervical trunk	Thyroid Artery, Right
	Thyroid Artery, Left
Thyroid cartilage	Larynx
Tibialis anterior muscle	Lower Leg Muscle, Right
	Lower Leg Muscle, Left
Tibialis posterior muscle	Lower Leg Muscle, Right
	Lower Leg Muscle, Left
Tibiofemoral joint	Knee Joint, Right
	Knee Joint, Left
	Knee Joint, Tibial Surface, Right
	Knee Joint, Tibial Surface, Left
Tongue, base of	Pharynx
Tracheobronchial lymph node	Lymphatic, Thorax
Tragus	External Ear, Right
	External Ear, Left
	External Ear, Bilateral
Transversalis fascia	Subcutaneous Tissue and Fascia, Trunk
Transverse (cutaneous) cervical nerve	Cervical Plexus
Transverse acetabular ligament	Hip Bursa and Ligament, Right
	Hip Bursa and Ligament, Left
Transverse facial artery	Temporal Artery, Right
	Temporal Artery, Left
Transverse foramen	Cervical Vertebra

Anatomical Term	ICD-10-PCS Value
Transverse humeral ligament	Shoulder Bursa and Ligament, Right
	Shoulder Bursa and Ligament, Left
Transverse ligament of atlas	Head and Neck Bursa and Ligament
Transverse process	Cervical Vertebra
	Thoracic Vertebra
	Lumbar Vertebra
Transverse scapular ligament	Shoulder Bursa and Ligament, Right
	Shoulder Bursa and Ligament, Left
Transverse thoracis muscle	Thorax Muscle, Right
	Thorax Muscle, Left
Transversospinalis muscle	Trunk Muscle, Right
	Trunk Muscle, Left
Transversus abdominis muscle	Abdomen Muscle, Right
	Abdomen Muscle, Left
Trapezium bone	Carpal, Right
	Carpal, Left
Trapezius muscle	Trunk Muscle, Right
	Trunk Muscle, Left
Trapezoid bone	Carpal, Right
	Carpal, Left
Triceps brachii muscle	Upper Arm Muscle, Right
	Upper Arm Muscle, Left
Tricuspid annulus	Tricuspid Valve
Trifacial nerve	Trigeminal Nerve
Trigone of bladder	Bladder
Triquetral bone	Carpal, Right
	Carpal, Left
Trochanteric bursa	Hip Bursa and Ligament, Right
	Hip Bursa and Ligament, Left
Twelfth cranial nerve	Hypoglossal Nerve
Tympanic cavity	Middle Ear, Right
	Middle Ear, Left
Tympanic nerve	Glossopharyngeal Nerve
Tympanic part of temporal bone	Temporal Bone, Right
	Temporal Bone, Left
Ulnar collateral carpal ligament	Wrist Bursa and Ligament, Right
	Wrist Bursa and Ligament, Left
Ulnar collateral ligament	Elbow Bursa and Ligament, Right
	Elbow Bursa and Ligament, Left
Ulnar notch	Radius, Right
	Radius, Left
Ulnar vein	Brachial Vein, Right
	Brachial Vein, Left

Anatomical Term	ICD-10-PCS Value
Umbilical artery	Internal Iliac Artery, Right
	Internal Iliac Artery, Left
	Lower Artery
Ureteral orifice	Ureter, Right
	Ureter, Left
	Ureters, Bilateral
	Ureter
Ureteropelvic junction (UPJ)	Kidney Pelvis, Right
	Kidney Pelvis, Left
Ureterovesical orifice	Ureter, Right
	Ureter, Left
	Ureters, Bilateral
	Ureter
Uterine Artery	Internal Iliac Artery, Right
	Internal Iliac Artery, Left
Uterine cornu	Uterus
Uterine tube	Fallopian Tube, Right
	Fallopian Tube, Left
Uterine vein	Hypogastric Vein, Right
	Hypogastric Vein, Left
Vaginal artery	Internal Iliac Artery, Right
	Internal Iliac Artery, Left
Vaginal vein	Hypogastric Vein, Right
	Hypogastric Vein, Left
Vastus intermedius muscle	Upper Leg Muscle, Right
	Upper Leg Muscle, Left
Vastus lateralis muscle	Upper Leg Muscle, Right
	Upper Leg Muscle, Left
Vastus medialis muscle	Upper Leg Muscle, Right
	Upper Leg Muscle, Left
Ventricular fold	Larynx
Vermiform appendix	Appendix
Vermilion border	Upper Lip
	Lower Lip
Vertebral arch	Cervical Vertebra
	Thoracic Vertebra
	Lumbar Vertebra
Vertebral body	Cervical Vertebra
	Thoracic Vertebra
	Lumbar Vertebra
Vertebral canal	Spinal Canal
Vertebral foramen	Cervical Vertebra
	Thoracic Vertebra
	Lumbar Vertebra

Anatomical Term	ICD-10-PCS Value
Vertebral lamina	Cervical Vertebra
	Thoracic Vertebra
	Lumbar Vertebra
Vertebral pedicle	Cervical Vertebra
	Thoracic Vertebra
	Lumbar Vertebra
Vesical vein	Hypogastric Vein, Right
	Hypogastric Vein, Left
Vestibular (Scarpa's) ganglion	Acoustic Nerve
Vestibular nerve	Acoustic Nerve
Vestibulocochlear nerve	Acoustic Nerve
Virchow's (supraclavicular) lymph node	Lymphatic, Right Neck
	Lymphatic, Left Neck
Vitreous body	Vitreous, Right
	Vitreous, Left
Vocal fold	Vocal Cord, Right
	Vocal Cord, Left
Volar (palmar) digital vein	Hand Vein, Right
	Hand Vein, Left
Volar (palmar) metacarpal vein	Hand Vein, Right
	Hand Vein, Left
Vomer bone	Nasal Septum
Vomer of nasal septum	Nasal Bone
Xiphoid process	Sternum
Zonule of Zinn	Lens, Right
	Lens, Left
Zygomatic process of frontal bone	Frontal Bone
Zygomatic process of temporal bone	Temporal Bone, Right
	Temporal Bone, Left
Zygomaticus muscle	Facial Muscle

This page intentionally left blank

Appendix C: Device Key

Device Term	ICD-10-PCS Value
3f® (Aortic) Bioprosthesis valve	Zooplastic Tissue in Heart and Great Vessels
AbioCor® Total Replacement Heart	Synthetic Substitute
Absolute Pro® Vascular (OTW) Self-Expanding Stent System	Intraluminal Device
Acculink™ (RX) Carotid Stent System	Intraluminal Device
Acellular Hydrated Dermis	Nonautologous Tissue Substitute
Acetabular cup	Liner in Lower Joints
Activa PC® neurostimulator	Stimulator Generator, Multiple Array for Insertion in Subcutaneous Tissue and Fascia
Activa RC® neurostimulator	Stimulator Generator, Multiple Array Rechargeable for Insertion in Subcutaneous Tissue and Fascia
Activa SC® neurostimulator	Stimulator Generator, Single Array for Insertion in Subcutaneous Tissue and Fascia
ACUITY™ Steerable Lead	Cardiac Lead, Pacemaker for Insertion in Heart and Great Vessels
	Cardiac Lead, Defibrillator for Insertion in Heart and Great Vessels
Advisa MRI™	Pacemaker, Dual Chamber for Insertion in Subcutaneous Tissue and Fascia
AFX® Endovascular AAA System	Intraluminal Device
AMPLATZER® Muscular VSD Occluder	Synthetic Substitute
AMS 800® Urinary Control System	Artificial Sphincter in Urinary System
AneuRx® AAA Advantage®	Intraluminal Device
Annuloplasty ring	Synthetic Substitute
Articulating Spacer (Antibiotic)	Articulating Spacer in Lower Joints
Artificial anal sphincter (AAS)	Artificial Sphincter in Gastrointestinal System
Artificial bowel sphincter (neosphincter)	Artificial Sphincter in Gastrointestinal System
Artificial urinary sphincter (AUS)	Artificial Sphincter in Urinary System
Ascenda® Intrathecal Catheter	Infusion Device
Assurant (Cobalt)® stent	Intraluminal Device
AtriClip® LAA Exclusion System	Extraluminal Device
Attain Ability® lead	Cardiac Lead, Pacemaker for Insertion in Heart and Great Vessels
	Cardiac Lead, Defibrillator for Insertion in Heart and Great Vessels
Attain StarFix® (OTW) lead	Cardiac Lead, Pacemaker for Insertion in Heart and Great Vessels
	Cardiac Lead, Defibrillator for Insertion in Heart and Great Vessels

Device Term	ICD-10-PCS Value
Autograft	Autologous Tissue Substitute
Autologous artery graft	Autologous Arterial Tissue in Heart and Great Vessels
	Autologous Arterial Tissue in Upper Arteries
	Autologous Arterial Tissue in Lower Arteries
	Autologous Arterial Tissue in Upper Veins
	Autologous Arterial Tissue in Lower Veins
Autologous vein graft	Autologous Venous Tissue in Heart and Great Vessels
	Autologous Venous Tissue in Upper Arteries
	Autologous Venous Tissue in Lower Arteries
	Autologous Venous Tissue in Upper Veins
	Autologous Venous Tissue in Lower Veins
Axial Lumbar Interbody Fusion System	Interbody Fusion Device in Lower Joints
AxiaLIF® System	Interbody Fusion Device in Lower Joints
BAK/C® Interbody Cervical Fusion System	Interbody Fusion Device in Upper Joints
Bard® Composix® (E/X) (LP) mesh	Synthetic Substitute
Bard® Composix® Kugel® patch	Synthetic Substitute
Bard® Dulex™ mesh	Synthetic Substitute
Bard® Ventralex™ hernia patch	Synthetic Substitute
Baroreflex Activation Therapy®(BAT®)	Stimulator Lead in Upper Arteries
	Stimulator Generator in Subcutaneous Tissue and Fascia
Berlin Heart® Ventricular Assist Device	Implantable Heart Assist System in Heart and Great Vessels
Bioactive embolization coil(s)	Intraluminal Device, Bioactive in Upper Arteries
Biventricular external heart assist system	Short-term External Heart Assist System in Heart and Great Vessels
Blood glucose monitoring system	Monitoring Device
Bone anchored hearing device	Hearing Device, Bone Conduction for Insertion in Ear, Nose, Sinus
	Hearing Device in Head and Facial Bones
Bone bank bone graft	Nonautologous Tissue Substitute
Bone screw(interlocking) (lag) (pedicle) (recessed)	Internal Fixation Device in Head and Facial Bones
	Internal Fixation Device in Upper Bones
	Internal Fixation Device in Lower Bones

Device Term	ICD-10-PCS Value
Bovine pericardial valve	Zooplastic Tissue in Heart and Great Vessels
Bovine pericardium graft	Zooplastic Tissue in Heart and Great Vessels
Brachytherapy seeds	Radioactive Element
BRYAN® Cervical Disc System	Synthetic Substitute
BVS 5000® Ventricular Assist Device	Short-term External Heart Assist System in Heart and Great Vessels
Cardiac contractility modulation lead	Cardiac Lead in Heart and Great Vessels
Cardiac event recorder	Monitoring Device
Cardiac resynchronization therapy (CRT) lead	Cardiac Lead, Pacemaker for Insertion in Heart and Great Vessels
	Cardiac Lead, Defibrillator for Insertion in Heart and Great Vessels
CardioMEMS® pressure sensor	Monitoring Device, Pressure Sensor for Insertion in Heart and Great Vessels
Carotid (artery) sinus (baroreceptor) lead	Stimulator Lead in Upper Arteries
Carotid WALLSTENT® Monorail® Endoprosthesis	Intraluminal Device
Centrimag® Blood Pump	Short-term External Heart Assist System in Heart and Great Vessels
Ceramic on ceramic bearing surface	Synthetic Substitute, Ceramic for Replacement in Lower Joints
Cesium-131 Collagen Implant	Radioactive Element, Cesium-131 Collagen Implant for Insertion in Central Nervous System and Cranial Nerves
Clamp and rod internal fixation system (CRIF)	Internal Fixation Device in Upper Bones
	Internal Fixation Device in Lower Bones
COALESCE® radiolucent interbody fusion device	Interbody Fusion Device, Radiolucent Porous in New Technology
CoAxia NeuroFlo™ catheter	Intraluminal Device
Cobalt/chromium head and polyethylene socket	Synthetic Substitute, Metal on Polyethylene for Replacement in Lower Joints
Cobalt/chromium head and socket	Synthetic Substitute, Metal for Replacement in Lower Joints
Cochlear implant (CI), multiple channel (electrode)	Hearing Device, Multiple Channel Cochlear Prosthesis for Insertion in Ear, Nose, Sinus
Cochlear implant (CI), single channel (electrode)	Hearing Device, Single Channel Cochlear Prosthesis for Insertion in Ear, Nose, Sinus
COGNIS® CRT-D	Cardiac Resynchronization Defibrillator Pulse Generator for Insertion in Subcutaneous Tissue and Fascia
COHERE® radiolucent interbody fusion device	Interbody Fusion Device, Radiolucent Porous in New Technology
Colonic Z-Stent®	Intraluminal Device
Complete® (SE) stent	Intraluminal Device
Concerto® II CRT-D	Cardiac Resynchronization Defibrillator Pulse Generator for Insertion in Subcutaneous Tissue and Fascia
CONSERVE® PLUS Total Resurfacing Hip System	Resurfacing Device in Lower Joints
Consulta® CRT-D	Cardiac Resynchronization Defibrillator Pulse Generator for Insertion in Subcutaneous Tissue and Fascia
Consulta® CRT-P	Cardiac Resynchronization Pacemaker Pulse Generator for Insertion in Subcutaneous Tissue and Fascia
CONTAK RENEWAL® 3 RF (HE) CRT-D	Cardiac Resynchronization Defibrillator Pulse Generator for Insertion in Subcutaneous Tissue and Fascia
Contegra® Pulmonary Valved Conduit	Zooplastic Tissue in Heart and Great Vessels
Continuous Glucose Monitoring (CGM) device	Monitoring Device
Cook Biodesign® Fistula Plug(s)	Nonautologous Tissue Substitute
Cook Biodesign® Hernia Graft(s)	Nonautologous Tissue Substitute
Cook Biodesign® Layered Graft(s)	Nonautologous Tissue Substitute
Cook Zenapro™ Layered Graft(s)	Nonautologous Tissue Substitute
Cook Zenith® AAA Endovascular Graft	Intraluminal Device, Branched or Fenestrated, One or Two Arteries for Restriction in Lower Arteries
	Intraluminal Device, Branched or Fenestrated, Three or More Arteries for Restriction in Lower Arteries
	Intraluminal Device
CoreValve™ transcatheter aortic valve	Zooplastic Tissue in Heart and Great Vessels
Cormet™ Hip Resurfacing System	Resurfacing Device in Lower Joints
CoRoent® XL	Interbody Fusion Device in Lower Joints
Corox® (OTW) Bipolar Lead	Cardiac Lead, Pacemaker for Insertion in Heart and Great Vessels
	Cardiac Lead, Defibrillator for Insertion in Heart and Great Vessels
Cortical strip neurostimulator lead	Neurostimulator Lead in Central Nervous System and Cranial Nerves
Cultured epidermal cell autograft	Autologous Tissue Substitute
CYPHER® Stent	Intraluminal Device, Drug-eluting in Heart and Great Vessels
Cystostomy tube	Drainage Device
DBS™ lead	Neurostimulator Lead in Central Nervous System and Cranial Nerves

Device Term	ICD-10-PCS Value
DeBakey® Left Ventricular Assist Device	Implantable Heart Assist System in Heart and Great Vessels
Deep brain neurostimulator lead	Neurostimulator Lead in Central Nervous System and Cranial Nerves
Delta frame external fixator	External Fixation Device, Hybrid for Insertion in Upper Bones
	External Fixation Device, Hybrid for Reposition in Upper Bones
	External Fixation Device, Hybrid for Insertion in Lower Bones
	External Fixation Device, Hybrid for Reposition in Lower Bones
Delta III™ Reverse shoulder prosthesis	Synthetic Substitute, Reverse Ball and Socket for Replacement in Upper Joints
Diaphragmatic pacemaker generator	Stimulator Generator in Subcutaneous Tissue and Fascia
Direct Lateral Interbody Fusion (DLIF) device	Interbody Fusion Device in Lower Joints
Driver® stent (RX) (OTW)	Intraluminal Device
DuraHeart® Left Ventricular Assist System	Implantable Heart Assist System in Heart and Great Vessels
Durata® Defibrillation Lead	Cardiac Lead, Defibrillator for Insertion in Heart and Great Vessels
Dynesys® Dynamic Stabilization System	Spinal Stabilization Device, Pedicle-Based for Insertion in Upper Joints
	Spinal Stabilization Device, Pedicle-Based for Insertion in Lower Joints
E-Luminexx™ (Biliary) (Vascular) Stent	Intraluminal Device
EDWARDS INTUITY Elite™ valve system	Zooplastic Tissue, Rapid Deployment Technique in New Technology
Electrical bone growth stimulator (EBGS)	Bone Growth Stimulator in Head and Facial Bones
	Bone Growth Stimulator in Upper Bones
	Bone Growth Stimulator in Lower Bones
Electrical muscle stimulation (EMS) lead	Stimulator Lead in Muscles
Electronic muscle stimulator lead	Stimulator Lead in Muscles
Embolization coil(s)	Intraluminal Device
Endeavor® (III) (IV) (Sprint) Zotarolimus-eluting Coronary Stent System	Intraluminal Device, Drug-eluting in Heart and Great Vessels
Endologix AFX® Endovascular AAA System	Intraluminal Device
EndoSure® sensor	Monitoring Device, Pressure Sensor for Insertion in Heart and Great Vessels
ENDOTAK RELIANCE® (G) Defibrillation Lead	Cardiac Lead, Defibrillator for Insertion in Heart and Great Vessels

Device Term	ICD-10-PCS Value
Endotracheal tube (cuffed) (double-lumen)	Intraluminal Device, Endotracheal Airway in Respiratory System
Endurant® Endovascular Stent Graft	Intraluminal Device
Endurant® II AAA stent graft system	Intraluminal Device
EnRhythm®	Pacemaker, Dual Chamber for Insertion in Subcutaneous Tissue and Fascia
Enterra® gastric neurostimulator	Stimulator Generator, Multiple Array for Insertion in Subcutaneous Tissue and Fascia
Epic™ Stented Tissue Valve (aortic)	Zooplastic Tissue in Heart and Great Vessels
Epicel® cultured epidermal autograft	Autologous Tissue Substitute
Esophageal obturator airway (EOA)	Intraluminal Device, Airway in Gastrointestinal System
Esteem® implantable hearing system	Hearing Device in Ear, Nose, Sinus
Evera™ (XT) (S) (DR/VR)	Defibrillator Generator for Insertion in Subcutaneous Tissue and Fascia
Everolimus-eluting coronary stent	Intraluminal Device, Drug-eluting in Heart and Great Vessels
Ex-PRESS™ mini glaucoma shunt	Synthetic Substitute
EXCLUDER® AAA Endoprosthesis	Intraluminal Device, Branched or Fenestrated, One or Two Arteries for Restriction in Lower Arteries
	Intraluminal Device, Branched or Fenestrated, Three or More Arteries for Restriction in Lower Arteries
	Intraluminal Device
EXCLUDER® IBE Endoprosthesis	Intraluminal Device, Branched or Fenestrated, One or Two Arteries for Restriction in Lower Arteries
Express® (LD) Premounted Stent System	Intraluminal Device
Express® Biliary SD Monorail® Premounted Stent System	Intraluminal Device
Express® SD Renal Monorail® Premounted Stent System	Intraluminal Device
External fixator	External Fixation Device in Head and Facial Bones
	External Fixation Device in Upper Bones
	External Fixation Device in Lower Bones
	External Fixation Device in Upper Joints
	External Fixation Device in Lower Joints
EXtreme Lateral Interbody Fusion(XLIF) device	Interbody Fusion Device in Lower Joints
Facet replacement spinal stabilization device	Spinal Stabilization Device, Facet Replacement for Insertion in Upper Joints
	Spinal Stabilization Device, Facet Replacement for Insertion in Lower Joints

Device Term	ICD-10-PCS Value
FLAIR® Endovascular Stent Graft	Intraluminal Device
Flexible Composite Mesh	Synthetic Substitute
Foley catheter	Drainage Device
Formula™ Balloon-Expandable Renal Stent System	Intraluminal Device
Freestyle® (Stentless) Aortic Root Bioprosthesis	Zooplastic Tissue in Heart and Great Vessels
Fusion screw (compression) (lag) (locking)	Internal Fixation Device in Upper Joints
Fusion screw (compression) (lag) (locking)	Internal Fixation Device in Lower Joints
GammaTile™	Radioactive Element, Cesium-131 Collagen Implant for Insertion in Central Nervous System and Cranial Nerves
Gastric electrical stimulation (GES) lead	Stimulator Lead in Gastrointestinal System
Gastric pacemaker lead	Stimulator Lead in Gastrointestinal System
GORE EXCLUDER® AAA Endoprosthesis	Intraluminal Device, Branched or Fenestrated, One or Two Arteries for Restriction in Lower Arteries
GORE EXCLUDER® AAA Endoprosthesis	Intraluminal Device, Branched or Fenestrated, Three or More Arteries for Restriction in Lower Arteries
GORE EXCLUDER® AAA Endoprosthesis	Intraluminal Device
GORE EXCLUDER® IBE Endoprosthesis	Intraluminal Device, Branched or Fenestrated, One or Two Arteries for Restriction in Lower Arteries
GORE TAG® Thoracic Endoprosthesis	Intraluminal Device
GORE® DUALMESH®	Synthetic Substitute
Guedel airway	Intraluminal Device, Airway in Mouth and Throat
Hancock® Bioprosthesis (aortic) (mitral) valve	Zooplastic Tissue in Heart and Great Vessels
Hancock® Bioprosthetic Valved Conduit	Zooplastic Tissue in Heart and Great Vessels
HeartMate 3™ LVAS	Implantable Heart Assist System in Heart and Great Vessels
HeartMate II® Left Ventricular Assist Device (LVAD)	Implantable Heart Assist System in Heart and Great Vessels
HeartMate XVE® Left Ventricular Assist Device (LVAD)	Implantable Heart Assist System in Heart and Great Vessels
Herculink® (RX) Elite Renal Stent System	Intraluminal Device
Hip (joint) liner	Liner in Lower Joints
Holter valve ventricular shunt	Synthetic Substitute
Ilizarov external fixator	External Fixation Device, Ring for Insertion in Upper Bones
Ilizarov external fixator	External Fixation Device, Ring for Reposition in Upper Bones
Ilizarov external fixator	External Fixation Device, Ring for Insertion in Lower Bones
Ilizarov external fixator	External Fixation Device, Ring for Reposition in Lower Bones

Device Term	ICD-10-PCS Value
Ilizarov-Vecklich device	External Fixation Device, Limb Lengthening for Insertion in Upper Bones
Ilizarov-Vecklich device	External Fixation Device, Limb Lengthening for Insertion in Lower Bones
Impella® heart pump	Short-term External Heart Assist System in Heart and Great Vessels
Implantable cardioverter-defibrillator (ICD)	Defibrillator Generator for Insertion in Subcutaneous Tissue and Fascia
Implantable drug infusion pump (anti-spasmodic) (chemotherapy) (pain)	Infusion Device, Pump in Subcutaneous Tissue and Fascia
Implantable glucose monitoring device	Monitoring Device
Implantable hemodynamic monitor (IHM)	Monitoring Device, Hemodynamic for Insertion in Subcutaneous Tissue and Fascia
Implantable hemodynamic monitoring system (IHMS)	Monitoring Device, Hemodynamic for Insertion in Subcutaneous Tissue and Fascia
Implantable Miniature Telescope™(IMT)	Synthetic Substitute, Intraocular Telescope for Replacement in Eye
Implanted (venous) (access) port	Vascular Access Device, Totally Implantable in Subcutaneous Tissue and Fascia
InDura®, intrathecal catheter (1P) (spinal)	Infusion Device
Injection reservoir, port	Vascular Access Device, Totally Implantable in Subcutaneous Tissue and Fascia
Injection reservoir, pump	Infusion Device, Pump in Subcutaneous Tissue and Fascia
Interbody fusion (spine) cage	Interbody Fusion Device in Upper Joints
Interbody fusion (spine) cage	Interbody Fusion Device in Lower Joints
Interspinous process spinal stabilization device	Spinal Stabilization Device, Interspinous Process for Insertion in Upper Joints
Interspinous process spinal stabilization device	Spinal Stabilization Device, Interspinous Process for Insertion in Lower Joints
InterStim® Therapy lead	Neurostimulator Lead in Peripheral Nervous System
InterStim® Therapy neurostimulator	Stimulator Generator, Single Array for Insertion in Subcutaneous Tissue and Fascia
Intramedullary (IM) rod (nail)	Internal Fixation Device, Intramedullary in Upper Bones
Intramedullary (IM) rod (nail)	Internal Fixation Device, Intramedullary in Lower Bones
Intramedullary skeletal kinetic distractor (ISKD)	Internal Fixation Device, Intramedullary in Upper Bones
Intramedullary skeletal kinetic distractor (ISKD)	Internal Fixation Device, Intramedullary in Lower Bones

Device Term	ICD-10-PCS Value
Intrauterine device (IUD)	Contraceptive Device in Female Reproductive System
INTUITY Elite® valve system, EDWARDS	Zooplastic Tissue, Rapid Deployment Technique in New Technology
Itrel® (3) (4) neurostimulator	Stimulator Generator, Single Array for Insertion in Subcutaneous Tissue and Fascia
Joint fixation plate	Internal Fixation Device in Upper Joints
	Internal Fixation Device in Lower Joints
Joint liner (insert)	Liner in Lower Joints
Joint spacer (antibiotic)	Spacer in Upper Joints
	Spacer in Lower Joints
Kappa®	Pacemaker, Dual Chamber for Insertion in Subcutaneous Tissue and Fascia
Kirschner wire (K-wire)	Internal Fixation Device in Head and Facial Bones
	Internal Fixation Device in Upper Bones
	Internal Fixation Device in Lower Bones
	Internal Fixation Device in Upper Joints
	Internal Fixation Device in Lower Joints
Knee (implant) insert	Liner in Lower Joints
Kuntscher nail	Internal Fixation Device, Intramedullary in Upper Bones
	Internal Fixation Device, Intramedullary in Lower Bones
LAP-BAND® adjustable gastric banding system	Extraluminal Device
LifeStent® (Flexstar) (XL) Vascular Stent System	Intraluminal Device
LIVIAN™ CRT-D	Cardiac Resynchronization Defibrillator Pulse Generator for Insertion in Subcutaneous Tissue and Fascia
Loop recorder, implantable	Monitoring Device
MAGEC® Spinal Bracing and Distraction System	Magnetically Controlled Growth Rod(s) in New Technology
Mark IV™ Breathing Pacemaker System	Stimulator Generator in Subcutaneous Tissue and Fascia
Maximo® II DR (VR)	Defibrillator Generator for Insertion in Subcutaneous Tissue and Fascia
Maximo® II DR CRT-D	Cardiac Resynchronization Defibrillator Pulse Generator for Insertion in Subcutaneous Tissue and Fascia
Medtronic Endurant® II AAA stent graft system	Intraluminal Device
Melody® transcatheter pulmonary valve	Zooplastic Tissue in Heart and Great Vessels
Metal on metal bearing surface	Synthetic Substitute, Metal for Replacement in Lower Joints
Micro-Driver® stent (RX) (OTW)	Intraluminal Device
MicroMed HeartAssist™	Implantable Heart Assist System in Heart and Great Vessels
Micrus CERECYTE® microcoil	Intraluminal Device, Bioactive in Upper Arteries
MIRODERM™ Biologic Wound Matrix	Skin Substitute, Porcine Liver Derived in New Technology
MitraClip® valve repair system	Synthetic Substitute
Mitroflow® Aortic Pericardial Heart Valve	Zooplastic Tissue in Heart and Great Vessels
Mosaic® Bioprosthesis (aortic) (mitral) valve	Zooplastic Tissue in Heart and Great Vessels
MULTI-LINK (VISION®) (MINI-VISION VISION®) (ULTRA™) Coronary Stent System	Intraluminal Device
nanoLOCK™ interbody fusion device	Interbody Fusion Device, Nanotextured Surface in New Technology
Nasopharyngeal airway (NPA)	Intraluminal Device, Airway in Ear, Nose, Sinus
Neuromuscular electrical stimulation (NEMS) lead	Stimulator Lead in Muscles
Neurostimulator generator, multiple channel	Stimulator Generator, Multiple Array for Insertion in Subcutaneous Tissue and Fascia
Neurostimulator generator, multiple channel rechargeable	Stimulator Generator, Multiple Array Rechargeable for Insertion in Subcutaneous Tissue and Fascia
Neurostimulator generator, single channel	Stimulator Generator, Single Array for Insertion in Subcutaneous Tissue and Fascia
Neurostimulator generator, single channel rechargeable	Stimulator Generator, Single Array Rechargeable for Insertion in Subcutaneous Tissue and Fascia
Neutralization plate	Internal Fixation Device in Head and Facial Bones
	Internal Fixation Device in Upper Bones
	Internal Fixation Device in Lower Bones
Nitinol framed polymer mesh	Synthetic Substitute
Non-tunneled central venous catheter	Infusion Device
Novacor® Left Ventricular Assist Device	Implantable Heart Assist System in Heart and Great Vessels
Novation® Ceramic AHS® (Articulation Hip System)	Synthetic Substitute, Ceramic for Replacement in Lower Joints
Omnilink Elite® Vascular Balloon Expandable Stent System	Intraluminal Device
Open Pivot™ (mechanical) valve	Synthetic Substitute
Open Pivot™ Aortic Valve Graft (AVG)	Synthetic Substitute

Device Term	ICD-10-PCS Value
Optimizer™ III implantable pulse generator	Contractility Modulation Device for Insertion in Subcutaneous Tissue and Fascia
Oropharyngeal airway (OPA)	Intraluminal Device, Airway in Mouth and Throat
Ovatio™ CRT-D	Cardiac Resynchronization Defibrillator Pulse Generator for Insertion in Subcutaneous Tissue and Fascia
OXINIUM™	Synthetic Substitute, Oxidized Zirconium on Polyethylene for Replacement in Lower Joints
Paclitaxel-eluting coronary stent	Intraluminal Device, Drug-eluting in Heart and Great Vessels
Paclitaxel-eluting peripheral stent	Intraluminal Device, Drug-eluting in Upper Arteries
	Intraluminal Device, Drug-eluting in Lower Arteries
Partially absorbable mesh	Synthetic Substitute
Pedicle-based dynamic stabilization device	Spinal Stabilization Device, Pedicle-Based for Insertion in Upper Joints
	Spinal Stabilization Device, Pedicle-Based for Insertion in Lower Joints
Perceval sutureless valve	Zooplastic Tissue, Rapid Deployment Technique in New Technology
Percutaneous endoscopic gastrojejunostomy (PEG/J) tube	Feeding Device in Gastrointestinal System
Percutaneous endoscopic gastrostomy (PEG) tube	Feeding Device in Gastrointestinal System
Percutaneous nephrostomy catheter	Drainage Device
Peripherally inserted central catheter (PICC)	Infusion Device
Pessary ring	Intraluminal Device, Pessary in Female Reproductive System
Phrenic nerve stimulator generator	Stimulator Generator in Subcutaneous Tissue and Fascia
Phrenic nerve stimulator lead	Diaphragmatic Pacemaker Lead in Respiratory System
PHYSIOMESH™ Flexible Composite Mesh	Synthetic Substitute
Pipeline™ Embolization device (PED)	Intraluminal Device
Polyethylene socket	Synthetic Substitute, Polyethylene for Replacement in Lower Joints
Polymethylmethacrylate (PMMA)	Synthetic Substitute
Polypropylene mesh	Synthetic Substitute
Porcine (bioprosthetic) valve	Zooplastic Tissue in Heart and Great Vessels
PRESTIGE® Cervical Disc	Synthetic Substitute
PrimeAdvanced® neurostimulator (SureScan®) (MRI Safe)	Stimulator Generator, Multiple Array for Insertion in Subcutaneous Tissue and Fascia
PROCEED™ Ventral Patch	Synthetic Substitute

Device Term	ICD-10-PCS Value
Prodisc-C™	Synthetic Substitute
Prodisc-L™	Synthetic Substitute
PROLENE® Polypropylene Hernia System (PHS)	Synthetic Substitute
Protecta™ XT CRT-D	Cardiac Resynchronization Defibrillator Pulse Generator for Insertion in Subcutaneous Tissue and Fascia
Protecta™ XT DR (XT VR)	Defibrillator Generator for Insertion in Subcutaneous Tissue and Fascia
Protege® RX Carotid Stent System	Intraluminal Device
Pump reservoir	Infusion Device, Pump in Subcutaneous Tissue and Fascia
REALIZE® Adjustable Gastric Band	Extraluminal Device
Rebound HRD® (Hernia Repair Device)	Synthetic Substitute
RestoreAdvanced® neurostimulator (SureScan®) (MRI Safe)	Stimulator Generator, Multiple Array Rechargeable for Insertion in Subcutaneous Tissue and Fascia
RestoreSensor® neurostimulator (SureScan®) (MRI Safe)	Stimulator Generator, Multiple Array Rechargeable for Insertion in Subcutaneous Tissue and Fascia
RestoreUltra® neurostimulator (SureScan®) (MRI Safe)	Stimulator Generator, Multiple Array Rechargeable for Insertion in Subcutaneous Tissue and Fascia
Reveal® (DX) (XT)	Monitoring Device
Reverse® Shoulder Prosthesis	Synthetic Substitute, Reverse Ball and Socket for Replacement in Upper Joints
Revo MRI™ SureScan® pacemaker	Pacemaker, Dual Chamber for Insertion in Subcutaneous Tissue and Fascia
Rheos® System device	Stimulator Generator in Subcutaneous Tissue and Fascia
Rheos® System lead	Stimulator Lead in Upper Arteries
RNS® System lead	Neurostimulator Lead in Central Nervous System and Cranial Nerves
RNS® system neurostimulator generator	Neurostimulator Generator in Head and Facial Bones
Sacral nerve modulation (SNM) lead	Stimulator Lead in Urinary System
Sacral neuromodulation lead	Stimulator Lead in Urinary System
SAPIEN® transcatheter aortic valve	Zooplastic Tissue in Heart and Great Vessels
Secura™ (DR) (VR)	Defibrillator Generator for Insertion in Subcutaneous Tissue and Fascia
Sheffield hybrid external fixator	External Fixation Device, Hybrid for Insertion in Upper Bones
	External Fixation Device, Hybrid for Reposition in Upper Bones
	External Fixation Device, Hybrid for Insertion in Lower Bones
	External Fixation Device, Hybrid for Reposition in Lower Bones

Device Term	ICD-10-PCS Value
Sheffield ring external fixator	External Fixation Device, Ring for Insertion in Upper Bones
	External Fixation Device, Ring for Reposition in Upper Bones
	External Fixation Device, Ring for Insertion in Lower Bones
	External Fixation Device, Ring for Reposition in Lower Bones
Single lead pacemaker (atrium) (ventricle)	Pacemaker, Single Chamber for Insertion in Subcutaneous Tissue and Fascia
Single lead rate responsive pacemaker (atrium) (ventricle)	Pacemaker, Single Chamber Rate Responsive for Insertion in Subcutaneous Tissue and Fascia
Sirolimus-eluting coronary stent	Intraluminal Device, Drug-eluting in Heart and Great Vessels
SJM Biocor® Stented Valve System	Zooplastic Tissue in Heart and Great Vessels
Spacer, Articulating (Antibiotic)	Articulating Spacer in Lower Joints
Spacer, Static (Antibiotic)	Spacer in Lower Joints
Spinal cord neurostimulator lead	Neurostimulator Lead in Central Nervous System and Cranial Nerves
Spinal growth rods, magnetically controlled	Magnetically Controlled Growth Rod(s) in New Technology
Spiration IBV™ Valve System	Intraluminal Device, Endobronchial Valve in Respiratory System
Static Spacer (Antibiotic)	Spacer in Lower Joints
Stent, intraluminal (cardiovascular) (gastrointestinal) (hepatobiliary) (urinary)	Intraluminal Device
Stented tissue valve	Zooplastic Tissue in Heart and Great Vessels
Stratos LV®	Cardiac Resynchronization Pacemaker Pulse Generator for Insertion in Subcutaneous Tissue and Fascia
Subcutaneous injection reservoir, port	Vascular Access Device, Totally Implantable in Subcutaneous Tissue and Fascia
Subcutaneous injection reservoir, pump	Infusion Device, Pump in Subcutaneous Tissue and Fascia
Subdermal progesterone implant	Contraceptive Device in Subcutaneous Tissue and Fascia
Sutureless valve, Perceval™	Zooplastic Tissue, Rapid Deployment Technique in New Technology
SynCardia™ Total Artificial Heart	Synthetic Substitute
Synchra™ CRT-P	Cardiac Resynchronization Pacemaker Pulse Generator for Insertion in Subcutaneous Tissue and Fascia

Device Term	ICD-10-PCS Value
SynchroMed® pump	Infusion Device, Pump in Subcutaneous Tissue and Fascia
Talent® Converter	Intraluminal Device
Talent® Occluder	Intraluminal Device
Talent® Stent Graft (abdominal) (thoracic)	Intraluminal Device
TandemHeart® System	Short-term External Heart Assist System in Heart and Great Vessels
TAXUS® Liberte® Paclitaxel-eluting Coronary Stent System	Intraluminal Device, Drug-eluting in Heart and Great Vessels
Therapeutic occlusion coil(s)	Intraluminal Device
Thoracostomy tube	Drainage Device
Thoratec® IVAD (Implantable Ventricular Assist Device)	Implantable Heart Assist System in Heart and Great Vessels
Thoratec Paracorporeal Ventricular Assist Device	Short-term External Heart Assist System in Heart and Great Vessels
Tibial insert	Liner in Lower Joints
Tissue bank graft	Nonautologous Tissue Substitute
Tissue expander (inflatable) (injectable)	Tissue Expander in Skin and Breast
	Tissue Expander in Subcutaneous Tissue and Fascia
Titanium Sternal Fixation System (TSFS)	Internal Fixation Device, Rigid Plate for Insertion in Upper Bones
	Internal Fixation Device, Rigid Plate for Reposition in Upper Bones
Total artificial (replacement) heart	Synthetic Substitute
Tracheostomy tube	Tracheostomy Device in Respiratory System
Trifecta™ Valve (aortic)	Zooplastic Tissue in Heart and Great Vessels
Tunneled central venous catheter	Vascular Access Device, Tunneled in Subcutaneous Tissue and Fascia
Tunneled spinal (intrathecal) catheter	Infusion Device
Two lead pacemaker	Pacemaker, Dual Chamber for Insertion in Subcutaneous Tissue and Fascia
Ultraflex™ Precision Colonic Stent System	Intraluminal Device
ULTRAPRO® Hernia System (UHS)	Synthetic Substitute
ULTRAPRO® Partially Absorbable Lightweight Mesh	Synthetic Substitute
ULTRAPRO® Plug	Synthetic Substitute
Ultrasonic osteogenic stimulator	Bone Growth Stimulator in Head and Facial Bones
	Bone Growth Stimulator in Upper Bones
	Bone Growth Stimulator in Lower Bones

Device Term	ICD-10-PCS Value
Ultrasound bone healing system	Bone Growth Stimulator in Head and Facial Bones
	Bone Growth Stimulator in Upper Bones
	Bone Growth Stimulator in Lower Bones
Uniplanar external fixator	External Fixation Device, Monoplanar for Insertion in Upper Bones
	External Fixation Device, Monoplanar for Reposition in Upper Bones
	External Fixation Device, Monoplanar for Insertion in Lower Bones
	External Fixation Device, Monoplanar for Reposition in Lower Bones
Urinary incontinence stimulator lead	Stimulator Lead in Urinary System
Vaginal pessary	Intraluminal Device, Pessary in Female Reproductive System
Valiant® Thoracic Stent Graft	Intraluminal Device
Vectra® Vascular Access Graft	Vascular Access Device, Tunneled in Subcutaneous Tissue and Fascia
Ventrio™ Hernia Patch	Synthetic Substitute
Versa®	Pacemaker, Dual Chamber for Insertion in Subcutaneous Tissue and Fascia
Virtuoso® (II) (DR) (VR)	Defibrillator Generator for Insertion in Subcutaneous Tissue and Fascia
Viva™ (XT) (S)	Cardiac Resynchronization Defibrillator Pulse Generator for Insertion in Subcutaneous Tissue and Fascia
WALLSTENT® Endoprosthesis	Intraluminal Device

Device Term	ICD-10-PCS Value
X-STOP® Spacer	Spinal Stabilization Device, Interspinous Process for Insertion in Upper Joints
	Spinal Stabilization Device, Interspinous Process for Insertion in Lower Joints
Xact® Carotid Stent System	Intraluminal Device
Xenograft	Zooplastic Tissue in Heart and Great Vessels
XIENCE™ Everolimus Eluting Coronary Stent System	Intraluminal Device, Drug-eluting in Heart and Great Vessels
XLIF® System	Interbody Fusion Device in Lower Joints
Zenith® AAA Endovascular Graft	Intraluminal Device, Branched or Fenestrated, One or Two Arteries for Restriction in Lower Arteries
	Intraluminal Device, Branched or Fenestrated, Three or More Arteries for Restriction in Lower Arteries
	Intraluminal Device
Zenith Flex® AAA Endovascular Graft	Intraluminal Device
Zenith TX2® TAA Endovascular Graft	Intraluminal Device
Zenith® Renu™ AAA Ancillary Graft	Intraluminal Device
Zilver® PTX® (paclitaxel) Drug-eluting Peripheral Stent	Intraluminal Device, Drug-eluting in Upper Arteries
	Intraluminal Device, Drug-eluting in Lower Arteries
Zimmer® NexGen® LPS Mobile Bearing Knee	Synthetic Substitute
Zimmer® NexGen® LPS-Flex Mobile Knee	Synthetic Substitute
Zotarolimus-eluting coronary stent	Intraluminal Device, Drug-eluting in Heart and Great Vessels

Appendix D: Device Aggregation Table

Specific Device	For Operation	In Body System	General Device
Autologous Arterial Tissue	All applicable	Heart and Great Vessels	**7** Autologous Tissue Substitute
		Lower Arteries	
		Lower Veins	
		Upper Arteries	
		Upper Veins	
Autologous Venous Tissue	All applicable	Heart and Great Vessels	**7** Autologous Tissue Substitute
		Lower Arteries	
		Lower Veins	
		Upper Arteries	
		Upper Veins	
Cardiac Lead, Defibrillator	Insertion	Heart and Great Vessels	**M** Cardiac Lead
Cardiac Lead, Pacemaker	Insertion	Heart and Great Vessels	**M** Cardiac Lead
Cardiac Resynchronization Defibrillator Pulse Generator	Insertion	Subcutaneous Tissue and Fascia	**P** Cardiac Rhythm Related Device
Cardiac Resynchronization Pacemaker Pulse Generator	Insertion	Subcutaneous Tissue and Fascia	**P** Cardiac Rhythm Related Device
Contractility Modulation Device	Insertion	Subcutaneous Tissue and Fascia	**P** Cardiac Rhythm Related Device
Defibrillator Generator	Insertion	Subcutaneous Tissue and Fascia	**P** Cardiac Rhythm Related Device
Epiretinal Visual Prosthesis	All applicable	Eye	**J** Synthetic Substitute
External Fixation Device, Hybrid	Insertion	Lower Bones	**5** External Fixation Device
		Upper Bones	
External Fixation Device, Hybrid	Reposition	Lower Bones	**5** External Fixation Device
		Upper Bones	
External Fixation Device, Limb Lengthening	Insertion	Lower Bones	**5** External Fixation Device
		Upper Bones	
External Fixation Device, Monoplanar	Insertion	Lower Bones	**5** External Fixation Device
		Upper Bones	
External Fixation Device, Monoplanar	Reposition	Lower Bones	**5** External Fixation Device
		Upper Bones	
External Fixation Device, Ring	Insertion	Lower Bones	**5** External Fixation Device
		Upper Bones	
External Fixation Device, Ring	Reposition	Lower Bones	**5** External Fixation Device
		Upper Bones	
Hearing Device, Bone Conduction	Insertion	Ear, Nose, Sinus	**S** Hearing Device
Hearing Device, Multiple Channel Cochlear Prosthesis	Insertion	Ear, Nose, Sinus	**S** Hearing Device
Hearing Device, Single Channel Cochlear Prosthesis	Insertion	Ear, Nose, Sinus	**S** Hearing Device
Internal Fixation Device, Intramedullary	All applicable	Lower Bones	**4** Internal Fixation Device
		Upper Bones	
Internal Fixation Device, Rigid Plate	Insertion	Upper Bones	**4** Internal Fixation Device
Internal Fixation Device, Rigid Plate	Reposition	Upper Bones	**4** Internal Fixation Device
Intraluminal Device, Airway	All applicable	Ear, Nose, Sinus Gastrointestinal System Mouth and Throat	**D** Intraluminal Device
Intraluminal Device, Bioactive	All applicable	Upper Arteries	**D** Intraluminal Device

Specific Device	For Operation	In Body System	General Device
Intraluminal Device, Branched or Fenestrated, One or Two Arteries	Restriction	Heart and Great Vessels	**D** Intraluminal Device
		Lower Arteries	
Intraluminal Device, Branched or Fenestrated, Three or More Arteries	Restriction	Heart and Great Vessels	**D** Intraluminal Device
		Lower Arteries	
Intraluminal Device, Drug-eluting	All applicable	Heart and Great Vessels	**D** Intraluminal Device
		Lower Arteries	
		Upper Arteries	
Intraluminal Device, Drug-eluting, Four or More	All applicable	Heart and Great Vessels	**D** Intraluminal Device
		Lower Arteries	
		Upper Arteries	
Intraluminal Device, Drug-eluting, Three	All applicable	Heart and Great Vessels	**D** Intraluminal Device
		Lower Arteries	
		Upper Arteries	
Intraluminal Device, Drug-eluting, Two	All applicable	Heart and Great Vessels	**D** Intraluminal Device
		Lower Arteries	
		Upper Arteries	
Intraluminal Device, Endobronchial Valve	All applicable	Respiratory System	**D** Intraluminal Device
Intraluminal Device, Endotracheal Airway	All applicable	Respiratory System	**D** Intraluminal Device
Intraluminal Device, Four or More	All applicable	Heart and Great Vessels	**D** Intraluminal Device
		Lower Arteries	
		Upper Arteries	
Intraluminal Device, Pessary	All applicable	Female Reproductive System	**D** Intraluminal Device
Intraluminal Device, Radioactive	All applicable	Heart and Great Vessels	**D** Intraluminal Device
Intraluminal Device, Three	All applicable	Heart and Great Vessels	**D** Intraluminal Device
		Lower Arteries	
		Upper Arteries	
Intraluminal Device, Two	All applicable	Heart and Great Vessels	**D** Intraluminal Device
		Lower Arteries	
		Upper Arteries	
Monitoring Device, Hemodynamic	Insertion	Subcutaneous Tissue and Fascia	**2** Monitoring Device
Monitoring Device, Pressure Sensor	Insertion	Heart and Great Vessels	**2** Monitoring Device
Pacemaker, Dual Chamber	Insertion	Subcutaneous Tissue and Fascia	**P** Cardiac Rhythm Related Device
Pacemaker, Single Chamber	Insertion	Subcutaneous Tissue and Fascia	**P** Cardiac Rhythm Related Device
Pacemaker, Single Chamber Rate Responsive	Insertion	Subcutaneous Tissue and Fascia	**P** Cardiac Rhythm Related Device
Spinal Stabilization Device, Facet Replacement	Insertion	Lower Joints	**4** Internal Fixation Device
		Upper Joints	
Spinal Stabilization Device, Interspinous Process	Insertion	Lower Joints	**4** Internal Fixation Device
		Upper Joints	
Spinal Stabilization Device, Pedicle-Based	Insertion	Lower Joints	**4** Internal Fixation Device
		Upper Joints	
Stimulator Generator, Multiple Array	Insertion	Subcutaneous Tissue and Fascia	**M** Stimulator Generator
Stimulator Generator, Multiple Array Rechargeable	Insertion	Subcutaneous Tissue and Fascia	**M** Stimulator Generator
Stimulator Generator, Single Array	Insertion	Subcutaneous Tissue and Fascia	**M** Stimulator Generator

Specific Device	For Operation	In Body System	General Device
Stimulator Generator, Single Array Rechargeable	Insertion	Subcutaneous Tissue and Fascia	**M** Stimulator Generator
Synthetic Substitute, Ceramic	Replacement	Lower Joints	**J** Synthetic Substitute
Synthetic Substitute, Ceramic on Polyethylene	Replacement	Lower Joints	**J** Synthetic Substitute
Synthetic Substitute, Intraocular Telescope	Replacement	Eye	**J** Synthetic Substitute
Synthetic Substitute, Metal	Replacement	Lower Joints	**J** Synthetic Substitute
Synthetic Substitute, Metal on Polyethylene	Replacement	Lower Joints	**J** Synthetic Substitute
Synthetic Substitute, Oxidized Zirconium on Polyethylene	Replacement	Lower Joints	**J** Synthetic Substitute
Synthetic Substitute, Polyethylene	Replacement	Lower Joints	**J** Synthetic Substitute
Synthetic Substitute, Reverse Ball and Socket	Replacement	Upper Joints	**J** Synthetic Substitute

This page intentionally left blank

Appendix E: Character Meaning

0: Medical and Surgical
0: Central Nervous System and Cranial Nerves

Operation-Character 3	Body Part-Character 4	Approach-Character 5	Device-Character 6	Qualifier-Character 7
1 Bypass	**0** Brain	**0** Open	**0** Drainage Device	**0** Nasopharynx
2 Change	**1** Cerebral Meninges	**3** Percutaneous	**2** Monitoring Device	**1** Mastoid Sinus
5 Destruction	**2** Dura Mater	**4** Percutaneous Endoscopic	**3** Infusion Device	**2** Atrium
7 Dilation	**3** Epidural Space, Intracranial	**X** External	**4** Radioactive Element,Cesium-131 Collagen Implant	**3** Blood Vessel
8 Division	**4** Subdural Space, Intracranial		**7** Autologous Tissue Substitute	**4** Pleural Cavity
9 Drainage	**5** Subarachnoid Space, Intracranial		**J** Synthetic Substitute	**5** Intestine
B Excision	**6** Cerebral Ventricle		**K** Nonautologous Tissue Substitute	**6** Peritoneal Cavity
C Extirpation	**7** Cerebral Hemisphere		**M** Neurostimulator Lead	**7** Urinary Tract
D Extraction	**8** Basal Ganglia		**Y** Other Device	**8** Bone Marrow
F Fragmentation	**9** Thalamus		**Z** No Device	**9** Fallopian Tube
H Insertion	**A** Hypothalamus			**B** Cerebral Cisterns
J Inspection	**B** Pons			**F** Olfactory Nerve
K Map	**C** Cerebellum			**G** Optic Nerve
N Release	**D** Medulla Oblongata			**H** Oculomotor Nerve
P Removal	**E** Cranial Nerve			**J** Trochlear Nerve
Q Repair	**F** Olfactory Nerve			**K** Trigeminal Nerve
R Replacement	**G** Optic Nerve			**L** Abducens Nerve
S Reposition	**H** Oculomotor Nerve			**M** Facial Nerve
T Resection	**J** Trochlear Nerve			**N** Acoustic Nerve
U Supplement	**K** Trigeminal Nerve			**P** Glossopharyngeal Nerve
W Revision	**L** Abducens Nerve			**Q** Vagus Nerve
X Transfer	**M** Facial Nerve			**R** Accessory Nerve
	N Acoustic Nerve			**S** Hypoglossal Nerve
	P Glossopharyngeal Nerve			**X** Diagnostic
	Q Vagus Nerve			**Z** No Qualifier
	R Accessory Nerve			
	S Hypoglossal Nerve			
	T Spinal Meninges			
	U Spinal Canal			
	V Spinal Cord			
	W Cervical Spinal Cord			
	X Thoracic Spinal Cord			
	Y Lumbar Spinal Cord			

0: Medical and Surgical
1: Peripheral Nervous System and Cranial Nerves

Operation-Character 3	Body Part-Character 4	Approach-Character 5	Device-Character 6	Qualifier-Character 7
2 Change	**0** Cervical Plexus	**0** Open	**0** Drainage Device	**1** Cervical Nerve
5 Destruction	**1** Cervical Nerve	**3** Percutaneous	**2** Monitoring Device	**2** Phrenic Nerve
8 Division	**2** Phrenic Nerve	**4** Percutaneous Endoscopic	**7** Autologous Tissue Substitute	**4** Ulnar Nerve
9 Drainage	**3** Brachial Plexus	**X** External	**J** Synthetic Substitute	**5** Median Nerve
B Excision	**4** Ulnar Nerve		**K** Nonautologous Tissue Substitute	**6** Radial Nerve
C Extirpation	**5** Median Nerve		**M** Neurostimulator Lead	**8** Thoracic Nerve
D Extraction	**6** Radial Nerve		**Y** Other Device	**B** Lumbar Nerve
H Insertion	**8** Thoracic Nerve		**Z** No Device	**C** Perineal Nerve
J Inspection	**9** Lumbar Plexus			**D** Femoral Nerve
N Release	**A** Lumbosacral Plexus			**F** Sciatic Nerve
P Removal	**B** Lumbar Nerve			**G** Tibial Nerve
Q Repair	**C** Pudendal Nerve			**H** Peroneal Nerve
R Replacement	**D** Femoral Nerve			**X** Diagnostic
S Reposition	**F** Sciatic Nerve			**Z** No Qualifier
U Supplement	**G** Tibial Nerve			
W Revision	**H** Peroneal Nerve			
X Transfer	**K** Head and Neck Sympathetic Nerve			
	L Thoracic Sympathetic Nerve			
	M Abdominal Sympathetic Nerve			
	N Lumbar Sympathetic Nerve			
	P Sacral Sympathetic Nerve			
	Q Sacral Plexus			
	R Sacral Nerve			
	Y Peripheral Nerve			

0: Medical and Surgical
2: Heart and Great Vessels

Operation-Character 3	Body Part-Character 4	Approach-Character 5	Device-Character 6	Qualifier-Character 7
1 Bypass	**0** Coronary Artery, One Artery	**0** Open	**0** Monitoring Device, Pressure Sensor	**0** Allogeneic
4 Creation	**1** Coronary Artery, Two Arteries	**3** Percutaneous	**2** Monitoring Device	**1** Syngeneic
5 Destruction	**2** Coronary Artery, Three Arteries	**4** Percutaneous Endoscopic	**3** Infusion Device	**2** Zooplastic
7 Dilation	**3** Coronary Artery, Four or More Arteries	**X** External	**4** Intraluminal Device, Drug-eluting	**2** Common Atrioventricular Valve
8 Division	**4** Coronary Vein		**5** Intraluminal Device, Drug-eluting, Two	**3** Coronary Artery
B Excision	**5** Atrial Septum		**6** Intraluminal Device, Drug-eluting, Three	**4** Coronary Vein
C Extirpation	**6** Atrium, Right		**7** Intraluminal Device, Drug-eluting, Four or More	**5** Coronary Circulation
F Fragmentation	**7** Atrium, Left		**7** Autologous Tissue Substitute	**6** Bifurcation
H Insertion	**8** Conduction Mechanism		**8** Zooplastic Tissue	**7** Atrium, Left
J Inspection	**9** Chordae Tendineae		**9** Autologous Venous Tissue	**8** Internal Mammary, Right
K Map	**A** Heart		**A** Autologous Arterial Tissue	**9** Internal Mammary, Left
L Occlusion	**B** Heart, Right		**C** Extraluminal Device	**A** Innominate Artery
N Release	**C** Heart, Left		**D** Intraluminal Device	**B** Subclavian
P Removal	**D** Papillary Muscle		**E** Intraluminal Device, Two	**C** Thoracic Artery
Q Repair	**F** Aortic Valve		**E** Intraluminal Device, Branched or Fenestrated, One or Two Arteries	**D** Carotid
R Replacement	**G** Mitral Valve		**F** Intraluminal Device, Three	**E** Atrioventricular Valve, Left
S Reposition	**H** Pulmonary Valve		**F** Intraluminal Device, Branched or Fenestrated, Three or More Arteries	**F** Abdominal Artery
T Resection	**J** Tricuspid Valve		**G** Intraluminal Device, Four or More	**G** Atrioventricular Valve, Right
U Supplement	**K** Ventricle, Right		**J** Cardiac Lead, Pacemaker	**G** Axillary Artery
V Restriction	**L** Ventricle, Left		**J** Synthetic Substitute	**H** Transapical
W Revision	**M** Ventricular Septum		**K** Cardiac Lead, Defibrillator	**H** Brachial Artery
Y Transplantation	**N** Pericardium		**K** Nonautologous Tissue Substitute	**J** Intraoperative
	P Pulmonary Trunk		**M** Cardiac Lead	**J** Temporary
	Q Pulmonary Artery, Right		**N** Intracardiac Pacemaker	**J** Truncal Valve
	R Pulmonary Artery, Left		**Q** Implantable Heart Assist System	**K** Left Atrial Appendage
	S Pulmonary Vein, Right		**R** Short-term External Heart Assist System	**P** Pulmonary Trunk
	T Pulmonary Vein, Left		**T** Intraluminal Device, Radioactive	**Q** Pulmonary Artery, Right
	V Superior Vena Cava		**Y** Other Device	**R** Pulmonary Artery, Left
	W Thoracic Aorta, Descending		**Z** No Device	**S** Biventricular
	X Thoracic Aorta, Ascending/Arch			**S** Pulmonary Vein, Right
	Y Great Vessel			**T** Pulmonary Vein, Left
				T Ductus Arteriosus
				U Pulmonary Vein, Confluence
				V Lower Extremity Artery
				W Aorta
				X Diagnostic
				Z No Qualifier

0: Medical and Surgical
3: Upper Arteries

Operation-Character 3	Body Part-Character 4	Approach-Character 5	Device-Character 6	Qualifier-Character 7
1 Bypass	**0** Internal Mammary Artery, Right	**0** Open	**0** Drainage Device	**0** Upper Arm Artery, Right
5 Destruction	**1** Internal Mammary Artery, Left	**3** Percutaneous	**2** Monitoring Device	**1** Drug-Coated Balloon
7 Dilation	**2** Innominate Artery	**4** Percutaneous Endoscopic	**3** Infusion Device	**1** Upper Arm Artery, Left
9 Drainage	**3** Subclavian Artery, Right	**X** External	**4** Intraluminal Device, Drug-eluting	**2** Upper Arm Artery, Bilateral
B Excision	**4** Subclavian Artery, Left		**5** Intraluminal Device, Drug-eluting, Two	**3** Lower Arm Artery, Right
C Extirpation	**5** Axillary Artery, Right		**6** Intraluminal Device, Drug-eluting, Three	**4** Lower Arm Artery, Left
H Insertion	**6** Axillary Artery, Left		**7** Autologous Tissue Substitute	**5** Lower Arm Artery, Bilateral
J Inspection	**7** Brachial Artery, Right		**7** Intraluminal Device, Drug-eluting, Four or More	**6** Bifurcation
L Occlusion	**8** Brachial Artery, Left		**9** Autologous Venous Tissue	**6** Upper Leg Artery, Right
N Release	**9** Ulnar Artery, Right		**A** Autologous Arterial Tissue	**7** Stent Retriever
P Removal	**A** Ulnar Artery, Left		**B** Intraluminal Device, Bioactive	**7** Upper Leg Artery, Left
Q Repair	**B** Radial Artery, Right		**C** Extraluminal Device	**8** Upper Leg Artery, Bilateral
R Replacement	**C** Radial Artery, Left		**D** Intraluminal Device	**9** Lower Leg Artery, Right
S Reposition	**D** Hand Artery, Right		**E** Intraluminal Device, Two	**B** Lower Leg Artery, Left
U Supplement	**F** Hand Artery, Left		**F** Intraluminal Device, Three	**C** Lower Leg Artery, Bilateral
V Restriction	**G** Intracranial Artery		**G** Intraluminal Device, Four or More	**D** Upper Arm Vein
W Revision	**H** Common Carotid Artery, Right		**J** Synthetic Substitute	**F** Lower Arm Vein
	J Common Carotid Artery, Left		**K** Nonautologous Tissue Substitute	**G** Intracranial Artery
	K Internal Carotid Artery, Right		**M** Stimulator Lead	**J** Extracranial Artery, Right
	L Internal Carotid Artery, Left		**Y** Other Device	**K** Extracranial Artery, Left
	M External Carotid Artery, Right		**Z** No Device	**M** Pulmonary Artery, Right
	N External Carotid Artery, Left			**N** Pulmonary Artery, Left
	P Vertebral Artery, Right			**T** Abdominal Artery
	Q Vertebral Artery, Left			**V** Superior Vena Cava
	R Face Artery			**X** Diagnostic
	S Temporal Artery, Right			**Y** Upper Artery
	T Temporal Artery, Left			**Z** No Qualifier
	U Thyroid Artery, Right			
	V Thyroid Artery, Left			
	Y Upper Artery			

0: Medical and Surgical
4: Lower Arteries

Operation-Character 3	Body Part-Character 4	Approach-Character 5	Device-Character 6	Qualifier-Character 7
1 Bypass	**0** Abdominal Aorta	**0** Open	**0** Drainage Device	**0** Abdominal Aorta
5 Destruction	**1** Celiac Artery	**3** Percutaneous	**1** Radioactive Element	**1** Celiac Artery
7 Dilation	**2** Gastric Artery	**4** Percutaneous Endoscopic	**2** Monitoring Device	**1** Drug-Coated Balloon
9 Drainage	**3** Hepatic Artery	**X** External	**3** Infusion Device	**2** Mesenteric Artery
B Excision	**4** Splenic Artery		**4** Intraluminal Device, Drug-eluting	**3** Renal Artery, Right
C Extirpation	**5** Superior Mesenteric Artery		**5** Intraluminal Device, Drug-eluting, Two	**4** Renal Artery, Left
H Insertion	**6** Colic Artery, Right		**6** Intraluminal Device, Drug-eluting, Three	**5** Renal Artery, Bilateral
J Inspection	**7** Colic Artery, Left		**7** Autologous Tissue Substitute	**6** Bifurcation
L Occlusion	**8** Colic Artery, Middle		**7** Intraluminal Device, Drug-eluting, Four or More	**6** Common Iliac Artery, Right
N Release	**9** Renal Artery, Right		**9** Autologous Venous Tissue	**7** Common Iliac Artery, Left
P Removal	**A** Renal Artery, Left		**A** Autologous Arterial Tissue	**8** Common Iliac Arteries, Bilateral
Q Repair	**B** Inferior Mesenteric Artery		**C** Extraluminal Device	**9** Internal Iliac Artery, Right
R Replacement	**C** Common Iliac Artery, Right		**D** Intraluminal Device	**B** Internal Iliac Artery, Left
S Reposition	**D** Common Iliac Artery, Left		**E** Intraluminal Device, Branched or Fenestrated, One or Two Arteries	**C** Internal Iliac Arteries, Bilateral
U Supplement	**E** Internal Iliac Artery, Right		**E** Intraluminal Device, Two	**D** External Iliac Artery, Right
V Restriction	**F** Internal Iliac Artery, Left		**F** Intraluminal Device, Branched or Fenestrated, Three or More Arteries	**F** External Iliac Artery, Left
W Revision	**H** External Iliac Artery, Right		**F** Intraluminal Device, Three	**G** External Iliac Arteries, Bilateral
	J External Iliac Artery, Left		**G** Intraluminal Device, Four or More	**H** Femoral Artery, Right
	K Femoral Artery, Right		**J** Synthetic Substitute	**J** Femoral Artery, Left
	L Femoral Artery, Left		**K** Nonautologous Tissue Substitute	**J** Temporary
	M Popliteal Artery, Right		**Y** Other Device	**K** Femoral Arteries, Bilateral
	N Popliteal Artery, Left		**Z** No Device	**L** Popliteal Artery
	P Anterior Tibial Artery, Right			**M** Peroneal Artery
	Q Anterior Tibial Artery, Left			**N** Posterior Tibial Artery
	R Posterior Tibial Artery, Right			**P** Foot Artery
	S Posterior Tibial Artery, Left			**Q** Lower Extremity Artery
	T Peroneal Artery, Right			**R** Lower Artery
	U Peroneal Artery, Left			**S** Lower Extremity Vein
	V Foot Artery, Right			**T** Uterine Artery, Right
	W Foot Artery, Left			**U** Uterine Artery, Left
	Y Lower Artery			**X** Diagnostic
				Z No Qualifier

0: Medical and Surgical
5: Upper Veins

Operation-Character 3	Body Part-Character 4	Approach-Character 5	Device-Character 6	Qualifier-Character 7
1 Bypass	**0** Azygos Vein	**0** Open	**0** Drainage Device	**1** Drug-Coated Balloon
5 Destruction	**1** Hemiazygos Vein	**3** Percutaneous	**2** Monitoring Device	**X** Diagnostic
7 Dilation	**3** Innominate Vein, Right	**4** Percutaneous Endoscopic	**3** Infusion Device	**Y** Upper Vein
9 Drainage	**4** Innominate Vein, Left	**X** External	**7** Autologous Tissue Substitute	**Z** No Qualifier
B Excision	**5** Subclavian Vein, Right		**9** Autologous Venous Tissue	
C Extirpation	**6** Subclavian Vein, Left		**A** Autologous Arterial Tissue	
D Extraction	**7** Axillary Vein, Right		**C** Extraluminal Device	
H Insertion	**8** Axillary Vein, Left		**D** Intraluminal Device	
J Inspection	**9** Brachial Vein, Right		**J** Synthetic Substitute	
L Occlusion	**A** Brachial Vein, Left		**K** Nonautologous Tissue Substitute	
N Release	**B** Basilic Vein, Right		**M** Neurostimulator Lead	
P Removal	**C** Basilic Vein, Left		**Y** Other Device	
Q Repair	**D** Cephalic Vein, Right		**Z** No Device	
R Replacement	**F** Cephalic Vein, Left			
S Reposition	**G** Hand Vein, Right			
U Supplement	**H** Hand Vein, Left			
V Restriction	**L** Intracranial Vein			
W Revision	**M** Internal Jugular Vein, Right			
	N Internal Jugular Vein, Left			
	P External Jugular Vein, Right			
	Q External Jugular Vein, Left			
	R Vertebral Vein, Right			
	S Vertebral Vein, Left			
	T Face Vein, Right			
	V Face Vein, Left			
	Y Upper Vein			

0: Medical and Surgical
6: Lower Veins

Operation-Character 3	Body Part-Character 4	Approach-Character 5	Device-Character 6	Qualifier-Character 7
1 Bypass	**0** Inferior Vena Cava	**0** Open	**0** Drainage Device	**4** Hepatic Vein
5 Destruction	**1** Splenic Vein	**3** Percutaneous	**2** Monitoring Device	**5** Superior Mesenteric Vein
7 Dilation	**2** Gastric Vein	**4** Percutaneous Endoscopic	**3** Infusion Device	**6** Inferior Mesenteric Vein
9 Drainage	**3** Esophageal Vein	**7** Via Natural or Artificial Opening	**7** Autologous Tissue Substitute	**9** Renal Vein, Right
B Excision	**4** Hepatic Vein	**8** Via Natural or Artificial Opening Endoscopic	**9** Autologous Venous Tissue	**B** Renal Vein, Left
C Extirpation	**5** Superior Mesenteric Vein	**X** External	**A** Autologous Arterial Tissue	**C** Hemorrhoidal Plexus
D Extraction	**6** Inferior Mesenteric Vein		**C** Extraluminal Device	**P** Pulmonary Trunk
H Insertion	**7** Colic Vein		**D** Intraluminal Device	**Q** Pulmonary Artery, Right
J Inspection	**8** Portal Vein		**J** Synthetic Substitute	**R** Pulmonary Artery, Left
L Occlusion	**9** Renal Vein, Right		**K** Nonautologous Tissue Substitute	**T** Via Umbilical Vein
N Release	**B** Renal Vein, Left		**Y** Other Device	**X** Diagnostic
P Removal	**C** Common Iliac Vein, Right		**Z** No Device	**Y** Lower Vein
Q Repair	**D** Common Iliac Vein, Left			**Z** No Qualifier
R Replacement	**F** External Iliac Vein, Right			
S Reposition	**G** External Iliac Vein, Left			
U Supplement	**H** Hypogastric Vein, Right			
V Restriction	**J** Hypogastric Vein, Left			
W Revision	**M** Femoral Vein, Right			
	N Femoral Vein, Left			
	P Saphenous Vein, Right			
	Q Saphenous Vein, Left			
	T Foot Vein, Right			
	V Foot Vein, Left			
	Y Lower Vein			

0: Medical and Surgical
7: Lymphatic and Hemic Systems

Operation-Character 3	Body Part-Character 4	Approach-Character 5	Device-Character 6	Qualifier-Character 7
2 Change	**0** Lymphatic, Head	**0** Open	**0** Drainage Device	**0** Allogeneic
5 Destruction	**1** Lymphatic, Right Neck	**3** Percutaneous	**3** Infusion Device	**1** Syngeneic
9 Drainage	**2** Lymphatic, Left Neck	**4** Percutaneous Endoscopic	**7** Autologous Tissue Substitute	**2** Zooplastic
B Excision	**3** Lymphatic, Right Upper Extremity	**8** Via Natural or Artificial Opening Endoscopic	**C** Extraluminal Device	**X** Diagnostic
C Extirpation	**4** Lymphatic, Left Upper Extremity	**X** External	**D** Intraluminal Device	**Z** No Qualifier
D Extraction	**5** Lymphatic, Right Axillary		**J** Synthetic Substitute	
H Insertion	**6** Lymphatic, Left Axillary		**K** Nonautologous Tissue Substitute	
J Inspection	**7** Lymphatic, Thorax		**Y** Other Device	
L Occlusion	**8** Lymphatic, Internal Mammary, Right		**Z** No Device	
N Release	**9** Lymphatic, Internal Mammary, Left			
P Removal	**B** Lymphatic, Mesenteric			
Q Repair	**C** Lymphatic, Pelvis			
S Reposition	**D** Lymphatic, Aortic			
T Resection	**F** Lymphatic, Right Lower Extremity			
U Supplement	**G** Lymphatic, Left Lower Extremity			
V Restriction	**H** Lymphatic, Right Inguinal			
W Revision	**J** Lymphatic, Left Inguinal			
Y Transplantation	**K** Thoracic Duct			
	L Cisterna Chyli			
	M Thymus			
	N Lymphatic			
	P Spleen			
	Q Bone Marrow, Sternum			
	R Bone Marrow, Iliac			
	S Bone Marrow, Vertebral			
	T Bone Marrow			

0: Medical and Surgical
8: Eye

Operation-Character 3	Body Part-Character 4	Approach-Character 5	Device-Character 6	Qualifier-Character 7
0 Alteration	**0** Eye, Right	**0** Open	**0** Drainage Device	**3** Nasal Cavity
1 Bypass	**1** Eye, Left	**3** Percutaneous	**0** Synthetic Substitute, Intraocular Telescope	**4** Sclera
2 Change	**2** Anterior Chamber, Right	**7** Via Natural or Artificial Opening	**1** Radioactive Element	**X** Diagnostic
5 Destruction	**3** Anterior Chamber, Left	**8** Via Natural or Artificial Opening Endoscopic	**3** Infusion Device	**Z** No Qualifier
7 Dilation	**4** Vitreous, Right	**X** External	**5** Epiretinal Visual Prosthesis	
9 Drainage	**5** Vitreous, Left		**7** Autologous Tissue Substitute	
B Excision	**6** Sclera, Right		**C** Extraluminal Device	
C Extirpation	**7** Sclera, Left		**D** Intraluminal Device	
D Extraction	**8** Cornea, Right		**J** Synthetic Substitute	
F Fragmentation	**9** Cornea, Left		**K** Nonautologous Tissue Substitute	
H Insertion	**A** Choroid, Right		**Y** Other Device	
J Inspection	**B** Choroid, Left		**Z** No Device	
L Occlusion	**C** Iris, Right			
M Reattachment	**D** Iris, Left			
N Release	**E** Retina, Right			
P Removal	**F** Retina, Left			
Q Repair	**G** Retinal Vessel, Right			
R Replacement	**H** Retinal Vessel, Left			
S Reposition	**J** Lens, Right			
T Resection	**K** Lens, Left			
U Supplement	**L** Extraocular Muscle, Right			
V Restriction	**M** Extraocular Muscle, Left			
W Revision	**N** Upper Eyelid, Right			
X Transfer	**P** Upper Eyelid, Left			
	Q Lower Eyelid, Right			
	R Lower Eyelid, Left			
	S Conjunctiva, Right			
	T Conjunctiva, Left			
	V Lacrimal Gland, Right			
	W Lacrimal Gland, Left			
	X Lacrimal Duct, Right			
	Y Lacrimal Duct, Left			

0: Medical and Surgical
9: Ear, Nose, Sinus

Operation-Character 3	Body Part-Character 4	Approach-Character 5	Device-Character 6	Qualifier-Character 7
0 Alteration	**0** External Ear, Right	**0** Open	**0** Drainage Device	**0** Endolymphatic
1 Bypass	**1** External Ear, Left	**3** Percutaneous	**4** Hearing Device, Bone Conduction	**X** Diagnostic
2 Change	**2** External Ear, Bilateral	**4** Percutaneous Endoscopic	**5** Hearing Device, Single Channel Cochlear Prosthesis	**Z** No Qualifier
3 Control	**3** External Auditory Canal, Right	**7** Via Natural or Artificial Opening	**6** Hearing Device, Multiple Channel Cochlear Prosthesis	
5 Destruction	**4** External Auditory Canal, Left	**8** Via Natural or Artificial Opening Endoscopic	**7** Autologous Tissue Substitute	
7 Dilation	**5** Middle Ear, Right	**X** External	**B** Intraluminal Device, Airway	
8 Division	**6** Middle Ear, Left		**D** Intraluminal Device	
9 Drainage	**7** Tympanic Membrane, Right		**J** Synthetic Substitute	
B Excision	**8** Tympanic Membrane, Left		**K** Nonautologous Tissue Substitute	
C Extirpation	**9** Auditory Ossicle, Right		**S** Hearing Device	
D Extraction	**A** Auditory Ossicle, Left		**Y** Other Device	
H Insertion	**B** Mastoid Sinus, Right		**Z** No Device	
J Inspection	**C** Mastoid Sinus, Left			
M Reattachment	**D** Inner Ear, Right			
N Release	**E** Inner Ear, Left			
P Removal	**F** Eustachian Tube, Right			
Q Repair	**G** Eustachian Tube, Left			
R Replacement	**H** Ear, Right			
S Reposition	**J** Ear, Left			
T Resection	**K** Nasal Mucosa and Soft Tissue			
U Supplement	**L** Nasal Turbinate			
W Revision	**M** Nasal Septum			
	N Nasopharynx			
	P Accessory Sinus			
	Q Maxillary Sinus, Right			
	R Maxillary Sinus, Left			
	S Frontal Sinus, Right			
	T Frontal Sinus, Left			
	U Ethmoid Sinus, Right			
	V Ethmoid Sinus, Left			
	W Sphenoid Sinus, Right			
	X Sphenoid Sinus, Left			
	Y Sinus			

0: Medical and Surgical
B: Respiratory System

Operation-Character 3	Body Part-Character 4	Approach-Character 5	Device-Character 6	Qualifier-Character 7
1 Bypass	**0** Tracheobronchial Tree	**0** Open	**0** Drainage Device	**0** Allogeneic
2 Change	**1** Trachea	**3** Percutaneous	**1** Radioactive Element	**1** Syngeneic
5 Destruction	**2** Carina	**4** Percutaneous Endoscopic	**2** Monitoring Device	**2** Zooplastic
7 Dilation	**3** Main Bronchus, Right	**7** Via Natural or Artificial Opening	**3** Infusion Device	**4** Cutaneous
9 Drainage	**4** Upper Lobe Bronchus, Right	**8** Via Natural or Artificial Opening Endoscopic	**7** Autologous Tissue Substitute	**6** Esophagus
B Excision	**5** Middle Lobe Bronchus, Right	**X** External	**C** Extraluminal Device	**X** Diagnostic
C Extirpation	**6** Lower Lobe Bronchus, Right		**D** Intraluminal Device	**Z** No Qualifier
D Extraction	**7** Main Bronchus, Left		**E** Intraluminal Device, Endotracheal Airway	
F Fragmentation	**8** Upper Lobe Bronchus, Left		**F** Tracheostomy Device	
H Insertion	**9** Lingula Bronchus		**G** Intraluminal Device, Endobronchial Valve	
J Inspection	**B** Lower Lobe Bronchus, Left		**J** Synthetic Substitute	
L Occlusion	**C** Upper Lung Lobe, Right		**K** Nonautologous Tissue Substitute	
M Reattachment	**D** Middle Lung Lobe, Right		**M** Diaphragmatic Pacemaker Lead	
N Release	**F** Lower Lung Lobe, Right		**Y** Other Device	
P Removal	**G** Upper Lung Lobe, Left		**Z** No Device	
Q Repair	**H** Lung Lingula			
R Replacement	**J** Lower Lung Lobe, Left			
S Reposition	**K** Lung, Right			
T Resection	**L** Lung, Left			
U Supplement	**M** Lungs, Bilateral			
V Restriction	**N** Pleura, Right			
W Revision	**P** Pleura, Left			
Y Transplantation	**Q** Pleura			
	T Diaphragm			

0: Medical and Surgical
C: Mouth and Throat

Operation-Character 3	Body Part-Character 4	Approach-Character 5	Device-Character 6	Qualifier-Character 7
0 Alteration	**0** Upper Lip	**0** Open	**0** Drainage Device	**0** Single
2 Change	**1** Lower Lip	**3** Percutaneous	**1** Radioactive Element	**1** Multiple
5 Destruction	**2** Hard Palate	**4** Percutaneous Endoscopic	**5** External Fixation Device	**2** All
7 Dilation	**3** Soft Palate	**7** Via Natural or Artificial Opening	**7** Autologous Tissue Substitute	**X** Diagnostic
9 Drainage	**4** Buccal Mucosa	**8** Via Natural or Artificial Opening Endoscopic	**B** Intraluminal Device, Airway	**Z** No Qualifier
B Excision	**5** Upper Gingiva	**X** External	**C** Extraluminal Device	
C Extirpation	**6** Lower Gingiva		**D** Intraluminal Device	
D Extraction	**7** Tongue		**J** Synthetic Substitute	
F Fragmentation	**8** Parotid Gland, Right		**K** Nonautologous Tissue Substitute	
H Insertion	**9** Parotid Gland, Left		**Y** Other Device	
J Inspection	**A** Salivary Gland		**Z** No Device	
L Occlusion	**B** Parotid Duct, Right			
M Reattachment	**C** Parotid Duct, Left			
N Release	**D** Sublingual Gland, Right			
P Removal	**F** Sublingual Gland, Left			
Q Repair	**G** Submaxillary Gland, Right			
R Replacement	**H** Submaxillary Gland, Left			
S Reposition	**J** Minor Salivary Gland			
T Resection	**M** Pharynx			
U Supplement	**N** Uvula			
V Restriction	**P** Tonsils			
W Revision	**Q** Adenoids			
X Transfer	**R** Epiglottis			
	S Larynx			
	T Vocal Cord, Right			
	V Vocal Cord, Left			
	W Upper Tooth			
	X Lower Tooth			
	Y Mouth and Throat			

0: Medical and Surgical
D: Gastrointestinal System

Operation-Character 3	Body Part-Character 4	Approach-Character 5	Device-Character 6	Qualifier-Character 7
1 Bypass	**0** Upper Intestinal Tract	**0** Open	**0** Drainage Device	**0** Allogeneic
2 Change	**1** Esophagus, Upper	**3** Percutaneous	**1** Radioactive Element	**1** Syngeneic
5 Destruction	**2** Esophagus, Middle	**4** Percutaneous Endoscopic	**2** Monitoring Device	**2** Zooplastic
7 Dilation	**3** Esophagus, Lower	**7** Via Natural or Artificial Opening	**3** Infusion Device	**3** Vertical
8 Division	**4** Esophagogastric Junction	**8** Via Natural or Artificial Opening Endoscopic	**7** Autologous Tissue Substitute	**4** Cutaneous
9 Drainage	**5** Esophagus	**X** External	**B** Intraluminal Device, Airway	**5** Esophagus
B Excision	**6** Stomach		**C** Extraluminal Device	**6** Stomach
C Extirpation	**7** Stomach, Pylorus		**D** Intraluminal Device	**9** Duodenum
D Extraction	**8** Small Intestine		**J** Synthetic Substitute	**A** Jejunum
F Fragmentation	**9** Duodenum		**K** Nonautologous Tissue Substitute	**B** Ileum
H Insertion	**A** Jejunum		**L** Artificial Sphincter	**H** Cecum
J Inspection	**B** Ileum		**M** Stimulator Lead	**K** Ascending Colon
L Occlusion	**C** Ileocecal Valve		**U** Feeding Device	**L** Transverse Colon
M Reattachment	**D** Lower Intestinal Tract		**Y** Other Device	**M** Descending Colon
N Release	**E** Large Intestine		**Z** No Device	**N** Sigmoid Colon
P Removal	**F** Large Intestine, Right			**P** Rectum
Q Repair	**G** Large Intestine, Left			**Q** Anus
R Replacement	**H** Cecum			**X** Diagnostic
S Reposition	**J** Appendix			**Z** No Qualifier
T Resection	**K** Ascending Colon			
U Supplement	**L** Transverse Colon			
V Restriction	**M** Descending Colon			
W Revision	**N** Sigmoid Colon			
X Transfer	**P** Rectum			
Y Transplantation	**Q** Anus			
	R Anal Sphincter			
	U Omentum			
	V Mesentery			
	W Peritoneum			

0: Medical and Surgical
F: Hepatobiliary System and Pancreas

Operation-Character 3	Body Part-Character 4	Approach-Character 5	Device-Character 6	Qualifier-Character 7
1 Bypass	**0** Liver	**0** Open	**0** Drainage Device	**0** Allogeneic
2 Change	**1** Liver, Right Lobe	**3** Percutaneous	**1** Radioactive Element	**1** Syngeneic
5 Destruction	**2** Liver, Left Lobe	**4** Percutaneous Endoscopic	**2** Monitoring Device	**2** Zooplastic
7 Dilation	**4** Gallbladder	**7** Via Natural or Artificial Opening	**3** Infusion Device	**3** Duodenum
8 Division	**5** Hepatic Duct, Right	**8** Via Natural or Artificial Opening Endoscopic	**7** Autologous Tissue Substitute	**4** Stomach
9 Drainage	**6** Hepatic Duct, Left	**X** External	**C** Extraluminal Device	**5** Hepatic Duct, Right
B Excision	**7** Hepatic Duct, Common		**D** Intraluminal Device	**6** Hepatic Duct, Left
C Extirpation	**8** Cystic Duct		**J** Synthetic Substitute	**7** Hepatic Duct, Caudate
D Extraction	**9** Common Bile Duct		**K** Nonautologous Tissue Substitute	**8** Cystic Duct
F Fragmentation	**B** Hepatobiliary Duct		**Y** Other Device	**9** Common Bile Duct
H Insertion	**C** Ampulla of Vater		**Z** No Device	**B** Small Intestine
J Inspection	**D** Pancreatic Duct			**C** Large Intestine
L Occlusion	**F** Pancreatic Duct, Accessory			**F** Irreversible Electroporation
M Reattachment	**G** Pancreas			**X** Diagnostic
N Release				**Z** No Qualifier
P Removal				
Q Repair				
R Replacement				
S Reposition				
T Resection				
U Supplement				
V Restriction				
W Revision				
Y Transplantation				

0: Medical and Surgical
G: Endocrine System

Operation-Character 3	Body Part-Character 4	Approach-Character 5	Device-Character 6	Qualifier-Character 7
2 Change	**0** Pituitary Gland	**0** Open	**0** Drainage Device	**X** Diagnostic
5 Destruction	**1** Pineal Body	**3** Percutaneous	**2** Monitoring Device	**Z** No Qualifier
8 Division	**2** Adrenal Gland, Left	**4** Percutaneous Endoscopic	**3** Infusion Device	
9 Drainage	**3** Adrenal Gland, Right	**X** External	**Y** Other Device	
B Excision	**4** Adrenal Glands, Bilateral		**Z** No Device	
C Extirpation	**5** Adrenal Gland			
H Insertion	**6** Carotid Body, Left			
J Inspection	**7** Carotid Body, Right			
M Reattachment	**8** Carotid Bodies, Bilateral			
N Release	**9** Para-aortic Body			
P Removal	**B** Coccygeal Glomus			
Q Repair	**C** Glomus Jugulare			
S Reposition	**D** Aortic Body			
T Resection	**F** Paraganglion Extremity			
W Revision	**G** Thyroid Gland Lobe, Left			
	H Thyroid Gland Lobe, Right			
	J Thyroid Gland Isthmus			
	K Thyroid Gland			
	L Superior Parathyroid Gland, Right			
	M Superior Parathyroid Gland, Left			
	N Inferior Parathyroid Gland, Right			
	P Inferior Parathyroid Gland, Left			
	Q Parathyroid Glands, Multiple			
	R Parathyroid Gland			
	S Endocrine Gland			

0: Medical and Surgical
H: Skin and Breast

Operation-Character 3	Body Part-Character 4	Approach-Character 5	Device-Character 6	Qualifier-Character 7
0 Alteration	**0** Skin, Scalp	**0** Open	**0** Drainage Device	**3** Full Thickness
2 Change	**1** Skin, Face	**3** Percutaneous	**1** Radioactive Element	**4** Partial Thickness
5 Destruction	**2** Skin, Right Ear	**7** Via Natural or Artificial Opening	**7** Autologous Tissue Substitute	**5** Latissimus Dorsi Myocutaneous Flap
8 Division	**3** Skin, Left Ear	**8** Via Natural or Artificial Opening Endoscopic	**J** Synthetic Substitute	**6** Transverse Rectus Abdominis Myocutaneous Flap
9 Drainage	**4** Skin, Neck	**X** External	**K** Nonautologous Tissue Substitute	**7** Deep Inferior Epigastric Artery Perforator Flap
B Excision	**5** Skin, Chest		**N** Tissue Expander	**8** Superficial Inferior Epigastric Artery Flap
C Extirpation	**6** Skin, Back		**Y** Other Device	**9** Gluteal Artery Perforator Flap
D Extraction	**7** Skin, Abdomen		**Z** No Device	**D** Multiple
H Insertion	**8** Skin, Buttock			**X** Diagnostic
J Inspection	**9** Skin, Perineum			**Z** No Qualifier
M Reattachment	**A** Skin, Inguinal			
N Release	**B** Skin, Right Upper Arm			
P Removal	**C** Skin, Left Upper Arm			
Q Repair	**D** Skin, Right Lower Arm			
R Replacement	**E** Skin, Left Lower Arm			
S Reposition	**F** Skin, Right Hand			
T Resection	**G** Skin, Left Hand			
U Supplement	**H** Skin, Right Upper Leg			
W Revision	**J** Skin, Left Upper Leg			
X Transfer	**K** Skin, Right Lower Leg			
	L Skin, Left Lower Leg			
	M Skin, Right Foot			
	N Skin, Left Foot			
	P Skin			
	Q Finger Nail			
	R Toe Nail			
	S Hair			
	T Breast, Right			
	U Breast, Left			
	V Breast, Bilateral			
	W Nipple, Right			
	X Nipple, Left			
	Y Supernumerary Breast			

0: Medical and Surgical
J: Subcutaneous Tissue and Fascia

Operation-Character 3	Body Part-Character 4	Approach-Character 5	Device-Character 6	Qualifier-Character 7
0 Alteration	**0** Subcutaneous Tissue and Fascia, Scalp	**0** Open	**0** Drainage Device	**B** Skin and Subcutaneous Tissue
2 Change	**1** Subcutaneous Tissue and Fascia, Face	**3** Percutaneous	**0** Monitoring Device, Hemodynamic	**C** Skin, Subcutaneous Tissue and Fascia
5 Destruction	**4** Subcutaneous Tissue and Fascia, Right Neck	**X** External	**1** Radioactive Element	**X** Diagnostic
8 Division	**5** Subcutaneous Tissue and Fascia, Left Neck		**2** Monitoring Device	**Z** No Qualifier
9 Drainage	**6** Subcutaneous Tissue and Fascia, Chest		**3** Infusion Device	
B Excision	**7** Subcutaneous Tissue and Fascia, Back		**4** Pacemaker, Single Chamber	
C Extirpation	**8** Subcutaneous Tissue and Fascia, Abdomen		**5** Pacemaker, Single Chamber Rate Responsive	
D Extraction	**9** Subcutaneous Tissue and Fascia, Buttock		**6** Pacemaker, Dual Chamber	
H Insertion	**B** Subcutaneous Tissue and Fascia, Perineum		**7** Autologous Tissue Substitute	
J Inspection	**C** Subcutaneous Tissue and Fascia, Pelvic Region		**7** Cardiac Resynchronization Pacemaker Pulse Generator	
N Release	**D** Subcutaneous Tissue and Fascia, Right Upper Arm		**8** Defibrillator Generator	
P Removal	**F** Subcutaneous Tissue and Fascia, Left Upper Arm		**9** Cardiac Resynchronization Defibrillator Pulse Generator	
Q Repair	**G** Subcutaneous Tissue and Fascia, Right Lower Arm		**A** Contractility Modulation Device	
R Replacement	**H** Subcutaneous Tissue and Fascia, Left Lower Arm		**B** Stimulator Generator, Single Array	
U Supplement	**J** Subcutaneous Tissue and Fascia, Right Hand		**C** Stimulator Generator, Single Array Rechargeable	
W Revision	**K** Subcutaneous Tissue and Fascia, Left Hand		**D** Stimulator Generator, Multiple Array	
X Transfer	**L** Subcutaneous Tissue and Fascia, Right Upper Leg		**E** Stimulator Generator, Multiple Array Rechargeable	
	M Subcutaneous Tissue and Fascia, Left Upper Leg		**H** Contraceptive Device	
	N Subcutaneous Tissue and Fascia, Right Lower Leg		**J** Synthetic Substitute	
	P Subcutaneous Tissue and Fascia, Left Lower Leg		**K** Nonautologous Tissue Substitute	
	Q Subcutaneous Tissue and Fascia, Right Foot		**M** Stimulator Generator	
	R Subcutaneous Tissue and Fascia, Left Foot		**N** Tissue Expander	
	S Subcutaneous Tissue and Fascia, Head and Neck		**P** Cardiac Rhythm Related Device	
	T Subcutaneous Tissue and Fascia, Trunk		**V** Infusion Device, Pump	
	V Subcutaneous Tissue and Fascia, Upper Extremity		**W** Vascular Access Device, Totally Implantable	
	W Subcutaneous Tissue and Fascia, Lower Extremity		**X** Vascular Access Device, Tunneled	
			Y Other Device	
			Z No Device	

0: Medical and Surgical
K: Muscles

Operation-Character 3	Body Part-Character 4	Approach-Character 5	Device-Character 6	Qualifier-Character 7
2 Change	**0** Head Muscle	**0** Open	**0** Drainage Device	**0** Skin
5 Destruction	**1** Facial Muscle	**3** Percutaneous	**7** Autologous Tissue Substitute	**1** Subcutaneous Tissue
8 Division	**2** Neck Muscle, Right	**4** Percutaneous Endoscopic	**J** Synthetic Substitute	**2** Skin and Subcutaneous Tissue
9 Drainage	**3** Neck Muscle, Left	**X** External	**K** Nonautologous Tissue Substitute	**5** Latissimus Dorsi Myocutaneous Flap
B Excision	**4** Tongue, Palate, Pharynx Muscle		**M** Stimulator Lead	**6** Transverse Rectus Abdominis Myocutaneous Flap
C Extirpation	**5** Shoulder Muscle, Right		**Y** Other Device	**7** Deep Inferior Epigastric Artery Perforator Flap
D Extraction	**6** Shoulder Muscle, Left		**Z** No Device	**8** Superficial Inferior Epigastric Artery Flap
H Insertion	**7** Upper Arm Muscle, Right			**9** Gluteal Artery Perforator Flap
J Inspection	**8** Upper Arm Muscle, Left			**X** Diagnostic
M Reattachment	**9** Lower Arm and Wrist Muscle, Right			**Z** No Qualifier
N Release	**B** Lower Arm and Wrist Muscle, Left			
P Removal	**C** Hand Muscle, Right			
Q Repair	**D** Hand Muscle, Left			
R Replacement	**F** Trunk Muscle, Right			
S Reposition	**G** Trunk Muscle, Left			
T Resection	**H** Thorax Muscle, Right			
U Supplement	**J** Thorax Muscle, Left			
W Revision	**K** Abdomen Muscle, Right			
X Transfer	**L** Abdomen Muscle, Left			
	M Perineum Muscle			
	N Hip Muscle, Right			
	P Hip Muscle, Left			
	Q Upper Leg Muscle, Right			
	R Upper Leg Muscle, Left			
	S Lower Leg Muscle, Right			
	T Lower Leg Muscle, Left			
	V Foot Muscle, Right			
	W Foot Muscle, Left			
	X Upper Muscle			
	Y Lower Muscle			

0: Medical and Surgical
L: Tendons

Operation-Character 3	Body Part-Character 4	Approach-Character 5	Device-Character 6	Qualifier-Character 7
2 Change	**0** Head and Neck Tendon	**0** Open	**0** Drainage Device	**X** Diagnostic
5 Destruction	**1** Shoulder Tendon, Right	**3** Percutaneous	**7** Autologous Tissue Substitute	**Z** No Qualifier
8 Division	**2** Shoulder Tendon, Left	**4** Percutaneous Endoscopic	**J** Synthetic Substitute	
9 Drainage	**3** Upper Arm Tendon, Right	**X** External	**K** Nonautologous Tissue Substitute	
B Excision	**4** Upper Arm Tendon, Left		**Y** Other Device	
C Extirpation	**5** Lower Arm and Wrist Tendon, Right		**Z** No Device	
D Extraction	**6** Lower Arm and Wrist Tendon, Left			
H Insertion	**7** Hand Tendon, Right			
J Inspection	**8** Hand Tendon, Left			
M Reattachment	**9** Trunk Tendon, Right			
N Release	**B** Trunk Tendon, Left			
P Removal	**C** Thorax Tendon, Right			
Q Repair	**D** Thorax Tendon, Left			
R Replacement	**F** Abdomen Tendon, Right			
S Reposition	**G** Abdomen Tendon, Left			
T Resection	**H** Perineum Tendon			
U Supplement	**J** Hip Tendon, Right			
W Revision	**K** Hip Tendon, Left			
X Transfer	**L** Upper Leg Tendon, Right			
	M Upper Leg Tendon, Left			
	N Lower Leg Tendon, Right			
	P Lower Leg Tendon, Left			
	Q Knee Tendon, Right			
	R Knee Tendon, Left			
	S Ankle Tendon, Right			
	T Ankle Tendon, Left			
	V Foot Tendon, Right			
	W Foot Tendon, Left			
	X Upper Tendon			
	Y Lower Tendon			

0: Medical and Surgical
M: Bursae and Ligaments

Operation-Character 3	Body Part-Character 4	Approach-Character 5	Device-Character 6	Qualifier-Character 7
2 Change	**0** Head and Neck Bursa and Ligament	**0** Open	**0** Drainage Device	**X** Diagnostic
5 Destruction	**1** Shoulder Bursa and Ligament, Right	**3** Percutaneous	**7** Autologous Tissue Substitute	**Z** No Qualifier
8 Division	**2** Shoulder Bursa and Ligament, Left	**4** Percutaneous Endoscopic	**J** Synthetic Substitute	
9 Drainage	**3** Elbow Bursa and Ligament, Right	**X** External	**K** Nonautologous Tissue Substitute	
B Excision	**4** Elbow Bursa and Ligament, Left		**Y** Other Device	
C Extirpation	**5** Wrist Bursa and Ligament, Right		**Z** No Device	
D Extraction	**6** Wrist Bursa and Ligament, Left			
H Insertion	**7** Hand Bursa and Ligament, Right			
J Inspection	**8** Hand Bursa and Ligament, Left			
M Reattachment	**9** Upper Extremity Bursa and Ligament, Right			
N Release	**B** Upper Extremity Bursa and Ligament, Left			
P Removal	**C** Upper Spine Bursa and Ligament			
Q Repair	**D** Lower Spine Bursa and Ligament			
R Replacement	**F** Sternum Bursa and Ligament			
S Reposition	**G** Rib(s) Bursa and Ligament			
T Resection	**H** Abdomen Bursa and Ligament, Right			
U Supplement	**J** Abdomen Bursa and Ligament, Left			
W Revision	**K** Perineum Bursa and Ligament			
X Transfer	**L** Hip Bursa and Ligament, Right			
	M Hip Bursa and Ligament, Left			
	N Knee Bursa and Ligament, Right			
	P Knee Bursa and Ligament, Left			
	Q Ankle Bursa and Ligament, Right			
	R Ankle Bursa and Ligament, Left			
	S Foot Bursa and Ligament, Right			
	T Foot Bursa and Ligament, Left			
	V Lower Extremity Bursa and Ligament, Right			
	W Lower Extremity Bursa and Ligament, Left			
	X Upper Bursa and Ligament			
	Y Lower Bursa and Ligament			

0: Medical and Surgical
N: Head and Facial Bones

Operation-Character 3	Body Part-Character 4	Approach-Character 5	Device-Character 6	Qualifier-Character 7
2 Change	**0** Skull	**0** Open	**0** Drainage Device	**X** Diagnostic
5 Destruction	**1** Frontal Bone	**3** Percutaneous	**4** Internal Fixation Device	**Z** No Qualifier
8 Division	**3** Parietal Bone, Right	**4** Percutaneous Endoscopic	**5** External Fixation Device	
9 Drainage	**4** Parietal Bone, Left	**X** External	**7** Autologous Tissue Substitute	
B Excision	**5** Temporal Bone, Right		**J** Synthetic Substitute	
C Extirpation	**6** Temporal Bone, Left		**K** Nonautologous Tissue Substitute	
D Extraction	**7** Occipital Bone		**M** Bone Growth Stimulator	
H Insertion	**B** Nasal Bone		**N** Neurostimulator Generator	
J Inspection	**C** Sphenoid Bone		**S** Hearing Device	
N Release	**F** Ethmoid Bone, Right		**Y** Other Device	
P Removal	**G** Ethmoid Bone, Left		**Z** No Device	
Q Repair	**H** Lacrimal Bone, Right			
R Replacement	**J** Lacrimal Bone, Left			
S Reposition	**K** Palatine Bone, Right			
T Resection	**L** Palatine Bone, Left			
U Supplement	**M** Zygomatic Bone, Right			
W Revision	**N** Zygomatic Bone, Left			
	P Orbit, Right			
	Q Orbit, Left			
	R Maxilla			
	T Mandible, Right			
	V Mandible, Left			
	W Facial Bone			
	X Hyoid Bone			

0: Medical and Surgical
P: Upper Bones

Operation-Character 3	Body Part-Character 4	Approach-Character 5	Device-Character 6	Qualifier-Character 7
2 Change	**0** Sternum	**0** Open	**0** Drainage Device	**X** Diagnostic
5 Destruction	**1** Ribs, 1 to 2	**3** Percutaneous	**0** Internal Fixation Device, Rigid Plate	**Z** No Qualifier
8 Division	**2** Ribs, 3 or More	**4** Percutaneous Endoscopic	**4** Internal Fixation Device	
9 Drainage	**3** Cervical Vertebra	**X** External	**5** External Fixation Device	
B Excision	**4** Thoracic Vertebra		**6** Internal Fixation Device, Intramedullary	
C Extirpation	**5** Scapula, Right		**7** Autologous Tissue Substitute	
D Extraction	**6** Scapula, Left		**8** External Fixation Device, Limb Lengthening	
H Insertion	**7** Glenoid Cavity, Right		**B** External Fixation Device, Monoplanar	
J Inspection	**8** Glenoid Cavity, Left		**C** External Fixation Device, Ring	
N Release	**9** Clavicle, Right		**D** External Fixation Device, Hybrid	
P Removal	**B** Clavicle, Left		**J** Synthetic Substitute	
Q Repair	**C** Humeral Head, Right		**K** Nonautologous Tissue Substitute	
R Replacement	**D** Humeral Head, Left		**M** Bone Growth Stimulator	
S Reposition	**F** Humeral Shaft, Right		**Y** Other Device	
T Resection	**G** Humeral Shaft, Left		**Z** No Device	
U Supplement	**H** Radius, Right			
W Revision	**J** Radius, Left			
	K Ulna, Right			
	L Ulna, Left			
	M Carpal, Right			
	N Carpal, Left			
	P Metacarpal, Right			
	Q Metacarpal, Left			
	R Thumb Phalanx, Right			
	S Thumb Phalanx, Left			
	T Finger Phalanx, Right			
	V Finger Phalanx, Left			
	Y Upper Bone			

0: Medical and Surgical
Q: Lower Bones

Operation-Character 3	Body Part-Character 4	Approach-Character 5	Device-Character 6	Qualifier-Character 7
2 Change	**0** Lumbar Vertebra	**0** Open	**0** Drainage Device	**2** Sesamoid Bone(s) 1st Toe
5 Destruction	**1** Sacrum	**3** Percutaneous	**4** Internal Fixation Device	**X** Diagnostic
8 Division	**2** Pelvic Bone, Right	**4** Percutaneous Endoscopic	**5** External Fixation Device	**Z** No Qualifier
9 Drainage	**3** Pelvic Bone, Left	**X** External	**6** Internal Fixation Device, Intramedullary	
B Excision	**4** Acetabulum, Right		**7** Autologous Tissue Substitute	
C Extirpation	**5** Acetabulum, Left		**8** External Fixation Device, Limb Lengthening	
D Extraction	**6** Upper Femur, Right		**B** External Fixation Device, Monoplanar	
H Insertion	**7** Upper Femur, Left		**C** External Fixation Device, Ring	
J Inspection	**8** Femoral Shaft, Right		**D** External Fixation Device, Hybrid	
N Release	**9** Femoral Shaft, Left		**J** Synthetic Substitute	
P Removal	**B** Lower Femur, Right		**K** Nonautologous Tissue Substitute	
Q Repair	**C** Lower Femur, Left		**M** Bone Growth Stimulator	
R Replacement	**D** Patella, Right		**Y** Other Device	
S Reposition	**F** Patella, Left		**Z** No Device	
T Resection	**G** Tibia, Right			
U Supplement	**H** Tibia, Left			
W Revision	**J** Fibula, Right			
	K Fibula, Left			
	L Tarsal, Right			
	M Tarsal, Left			
	N Metatarsal, Right			
	P Metatarsal, Left			
	Q Toe Phalanx, Right			
	R Toe Phalanx, Left			
	S Coccyx			
	Y Lower Bone			

0: Medical and Surgical
R: Upper Joints

Operation-Character 3	Body Part-Character 4	Approach-Character 5	Device-Character 6	Qualifier-Character 7
2 Change	**0** Occipital-cervical Joint	**0** Open	**0** Drainage Device	**0** Anterior Approach, Anterior Column
5 Destruction	**1** Cervical Vertebral Joint	**3** Percutaneous	**0** Synthetic Substitute, Reverse Ball and Socket	**1** Posterior Approach, Posterior Column
9 Drainage	**2** Cervical Vertebral Joints, 2 or more	**4** Percutaneous Endoscopic	**3** Infusion Device	**6** Humeral Surface
B Excision	**3** Cervical Vertebral Disc	**X** External	**4** Internal Fixation Device	**7** Glenoid Surface
C Extirpation	**4** Cervicothoracic Vertebral Joint		**5** External Fixation Device	**J** Posterior Approach, Anterior Column
G Fusion	**5** Cervicothoracic Vertebral Disc		**7** Autologous Tissue Substitute	**X** Diagnostic
H Insertion	**6** Thoracic Vertebral Joint		**8** Spacer	**Z** No Qualifier
J Inspection	**7** Thoracic Vertebral Joints, 2 to 7		**A** Interbody Fusion Device	
N Release	**8** Thoracic Vertebral Joints, 8 or more		**B** Spinal Stabilization Device, Interspinous Process	
P Removal	**9** Thoracic Vertebral Disc		**C** Spinal Stabilization Device, Pedicle-Based	
Q Repair	**A** Thoracolumbar Vertebral Joint		**D** Spinal Stabilization Device, Facet Replacement	
R Replacement	**B** Thoracolumbar Vertebral Disc		**J** Synthetic Substitute	
S Reposition	**C** Temporomandibular Joint, Right		**K** Nonautologous Tissue Substitute	
T Resection	**D** Temporomandibular Joint, Left		**Y** Other Device	
U Supplement	**E** Sternoclavicular Joint, Right		**Z** No Device	
W Revision	**F** Sternoclavicular Joint, Left			
	G Acromioclavicular Joint, Right			
	H Acromioclavicular Joint, Left			
	J Shoulder Joint, Right			
	K Shoulder Joint, Left			
	L Elbow Joint, Right			
	M Elbow Joint, Left			
	N Wrist Joint, Right			
	P Wrist Joint, Left			
	Q Carpal Joint, Right			
	R Carpal Joint, Left			
	S Carpometacarpal Joint, Right			
	T Carpometacarpal Joint, Left			
	U Metacarpophalangeal Joint, Right			
	V Metacarpophalangeal Joint, Left			
	W Finger Phalangeal Joint, Right			
	X Finger Phalangeal Joint, Left			
	Y Upper Joint			

0: Medical and Surgical
S: Lower Joints

Operation-Character 3	Body Part-Character 4	Approach-Character 5	Device-Character 6	Qualifier-Character 7
2 Change	**0** Lumbar Vertebral Joint	**0** Open	**0** Drainage Device	**0** Anterior Approach, Anterior Column
5 Destruction	**1** Lumbar Vertebral Joints, 2 or more	**3** Percutaneous	**0** Synthetic Substitute, Polyethylene	**1** Posterior Approach, Posterior Column
9 Drainage	**2** Lumbar Vertebral Disc	**4** Percutaneous Endoscopic	**1** Synthetic Substitute, Metal	**9** Cemented
B Excision	**3** Lumbosacral Joint	**X** External	**2** Synthetic Substitute, Metal on Polyethylene	**A** Uncemented
C Extirpation	**4** Lumbosacral Disc		**3** Infusion Device	**C** Patellar Surface
G Fusion	**5** Sacrococcygeal Joint		**3** Synthetic Substitute, Ceramic	**J** Posterior Approach, Anterior Column
H Insertion	**6** Coccygeal Joint		**4** Internal Fixation Device	**X** Diagnostic
J Inspection	**7** Sacroiliac Joint, Right		**4** Synthetic Substitute, Ceramic on Polyethylene	**Z** No Qualifier
N Release	**8** Sacroiliac Joint, Left		**5** External Fixation Device	
P Removal	**9** Hip Joint, Right		**6** Synthetic Substitute, Oxidized Zirconium on Polyethylene	
Q Repair	**A** Hip Joint, Acetabular Surface, Right		**7** Autologous Tissue Substitute	
R Replacement	**B** Hip Joint, Left		**8** Spacer	
S Reposition	**C** Knee Joint, Right		**9** Liner	
T Resection	**D** Knee Joint, Left		**A** Interbody Fusion Device	
U Supplement	**E** Hip Joint, Acetabular Surface, Left		**B** Resurfacing Device	
W Revision	**F** Ankle Joint, Right		**B** Spinal Stabilization Device, Interspinous Process	
	G Ankle Joint, Left		**C** Spinal Stabilization Device, Pedicle-Based	
	H Tarsal Joint, Right		**D** Spinal Stabilization Device, Facet Replacement	
	J Tarsal Joint, Left		**E** Articulating Spacer	
	K Tarsometatarsal Joint, Right		**J** Synthetic Substitute	
	L Tarsometatarsal Joint, Left		**K** Nonautologous Tissue Substitute	
	M Metatarsal-Phalangeal Joint, Right		**L** Synthetic Substitute, Unicondylar Medial	
	N Metatarsal-Phalangeal Joint, Left		**M** Synthetic Substitute, Unicondylar Lateral	
	P Toe Phalangeal Joint, Right		**N** Synthetic Substitute, Patellofemoral	
	Q Toe Phalangeal Joint, Left		**Y** Other Device	
	R Hip Joint, Femoral Surface, Right		**Z** No Device	
	S Hip Joint, Femoral Surface, Left			
	T Knee Joint, Femoral Surface, Right			
	U Knee Joint, Femoral Surface, Left			
	V Knee Joint, Tibial Surface, Right			
	W Knee Joint, Tibial Surface, Left			
	Y Lower Joint			

0: Medical and Surgical
T: Urinary System

Operation-Character 3	Body Part-Character 4	Approach-Character 5	Device-Character 6	Qualifier-Character 7
1 Bypass	**0** Kidney, Right	**0** Open	**0** Drainage Device	**0** Allogeneic
2 Change	**1** Kidney, Left	**3** Percutaneous	**2** Monitoring Device	**1** Syngeneic
5 Destruction	**2** Kidneys, Bilateral	**4** Percutaneous Endoscopic	**3** Infusion Device	**2** Zooplastic
7 Dilation	**3** Kidney Pelvis, Right	**7** Via Natural or Artificial Opening	**7** Autologous Tissue Substitute	**3** Kidney Pelvis, Right
8 Division	**4** Kidney Pelvis, Left	**8** Via Natural or Artificial Opening Endoscopic	**C** Extraluminal Device	**4** Kidney Pelvis, Left
9 Drainage	**5** Kidney	**X** External	**D** Intraluminal Device	**6** Ureter, Right
B Excision	**6** Ureter, Right		**J** Synthetic Substitute	**7** Ureter, Left
C Extirpation	**7** Ureter, Left		**K** Nonautologous Tissue Substitute	**8** Colon
D Extraction	**8** Ureters, Bilateral		**L** Artificial Sphincter	**9** Colocutaneous
F Fragmentation	**9** Ureter		**M** Stimulator Lead	**A** Ileum
H Insertion	**B** Bladder		**Y** Other Device	**B** Bladder
J Inspection	**C** Bladder Neck		**Z** No Device	**C** Ileocutaneous
L Occlusion	**D** Urethra			**D** Cutaneous
M Reattachment				**X** Diagnostic
N Release				**Z** No Qualifier
P Removal				
Q Repair				
R Replacement				
S Reposition				
T Resection				
U Supplement				
V Restriction				
W Revision				
Y Transplantation				

0: Medical and Surgical
U: Female Reproductive System

Operation-Character 3	Body Part-Character 4	Approach-Character 5	Device-Character 6	Qualifier-Character 7
1 Bypass	**0** Ovary, Right	**0** Open	**0** Drainage Device	**0** Allogeneic
2 Change	**1** Ovary, Left	**3** Percutaneous	**1** Radioactive Element	**1** Syngeneic
5 Destruction	**2** Ovaries, Bilateral	**4** Percutaneous Endoscopic	**3** Infusion Device	**2** Zooplastic
7 Dilation	**3** Ovary	**7** Via Natural or Artificial Opening	**7** Autologous Tissue Substitute	**5** Fallopian Tube, Right
8 Division	**4** Uterine Supporting Structure	**8** Via Natural or Artificial Opening Endoscopic	**C** Extraluminal Device	**6** Fallopian Tube, Left
9 Drainage	**5** Fallopian Tube, Right	**F** Via Natural or Artificial Opening With Percutaneous Endoscopic Assistance	**D** Intraluminal Device	**9** Uterus
B Excision	**6** Fallopian Tube, Left	**X** External	**G** Intraluminal Device, Pessary	**L** Supracervical
C Extirpation	**7** Fallopian Tubes, Bilateral		**H** Contraceptive Device	**X** Diagnostic
D Extraction	**8** Fallopian Tube		**J** Synthetic Substitute	**Z** No Qualifier
F Fragmentation	**9** Uterus		**K** Nonautologous Tissue Substitute	
H Insertion	**B** Endometrium		**Y** Other Device	
J Inspection	**C** Cervix		**Z** No Device	
L Occlusion	**D** Uterus and Cervix			
M Reattachment	**F** Cul-de-sac			
N Release	**G** Vagina			
P Removal	**H** Vagina and Cul-de-sac			
Q Repair	**J** Clitoris			
S Reposition	**K** Hymen			
T Resection	**L** Vestibular Gland			
U Supplement	**M** Vulva			
V Restriction	**N** Ova			
W Revision				
Y Transplantation				

0: Medical and Surgical
V: Male Reproductive System

Operation-Character 3	Body Part-Character 4	Approach-Character 5	Device-Character 6	Qualifier-Character 7
1 Bypass	**0** Prostate	**0** Open	**0** Drainage Device	**D** Urethra
2 Change	**1** Seminal Vesicle, Right	**3** Percutaneous	**1** Radioactive Element	**J** Epididymis, Right
5 Destruction	**2** Seminal Vesicle, Left	**4** Percutaneous Endoscopic	**3** Infusion Device	**K** Epididymis, Left
7 Dilation	**3** Seminal Vesicles, Bilateral	**7** Via Natural or Artificial Opening	**7** Autologous Tissue Substitute	**N** Vas Deferens, Right
9 Drainage	**4** Prostate and Seminal Vesicles	**8** Via Natural or Artificial Opening Endoscopic	**C** Extraluminal Device	**P** Vas Deferens, Left
B Excision	**5** Scrotum	**X** External	**D** Intraluminal Device	**S** Penis
C Extirpation	**6** Tunica Vaginalis, Right		**J** Synthetic Substitute	**X** Diagnostic
H Insertion	**7** Tunica Vaginalis, Left		**K** Nonautologous Tissue Substitute	**Z** No Qualifier
J Inspection	**8** Scrotum and Tunica Vaginalis		**Y** Other Device	
L Occlusion	**9** Testis, Right		**Z** No Device	
M Reattachment	**B** Testis, Left			
N Release	**C** Testes, Bilateral			
P Removal	**D** Testis			
Q Repair	**F** Spermatic Cord, Right			
R Replacement	**G** Spermatic Cord, Left			
S Reposition	**H** Spermatic Cords, Bilateral			
T Resection	**J** Epididymis, Right			
U Supplement	**K** Epididymis, Left			
W Revision	**L** Epididymis, Bilateral			
X Transfer	**M** Epididymis and Spermatic Cord			
	N Vas Deferens, Right			
	P Vas Deferens, Left			
	Q Vas Deferens, Bilateral			
	R Vas Deferens			
	S Penis			
	T Prepuce			

0: Medical and Surgical
W: Anatomical Regions, General

Operation-Character 3	Body Part-Character 4	Approach-Character 5	Device-Character 6	Qualifier-Character 7
0 Alteration	**0** Head	**0** Open	**0** Drainage Device	**0** Allogeneic
1 Bypass	**1** Cranial Cavity	**3** Percutaneous	**1** Radioactive Element	**0** Vagina
2 Change	**2** Face	**4** Percutaneous Endoscopic	**3** Infusion Device	**1** Penis
3 Control	**3** Oral Cavity and Throat	**7** Via Natural or Artificial Opening	**7** Autologous Tissue Substitute	**1** Syngeneic
4 Creation	**4** Upper Jaw	**8** Via Natural or Artificial Opening Endoscopic	**J** Synthetic Substitute	**2** Stoma
8 Division	**5** Lower Jaw	**X** External	**K** Nonautologous Tissue Substitute	**4** Cutaneous
9 Drainage	**6** Neck		**Y** Other Device	**9** Pleural Cavity, Right
B Excision	**8** Chest Wall		**Z** No Device	**B** Pleural Cavity, Left
C Extirpation	**9** Pleural Cavity, Right			**G** Peritoneal Cavity
F Fragmentation	**B** Pleural Cavity, Left			**J** Pelvic Cavity
H Insertion	**C** Mediastinum			**W** Upper Vein
J Inspection	**D** Pericardial Cavity			**X** Diagnostic
M Reattachment	**F** Abdominal Wall			**Y** Lower Vein
P Removal	**G** Peritoneal Cavity			**Z** No Qualifier
Q Repair	**H** Retroperitoneum			
U Supplement	**J** Pelvic Cavity			
W Revision	**K** Upper Back			
Y Transplantation	**L** Lower Back			
	M Perineum, Male			
	N Perineum, Female			
	P Gastrointestinal Tract			
	Q Respiratory Tract			
	R Genitourinary Tract			

0: Medical and Surgical
X: Anatomical Regions, Upper Extremities

Operation-Character 3	Body Part-Character 4	Approach-Character 5	Device-Character 6	Qualifier-Character 7
0 Alteration	**0** Forequarter, Right	**0** Open	**0** Drainage Device	**0** Allogeneic
2 Change	**1** Forequarter, Left	**3** Percutaneous	**1** Radioactive Element	**0** Complete
3 Control	**2** Shoulder Region, Right	**4** Percutaneous Endoscopic	**3** Infusion Device	**1** High
6 Detachment	**3** Shoulder Region, Left	**X** External	**7** Autologous Tissue Substitute	**1** Syngeneic
9 Drainage	**4** Axilla, Right		**J** Synthetic Substitute	**2** Mid
B Excision	**5** Axilla, Left		**K** Nonautologous Tissue Substitute	**3** Low
H Insertion	**6** Upper Extremity, Right		**Y** Other Device	**4** Complete 1st Ray
J Inspection	**7** Upper Extremity, Left		**Z** No Device	**5** Complete 2nd Ray
M Reattachment	**8** Upper Arm, Right			**6** Complete 3rd Ray
P Removal	**9** Upper Arm, Left			**7** Complete 4th Ray
Q Repair	**B** Elbow Region, Right			**8** Complete 5th Ray
R Replacement	**C** Elbow Region, Left			**9** Partial 1st Ray
U Supplement	**D** Lower Arm, Right			**B** Partial 2nd Ray
W Revision	**F** Lower Arm, Left			**C** Partial 3rd Ray
X Transfer	**G** Wrist Region, Right			**D** Partial 4th Ray
Y Transplantation	**H** Wrist Region, Left			**F** Partial 5th Ray
	J Hand, Right			**L** Thumb, Right
	K Hand, Left			**M** Thumb, Left
	L Thumb, Right			**N** Toe, Right
	M Thumb, Left			**P** Toe, Left
	N Index Finger, Right			**X** Diagnostic
	P Index Finger, Left			**Z** No Qualifier
	Q Middle Finger, Right			
	R Middle Finger, Left			
	S Ring Finger, Right			
	T Ring Finger, Left			
	V Little Finger, Right			
	W Little Finger, Left			

0: Medical and Surgical
Y: Anatomical Regions, Lower Extremities

Operation-Character 3	Body Part-Character 4	Approach-Character 5	Device-Character 6	Qualifier-Character 7
0 Alteration	**0** Buttock, Right	**0** Open	**0** Drainage Device	**0** Complete
2 Change	**1** Buttock, Left	**3** Percutaneous	**1** Radioactive Element	**1** High
3 Control	**2** Hindquarter, Right	**4** Percutaneous Endoscopic	**3** Infusion Device	**2** Mid
6 Detachment	**3** Hindquarter, Left	**X** External	**7** Autologous Tissue Substitute	**3** Low
9 Drainage	**4** Hindquarter, Bilateral		**J** Synthetic Substitute	**4** Complete 1st Ray
B Excision	**5** Inguinal Region, Right		**K** Nonautologous Tissue Substitute	**5** Complete 2nd Ray
H Insertion	**6** Inguinal Region, Left		**Y** Other Device	**6** Complete 3rd Ray
J Inspection	**7** Femoral Region, Right		**Z** No Device	**7** Complete 4th Ray
M Reattachment	**8** Femoral Region, Left			**8** Complete 5th Ray
P Removal	**9** Lower Extremity, Right			**9** Partial 1st Ray
Q Repair	**A** Inguinal Region, Bilateral			**B** Partial 2nd Ray
U Supplement	**B** Lower Extremity, Left			**C** Partial 3rd Ray
W Revision	**C** Upper Leg, Right			**D** Partial 4th Ray
	D Upper Leg, Left			**F** Partial 5th Ray
	E Femoral Region, Bilateral			**X** Diagnostic
	F Knee Region, Right			**Z** No Qualifier
	G Knee Region, Left			
	H Lower Leg, Right			
	J Lower Leg, Left			
	K Ankle Region, Right			
	L Ankle Region, Left			
	M Foot, Right			
	N Foot, Left			
	P 1st Toe, Right			
	Q 1st Toe, Left			
	R 2nd Toe, Right			
	S 2nd Toe, Left			
	T 3rd Toe, Right			
	U 3rd Toe, Left			
	V 4th Toe, Right			
	W 4th Toe, Left			
	X 5th Toe, Right			
	Y 5th Toe, Left			

1: Obstetrics
0: Pregnancy

Operation-Character 3	Body Part-Character 4	Approach-Character 5	Device-Character 6	Qualifier-Character 7
2 Change	**0** Products of Conception	**0** Open	**3** Monitoring Electrode	**0** High
9 Drainage	**1** Products of Conception, Retained	**3** Percutaneous	**Y** Other Device	**1** Low
A Abortion	**2** Products of Conception, Ectopic	**4** Percutaneous Endoscopic	**Z** No Device	**2** Extraperitoneal
D Extraction		**7** Via Natural or Artificial Opening		**3** Low Forceps
E Delivery		**8** Via Natural or Artificial Opening Endoscopic		**4** Mid Forceps
H Insertion		**X** External		**5** High Forceps
J Inspection				**6** Vacuum
P Removal				**7** Internal Version
Q Repair				**8** Other
S Reposition				**9** Fetal Blood
T Resection				**9** Manual
Y Transplantation				**A** Fetal Cerebrospinal Fluid
				B Fetal Fluid, Other
				C Amniotic Fluid, Therapeutic
				D Fluid, Other
				E Nervous System
				F Cardiovascular System
				G Lymphatics and Hemic
				H Eye
				J Ear, Nose and Sinus
				K Respiratory System
				L Mouth and Throat
				M Gastrointestinal System
				N Hepatobiliary and Pancreas
				P Endocrine System
				Q Skin
				R Musculoskeletal System
				S Urinary System
				T Female Reproductive System
				U Amniotic Fluid, Diagnostic
				V Male Reproductive System
				W Laminaria
				X Abortifacient
				Y Other Body System
				Z No Qualifier

2: Placement
W: Anatomical Regions

Operation-Character 3	Body Region-Character 4	Approach-Character 5	Device-Character 6	Qualifier-Character 7
0 Change	**0** Head	**X** External	**0** Traction Apparatus	**Z** No Qualifier
1 Compression	**1** Face		**1** Splint	
2 Dressing	**2** Neck		**2** Cast	
3 Immobilization	**3** Abdominal Wall		**3** Brace	
4 Packing	**4** Chest Wall		**4** Bandage	
5 Removal	**5** Back		**5** Packing Material	
6 Traction	**6** Inguinal Region, Right		**6** Pressure Dressing	
	7 Inguinal Region, Left		**7** Intermittent Pressure Device	
	8 Upper Extremity, Right		**9** Wire	
	9 Upper Extremity, Left		**Y** Other Device	
	A Upper Arm, Right		**Z** No Device	
	B Upper Arm, Left			
	C Lower Arm, Right			
	D Lower Arm, Left			
	E Hand, Right			
	F Hand, Left			
	G Thumb, Right			
	H Thumb, Left			
	J Finger, Right			
	K Finger, Left			
	L Lower Extremity, Right			
	M Lower Extremity, Left			
	N Upper Leg, Right			
	P Upper Leg, Left			
	Q Lower Leg, Right			
	R Lower Leg, Left			
	S Foot, Right			
	T Foot, Left			
	U Toe, Right			
	V Toe, Left			

2: Placement
Y: Anatomical Orifices

Operation-Character 3	Body Region-Character 4	Approach-Character 5	Device-Character 6	Qualifier-Character 7
0 Change	**0** Mouth and Pharynx	**X** External	**5** Packing Material	**Z** No Qualifier
4 Packing	**1** Nasal			
5 Removal	**2** Ear			
	3 Anorectal			
	4 Female Genital Tract			
	5 Urethra			

3: Administration
0: Circulatory

Operation-Character 3	Body System/Region-Character 4	Approach-Character 5	Substance-Character 6	Qualifier-Character 7
2 Transfusion	**3** Peripheral Vein	**0** Open	**A** Stem Cells, Embryonic	**0** Autologous
	4 Central Vein	**3** Percutaneous	**B** 4-Factor Prothrombin Complex Concentrate	**1** Nonautologous
	5 Peripheral Artery	**7** Via Natural or Artificial Opening	**G** Bone Marrow	**2** Allogeneic, Related
	6 Central Artery		**H** Whole Blood	**3** Allogeneic, Unrelated
	7 Products of Conception, Circulatory		**J** Serum Albumin	**4** Allogeneic, Unspecified
	8 Vein		**K** Frozen Plasma	**Z** No Qualifier
			L Fresh Plasma	
			M Plasma Cryoprecipitate	
			N Red Blood Cells	
			P Frozen Red Cells	
			Q White Cells	
			R Platelets	
			S Globulin	
			T Fibrinogen	
			V Antihemophilic Factors	
			W Factor IX	
			X Stem Cells, Cord Blood	
			Y Stem Cells, Hematopoietic	

3: Administration
C: Indwelling Device

Operation-Character 3	Body System/Region-Character 4	Approach-Character 5	Substance-Character 6	Qualifier-Character 7
1 Irrigation	**Z** None	**X** External	**8** Irrigating Substance	**Z** No Qualifier

3: Administration
E: Physiological Systems and Anatomical Regions

Operation-Character 3	Body System/Region-Character 4	Approach-Character 5	Substance-Character 6	Qualifier-Character 7
0 Introduction	**0** Skin and Mucous Membranes	**0** Open	**0** Antineoplastic	**0** Autologous
1 Irrigation	**1** Subcutaneous Tissue	**3** Percutaneous	**1** Thrombolytic	**0** Influenza Vaccine
	2 Muscle	**7** Via Natural or Artificial Opening	**2** Anti-infective	**1** Nonautologous
	3 Peripheral Vein	**8** Via Natural or Artificial Opening Endoscopic	**3** Anti-inflammatory	**2** High-dose Interleukin-2
	4 Central Vein	**X** External	**4** Serum, Toxoid and Vaccine	**3** Low-dose Interleukin-2
	5 Peripheral Artery		**5** Adhesion Barrier	**4** Liquid Brachytherapy Radioisotope
	6 Central Artery		**6** Nutritional Substance	**5** Other Antineoplastic
	7 Coronary Artery		**7** Electrolytic and Water Balance Substance	**6** Recombinant Human activated Protein C
	8 Heart		**8** Irrigating Substance	**7** Other Thrombolytic
	9 Nose		**9** Dialysate	**8** Oxazolidinones
	A Bone Marrow		**A** Stem Cells, Embryonic	**9** Other Anti-infective
	B Ear		**B** Anesthetic Agent	**A** Anti-Infective Envelope
	C Eye		**E** Stem Cells, Somatic	**B** Recombinant Bone Morphogenetic Protein
	D Mouth and Pharynx		**F** Intracirculatory Anesthetic	**C** Other Substance
	E Products of Conception		**G** Other Therapeutic Substance	**D** Nitric Oxide
	F Respiratory Tract		**H** Radioactive Substance	**F** Other Gas
	G Upper GI		**K** Other Diagnostic Substance	**G** Insulin
	H Lower GI		**L** Sperm	**H** Human B-type Natriuretic Peptide
	J Biliary and Pancreatic Tract		**M** Pigment	**J** Other Hormone
	K Genitourinary Tract		**N** Analgesics, Hypnotics, Sedatives	**K** Immunostimulator
	L Pleural Cavity		**P** Platelet Inhibitor	**L** Immunosuppressive
	M Peritoneal Cavity		**Q** Fertilized Ovum	**M** Monoclonal Antibody
	N Male Reproductive		**R** Antiarrhythmic	**N** Blood Brain Barrier Disruption
	P Female Reproductive		**S** Gas	**P** Clofarabine
	Q Cranial Cavity and Brain		**T** Destructive Agent	**Q** Glucarpidase
	R Spinal Canal		**U** Pancreatic Islet Cells	**Z** No Qualifier
	S Epidural Space		**V** Hormone	
	T Peripheral Nerves and Plexi		**W** Immunotherapeutic	
	U Joints		**X** Vasopressor	
	V Bones			
	W Lymphatics			
	X Cranial Nerves			
	Y Pericardial Cavity			

4: Measurement and Monitoring
A: Physiological Systems

Operation-Character 3	Body System-Character 4	Approach-Character 5	Function/Device-Character 6	Qualifier-Character 7
0 Measurement	**0** Central Nervous	**0** Open	**0** Acuity	**0** Central
1 Monitoring	**1** Peripheral Nervous	**3** Percutaneous	**1** Capacity	**1** Peripheral
	2 Cardiac	**7** Via Natural or Artificial Opening	**2** Conductivity	**2** Portal
	3 Arterial	**8** Via Natural or Artificial Opening Endoscopic	**3** Contractility	**3** Pulmonary
	4 Venous	**X** External	**4** Electrical Activity	**4** Stress
	5 Circulatory		**5** Flow	**5** Ambulatory
	6 Lymphatic		**6** Metabolism	**6** Right Heart
	7 Visual		**7** Mobility	**7** Left Heart
	8 Olfactory		**8** Motility	**8** Bilateral
	9 Respiratory		**9** Output	**9** Sensory
	B Gastrointestinal		**B** Pressure	**A** Guidance
	C Biliary		**C** Rate	**B** Motor
	D Urinary		**D** Resistance	**C** Coronary
	F Musculoskeletal		**F** Rhythm	**D** Intracranial
	G Skin and Breast		**G** Secretion	**F** Other Thoracic
	H Products of Conception, Cardiac		**H** Sound	**G** Intraoperative
	J Products of Conception, Nervous		**J** Pulse	**H** Indocyanine Green Dye
	Z None		**K** Temperature	**Z** No Qualifier
			L Volume	
			M Total Activity	
			N Sampling and Pressure	
			P Action Currents	
			Q Sleep	
			R Saturation	
			S Vascular Perfusion	

4: Measurement and Monitoring
B: Physiological Devices

Operation-Character 3	Body System-Character 4	Approach-Character 5	Function/Device-Character 6	Qualifier-Character 7
0 Measurement	**0** Central Nervous	**X** External	**S** Pacemaker	**Z** No Qualifier
	1 Peripheral Nervous		**T** Defibrillator	
	2 Cardiac		**V** Stimulator	
	9 Respiratory			
	F Musculoskeletal			

5: Extracorporeal Assistance and Performance
A: Physiological Systems

Operation-Character 3	Body System-Character 4	Duration-Character 5	Function-Character 6	Qualifier-Character 7
0 Assistance	**2** Cardiac	**0** Single	**0** Filtration	**0** Balloon Pump
1 Performance	**5** Circulatory	**1** Intermittent	**1** Output	**1** Hyperbaric
2 Restoration	**9** Respiratory	**2** Continuous	**2** Oxygenation	**2** Manual
	C Biliary	**3** Less than 24 Consecutive Hours	**3** Pacing	**4** Nonmechanical
	D Urinary	**4** 24-96 Consecutive Hours	**4** Rhythm	**5** Pulsatile Compression
		5 Greater than 96 Consecutive Hours	**5** Ventilation	**6** Other Pump
		6 Multiple		**7** Continuous Positive Airway Pressure
				8 Intermittent Positive Airway Pressure
				9 Continuous Negative Airway Pressure
				B Intermittent Negative Airway Pressure
				C Supersaturated
				D Impeller Pump
				F Membrane, Central
				G Membrane, PeripheralVeno-arterial
				H Membrane, PeripheralVeno-venous
				Z No Qualifier

6: Extracorporeal Therapies
A: Physiological Systems

Operation-Character 3	Body System-Character 4	Duration-Character 5	Qualifier-Character 6	Qualifier-Character 7
0 Atmospheric Control	**0** Skin	**0** Single	**B** Donor Organ	**0** Erythrocytes
1 Decompression	**1** Urinary	**1** Multiple	**Z** No Qualifier	**1** Leukocytes
2 Electromagnetic Therapy	**2** Central Nervous			**2** Platelets
3 Hyperthermia	**3** Musculoskeletal			**3** Plasma
4 Hypothermia	**5** Circulatory			**4** Head and Neck Vessels
5 Pheresis	**B** Respiratory System			**5** Heart
6 Phototherapy	**F** Hepatobiliary System and Pancreas			**6** Peripheral Vessels
7 Ultrasound Therapy	**T** Urinary System			**7** Other Vessels
8 Ultraviolet Light Therapy	**Z** None			**T** Stem Cells, Cord Blood
9 Shock Wave Therapy				**V** Stem Cells, Hematopoietic
B Perfusion				**Z** No Qualifier

7: Osteopathic
W: Anatomical Regions

Operation-Character 3	Body Region-Character 4	Approach-Character 5	Method-Character 6	Qualifier-Character 7
0 Treatment	**0** Head	**X** External	**0** Articulatory-Raising	**Z** None
	1 Cervical		**1** Fascial Release	
	2 Thoracic		**2** General Mobilization	
	3 Lumbar		**3** High Velocity-Low Amplitude	
	4 Sacrum		**4** Indirect	
	5 Pelvis		**5** Low Velocity-High Amplitude	
	6 Lower Extremities		**6** Lymphatic Pump	
	7 Upper Extremities		**7** Muscle Energy-Isometric	
	8 Rib Cage		**8** Muscle Energy-Isotonic	
	9 Abdomen		**9** Other Method	

8: Other Procedures
C: Indwelling Device

Operation-Character 3	Body Region-Character 4	Approach-Character 5	Method-Character 6	Qualifier-Character 7
0 Other Procedures	**1** Nervous System	**X** External	**6** Collection	**J** Cerebrospinal Fluid
	2 Circulatory System			**K** Blood
				L Other Fluid

8: Other Procedures
E: Physiological Systems and Anatomical Regions

Operation-Character 3	Body Region-Character 4	Approach-Character 5	Method-Character 6	Qualifier-Character 7
0 Other Procedures	**1** Nervous System	**0** Open	**0** Acupuncture	**0** Anesthesia
	2 Circulatory System	**3** Percutaneous	**1** Therapeutic Massage	**1** In Vitro Fertilization
	9 Head and Neck Region	**7** Via Natural or Artificial Opening	**6** Collection	**2** Breast Milk
	H Integumentary System and Breast	**8** Via Natural or Artificial Opening Endoscopic	**B** Computer Assisted Procedure	**3** Sperm
	K Musculoskeletal System	**X** External	**C** Robotic Assisted Procedure	**4** Yoga Therapy
	U Female Reproductive System		**D** Near Infrared Spectroscopy	**5** Meditation
	V Male Reproductive System		**Y** Other Method	**6** Isolation
	W Trunk Region			**7** Examination
	X Upper Extremity			**8** Suture Removal
	Y Lower Extremity			**9** Piercing
	Z None			**C** Prostate
				D Rectum
				F With Fluoroscopy
				G With Computerized Tomography
				H With Magnetic Resonance Imaging
				Z No Qualifier

9: Chiropractic
W: Anatomical Regions

Operation-Character 3	Body Region-Character 4	Approach-Character 5	Method-Character 6	Qualifier-Character 7
B Manipulation	**0** Head	**X** External	**B** Non-Manual	**Z** None
	1 Cervical		**C** Indirect Visceral	
	2 Thoracic		**D** Extra-Articular	
	3 Lumbar		**F** Direct Visceral	
	4 Sacrum		**G** Long Lever Specific Contact	
	5 Pelvis		**H** Short Lever Specific Contact	
	6 Lower Extremities		**J** Long and Short Lever Specific Contact	
	7 Upper Extremities		**K** Mechanically Assisted	
	8 Rib Cage		**L** Other Method	
	9 Abdomen			

B: Imaging
0: Central Nervous System

Type-Character 3	Body Part-Character 4	Contrast-Character 5	Qualifier-Character 6	Qualifier-Character 7
0 Plain Radiography	**0** Brain	**0** High Osmolar	**0** Unenhanced and Enhanced	**Z** None
1 Fluoroscopy	**7** Cisterna	**1** Low Osmolar	**Z** None	
2 Computerized Tomography (CT Scan)	**8** Cerebral Ventricle(s)	**Y** Other Contrast		
3 Magnetic Resonance Imaging (MRI)	**9** Sella Turcica/Pituitary Gland	**Z** None		
4 Ultrasonography	**B** Spinal Cord			
	C Acoustic Nerves			

B: Imaging
2: Heart

Type-Character 3	Body Part-Character 4	Contrast-Character 5	Qualifier-Character 6	Qualifier-Character 7
0 Plain Radiography	**0** Coronary Artery, Single	**0** High Osmolar	**0** Unenhanced and Enhanced	**0** Intraoperative
1 Fluoroscopy	**1** Coronary Arteries, Multiple	**1** Low Osmolar	**1** Laser	**3** Intravascular
2 Computerized Tomography (CT Scan)	**2** Coronary Artery Bypass Graft, Single	**Y** Other Contrast	**2** Intravascular Optical Coherence	**4** Transesophageal
3 Magnetic Resonance Imaging (MRI)	**3** Coronary Artery Bypass Grafts, Multiple	**Z** None	**Z** None	**Z** None
4 Ultrasonography	**4** Heart, Right			
	5 Heart, Left			
	6 Heart, Right and Left			
	7 Internal Mammary Bypass Graft, Right			
	8 Internal Mammary Bypass Graft, Left			
	B Heart with Aorta			
	C Pericardium			
	D Pediatric Heart			
	F Bypass Graft, Other			

B: Imaging
3: Upper Arteries

Type-Character 3	Body Part-Character 4	Contrast-Character 5	Qualifier-Character 6	Qualifier-Character 7
0 Plain Radiography	**0** Thoracic Aorta	**0** High Osmolar	**0** Unenhanced and Enhanced	**0** Intraoperative
1 Fluoroscopy	**1** Brachiocephalic-Subclavian Artery, Right	**1** Low Osmolar	**1** Laser	**3** Intravascular
2 Computerized Tomography (CT Scan)	**2** Subclavian Artery, Left	**Y** Other Contrast	**2** Intravascular Optical Coherence	**Z** None
3 Magnetic Resonance Imaging (MRI)	**3** Common Carotid Artery, Right	**Z** None	**Z** None	
4 Ultrasonography	**4** Common Carotid Artery, Left			
	5 Common Carotid Arteries, Bilateral			
	6 Internal Carotid Artery, Right			
	7 Internal Carotid Artery, Left			
	8 Internal Carotid Arteries, Bilateral			
	9 External Carotid Artery, Right			
	B External Carotid Artery, Left			
	C External Carotid Arteries, Bilateral			
	D Vertebral Artery, Right			
	F Vertebral Artery, Left			
	G Vertebral Arteries, Bilateral			
	H Upper Extremity Arteries, Right			
	J Upper Extremity Arteries, Left			
	K Upper Extremity Arteries, Bilateral			
	L Intercostal and Bronchial Arteries			
	M Spinal Arteries			
	N Upper Arteries, Other			
	P Thoraco-Abdominal Aorta			
	Q Cervico-Cerebral Arch			
	R Intracranial Arteries			
	S Pulmonary Artery, Right			
	T Pulmonary Artery, Left			
	U Pulmonary Trunk			
	V Ophthalmic Arteries			

B: Imaging
4: Lower Arteries

Type-Character 3	Body Part-Character 4	Contrast-Character 5	Qualifier-Character 6	Qualifier-Character 7
0 Plain Radiography	**0** Abdominal Aorta	**0** High Osmolar	**0** Unenhanced and Enhanced	**0** Intraoperative
1 Fluoroscopy	**1** Celiac Artery	**1** Low Osmolar	**1** Laser	**3** Intravascular
2 Computerized Tomography (CT Scan)	**2** Hepatic Artery	**Y** Other Contrast	**2** Intravascular Optical Coherence	**Z** None
3 Magnetic Resonance Imaging (MRI)	**3** Splenic Arteries	**Z** None	**Z** None	
4 Ultrasonography	**4** Superior Mesenteric Artery			
	5 Inferior Mesenteric Artery			
	6 Renal Artery, Right			
	7 Renal Artery, Left			
	8 Renal Arteries, Bilateral			
	9 Lumbar Arteries			
	B Intra-Abdominal Arteries, Other			
	C Pelvic Arteries			
	D Aorta and Bilateral Lower Extremity Arteries			
	F Lower Extremity Arteries, Right			
	G Lower Extremity Arteries, Left			
	H Lower Extremity Arteries, Bilateral			
	J Lower Arteries, Other			
	K Celiac and Mesenteric Arteries			
	L Femoral Artery			
	M Renal Artery Transplant			
	N Penile Arteries			

B: Imaging
5: Veins

Type-Character 3	Body Part-Character 4	Contrast-Character 5	Qualifier-Character 6	Qualifier-Character 7
0 Plain Radiography	**0** Epidural Veins	**0** High Osmolar	**0** Unenhanced and Enhanced	**3** Intravascular
1 Fluoroscopy	**1** Cerebral and Cerebellar Veins	**1** Low Osmolar	**2** Intravascular Optical Coherence	**A** Guidance
2 Computerized Tomography (CT Scan)	**2** Intracranial Sinuses	**Y** Other Contrast	**Z** None	**Z** None
3 Magnetic Resonance Imaging (MRI)	**3** Jugular Veins, Right	**Z** None		
4 Ultrasonography	**4** Jugular Veins, Left			
	5 Jugular Veins, Bilateral			
	6 Subclavian Vein, Right			
	7 Subclavian Vein, Left			
	8 Superior Vena Cava			
	9 Inferior Vena Cava			
	B Lower Extremity Veins, Right			
	C Lower Extremity Veins, Left			
	D Lower Extremity Veins, Bilateral			
	F Pelvic (Iliac) Veins, Right			
	G Pelvic (Iliac) Veins, Left			
	H Pelvic (Iliac) Veins, Bilateral			
	J Renal Vein, Right			
	K Renal Vein, Left			
	L Renal Veins, Bilateral			
	M Upper Extremity Veins, Right			
	N Upper Extremity Veins, Left			
	P Upper Extremity Veins, Bilateral			
	Q Pulmonary Vein, Right			
	R Pulmonary Vein, Left			
	S Pulmonary Veins, Bilateral			
	T Portal and Splanchnic Veins			
	V Veins, Other			
	W Dialysis Shunt/Fistula			

B: Imaging
7: Lymphatic System

Type-Character 3	Body Part-Character 4	Contrast-Character 5	Qualifier-Character 6	Qualifier-Character 7
0 Plain Radiography	**0** Abdominal/Retroperitoneal Lymphatics, Unilateral	**0** High Osmolar	**Z** None	**Z** None
	1 Abdominal/Retroperitoneal Lymphatics, Bilateral	**1** Low Osmolar		
	4 Lymphatics, Head and Neck	**Y** Other Contrast		
	5 Upper Extremity Lymphatics, Right			
	6 Upper Extremity Lymphatics, Left			
	7 Upper Extremity Lymphatics, Bilateral			
	8 Lower Extremity Lymphatics, Right			
	9 Lower Extremity Lymphatics, Left			
	B Lower Extremity Lymphatics, Bilateral			
	C Lymphatics, Pelvic			

B: Imaging
8: Eye

Type-Character 3	Body Part-Character 4	Contrast-Character 5	Qualifier-Character 6	Qualifier-Character 7
0 Plain Radiography	**0** Lacrimal Duct, Right	**0** High Osmolar	**0** Unenhanced and Enhanced	**Z** None
2 Computerized Tomography (CT Scan)	**1** Lacrimal Duct, Left	**1** Low Osmolar	**Z** None	
3 Magnetic Resonance Imaging (MRI)	**2** Lacrimal Ducts, Bilateral	**Y** Other Contrast		
4 Ultrasonography	**3** Optic Foramina, Right	**Z** None		
	4 Optic Foramina, Left			
	5 Eye, Right			
	6 Eye, Left			
	7 Eyes, Bilateral			

B: Imaging
9: Ear, Nose, Mouth and Throat

Type-Character 3	Body Part-Character 4	Contrast-Character 5	Qualifier-Character 6	Qualifier-Character 7
0 Plain Radiography	**0** Ear	**0** High Osmolar	**0** Unenhanced and Enhanced	**Z** None
1 Fluoroscopy	**2** Paranasal Sinuses	**1** Low Osmolar	**Z** None	
2 Computerized Tomography (CT Scan)	**4** Parotid Gland, Right	**Y** Other Contrast		
3 Magnetic Resonance Imaging (MRI)	**5** Parotid Gland, Left	**Z** None		
	6 Parotid Glands, Bilateral			
	7 Submandibular Gland, Right			
	8 Submandibular Gland, Left			
	9 Submandibular Glands, Bilateral			
	B Salivary Gland, Right			
	C Salivary Gland, Left			
	D Salivary Glands, Bilateral			
	F Nasopharynx/Oropharynx			
	G Pharynx and Epiglottis			
	H Mastoids			
	J Larynx			

B: Imaging
B: Respiratory System

Type-Character 3	Body Part-Character 4	Contrast-Character 5	Qualifier-Character 6	Qualifier-Character 7
0 Plain Radiography	**2** Lung, Right	**0** High Osmolar	**0** Unenhanced and Enhanced	**Z** None
1 Fluoroscopy	**3** Lung, Left	**1** Low Osmolar	**Z** None	
2 Computerized Tomography (CT Scan)	**4** Lungs, Bilateral	**Y** Other Contrast		
3 Magnetic Resonance Imaging (MRI)	**6** Diaphragm	**Z** None		
4 Ultrasonography	**7** Tracheobronchial Tree, Right			
	8 Tracheobronchial Tree, Left			
	9 Tracheobronchial Trees, Bilateral			
	B Pleura			
	C Mediastinum			
	D Upper Airways			
	F Trachea/Airways			
	G Lung Apices			

B: Imaging
D: Gastrointestinal System

Type-Character 3	Body Part-Character 4	Contrast-Character 5	Qualifier-Character 6	Qualifier-Character 7
1 Fluoroscopy	**1** Esophagus	**0** High Osmolar	**0** Unenhanced and Enhanced	**Z** None
2 Computerized Tomography (CT Scan)	**2** Stomach	**1** Low Osmolar	**Z** None	
4 Ultrasonography	**3** Small Bowel	**Y** Other Contrast		
	4 Colon	**Z** None		
	5 Upper GI			
	6 Upper GI and Small Bowel			
	7 Gastrointestinal Tract			
	8 Appendix			
	9 Duodenum			
	B Mouth/Oropharynx			
	C Rectum			

B: Imaging
F: Hepatobiliary System and Pancreas

Type-Character 3	Body Part-Character 4	Contrast-Character 5	Qualifier-Character 6	Qualifier-Character 7
0 Plain Radiography	**0** Bile Ducts	**0** High Osmolar	**0** Unenhanced and Enhanced	**Z** None
1 Fluoroscopy	**1** Biliary and Pancreatic Ducts	**1** Low Osmolar	**Z** None	
2 Computerized Tomography (CT Scan)	**2** Gallbladder	**Y** Other Contrast		
3 Magnetic Resonance Imaging (MRI)	**3** Gallbladder and Bile Ducts	**Z** None		
4 Ultrasonography	**4** Gallbladder, Bile Ducts and Pancreatic Ducts			
	5 Liver			
	6 Liver and Spleen			
	7 Pancreas			
	8 Pancreatic Ducts			
	C Hepatobiliary System, All			

B: Imaging
G: Endocrine System

Type-Character 3	Body Part-Character 4	Contrast-Character 5	Qualifier-Character 6	Qualifier-Character 7
2 Computerized Tomography (CT Scan)	**0** Adrenal Gland, Right	**0** High Osmolar	**0** Unenhanced and Enhanced	**Z** None
3 Magnetic Resonance Imaging (MRI)	**1** Adrenal Gland, Left	**1** Low Osmolar	**Z** None	
4 Ultrasonography	**2** Adrenal Glands, Bilateral	**Y** Other Contrast		
	3 Parathyroid Glands	**Z** None		
	4 Thyroid Gland			

B: Imaging
H: Skin, Subcutaneous Tissue and Breast

Type-Character 3	Body Part-Character 4	Contrast-Character 5	Qualifier-Character 6	Qualifier-Character 7
0 Plain Radiography	**0** Breast, Right	**0** High Osmolar	**0** Unenhanced and Enhanced	**Z** None
3 Magnetic Resonance Imaging (MRI)	**1** Breast, Left	**1** Low Osmolar	**Z** None	
4 Ultrasonography	**2** Breasts, Bilateral	**Y** Other Contrast		
	3 Single Mammary Duct, Right	**Z** None		
	4 Single Mammary Duct, Left			
	5 Multiple Mammary Ducts, Right			
	6 Multiple Mammary Ducts, Left			
	7 Extremity, Upper			
	8 Extremity, Lower			
	9 Abdominal Wall			
	B Chest Wall			
	C Head and Neck			
	D Subcutaneous Tissue, Head/Neck			
	F Subcutaneous Tissue, Upper Extremity			
	G Subcutaneous Tissue, Thorax			
	H Subcutaneous Tissue, Abdomen and Pelvis			
	J Subcutaneous Tissue, Lower Extremity			

B: Imaging
L: Connective Tissue

Type-Character 3	Body Part-Character 4	Contrast-Character 5	Qualifier-Character 6	Qualifier-Character 7
3 Magnetic Resonance Imaging (MRI)	**0** Connective Tissue, Upper Extremity	**Y** Other Contrast	**0** Unenhanced and Enhanced	**Z** None
4 Ultrasonography	**1** Connective Tissue, Lower Extremity	**Z** None	**Z** None	
	2 Tendons, Upper Extremity			
	3 Tendons, Lower Extremity			

B: Imaging
N: Skull and Facial Bones

Type-Character 3	Body Part-Character 4	Contrast-Character 5	Qualifier-Character 6	Qualifier-Character 7
0 Plain Radiography	**0** Skull	**0** High Osmolar	**Z** None	**Z** None
1 Fluoroscopy	**1** Orbit, Right	**1** Low Osmolar		
2 Computerized Tomography (CT Scan)	**2** Orbit, Left	**Y** Other Contrast		
3 Magnetic Resonance Imaging (MRI)	**3** Orbits, Bilateral	**Z** None		
	4 Nasal Bones			
	5 Facial Bones			
	6 Mandible			
	7 Temporomandibular Joint, Right			
	8 Temporomandibular Joint, Left			
	9 Temporomandibular Joints, Bilateral			
	B Zygomatic Arch, Right			
	C Zygomatic Arch, Left			
	D Zygomatic Arches, Bilateral			
	F Temporal Bones			
	G Tooth, Single			
	H Teeth, Multiple			
	J Teeth, All			

B: Imaging
P: Non-Axial Upper Bones

Type-Character 3	Body Part-Character 4	Contrast-Character 5	Qualifier-Character 6	Qualifier-Character 7
0 Plain Radiography	**0** Sternoclavicular Joint, Right	**0** High Osmolar	**0** Unenhanced and Enhanced	**1** Densitometry
1 Fluoroscopy	**1** Sternoclavicular Joint, Left	**1** Low Osmolar	**Z** None	**Z** None
2 Computerized Tomography (CT Scan)	**2** Sternoclavicular Joints, Bilateral	**Y** Other Contrast		
3 Magnetic Resonance Imaging (MRI)	**3** Acromioclavicular Joints, Bilateral	**Z** None		
4 Ultrasonography	**4** Clavicle, Right			
	5 Clavicle, Left			
	6 Scapula, Right			
	7 Scapula, Left			
	8 Shoulder, Right			
	9 Shoulder, Left			
	A Humerus, Right			
	B Humerus, Left			
	C Hand/Finger Joint, Right			
	D Hand/Finger Joint, Left			
	E Upper Arm, Right			
	F Upper Arm, Left			
	G Elbow, Right			
	H Elbow, Left			
	J Forearm, Right			
	K Forearm, Left			
	L Wrist, Right			
	M Wrist, Left			
	N Hand, Right			
	P Hand, Left			
	Q Hands and Wrists, Bilateral			
	R Finger(s), Right			
	S Finger(s), Left			
	T Upper Extremity, Right			
	U Upper Extremity, Left			
	V Upper Extremities, Bilateral			
	W Thorax			
	X Ribs, Right			
	Y Ribs, Left			

B: Imaging
Q: Non-Axial Lower Bones

Type-Character 3	Body Part-Character 4	Contrast-Character 5	Qualifier-Character 6	Qualifier-Character 7
0 Plain Radiography	**0** Hip, Right	**0** High Osmolar	**0** Unenhanced and Enhanced	**1** Densitometry
1 Fluoroscopy	**1** Hip, Left	**1** Low Osmolar	**Z** None	**Z** None
2 Computerized Tomography (CT Scan)	**2** Hips, Bilateral	**Y** Other Contrast		
3 Magnetic Resonance Imaging (MRI)	**3** Femur, Right	**Z** None		
4 Ultrasonography	**4** Femur, Left			
	7 Knee, Right			
	8 Knee, Left			
	9 Knees, Bilateral			
	B Tibia/Fibula, Right			
	C Tibia/Fibula, Left			
	D Lower Leg, Right			
	F Lower Leg, Left			
	G Ankle, Right			
	H Ankle, Left			
	J Calcaneus, Right			
	K Calcaneus, Left			
	L Foot, Right			
	M Foot, Left			
	P Toe(s), Right			
	Q Toe(s), Left			
	R Lower Extremity, Right			
	S Lower Extremity, Left			
	V Patella, Right			
	W Patella, Left			
	X Foot/Toe Joint, Right			
	Y Foot/Toe Joint, Left			

B: Imaging
R: Axial Skeleton, Except Skull and Facial Bones

Type-Character 3	Body Part-Character 4	Contrast-Character 5	Qualifier-Character 6	Qualifier-Character 7
0 Plain Radiography	**0** Cervical Spine	**0** High Osmolar	**0** Unenhanced and Enhanced	**1** Densitometry
1 Fluoroscopy	**1** Cervical Disc(s)	**1** Low Osmolar	**Z** None	**Z** None
2 Computerized Tomography (CT Scan)	**2** Thoracic Disc(s)	**Y** Other Contrast		
3 Magnetic Resonance Imaging (MRI)	**3** Lumbar Disc(s)	**Z** None		
4 Ultrasonography	**4** Cervical Facet Joint(s)			
	5 Thoracic Facet Joint(s)			
	6 Lumbar Facet Joint(s)			
	7 Thoracic Spine			
	8 Thoracolumbar Joint			
	9 Lumbar Spine			
	B Lumbosacral Joint			
	C Pelvis			
	D Sacroiliac Joints			
	F Sacrum and Coccyx			
	G Whole Spine			
	H Sternum			

B: Imaging
T: Urinary System

Type-Character 3	Body Part-Character 4	Contrast-Character 5	Qualifier-Character 6	Qualifier-Character 7
0 Plain Radiography	**0** Bladder	**0** High Osmolar	**0** Unenhanced and Enhanced	**Z** None
1 Fluoroscopy	**1** Kidney, Right	**1** Low Osmolar	**Z** None	
2 Computerized Tomography (CT Scan)	**2** Kidney, Left	**Y** Other Contrast		
3 Magnetic Resonance Imaging (MRI)	**3** Kidneys, Bilateral	**Z** None		
4 Ultrasonography	**4** Kidneys, Ureters and Bladder			
	5 Urethra			
	6 Ureter, Right			
	7 Ureter, Left			
	8 Ureters, Bilateral			
	9 Kidney Transplant			
	B Bladder and Urethra			
	C Ileal Diversion Loop			
	D Kidney, Ureter and Bladder, Right			
	F Kidney, Ureter and Bladder, Left			
	G Ileal Loop, Ureters and Kidneys			
	J Kidneys and Bladder			

B: Imaging
U: Female Reproductive System

Type-Character 3	Body Part-Character 4	Contrast-Character 5	Qualifier-Character 6	Qualifier-Character 7
0 Plain Radiography	**0** Fallopian Tube, Right	**0** High Osmolar	**0** Unenhanced and Enhanced	**Z** None
1 Fluoroscopy	**1** Fallopian Tube, Left	**1** Low Osmolar	**Z** None	
3 Magnetic Resonance Imaging (MRI)	**2** Fallopian Tubes, Bilateral	**Y** Other Contrast		
4 Ultrasonography	**3** Ovary, Right	**Z** None		
	4 Ovary, Left			
	5 Ovaries, Bilateral			
	6 Uterus			
	8 Uterus and Fallopian Tubes			
	9 Vagina			
	B Pregnant Uterus			
	C Uterus and Ovaries			

B: Imaging
V: Male Reproductive System

Type-Character 3	Body Part-Character 4	Contrast-Character 5	Qualifier-Character 6	Qualifier-Character 7
0 Plain Radiography	**0** Corpora Cavernosa	**0** High Osmolar	**0** Unenhanced and Enhanced	**Z** None
1 Fluoroscopy	**1** Epididymis, Right	**1** Low Osmolar	**Z** None	
2 Computerized Tomography (CT Scan)	**2** Epididymis, Left	**Y** Other Contrast		
3 Magnetic Resonance Imaging (MRI)	**3** Prostate	**Z** None		
4 Ultrasonography	**4** Scrotum			
	5 Testicle, Right			
	6 Testicle, Left			
	7 Testicles, Bilateral			
	8 Vasa Vasorum			
	9 Prostate and Seminal Vesicles			
	B Penis			

B: Imaging
W: Anatomical Regions

Type-Character 3	Body Part-Character 4	Contrast-Character 5	Qualifier-Character 6	Qualifier-Character 7
0 Plain Radiography	**0** Abdomen	**0** High Osmolar	**0** Unenhanced and Enhanced	**Z** None
1 Fluoroscopy	**1** Abdomen and Pelvis	**1** Low Osmolar	**Z** None	
2 Computerized Tomography (CT Scan)	**3** Chest	**Y** Other Contrast		
3 Magnetic Resonance Imaging (MRI)	**4** Chest and Abdomen	**Z** None		
4 Ultrasonography	**5** Chest, Abdomen and Pelvis			
	8 Head			
	9 Head and Neck			
	B Long Bones, All			
	C Lower Extremity			
	F Neck			
	G Pelvic Region			
	H Retroperitoneum			
	J Upper Extremity			
	K Whole Body			
	L Whole Skeleton			
	M Whole Body, Infant			
	P Brachial Plexus			

B: Imaging
Y: Fetus and Obstetrical

Type-Character 3	Body Part-Character 4	Contrast-Character 5	Qualifier-Character 6	Qualifier-Character 7
3 Magnetic Resonance Imaging (MRI)	**0** Fetal Head	**Y** Other Contrast	**0** Unenhanced and Enhanced	**Z** None
4 Ultrasonography	**1** Fetal Heart	**Z** None	**Z** None	
	2 Fetal Thorax			
	3 Fetal Abdomen			
	4 Fetal Spine			
	5 Fetal Extremities			
	6 Whole Fetus			
	7 Fetal Umbilical Cord			
	8 Placenta			
	9 First Trimester, Single Fetus			
	B First Trimester, Multiple Gestation			
	C Second Trimester, Single Fetus			
	D Second Trimester, Multiple Gestation			
	F Third Trimester, Single Fetus			
	G Third Trimester, Multiple Gestation			

C: Nuclear Medicine
0: Central Nervous System

Type-Character 3	Body Part-Character 4	Radionuclide-Character 5	Qualifier-Character 6	Qualifier-Character 7
1 Planar Nuclear Medicine Imaging	**0** Brain	**1** Technetium 99m (Tc-99m)	**Z** None	**Z** None
2 Tomographic (Tomo) Nuclear Medicine Imaging	**5** Cerebrospinal Fluid	**B** Carbon 11 (C-11)		
3 Positron Emission Tomographic (PET) Imaging	**Y** Central Nervous System	**D** Indium 111 (In-111)		
5 Nonimaging Nuclear Medicine Probe		**F** Iodine 123 (I-123)		
		K Fluorine 18 (F-18)		
		M Oxygen 15 (O-15)		
		S Thallium 201 (Tl-201)		
		V Xenon 133 (Xe-133)		
		Y Other Radionuclide		

C: Nuclear Medicine
2: Heart

Type-Character 3	Body Part-Character 4	Radionuclide-Character 5	Qualifier-Character 6	Qualifier-Character 7
1 Planar Nuclear Medicine Imaging	**6** Heart, Right and Left	**1** Technetium 99m (Tc-99m)	**Z** None	**Z** None
2 Tomographic (Tomo) Nuclear Medicine Imaging	**G** Myocardium	**D** Indium 111 (In-111)		
3 Positron Emission Tomographic (PET) Imaging	**Y** Heart	**K** Fluorine 18 (F-18)		
5 Nonimaging Nuclear Medicine Probe		**M** Oxygen 15 (O-15)		
		Q Rubidium 82 (Rb-82)		
		R Nitrogen 13 (N-13)		
		S Thallium 201 (Tl-201)		
		Y Other Radionuclide		
		Z None		

C: Nuclear Medicine
5: Veins

Type-Character 3	Body Part-Character 4	Radionuclide-Character 5	Qualifier-Character 6	Qualifier-Character 7
1 Planar Nuclear Medicine Imaging	**B** Lower Extremity Veins, Right	**1** Technetium 99m (Tc-99m)	**Z** None	**Z** None
	C Lower Extremity Veins, Left	**Y** Other Radionuclide		
	D Lower Extremity Veins, Bilateral			
	N Upper Extremity Veins, Right			
	P Upper Extremity Veins, Left			
	Q Upper Extremity Veins, Bilateral			
	R Central Veins			
	Y Veins			

C: Nuclear Medicine
7: Lymphatic and Hematologic System

Type-Character 3	Body Part-Character 4	Radionuclide-Character 5	Qualifier-Character 6	Qualifier-Character 7
1 Planar Nuclear Medicine Imaging	**0** Bone Marrow	**1** Technetium 99m (Tc-99m)	**Z** None	**Z** None
2 Tomographic (Tomo) Nuclear Medicine Imaging	**2** Spleen	**7** Cobalt 58 (Co-58)		
5 Nonimaging Nuclear Medicine Probe	**3** Blood	**C** Cobalt 57 (Co-57)		
6 Nonimaging Nuclear Medicine Assay	**5** Lymphatics, Head and Neck	**D** Indium 111 (In-111)		
	D Lymphatics, Pelvic	**H** Iodine 125 (I-125)		
	J Lymphatics, Head	**W** Chromium (Cr-51)		
	K Lymphatics, Neck	**Y** Other Radionuclide		
	L Lymphatics, Upper Chest			
	M Lymphatics, Trunk			
	N Lymphatics, Upper Extremity			
	P Lymphatics, Lower Extremity			
	Y Lymphatic and Hematologic System			

C: Nuclear Medicine
8: Eye

Type-Character 3	Body Part-Character 4	Radionuclide-Character 5	Qualifier-Character 6	Qualifier-Character 7
1 Planar Nuclear Medicine Imaging	**9** Lacrimal Ducts, Bilateral	**1** Technetium 99m (Tc-99m)	**Z** None	**Z** None
	Y Eye	**Y** Other Radionuclide		

C: Nuclear Medicine
9: Ear, Nose, Mouth and Throat

Type-Character 3	Body Part-Character 4	Radionuclide-Character 5	Qualifier-Character 6	Qualifier-Character 7
1 Planar Nuclear Medicine Imaging	**B** Salivary Glands, Bilateral	**1** Technetium 99m (Tc-99m)	**Z** None	**Z** None
	Y Ear, Nose, Mouth and Throat	**Y** Other Radionuclide		

C: Nuclear Medicine
B: Respiratory System

Type-Character 3	Body Part-Character 4	Radionuclide-Character 5	Qualifier-Character 6	Qualifier-Character 7
1 Planar Nuclear Medicine Imaging	**2** Lungs and Bronchi	**1** Technetium 99m (Tc-99m)	**Z** None	**Z** None
2 Tomographic (Tomo) Nuclear Medicine Imaging	**Y** Respiratory System	**9** Krypton (Kr-81m)		
3 Positron Emission Tomographic (PET) Imaging		**K** Fluorine 18 (F-18)		
		T Xenon 127 (Xe-127)		
		V Xenon 133 (Xe-133)		
		Y Other Radionuclide		

C: Nuclear Medicine
D: Gastrointestinal System

Type-Character 3	Body Part-Character 4	Radionuclide-Character 5	Qualifier-Character 6	Qualifier-Character 7
1 Planar Nuclear Medicine Imaging	**5** Upper Gastrointestinal Tract	**1** Technetium 99m (Tc-99m)	**Z** None	**Z** None
2 Tomographic (Tomo) Nuclear Medicine Imaging	**7** Gastrointestinal Tract	**D** Indium 111 (In-111)		
	Y Digestive System	**Y** Other Radionuclide		

C: Nuclear Medicine
F: Hepatobiliary System and Pancreas

Type-Character 3	Body Part-Character 4	Radionuclide-Character 5	Qualifier-Character 6	Qualifier-Character 7
1 Planar Nuclear Medicine Imaging	**4** Gallbladder	**1** Technetium 99m (Tc-99m)	**Z** None	**Z** None
2 Tomographic (Tomo) Nuclear Medicine Imaging	**5** Liver	**Y** Other Radionuclide		
	6 Liver and Spleen			
	C Hepatobiliary System, All			
	Y Hepatobiliary System and Pancreas			

C: Nuclear Medicine
G: Endocrine System

Type-Character 3	Body Part-Character 4	Radionuclide-Character 5	Qualifier-Character 6	Qualifier-Character 7
1 Planar Nuclear Medicine Imaging	**1** Parathyroid Glands	**1** Technetium 99m (Tc-99m)	**Z** None	**Z** None
2 Tomographic (Tomo) Nuclear Medicine Imaging	**2** Thyroid Gland	**F** Iodine 123 (I-123)		
4 Nonimaging Nuclear Medicine Uptake	**4** Adrenal Glands, Bilateral	**G** Iodine 131 (I-131)		
	Y Endocrine System	**S** Thallium 201 (Tl-201)		
		Y Other Radionuclide		

C: Nuclear Medicine
H: Skin, Subcutaneous Tissue and Breast

Type-Character 3	Body Part-Character 4	Radionuclide-Character 5	Qualifier-Character 6	Qualifier-Character 7
1 Planar Nuclear Medicine Imaging	**0** Breast, Right	**1** Technetium 99m (Tc-99m)	**Z** None	**Z** None
2 Tomographic (Tomo) Nuclear Medicine Imaging	**1** Breast, Left	**S** Thallium 201 (Tl-201)		
	2 Breasts, Bilateral	**Y** Other Radionuclide		
	Y Skin, Subcutaneous Tissue and Breast			

C: Nuclear Medicine
P: Musculoskeletal System

Type-Character 3	Body Part-Character 4	Radionuclide-Character 5	Qualifier-Character 6	Qualifier-Character 7
1 Planar Nuclear Medicine Imaging	**1** Skull	**1** Technetium 99m (Tc-99m)	**Z** None	**Z** None
2 Tomographic (Tomo) Nuclear Medicine Imaging	**2** Cervical Spine	**Y** Other Radionuclide		
5 Nonimaging Nuclear Medicine Probe	**3** Skull and Cervical Spine	**Z** None		
	4 Thorax			
	5 Spine			
	6 Pelvis			
	7 Spine and Pelvis			
	8 Upper Extremity, Right			
	9 Upper Extremity, Left			
	B Upper Extremities, Bilateral			
	C Lower Extremity, Right			
	D Lower Extremity, Left			
	F Lower Extremities, Bilateral			
	G Thoracic Spine			
	H Lumbar Spine			
	J Thoracolumbar Spine			
	N Upper Extremities			
	P Lower Extremities			
	Y Musculoskeletal System, Other			
	Z Musculoskeletal System, All			

C: Nuclear Medicine
T: Urinary System

Type-Character 3	Body Part-Character 4	Radionuclide-Character 5	Qualifier-Character 6	Qualifier-Character 7
1 Planar Nuclear Medicine Imaging	**3** Kidneys, Ureters and Bladder	**1** Technetium 99m (Tc-99m)	**Z** None	**Z** None
2 Tomographic (Tomo) Nuclear Medicine Imaging	**H** Bladder and Ureters	**F** Iodine 123 (I-123)		
6 Nonimaging Nuclear Medicine Assay	**Y** Urinary System	**G** Iodine 131 (I-131)		
		H Iodine 125 (I-125)		
		Y Other Radionuclide		

C: Nuclear Medicine
V: Male Reproductive System

Type-Character 3	Body Part-Character 4	Radionuclide-Character 5	Qualifier-Character 6	Qualifier-Character 7
1 Planar Nuclear Medicine Imaging	**9** Testicles, Bilateral	**1** Technetium 99m (Tc-99m)	**Z** None	**Z** None
	Y Male Reproductive System	**Y** Other Radionuclide		

C: Nuclear Medicine
W: Anatomical Regions

Type-Character 3	Body Part-Character 4	Radionuclide-Character 5	Qualifier-Character 6	Qualifier-Character 7
1 Planar Nuclear Medicine Imaging	**0** Abdomen	**1** Technetium 99m (Tc-99m)	**Z** None	**Z** None
2 Tomographic (Tomo) Nuclear Medicine Imaging	**1** Abdomen and Pelvis	**8** Samarium 153 (Sm-153)		
3 Positron Emission Tomographic (PET) Imaging	**3** Chest	**D** Indium 111 (In-111)		
5 Nonimaging Nuclear Medicine Probe	**4** Chest and Abdomen	**F** Iodine 123 (I-123)		
7 Systemic Nuclear Medicine Therapy	**6** Chest and Neck	**G** Iodine 131 (I-131)		
	B Head and Neck	**K** Fluorine 18 (F-18)		
	D Lower Extremity	**L** Gallium 67 (Ga-67)		
	G Thyroid	**N** Phosphorus 32 (P-32)		
	J Pelvic Region	**P** Strontium 89 (Sr-89)		
	M Upper Extremity	**S** Thallium 201 (Tl-201)		
	N Whole Body	**Y** Other Radionuclide		
	Y Anatomical Regions, Multiple	**Z** None		
	Z Anatomical Region, Other			

D: Radiation Therapy
0: Central and Peripheral Nervous System

Modality-Character 3	Treatment Site -Character 4	Modality Qualifier-Character 5	Isotope -Character 6	Qualifier-Character 7
0 Beam Radiation	**0** Brain	**0** Photons <1 MeV	**7** Cesium 137 (Cs-137)	**0** Intraoperative
1 Brachytherapy	**1** Brain Stem	**1** Photons 1 - 10 MeV	**8** Iridium 192 (Ir-192)	**Z** None
2 Stereotactic Radiosurgery	**6** Spinal Cord	**2** Photons >10 MeV	**9** Iodine 125 (I-125)	
Y Other Radiation	**7** Peripheral Nerve	**3** Electrons	**B** Palladium 103 (Pd-103)	
		4 Heavy Particles (Protons, Ions)	**C** Californium 252 (Cf-252)	
		5 Neutrons	**Y** Other Isotope	
		6 Neutron Capture	**Z** None	
		7 Contact Radiation		
		8 Hyperthermia		
		9 High Dose Rate (HDR)		
		B Low Dose Rate (LDR)		
		D Stereotactic Other Photon Radiosurgery		
		F Plaque Radiation		
		H Stereotactic Particulate Radiosurgery		
		J Stereotactic Gamma Beam Radiosurgery		
		K Laser Interstitial Thermal Therapy		

D: Radiation Therapy
7: Lymphatic and Hematologic System

Modality-Character 3	Treatment Site -Character 4	Modality Qualifier-Character 5	Isotope -Character 6	Qualifier-Character 7
0 Beam Radiation	**0** Bone Marrow	**0** Photons <1 MeV	**7** Cesium 137 (Cs-137)	**0** Intraoperative
1 Brachytherapy	**1** Thymus	**1** Photons 1 - 10 MeV	**8** Iridium 192 (Ir-192)	**Z** None
2 Stereotactic Radiosurgery	**2** Spleen	**2** Photons >10 MeV	**9** Iodine 125 (I-125)	
Y Other Radiation	**3** Lymphatics, Neck	**3** Electrons	**B** Palladium 103 (Pd-103)	
	4 Lymphatics, Axillary	**4** Heavy Particles (Protons, Ions)	**C** Californium 252 (Cf-252)	
	5 Lymphatics, Thorax	**5** Neutrons	**Y** Other Isotope	
	6 Lymphatics, Abdomen	**6** Neutron Capture	**Z** None	
	7 Lymphatics, Pelvis	**8** Hyperthermia		
	8 Lymphatics, Inguinal	**9** High Dose Rate (HDR)		
		B Low Dose Rate (LDR)		
		D Stereotactic Other Photon Radiosurgery		
		F Plaque Radiation		
		H Stereotactic Particulate Radiosurgery		
		J Stereotactic Gamma Beam Radiosurgery		

D: Radiation Therapy
8: Eye

Modality-Character 3	Treatment Site -Character 4	Modality Qualifier-Character 5	Isotope -Character 6	Qualifier-Character 7
0 Beam Radiation	**0** Eye	**0** Photons <1 MeV	**7** Cesium 137 (Cs-137)	**0** Intraoperative
1 Brachytherapy		**1** Photons 1 - 10 MeV	**8** Iridium 192 (Ir-192)	**Z** None
2 Stereotactic Radiosurgery		**2** Photons >10 MeV	**9** Iodine 125 (I-125)	
Y Other Radiation		**3** Electrons	**B** Palladium 103 (Pd-103)	
		4 Heavy Particles (Protons, Ions)	**C** Californium 252 (Cf-252)	
		5 Neutrons	**Y** Other Isotope	
		6 Neutron Capture	**Z** None	
		7 Contact Radiation		
		8 Hyperthermia		
		9 High Dose Rate (HDR)		
		B Low Dose Rate (LDR)		
		D Stereotactic Other Photon Radiosurgery		
		F Plaque Radiation		
		H Stereotactic Particulate Radiosurgery		
		J Stereotactic Gamma Beam Radiosurgery		

D: Radiation Therapy
9: Ear, Nose, Mouth and Throat

Modality-Character 3	Treatment Site -Character 4	Modality Qualifier-Character 5	Isotope -Character 6	Qualifier-Character 7
0 Beam Radiation	**0** Ear	**0** Photons <1 MeV	**7** Cesium 137 (Cs-137)	**0** Intraoperative
1 Brachytherapy	**1** Nose	**1** Photons 1 - 10 MeV	**8** Iridium 192 (Ir-192)	**Z** None
2 Stereotactic Radiosurgery	**3** Hypopharynx	**2** Photons >10 MeV	**9** Iodine 125 (I-125)	
Y Other Radiation	**4** Mouth	**3** Electrons	**B** Palladium 103 (Pd-103)	
	5 Tongue	**4** Heavy Particles (Protons, Ions)	**C** Californium 252 (Cf-252)	
	6 Salivary Glands	**5** Neutrons	**Y** Other Isotope	
	7 Sinuses	**6** Neutron Capture	**Z** None	
	8 Hard Palate	**7** Contact Radiation		
	9 Soft Palate	**8** Hyperthermia		
	B Larynx	**9** High Dose Rate (HDR)		
	C Pharynx	**B** Low Dose Rate (LDR)		
	D Nasopharynx	**C** Intraoperative Radiation Therapy (IORT)		
	F Oropharynx	**D** Stereotactic Other Photon Radiosurgery		
		F Plaque Radiation		
		H Stereotactic Particulate Radiosurgery		
		J Stereotactic Gamma Beam Radiosurgery		

D: Radiation Therapy
B: Respiratory System

Modality-Character 3	Treatment Site -Character 4	Modality Qualifier-Character 5	Isotope -Character 6	Qualifier-Character 7
0 Beam Radiation	**0** Trachea	**0** Photons <1 MeV	**7** Cesium 137 (Cs-137)	**0** Intraoperative
1 Brachytherapy	**1** Bronchus	**1** Photons 1 - 10 MeV	**8** Iridium 192 (Ir-192)	**Z** None
2 Stereotactic Radiosurgery	**2** Lung	**2** Photons >10 MeV	**9** Iodine 125 (I-125)	
Y Other Radiation	**5** Pleura	**3** Electrons	**B** Palladium 103 (Pd-103)	
	6 Mediastinum	**4** Heavy Particles (Protons, Ions)	**C** Californium 252 (Cf-252)	
	7 Chest Wall	**5** Neutrons	**Y** Other Isotope	
	8 Diaphragm	**6** Neutron Capture	**Z** None	
		7 Contact Radiation		
		8 Hyperthermia		
		9 High Dose Rate (HDR)		
		B Low Dose Rate (LDR)		
		D Stereotactic Other Photon Radiosurgery		
		F Plaque Radiation		
		H Stereotactic Particulate Radiosurgery		
		J Stereotactic Gamma Beam Radiosurgery		
		K Laser Interstitial Thermal Therapy		

D: Radiation Therapy
D: Gastrointestinal System

Modality-Character 3	Treatment Site -Character 4	Modality Qualifier-Character 5	Isotope -Character 6	Qualifier-Character 7
0 Beam Radiation	**0** Esophagus	**0** Photons <1 MeV	**7** Cesium 137 (Cs-137)	**0** Intraoperative
1 Brachytherapy	**1** Stomach	**1** Photons 1 - 10 MeV	**8** Iridium 192 (Ir-192)	**Z** None
2 Stereotactic Radiosurgery	**2** Duodenum	**2** Photons >10 MeV	**9** Iodine 125 (I-125)	
Y Other Radiation	**3** Jejunum	**3** Electrons	**B** Palladium 103 (Pd-103)	
	4 Ileum	**4** Heavy Particles (Protons, Ions)	**C** Californium 252 (Cf-252)	
	5 Colon	**5** Neutrons	**Y** Other Isotope	
	7 Rectum	**6** Neutron Capture	**Z** None	
	8 Anus	**7** Contact Radiation		
		8 Hyperthermia		
		9 High Dose Rate (HDR)		
		B Low Dose Rate (LDR)		
		C Intraoperative Radiation Therapy (IORT)		
		D Stereotactic Other Photon Radiosurgery		
		F Plaque Radiation		
		H Stereotactic Particulate Radiosurgery		
		J Stereotactic Gamma Beam Radiosurgery		
		K Laser Interstitial Thermal Therapy		

D: Radiation Therapy
F: Hepatobiliary System and Pancreas

Modality-Character 3	Treatment Site -Character 4	Modality Qualifier-Character 5	Isotope -Character 6	Qualifier-Character 7
0 Beam Radiation	**0** Liver	**0** Photons <1 MeV	**7** Cesium 137 (Cs-137)	**0** Intraoperative
1 Brachytherapy	**1** Gallbladder	**1** Photons 1 - 10 MeV	**8** Iridium 192 (Ir-192)	**Z** None
2 Stereotactic Radiosurgery	**2** Bile Ducts	**2** Photons >10 MeV	**9** Iodine 125 (I-125)	
Y Other Radiation	**3** Pancreas	**3** Electrons	**B** Palladium 103 (Pd-103)	
		4 Heavy Particles (Protons, Ions)	**C** Californium 252 (Cf-252)	
		5 Neutrons	**Y** Other Isotope	
		6 Neutron Capture	**Z** None	
		7 Contact Radiation		
		8 Hyperthermia		
		9 High Dose Rate (HDR)		
		B Low Dose Rate (LDR)		
		C Intraoperative Radiation Therapy (IORT)		
		D Stereotactic Other Photon Radiosurgery		
		F Plaque Radiation		
		H Stereotactic Particulate Radiosurgery		
		J Stereotactic Gamma Beam Radiosurgery		
		K Laser Interstitial Thermal Therapy		

D: Radiation Therapy
G: Endocrine System

Modality-Character 3	Treatment Site -Character 4	Modality Qualifier-Character 5	Isotope -Character 6	Qualifier-Character 7
0 Beam Radiation	**0** Pituitary Gland	**0** Photons <1 MeV	**7** Cesium 137 (Cs-137)	**0** Intraoperative
1 Brachytherapy	**1** Pineal Body	**1** Photons 1 - 10 MeV	**8** Iridium 192 (Ir-192)	**Z** None
2 Stereotactic Radiosurgery	**2** Adrenal Glands	**2** Photons >10 MeV	**9** Iodine 125 (I-125)	
Y Other Radiation	**4** Parathyroid Glands	**3** Electrons	**B** Palladium 103 (Pd-103)	
	5 Thyroid	**5** Neutrons	**C** Californium 252 (Cf-252)	
		6 Neutron Capture	**Y** Other Isotope	
		7 Contact Radiation	**Z** None	
		8 Hyperthermia		
		9 High Dose Rate (HDR)		
		B Low Dose Rate (LDR)		
		D Stereotactic Other Photon Radiosurgery		
		F Plaque Radiation		
		H Stereotactic Particulate Radiosurgery		
		J Stereotactic Gamma Beam Radiosurgery		
		K Laser Interstitial Thermal Therapy		

D: Radiation Therapy
H: Skin

Modality-Character 3	Treatment Site -Character 4	Modality Qualifier-Character 5	Isotope -Character 6	Qualifier-Character 7
0 Beam Radiation	**2** Skin, Face	**0** Photons <1 MeV	**Z** None	**0** Intraoperative
Y Other Radiation	**3** Skin, Neck	**1** Photons 1 - 10 MeV		**Z** None
	4 Skin, Arm	**2** Photons >10 MeV		
	5 Skin, Hand	**3** Electrons		
	6 Skin, Chest	**4** Heavy Particles (Protons, Ions)		
	7 Skin, Back	**5** Neutrons		
	8 Skin, Abdomen	**6** Neutron Capture		
	9 Skin, Buttock	**7** Contact Radiation		
	B Skin, Leg	**8** Hyperthermia		
	C Skin, Foot	**F** Plaque Radiation		

D: Radiation Therapy
M: Breast

Modality-Character 3	Treatment Site -Character 4	Modality Qualifier-Character 5	Isotope -Character 6	Qualifier-Character 7
0 Beam Radiation	**0** Breast, Left	**0** Photons <1 MeV	**7** Cesium 137 (Cs-137)	**0** Intraoperative
1 Brachytherapy	**1** Breast, Right	**1** Photons 1 - 10 MeV	**8** Iridium 192 (Ir-192)	**Z** None
2 Stereotactic Radiosurgery		**2** Photons >10 MeV	**9** Iodine 125 (I-125)	
Y Other Radiation		**3** Electrons	**B** Palladium 103 (Pd-103)	
		4 Heavy Particles (Protons, Ions)	**C** Californium 252 (Cf-252)	
		5 Neutrons	**Y** Other Isotope	
		6 Neutron Capture	**Z** None	
		7 Contact Radiation		
		8 Hyperthermia		
		9 High Dose Rate (HDR)		
		B Low Dose Rate (LDR)		
		D Stereotactic Other Photon Radiosurgery		
		F Plaque Radiation		
		H Stereotactic Particulate Radiosurgery		
		J Stereotactic Gamma Beam Radiosurgery		
		K Laser Interstitial Thermal Therapy		

D: Radiation Therapy
P: Musculoskeletal System

Modality-Character 3	Treatment Site -Character 4	Modality Qualifier-Character 5	Isotope -Character 6	Qualifier-Character 7
0 Beam Radiation	**0** Skull	**0** Photons <1 MeV	**Z** None	**0** Intraoperative
Y Other Radiation	**2** Maxilla	**1** Photons 1 - 10 MeV		**Z** None
	3 Mandible	**2** Photons >10 MeV		
	4 Sternum	**3** Electrons		
	5 Rib(s)	**4** Heavy Particles (Protons, Ions)		
	6 Humerus	**5** Neutrons		
	7 Radius/Ulna	**6** Neutron Capture		
	8 Pelvic Bones	**7** Contact Radiation		
	9 Femur	**8** Hyperthermia		
	B Tibia/Fibula	**F** Plaque Radiation		
	C Other Bone			

D: Radiation Therapy
T: Urinary System

Modality-Character 3	Treatment Site -Character 4	Modality Qualifier-Character 5	Isotope -Character 6	Qualifier-Character 7
0 Beam Radiation	**0** Kidney	**0** Photons <1 MeV	**7** Cesium 137 (Cs-137)	**0** Intraoperative
1 Brachytherapy	**1** Ureter	**1** Photons 1 - 10 MeV	**8** Iridium 192 (Ir-192)	**Z** None
2 Stereotactic Radiosurgery	**2** Bladder	**2** Photons >10 MeV	**9** Iodine 125 (I-125)	
Y Other Radiation	**3** Urethra	**3** Electrons	**B** Palladium 103 (Pd-103)	
		4 Heavy Particles (Protons, Ions)	**C** Californium 252 (Cf-252)	
		5 Neutrons	**Y** Other Isotope	
		6 Neutron Capture	**Z** None	
		7 Contact Radiation		
		8 Hyperthermia		
		9 High Dose Rate (HDR)		
		B Low Dose Rate (LDR)		
		C Intraoperative Radiation Therapy (IORT)		
		D Stereotactic Other Photon Radiosurgery		
		F Plaque Radiation		
		H Stereotactic Particulate Radiosurgery		
		J Stereotactic Gamma Beam Radiosurgery		

D: Radiation Therapy
U: Female Reproductive System

Modality-Character 3	Treatment Site -Character 4	Modality Qualifier-Character 5	Isotope -Character 6	Qualifier-Character 7
0 Beam Radiation	**0** Ovary	**0** Photons <1 MeV	**7** Cesium 137 (Cs-137)	**0** Intraoperative
1 Brachytherapy	**1** Cervix	**1** Photons 1 - 10 MeV	**8** Iridium 192 (Ir-192)	**Z** None
2 Stereotactic Radiosurgery	**2** Uterus	**2** Photons >10 MeV	**9** Iodine 125 (I-125)	
Y Other Radiation		**3** Electrons	**B** Palladium 103 (Pd-103)	
		4 Heavy Particles (Protons, Ions)	**C** Californium 252 (Cf-252)	
		5 Neutrons	**Y** Other Isotope	
		6 Neutron Capture	**Z** None	
		7 Contact Radiation		
		8 Hyperthermia		
		9 High Dose Rate (HDR)		
		B Low Dose Rate (LDR)		
		C Intraoperative Radiation Therapy (IORT)		
		D Stereotactic Other Photon Radiosurgery		
		F Plaque Radiation		
		H Stereotactic Particulate Radiosurgery		
		J Stereotactic Gamma Beam Radiosurgery		

D: Radiation Therapy
V: Male Reproductive System

Modality-Character 3	Treatment Site -Character 4	Modality Qualifier-Character 5	Isotope -Character 6	Qualifier-Character 7
0 Beam Radiation	**0** Prostate	**0** Photons <1 MeV	**7** Cesium 137 (Cs-137)	**0** Intraoperative
1 Brachytherapy	**1** Testis	**1** Photons 1 - 10 MeV	**8** Iridium 192 (Ir-192)	**Z** None
2 Stereotactic Radiosurgery		**2** Photons >10 MeV	**9** Iodine 125 (I-125)	
Y Other Radiation		**3** Electrons	**B** Palladium 103 (Pd-103)	
		4 Heavy Particles (Protons, Ions)	**C** Californium 252 (Cf-252)	
		5 Neutrons	**Y** Other Isotope	
		6 Neutron Capture	**Z** None	
		7 Contact Radiation		
		8 Hyperthermia		
		9 High Dose Rate (HDR)		
		B Low Dose Rate (LDR)		
		C Intraoperative Radiation Therapy (IORT)		
		D Stereotactic Other Photon Radiosurgery		
		F Plaque Radiation		
		H Stereotactic Particulate Radiosurgery		
		J Stereotactic Gamma Beam Radiosurgery		

D: Radiation Therapy
W: Anatomical Regions

Modality-Character 3	Treatment Site -Character 4	Modality Qualifier-Character 5	Isotope -Character 6	Qualifier-Character 7
0 Beam Radiation	**1** Head and Neck	**0** Photons <1 MeV	**7** Cesium 137 (Cs-137)	**0** Intraoperative
1 Brachytherapy	**2** Chest	**1** Photons 1 - 10 MeV	**8** Iridium 192 (Ir-192)	**Z** None
2 Stereotactic Radiosurgery	**3** Abdomen	**2** Photons >10 MeV	**9** Iodine 125 (I-125)	
Y Other Radiation	**4** Hemibody	**3** Electrons	**B** Palladium 103 (Pd-103)	
	5 Whole Body	**4** Heavy Particles (Protons, Ions)	**C** Californium 252 (Cf-252)	
	6 Pelvic Region	**5** Neutrons	**D** Iodine 131 (I-131)	
		6 Neutron Capture	**F** Phosphorus 32 (P-32)	
		7 Contact Radiation	**G** Strontium 89 (Sr-89)	
		8 Hyperthermia	**H** Strontium 90 (Sr-90)	
		9 High Dose Rate (HDR)	**Y** Other Isotope	
		B Low Dose Rate (LDR)	**Z** None	
		D Stereotactic Other Photon Radiosurgery		
		F Plaque Radiation		
		G Isotope Administration		
		H Stereotactic Particulate Radiosurgery		
		J Stereotactic Gamma Beam Radiosurgery		

F: Physical Rehabilitation and Diagnostic Audiology
0: Rehabilitation

Type-Character 3	Body System/Region-Character 4	Type Qualifier-Character 5	Equipment-Character 6	Qualifier-Character 7
0 Speech Assessment	**0** Neurological System - Head and Neck	**0** Bathing/Showering	**1** Audiometer	**Z** None
1 Motor and/or Nerve Function Assessment	**1** Neurological System - Upper Back / Upper Extremity	**0** Bathing/Showering Technique	**2** Sound Field / Booth	
2 Activities of Daily Living Assessment	**2** Neurological System - Lower Back / Lower Extremity	**0** Bathing/Showering Techniques	**4** Electroacoustic Immittance / Acoustic Reflex	
6 Speech Treatment	**3** Neurological System - Whole Body	**0** Cochlear Implant Rehabilitation	**5** Hearing Aid Selection / Fitting / Test	
7 Motor Treatment	**4** Circulatory System - Head and Neck	**0** Filtered Speech	**7** Electrophysiologic	
8 Activities of Daily Living Treatment	**5** Circulatory System - Upper Back / Upper Extremity	**0** Hearing and Related Disorders Counseling	**8** Vestibular / Balance	
9 Hearing Treatment	**6** Circulatory System - Lower Back / Lower Extremity	**0** Muscle Performance	**9** Cochlear Implant	
B Cochlear Implant Treatment	**7** Circulatory System - Whole Body	**0** Nonspoken Language	**B** Physical Agents	
C Vestibular Treatment	**8** Respiratory System - Head and Neck	**0** Range of Motion and Joint Mobility	**C** Mechanical	
D Device Fitting	**9** Respiratory System - Upper Back / Upper Extremity	**0** Tinnitus Masker	**D** Electrotherapeutic	
F Caregiver Training	**B** Respiratory System - Lower Back / Lower Extremity	**0** Vestibular	**E** Orthosis	
	C Respiratory System - Whole Body	**1** Dressing	**F** Assistive, Adaptive, Supportive or Protective	
	D Integumentary System - Head and Neck	**1** Dressing Techniques	**G** Aerobic Endurance and Conditioning	
	F Integumentary System - Upper Back / Upper Extremity	**1** Hearing and Related Disorders Prevention	**H** Mechanical or Electromechanical	
	G Integumentary System -Lower Back / Lower Extremity	**1** Integumentary Integrity	**J** Somatosensory	
	H Integumentary System - Whole Body	**1** Monaural Hearing Aid	**K** Audiovisual	
	J Musculoskeletal System - Head and Neck	**1** Muscle Performance	**L** Assistive Listening	
	K Musculoskeletal System - Upper Back / Upper Extremity	**1** Perceptual Processing	**M** Augmentative / Alternative Communication	
	L Musculoskeletal System - Lower Back / Lower Extremity	**1** Speech Threshold	**N** Biosensory Feedback	
	M Musculoskeletal System - Whole Body	**1** Speech-Language Pathology and Related Disorders Counseling	**P** Computer	
	N Genitourinary System	**2** Auditory Processing	**Q** Speech Analysis	
	Z None	**2** Binaural Hearing Aid	**S** Voice Analysis	
		2 Coordination/Dexterity	**T** Aerodynamic Function	
		2 Feeding and Eating	**U** Prosthesis	
		2 Feeding/Eating	**V** Speech Prosthesis	
		2 Grooming/Personal Hygiene	**W** Swallowing	
		2 Speech/Word Recognition	**X** Cerumen Management	
		2 Speech-Language Pathology and Related Disorders Prevention	**Y** Other Equipment	
		2 Visual Motor Integration	**Z** None	
		3 Aphasia		
		3 Augmentative/Alternative Communication System		
		3 Cerumen Management		
		3 Coordination/Dexterity		
		3 Feeding/Eating		

Type-Character 3	Body System/Region-Character 4	Type Qualifier-Character 5	Equipment-Character 6	Qualifier-Character 7
		3 Grooming/Personal Hygiene		
		3 Motor Function		
		3 Postural Control		
		3 Staggered Spondaic Word		
		4 Articulation/Phonology		
		4 Bed Mobility		
		4 Home Management		
		4 Motor Function		
		4 Sensorineural Acuity Level		
		4 Voice Prosthetic		
		4 Wheelchair Mobility		
		5 Assistive Listening Device		
		5 Aural Rehabilitation		
		5 Bed Mobility		
		5 Perceptual Processing		
		5 Range of Motion and Joint Integrity		
		5 Synthetic Sentence Identification		
		5 Transfer		
		5 Wound Management		
		6 Communicative/Cognitive Integration Skills		
		6 Dynamic Orthosis		
		6 Psychosocial Skills		
		6 Sensory Awareness/Processing/Integrity		
		6 Speech and/or Language Screening		
		6 Therapeutic Exercise		
		6 Wheelchair Mobility		
		7 Aerobic Capacity and Endurance		
		7 Facial Nerve Function		
		7 Fluency		
		7 Manual Therapy Techniques		
		7 Nonspoken Language		
		7 Static Orthosis		
		7 Therapeutic Exercise		
		7 Vocational Activities and Functional Community or Work Reintegration Skills		
		8 Airway Clearance Techniques		
		8 Anthropometric Characteristics		
		8 Motor Speech		
		8 Prosthesis		
		8 Receptive/Expressive Language		
		8 Transfer Training		
		9 Articulation/Phonology		
		9 Assistive, Adaptive, Supportive or Protective Devices		
		9 Cranial Nerve Integrity		
		9 Gait Training/Functional Ambulation		
		9 Orofacial Myofunctional		
		9 Somatosensory Evoked Potentials		
		9 Wound Management		
		B Bed Mobility		

Type-Character 3	Body System/Region-Character 4	Type Qualifier-Character 5	Equipment-Character 6	Qualifier-Character 7
		B Environmental, Home and Work Barriers		
		B Motor Speech		
		B Receptive/Expressive Language		
		B Vocational Activities and Functional Community or Work Reintegration Skills		
		C Aphasia		
		C Ergonomics and Body Mechanics		
		C Gait Training/Functional Ambulation		
		C Transfer		
		C Voice		
		D Application, Proper Use and Care of Devices		
		D Fluency		
		D Gait and/or Balance		
		D Neuromotor Development		
		D Swallowing Dysfunction		
		F Application, Proper Use and Care of Orthoses		
		F Pain		
		F Voice		
		F Wheelchair Mobility		
		G Application, Proper Use and Care of Prosthesis		
		G Communicative/Cognitive Integration Skills		
		G Reflex Integrity		
		G Ventilation, Respiration and Circulation		
		H Bedside Swallowing and Oral Function		
		H Home Management		
		H Vocational Activities and Functional Community or Work Reintegration Skills		
		J Communication Skills		
		J Instrumental Swallowing and Oral Function		
		K Orofacial Myofunctional		
		L Augmentative/Alternative Communication System		
		M Voice Prosthetic		
		N Non-invasive Instrumental Status		
		P Oral Peripheral Mechanism		
		Q Performance Intensity Phonetically Balanced Speech Discrimination		
		R Brief Tone Stimuli		
		S Distorted Speech		
		T Dichotic Stimuli		
		V Temporal Ordering of Stimuli		
		W Masking Patterns		
		X Other Specified Central Auditory Processing		

F: Physical Rehabilitation and Diagnostic Audiology
1: Diagnostic Audiology

Type-Character 3	Body System/Region-Character 4	Type Qualifier-Character 5	Equipment-Character 6	Qualifier-Character 7
3 Hearing Assessment	**Z** None	**0** Bithermal, Binaural Caloric Irrigation	**0** Occupational Hearing	**Z** None
4 Hearing Aid Assessment		**0** Cochlear Implant	**1** Audiometer	
5 Vestibular Assessment		**0** Hearing Screening	**2** Sound Field / Booth	
		1 Bithermal, Monaural Caloric Irrigation	**3** Tympanometer	
		1 Ear Canal Probe Microphone	**4** Electroacoustic Immittance / Acoustic Reflex	
		1 Pure Tone Audiometry, Air	**5** Hearing Aid Selection / Fitting / Test	
		2 Monaural Hearing Aid	**6** Otoacoustic Emission (OAE)	
		2 Pure Tone Audiometry, Air and Bone	**7** Electrophysiologic	
		2 Unithermal Binaural Screen	**8** Vestibular / Balance	
		3 Bekesy Audiometry	**9** Cochlear Implant	
		3 Binaural Hearing Aid	**K** Audiovisual	
		3 Oscillating Tracking	**L** Assistive Listening	
		4 Assistive Listening System/Device Selection	**P** Computer	
		4 Conditioned Play Audiometry	**Y** Other Equipment	
		4 Sinusoidal Vertical Axis Rotational	**Z** None	
		5 Dix-Hallpike Dynamic		
		5 Select Picture Audiometry		
		5 Sensory Aids		
		6 Binaural Electroacoustic Hearing Aid Check		
		6 Computerized Dynamic Posturography		
		6 Visual Reinforcement Audiometry		
		7 Alternate Binaural or Monaural Loudness Balance		
		7 Ear Protector Attenuation		
		7 Tinnitus Masker		
		8 Monaural Electroacoustic Hearing Aid Check		
		8 Tone Decay		
		9 Short Increment Sensitivity Index		
		B Stenger		
		C Pure Tone Stenger		
		D Tympanometry		
		F Eustachian Tube Function		
		G Acoustic Reflex Patterns		
		H Acoustic Reflex Threshold		
		J Acoustic Reflex Decay		
		K Electrocochleography		
		L Auditory Evoked Potentials		
		M Evoked Otoacoustic Emissions, Screening		
		N Evoked Otoacoustic Emissions, Diagnostic		
		P Aural Rehabilitation Status		
		Q Auditory Processing		

G: Mental Health
Z: None

Type-Character 3	Qualifier-Character 4	Qualifier-Character 5	Qualifier-Character 6	Qualifier-Character 7
1 Psychological Tests	**0** Developmental	**Z** None	**Z** None	**Z** None
2 Crisis Intervention	**0** Educational			
3 Medication Management	**0** Interactive			
5 Individual Psychotherapy	**0** Unilateral-Single Seizure			
6 Counseling	**1** Behavioral			
7 Family Psychotherapy	**1** Personality and Behavioral			
B Electroconvulsive Therapy	**1** Unilateral-Multiple Seizure			
C Biofeedback	**1** Vocational			
F Hypnosis	**2** Bilateral-Single Seizure			
G Narcosynthesis	**2** Cognitive			
H Group Psychotherapy	**2** Intellectual and Psychoeducational			
J Light Therapy	**2** Other Family Psychotherapy			
	3 Bilateral-Multiple Seizure			
	3 Interpersonal			
	3 Neuropsychological			
	3 Other Counseling			
	4 Neurobehavioral and Cognitive Status			
	4 Other Electroconvulsive Therapy			
	4 Psychoanalysis			
	5 Psychodynamic			
	6 Supportive			
	8 Cognitive-Behavioral			
	9 Other Biofeedback			
	9 Psychophysiological			
	Z None			

H: Substance Abuse Treatment
Z: None

Type-Character 3	Qualifier-Character 4	Qualifier-Character 5	Qualifier-Character 6	Qualifier-Character 7
2 Detoxification Services	**0** Cognitive	**Z** None	**Z** None	**Z** None
3 Individual Counseling	**0** Nicotine Replacement			
4 Group Counseling	**1** Behavioral			
5 Individual Psychotherapy	**1** Methadone Maintenance			
6 Family Counseling	**2** Cognitive-Behavioral			
8 Medication Management	**2** Levo-alpha-acetylmethadol (LAAM)			
9 Pharmacotherapy	**3** 12-Step			
	3 Antabuse			
	3 Other Family Counseling			
	4 Interpersonal			
	4 Naltrexone			
	5 Interactive			
	5 Naloxone			
	5 Vocational			
	6 Clonidine			
	6 Psychoeducation			
	7 Bupropion			
	7 Motivational Enhancement			
	8 Confrontational			
	8 Psychiatric Medication			
	9 Continuing Care			
	9 Other Replacement Medication			
	9 Supportive			
	B Psychoanalysis			
	B Spiritual			
	C Pre/Post-Test Infectious Disease			
	C Psychodynamic			
	D Psychophysiological			
	Z None			

X: New Technology
2: Cardiovascular System

Operation-Character 3	Body Part-Character 4	Approach-Character 5	Device-Character 6	Qualifier-Character 7
A Assistance	**0** Coronary Artery, One Artery	**0** Open	**1** Cerebral Embolic Filtration, Dual Filter	**1** New Technology Group 1
C Extirpation	**1** Coronary Artery, Two Arteries	**3** Percutaneous	**3** Zooplastic Tissue, Rapid Deployment Technique	**2** New Technology Group 2
R Replacement	**2** Coronary Artery, Three Arteries	**4** Percutaneous Endoscopic	**6** Orbital Atherectomy Technology	
	3 Coronary Artery, Four or More Arteries			
	5 Innominate Artery and Left Common Carotid Artery			
	F Aortic Valve			

X: New Technology
H: Skin, Subcutaneous Tissue, Fascia and Breast

Operation-Character 3	Body Part-Character 4	Approach-Character 5	Device-Character 6	Qualifier-Character 7
R Replacement	**P** Skin	**X** External	**L** Skin Substitute, Porcine Liver Derived	**2** New Technology Group 2

X: New Technology
K: Muscles, Tendons, Bursae and Ligaments

Operation-Character 3	Body Part-Character 4	Approach-Character 5	Device-Character 6	Qualifier-Character 7
0 Introduction	**2** Muscle	**3** Percutaneous	**0** Concentrated Bone Marrow Aspirate	**3** New Technology Group 3

X: New Technology
N: Bones

Operation-Character 3	Body Part-Character 4	Approach-Character 5	Device-Character 6	Qualifier-Character 7
S Reposition	**0** Lumbar Vertebra	**0** Open	**3** Magnetically Controlled Growth Rod(s)	**2** New Technology Group 2
	3 Cervical Vertebra	**3** Percutaneous		
	4 Thoracic Vertebra			

X: New Technology
R: Joints

Operation-Character 3	Body Part-Character 4	Approach-Character 5	Device-Character 6	Qualifier-Character 7
2 Monitoring	**0** Occipital-cervical Joint	**0** Open	**2** Intraoperative Knee Replacement Sensor	**1** New Technology Group 1
G Fusion	**1** Cervical Vertebral Joint		**9** Interbody Fusion Device, Nanotextured Surface	**2** New Technology Group 2
	2 Cervical Vertebral Joints, 2 or more		**F** Interbody Fusion Device, Radiolucent Porous	**3** New Technology Group 3
	4 Cervicothoracic Vertebral Joint			
	6 Thoracic Vertebral Joint			
	7 Thoracic Vertebral Joints, 2 to 7			
	8 Thoracic Vertebral Joints, 8 or more			
	A Thoracolumbar Vertebral Joint			
	B Lumbar Vertebral Joint			
	C Lumbar Vertebral Joints, 2 or more			
	D Lumbosacral Joint			
	G Knee Joint, Right			
	H Knee Joint, Left			

X: New Technology
V: Male Reproductive System

Operation-Character 3	Body Part-Character 4	Approach-Character 5	Device-Character 6	Qualifier-Character 7
5 Destruction	**0** Prostate	**8** Via Natural or Artificial Opening Endoscopic	**A** Robotic Waterjet Ablation	**4** New Technology Group 4

X: New Technology
W: Anatomical Regions

Operation-Character 3	Body Part-Character 4	Approach-Character 5	Device-Character 6	Qualifier-Character 7
0 Introduction	**3** Peripheral Vein	**3** Percutaneous	**2** Ceftazidime-Avibactam Anti-infective	**1** New Technology Group 1
	4 Central Vein	**X** External	**3** Idarucizumab, Dabigatran Reversal Agent	**2** New Technology Group 2
	D Mouth and Pharynx		**4** Isavuconazole Antiinfective	**3** New Technology Group 3
			5 Blinatumomab Antineoplastic Immunotherapy	**4** New Technology Group 4
			7 Andexanet Alfa, Factor Xa Inhibitor Reversal Agent	
			8 Uridine Triacetate	
			9 Defibrotide Sodium Anticoagulant	
			A Bezlotoxumab Monoclonal Antibody	
			B Cytarabine and Daunorubicin Liposome Antineoplastic	
			C Engineered Autologous Chimeric Antigen Receptor T-cell Immunotherapy	
			F Other New Technology Therapeutic Substance	
			G Plazomicin Anti-infective	
			H Synthetic Human Angiotensin II	

X: New Technology
Y: Extracorporeal

Operation-Character 3	Body Part-Character 4	Approach-Character 5	Device-Character 6	Qualifier-Character 7
0 Introduction	**V** Vein Graft	**X** External	**8** Endothelial Damage Inhibitor	**3** New Technology Group 3

This page intentionally left blank

Appendix F: Substance Key

Substance Term	ICD-10-PCS Value
AIGISRx® Antibacterial Envelope	Anti-Infective Envelope
Angiotensin II	Synthetic Human Angiotensin II
Antimicrobial envelope	Anti-Infective Envelope
Axicabtagene Ciloeucel	Engineered Autologous Chimeric Antigen Receptor T-cell Immunotherapy
Bone morphogenetic protein 2 (BMP 2)	Recombinant Bone Morphogenetic Protein
CBMA (Concentrated Bone Marrow Aspirate)	Concentrated Bone Marrow Aspirate
Clolar®	Clofarabine
Defitelio®	Defibrotide Sodium Anticoagulant
DuraGraft® Endothelial Damage Inhibitor	Endothelial Damage Inhibitor
Factor Xa Inhibitor Reversal Agent, Andexanet Alfa	Andexanet Alfa, Factor Xa Inhibitor Reversal Agent
GIAPREZA™	Synthetic Human Angiotensin II
Human angiotensin II, synthetic	Synthetic Human Angiotensin II
Kcentra®	4-Factor Prothrombin Complex Concentrate
KYMRIAH	Engineered Autologous Chimeric Antigen Receptor T-cell Immunotherapy
Nesiritide®	Human B-type Natriuretic Peptide
rhBMP-2	Recombinant Bone Morphogenetic Protein
Seprafilm®	Adhesion Barrier
STELARA®	Other New Technology Therapeutic Substance
Tisagenlecleucel	Engineered Autologous Chimeric Antigen Receptor T-cell Immunotherapy
Tissue Plasminogen Activator (tPA)(r- tPA)	Other Thrombolytic
Ustekinumab	Other New Technology Therapeutic Substance
Vistogard®	Uridine Triacetate
Voraxaze®	Glucarpidase
VYXEOS™	Cytarabine and Daunorubicin Liposome Antineoplastic
ZINPLAVA™	Bezlotoxumab Monoclonal Antibody
Zyvox®	Oxazolidinones

This page intentionally left blank

Appendix G: Combination Clusters

Due to the nature of a specific procedure, the first code in the cluster needs to be reported with one or more of the additional codes listed for all codes to be considered valid. The example below is for insertion of a cardiac defibrillator lead into the right ventricle (highlighted code). The additional procedure describes the exact location of where the lead is inserted, which is required for correct reporting:

02HK0KZ
and 0JH609Z

You would need to review the first procedure in the combination/cluster to determine whether you need to report the additional code.

The CMS site also provides additional information on combinations/clusters.

02H60KZ
and 0JH608Z

02H60KZ
and 0JH638Z

02H60KZ
and 0JH808Z

02H60KZ
and 0JH838Z

02H63KZ
and 0JH608Z

02H63KZ
and 0JH638Z

02H63KZ
and 0JH808Z

02H63KZ
and 0JH838Z

02H64KZ
and 0JH608Z

02H64KZ
and 0JH638Z

02H64KZ
and 0JH808Z

02H64KZ
and 0JH838Z

02H70KZ
and 0JH608Z

02H70KZ
and 0JH638Z

02H70KZ
and 0JH808Z

02H70KZ
and 0JH838Z

02H73KZ
and 0JH608Z

02H73KZ
and 0JH638Z

02H73KZ
and 0JH808Z

02H73KZ
and 0JH838Z

02H74KZ
and 0JH608Z

02H74KZ
and 0JH638Z

02H74KZ
and 0JH808Z

02H74KZ
and 0JH838Z

02HA0RS
and 02PA0RZ

02HA0RS
and 02PA3RZ

02HA0RS
and 02PA4RZ

02HA0RZ
and 02PA0RZ

02HA0RZ
and 02PA3RZ

02HA0RZ
and 02PA4RZ

02HA3RS
and 02PA0RZ

02HA3RS
and 02PA3RZ

02HA3RS
and 02PA4RZ

02HA4RS
and 02PA0RZ

02HA4RS
and 02PA3RZ

02HA4RS
and 02PA4RZ

02HA4RZ
and 02PA0RZ

02HA4RZ
and 02PA3RZ

02HA4RZ
and 02PA4RZ

02HK0KZ
and 0JH608Z

02HK0KZ
and 0JH609Z

02HK0KZ
and 0JH638Z

02HK0KZ
and 0JH639Z

02HK0KZ
and 0JH808Z

02HK0KZ
and 0JH809Z

02HK0KZ
and 0JH838Z

02HK0KZ
and 0JH839Z

02HK3KZ
and 0JH608Z

02HK3KZ
and 0JH609Z

02HK3KZ
and 0JH638Z

02HK3KZ
and 0JH639Z

02HK3KZ
and 0JH808Z

02HK3KZ
and 0JH809Z

02HK3KZ
and 0JH838Z

02HK3KZ
and 0JH839Z

02HK4KZ
and 0JH608Z

02HK4KZ
and 0JH609Z

02HK4KZ
and 0JH638Z

02HK4KZ
and 0JH639Z

02HK4KZ
and 0JH808Z

02HK4KZ
and 0JH809Z

02HK4KZ
and 0JH838Z

02HK4KZ
and 0JH839Z

02HL0KZ
and 0JH608Z

02HL0KZ
and 0JH609Z

02HL0KZ
and 0JH638Z

02HL0KZ
and 0JH639Z

02HL0KZ
and 0JH808Z

02HL0KZ
and 0JH809Z

02HL0KZ
and 0JH838Z

02HL0KZ
and 0JH839Z

02HL0MZ
and 0JH60AZ

02HL0MZ
and 0JH63AZ

02HL0MZ
and 0JH80AZ

02HL0MZ
and 0JH83AZ

02HL3KZ
and 0JH608Z

02HL3KZ
and 0JH609Z

02HL3KZ
and 0JH638Z

02HL3KZ
and 0JH639Z

02HL3KZ
and 0JH808Z

02HL3KZ
and 0JH809Z

02HL3KZ
and 0JH838Z

02HL3KZ
and 0JH839Z

02HL3MZ
and 0JH60AZ

02HL3MZ
and 0JH63AZ

02HL3MZ
and 0JH80AZ

02HL3MZ
and 0JH83AZ

02HL4KZ
and 0JH608Z

02HL4KZ
and 0JH609Z

02HL4KZ
and 0JH638Z

02HL4KZ
and 0JH639Z

02HL4KZ
and 0JH808Z

02HL4KZ
and 0JH809Z

02HL4KZ
and 0JH838Z

02HL4KZ
and 0JH839Z

02HL4MZ
and 0JH60AZ

02HL4MZ
and 0JH63AZ

02HL4MZ
and 0JH80AZ

02HL4MZ
and 0JH83AZ

02RK0JZ
and 02RL0JZ

02WA0QZ
and 02PA0RZ

02WA0QZ
and 02PA3RZ

02WA0QZ
and 02PA4RZ

02WA0RZ
and 02PA0RZ

02WA0RZ
and 02PA3RZ

02WA0RZ
and 02PA4RZ

02WA3QZ
and 02PA0RZ

02WA3QZ
and 02PA3RZ

02WA3QZ
and 02PA4RZ

02WA3RZ
and 02PA0RZ

02WA3RZ
and 02PA3RZ

02WA3RZ
and 02PA4RZ

02WA4QZ
and 02PA0RZ

02WA4QZ
and 02PA3RZ

02WA4QZ
and 02PA4RZ

02WA4RZ
and 02PA0RZ

02WA4RZ
and 02PA3RZ

02WA4RZ
and 02PA4RZ

07BH0ZZ
and 0UTM0ZZ

07BH0ZZ
and 0UTMXZZ

07BH4ZZ
and 0UTM0ZZ

07BH4ZZ
and 0UTMXZZ

07BJ0ZZ
and 0UTM0ZZ

07BJ0ZZ
and 0UTMXZZ

07BJ4ZZ
and 0UTM0ZZ

07BJ4ZZ
and 0UTMXZZ

07T50ZZ
and 07T60ZZ
and 07T70ZZ
and 07T80ZZ
and 07T90ZZ
and 0HTV0ZZ
and 0KTH0ZZ
and 0KTJ0ZZ

07T50ZZ
and 07T60ZZ
and 0HTV0ZZ

07T50ZZ
and 07T60ZZ
and 0HTV0ZZ
and 0KTH0ZZ
and 0KTJ0ZZ

07T50ZZ
and 07T70ZZ
and 07T80ZZ
and 0HTT0ZZ
and 0KTH0ZZ

07T50ZZ
and 0HTT0ZZ

07T50ZZ
and 0HTT0ZZ
and 0KTH0ZZ

07T60ZZ
and 07T70ZZ
and 07T90ZZ
and 0HTU0ZZ
and 0KTJ0ZZ

07T60ZZ
and 0HTU0ZZ

07T60ZZ
and 0HTU0ZZ
and 0KTJ0ZZ

0DQ80ZZ
and 0WQFXZ2

0DQ90ZZ
and 0WQFXZ2

0DQA0ZZ
and 0WQFXZ2

0DQB0ZZ
and 0WQFXZ2

0DQE0ZZ
and 0WQFXZ2

0DQF0ZZ
and 0WQFXZ2

0DQG0ZZ
and 0WQFXZ2

0DQH0ZZ
and 0WQFXZ2

0DQK0ZZ
and 0WQFXZ2

0DQL0ZZ
and 0WQFXZ2

0DQM0ZZ
and 0WQFXZ2

0DQN0ZZ
and 0WQFXZ2

0DT90ZZ
and 0FTG0ZZ

0HRT37Z
and 0JD63ZZ

0HRT37Z
and 0JD73ZZ

0HRT37Z
and 0JD83ZZ

0HRT37Z
and 0JD93ZZ

0HRT37Z
and 0JDL3ZZ

0HRT37Z
and 0JDM3ZZ

0HRU37Z
and 0JD63ZZ

0HRU37Z
and 0JD73ZZ

0HRU37Z
and 0JD83ZZ

0HRU37Z
and 0JD93ZZ

0HRU37Z
and 0JDL3ZZ

0HRU37Z
and 0JDM3ZZ

0HRV37Z
and 0JD63ZZ

0HRV37Z
and 0JD73ZZ

0HRV37Z
and 0JD83ZZ

0HRV37Z
and 0JD93ZZ

0HRV37Z
and 0JDL3ZZ

0HRV37Z
and 0JDM3ZZ

0JH608Z
and 02H40KZ

0JH608Z
and 02H44KZ

0JH608Z
and 02HN0JZ

0JH608Z
and 02HN0KZ

0JH608Z
and 02HN0MZ

0JH608Z
and 02HN3JZ

0JH608Z
and 02HN3KZ

0JH608Z
and 02HN3MZ

0JH608Z
and 02HN4JZ

0JH608Z
and 02HN4KZ

0JH608Z
and 02HN4MZ

0JH609Z
and 02H40KZ

0JH609Z
and 02H43JZ

0JH609Z
and 02H43KZ

0JH609Z
and 02H43MZ

0JH609Z
and 02H44KZ

0JH609Z
and 02H60KZ

0JH609Z
and 02H63KZ

0JH609Z
and 02H64KZ

0JH609Z
and 02H70KZ

0JH609Z
and 02H73KZ

0JH609Z
and 02H74KZ

0JH609Z
and 02HN0JZ

0JH609Z
and 02HN0KZ

0JH609Z
and 02HN0MZ

0JH609Z
and 02HN3JZ

0JH609Z
and 02HN3KZ

0JH609Z
and 02HN3MZ

0JH609Z
and 02HN4JZ

0JH609Z
and 02HN4KZ

0JH609Z
and 02HN4MZ

0JH60BZ
and 00HE0MZ

0JH60BZ
and 00HE3MZ

0JH60BZ
and 00HE4MZ

0JH60BZ
and 00HU0MZ

0JH60BZ
and 00HU3MZ

0JH60BZ
and 00HU4MZ

0JH60BZ
and 00HV0MZ

0JH60BZ
and 00HV3MZ

0JH60BZ
and 00HV4MZ

0JH60BZ
and 01HY0MZ

0JH60BZ
and 01HY3MZ

0JH60BZ
and 01HY4MZ

0JH60BZ
and 05H00MZ

0JH60BZ
and 05H03MZ

0JH60BZ
and 05H04MZ

0JH60BZ
and 05H30MZ

0JH60BZ
and 05H33MZ

0JH60BZ
and 05H34MZ

0JH60BZ
and 05H40MZ

0JH60BZ
and 05H43MZ

0JH60BZ
and 05H44MZ

0JH60BZ
and 0DH60MZ

0JH60BZ
and 0DH63MZ

0JH60BZ
and 0DH64MZ

0JH60CZ
and 00HE0MZ

0JH60CZ
and 00HE3MZ

0JH60CZ
and 00HE4MZ

0JH60CZ
and 00HU0MZ

0JH60CZ
and 00HU3MZ

0JH60CZ
and 00HU4MZ

0JH60CZ
and 00HV0MZ

0JH60CZ
and 00HV3MZ

0JH60CZ
and 00HV4MZ

0JH60CZ
and 01HY0MZ

0JH60CZ
and 01HY3MZ

0JH60CZ
and 01HY4MZ

0JH60CZ
and 05H00MZ

0JH60CZ
and 05H03MZ

0JH60CZ
and 05H04MZ

0JH60CZ
and 05H30MZ

0JH60CZ
and 05H33MZ

0JH60CZ
and 05H34MZ

0JH60CZ
and 05H40MZ

0JH60CZ
and 05H43MZ

0JH60CZ
and 05H44MZ

0JH60CZ
and 0DH60MZ

0JH60CZ
and 0DH63MZ

0JH60CZ
and 0DH64MZ

0JH60DZ
and 00H00MZ

0JH60DZ
and 00H03MZ

0JH60DZ
and 00H04MZ

0JH60DZ
and 00H60MZ

0JH60DZ
and 00H63MZ

0JH60DZ
and 00H64MZ

0JH60DZ
and 00HE0MZ

0JH60DZ
and 00HE3MZ

0JH60DZ
and 00HE4MZ

0JH60DZ
and 00HU0MZ

0JH60DZ
and 00HU3MZ

0JH60DZ
and 00HU4MZ

0JH60DZ
and 00HV0MZ

0JH60DZ
and 00HV3MZ

0JH60DZ
and 00HV4MZ

0JH60DZ
and 01HY0MZ

0JH60DZ
and 01HY3MZ

0JH60DZ
and 01HY4MZ

0JH60DZ
and 05H00MZ

0JH60DZ
and 05H03MZ

0JH60DZ
and 05H04MZ

0JH60DZ
and 05H30MZ

0JH60DZ and 05H33MZ

0JH60DZ and 05H34MZ

0JH60DZ and 05H40MZ

0JH60DZ and 05H43MZ

0JH60DZ and 05H44MZ

0JH60DZ and 0DH60MZ

0JH60DZ and 0DH63MZ

0JH60DZ and 0DH64MZ

0JH60EZ and 00H00MZ

0JH60EZ and 00H03MZ

0JH60EZ and 00H04MZ

0JH60EZ and 00H60MZ

0JH60EZ and 00H63MZ

0JH60EZ and 00H64MZ

0JH60EZ and 00HE0MZ

0JH60EZ and 00HE3MZ

0JH60EZ and 00HE4MZ

0JH60EZ and 00HU0MZ

0JH60EZ and 00HU3MZ

0JH60EZ and 00HU4MZ

0JH60EZ and 00HV0MZ

0JH60EZ and 00HV3MZ

0JH60EZ and 00HV4MZ

0JH60EZ and 01HY0MZ

0JH60EZ and 01HY3MZ

0JH60EZ and 01HY4MZ

0JH60EZ and 05H00MZ

0JH60EZ and 05H03MZ

0JH60EZ and 05H04MZ

0JH60EZ and 05H30MZ

0JH60EZ and 05H33MZ

0JH60EZ and 05H34MZ

0JH60EZ and 05H40MZ

0JH60EZ and 05H43MZ

0JH60EZ and 05H44MZ

0JH60EZ and 0DH60MZ

0JH60EZ and 0DH63MZ

0JH60EZ and 0DH64MZ

0JH638Z and 02H40KZ

0JH638Z and 02H44KZ

0JH638Z and 02HN0JZ

0JH638Z and 02HN0KZ

0JH638Z and 02HN0MZ

0JH638Z and 02HN3JZ

0JH638Z and 02HN3KZ

0JH638Z and 02HN3MZ

0JH638Z and 02HN4JZ

0JH638Z and 02HN4KZ

0JH638Z and 02HN4MZ

0JH639Z and 02H40KZ

0JH639Z and 02H43JZ

0JH639Z and 02H43KZ

0JH639Z and 02H43MZ

0JH639Z and 02H44KZ

0JH639Z and 02H60KZ

0JH639Z and 02H63KZ

0JH639Z and 02H64KZ

0JH639Z and 02H70KZ

0JH639Z and 02H73KZ

0JH639Z and 02H74KZ

0JH639Z and 02HN0JZ

0JH639Z and 02HN0KZ

0JH639Z and 02HN0MZ

0JH639Z and 02HN3JZ

0JH639Z and 02HN3KZ

0JH639Z and 02HN3MZ

0JH639Z and 02HN4JZ

0JH639Z and 02HN4KZ

0JH639Z and 02HN4MZ

0JH63BZ and 00HE0MZ

0JH63BZ and 00HE3MZ

0JH63BZ and 00HE4MZ

0JH63BZ and 00HU0MZ

0JH63BZ and 00HU3MZ

0JH63BZ and 00HU4MZ

0JH63BZ and 00HV0MZ

0JH63BZ and 00HV3MZ

0JH63BZ and 00HV4MZ

0JH63BZ and 01HY0MZ

0JH63BZ and 01HY3MZ

0JH63BZ and 01HY4MZ

0JH63BZ and 05H00MZ

0JH63BZ and 05H03MZ

0JH63BZ and 05H04MZ

0JH63BZ and 05H30MZ

0JH63BZ and 05H33MZ

0JH63BZ and 05H34MZ

0JH63BZ and 05H40MZ

0JH63BZ and 05H43MZ

0JH63BZ and 05H44MZ

0JH63BZ and 0DH60MZ

0JH63BZ and 0DH63MZ

0JH63BZ and 0DH64MZ

0JH63CZ and 00HE0MZ

0JH63CZ and 00HE3MZ

0JH63CZ and 00HE4MZ

0JH63CZ and 00HU0MZ

0JH63CZ and 00HU3MZ

0JH63CZ and 00HU4MZ

0JH63CZ and 00HV0MZ

0JH63CZ and 00HV3MZ

0JH63CZ and 00HV4MZ

0JH63CZ and 01HY0MZ

0JH63CZ and 01HY3MZ

0JH63CZ and 01HY4MZ

0JH63CZ and 05H00MZ

0JH63CZ and 05H03MZ

0JH63CZ and 05H04MZ

0JH63CZ and 05H30MZ

0JH63CZ and 05H33MZ

0JH63CZ and 05H34MZ

0JH63CZ and 05H40MZ

0JH63CZ and 05H43MZ

0JH63CZ and 05H44MZ

0JH63CZ and 0DH60MZ

0JH63CZ and 0DH63MZ

0JH63CZ and 0DH64MZ

0JH63DZ and 00H00MZ

0JH63DZ and 00H03MZ

0JH63DZ and 00H04MZ

0JH63DZ and 00H60MZ

0JH63DZ and 00H63MZ

0JH63DZ and 00H64MZ

0JH63DZ and 00HE0MZ

0JH63DZ and 00HE3MZ

0JH63DZ and 00HE4MZ

0JH63DZ and 00HU0MZ

0JH63DZ and 00HU3MZ

0JH63DZ and 00HU4MZ

0JH63DZ and 00HV0MZ

0JH63DZ and 00HV3MZ

0JH63DZ and 00HV4MZ

0JH63DZ and 01HY0MZ

0JH63DZ and 01HY3MZ

0JH63DZ and 01HY4MZ

0JH63DZ and 05H00MZ

0JH63DZ and 05H03MZ

0JH63DZ and 05H04MZ

0JH63DZ and 05H30MZ

0JH63DZ and 05H33MZ

0JH63DZ and 05H34MZ

0JH63DZ and 05H40MZ

0JH63DZ and 05H43MZ

0JH63DZ and 05H44MZ

0JH63DZ and 0DH60MZ

0JH63DZ and 0DH63MZ

0JH63DZ and 0DH64MZ

0JH63EZ and 00H00MZ

0JH63EZ and 00H03MZ

0JH63EZ and 00H04MZ

0JH63EZ and 00H60MZ

0JH63EZ and 00H63MZ

0JH63EZ and 00H64MZ

0JH63EZ and 00HE0MZ

0JH63EZ and 00HE3MZ

0JH63EZ and 00HE4MZ

0JH63EZ and 00HU0MZ

0JH63EZ and 00HU3MZ

0JH63EZ and 00HU4MZ

0JH63EZ and 00HV0MZ

0JH63EZ and 00HV3MZ

0JH63EZ and 00HV4MZ

0JH63EZ and 01HY0MZ

0JH63EZ and 01HY3MZ

0JH63EZ and 01HY4MZ

0JH63EZ and 05H00MZ

0JH63EZ and 05H03MZ

0JH63EZ and 05H04MZ

0JH63EZ and 05H30MZ

0JH63EZ and 05H33MZ

0JH63EZ and 05H34MZ

0JH63EZ and 05H40MZ

0JH63EZ and 05H43MZ

0JH63EZ and 05H44MZ

0JH63EZ and 0DH60MZ

0JH63EZ and 0DH63MZ

0JH63EZ and 0DH64MZ

0JH70BZ and 00HE0MZ

0JH70BZ and 00HE3MZ

0JH70BZ and 00HE4MZ

0JH70BZ and 00HU0MZ

0JH70BZ and 00HU3MZ

0JH70BZ and 00HU4MZ

0JH70BZ and 00HV0MZ

0JH70BZ and 00HV3MZ

0JH70BZ and 00HV4MZ

0JH70BZ and 01HY0MZ

0JH70BZ and 01HY3MZ

0JH70BZ and 01HY4MZ

0JH70BZ and 05H00MZ

0JH70BZ and 05H03MZ

0JH70BZ and 05H04MZ

0JH70BZ and 05H30MZ

0JH70BZ and 05H33MZ

0JH70BZ and 05H34MZ

0JH70BZ and 05H40MZ

0JH70BZ and 05H43MZ

0JH70BZ and 05H44MZ

0JH70BZ and 0DH60MZ

0JH70BZ and 0DH63MZ

0JH70BZ and 0DH64MZ

0JH70CZ and 00HE0MZ

0JH70CZ and 00HE3MZ

0JH70CZ and 00HE4MZ

0JH70CZ and 00HU0MZ

0JH70CZ and 00HU3MZ

0JH70CZ and 00HU4MZ

0JH70CZ and 00HV0MZ

0JH70CZ and 00HV3MZ

0JH70CZ and 00HV4MZ

0JH70CZ and 01HY0MZ

0JH70CZ and 01HY3MZ

0JH70CZ and 01HY4MZ

0JH70CZ and 05H00MZ

0JH70CZ and 05H03MZ

0JH70CZ and 05H04MZ

0JH70CZ and 05H30MZ

0JH70CZ and 05H33MZ

0JH70CZ and 05H34MZ

0JH70CZ and 05H40MZ

0JH70CZ and 05H43MZ

0JH70CZ and 05H44MZ

0JH70CZ and 0DH60MZ

0JH70CZ and 0DH63MZ

0JH70CZ and 0DH64MZ

0JH70DZ and 00H00MZ

0JH70DZ and 00H03MZ

0JH70DZ and 00H04MZ

0JH70DZ and 00H60MZ

0JH70DZ and 00H63MZ

0JH70DZ and 00H64MZ

0JH70DZ and 00HE0MZ

0JH70DZ and 00HE3MZ

0JH70DZ and 00HE4MZ

0JH70DZ and 00HU0MZ

0JH70DZ and 00HU3MZ

0JH70DZ and 00HU4MZ

0JH70DZ and 00HV0MZ

0JH70DZ and 00HV3MZ

0JH70DZ and 00HV4MZ

0JH70DZ and 01HY0MZ

0JH70DZ and 01HY3MZ

0JH70DZ and 01HY4MZ

0JH70DZ and 05H00MZ

0JH70DZ and 05H03MZ

0JH70DZ and 05H04MZ

0JH70DZ and 05H30MZ

0JH70DZ and 05H33MZ

0JH70DZ and 05H34MZ

0JH70DZ and 05H40MZ

0JH70DZ and 05H43MZ

0JH70DZ and 05H44MZ

0JH70DZ and 0DH60MZ

0JH70DZ and 0DH63MZ

0JH70DZ and 0DH64MZ

0JH70EZ and 00H00MZ

0JH70EZ and 00H03MZ

0JH70EZ and 00H04MZ

0JH70EZ and 00H60MZ

0JH70EZ and 00H63MZ

0JH70EZ and 00H64MZ

0JH70EZ and 00HE0MZ

0JH70EZ and 00HE3MZ

0JH70EZ and 00HE4MZ

0JH70EZ and 00HU0MZ

0JH70EZ and 00HU3MZ

0JH70EZ and 00HU4MZ

0JH70EZ and 00HV0MZ

0JH70EZ and 00HV3MZ

0JH70EZ and 00HV4MZ

0JH70EZ and 01HY0MZ

0JH70EZ and 01HY3MZ

0JH70EZ and 01HY4MZ

0JH70EZ and 05H00MZ

0JH70EZ and 05H03MZ

0JH70EZ and 05H04MZ

0JH70EZ and 05H30MZ

0JH70EZ and 05H33MZ

0JH70EZ and 05H34MZ

0JH70EZ and 05H40MZ

0JH70EZ and 05H43MZ

0JH70EZ and 05H44MZ

0JH70EZ and 0DH60MZ

0JH70EZ and 0DH63MZ

0JH70EZ and 0DH64MZ

0JH73BZ and 00HE0MZ

0JH73BZ and 00HE3MZ

0JH73BZ and 00HE4MZ

0JH73BZ and 00HU0MZ

0JH73BZ and 00HU3MZ

0JH73BZ and 00HU4MZ

0JH73BZ and 00HV0MZ

0JH73BZ and 00HV3MZ

0JH73BZ and 00HV4MZ

0JH73BZ and 01HY0MZ

0JH73BZ and 01HY3MZ

0JH73BZ and 01HY4MZ

0JH73BZ and 05H00MZ

0JH73BZ and 05H03MZ

0JH73BZ and 05H04MZ

0JH73BZ and 05H30MZ

0JH73BZ and 05H33MZ

0JH73BZ and 05H34MZ

0JH73BZ and 05H40MZ

0JH73BZ and 05H43MZ

0JH73BZ and 05H44MZ

0JH73BZ and 0DH60MZ

0JH73BZ and 0DH63MZ

0JH73BZ and 0DH64MZ

0JH73CZ and 00HE0MZ

0JH73CZ and 00HE3MZ

0JH73CZ and 00HE4MZ

0JH73CZ and 00HU0MZ

0JH73CZ and 00HU3MZ

0JH73CZ and 00HU4MZ

0JH73CZ and 00HV0MZ

0JH73CZ and 00HV3MZ

0JH73CZ and 00HV4MZ

0JH73CZ and 01HY0MZ

0JH73CZ and 01HY3MZ

0JH73CZ and 01HY4MZ

0JH73CZ and 05H00MZ

0JH73CZ and 05H03MZ

0JH73CZ and 05H04MZ

0JH73CZ and 05H30MZ

0JH73CZ and 05H33MZ

0JH73CZ and 05H34MZ

0JH73CZ and 05H40MZ

0JH73CZ and 05H43MZ

0JH73CZ and 05H44MZ

0JH73CZ and 0DH60MZ

0JH73CZ and 0DH63MZ

0JH73CZ and 0DH64MZ

0JH73DZ and 00H00MZ

0JH73DZ and 00H03MZ

0JH73DZ and 00H04MZ

0JH73DZ and 00H60MZ

0JH73DZ and 00H63MZ

0JH73DZ and 00H64MZ

0JH73DZ and 00HE0MZ

0JH73DZ and 00HE3MZ

0JH73DZ and 00HE4MZ

0JH73DZ and 00HU0MZ

0JH73DZ and 00HU3MZ

0JH73DZ and 00HU4MZ

0JH73DZ and 00HV0MZ

0JH73DZ and 00HV3MZ

0JH73DZ and 00HV4MZ

0JH73DZ and 01HY0MZ

0JH73DZ and 01HY3MZ

0JH73DZ and 01HY4MZ

0JH73DZ and 05H00MZ

0JH73DZ and 05H03MZ

0JH73DZ and 05H04MZ

0JH73DZ and 05H30MZ

0JH73DZ and 05H33MZ

0JH73DZ and 05H34MZ

0JH73DZ and 05H40MZ

0JH73DZ and 05H43MZ

0JH73DZ and 05H44MZ

0JH73DZ and 0DH60MZ

0JH73DZ and 0DH63MZ

0JH73DZ and 0DH64MZ

0JH73EZ and 00H00MZ

0JH73EZ and 00H03MZ

0JH73EZ and 00H04MZ

0JH73EZ and 00H60MZ

0JH73EZ and 00H63MZ

0JH73EZ and 00H64MZ

0JH73EZ and 00HE0MZ

0JH73EZ and 00HE3MZ

0JH73EZ and 00HE4MZ

0JH73EZ and 00HU0MZ

0JH73EZ and 00HU3MZ

0JH73EZ and 00HU4MZ

0JH73EZ and 00HV0MZ

0JH73EZ and 00HV3MZ

0JH73EZ and 00HV4MZ

0JH73EZ and 01HY0MZ

0JH73EZ and 01HY3MZ

0JH73EZ and 01HY4MZ

0JH73EZ and 05H00MZ

0JH73EZ and 05H03MZ

0JH73EZ and 05H04MZ

0JH73EZ and 05H30MZ

0JH73EZ and 05H33MZ

0JH73EZ and 05H34MZ

0JH73EZ and 05H40MZ

0JH73EZ and 05H43MZ

0JH73EZ and 05H44MZ

0JH73EZ and 0DH60MZ

0JH73EZ and 0DH63MZ

0JH73EZ and 0DH64MZ

0JH808Z and 02H40KZ

0JH808Z and 02H44KZ

0JH808Z and 02HN0JZ

0JH808Z and 02HN0KZ

0JH808Z and 02HN0MZ

0JH808Z and 02HN3JZ

0JH808Z and 02HN3KZ

0JH808Z and 02HN3MZ

0JH808Z and 02HN4JZ

0JH808Z and 02HN4KZ

0JH808Z and 02HN4MZ

0JH809Z and 02H40KZ

0JH809Z and 02H43JZ

0JH809Z and 02H43KZ

0JH809Z and 02H43MZ

0JH809Z and 02H44KZ

0JH809Z and 02H60KZ

0JH809Z and 02H63KZ

0JH809Z and 02H64KZ

0JH809Z and 02H70KZ

0JH809Z and 02H73KZ

0JH809Z and 02H74KZ

0JH809Z and 02HN0JZ

0JH809Z and 02HN0KZ

0JH809Z and 02HN0MZ

0JH809Z and 02HN3JZ

0JH809Z and 02HN3KZ

0JH809Z and 02HN3MZ

0JH809Z and 02HN4JZ

0JH809Z and 02HN4KZ

0JH809Z and 02HN4MZ

0JH80BZ and 00HE0MZ

0JH80BZ and 00HE3MZ

0JH80BZ and 00HE4MZ

0JH80BZ and 00HU0MZ

0JH80BZ and 00HU3MZ

0JH80BZ and 00HU4MZ

0JH80BZ and 00HV0MZ

0JH80BZ and 00HV3MZ

0JH80BZ and 00HV4MZ

0JH80BZ and 01HY0MZ

0JH80BZ and 01HY3MZ

0JH80BZ and 01HY4MZ

0JH80BZ and 05H00MZ

0JH80BZ and 05H03MZ

0JH80BZ and 05H04MZ

0JH80BZ and 05H30MZ

0JH80BZ and 05H33MZ

0JH80BZ and 05H34MZ

0JH80BZ and 05H40MZ

0JH80BZ and 05H43MZ

0JH80BZ and 05H44MZ

0JH80BZ and 0DH60MZ

0JH80BZ and 0DH63MZ

0JH80BZ and 0DH64MZ

0JH80CZ and 00HE0MZ

0JH80CZ and 00HE3MZ

0JH80CZ and 00HE4MZ

0JH80CZ and 00HU0MZ

0JH80CZ and 00HU3MZ

0JH80CZ and 00HU4MZ

0JH80CZ and 00HV0MZ

0JH80CZ and 00HV3MZ

0JH80CZ and 00HV4MZ

0JH80CZ and 01HY0MZ

0JH80CZ and 01HY3MZ

0JH80CZ and 01HY4MZ

0JH80CZ and 05H00MZ

0JH80CZ and 05H03MZ

0JH80CZ and 05H04MZ

0JH80CZ and 05H30MZ

0JH80CZ and 05H33MZ

0JH80CZ and 05H34MZ

0JH80CZ and 05H40MZ

0JH80CZ and 05H43MZ

0JH80CZ and 05H44MZ

0JH80CZ and 0DH60MZ

0JH80CZ and 0DH63MZ

0JH80CZ and 0DH64MZ

0JH80DZ and 00H00MZ

0JH80DZ and 00H03MZ

0JH80DZ and 00H04MZ

0JH80DZ and 00H60MZ

0JH80DZ and 00H63MZ

0JH80DZ and 00H64MZ

0JH80DZ and 00HE0MZ

0JH80DZ and 00HE3MZ

0JH80DZ and 00HE4MZ

0JH80DZ and 00HU0MZ

0JH80DZ and 00HU3MZ

0JH80DZ and 00HU4MZ

0JH80DZ and 00HV0MZ

0JH80DZ and 00HV3MZ

0JH80DZ and 00HV4MZ

0JH80DZ and 01HY0MZ

0JH80DZ and 01HY3MZ

0JH80DZ and 01HY4MZ

0JH80DZ and 05H00MZ

0JH80DZ and 05H03MZ

0JH80DZ and 05H04MZ

0JH80DZ and 05H30MZ

0JH80DZ and 05H33MZ

0JH80DZ and 05H34MZ

0JH80DZ and 05H40MZ

0JH80DZ and 05H43MZ

0JH80DZ and 05H44MZ

0JH80DZ and 0DH60MZ

0JH80DZ and 0DH63MZ

0JH80DZ and 0DH64MZ

0JH80EZ and 00H00MZ

0JH80EZ and 00H03MZ

0JH80EZ and 00H04MZ

0JH80EZ and 00H60MZ

0JH80EZ and 00H63MZ

0JH80EZ and 00H64MZ

0JH80EZ and 00HE0MZ

0JH80EZ and 00HE3MZ

0JH80EZ and 00HE4MZ

0JH80EZ and 00HU0MZ

0JH80EZ and 00HU3MZ

0JH80EZ and 00HU4MZ

0JH80EZ and 00HV0MZ

0JH80EZ and 00HV3MZ

0JH80EZ and 00HV4MZ

0JH80EZ and 01HY0MZ

0JH80EZ and 01HY3MZ

0JH80EZ and 01HY4MZ

0JH80EZ and 05H00MZ

0JH80EZ and 05H03MZ

0JH80EZ and 05H04MZ

0JH80EZ and 05H30MZ

0JH80EZ and 05H33MZ

0JH80EZ and 05H34MZ

0JH80EZ and 05H40MZ

0JH80EZ and 05H43MZ

0JH80EZ and 05H44MZ

0JH80EZ and 0DH60MZ

0JH80EZ and 0DH63MZ

0JH80EZ and 0DH64MZ

0JH838Z and 02H40KZ

0JH838Z and 02H44KZ

0JH838Z and 02HN0JZ

0JH838Z and 02HN0KZ

0JH838Z and 02HN0MZ

0JH838Z and 02HN3JZ

0JH838Z and 02HN3KZ

0JH838Z and 02HN3MZ

0JH838Z and 02HN4JZ

0JH838Z and 02HN4KZ

0JH838Z and 02HN4MZ

0JH839Z and 02H40KZ

0JH839Z and 02H43JZ

0JH839Z and 02H43KZ

0JH839Z and 02H43MZ

0JH839Z and 02H44KZ

0JH839Z and 02H60KZ

0JH839Z and 02H63KZ

0JH839Z and 02H64KZ

0JH839Z and 02H70KZ

0JH839Z and 02H73KZ

0JH839Z and 02H74KZ

0JH839Z and 02HN0JZ

0JH839Z and 02HN0KZ

0JH839Z and 02HN0MZ

0JH839Z and 02HN3JZ

0JH839Z and 02HN3KZ

0JH839Z and 02HN3MZ

0JH839Z and 02HN4JZ

0JH839Z and 02HN4KZ

0JH839Z and 02HN4MZ

0JH83BZ and 00HE0MZ

0JH83BZ and 00HE3MZ

0JH83BZ and 00HE4MZ

0JH83BZ and 00HU0MZ

0JH83BZ and 00HU3MZ

0JH83BZ and 00HU4MZ

0JH83BZ and 00HV0MZ

0JH83BZ and 00HV3MZ

0JH83BZ and 00HV4MZ

0JH83BZ and 01HY0MZ

0JH83BZ and 01HY3MZ

0JH83BZ and 01HY4MZ

0JH83BZ and 05H00MZ

0JH83BZ and 05H03MZ

0JH83BZ and 05H04MZ

0JH83BZ and 05H30MZ

0JH83BZ and 05H33MZ

0JH83BZ and 05H34MZ

0JH83BZ and 05H40MZ

0JH83BZ and 05H43MZ

0JH83BZ and 05H44MZ

0JH83BZ and 0DH60MZ

0JH83BZ and 0DH63MZ

0JH83BZ and 0DH64MZ

0JH83CZ and 00HE0MZ

0JH83CZ and 00HE3MZ

0JH83CZ and 00HE4MZ

0JH83CZ and 00HU0MZ

0JH83CZ and 00HU3MZ

0JH83CZ and 00HU4MZ

0JH83CZ and 00HV0MZ

0JH83CZ and 00HV3MZ

0JH83CZ and 00HV4MZ

0JH83CZ and 01HY0MZ

0JH83CZ and 01HY3MZ

0JH83CZ and 01HY4MZ

0JH83CZ and 05H00MZ

0JH83CZ and 05H03MZ

0JH83CZ and 05H04MZ

0JH83CZ and 05H30MZ

0JH83CZ and 05H33MZ

0JH83CZ and 05H34MZ

0JH83CZ and 05H40MZ

0JH83CZ and 05H43MZ

0JH83CZ and 05H44MZ

0JH83CZ and 0DH60MZ

0JH83CZ and 0DH63MZ

0JH83CZ and 0DH64MZ

0JH83DZ and 00H00MZ

0JH83DZ and 00H03MZ

0JH83DZ and 00H04MZ

0JH83DZ and 00H60MZ

0JH83DZ and 00H63MZ

0JH83DZ
and 00H64MZ

0JH83DZ
and 00HE0MZ

0JH83DZ
and 00HE3MZ

0JH83DZ
and 00HE4MZ

0JH83DZ
and 00HU0MZ

0JH83DZ
and 00HU3MZ

0JH83DZ
and 00HU4MZ

0JH83DZ
and 00HV0MZ

0JH83DZ
and 00HV3MZ

0JH83DZ
and 00HV4MZ

0JH83DZ
and 01HY0MZ

0JH83DZ
and 01HY3MZ

0JH83DZ
and 01HY4MZ

0JH83DZ
and 05H00MZ

0JH83DZ
and 05H03MZ

0JH83DZ
and 05H04MZ

0JH83DZ
and 05H30MZ

0JH83DZ
and 05H33MZ

0JH83DZ
and 05H34MZ

0JH83DZ
and 05H40MZ

0JH83DZ
and 05H43MZ

0JH83DZ
and 05H44MZ

0JH83DZ
and 0DH60MZ

0JH83DZ
and 0DH63MZ

0JH83DZ
and 0DH64MZ

0JH83EZ
and 00H00MZ

0JH83EZ
and 00H03MZ

0JH83EZ
and 00H04MZ

0JH83EZ
and 00H60MZ

0JH83EZ
and 00H63MZ

0JH83EZ
and 00H64MZ

0JH83EZ
and 00HE0MZ

0JH83EZ
and 00HE3MZ

0JH83EZ
and 00HE4MZ

0JH83EZ
and 00HU0MZ

0JH83EZ
and 00HU3MZ

0JH83EZ
and 00HU4MZ

0JH83EZ
and 00HV0MZ

0JH83EZ
and 01HY0MZ

0JH83EZ
and 01HY3MZ

0JH83EZ
and 01HY4MZ

0JH83EZ
and 05H00MZ

0JH83EZ
and 05H03MZ

0JH83EZ
and 05H04MZ

0JH83EZ
and 05H30MZ

0JH83EZ
and 05H33MZ

0JH83EZ
and 05H34MZ

0JH83EZ
and 05H40MZ

0JH83EZ
and 05H43MZ

0JH83EZ
and 05H44MZ

0JH83EZ
and 0DH60MZ

0JH83EZ
and 0DH63MZ

0JH83EZ
and 0DH64MZ

0NH00NZ
and 00H00MZ

0NH00NZ
and 00H03MZ

0NH00NZ
and 00H04MZ

0NH00NZ
and 00H60MZ

0NH00NZ
and 00H63MZ

0NH00NZ
and 00H64MZ

0PS33ZZ
and 0PU33JZ

0PS43ZZ
and 0PU43JZ

0QS03ZZ
and 0QU03JZ

0QS13ZZ
and 0QU13JZ

0QSS3ZZ
and 0QUS3JZ

One of
0RG7070
0RG70A0
0RG70J0
0RG70K0
0RG7370
0RG73A0
0RG73J0
0RG73K0
0RG7470
0RG74A0
0RG74J0
0RG74K0
XRG70F3

with one of
0SG1070
0SG10A0
0SG10J0
0SG10K0
0SG1370
0SG13A0
0SG13J0
0SG13K0
0SG1470
0SG14A0
0SG14J0
0SG14K0
XRGC0F3

One of
0RG7071
0RG707J
0RG70AJ
0RG70J1
0RG70JJ
0RG70K1
0RG70KJ
0RG7371
0RG737J
0RG73AJ
0RG73J1
0RG73JJ
0RG73K1
0RG73KJ
0RG7471
0RG747J
0RG74AJ
0RG74J1
0RG74JJ
0RG74K1
0RG74KJ
XRG7092
XRG70F3

with one of
0SG1071
0SG107J
0SG10AJ
0SG10J1
0SG10JJ
0SG10K1
0SG10KJ
0SG1371
0SG137J
0SG13AJ
0SG13J1
0SG13JJ
0SG13K1
0SG13KJ
0SG1471
0SG147J
0SG14AJ
0SG14J1
0SG14JJ
0SG14K1
0SG14KJ
XRGC092
XRGC0F3

0SP908Z
and 0SR9019

0SP908Z
and 0SR901A

0SP908Z
and 0SR901Z

0SP908Z
and 0SR9029

0SP908Z
and 0SR902A

0SP908Z
and 0SR902Z

0SP908Z
and 0SR9039

0SP908Z
and 0SR903A

0SP908Z
and 0SR903Z

0SP908Z
and 0SR9049

0SP908Z
and 0SR904A

0SP908Z
and 0SR904Z

0SP908Z
and 0SR9069

0SP908Z
and 0SR906A

0SP908Z
and 0SR906Z

0SP908Z
and 0SR90J9

0SP908Z
and 0SR90JA

0SP908Z
and 0SR90JZ

0SP908Z
and 0SRA009

0SP908Z
and 0SRA00A

0SP908Z
and 0SRA00Z

0SP908Z
and 0SRA019

0SP908Z
and 0SRA01A

0SP908Z
and 0SRA01Z

0SP908Z
and 0SRA039

0SP908Z
and 0SRA03A

0SP908Z
and 0SRA03Z

0SP908Z
and 0SRA0J9

0SP908Z
and 0SRA0JA

0SP908Z
and 0SRA0JZ

0SP908Z
and 0SRR019

0SP908Z
and 0SRR01A

0SP908Z
and 0SRR01Z

0SP908Z
and 0SRR039

0SP908Z
and 0SRR03A

0SP908Z
and 0SRR03Z

0SP908Z
and 0SRR0J9

0SP908Z
and 0SRR0JA

0SP908Z
and 0SRR0JZ

0SP908Z
and 0SU909Z

0SP908Z
and 0SUA09Z

0SP908Z
and 0SUR09Z

0SP909Z
and 0SR9019

0SP909Z
and 0SR901A

0SP909Z
and 0SR901Z

0SP909Z
and 0SR9029

0SP909Z
and 0SR902A

0SP909Z
and 0SR902Z

0SP909Z
and 0SR9039

0SP909Z
and 0SR903A

0SP909Z
and 0SR903Z

0SP909Z
and 0SR9049

0SP909Z
and 0SR904A

0SP909Z
and 0SR904Z

0SP909Z
and 0SR9069

0SP909Z
and 0SR906A

0SP909Z
and 0SR906Z

0SP909Z
and 0SR90J9

0SP909Z
and 0SR90JA

0SP909Z
and 0SR90JZ

0SP909Z
and 0SRA009

0SP909Z
and 0SRA00A

0SP909Z
and 0SRA00Z

0SP909Z
and 0SRA019

0SP909Z and 0SRA01A

0SP909Z and 0SRA01Z

0SP909Z and 0SRA039

0SP909Z and 0SRA03A

0SP909Z and 0SRA03Z

0SP909Z and 0SRA0J9

0SP909Z and 0SRA0JA

0SP909Z and 0SRA0JZ

0SP909Z and 0SRR019

0SP909Z and 0SRR01A

0SP909Z and 0SRR01Z

0SP909Z and 0SRR039

0SP909Z and 0SRR03A

0SP909Z and 0SRR03Z

0SP909Z and 0SRR0J9

0SP909Z and 0SRR0JA

0SP909Z and 0SRR0JZ

0SP909Z and 0SU909Z

0SP909Z and 0SU909Z

0SP909Z and 0SUA09Z

0SP909Z and 0SUA09Z

0SP909Z and 0SUR09Z

0SP909Z and 0SUR09Z

0SP90BZ and 0SR9019

0SP90BZ and 0SR901A

0SP90BZ and 0SR901Z

0SP90BZ and 0SR9029

0SP90BZ and 0SR902A

0SP90BZ and 0SR902Z

0SP90BZ and 0SR9039

0SP90BZ and 0SR903A

0SP90BZ and 0SR903Z

0SP90BZ and 0SR9049

0SP90BZ and 0SR904A

0SP90BZ and 0SR904Z

0SP90BZ and 0SR9069

0SP90BZ and 0SR906A

0SP90BZ and 0SR906Z

0SP90BZ and 0SR90J9

0SP90BZ and 0SR90JA

0SP90BZ and 0SR90JZ

0SP90BZ and 0SRA009

0SP90BZ and 0SRA00A

0SP90BZ and 0SRA00Z

0SP90BZ and 0SRA019

0SP90BZ and 0SRA01A

0SP90BZ and 0SRA01Z

0SP90BZ and 0SRA039

0SP90BZ and 0SRA03A

0SP90BZ and 0SRA03Z

0SP90BZ and 0SRA0J9

0SP90BZ and 0SRA0JA

0SP90BZ and 0SRA0JZ

0SP90BZ and 0SRR019

0SP90BZ and 0SRR01A

0SP90BZ and 0SRR01Z

0SP90BZ and 0SRR039

0SP90BZ and 0SRR03A

0SP90BZ and 0SRR03Z

0SP90BZ and 0SRR0J9

0SP90BZ and 0SRR0JA

0SP90BZ and 0SRR0JZ

0SP90BZ and 0SU909Z

0SP90BZ and 0SUA09Z

0SP90BZ and 0SUR09Z

0SP90JZ and 0SR9019

0SP90JZ and 0SR901A

0SP90JZ and 0SR901Z

0SP90JZ and 0SR9029

0SP90JZ and 0SR902A

0SP90JZ and 0SR902Z

0SP90JZ and 0SR9039

0SP90JZ and 0SR903A

0SP90JZ and 0SR903Z

0SP90JZ and 0SR9049

0SP90JZ and 0SR904A

0SP90JZ and 0SR904Z

0SP90JZ and 0SR9069

0SP90JZ and 0SR906A

0SP90JZ and 0SR906Z

0SP90JZ and 0SR90J9

0SP90JZ and 0SR90JA

0SP90JZ and 0SR90JZ

0SP90JZ and 0SRA009

0SP90JZ and 0SRA00A

0SP90JZ and 0SRA00Z

0SP90JZ and 0SRA019

0SP90JZ and 0SRA01A

0SP90JZ and 0SRA01Z

0SP90JZ and 0SRA039

0SP90JZ and 0SRA03A

0SP90JZ and 0SRA03Z

0SP90JZ and 0SRA0J9

0SP90JZ and 0SRA0JA

0SP90JZ and 0SRA0JZ

0SP90JZ and 0SRR019

0SP90JZ and 0SRR01A

0SP90JZ and 0SRR01Z

0SP90JZ and 0SRR039

0SP90JZ and 0SRR03A

0SP90JZ and 0SRR03Z

0SP90JZ and 0SRR0J9

0SP90JZ and 0SRR0JA

0SP90JZ and 0SRR0JZ

0SP948Z and 0SR9019

0SP948Z and 0SR901A

0SP948Z and 0SR901Z

0SP948Z and 0SR9029

0SP948Z and 0SR902A

0SP948Z and 0SR902Z

0SP948Z and 0SR9039

0SP948Z and 0SR903A

0SP948Z and 0SR903Z

0SP948Z and 0SR9049

0SP948Z and 0SR904A

0SP948Z and 0SR904Z

0SP948Z and 0SR9069

0SP948Z and 0SR906A

0SP948Z and 0SR906Z

0SP948Z and 0SR90J9

0SP948Z and 0SR90JA

0SP948Z and 0SR90JZ

0SP948Z and 0SRA009

0SP948Z and 0SRA00A

0SP948Z and 0SRA00Z

0SP948Z and 0SRA019

0SP948Z and 0SRA01A

0SP948Z and 0SRA01Z

0SP948Z and 0SRA039

0SP948Z and 0SRA03A

0SP948Z and 0SRA03Z

0SP948Z and 0SRA0J9

0SP948Z and 0SRA0JA

0SP948Z and 0SRA0JZ

0SP948Z and 0SRR019

0SP948Z and 0SRR01A

0SP948Z and 0SRR01Z

0SP948Z and 0SRR039

0SP948Z and 0SRR03A

0SP948Z and 0SRR03Z

0SP948Z and 0SRR0J9

0SP948Z and 0SRR0JA

0SP948Z and 0SRR0JZ

0SP948Z and 0SU909Z

0SP948Z and 0SUA09Z

0SP948Z and 0SUR09Z

0SP94JZ and 0SR9019

0SP94JZ and 0SR901A

0SP94JZ and 0SR901Z

0SP94JZ and 0SR9029

0SP94JZ and 0SR902A

0SP94JZ and 0SR902Z

0SP94JZ and 0SR9039

0SP94JZ and 0SR903A

0SP94JZ and 0SR903Z

0SP94JZ and 0SR9049

0SP94JZ and 0SR904A

0SP94JZ and 0SR904Z

0SP94JZ and 0SR9069

0SP94JZ and 0SR906A

0SP94JZ and 0SR906Z

0SP94JZ and 0SR90J9

0SP94JZ and 0SR90JA

0SP94JZ and 0SR90JZ

0SP94JZ and 0SRA009

0SP94JZ and 0SRA00A

0SP94JZ and 0SRA00Z

0SP94JZ and 0SRA019

0SP94JZ and 0SRA01A

0SP94JZ and 0SRA01Z

0SP94JZ and 0SRA039

0SP94JZ and 0SRA03A

0SP94JZ and 0SRA03Z

0SP94JZ and 0SRA0J9

0SP94JZ and 0SRA0JA

0SP94JZ and 0SRA0JZ

0SP94JZ and 0SRR019

0SP94JZ and 0SRR01A

0SP94JZ and 0SRR01Z

0SP94JZ and 0SRR039

0SP94JZ and 0SRR03A

0SP94JZ and 0SRR03Z

0SP94JZ and 0SRR0J9

0SP94JZ and 0SRR0JA

0SP94JZ and 0SRR0JZ

0SP94JZ and 0SU909Z

0SP94JZ and 0SUA09Z

0SP94JZ and 0SUR09Z

0SPA0JZ and 0SR9019

0SPA0JZ and 0SR901A

0SPA0JZ and 0SR901Z

0SPA0JZ and 0SR9029

0SPA0JZ and 0SR902A

0SPA0JZ and 0SR902Z

0SPA0JZ and 0SR9039

0SPA0JZ and 0SR903A

0SPA0JZ and 0SR903Z

0SPA0JZ and 0SR9049

0SPA0JZ and 0SR904A

0SPA0JZ and 0SR904Z

0SPA0JZ and 0SR9069

0SPA0JZ and 0SR906A

0SPA0JZ and 0SR906Z

0SPA0JZ and 0SR90J9

0SPA0JZ and 0SR90JA

0SPA0JZ and 0SR90JZ

0SPA0JZ and 0SRA009

0SPA0JZ and 0SRA00A

0SPA0JZ and 0SRA00Z

0SPA0JZ and 0SRA019

0SPA0JZ and 0SRA01A

0SPA0JZ and 0SRA01Z

0SPA0JZ and 0SRA039

0SPA0JZ and 0SRA03A

0SPA0JZ and 0SRA03Z

0SPA0JZ and 0SRA0J9

0SPA0JZ and 0SRA0JA

0SPA0JZ and 0SRA0JZ

0SPA0JZ and 0SRR019

0SPA0JZ and 0SRR01A

0SPA0JZ and 0SRR01Z

0SPA0JZ and 0SRR039

0SPA0JZ and 0SRR03A

0SPA0JZ and 0SRR03Z

0SPA0JZ and 0SRR0J9

0SPA0JZ and 0SRR0JA

0SPA0JZ and 0SRR0JZ

0SPA4JZ and 0SR9019

0SPA4JZ and 0SR901A

0SPA4JZ and 0SR901Z

0SPA4JZ and 0SR9029

0SPA4JZ and 0SR902A

0SPA4JZ and 0SR902Z

0SPA4JZ and 0SR9039

0SPA4JZ and 0SR903A

0SPA4JZ and 0SR903Z

0SPA4JZ and 0SR9049

0SPA4JZ and 0SR904A

0SPA4JZ and 0SR904Z

0SPA4JZ and 0SR9069

0SPA4JZ and 0SR906A

0SPA4JZ and 0SR906Z

0SPA4JZ and 0SR90J9

0SPA4JZ and 0SR90JA

0SPA4JZ and 0SR90JZ

0SPA4JZ and 0SRA009

0SPA4JZ and 0SRA00A

0SPA4JZ and 0SRA00Z

0SPA4JZ and 0SRA019

0SPA4JZ and 0SRA01A

0SPA4JZ and 0SRA01Z

0SPA4JZ and 0SRA039

0SPA4JZ and 0SRA03A

0SPA4JZ and 0SRA03Z

0SPA4JZ and 0SRA0J9

0SPA4JZ and 0SRA0JA

0SPA4JZ and 0SRA0JZ

0SPA4JZ and 0SRR019

0SPA4JZ and 0SRR01A

0SPA4JZ and 0SRR01Z

0SPA4JZ and 0SRR039

0SPA4JZ and 0SRR03A

0SPA4JZ and 0SRR03Z

0SPA4JZ and 0SRR0J9

0SPA4JZ and 0SRR0JA

0SPA4JZ and 0SRR0JZ

0SPA4JZ and 0SU909Z

0SPA4JZ and 0SUA09Z

0SPA4JZ and 0SUR09Z

0SPB08Z and 0SRB019

0SPB08Z and 0SRB01A

0SPB08Z and 0SRB01Z

0SPB08Z and 0SRB029

0SPB08Z and 0SRB02A

0SPB08Z and 0SRB02Z

0SPB08Z and 0SRB039

0SPB08Z and 0SRB03A

0SPB08Z and 0SRB03Z

0SPB08Z and 0SRB049

0SPB08Z and 0SRB04A

0SPB08Z and 0SRB04Z

0SPB08Z and 0SRB069

0SPB08Z and 0SRB06A

0SPB08Z and 0SRB06Z

0SPB08Z and 0SRB0J9

0SPB08Z and 0SRB0JA

0SPB08Z and 0SRB0JZ

0SPB08Z and 0SRE009

0SPB08Z and 0SRE00A

0SPB08Z and 0SRE00Z

0SPB08Z and 0SRE019

0SPB08Z and 0SRE01A

0SPB08Z and 0SRE01Z

0SPB08Z and 0SRE039

0SPB08Z and 0SRE03A

0SPB08Z and 0SRE03Z

0SPB08Z and 0SRE0J9

0SPB08Z and 0SRE0JA

0SPB08Z and 0SRE0JZ

0SPB08Z and 0SRS019

0SPB08Z and 0SRS01A

0SPB08Z and 0SRS01Z

0SPB08Z and 0SRS039

0SPB08Z and 0SRS03A

0SPB08Z and 0SRS03Z

0SPB08Z and 0SRS0J9

0SPB08Z and 0SRS0JA

0SPB08Z and 0SRS0JZ

0SPB08Z and 0SUB09Z
0SPB08Z and 0SUE09Z
0SPB08Z and 0SUS09Z
0SPB09Z and 0SRB019
0SPB09Z and 0SRB01A
0SPB09Z and 0SRB01Z
0SPB09Z and 0SRB029
0SPB09Z and 0SRB02A
0SPB09Z and 0SRB02Z
0SPB09Z and 0SRB039
0SPB09Z and 0SRB03A
0SPB09Z and 0SRB03Z
0SPB09Z and 0SRB049
0SPB09Z and 0SRB04A
0SPB09Z and 0SRB04Z
0SPB09Z and 0SRB069
0SPB09Z and 0SRB06A
0SPB09Z and 0SRB06Z
0SPB09Z and 0SRB0J9
0SPB09Z and 0SRB0JA
0SPB09Z and 0SRB0JZ
0SPB09Z and 0SRE009
0SPB09Z and 0SRE00A
0SPB09Z and 0SRE00Z
0SPB09Z and 0SRE019
0SPB09Z and 0SRE01A
0SPB09Z and 0SRE01Z
0SPB09Z and 0SRE039
0SPB09Z and 0SRE03A
0SPB09Z and 0SRE03Z
0SPB09Z and 0SRE0J9
0SPB09Z and 0SRE0JA
0SPB09Z and 0SRE0JZ
0SPB09Z and 0SRS019
0SPB09Z and 0SRS01A
0SPB09Z and 0SRS01Z
0SPB09Z and 0SRS039
0SPB09Z and 0SRS03A
0SPB09Z and 0SRS03Z
0SPB09Z and 0SRS0J9
0SPB09Z and 0SRS0JA
0SPB09Z and 0SRS0JZ
0SPB09Z and 0SUB09Z
0SPB09Z and 0SUB09Z
0SPB09Z and 0SUE09Z
0SPB09Z and 0SUE09Z
0SPB09Z and 0SUS09Z
0SPB09Z and 0SUS09Z
0SPB0BZ and 0SRB019
0SPB0BZ and 0SRB01A
0SPB0BZ and 0SRB01Z
0SPB0BZ and 0SRB029
0SPB0BZ and 0SRB02A
0SPB0BZ and 0SRB02Z
0SPB0BZ and 0SRB039
0SPB0BZ and 0SRB03A
0SPB0BZ and 0SRB03Z
0SPB0BZ and 0SRB049
0SPB0BZ and 0SRB04A
0SPB0BZ and 0SRB04Z
0SPB0BZ and 0SRB069
0SPB0BZ and 0SRB06A
0SPB0BZ and 0SRB06Z
0SPB0BZ and 0SRB0J9
0SPB0BZ and 0SRB0JA
0SPB0BZ and 0SRB0JZ
0SPB0BZ and 0SRE009
0SPB0BZ and 0SRE00A
0SPB0BZ and 0SRE00Z
0SPB0BZ and 0SRE019
0SPB0BZ and 0SRE01A
0SPB0BZ and 0SRE01Z
0SPB0BZ and 0SRE039
0SPB0BZ and 0SRE03A
0SPB0BZ and 0SRE03Z
0SPB0BZ and 0SRE0J9
0SPB0BZ and 0SRE0JA
0SPB0BZ and 0SRE0JZ
0SPB0BZ and 0SRS019
0SPB0BZ and 0SRS01A
0SPB0BZ and 0SRS01Z
0SPB0BZ and 0SRS039
0SPB0BZ and 0SRS03A
0SPB0BZ and 0SRS03Z
0SPB0BZ and 0SRS0J9
0SPB0BZ and 0SRS0JA
0SPB0BZ and 0SRS0JZ
0SPB0BZ and 0SUB09Z
0SPB0BZ and 0SUE09Z
0SPB0BZ and 0SUS09Z
0SPB0JZ and 0SRB019
0SPB0JZ and 0SRB01A
0SPB0JZ and 0SRB01Z
0SPB0JZ and 0SRB029
0SPB0JZ and 0SRB02A
0SPB0JZ and 0SRB02Z
0SPB0JZ and 0SRB039
0SPB0JZ and 0SRB03A
0SPB0JZ and 0SRB03Z
0SPB0JZ and 0SRB049
0SPB0JZ and 0SRB04A
0SPB0JZ and 0SRB04Z
0SPB0JZ and 0SRB069
0SPB0JZ and 0SRB06A
0SPB0JZ and 0SRB06Z
0SPB0JZ and 0SRB0J9
0SPB0JZ and 0SRB0JA
0SPB0JZ and 0SRB0JZ
0SPB0JZ and 0SRE009
0SPB0JZ and 0SRE00A
0SPB0JZ and 0SRE00Z
0SPB0JZ and 0SRE019
0SPB0JZ and 0SRE01A
0SPB0JZ and 0SRE01Z
0SPB0JZ and 0SRE039
0SPB0JZ and 0SRE03A
0SPB0JZ and 0SRE03Z
0SPB0JZ and 0SRE0J9
0SPB0JZ and 0SRE0JA
0SPB0JZ and 0SRE0JZ
0SPB0JZ and 0SRS019
0SPB0JZ and 0SRS01A
0SPB0JZ and 0SRS01Z
0SPB0JZ and 0SRS039
0SPB0JZ and 0SRS03A
0SPB0JZ and 0SRS03Z
0SPB0JZ and 0SRS0J9
0SPB0JZ and 0SRS0JA
0SPB0JZ and 0SRS0JZ
0SPB48Z and 0SRB019
0SPB48Z and 0SRB01A
0SPB48Z and 0SRB01Z
0SPB48Z and 0SRB029
0SPB48Z and 0SRB02A
0SPB48Z and 0SRB02Z
0SPB48Z and 0SRB039
0SPB48Z and 0SRB03A
0SPB48Z and 0SRB03Z
0SPB48Z and 0SRB049
0SPB48Z and 0SRB04A
0SPB48Z and 0SRB04Z
0SPB48Z and 0SRB069
0SPB48Z and 0SRB06A
0SPB48Z and 0SRB06Z
0SPB48Z and 0SRB0J9
0SPB48Z and 0SRB0JA
0SPB48Z and 0SRB0JZ
0SPB48Z and 0SRE009
0SPB48Z and 0SRE00A
0SPB48Z and 0SRE00Z
0SPB48Z and 0SRE019
0SPB48Z and 0SRE01A
0SPB48Z and 0SRE01Z
0SPB48Z and 0SRE039

0SPB48Z and 0SRE03A
0SPB48Z and 0SRE03Z
0SPB48Z and 0SRE0J9
0SPB48Z and 0SRE0JA
0SPB48Z and 0SRE0JZ
0SPB48Z and 0SRS019
0SPB48Z and 0SRS01A
0SPB48Z and 0SRS01Z
0SPB48Z and 0SRS039
0SPB48Z and 0SRS03A
0SPB48Z and 0SRS03Z
0SPB48Z and 0SRS0J9
0SPB48Z and 0SRS0JA
0SPB48Z and 0SRS0JZ
0SPB48Z and 0SUB09Z
0SPB48Z and 0SUE09Z
0SPB48Z and 0SUS09Z
0SPB4JZ and 0SRB019
0SPB4JZ and 0SRB01A
0SPB4JZ and 0SRB01Z
0SPB4JZ and 0SRB029
0SPB4JZ and 0SRB02A
0SPB4JZ and 0SRB02Z
0SPB4JZ and 0SRB039
0SPB4JZ and 0SRB03A
0SPB4JZ and 0SRB03Z
0SPB4JZ and 0SRB049
0SPB4JZ and 0SRB04A
0SPB4JZ and 0SRB04Z
0SPB4JZ and 0SRB069
0SPB4JZ and 0SRB06A
0SPB4JZ and 0SRB06Z
0SPB4JZ and 0SRB0J9
0SPB4JZ and 0SRB0JA
0SPB4JZ and 0SRB0JZ
0SPB4JZ and 0SRE009
0SPB4JZ and 0SRE00A
0SPB4JZ and 0SRE00Z
0SPB4JZ and 0SRE019
0SPB4JZ and 0SRE01A
0SPB4JZ and 0SRE01Z
0SPB4JZ and 0SRE039
0SPB4JZ and 0SRE03A
0SPB4JZ and 0SRE03Z
0SPB4JZ and 0SRE0J9
0SPB4JZ and 0SRE0JA
0SPB4JZ and 0SRE0JZ
0SPB4JZ and 0SRS019
0SPB4JZ and 0SRS01A
0SPB4JZ and 0SRS01Z
0SPB4JZ and 0SRS039
0SPB4JZ and 0SRS03A
0SPB4JZ and 0SRS03Z
0SPB4JZ and 0SRS0J9
0SPB4JZ and 0SRS0JA
0SPB4JZ and 0SRS0JZ
0SPB4JZ and 0SUB09Z
0SPB4JZ and 0SUE09Z
0SPB4JZ and 0SUS09Z
0SPC08Z and 0SRC069
0SPC08Z and 0SRC06A
0SPC08Z and 0SRC06Z
0SPC08Z and 0SRC0J9
0SPC08Z and 0SRC0JA
0SPC08Z and 0SRC0JZ
0SPC08Z and 0SRT0J9
0SPC08Z and 0SRT0JA
0SPC08Z and 0SRT0JZ
0SPC08Z and 0SRV0J9
0SPC08Z and 0SRV0JA
0SPC08Z and 0SRV0JZ
0SPC09Z and 0SRC069
0SPC09Z and 0SRC06A
0SPC09Z and 0SRC06Z
0SPC09Z and 0SRC0J9
0SPC09Z and 0SRC0JA
0SPC09Z and 0SRC0JZ
0SPC09Z and 0SRC0L9
0SPC09Z and 0SRC0LA
0SPC09Z and 0SRC0LZ
0SPC09Z and 0SRT0J9
0SPC09Z and 0SRT0JA
0SPC09Z and 0SRT0JZ
0SPC09Z and 0SRV0J9
0SPC09Z and 0SRV0JA
0SPC09Z and 0SRV0JZ
0SPC09Z and 0SUV09Z
0SPC0JC and 0SRC069
0SPC0JC and 0SRC06A
0SPC0JC and 0SRC06Z
0SPC0JC and 0SRC0J9
0SPC0JC and 0SRC0JA
0SPC0JC and 0SRC0JZ
0SPC0JC and 0SRT0J9
0SPC0JC and 0SRT0JA
0SPC0JC and 0SRT0JZ
0SPC0JC and 0SRV0J9
0SPC0JC and 0SRV0JA
0SPC0JC and 0SRV0JZ
0SPC0JZ and 0SRC069
0SPC0JZ and 0SRC06A
0SPC0JZ and 0SRC06Z
0SPC0JZ and 0SRC0J9
0SPC0JZ and 0SRC0JA
0SPC0JZ and 0SRC0JZ
0SPC0JZ and 0SRC0L9
0SPC0JZ and 0SRC0LA
0SPC0JZ and 0SRC0LZ
0SPC0JZ and 0SRT0J9
0SPC0JZ and 0SRT0JA
0SPC0JZ and 0SRT0JZ
0SPC0JZ and 0SRV0J9
0SPC0JZ and 0SRV0JA
0SPC0JZ and 0SRV0JZ
0SPC38Z and 0SRC069
0SPC38Z and 0SRC06A
0SPC38Z and 0SRC06Z
0SPC38Z and 0SRC0J9
0SPC38Z and 0SRC0JA
0SPC38Z and 0SRC0JZ
0SPC38Z and 0SRT0J9
0SPC38Z and 0SRT0JA
0SPC38Z and 0SRT0JZ
0SPC38Z and 0SRV0J9
0SPC38Z and 0SRV0JA
0SPC38Z and 0SRV0JZ
0SPC48Z and 0SRC069
0SPC48Z and 0SRC06A
0SPC48Z and 0SRC06Z
0SPC48Z and 0SRC0J9
0SPC48Z and 0SRC0JA
0SPC48Z and 0SRC0JZ
0SPC48Z and 0SRT0J9
0SPC48Z and 0SRT0JA
0SPC48Z and 0SRT0JZ
0SPC48Z and 0SRV0J9
0SPC48Z and 0SRV0JA
0SPC48Z and 0SRV0JZ
0SPC4JC and 0SRC069
0SPC4JC and 0SRC06A
0SPC4JC and 0SRC06Z
0SPC4JC and 0SRC0J9
0SPC4JC and 0SRC0JA
0SPC4JC and 0SRC0JZ
0SPC4JC and 0SRT0J9
0SPC4JC and 0SRT0JA
0SPC4JC and 0SRV0J9
0SPC4JC and 0SRV0JA
0SPC4JZ and 0SRC069
0SPC4JZ and 0SRC06A
0SPC4JZ and 0SRC06Z
0SPC4JZ and 0SRC0J9
0SPC4JZ and 0SRC0JA
0SPC4JZ and 0SRC0JZ

0SPC4JZ and 0SRC0L9

0SPC4JZ and 0SRC0LA

0SPC4JZ and 0SRC0LZ

0SPC4JZ and 0SRT0J9

0SPC4JZ and 0SRT0JA

0SPC4JZ and 0SRT0JZ

0SPC4JZ and 0SRV0J9

0SPC4JZ and 0SRV0JA

0SPC4JZ and 0SRV0JZ

0SPD08Z and 0SRD069

0SPD08Z and 0SRD06A

0SPD08Z and 0SRD06Z

0SPD08Z and 0SRD0J9

0SPD08Z and 0SRD0JA

0SPD08Z and 0SRD0JZ

0SPD08Z and 0SRU0J9

0SPD08Z and 0SRU0JA

0SPD08Z and 0SRU0JZ

0SPD08Z and 0SRW0J9

0SPD08Z and 0SRW0JA

0SPD08Z and 0SRW0JZ

0SPD09Z and 0SRD069

0SPD09Z and 0SRD06A

0SPD09Z and 0SRD06Z

0SPD09Z and 0SRD0J9

0SPD09Z and 0SRD0JA

0SPD09Z and 0SRD0JZ

0SPD09Z and 0SRD0L9

0SPD09Z and 0SRD0LA

0SPD09Z and 0SRD0LZ

0SPD09Z and 0SRU0J9

0SPD09Z and 0SRU0JA

0SPD09Z and 0SRU0JZ

0SPD09Z and 0SRW0J9

0SPD09Z and 0SRW0JA

0SPD09Z and 0SRW0JZ

0SPD09Z and 0SUW09Z

0SPD0JC and 0SRD069

0SPD0JC and 0SRD06A

0SPD0JC and 0SRD06Z

0SPD0JC and 0SRD0J9

0SPD0JC and 0SRD0JA

0SPD0JC and 0SRD0JZ

0SPD0JC and 0SRU0J9

0SPD0JC and 0SRU0JA

0SPD0JC and 0SRU0JZ

0SPD0JC and 0SRW0J9

0SPD0JC and 0SRW0JA

0SPD0JC and 0SRW0JZ

0SPD0JZ and 0SRD069

0SPD0JZ and 0SRD06A

0SPD0JZ and 0SRD06Z

0SPD0JZ and 0SRD0J9

0SPD0JZ and 0SRD0JA

0SPD0JZ and 0SRD0JZ

0SPD0JZ and 0SRD0L9

0SPD0JZ and 0SRD0LA

0SPD0JZ and 0SRD0LZ

0SPD0JZ and 0SRU0J9

0SPD0JZ and 0SRU0JA

0SPD0JZ and 0SRU0JZ

0SPD0JZ and 0SRW0J9

0SPD0JZ and 0SRW0JA

0SPD0JZ and 0SRW0JZ

0SPD38Z and 0SRD069

0SPD38Z and 0SRD06A

0SPD38Z and 0SRD06Z

0SPD38Z and 0SRD0J9

0SPD38Z and 0SRD0JA

0SPD38Z and 0SRD0JZ

0SPD38Z and 0SRU0J9

0SPD38Z and 0SRU0JA

0SPD38Z and 0SRU0JZ

0SPD38Z and 0SRW0J9

0SPD38Z and 0SRW0JA

0SPD38Z and 0SRW0JZ

0SPD48Z and 0SRD069

0SPD48Z and 0SRD06A

0SPD48Z and 0SRD06Z

0SPD48Z and 0SRD0J9

0SPD48Z and 0SRD0JA

0SPD48Z and 0SRD0JZ

0SPD48Z and 0SRU0J9

0SPD48Z and 0SRU0JA

0SPD48Z and 0SRU0JZ

0SPD48Z and 0SRW0J9

0SPD48Z and 0SRW0JA

0SPD48Z and 0SRW0JZ

0SPD4JC and 0SRD069

0SPD4JC and 0SRD06A

0SPD4JC and 0SRD06Z

0SPD4JC and 0SRD0J9

0SPD4JC and 0SRD0JA

0SPD4JC and 0SRD0JZ

0SPD4JC and 0SRU0J9

0SPD4JC and 0SRU0JA

0SPD4JC and 0SRW0J9

0SPD4JC and 0SRW0JA

0SPD4JC and 0SRW0JZ

0SPD4JZ and 0SRD069

0SPD4JZ and 0SRD06A

0SPD4JZ and 0SRD06Z

0SPD4JZ and 0SRD0J9

0SPD4JZ and 0SRD0JA

0SPD4JZ and 0SRD0JZ

0SPD4JZ and 0SRD0L9

0SPD4JZ and 0SRD0LA

0SPD4JZ and 0SRD0LZ

0SPD4JZ and 0SRU0J9

0SPD4JZ and 0SRU0JA

0SPD4JZ and 0SRU0JZ

0SPD4JZ and 0SRW0J9

0SPD4JZ and 0SRW0JA

0SPD4JZ and 0SRW0JZ

0SPE0JZ and 0SRB019

0SPE0JZ and 0SRB01A

0SPE0JZ and 0SRB01Z

0SPE0JZ and 0SRB029

0SPE0JZ and 0SRB02A

0SPE0JZ and 0SRB02Z

0SPE0JZ and 0SRB039

0SPE0JZ and 0SRB03A

0SPE0JZ and 0SRB03Z

0SPE0JZ and 0SRB049

0SPE0JZ and 0SRB04A

0SPE0JZ and 0SRB04Z

0SPE0JZ and 0SRB069

0SPE0JZ and 0SRB06A

0SPE0JZ and 0SRB06Z

0SPE0JZ and 0SRB0J9

0SPE0JZ and 0SRB0JA

0SPE0JZ and 0SRB0JZ

0SPE0JZ and 0SRE009

0SPE0JZ and 0SRE00A

0SPE0JZ and 0SRE00Z

0SPE0JZ and 0SRE019

0SPE0JZ and 0SRE01A

0SPE0JZ and 0SRE01Z

0SPE0JZ and 0SRE039

0SPE0JZ and 0SRE03A

0SPE0JZ and 0SRE03Z

0SPE0JZ and 0SRE0J9

0SPE0JZ and 0SRE0JA

0SPE0JZ and 0SRE0JZ

0SPE0JZ and 0SRS019

0SPE0JZ and 0SRS01A

0SPE0JZ and 0SRS01Z

0SPE0JZ and 0SRS039

0SPE0JZ and 0SRS03A

0SPE0JZ and 0SRS03Z

0SPE0JZ and 0SRS0J9

0SPE0JZ and 0SRS0JA

0SPE0JZ and 0SRS0JZ

0SPE4JZ and 0SRB019

0SPE4JZ and 0SRB01A

0SPE4JZ and 0SRB01Z

0SPE4JZ and 0SRB029

0SPE4JZ and 0SRB02A

0SPE4JZ and 0SRB02Z

0SPE4JZ and 0SRB039

0SPE4JZ and 0SRB03A

0SPE4JZ and 0SRB03Z

0SPE4JZ and 0SRB049

0SPE4JZ and 0SRB04A

0SPE4JZ and 0SRB04Z

0SPE4JZ and 0SRB069

0SPE4JZ and 0SRB06A

0SPE4JZ and 0SRB06Z

0SPE4JZ and 0SRB0J9

0SPE4JZ and 0SRB0JA

0SPE4JZ and 0SRB0JZ

0SPE4JZ and 0SRE009

0SPE4JZ and 0SRE00A

0SPE4JZ and 0SRE00Z

0SPE4JZ and 0SRE019

0SPE4JZ and 0SRE01A

0SPE4JZ and 0SRE01Z

0SPE4JZ and 0SRE039

0SPE4JZ and 0SRE03A

0SPE4JZ and 0SRE03Z

0SPE4JZ and 0SRE0J9

0SPE4JZ and 0SRE0JA

0SPE4JZ and 0SRE0JZ

0SPE4JZ and 0SRS019

0SPE4JZ and 0SRS01A

0SPE4JZ and 0SRS01Z

0SPE4JZ and 0SRS039

0SPE4JZ and 0SRS03A

0SPE4JZ and 0SRS03Z

0SPE4JZ and 0SRS0J9

0SPE4JZ and 0SRS0JA

0SPE4JZ and 0SRS0JZ

0SPE4JZ and 0SUB09Z

0SPE4JZ and 0SUE09Z

0SPE4JZ and 0SUS09Z

0SPR0JZ and 0SR9019

0SPR0JZ and 0SR901A

0SPR0JZ and 0SR901Z

0SPR0JZ and 0SR9029

0SPR0JZ and 0SR902A

0SPR0JZ and 0SR902Z

0SPR0JZ and 0SR9039

0SPR0JZ and 0SR903A

0SPR0JZ and 0SR903Z

0SPR0JZ and 0SR9049

0SPR0JZ and 0SR904A

0SPR0JZ and 0SR904Z

0SPR0JZ and 0SR9069

0SPR0JZ and 0SR906A

0SPR0JZ and 0SR906Z

0SPR0JZ and 0SR90J9

0SPR0JZ and 0SR90JA

0SPR0JZ and 0SR90JZ

0SPR0JZ and 0SRA009

0SPR0JZ and 0SRA00A

0SPR0JZ and 0SRA00Z

0SPR0JZ and 0SRA019

0SPR0JZ and 0SRA01A

0SPR0JZ and 0SRA01Z

0SPR0JZ and 0SRA039

0SPR0JZ and 0SRA03A

0SPR0JZ and 0SRA03Z

0SPR0JZ and 0SRA0J9

0SPR0JZ and 0SRA0JA

0SPR0JZ and 0SRA0JZ

0SPR0JZ and 0SRR019

0SPR0JZ and 0SRR01A

0SPR0JZ and 0SRR01Z

0SPR0JZ and 0SRR039

0SPR0JZ and 0SRR03A

0SPR0JZ and 0SRR03Z

0SPR0JZ and 0SRR0J9

0SPR0JZ and 0SRR0JA

0SPR0JZ and 0SRR0JZ

0SPR4JZ and 0SR9019

0SPR4JZ and 0SR901A

0SPR4JZ and 0SR901Z

0SPR4JZ and 0SR9029

0SPR4JZ and 0SR902A

0SPR4JZ and 0SR902Z

0SPR4JZ and 0SR9039

0SPR4JZ and 0SR903A

0SPR4JZ and 0SR903Z

0SPR4JZ and 0SR9049

0SPR4JZ and 0SR904A

0SPR4JZ and 0SR904Z

0SPR4JZ and 0SR9069

0SPR4JZ and 0SR906A

0SPR4JZ and 0SR906Z

0SPR4JZ and 0SR90J9

0SPR4JZ and 0SR90JA

0SPR4JZ and 0SR90JZ

0SPR4JZ and 0SRA009

0SPR4JZ and 0SRA00A

0SPR4JZ and 0SRA00Z

0SPR4JZ and 0SRA019

0SPR4JZ and 0SRA01A

0SPR4JZ and 0SRA01Z

0SPR4JZ and 0SRA039

0SPR4JZ and 0SRA03A

0SPR4JZ and 0SRA03Z

0SPR4JZ and 0SRA0J9

0SPR4JZ and 0SRA0JA

0SPR4JZ and 0SRA0JZ

0SPR4JZ and 0SRR019

0SPR4JZ and 0SRR01A

0SPR4JZ and 0SRR01Z

0SPR4JZ and 0SRR039

0SPR4JZ and 0SRR03A

0SPR4JZ and 0SRR03Z

0SPR4JZ and 0SRR0J9

0SPR4JZ and 0SRR0JA

0SPR4JZ and 0SRR0JZ

0SPR4JZ and 0SU909Z

0SPR4JZ and 0SUA09Z

0SPR4JZ and 0SUR09Z

0SPS0JZ and 0SRB019

0SPS0JZ and 0SRB01A

0SPS0JZ and 0SRB01Z

0SPS0JZ and 0SRB029

0SPS0JZ and 0SRB02A

0SPS0JZ and 0SRB02Z

0SPS0JZ and 0SRB039

0SPS0JZ and 0SRB03A

0SPS0JZ and 0SRB03Z

0SPS0JZ and 0SRB049

0SPS0JZ and 0SRB04A

0SPS0JZ and 0SRB04Z

0SPS0JZ and 0SRB069

0SPS0JZ and 0SRB06A

0SPS0JZ and 0SRB06Z

0SPS0JZ and 0SRB0J9

0SPS0JZ and 0SRB0JA

0SPS0JZ and 0SRB0JZ

0SPS0JZ and 0SRE009

0SPS0JZ and 0SRE00A

0SPS0JZ and 0SRE00Z

0SPS0JZ and 0SRE019

0SPS0JZ and 0SRE01A

0SPS0JZ and 0SRE01Z

0SPS0JZ and 0SRE039

0SPS0JZ and 0SRE03A

0SPS0JZ and 0SRE03Z

0SPS0JZ and 0SRE0J9

0SPS0JZ and 0SRE0JA

0SPS0JZ and 0SRE0JZ

0SPS0JZ and 0SRS019

0SPS0JZ and 0SRS01A

0SPS0JZ and 0SRS01Z

0SPS0JZ and 0SRS039

0SPS0JZ and 0SRS03A

0SPS0JZ and 0SRS03Z

0SPS0JZ and 0SRS0J9

0SPS0JZ and 0SRS0JA

0SPS0JZ and 0SRS0JZ

0SPS4JZ and 0SRB019

0SPS4JZ and 0SRB01A

0SPS4JZ and 0SRB01Z

0SPS4JZ and 0SRB029

0SPS4JZ and 0SRB02A

0SPS4JZ and 0SRB02Z

0SPS4JZ and 0SRB039

0SPS4JZ and 0SRB03A

0SPS4JZ and 0SRB03Z

0SPS4JZ and 0SRB049

0SPS4JZ and 0SRB04A

0SPS4JZ and 0SRB04Z

0SPS4JZ and 0SRB069

0SPS4JZ and 0SRB06A

0SPS4JZ and 0SRB06Z

0SPS4JZ and 0SRB0J9

0SPS4JZ and 0SRB0JA

0SPS4JZ and 0SRB0JZ

0SPS4JZ and 0SRE009

0SPS4JZ and 0SRE00A

0SPS4JZ and 0SRE00Z

0SPS4JZ and 0SRE019

0SPS4JZ and 0SRE01A

0SPS4JZ and 0SRE01Z

0SPS4JZ and 0SRE039

0SPS4JZ and 0SRE03A

0SPS4JZ and 0SRE03Z

0SPS4JZ and 0SRE0J9

0SPS4JZ and 0SRE0JA

0SPS4JZ and 0SRE0JZ

0SPS4JZ and 0SRS019

0SPS4JZ and 0SRS01A

0SPS4JZ and 0SRS01Z

0SPS4JZ and 0SRS039

0SPS4JZ and 0SRS03A

0SPS4JZ and 0SRS03Z

0SPS4JZ and 0SRS0J9

0SPS4JZ and 0SRS0JA

0SPS4JZ and 0SRS0JZ

0SPS4JZ and 0SUB09Z

0SPS4JZ and 0SUE09Z

0SPS4JZ and 0SUS09Z

0SPT0JZ and 0SRC069

0SPT0JZ and 0SRC06A

0SPT0JZ and 0SRC06Z

0SPT0JZ and 0SRC0J9

0SPT0JZ and 0SRC0JA

0SPT0JZ and 0SRC0JZ

0SPT0JZ and 0SRT0J9

0SPT0JZ and 0SRT0JA

0SPT0JZ and 0SRT0JZ

0SPT0JZ and 0SRV0J9

0SPT0JZ and 0SRV0JA

0SPT0JZ and 0SRV0JZ

0SPT4JZ and 0SRC069

0SPT4JZ and 0SRC06A

0SPT4JZ and 0SRC06Z

0SPT4JZ and 0SRC0J9

0SPT4JZ and 0SRC0JA

0SPT4JZ and 0SRC0JZ

0SPT4JZ and 0SRT0J9

0SPT4JZ and 0SRT0JA

0SPT4JZ and 0SRV0J9

0SPT4JZ and 0SRV0JA

0SPU0JZ and 0SRD069

0SPU0JZ and 0SRD06A

0SPU0JZ and 0SRD06Z

0SPU0JZ and 0SRD0J9

0SPU0JZ and 0SRD0JA

0SPU0JZ and 0SRD0JZ

0SPU0JZ and 0SRU0J9

0SPU0JZ and 0SRU0JA

0SPU0JZ and 0SRU0JZ

0SPU0JZ and 0SRW0J9

0SPU0JZ and 0SRW0JA

0SPU0JZ and 0SRW0JZ

0SPU4JZ and 0SRD069

0SPU4JZ and 0SRD06A

0SPU4JZ and 0SRD06Z

0SPU4JZ and 0SRD0J9

0SPU4JZ and 0SRD0JA

0SPU4JZ and 0SRD0JZ

0SPU4JZ and 0SRU0J9

0SPU4JZ and 0SRU0JA

0SPU4JZ and 0SRW0J9

0SPU4JZ and 0SRW0JA

0SPU4JZ and 0SRW0JZ

0SPV0JZ and 0SRC069

0SPV0JZ and 0SRC06A

0SPV0JZ and 0SRC06Z

0SPV0JZ and 0SRC0J9

0SPV0JZ and 0SRC0JA

0SPV0JZ and 0SRC0JZ

0SPV0JZ and 0SRT0J9

0SPV0JZ and 0SRT0JA

0SPV0JZ and 0SRT0JZ

0SPV0JZ and 0SRV0J9

0SPV0JZ and 0SRV0JA

0SPV0JZ and 0SRV0JZ

0SPV4JZ and 0SRC069

0SPV4JZ and 0SRC06A

0SPV4JZ and 0SRC06Z

0SPV4JZ and 0SRC0J9

0SPV4JZ and 0SRC0JA

0SPV4JZ and 0SRC0JZ

0SPV4JZ and 0SRT0J9

0SPV4JZ and 0SRT0JA

0SPV4JZ and 0SRV0J9

0SPV4JZ and 0SRV0JA

0SPW0JZ and 0SRD069

0SPW0JZ and 0SRD06A

0SPW0JZ and 0SRD06Z

0SPW0JZ and 0SRD0J9

0SPW0JZ and 0SRD0JA

0SPW0JZ and 0SRD0JZ

0SPW0JZ and 0SRU0J9

0SPW0JZ and 0SRU0JA

0SPW0JZ and 0SRU0JZ

0SPW0JZ and 0SRW0J9

0SPW0JZ and 0SRW0JA

0SPW0JZ and 0SRW0JZ

0SPW4JZ and 0SRD069

0SPW4JZ and 0SRD06A

0SPW4JZ and 0SRD06Z

0SPW4JZ and 0SRD0J9

0SPW4JZ and 0SRD0JA

0SPW4JZ and 0SRD0JZ

0SPW4JZ and 0SRU0J9

0SPW4JZ and 0SRU0JA

0SPW4JZ and 0SRW0J9

0SPW4JZ and 0SRW0JA

0SPW4JZ and 0SRW0JZ

0TQB0ZZ and 0WQFXZ2

0TQB0ZZ and 0WQFXZZ

0TQB3ZZ and 0WQFXZ2

0TQB3ZZ and 0WQFXZZ

0TQB4ZZ and 0WQFXZ2

0TQB4ZZ and 0WQFXZZ

0TTB0ZZ
and 0TTD0ZZ
and 0UT20ZZ
and 0UT70ZZ
and 0UT90ZZ
and 0UTC0ZZ
and 0UTG0ZZ

0TY00Z0 and 0FYG0Z0

0TY00Z0 and 0FYG0Z1

0TY00Z0 and 0FYG0Z2

0TY00Z1 and 0FYG0Z0

0TY00Z1 and 0FYG0Z1

0TY00Z1
and 0FYG0Z2

0TY00Z2
and 0FYG0Z0

0TY00Z2
and 0FYG0Z1

0TY00Z2
and 0FYG0Z2

0TY10Z0
and 0FYG0Z0

0TY10Z0
and 0FYG0Z1

0TY10Z0
and 0FYG0Z2

0TY10Z1
and 0FYG0Z0

0TY10Z1
and 0FYG0Z1

0TY10Z1
and 0FYG0Z2

0TY10Z2
and 0FYG0Z0

0TY10Z2
and 0FYG0Z1

0TY10Z2
and 0FYG0Z2

0UT40ZZ
and 0UT90ZZ
and 0UTC0ZZ

0UT44ZZ
and 0UT94ZZ
and 0UTC4ZZ

0UT44ZZ
and 0UT9FZZ
and 0UTC4ZZ

0UT47ZZ
and 0UT97ZZ
and 0UTC7ZZ

0UT47ZZ
and 0UT97ZZ
and 0UTC8ZZ

0UT47ZZ
and 0UT98ZZ
and 0UTC7ZZ

0UT47ZZ
and 0UT98ZZ
and 0UTC8ZZ

0UT48ZZ
and 0UT97ZZ
and 0UTC7ZZ

0UT48ZZ
and 0UT97ZZ
and 0UTC8ZZ

0UT48ZZ
and 0UT98ZZ
and 0UTC7ZZ

0UT48ZZ
and 0UT98ZZ
and 0UTC8ZZ

0VT00ZZ
and 0VT30ZZ

0VT00ZZ
and 0VT34ZZ

0VT04ZZ
and 0VT30ZZ

0VT04ZZ
and 0VT34ZZ

0VT07ZZ
and 0VT30ZZ

0VT07ZZ
and 0VT34ZZ

0VT08ZZ
and 0VT30ZZ

0VT08ZZ
and 0VT34ZZ

This page intentionally left blank

Appendix H: Non-OR Not Affecting MS-DRG Assignment

00164JB
00164K0
00164K1
00164K2
00164K3
00164K4
00164K5
00164K6
00164K7
00164K8
00164KB
00164ZB
001U072
001U074
001U076
001U077
001U079
001U0J2
001U0J4
001U0J6
001U0J7
001U0J9
001U0K2
001U0K4
001U0K6
001U0K7
001U0K9
001U372
001U374
001U376
001U377
001U379
001U3J2
001U3J4
001U3J6
001U3J7
001U3J9
001U3K2
001U3K4
001U3K6
001U3K7
001U3K9
001U472
001U474
001U476
001U477
001U479
001U4J2
001U4J4
001U4J6
001U4J7
001U4J9
001U4K2
001U4K4
001U4K6
001U4K7
001U4K9
0020X0Z
0020XYZ
002EX0Z
002EXYZ
002UX0Z
002UXYZ
00500ZZ
00503ZZ
00504ZZ
00510ZZ
00513ZZ
00514ZZ
00520ZZ
00523ZZ
00524ZZ
00560ZZ
00563ZZ
00564ZZ
00570ZZ
00573ZZ
00574ZZ
00580ZZ
00583ZZ
00584ZZ
00590ZZ
00593ZZ
00594ZZ
005A0ZZ
005A3ZZ
005A4ZZ
005B0ZZ
005B3ZZ
005B4ZZ
005C0ZZ
005C3ZZ
005C4ZZ
005D0ZZ
005D3ZZ
005D4ZZ
005F0ZZ
005F3ZZ
005F4ZZ
005G0ZZ
005G3ZZ
005G4ZZ
005H0ZZ
005H3ZZ
005H4ZZ
005J0ZZ
005J3ZZ
005J4ZZ
005K0ZZ
005K3ZZ
005K4ZZ
005L0ZZ
005L3ZZ
005L4ZZ
005M0ZZ
005M3ZZ
005M4ZZ
005N0ZZ
005N3ZZ
005N4ZZ
005P0ZZ
005P3ZZ
005P4ZZ
005Q0ZZ
005Q3ZZ
005Q4ZZ
005R0ZZ
005R3ZZ
005R4ZZ
005S0ZZ
005S3ZZ
005S4ZZ
005T0ZZ
005T3ZZ
005T4ZZ
005W0ZZ
005W3ZZ
005W4ZZ
005X0ZZ
005X3ZZ
005X4ZZ
005Y0ZZ
005Y3ZZ
005Y4ZZ
00760ZZ
00763ZZ
00764ZZ
00800ZZ
00803ZZ
00804ZZ
00870ZZ
00873ZZ
00874ZZ
00880ZZ
00883ZZ
00884ZZ
008F0ZZ
008F3ZZ
008F4ZZ
008G0ZZ
008G3ZZ
008G4ZZ
008H0ZZ
008H3ZZ
008H4ZZ
008J0ZZ
008J3ZZ
008J4ZZ
008K0ZZ
008K3ZZ
008K4ZZ
008L0ZZ
008L3ZZ
008L4ZZ
008M0ZZ
008M3ZZ
008M4ZZ
008N0ZZ
008N3ZZ
008N4ZZ
008P0ZZ
008P3ZZ
008P4ZZ
008Q0ZZ
008Q3ZZ
008Q4ZZ
008R0ZZ
008R3ZZ
008R4ZZ
008S0ZZ
008S3ZZ
008S4ZZ
008W0ZZ
008W3ZZ
008W4ZZ
008X0ZZ
008X3ZZ
008X4ZZ
008Y0ZZ
008Y3ZZ
008Y4ZZ
009000Z
00900ZX
00900ZZ
009030Z
00903ZX
00903ZZ
009040Z
00904ZX
00904ZZ
009100Z
00910ZX
00910ZZ
009130Z
00913ZX
00913ZZ
009140Z
00914ZX
00914ZZ
009200Z
00920ZX
00920ZZ
009230Z
00923ZX
00923ZZ
009240Z
00924ZX
00924ZZ
009300Z
00930ZX
00930ZZ
009330Z
00933ZX
00933ZZ
009340Z
00934ZX
00934ZZ
009400Z
00940ZX
00940ZZ
009430Z
00943ZX
00943ZZ
009440Z
00944ZX
00944ZZ
009500Z
00950ZX
00950ZZ
009530Z
00953ZX
00953ZZ
009540Z
00954ZX
00954ZZ
009600Z
00960ZX
00960ZZ
009630Z
00963ZX
00963ZZ
009640Z
00964ZX
00964ZZ
009700Z
00970ZX
00970ZZ
009730Z
00973ZX
00973ZZ
009740Z
00974ZX
00974ZZ
009800Z
00980ZX
00980ZZ
009830Z
00983ZX
00983ZZ
009840Z
00984ZX
00984ZZ
009900Z
00990ZX
00990ZZ
009930Z
00993ZX
00993ZZ
009940Z
00994ZX
009A3ZX
009A4ZX
009B3ZX
009B4ZX
009C3ZX
009C4ZX
009D3ZX
009D4ZX
009F3ZX
009F4ZX
009G3ZX
009G4ZX
009H3ZX
009H4ZX
009J3ZX
009J4ZX
009K3ZX
009K4ZX
009L3ZX
009L4ZX
009M3ZX
009M4ZX
009N3ZX
009N4ZX
009P3ZX
009P4ZX
009Q3ZX
009Q4ZX
009R3ZX
009R4ZX
009S3ZX
009S4ZX
009T30Z
009T3ZX
009T3ZZ
009U30Z
009U3ZX
009U3ZZ
009U40Z
009U4ZX
009U4ZZ
009W30Z
009W3ZX
009W3ZZ
009X30Z
009X3ZX
009X3ZZ
009Y30Z
009Y3ZX
009Y3ZZ
00B03ZX
00B04ZX
00B13ZX
00B13ZZ
00B14ZX
00B14ZZ
00B20ZX
00B20ZZ
00B23ZX
00B23ZZ
00B24ZX
00B24ZZ
00B60ZX
00B60ZZ
00B63ZX
00B63ZZ
00B64ZX
00B64ZZ
00B70ZX
00B70ZZ
00B73ZX
00B73ZZ
00B74ZX
00B74ZZ
00B80ZX
00B80ZZ
00B83ZX
00B83ZZ
00B84ZX
00B84ZZ
00B90ZX
00B90ZZ
00B93ZX
00B93ZZ
00B94ZX
00B94ZZ
00BA0ZX
00BA0ZZ
00BA3ZX
00BA3ZZ
00BA4ZX
00BA4ZZ
00BB0ZX
00BB0ZZ
00BB3ZX
00BB3ZZ
00BB4ZX
00BB4ZZ
00BC0ZX
00BC0ZZ
00BC3ZX
00BC3ZZ
00BC4ZX
00BC4ZZ
00BD0ZX
00BD0ZZ
00BD3ZX
00BD3ZZ
00BD4ZX
00BD4ZZ
00BF0ZX
00BF0ZZ
00BF3ZX
00BF3ZZ
00BF4ZX
00BF4ZZ
00BG0ZX
00BG0ZZ
00BG3ZX
00BG3ZZ
00BG4ZX
00BG4ZZ
00BH0ZX
00BH0ZZ
00BH3ZX
00BH3ZZ
00BH4ZX
00BH4ZZ
00BJ0ZX
00BJ0ZZ
00BJ3ZX
00BJ3ZZ
00BJ4ZX
00BJ4ZZ
00BK0ZX
00BK0ZZ
00BK3ZX
00BK3ZZ
00BK4ZX
00BK4ZZ
00BL0ZX
00BL0ZZ
00BL3ZX
00BL3ZZ
00BL4ZX
00BL4ZZ
00BM0ZX
00BM0ZZ
00BM3ZX
00BM3ZZ
00BM4ZX
00BM4ZZ
00BN0ZX
00BN0ZZ
00BN3ZX
00BN3ZZ
00BN4ZX
00BN4ZZ
00BP0ZX
00BP0ZZ
00BP3ZX
00BP3ZZ
00BP4ZX
00BP4ZZ
00BQ0ZX
00BQ0ZZ
00BQ3ZX
00BQ3ZZ
00BQ4ZX
00BQ4ZZ
00BR0ZX
00BR0ZZ
00BR3ZX
00BR3ZZ
00BR4ZX
00BR4ZZ
00BS0ZX
00BS0ZZ
00BS3ZX
00BS3ZZ
00BS4ZX
00BS4ZZ
00BT0ZX
00BT0ZZ
00BT3ZX
00BT3ZZ
00BT4ZX
00BT4ZZ
00BW0ZX
00BW0ZZ
00BW3ZX
00BW3ZZ
00BW4ZX
00BW4ZZ
00BX0ZX
00BX0ZZ
00BX3ZX
00BX3ZZ
00BX4ZX
00BX4ZZ
00BY0ZX
00BY0ZZ
00BY3ZX
00BY3ZZ
00BY4ZX
00BY4ZZ
00C00ZZ
00C03ZZ
00C04ZZ
00C10ZZ
00C13ZZ
00C14ZZ
00C20ZZ
00C23ZZ
00C24ZZ
00C30ZZ
00C33ZZ
00C34ZZ
00C40ZZ
00C43ZZ
00C44ZZ
00C50ZZ
00C53ZZ
00C54ZZ
00C60ZZ
00C63ZZ
00C64ZZ
00C70ZZ
00C73ZZ
00C74ZZ
00C80ZZ
00C83ZZ
00C84ZZ
00C90ZZ
00C93ZZ
00C94ZZ
00CA0ZZ
00CA3ZZ
00CA4ZZ
00CB0ZZ
00CB3ZZ
00CB4ZZ
00CC0ZZ
00CC3ZZ
00CC4ZZ
00CD0ZZ
00CD3ZZ
00CD4ZZ
00CF0ZZ
00CF3ZZ
00CF4ZZ
00CG0ZZ
00CG3ZZ
00CG4ZZ
00CH0ZZ
00CH3ZZ
00CH4ZZ
00CJ0ZZ
00CJ3ZZ
00CJ4ZZ
00CK0ZZ
00CK3ZZ
00CK4ZZ
00CL0ZZ
00CL3ZZ
00CL4ZZ
00CM0ZZ
00CM3ZZ
00CM4ZZ
00CN0ZZ
00CN3ZZ
00CN4ZZ
00CP0ZZ
00CP3ZZ
00CP4ZZ
00CQ0ZZ
00CQ3ZZ
00CQ4ZZ
00CR0ZZ
00CR3ZZ
00CR4ZZ
00CS0ZZ
00CS3ZZ
00CS4ZZ
00CT0ZZ
00CT3ZZ
00CT4ZZ
00CU0ZZ
00CU3ZZ
00CU4ZZ
00CW0ZZ
00CW3ZZ
00CW4ZZ
00CX0ZZ
00CX3ZZ
00CX4ZZ
00CY0ZZ
00CY3ZZ
00CY4ZZ
00D10ZZ
00D13ZZ
00D14ZZ
00D20ZZ
00D23ZZ
00D24ZZ
00DF0ZZ
00DF3ZZ
00DF4ZZ
00DG0ZZ
00DG3ZZ
00DG4ZZ
00DH0ZZ
00DH3ZZ
00DH4ZZ
00DJ0ZZ
00DJ3ZZ
00DJ4ZZ
00DK0ZZ
00DK3ZZ
00DK4ZZ
00DL0ZZ
00DL3ZZ
00F3XZZ
00F4XZZ
00F5XZZ
00F6XZZ
00H00MZ
00H03MZ
00H04MZ
00H60MZ
00H63MZ
00H64MZ
00HE0MZ
00HE32Z
00HE3MZ
00HE3YZ
00HE4MZ
00HE4YZ
00HU03Z
00HU0MZ
00HU32Z
00HU33Z
00HU3MZ
00HU3YZ
00HU43Z
00HU4MZ
00HU4YZ
00HV03Z
00HV0MZ
00HV32Z
00HV33Z
00HV3MZ
00HV43Z
00HV4MZ
00J03ZZ
00JE3ZZ
00JU3ZZ
00JV3ZZ
00JV4ZZ
00K00ZZ
00K03ZZ
00K04ZZ
00K70ZZ
00K73ZZ
00K74ZZ
00K80ZZ
00K83ZZ
00K84ZZ
00K90ZZ
00K93ZZ
00K94ZZ
00KA0ZZ
00KA3ZZ
00KA4ZZ
00KB0ZZ
00KB3ZZ
00KB4ZZ
00KC0ZZ
00KC3ZZ
00KC4ZZ
00KD0ZZ
00KD3ZZ
00KD4ZZ
00N00ZZ
00N03ZZ
00N04ZZ
00N10ZZ
00N13ZZ
00N14ZZ
00N20ZZ
00N23ZZ
00N24ZZ
00N60ZZ
00N63ZZ
00N64ZZ
00N70ZZ
00N73ZZ
00N74ZZ
00N80ZZ
00N83ZZ
00N84ZZ
00N90ZZ
00N93ZZ

00N94ZZ
00NA0ZZ
00NA3ZZ
00NA4ZZ
00NB0ZZ
00NB3ZZ
00NB4ZZ
00NC0ZZ
00NC3ZZ
00NC4ZZ
00ND0ZZ
00ND3ZZ
00ND4ZZ
00NF0ZZ
00NF3ZZ
00NF4ZZ
00NG0ZZ
00NG3ZZ
00NG4ZZ
00NH0ZZ
00NH3ZZ
00NH4ZZ
00NJ0ZZ
00NJ3ZZ
00NJ4ZZ
00NK0ZZ
00NK3ZZ
00NK4ZZ
00NL0ZZ
00NL3ZZ
00NL4ZZ
00NM0ZZ
00NM3ZZ
00NM4ZZ
00NN0ZZ
00NN3ZZ
00NN4ZZ
00NP0ZZ
00NP3ZZ
00NP4ZZ
00NQ0ZZ
00NQ3ZZ
00NQ4ZZ
00NR0ZZ
00NR3ZZ
00NR4ZZ
00NS0ZZ
00NS3ZZ
00NS4ZZ
00NT0ZZ
00NT3ZZ
00NT4ZZ
00NW0ZZ
00NW3ZZ
00NW4ZZ
00NX0ZZ
00NX3ZZ
00NX4ZZ
00NY0ZZ
00NY3ZZ
00NY4ZZ
00P000Z
00P002Z
00P003Z
00P007Z
00P00JZ
00P00KZ
00P00MZ
00P00YZ
00P030Z
00P032Z
00P033Z
00P037Z
00P03JZ
00P03KZ
00P03MZ
00P03YZ
00P040Z
00P042Z
00P043Z
00P047Z
00P04JZ
00P04KZ
00P04MZ
00P04YZ
00P0X0Z
00P0X2Z
00P0X3Z
00P0XMZ
00P600Z
00P602Z
00P603Z
00P60JZ
00P60MZ
00P60YZ
00P630Z
00P632Z
00P633Z
00P63JZ
00P63MZ
00P63YZ
00P640Z
00P642Z
00P643Z
00P64JZ
00P64MZ
00P64YZ
00P6X0Z
00P6X2Z
00P6X3Z
00P6XMZ
00PE00Z
00PE02Z
00PE03Z
00PE07Z
00PE0MZ
00PE0YZ
00PE30Z
00PE32Z
00PE33Z
00PE37Z
00PE3MZ
00PE3YZ
00PE40Z
00PE42Z
00PE43Z
00PE47Z
00PE4MZ
00PE4YZ
00PEX0Z
00PEX2Z
00PEX3Z
00PEXMZ
00PU00Z
00PU02Z
00PU03Z
00PU0JZ
00PU0MZ
00PU0YZ
00PU30Z
00PU32Z
00PU33Z
00PU3JZ
00PU3MZ
00PU3YZ
00PU40Z
00PU42Z
00PU43Z
00PU4JZ
00PU4MZ
00PU4YZ
00PUX0Z
00PUX2Z
00PUX3Z
00PUXMZ
00PV00Z
00PV02Z
00PV03Z
00PV07Z
00PV0JZ
00PV0KZ
00PV0MZ
00PV0YZ
00PV30Z
00PV32Z
00PV33Z
00PV37Z
00PV3JZ
00PV3KZ
00PV3MZ
00PV3YZ
00PV40Z
00PV42Z
00PV43Z
00PV47Z
00PV4JZ
00PV4KZ
00PV4MZ
00PV4YZ
00PVX0Z
00PVX2Z
00PVX3Z
00PVXMZ
00Q00ZZ
00Q03ZZ
00Q04ZZ
00Q10ZZ
00RG0KZ
00RG47Z
00RG4JZ
00RG4KZ
00RH07Z
00RH0JZ
00RH0KZ
00RH47Z
00RH4JZ
00RH4KZ
00RJ07Z
00RJ0JZ
00RJ0KZ
00RJ47Z
00RJ4JZ
00RJ4KZ
00RK07Z
00RK0JZ
00RK0KZ
00RK47Z
00RK4JZ
00RK4KZ
00RL07Z
00RL0JZ
00RL0KZ
00RL47Z
00RL4JZ
00RL4KZ
00RM07Z
00RM0JZ
00RM0KZ
00RM47Z
00RM4JZ
00RM4KZ
00RN07Z
00RN0JZ
00RN0KZ
00RN47Z
00RN4JZ
00RN4KZ
00RP07Z
00RP0JZ
00RP0KZ
00RP47Z
00RP4JZ
00RP4KZ
00RQ07Z
00RQ0JZ
00RQ0KZ
00RQ47Z
00RQ4JZ
00RQ4KZ
00RR07Z
00RR0JZ
00RR0KZ
00RR47Z
00RR4JZ
00RR4KZ
00RS07Z
00RS0JZ
00RS0KZ
00RS47Z
00RS4JZ
00RS4KZ
00RT07Z
00RT0JZ
00RT0KZ
00RT47Z
00RT4JZ
00RT4KZ
00SF0ZZ
00SF3ZZ
00SF4ZZ
00SG0ZZ
00SG3ZZ
00SG4ZZ
00SH0ZZ
00SH3ZZ
00SH4ZZ
00SJ0ZZ
00SJ3ZZ
00SJ4ZZ
00SK0ZZ
00SK3ZZ
00SK4ZZ
00SL0ZZ
00SL3ZZ
00SL4ZZ
00SM0ZZ
00SM3ZZ
00SM4ZZ
00SN0ZZ
00SN3ZZ
00SN4ZZ
00SP0ZZ
00SP3ZZ
00SP4ZZ
00SQ0ZZ
00SQ3ZZ
00SQ4ZZ
00SR0ZZ
00SR3ZZ
00SR4ZZ
00SS0ZZ
00SS3ZZ
00SS4ZZ
00SW0ZZ
00SW3ZZ
00SW4ZZ
00SX0ZZ
00SX3ZZ
00SX4ZZ
00SY0ZZ
00SY3ZZ
00SY4ZZ
00T70ZZ
00T73ZZ
00T74ZZ
00U107Z
00U10JZ
00U10KZ
00U137Z
00U13JZ
00U13KZ
00U147Z
00U14JZ
00U14KZ
00U207Z
00U20JZ
00U20KZ
00U237Z
00U23JZ
00U23KZ
00U247Z
00U24JZ
00U24KZ
00U607Z
00U60JZ
00U60KZ
00U637Z
00U63JZ
00U63KZ
00U647Z
00U64JZ
00U64KZ
00UF07Z
00UF0JZ
00UF0KZ
00UF37Z
00UF3JZ
00UF3KZ
00UF47Z
00UF4JZ
00UF4KZ
00UG07Z
00UG0JZ
00UG0KZ
00UG37Z
00UG3JZ
00UG3KZ
00UG47Z
00UG4JZ
00UG4KZ
00UH07Z
00UH0JZ
00UH0KZ
00UH37Z
00UH3JZ
00UH3KZ
00UH47Z
00UH4JZ
00UH4KZ
00UJ07Z
00UJ0JZ
00UJ0KZ
00UJ37Z
00UJ3JZ
00UJ3KZ
00UJ47Z
00UJ4JZ
00UJ4KZ
00UK07Z
00UK0JZ
00UK0KZ
00UK37Z
00UK3JZ
00UK3KZ
00UK47Z
00UK4JZ
00UK4KZ
00UL07Z
00UL0JZ
00UL0KZ
00UL37Z
00UL3JZ
00UL3KZ
00UL47Z
00UL4JZ
00UL4KZ
00UM07Z
00UM0JZ
00UM0KZ
00UM37Z
00UM3JZ
00UM3KZ
00UM47Z
00UM4JZ
00UM4KZ
00UN07Z
00UN0JZ
00UN0KZ
00UN37Z
00UN3JZ
00UN3KZ
00UN47Z
00UN4JZ
00UN4KZ
00UP07Z
00UP0JZ
00UP0KZ
00UP37Z
00UP3JZ
00UP3KZ
00UP47Z
00UP4JZ
00W03YZ
00W04YZ
00W0X0Z
00W0X2Z
00W0X3Z
00W0X7Z
00W0XJZ
00W0XKZ
00W0XMZ
00W63YZ
00W64YZ
00W6X0Z
00W6X2Z
00W6X3Z
00W6XJZ
00W6XMZ
00WE3YZ
00WE4YZ
00WEX0Z
00WEX2Z
00WEX3Z
00WEX7Z
00WEXMZ
00WU3YZ
00WU4YZ
00WUX0Z
00WUX2Z
00WUX3Z
00WUXJZ
00WUXMZ
00WV07Z
00WV0JZ
00WV0KZ
00WV0MZ
00WV0YZ
00WV30Z
00WV32Z
00WV33Z
00WV37Z
00WV3JZ
00WV3KZ
00WV3MZ
00WV3YZ
00WV40Z
00WV42Z
00WV43Z
00WV47Z
00WV4JZ
00WV4KZ
00WV4MZ
00WV4YZ
00WVX0Z
00WVX2Z
00WVX3Z
00WVX7Z
00WVXJZ
00WVXKZ
00WVXMZ
00XF0ZF
00XF0ZG
00XF0ZH
00XF0ZJ
00XF0ZK
00XF0ZL
00XF0ZM
00XF0ZN
00XF0ZP
00XF0ZQ
00XF0ZR
00XF0ZS
00XF4ZF
00XF4ZG
00XF4ZH
00XF4ZJ
00XF4ZK
00XF4ZL
00XF4ZM
00XF4ZN
00XF4ZP
00XF4ZQ
00XF4ZR
00XF4ZS
00XG0ZF
00XG0ZG
00XG0ZH
00XG0ZJ
00XG0ZK
00XG0ZL
00XG0ZM
00XG0ZN
00XG0ZP
00XG0ZQ
00XG0ZR
00XG0ZS
00XG4ZF
00XG4ZG
00XG4ZH
00XG4ZJ
00XG4ZK
00XG4ZL
00XG4ZM
00XG4ZN
00XG4ZP
00XG4ZQ
00XG4ZR
00XG4ZS
00XH0ZF
00XH0ZG
00XH0ZH
00XH0ZJ
00XH0ZK
00XH0ZL
00XH0ZM
00XH0ZN
00XH0ZP
00XH0ZQ
00XH0ZR
00XH0ZS
00XH4ZF
00XH4ZG
00XH4ZH
00XH4ZJ
00XH4ZK
00XH4ZL
00XH4ZM
00XH4ZN
00XH4ZP
00XH4ZQ
00XH4ZR
00XH4ZS
00XJ0ZF
00XJ0ZG
00XJ0ZH
00XJ0ZJ
00XJ0ZK
00XJ0ZL
00XJ0ZM
00XJ0ZN
00XJ0ZP
00XJ0ZQ
00XJ0ZR
00XJ0ZS
00XJ4ZF
00XJ4ZG
00XJ4ZH
00XJ4ZJ
00XJ4ZK
00XJ4ZL
00XJ4ZM
00XJ4ZN
00XJ4ZP
00XJ4ZQ
00XJ4ZR
00XJ4ZS
00XK0ZF
00XK0ZG
00XK0ZH
00XK0ZJ
00XK0ZK
00XK0ZL
00XK0ZM
00XK0ZN
00XK0ZP
00XK0ZQ
00XK0ZR
00XK0ZS
00XK4ZF
00XK4ZG
00XK4ZH
00XK4ZJ
00XK4ZK
00XK4ZL
00XK4ZM
00XK4ZN
00XK4ZP
00XK4ZQ
00XK4ZR
00XK4ZS
00XL0ZF
00XL0ZG
00XL0ZH
00XL0ZJ
00XL0ZK
00XL0ZL
00XL0ZM
00XL0ZN
00XL0ZP
00XL0ZQ
00XL0ZR
00XL0ZS
00XL4ZF
00XL4ZG
00XL4ZH
00XL4ZJ
00XL4ZK
00XL4ZL
00XL4ZM
00XL4ZN
00XL4ZP
00XL4ZQ
00XL4ZR
00XL4ZS
00XM0ZF
00XM0ZG
00XM0ZH
00XM0ZJ
00XM0ZK
00XM0ZL
00XM0ZM
00XM0ZN
00XM0ZP
00XM0ZQ
00XM0ZR
00XM0ZS
00XM4ZF
00XM4ZG
00XM4ZH
00XM4ZJ
00XM4ZK
00XM4ZL
00XM4ZM
00XM4ZN
00XM4ZP
00XM4ZQ
00XM4ZR
00XM4ZS
00XN0ZF
00XN0ZG
00XN0ZH
00XN0ZJ
00XN0ZK
00XN0ZL
00XN0ZM
00XN0ZN
00XN0ZP
00XN0ZQ
00XN0ZR
00XN0ZS
00XN4ZF
00XN4ZG
00XN4ZH
00XN4ZJ
00XN4ZK
00XN4ZL
00XN4ZM
00XN4ZN
00XN4ZP
00XN4ZQ
00XN4ZR
00XN4ZS
00XP0ZF
00XP0ZG
00XP0ZH
00XP0ZJ
00XP0ZK
00XP0ZL
00XP0ZM
00XP0ZN
00XP0ZP
00XP0ZQ
00XP0ZR
00XP0ZS
00XP4ZF
00XP4ZG
00XP4ZH
00XP4ZJ
00XP4ZK
00XP4ZL
00XP4ZM
00XP4ZN
00XP4ZP
00XP4ZQ
00XP4ZR
00XP4ZS
00XQ0ZF
00XQ0ZG
00XQ0ZH
00XQ0ZJ
00XQ0ZK
00XQ0ZL
00XQ0ZM
00XQ0ZN
00XQ0ZP
00XQ0ZQ
00XQ0ZR
00XQ0ZS
00XQ4ZF
00XQ4ZG
012YX0Z
012YXYZ
01500ZZ
01503ZZ
01504ZZ
01513ZZ
01520ZZ
01523ZZ
01524ZZ
01530ZZ
01533ZZ
01534ZZ
01540ZZ
01543ZZ
01544ZZ
01550ZZ
01553ZZ
01554ZZ
01560ZZ
01563ZZ
01564ZZ
01583ZZ
01590ZZ
01593ZZ
01594ZZ
015A0ZZ

015A3ZZ
015A4ZZ
015B3ZZ
015C0ZZ
015C3ZZ
015C4ZZ
015D0ZZ
015D3ZZ
015D4ZZ
015F0ZZ
015F3ZZ
015F4ZZ
015G0ZZ
015G3ZZ
015G4ZZ
015H0ZZ
015H3ZZ
015H4ZZ
015Q0ZZ
015Q3ZZ
015Q4ZZ
015R3ZZ
018B3ZZ
018B4ZZ
018C0ZZ
018C3ZZ
018C4ZZ
018D0ZZ
018D3ZZ
018D4ZZ
018F0ZZ
018F3ZZ
018F4ZZ
018G0ZZ
018G3ZZ
018G4ZZ
018H0ZZ
018H3ZZ
018H4ZZ
018K0ZZ
018K3ZZ
018K4ZZ
018L0ZZ
018L3ZZ
018L4ZZ
018M0ZZ
018M3ZZ
018M4ZZ
018N0ZZ
018N3ZZ
018N4ZZ
018P0ZZ
018P3ZZ
018P4ZZ
018Q0ZZ
018Q3ZZ
018Q4ZZ
018R0ZZ
018R3ZZ
018R4ZZ
019000Z
01900ZX
01900ZZ
019030Z
01903ZX
01903ZZ
019040Z
01904ZX
01904ZZ
019100Z
01910ZX
01910ZZ
019130Z
01913ZX
01913ZZ
019140Z
01914ZX
01914ZZ
019200Z
01920ZX
01920ZZ
019230Z
01923ZX
01923ZZ
019240Z
01924ZX
01924ZZ
019300Z
01930ZX
01930ZZ
019330Z
01933ZX
01933ZZ
019340Z
01934ZX
01934ZZ
019400Z
01940ZX
01940ZZ
019430Z
01943ZX
01943ZZ
019440Z
01944ZX
01944ZZ
019500Z
01950ZX
01950ZZ
019530Z
01953ZX
01953ZZ
019540Z
01954ZX
01954ZZ
019600Z
01960ZX
01960ZZ
019630Z
01963ZX
01963ZZ
019640Z
01964ZX
01964ZZ
019800Z
01980ZX
01980ZZ
019830Z
01983ZX
01983ZZ
019840Z
01984ZX
01984ZZ
019900Z
01990ZX
01990ZZ
019930Z
01993ZX
01993ZZ
019940Z
01994ZX
01994ZZ
019A00Z
019A0ZX
019A0ZZ
019A30Z
019A3ZX
019A3ZZ
019A40Z
019A4ZX
019A4ZZ
019B00Z
019B0ZX
019B0ZZ
019B30Z
019B3ZX
019B3ZZ
019B40Z
019B4ZX
019B4ZZ
019C00Z
019C0ZX
019C0ZZ
019C30Z
019C3ZX
019C3ZZ
019C40Z
019C4ZX
019C4ZZ
019D00Z
019D0ZX
019D0ZZ
019D30Z
019D3ZX
019D3ZZ
019D40Z
019D4ZX
019D4ZZ
019F00Z
019F0ZX
019F0ZZ
019F30Z
019F3ZX
019F3ZZ
019F40Z
019F4ZX
019F4ZZ
019G00Z
019G0ZX
019G0ZZ
019G30Z
019G3ZX
019G3ZZ
019G40Z
019G4ZX
019G4ZZ
019H00Z
019H0ZX
019H0ZZ
019H30Z
019H3ZX
019H3ZZ
019H40Z
019H4ZX
019H4ZZ
019K00Z
019K0ZX
019K0ZZ
019K30Z
019K3ZX
019K3ZZ
019K40Z
019K4ZX
019K4ZZ
019L00Z
019L0ZX
019L0ZZ
019L30Z
019L3ZX
019L3ZZ
019L40Z
019L4ZX
019L4ZZ
019M00Z
019M0ZX
019M0ZZ
019M30Z
019M3ZX
019M3ZZ
019M40Z
019M4ZX
019M4ZZ
019N00Z
019N0ZX
019N0ZZ
019N30Z
019N3ZX
019N3ZZ
019N40Z
019N4ZX
019N4ZZ
019P00Z
019P0ZX
019P0ZZ
019P30Z
019P3ZX
019P3ZZ
019P40Z
019P4ZX
019P4ZZ
019Q00Z
019Q0ZX
019Q0ZZ
019Q30Z
019Q3ZX
019Q3ZZ
019Q40Z
019Q4ZX
019Q4ZZ
019R00Z
019R0ZX
019R0ZZ
019R30Z
019R3ZX
019R3ZZ
019R40Z
019R4ZX
019R4ZZ
01B00ZX
01B00ZZ
01B03ZX
01B03ZZ
01B04ZX
01B04ZZ
01B10ZX
01B10ZZ
01B13ZX
01B13ZZ
01B14ZX
01B14ZZ
01B20ZX
01B20ZZ
01B23ZX
01B23ZZ
01B24ZX
01B24ZZ
01B30ZX
01B30ZZ
01B33ZX
01B33ZZ
01B34ZX
01B34ZZ
01B40ZX
01B40ZZ
01B43ZX
01B43ZZ
01B44ZX
01B44ZZ
01B50ZX
01B50ZZ
01B53ZX
01B53ZZ
01B54ZX
01B54ZZ
01B60ZX
01B60ZZ
01B63ZX
01B63ZZ
01B64ZX
01B64ZZ
01B80ZX
01B80ZZ
01B83ZX
01B83ZZ
01B84ZX
01B84ZZ
01B90ZX
01B90ZZ
01B93ZX
01B93ZZ
01B94ZX
01B94ZZ
01BA0ZX
01BA0ZZ
01BA3ZX
01BA3ZZ
01BA4ZX
01BA4ZZ
01BB0ZX
01BB0ZZ
01BB3ZX
01BB3ZZ
01BB4ZX
01BB4ZZ
01BC0ZX
01BC0ZZ
01BC3ZX
01BC3ZZ
01BC4ZX
01BC4ZZ
01BD0ZX
01BD0ZZ
01BD3ZX
01BD3ZZ
01BD4ZX
01BD4ZZ
01BF0ZX
01BF0ZZ
01BF3ZX
01BF3ZZ
01BF4ZX
01BF4ZZ
01BG0ZX
01BG0ZZ
01BG3ZX
01BG3ZZ
01BG4ZX
01BG4ZZ
01BH0ZX
01BH0ZZ
01BH3ZX
01BH3ZZ
01BH4ZX
01BH4ZZ
01BK0ZX
01BK0ZZ
01BK3ZX
01BK3ZZ
01BK4ZX
01BK4ZZ
01BL0ZX
01BL0ZZ
01BL3ZX
01BL3ZZ
01BL4ZX
01BL4ZZ
01BM0ZX
01BM0ZZ
01BM3ZX
01BM3ZZ
01BM4ZX
01BM4ZZ
01BN0ZX
01BN0ZZ
01BN3ZX
01BN3ZZ
01BN4ZX
01BN4ZZ
01BP0ZX
01BP0ZZ
01BP3ZX
01BP3ZZ
01BP4ZX
01BP4ZZ
01BQ0ZX
01BQ0ZZ
01BQ3ZX
01BQ3ZZ
01BQ4ZX
01BQ4ZZ
01BR0ZX
01BR0ZZ
01BR3ZX
01BR3ZZ
01BR4ZX
01BR4ZZ
01C00ZZ
01C03ZZ
01C04ZZ
01C10ZZ
01C13ZZ
01C14ZZ
01C20ZZ
01C23ZZ
01C24ZZ
01C30ZZ
01C33ZZ
01C34ZZ
01C40ZZ
01C43ZZ
01C44ZZ
01C50ZZ
01C53ZZ
01C54ZZ
01C60ZZ
01C63ZZ
01C64ZZ
01C80ZZ
01C83ZZ
01C84ZZ
01C90ZZ
01C93ZZ
01C94ZZ
01CA0ZZ
01CA3ZZ
01CA4ZZ
01CB0ZZ
01CB3ZZ
01CB4ZZ
01CC0ZZ
01CC3ZZ
01CC4ZZ
01CD0ZZ
01CD3ZZ
01CD4ZZ
01CF0ZZ
01CF3ZZ
01CF4ZZ
01CG0ZZ
01CG3ZZ
01CG4ZZ
01CH0ZZ
01CH3ZZ
01CH4ZZ
01CK0ZZ
01CK3ZZ
01CK4ZZ
01CL0ZZ
01CL3ZZ
01CL4ZZ
01CM0ZZ
01CM3ZZ
01CM4ZZ
01CN0ZZ
01CN3ZZ
01CN4ZZ
01CP0ZZ
01CP3ZZ
01CP4ZZ
01CQ0ZZ
01CQ3ZZ
01CQ4ZZ
01CR0ZZ
01CR3ZZ
01CR4ZZ
01D00ZZ
01D03ZZ
01D04ZZ
01D10ZZ
01D13ZZ
01D14ZZ
01D20ZZ
01D23ZZ
01D24ZZ
01D30ZZ
01D33ZZ
01D34ZZ
01D40ZZ
01D43ZZ
01D44ZZ
01D50ZZ
01D53ZZ
01D54ZZ
01D60ZZ
01D63ZZ
01D64ZZ
01D80ZZ
01D83ZZ
01D84ZZ
01D90ZZ
01D93ZZ
01D94ZZ
01DA0ZZ
01DA3ZZ
01DA4ZZ
01DB0ZZ
01DB3ZZ
01DB4ZZ
01DC0ZZ
01HY0MZ
01HY3MZ
01HY3YZ
01HY4MZ
01HY4YZ
01JY3ZZ
01PY30Z
01PY32Z
01PY3YZ
01PY4YZ
01PYX0Z
01PYX2Z
01PYXMZ
01Q10ZZ
01Q13ZZ
01Q14ZZ
01Q20ZZ
01Q23ZZ
01Q24ZZ
01Q30ZZ
01Q33ZZ
01Q34ZZ
01Q40ZZ
01Q43ZZ
01Q44ZZ
01Q50ZZ
01Q53ZZ
01Q54ZZ
01Q60ZZ
01Q63ZZ
01Q64ZZ
01Q80ZZ
01Q83ZZ
01Q84ZZ
01Q90ZZ
01Q93ZZ
01Q94ZZ
01QA0ZZ
01QA3ZZ
01QA4ZZ
01QB0ZZ
01QB3ZZ
01QB4ZZ
01QC0ZZ
01QC3ZZ
01QC4ZZ
01QD0ZZ
01QD3ZZ
01QD4ZZ
01QF0ZZ
01QF3ZZ
01QF4ZZ
01QG0ZZ
01QG3ZZ
01QG4ZZ
01QH0ZZ
01QH3ZZ
01QH4ZZ
01QK0ZZ
01QK3ZZ
01QK4ZZ
01QL0ZZ
01QL3ZZ
01QL4ZZ
01QM0ZZ
01QM3ZZ
01QM4ZZ
01QN0ZZ
01QN3ZZ
01QN4ZZ
01QP0ZZ
01QP3ZZ
01QP4ZZ
01QQ0ZZ
01QQ3ZZ
01QQ4ZZ
01QR0ZZ
01QR3ZZ
01QR4ZZ
01R107Z
01R10JZ
01R10KZ
01R147Z
01R14JZ
01R14KZ
01R207Z
01R20JZ
01R20KZ
01R247Z
01R24JZ
01R24KZ
01R407Z
01R40JZ
01R40KZ
01R447Z
01R44JZ
01R44KZ
01R507Z
01R50JZ
01R50KZ
01R547Z
01R54JZ
01R54KZ
01R607Z
01R60JZ
01R60KZ
01R647Z
01R64JZ
01R64KZ
01R807Z
01R80JZ
01R80KZ
01R847Z
01R84JZ
01R84KZ
01RB07Z
01RB0JZ
01RB0KZ
01RB47Z
01RB4JZ
01RB4KZ
01RC07Z
01RC0JZ
01RC0KZ
01RC47Z
01RC4JZ
01RC4KZ
01RD07Z
01RD0JZ
01RD0KZ
01RD47Z
01RD4JZ
01RD4KZ
01RF07Z
01RF0JZ
01RF0KZ
01RF47Z
01RF4JZ
01RF4KZ
01RG07Z
01RG0JZ
01RG0KZ
01RG47Z
01RG4JZ
01RG4KZ
01RH07Z
01RH0JZ
01RH0KZ
01RH47Z
01RH4JZ
01RH4KZ
01RR07Z
01RR0JZ
01RR0KZ
01RR47Z
01RR4JZ
01RR4KZ
01S00ZZ
01S03ZZ
01S04ZZ
01S10ZZ
01S13ZZ
01S14ZZ
01S20ZZ
01S23ZZ
01S24ZZ
01S30ZZ
01S33ZZ
01S34ZZ
01S40ZZ
01S43ZZ
01S44ZZ
01S50ZZ
01S53ZZ
01S54ZZ
01S60ZZ
01S63ZZ
01S64ZZ
01S80ZZ
01S83ZZ
01S84ZZ
01S90ZZ
01S93ZZ
01S94ZZ
01SA0ZZ
01SA3ZZ
01SA4ZZ
01SB0ZZ
01SB3ZZ
01SB4ZZ
01SC0ZZ
01SC3ZZ
01SC4ZZ
01SD0ZZ
01SD3ZZ
01SD4ZZ
01SF0ZZ
01SF3ZZ
01SF4ZZ
01SG0ZZ
01SG3ZZ
01SG4ZZ
01SH0ZZ
01SH3ZZ
01SH4ZZ
01SQ0ZZ
01SQ3ZZ
01SQ4ZZ
01SR0ZZ
01SR3ZZ
01SR4ZZ
01U107Z
01U10JZ
01U10KZ
01U137Z
01U13JZ
01U13KZ
01U147Z

01U14JZ-0270056

01U14JZ
01U14KZ
01U207Z
01U20JZ
01U20KZ
01U237Z
01U23JZ
01U23KZ
01U247Z
01U24JZ
01U24KZ
01U407Z
01U40JZ
01U40KZ
01U437Z
01U43JZ
01U43KZ
01U447Z
01U44JZ
01U44KZ
01U507Z
01U50JZ
01U50KZ
01U537Z
01U53JZ
01U53KZ
01U547Z
01U54JZ
01U54KZ
01U607Z
01U60JZ
01U60KZ
01U637Z
01U63JZ
01U63KZ
01U647Z
01U64JZ
01U64KZ
01U807Z
01U80JZ
01U80KZ
01WY3YZ
01WY4YZ
01WYX0Z
01WYX2Z
01WYX7Z
01WYXMZ
02104ZF
0211083
0211088
0211089
021108C
021108F
021108W
0211093
0211098
0211099
021109C
021109F
021109W
02110A3
02110A8
02110A9
02110AC
02110AF
02110AW
02110J3
02110J8
02110J9
02110JC
02110JF
02110JW
02110K3
02110K8
02110K9
02110KC
02110KF
02110KW
02110Z3
02110Z8
02110Z9
02110ZC
02110ZF
0211344
02113D4
0211444
0211483
0211488
0211489
021148C
021148F
021148W
0211493
0211498
0211499
021149C
021149F
021149W
02114A3
02114A8
02114A9
02114AC
02114AF
02114AW
02114D4
02114J3
02114J8
02114J9
02114JC
02114JF
02114JW
02114K3
02114K8
02114K9
02114KC
02114KF
02114KW
02114Z3
02114Z8
02114Z9
02114ZC
02114ZF
0212083
0212088
0212089
021208C
021208F
021208W
0212093
0212098
0212099
021209C
021209F
021209W
02120A3
02120A8
02120A9
02120AC
02120AF
02120AW
02120J3
02120J8
02120J9
02120JC
02120JF
02120JW
02120K3
02120K8
02120K9
02120KC
02120KF
02120KW
02120Z3
02120Z8
02120Z9
02120ZC
02120ZF
0212344
02123D4
0212444
0212483
0212488
0212489
021248C
021248F
021248W
0212493
0212498
0212499
021249C
021249F
021249W
02124A3
02124A8
02124A9
02124AC
02124AF
02124AW
02124D4
02124J3
02124J8
02124J9
02124JC
02124JF
02124JW
02124K3
02124K8
02124K9
02124KC
02124KF
02124KW
02124Z3
02124Z8
02124Z9
02124ZC
02124ZF
0213083
0213088
0213089
021308C
021308F
021308W
0213093
0213098
0213099
021309C
021309F
021309W
02130A3
02130A8
02130A9
02130AC
02130AF
02130AW
02130J3
02130J8
02130J9
02130JC
02130JF
02130JW
02130K3
02130K8
02130K9
02130KC
02130KF
02130KW
02130Z3
02130Z8
02130Z9
02130ZC
02130ZF
0213344
02133D4
0213444
0213483
0213488
0213489
021348C
021348F
021348W
0213493
0213498
0213499
021349C
021349F
021349W
02134A3
02134A8
02134A9
02134AC
02134AF
02134AW
02134D4
02134J3
02134J8
02134J9
02134JC
02134JF
02134JW
02134K3
02134K8
02134K9
02134KC
02134KF
02134KW
02134Z3
02134Z8
02134Z9
02134ZC
02134ZF
021608P
021608Q
021608R
021609P
021609Q
021609R
02160AP
02160AQ
02160AR
02160JP
02160JQ
02160JR
02160KP
02160KQ
02160KR
02160Z7
02160ZP
02160ZQ
02160ZR
02163Z7
021648P
021648Q
021648R
021649P
021649Q
021649R
02164AP
02164AQ
02164AR
02164JP
02164JQ
02164JR
02164KP
02164KQ
02164KR
02164Z7
02164ZP
02164ZQ
02164ZR
021708P
021708Q
021708R
021708S
021708T
021708U
021709P
021709Q
021709R
021709S
021709T
021709U
02170AP
02170AQ
02170AR
02170AS
02170AT
02170AU
02170JP
02170JQ
02170JR
02170JS
02170JT
02170JU
02170KP
02170KQ
02170KR
02170KS
02170KT
02170KU
02170ZP
02170ZQ
02170ZR
02170ZS
02170ZT
02170ZU
021748P
021748Q
021748R
021748S
021748T
021748U
021749P
021749Q
021749R
021749S
021749T
021749U
02174AP
02174AQ
02174AR
02174AS
02174AT
02174AU
02174JP
02174JQ
02174JR
02174JS
02174JT
02174JU
02174KP
02174KQ
02174KR
02174KS
02174KT
02174KU
02174ZP
02174ZQ
02174ZR
02174ZS
02174ZT
02174ZU
021K08P
021K08Q
021K08R
021K09P
021K09Q
021K09R
021K0AP
021K0AQ
021K0AR
021K0JP
021K0JQ
021K0JR
021K0KP
021K0KQ
021K0KR
021K0Z5
021K0Z8
021K0Z9
021K0ZC
021K0ZF
021K0ZP
021K0ZQ
021K0ZR
021K0ZW
021K48P
021K48Q
021K48R
021K49P
021K49Q
021K49R
021K4AP
021K4AQ
021K4AR
021K4JP
021K4JQ
021K4JR
021K4KP
021K4KQ
021K4KR
021K4Z5
021K4Z8
021K4Z9
021K4ZC
021K4ZF
021K4ZP
021K4ZQ
021K4ZR
021K4ZW
021L08P
021L08Q
021L08R
021L09P
021L09Q
021L09R
021L0AP
021L0AQ
021L0AR
021L0JP
021L0JQ
021L0JR
021L0KP
021L0KQ
021L0KR
021L0Z5
021L0Z8
021L0Z9
021L0ZC
021L0ZF
021L0ZP
021L0ZQ
021L0ZR
021L0ZW
021L48P
021L48Q
021L48R
021L49P
021L49Q
021L49R
021L4AP
021L4AQ
021L4AR
021L4JP
021L4JQ
021L4JR
021L4KP
021L4KQ
021L4KR
021L4Z5
021L4Z8
021L4Z9
021L4ZC
021L4ZF
021L4ZP
021L4ZQ
021L4ZR
021L4ZW
021P08A
021P08B
021P08D
021P09A
021P09B
021P09D
021P0AA
021P0AB
021P0AD
021P0JA
021P0JB
021P0JD
021P0KA
021P0KB
021P0KD
021P0ZA
021P0ZB
021P0ZD
021P48A
021P48B
021P48D
021P49A
021P49B
021P49D
021P4AA
021P4AB
021P4AD
021P4JA
021P4JB
021P4JD
021P4KA
021P4KB
021P4KD
021P4ZA
021P4ZB
021P4ZD
021Q08A
021Q08B
021Q08D
021Q09A
021Q09B
021Q09D
021Q0AA
021Q0AB
021Q0AD
021Q0JA
021Q0JB
021Q0JD
021Q0KA
021Q0KB
021Q0KD
021Q0ZA
021Q0ZB
021Q0ZD
021Q48A
021Q48B
021Q48D
021Q49A
021Q49B
021Q49D
021Q4AA
021Q4AB
021Q4AD
021Q4JA
021Q4JB
021Q4JD
021Q4KA
021Q4KB
021Q4KD
021Q4ZA
021Q4ZB
021Q4ZD
021R08A
021R08B
021R08D
021W08F
021W08G
021W08H
021W08V
021W09F
021W09G
021W09H
021W09V
021W0AF
021W0AG
021W0AH
021W0AV
021W0JF
021W0JV
021W0KF
021W0KV
021W4JR
021W4KB
021W4KD
021W4KP
021W4KQ
021W4KR
021W4ZB
021W4ZD
021W4ZP
021W4ZQ
021W4ZR
021X08B
021X08D
021X08P
021X08Q
021X08R
021X09B
021X09D
021X09P
021X09Q
021X09R
021X0AB
021X0AD
021X0AP
021X0AQ
021X0AR
021X0JB
021X0JD
021X0JP
021X0JQ
021X0JR
021X0KB
021X0KD
021X0KP
021X0KQ
021X0KR
021X0ZB
021X0ZD
021X0ZP
021X0ZQ
021X0ZR
021X48B
021X48D
021X48P
021X48Q
021X48R
021X49B
021X49D
021X49P
021X49Q
021X49R
021X4AB
021X4AD
021X4AP
021X4AQ
021X4AR
021X4JB
021X4JD
021X4JP
021X4JQ
021X4JR
021X4KB
021X4KD
021X4KP
021X4KQ
021X4KR
021X4ZB
021X4ZD
021X4ZP
021X4ZQ
021X4ZR
024F07J
024F08J
024F0JJ
024F0KJ
024G072
024G082
024G0J2
024G0K2
024J072
024J082
024J0J2
024J0K2
02540ZZ
02543ZZ
02544ZZ
02550ZZ
02553ZZ
02554ZZ
02560ZZ
02563ZZ
02564ZZ
02570ZK
02570ZZ
02573ZK
02573ZZ
02574ZK
02574ZZ
02580ZZ
02583ZZ
02584ZZ
02590ZZ
02593ZZ
02594ZZ
025D0ZZ
025D3ZZ
025D4ZZ
025F0ZZ
025F3ZZ
025F4ZZ
025G0ZZ
025G3ZZ
025G4ZZ
025H0ZZ
025H3ZZ
025H4ZZ
025J0ZZ
025J3ZZ
025J4ZZ
025K0ZZ
025K3ZZ
025K4ZZ
025L0ZZ
025L3ZZ
025L4ZZ
025M0ZZ
025M3ZZ
025M4ZZ
025N0ZZ
025N3ZZ
025N4ZZ
025P0ZZ
025P3ZZ
025P4ZZ
025Q0ZZ
025Q3ZZ
025Q4ZZ
025R0ZZ
025R3ZZ
025R4ZZ
025S0ZZ
025S3ZZ
025S4ZZ
025T0ZZ
025T3ZZ
025T4ZZ
025V0ZZ
025V3ZZ
025V4ZZ
025W0ZZ
025W3ZZ
025W4ZZ
025X0ZZ
025X3ZZ
025X4ZZ
0270046
027004Z
0270056

APPENDIX H: NON-OR NOT AFFECTING MS-DRG ASSIGNMENT

027005Z
0270066
027006Z
0270076
027007Z
02700D6
02700DZ
02700E6
02700EZ
02700F6
02700FZ
02700G6
02700GZ
02700T6
02700TZ
02700Z6
02700ZZ
0270346
027034Z
0270356
027035Z
0270366
027036Z
0270376
027037Z
02703D6
02703DZ
02703E6
02703EZ
02703F6
02703FZ
02703G6
02703GZ
02703T6
02703TZ
02703Z6
02703ZZ
0270446
027044Z
0270456
027045Z
0270466
027046Z
0270476
027047Z
02704D6
02704DZ
02704E6
02704EZ
02704F6
02704FZ
02704G6
02704GZ
02704T6
02704TZ
02704Z6
02704ZZ
0271046
027104Z
0271056
027105Z
0271066
027106Z
0271076
027107Z
02710D6
02710DZ
02710E6
02710EZ
02710F6
02710FZ
02710G6
02710GZ
02710T6
02710TZ
02710Z6
02710ZZ
0271346
027134Z
0271356
027135Z
0271366
027136Z
0271376
027137Z
02713D6
02713DZ
02713E6
02713EZ
02713F6
02713FZ
02713G6
02713GZ
02713T6
02713TZ
02713Z6
02713ZZ
0271446
027144Z
0271456
027145Z
0271466
027146Z
0271476
027147Z
02714D6
02714DZ
02714E6
02714EZ
02714F6
02714FZ
02714G6
02714GZ
02714T6
02714TZ
02714Z6
02714ZZ
0272046
027204Z
0272056
027205Z
0272066
027206Z
0272076
027207Z
02720D6
02720DZ
02720E6
02720EZ
02720F6
02720FZ
02720G6
02720GZ
02720T6
02720TZ
02720Z6
02720ZZ
0272346
027234Z
0272356
027235Z
0272366
027236Z
0272376
027237Z
02723D6
02723DZ
02723E6
02723EZ
02723F6
02723FZ
02723G6
02723GZ
02723T6
02723TZ
02723Z6
02723ZZ
0272446
027244Z
0272456
027245Z
0272466
027246Z
0272476
027247Z
02724D6
02724DZ
02724E6
02724EZ
02724F6
02724FZ
02724G6
02724GZ
02724T6
02724TZ
02724Z6
02724ZZ
0273046
027304Z
0273056
027305Z
0273066
027306Z
0273076
027307Z
02730D6
02730DZ
02730E6
02730EZ
02730F6
02730FZ
02730G6
02730GZ
02730T6
02730TZ
02730Z6
02730ZZ
0273346
027334Z
0273356
027335Z
0273366
027336Z
0273376
027337Z
02733D6
02733DZ
02733E6
02733EZ
02733F6
02733FZ
02733G6
02733GZ
02733T6
02733TZ
02733Z6
02733ZZ
0273446
027344Z
0273456
027345Z
0273466
027346Z
0273476
027347Z
02734D6
02734DZ
02734E6
02734EZ
02734F6
02734FZ
02734G6
02734GZ
02734T6
02734TZ
02734Z6
02734ZZ
027F04Z
027F0DZ
027F0ZZ
027F34Z
027F3DZ
027F3ZZ
027F44Z
027F4DZ
027F4ZZ
027G04Z
027G0DZ
027G0ZZ
027G34Z
027G3DZ
027G3ZZ
027G44Z
027G4DZ
027G4ZZ
027H04Z
027H0DZ
027H0ZZ
027H34Z
027H3DZ
027H3ZZ
027H44Z
027H4DZ
027H4ZZ
027J04Z
027J0DZ
027J0ZZ
027J34Z
027J3DZ
027J3ZZ
027J44Z
027J4DZ
027J4ZZ
027K04Z
027K0DZ
027K0ZZ
027K34Z
027K3DZ
027K3ZZ
027K44Z
027K4DZ
027K4ZZ
027L04Z
027L0DZ
027L0ZZ
027L34Z
027L3DZ
027L3ZZ
027L44Z
027L4DZ
027L4ZZ
027P04Z
027P0DZ
027P0ZZ
027P34Z
027P3DZ
027P3ZZ
027P44Z
027P4DZ
027P4ZZ
027Q04Z
027Q0DZ
027Q0ZZ
027Q34Z
027Q3DZ
027Q3ZZ
027Q44Z
027Q4DZ
027Q4ZZ
027R04T
027R04Z
027R0DT
027R0DZ
027R0ZT
027R0ZZ
027R34T
02B40ZX
02B43ZX
02B44ZX
02B50ZX
02B53ZX
02B54ZX
02B60ZX
02B63ZX
02B64ZX
02B70ZX
02B73ZX
02B74ZX
02B80ZX
02B83ZX
02B84ZX
02B90ZX
02B93ZX
02B94ZX
02BD0ZX
02BD3ZX
02BD4ZX
02BF0ZX
02BF3ZX
02BF4ZX
02BG0ZX
02BG3ZX
02BG4ZX
02BH0ZX
02BH3ZX
02BH4ZX
02BJ0ZX
02BJ3ZX
02BJ4ZX
02BK0ZX
02BK3ZX
02BK4ZX
02BL0ZX
02BL3ZX
02BL4ZX
02BM0ZX
02BM3ZX
02BM4ZX
02CS4ZZ
02CT0ZZ
02CT3ZZ
02CT4ZZ
02CV0ZZ
02CV3ZZ
02CV4ZZ
02CW0ZZ
02CW3ZZ
02CW4ZZ
02CX0ZZ
02CX3ZZ
02CX4ZZ
02FN0ZZ
02FN3ZZ
02FN4ZZ
02FNXZZ
02H400Z
02H402Z
02H403Z
02H40DZ
02H40JZ
02H40KZ
02H40MZ
02H40NZ
02H40YZ
02H430Z
02H432Z
02H433Z
02H43DZ
02H43JZ
02H43KZ
02H43MZ
02H43NZ
02H43YZ
02H440Z
02H442Z
02H443Z
02H44DZ
02H44JZ
02H44KZ
02H44MZ
02H44NZ
02H44YZ
02H600Z
02H602Z
02H603Z
02H60DZ
02H60JZ
02H60KZ
02H60MZ
02H60NZ
02H60YZ
02H630Z
02H632Z
02H633Z
02H63DZ
02H63JZ
02H63KZ
02H63MZ
02H63NZ
02H63YZ
02H640Z
02H642Z
02H643Z
02H64DZ
02H64JZ
02H64KZ
02H64MZ
02H64NZ
02H64YZ
02H700Z
02H702Z
02H703Z
02H70DZ
02H70JZ
02H70KZ
02H70MZ
02H70NZ
02H70YZ
02H730Z
02H732Z
02H733Z
02H73DZ
02H73JZ
02H73KZ
02H73MZ
02H73NZ
02H73YZ
02H740Z
02H742Z
02H743Z
02H74DZ
02H74JZ
02H74KZ
02H74MZ
02H74NZ
02H74YZ
02HA0QZ
02HA0RJ
02HA0RS
02HA0RZ
02HA0YZ
02HA3QZ
02HA3RJ
02HA3RS
02HA3RZ
02HA3YZ
02HA4QZ
02HA4RJ
02HA4RS
02HA4RZ
02HA4YZ
02HK00Z
02HK02Z
02HK03Z
02HK0DZ
02HK0JZ
02HK0KZ
02HK0MZ
02HK0NZ
02HK0YZ
02HK30Z
02HK32Z
02HK33Z
02HK3DZ
02HK3JZ
02HK3KZ
02HK3MZ
02HK3NZ
02HK3YZ
02HK40Z
02HK42Z
02HK43Z
02HK4DZ
02HK4JZ
02HK4KZ
02HK4MZ
02HK4NZ
02HK4YZ
02HL00Z
02HL02Z
02HL03Z
02HL0DZ
02HL0JZ
02HL0KZ
02HL0MZ
02HL0NZ
02HL0YZ
02HL30Z
02HL32Z
02HL33Z
02HL3DZ
02HL3JZ
02HL3KZ
02HL3MZ
02HL3NZ
02HL3YZ
02HL40Z
02HL42Z
02HL43Z
02HL4DZ
02HL4JZ
02HL4KZ
02HL4MZ
02HL4NZ
02HL4YZ
02HN00Z
02HN02Z
02HN0JZ
02HN0KZ
02HN0MZ
02HN0YZ
02HN30Z
02HN32Z
02HN3JZ
02HN3KZ
02HN3MZ
02HN3YZ
02HN40Z
02HN42Z
02HN4JZ
02HN4KZ
02HN4MZ
02HN4YZ
02HP00Z
02HP02Z
02HP03Z
02HP0DZ
02HP0YZ
02HP30Z
02HP32Z
02HP33Z
02HP3DZ
02HP3YZ
02HP40Z
02HP42Z
02HP43Z
02HP4DZ
02HP4YZ
02HQ00Z
02HQ02Z
02HQ03Z
02HQ0DZ
02HQ0YZ
02HQ30Z
02HQ32Z
02HQ33Z
02HQ3DZ
02HQ3YZ
02HQ40Z
02HQ42Z
02HQ43Z
02HQ4DZ
02HQ4YZ
02HR00Z
02HR02Z
02HR03Z
02HR0DZ
02HR0YZ
02HR30Z
02HR32Z
02HR33Z
02HR3DZ
02HR3YZ
02HR40Z
02HR42Z
02HR43Z
02HR4DZ
02HR4YZ
02HS00Z
02HS02Z
02HS03Z
02HS0DZ
02HS0YZ
02HS30Z
02HS32Z
02HS33Z
02HS3DZ
02HS3YZ
02HS40Z
02HS42Z
02HS43Z
02HS4DZ
02HS4YZ
02HT00Z
02HT02Z
02HT03Z
02HT0DZ
02HT0YZ
02HT30Z
02HT32Z
02HT33Z
02HT3DZ
02HT3YZ
02HT40Z
02HT42Z
02HT43Z
02HT4DZ
02HT4YZ
02HV00Z
02HV02Z
02HV03Z
02HV0DZ
02HV0YZ
02HV30Z
02HV32Z
02HV33Z
02HV3DZ
02HV3YZ
02HV40Z
02HV42Z
02HV43Z
02HV4DZ
02HV4YZ
02HW00Z
02HW02Z
02HW03Z
02HW0DZ
02HW0YZ
02HW30Z
02HW32Z
02HW33Z
02HW3DZ
02HW3YZ
02HW40Z
02HW42Z
02HW43Z
02HW4DZ
02HW4YZ
02HX00Z
02HX02Z
02HX03Z
02HX0DZ
02HX30Z
02HX32Z
02HX33Z
02HX3DZ
02HX40Z
02HX42Z
02HX43Z
02HX4DZ
02JA0ZZ
02JA3ZZ
02JA4ZZ
02JY0ZZ
02JY3ZZ
02JY4ZZ
02K80ZZ
02K83ZZ
02K84ZZ
02L70CK
02L70DK
02L70ZK
02L73CK
02L73DK
02L73ZK
02L74CK
02L74DK
02L74ZK
02LH0CZ
02LH0DZ
02LH0ZZ
02LH3CZ
02LH3DZ
02LH3ZZ
02LH4CZ
02LH4DZ
02LH4ZZ
02LP0CZ
02LP0DZ
02LP0ZZ
02LP3CZ
02LP3DZ
02LP3ZZ
02LP4CZ
02LP4DZ
02LP4ZZ
02LQ0CZ
02LQ0DZ
02LQ0ZZ
02LQ3CZ
02LQ3DZ
02LQ3ZZ
02LQ4CZ
02LQ4DZ
02LQ4ZZ
02LR0CT
02LR0CZ
02LR0DT
02LR0DZ
02LR0ZT
02LR0ZZ
02LR3CT
02LR3CZ
02LR3DT
02LR3DZ
02LR3ZT
02LR3ZZ
02LR4CT
02LR4CZ
02LR4DT
02LR4DZ
02LR4ZT
02LR4ZZ
02LS0CZ
02LS0DZ
02LS0ZZ

02LS3CZ
02LS3DZ
02LS3ZZ
02LS4CZ
02LS4DZ
02LS4ZZ
02LT0CZ
02LT0DZ
02LT0ZZ
02LT3CZ
02LT3DZ
02LT3ZZ
02LT4CZ
02LT4DZ
02LT4ZZ
02LV0CZ
02LV0DZ
02LV0ZZ
02LV3CZ
02LV3DZ
02LV3ZZ
02LV4CZ
02LV4DZ
02LV4ZZ
02PA0RZ
02PA32Z
02PA33Z
02PA3DZ
02PA3RZ
02PA3YZ
02PA4RZ
02PA4YZ
02PAX2Z
02PAX3Z
02PAXDZ
02PAXMZ
02PY32Z
02PY33Z
02PY3DZ
02PY3YZ
02PY4YZ
02PYX2Z
02PYX3Z
02PYXDZ
02R748Z
02R74JZ
02R74KZ
02R907Z
02R908Z
02R90JZ
02R90KZ
02R947Z
02R948Z
02R94JZ
02R94KZ
02RD07Z
02RD08Z
02RD0JZ
02RD0KZ
02RD47Z
02RD48Z
02RD4JZ
02RD4KZ
02RF07Z
02RF08Z
02RF0JZ
02RF0KZ
02RF37H
02RF37Z
02RF38H
02RF38Z
02RF3JH
02RF3JZ
02RF3KH
02RF3KZ
02RF47Z
02RF48Z
02RF4JZ
02RF4KZ
02RG07Z
02RG08Z
02RG0JZ
02RG0KZ
02RG37H
02RG37Z
02RG38H
02RG38Z
02RG3JH
02RG3JZ
02RG3KH
02RG3KZ
02RG47Z
02RG48Z
02RG4JZ
02RG4KZ
02RH07Z
02RH08Z
02RH0JZ
02RH0KZ
02RH37H
02RH37Z
02RH38H
02RH38Z
02RH3JH
02RH3JZ
02RH3KH
02RH3KZ
02RH47Z
02RH48Z
02RH4JZ
02RH4KZ
02RJ07Z
02RJ08Z
02RJ0JZ
02RJ0KZ
02RJ37H
02RJ37Z
02RJ38H
02RJ38Z
02RJ3JH
02RJ3JZ
02RJ3KH
02RJ3KZ
02RJ47Z
02RJ48Z
02RJ4JZ
02RJ4KZ
02RK07Z
02RK08Z
02RK0JZ
02RK0KZ
02RK47Z
02RK48Z
02RK4JZ
02RK4KZ
02RL07Z
02RL08Z
02RL0JZ
02RL0KZ
02RL47Z
02RL48Z
02RL4JZ
02RL4KZ
02RM07Z
02RM08Z
02RM0JZ
02RM0KZ
02RM47Z
02RM48Z
02RM4JZ
02RM4KZ
02RN07Z
02RN08Z
02RN0JZ
02RN0KZ
02RN47Z
02RN48Z
02RN4JZ
02RN4KZ
02RP07Z
02RP08Z
02RP0JZ
02RP0KZ
02RP47Z
02RP48Z
02RP4JZ
02RP4KZ
02RQ07Z
02RQ08Z
02RQ0JZ
02RQ0KZ
02RQ47Z
02RQ48Z
02RQ4JZ
02RQ4KZ
02RR07Z
02RR08Z
02RR0JZ
02RR0KZ
02RR47Z
02RR48Z
02RR4JZ
02RR4KZ
02RS07Z
02RS08Z
02RS0JZ
02RS0KZ
02RS47Z
02RS48Z
02RS4JZ
02RS4KZ
02RT07Z
02RT08Z
02RT0JZ
02RT0KZ
02RT47Z
02RT48Z
02RT4JZ
02RT4KZ
02RV07Z
02RV08Z
02RV0JZ
02RV0KZ
02RV47Z
02RV48Z
02RV4JZ
02RV4KZ
02RW07Z
02RW08Z
02RW0JZ
02RW0KZ
02RW47Z
02RW48Z
02RW4JZ
02RW4KZ
02RX07Z
02RX08Z
02RX0JZ
02RX0KZ
02RX47Z
02RX48Z
02RX4JZ
02RX4KZ
02S00ZZ
02S10ZZ
02SP0ZZ
02SQ0ZZ
02SR0ZZ
02SS0ZZ
02ST0ZZ
02SV0ZZ
02SW0ZZ
02SX0ZZ
02T50ZZ
02T53ZZ
02T54ZZ
02T80ZZ
02T83ZZ
02T84ZZ
02T90ZZ
02T93ZZ
02T94ZZ
02TD0ZZ
02TD3ZZ
02TD4ZZ
02TH0ZZ
02TH3ZZ
02TH4ZZ
02TM0ZZ
02TM3ZZ
02TM4ZZ
02TN0ZZ
02TN3ZZ
02TN4ZZ
02U507Z
02U508Z
02U50JZ
02U50KZ
02U537Z
02U538Z
02U53JZ
02U53KZ
02U547Z
02U548Z
02U54JZ
02U54KZ
02U607Z
02U608Z
02U60JZ
02U60KZ
02U637Z
02U638Z
02U63JZ
02U63KZ
02U647Z
02U648Z
02U64JZ
02U64KZ
02U707Z
02U708Z
02U70JZ
02U70KZ
02U737Z
02U738Z
02U73JZ
02U73KZ
02U747Z
02U748Z
02U74JZ
02U74KZ
02U907Z
02U908Z
02U90JZ
02U90KZ
02U937Z
02U938Z
02U93JZ
02U93KZ
02U947Z
02U948Z
02U94JZ
02U94KZ
02UA07Z
02UA08Z
02UA0JZ
02UA0KZ
02UA37Z
02UA38Z
02UA3JZ
02UA3KZ
02UA47Z
02UA48Z
02UA4JZ
02UA4KZ
02UD07Z
02UD08Z
02UD0JZ
02UD0KZ
02UD37Z
02UD38Z
02UD3JZ
02UD3KZ
02UD47Z
02UD48Z
02UD4JZ
02UD4KZ
02UF07J
02UF07Z
02UF08J
02UF08Z
02UF0JJ
02UF0JZ
02UF0KJ
02UF0KZ
02UF37J
02UF37Z
02UF38J
02UF38Z
02UF3JJ
02UF3JZ
02UF3KJ
02UF3KZ
02UF47J
02UF47Z
02UF48J
02UF48Z
02UF4JJ
02UF4JZ
02UF4KJ
02UF4KZ
02UG07E
02UG07Z
02UG08E
02UG08Z
02UG0JE
02UG0JZ
02UG0KE
02UG0KZ
02UG37E
02UG37Z
02UG38E
02UG38Z
02UG3JE
02UG3JZ
02UG3KE
02UG3KZ
02UG47E
02UG47Z
02UG48E
02UG48Z
02UG4JE
02UG4JZ
02UG4KE
02UG4KZ
02UH07Z
02UH08Z
02UH0JZ
02UH0KZ
02UH37Z
02UH38Z
02UH3JZ
02UH3KZ
02UH47Z
02UH48Z
02UH4JZ
02UH4KZ
02UJ07G
02UJ07Z
02UJ08G
02UJ08Z
02UJ0JG
02UJ0JZ
02UJ0KG
02UJ0KZ
02UJ37G
02UJ37Z
02UJ38G
02UJ38Z
02UJ3JG
02UJ3JZ
02UJ3KG
02UJ3KZ
02UJ47G
02UJ47Z
02UJ48G
02UJ48Z
02UJ4JG
02UJ4JZ
02UJ4KG
02UJ4KZ
02UK07Z
02UK08Z
02UK0JZ
02UK0KZ
02UK37Z
02UK38Z
02UK3JZ
02UK3KZ
02UK47Z
02UK48Z
02UK4JZ
02UK4KZ
02UL07Z
02UL08Z
02UL0JZ
02UL0KZ
02UL37Z
02UL38Z
02UL3JZ
02UL3KZ
02UL47Z
02UL48Z
02UL4JZ
02UL4KZ
02UM07Z
02UM08Z
02UM0JZ
02UM0KZ
02UM37Z
02UM38Z
02UM3JZ
02UM3KZ
02UM47Z
02UM48Z
02UM4JZ
02UM4KZ
02UN07Z
02UN08Z
02UN0JZ
02UN0KZ
02UN37Z
02UN38Z
02UN3JZ
02UN3KZ
02UN47Z
02UN48Z
02UN4JZ
02UN4KZ
02UP07Z
02UP08Z
02UP0JZ
02UP0KZ
02UP37Z
02UP38Z
02UP3JZ
02UP3KZ
02UP47Z
02UP48Z
02UP4JZ
02UP4KZ
02UQ07Z
02UQ08Z
02UQ0JZ
02UQ0KZ
02UQ37Z
02UQ38Z
02UQ3JZ
02UQ3KZ
02UQ47Z
02UQ48Z
02UQ4JZ
02UQ4KZ
02UR07Z
02UR08Z
02UR0JZ
02UR0KZ
02UR37Z
02UR38Z
02UR3JZ
02UR3KZ
02UR47Z
02VW0CZ
02VW0DZ
02VW0EZ
02VW0FZ
02VW0ZZ
02VW3CZ
02VW3DZ
02VW3EZ
02VW3FZ
02VW3ZZ
02VW4CZ
02VW4DZ
02VW4EZ
02VW4FZ
02VW4ZZ
02VX0CZ
02VX0DZ
02VX0EZ
02VX0FZ
02VX0ZZ
02VX3CZ
02VX3DZ
02VX3EZ
02VX3FZ
02VX3ZZ
02VX4CZ
02VX4DZ
02VX4EZ
02VX4FZ
02VX4ZZ
02W50JZ
02W54JZ
02WA02Z
02WA03Z
02WA07Z
02WA08Z
02WA0CZ
02WA0DZ
02WA0JZ
02WA0KZ
02WA0MZ
02WA0NZ
02WA0QZ
02WA0RS
02WA0RZ
02WA0YZ
02WA32Z
02WA33Z
02WA37Z
02WA38Z
02WA3CZ
02WA3DZ
02WA3JZ
02WA3KZ
02WA3MZ
02WA3NZ
02WA3QZ
02WA3RS
02WA3RZ
02WA3YZ
02WA42Z
02WA43Z
02WA47Z
02WA48Z
02WA4CZ
02WA4DZ
02WA4JZ
02WA4KZ
02WA4MZ
02WA4NZ
02WA4QZ
02WA4RS
02WA4RZ
02WA4YZ
02WAX2Z
02WAX3Z
02WAX7Z
02WAX8Z
02WAXCZ
02WAXDZ
02WAXJZ
02WAXKZ
02WAXMZ
02WAXNZ
02WAXQZ
02WAXRS
02WAXRZ
02WF07Z
02WF08Z
02WF0JZ
02WF0KZ
02WF37Z
02WF38Z
02WF3JZ
02WF3KZ
02WF47Z
02WF48Z
02WF4JZ
02WF4KZ
02WG07Z
02WG08Z
02WG0JZ
02WG0KZ
02WG37Z
02WG38Z
02WG3JZ
02WG3KZ
02WG47Z
02WG48Z
02WG4JZ
02WG4KZ
02WH07Z
02WH08Z
02WH0JZ
02WH0KZ
02WH37Z
02WH38Z
02WH3JZ
02WH3KZ
02WH47Z
02WH48Z
02WH4JZ
02WH4KZ
02WJ07Z
02WJ08Z
02WJ0JZ
02WJ0KZ
02WJ37Z
02WJ38Z
02WJ3JZ
02WJ3KZ
02WJ47Z
02WJ48Z
02WJ4JZ
02WJ4KZ
02WM0JZ
02WM4JZ
02WY02Z
02WY03Z
02WY07Z
02WY08Z
02WY0CZ
02WY0DZ
02WY0JZ
02WY0KZ
02WY0YZ
02WY32Z
02WY33Z
02WY37Z
02WY38Z
02WY3CZ
02WY3DZ
02WY3JZ
02WY3KZ
02WY3YZ
02WY42Z
02WY43Z
02WY47Z
02WY48Z
02WY4CZ
02WY4DZ
02WY4JZ
02WY4KZ
02WY4YZ
02WYX2Z
02WYX3Z
02WYX7Z
02WYX8Z
02WYXCZ
02WYXDZ
02WYXJZ
02WYXKZ
02YA0Z0
02YA0Z1
02YA0Z2
0312090
0312091
0312092
0312093
0312094
0312095
0312096
0312097
0312098
0312099
031209B
031209C
031209D
031209F
031209J
031209K
03120A0
03120A1
03120A2
03120A3
03120A4
03120A5
03120A6
03120A7
03120A8
03120A9
03120AB
03120AC
03120AD
03120AF
03120AJ
03120AK
03120J0
03120J1
03120J2
03120J3
03120J4
03120J5
03120J6
03120J7
03120J8
03120J9
03120JB
03120JC
03120JD
03120JF
03120JJ
03120JK
03120K0
03120K1
03120K2
03120K3
03120K4
03120K5
03120K6
03120K7
03120K8
03120K9
03120KB
03120KC

03120KD-03724Z1
APPENDIX H: NON-OR NOT AFFECTING MS-DRG ASSIGNMENT

03120KD
03120KF
03120KJ
03120KK
03120Z0
03120Z1
03120Z2
03120Z3
03120Z4
03120Z5
03120Z6
03120Z7
03120Z8
03120Z9
03120ZB
03120ZC
03120ZD
03120ZF
03120ZJ
03120ZK
0313090
0313091
0313092
0313093
0313094
0313095
0313096
0313097
0313098
0313099
031309B
031309C
031309D
031309F
031309J
031309K
031309M
031309N
03130A0
03130A1
03130A2
03130A3
03130A4
03130A5
03130A6
03130A7
03130A8
03130A9
03130AB
03130AC
03130AD
03130AF
03130AJ
03130AK
03130AM
03130AN
03130J0
03130J1
03130J2
03130J3
03130J4
03130J5
03130J6
03130J7
03130J8
03130J9
03130JB
03130JC
03130JD
03130JF
03130JJ
03130JK
03130JM
03130JN
03130K0
03130K1
03130K2
03130K3
03130K4
03130K5
03130K6
03130K7
03130K8
03130K9
03130KB
03130KC
03130KD
03130KF
03130KJ
03130KK
03130KM
03130KN
03130Z0
03130Z1
03130Z2
03130Z3
03130Z4
03130Z5
03130Z6
03130Z7
03130Z8
03130Z9
03130ZB
03130ZC
03130ZD
03130ZF
03130ZJ
03130ZK
03130ZM
03130ZN
0314090
0314091
0314092
0314093
0314094
0314095
0314096
0314097
0314098
0314099
031409B
031409C
031409D
031409F
031409J
031409K
031409M
031409N
03140A0
03140A1
03140A2
03140A3
03140A4
03140A5
03140A6
03140A7
03140A8
03140A9
03140AB
03140AC
03140AD
03140AF
03140AJ
03140AK
03140AM
03140AN
03140J0
03140J1
03140J2
03140J3
03140J4
03140J5
03140J6
03140J7
03140J8
03140J9
03140JB
03140JC
03140JD
03140JF
03140JJ
03140JK
03140JM
03140JN
03140K0
03140K1
03140K2
03140K3
03140K4
03140K5
03140K6
03140K7
03140K8
03140K9
03140KB
03140KC
03140KD
03140KF
03140KJ
03140KK
03140KM
03140KN
03140Z0
03140Z1
03140Z2
03140Z3
03140Z4
03140Z5
03140Z6
03140Z7
03140Z8
03140Z9
03140ZB
03140ZC
03140ZD
03140ZF
03140ZJ
03140ZK
03140ZM
03140ZN
0315090
0315091
0315092
0315093
0315094
0315095
0315096
0315097
0315098
0315099
031509B
031509C
031509D
031509F
031509J
031509K
031509T
031509V
03150A0
03150A1
03150A2
03150A3
03150A4
03150A5
03150A6
03150A7
03150A8
03150A9
03150AB
03150AC
03150AD
03150AF
03150AJ
03150AK
03150AT
03150AV
03150J0
03150J1
03150J2
03150J3
03150J4
03150J5
03150J6
03150J7
03150J8
03150J9
03150JB
03150JC
03150JD
03150JF
03150JJ
03150JK
03150JT
03150JV
03150K0
03150K1
03150K2
03150K3
03150K4
03150K5
03150K6
03150K7
03150K8
03150K9
03150KB
03150KC
03150KD
03150KF
03150KJ
03150KK
03150KT
03150KV
03150Z0
03150Z1
03150Z2
03150Z3
03150Z4
03150Z5
03150Z6
03150Z7
03150Z8
03150Z9
03150ZB
03150ZC
03150ZD
03150ZF
03150ZJ
03150ZK
03150ZT
03150ZV
0316090
0316091
0316092
0316093
0316094
0316095
0316096
0316097
0316098
0316099
031609B
031609C
031609D
031609F
031609J
031609K
031609T
031609V
03160A0
03160A1
03160A2
03160A3
03160A4
03160A5
03160A6
03160A7
03160A8
03160A9
03160AB
03160AC
03160AD
03160AF
03160AJ
03160AK
03160AT
03160AV
03160J0
03160J1
03160J2
03160J3
03160J4
03160J5
03160J6
03160J7
03160J8
03160J9
03160JB
03160JC
03160JD
03160JF
03160JJ
03160JK
03160JT
03160JV
03160K0
03160K1
03160K2
03160K3
03160K4
03160K5
03160K6
03160K7
03160K8
03160K9
03160KB
03160KC
03160KD
03160KF
03160KJ
03160KK
03160KT
03160KV
03160Z0
03160Z1
03160Z2
03160Z3
03160Z4
03160Z5
03160Z6
03160Z7
03160Z8
03160Z9
03160ZB
03160ZC
03160ZD
03160ZF
03160ZJ
03160ZK
03160ZT
03160ZV
0317090
0317093
031709D
031709F
031709V
03170A0
03170A3
03170AD
03170AF
03170AV
03170J0
03170J3
03170JD
03170JF
03170JV
03170K0
03170K3
03170KD
03170KF
031H09Y
031H0AY
031H0JY
031H0KY
031H0ZY
031J09Y
031J0AY
031J0JY
031J0KY
031J0ZY
031K09K
031K0AJ
031K0AK
031K0JJ
031K0JK
031K0KJ
031K0KK
031K0ZJ
031K0ZK
031L09J
031L09K
031L0AJ
031L0AK
031L0JJ
031L0JK
031L0KJ
031L0KK
031L0ZJ
031L0ZK
031M09J
031M09K
031M0AJ
031M0AK
031M0JJ
031M0JK
031M0KJ
031M0KK
031M0ZJ
031M0ZK
031N09J
031N09K
031N0AJ
031N0AK
031N0JJ
031N0JK
031N0KJ
031N0KK
031N0ZJ
031N0ZK
031S09G
031S0AG
031S0JG
031S0KG
031S0ZG
031T09G
031T0AG
031T0JG
031T0KG
031T0ZG
03500ZZ
03503ZZ
03504ZZ
03510ZZ
03513ZZ
03514ZZ
03520ZZ
03523ZZ
03524ZZ
03530ZZ
03533ZZ
03534ZZ
03540ZZ
03543ZZ
03544ZZ
03550ZZ
03553ZZ
03554ZZ
03560ZZ
03563ZZ
03564ZZ
03570ZZ
03573ZZ
03574ZZ
03580ZZ
03583ZZ
03584ZZ
03590ZZ
03593ZZ
03594ZZ
035A0ZZ
035A3ZZ
035A4ZZ
035B0ZZ
035B3ZZ
035B4ZZ
035C0ZZ
035C3ZZ
035C4ZZ
035D0ZZ
035D3ZZ
035D4ZZ
035F0ZZ
035F3ZZ
035F4ZZ
035G0ZZ
035G3ZZ
035G4ZZ
035H0ZZ
035H3ZZ
035H4ZZ
035J0ZZ
035J3ZZ
035J4ZZ
035K0ZZ
035K3ZZ
035K4ZZ
035L0ZZ
035L3ZZ
035L4ZZ
035M0ZZ
035M3ZZ
035M4ZZ
035N0ZZ
035N3ZZ
035N4ZZ
035P0ZZ
035P3ZZ
035P4ZZ
035Q0ZZ
035Q3ZZ
035Q4ZZ
035R0ZZ
035R3ZZ
035R4ZZ
035S0ZZ
035S3ZZ
035S4ZZ
035T0ZZ
035T3ZZ
035T4ZZ
035U0ZZ
035U3ZZ
035U4ZZ
035V0ZZ
035V3ZZ
035V4ZZ
035Y0ZZ
035Y3ZZ
035Y4ZZ
0370046
037004Z
0370056
037005Z
0370066
037006Z
0370076
037007Z
03700D1
03700D6
03700DZ
03700E6
03700EZ
03700F6
03700FZ
03700G6
03700GZ
03700Z1
03700Z6
03700ZZ
0370346
037034Z
0370356
037035Z
0370366
037036Z
0370376
037037Z
03703D1
03703D6
03703DZ
03703E6
03703EZ
03703F6
03703FZ
03703G6
03703GZ
03703Z1
03703Z6
03703ZZ
0370446
037044Z
0370456
037045Z
0370466
037046Z
0370476
037047Z
03704D1
03704D6
03704DZ
03704E6
03704EZ
03704F6
03704FZ
03704G6
03704GZ
03704Z1
03704Z6
03704ZZ
0371046
037104Z
0371056
037105Z
0371066
037106Z
0371076
037107Z
03710D1
03710D6
03710DZ
03710E6
03710EZ
03710F6
03710FZ
03710G6
03710GZ
03710Z1
03710Z6
03710ZZ
0371346
037134Z
0371356
037135Z
0371366
037136Z
0371376
037137Z
03713D1
03713D6
03713DZ
03713E6
03713EZ
03713F6
03713FZ
03713G6
03713GZ
03713Z1
03713Z6
03713ZZ
0371446
037144Z
0371456
037145Z
0371466
037146Z
0371476
037147Z
03714D1
03714D6
03714DZ
03714E6
03714EZ
03714F6
03714FZ
03714G6
03714GZ
03714Z1
03714Z6
03714ZZ
0372046
037204Z
0372056
037205Z
0372066
037206Z
0372076
037207Z
03720D1
03720D6
03720DZ
03720E6
03720EZ
03720F6
03720FZ
03720G6
03720GZ
03720Z1
03720Z6
03720ZZ
0372346
037234Z
0372356
037235Z
0372366
037236Z
0372376
037237Z
03723D1
03723D6
03723DZ
03723E6
03723EZ
03723F6
03723FZ
03723G6
03723GZ
03723Z1
03723Z6
03723ZZ
0372446
037244Z
0372456
037245Z
0372466
037246Z
0372476
037247Z
03724D1
03724D6
03724DZ
03724E6
03724EZ
03724F6
03724FZ
03724G6
03724GZ
03724Z1

03724Z6
03724ZZ
0373046
037304Z
0373056
037305Z
0373066
037306Z
0373076
037307Z
03730D1
03730D6
03730DZ
03730E6
03730EZ
03730F6
03730FZ
03730G6
03730GZ
03730Z1
03730Z6
03730ZZ
0373346
037334Z
0373356
037335Z
0373366
037336Z
0373376
037337Z
03733D1
03733D6
03733Z1
03734D1
03734Z1
03740D1
03740Z1
03743D1
03743Z1
03744D1
03744Z1
03750D1
03750Z1
03753D1
03753Z1
03754D1
03754G6
03754GZ
03754Z1
03754Z6
03754ZZ
0376046
037604Z
0376056
037605Z
0376066
037606Z
0376076
037607Z
03760D1
03760D6
03760DZ
03760E6
03760EZ
03760F6
03760FZ
03760G6
03760GZ
03760Z1
03760Z6
03760ZZ
0376346
037634Z
0376356
037635Z
0376366
037636Z
0376376
037637Z
03763D1
03763D6
03763DZ
03763E6
03763EZ
03763F6
03763FZ
03763G6
03763GZ
03763Z1
03763Z6
03763ZZ
0376446
037644Z
0376456
037645Z
0376466
037646Z
0376476
037647Z
03764D1
03764D6
03764DZ
03764E6
03764EZ
03764F6
03764FZ
03764G6
03764GZ
03764Z1
03764Z6
03764ZZ
0377046
037704Z
0377056
037705Z
0377066
037706Z
0377076
037707Z
03770D1
03770D6
03770DZ
03770E6
03770EZ
03770F6
03770FZ
03770G6
03770GZ
03770Z1
03770Z6
03770ZZ
0377346
037734Z
0377356
037735Z
0377366
037736Z
0377376
037737Z
03773D1
03773D6
03773DZ
03773E6
03773EZ
03773F6
03773FZ
03773G6
03773GZ
03773Z1
03773Z6
03773ZZ
0377446
037744Z
0377456
037745Z
0377466
037746Z
0377476
037747Z
03774D1
03774D6
03774DZ
03774E6
03774EZ
03774F6
03774FZ
03774G6
03774GZ
03774Z1
03774Z6
03774ZZ
0378046
037804Z
0378056
037805Z
0378066
037806Z
0378076
037807Z
03780D1
03780D6
03780DZ
03780E6
03780EZ
03780F6
03780FZ
03780G6
03780GZ
03780Z1
03780Z6
03780ZZ
0378346
037834Z
0378356
037835Z
0378366
037836Z
0378376
037837Z
03783D1
03783D6
03783DZ
03783E6
03783EZ
03783F6
03783FZ
03783G6
03783GZ
03783Z1
03783Z6
03783ZZ
0378446
037844Z
0378456
037845Z
0378466
037846Z
0378476
037847Z
03784D1
03784D6
03784DZ
03784E6
03784EZ
03784F6
03784FZ
03784G6
03784GZ
03784Z1
03784Z6
03784ZZ
0379046
037904Z
0379056
037905Z
0379066
037906Z
0379076
037907Z
03790D1
03790D6
03790DZ
03790E6
03790EZ
03790F6
03790FZ
03790G6
03790GZ
03790Z1
03790Z6
03790ZZ
0379346
037934Z
0379356
037935Z
0379366
037936Z
0379376
037937Z
03793D1
03793D6
03793DZ
03793E6
03793EZ
03793F6
03793FZ
03793G6
03793GZ
03793Z1
03793Z6
03793ZZ
0379446
037944Z
0379456
037945Z
0379466
037946Z
0379476
037947Z
03794D1
03794D6
03794DZ
03794E6
03794EZ
03794F6
03794FZ
03794G6
03794GZ
03794Z1
03794Z6
03794ZZ
037A046
037A04Z
037A056
037A05Z
037A066
037A06Z
037A076
037A07Z
037A0D1
037A0D6
037A0DZ
037A0E6
037A0EZ
037A0F6
037A0FZ
037A0G6
037A0GZ
037A0Z1
037A0Z6
037A0ZZ
037A346
037A34Z
037A356
037A3D1
037A3Z1
037A4D1
037A4Z1
037B0D1
037B0Z1
037B3D1
037B3Z1
037B4D1
037B4Z1
037C0D1
037C0Z1
037C3D1
037C3Z1
037C4D1
037C4Z1
037G056
037G05Z
037G066
037G06Z
037G076
037G07Z
037G0D6
037G0DZ
037G0E6
037G0EZ
037G0F6
037G0FZ
037G0G6
037G0GZ
037G0Z6
037G0ZZ
037G346
037G34Z
037G356
037G35Z
037G366
037G36Z
037G376
037G37Z
037G3D6
037G3DZ
037G3E6
037G3EZ
037G3F6
037G3FZ
037G3G6
037G3GZ
037G3Z6
037G3ZZ
037G446
037G44Z
037G456
037G45Z
037G466
037G46Z
037G476
037G47Z
037G4D6
037G4DZ
037G4E6
037G4EZ
037G4F6
037G4FZ
037G4G6
037G4GZ
037G4Z6
037G4ZZ
037H046
037H04Z
037H056
037H05Z
037H066
037H06Z
037H076
037H07Z
037H0D6
037H0DZ
037H0E6
037H0EZ
037H0F6
037H0FZ
037H0G6
037H0GZ
037H0Z6
037H0ZZ
037H346
037H34Z
037H356
037H35Z
037H366
037H36Z
037H376
037H37Z
037H3D6
037H3DZ
037H3E6
037H3EZ
037H3F6
037H3FZ
037H3G6
037H3GZ
037H3Z6
037H3ZZ
037H446
037H44Z
037H456
037H45Z
037H466
037H46Z
037H476
037H47Z
037H4D6
037H4DZ
037H4E6
037H4EZ
037H4F6
037H4FZ
037H4G6
037H4GZ
037H4Z6
037H4ZZ
037J046
037J04Z
037J056
037J05Z
037J066
037J06Z
037J076
037J07Z
037J0D6
037J0DZ
037J0E6
037J0EZ
037J0F6
037J0FZ
037J0G6
037J0GZ
037J0Z6
037J0ZZ
037J346
037J34Z
037J356
037J35Z
037J366
037J36Z
037J376
037J37Z
037J3D6
037J3DZ
037J3E6
037J3EZ
037J3F6
037J3FZ
037J3G6
037J3GZ
037J3Z6
037J3ZZ
037J446
037J44Z
037J456
037J45Z
037J466
037J46Z
037J476
037J47Z
037J4D6
037J4DZ
037J4E6
037J4EZ
037J4F6
037J4FZ
037J4G6
037J4GZ
037J4Z6
037J4ZZ
037K046
037K04Z
037K056
037K05Z
037K066
037K06Z
037K076
037K07Z
037K0D6
037K0DZ
037K0E6
037K0EZ
037K0F6
037K0FZ
037K0G6
037K0GZ
037K0Z6
037K0ZZ
037K346
037K34Z
037K356
037K35Z
037K366
037K36Z
037K376
037K37Z
037K3D6
037K3DZ
037K3E6
037K3EZ
037K3F6
037K3FZ
037K3G6
037K3GZ
037K3Z6
037K3ZZ
037K446
037K44Z
037K456
037K45Z
037K466
037K46Z
037K476
037K47Z
037K4D6
037K4DZ
037K4E6
037K4EZ
037K4F6
037K4FZ
037K4G6
037K4GZ
037K4Z6
037K4ZZ
037L046
037L04Z
037L056
037L05Z
037L066
037L06Z
037L076
037L07Z
037L0D6
037L0DZ
037L0E6
037L0EZ
037L0F6
037L0FZ
037L0G6
037L0GZ
037L0Z6
037L0ZZ
037L346
037L34Z
037L356
037L35Z
037N366
037N36Z
037N376
037N37Z
037N3D6
037N3DZ
037N3E6
037N3EZ
037N3F6
037N3FZ
037N3G6
037N3GZ
037N3Z6
037N3ZZ
037N446
037N44Z
037N456
037N45Z
037N466
037N46Z
037N476
037N47Z
037N4D6
037N4DZ
037N4E6
037N4EZ
037N4F6
037N4FZ
037N4G6
037N4GZ
037N4Z6
037N4ZZ
037P046
037P04Z
037P056
037P05Z
037P066
037P06Z
037P076
037P07Z
037P0D6
037P0DZ
037P0E6
037P0EZ
037P0F6
037P0FZ
037P0G6
037P0GZ
037P0Z6
037P0ZZ
037P346
037P34Z
037P356
037P35Z
037P366
037P36Z
037P376
037P37Z
037P3D6
037P3DZ
037P3E6
037P3EZ
037P3F6
037P3FZ
037P3G6
037P3GZ
037P3Z6
037P3ZZ
037P446
037P44Z
037P456
037P45Z
037P466
037P46Z
037P476
037P47Z
037P4D6
037P4DZ
037P4E6
037P4EZ
037P4F6
037P4FZ
037P4G6
037P4GZ
037P4Z6
037P4ZZ
037Q046
037Q04Z
037Q056
037Q05Z
037Q066
037Q06Z
037Q076
037Q07Z
037Q0D6
037Q0DZ
037Q0E6
037Q0EZ
037Q0F6
037Q0FZ
037Q0G6
037Q0GZ
037Q0Z6
037Q0ZZ
037Q346
037Q34Z
037Q356
037Q35Z
037Q366
037Q36Z
037Q376
037Q37Z
037Q3D6
037Q3DZ
037Q3E6
037Q3EZ
037Q3F6
037Q3FZ
037Q3G6
037Q3GZ
037Q3Z6
037Q3ZZ
037Q446
037Q44Z
037Q456
037Q45Z
037Q466
037Q46Z
037Q476
037Q47Z
037Q4D6
037Q4DZ
037Q4E6
037Q4EZ
037Q4F6
037Q4FZ
037Q4G6
037Q4GZ
037Q4Z6
037Q4ZZ
037R046
037R04Z
037R056
037R05Z
037R066
037R06Z
037R076
037R07Z
037R0D6
037R0DZ
037R0E6
037R0EZ
037R0F6
037R0FZ
037R0G6
037R0GZ
037R0Z6
037R0ZZ
037R346
037R34Z

037R356
037R35Z
037R366
037R36Z
037R376
037R37Z
037R3D6
037R3DZ
037R3E6
037R3EZ
037R3F6
037R3FZ
037R3G6
037R3GZ
037R3Z6
037R3ZZ
037R446
037R44Z
037R456
037R45Z
037R466
037R46Z
037R476
037R47Z
037R4D6
037R4DZ
037R4E6
037R4EZ
037R4F6
037R4FZ
037R4G6
037R4GZ
037R4Z6
037R4ZZ
037S046
037S04Z
037S056
037S05Z
037S066
037S06Z
037S076
037S07Z
037S0D6
037S0DZ
037S0E6
037S0EZ
037S0F6
037S0FZ
037S0G6
037S0GZ
037S0Z6
037S0ZZ
037S346
037S34Z
037S356
037S35Z
037S366
037S36Z
037S376
037S37Z
037S3D6
037S3DZ
037S3E6
037S3EZ
037S3F6
037S3FZ
037S3G6
037S3GZ
037S3Z6
037S3ZZ
037S446
037S44Z
037S456
037S45Z
037S466
037S46Z
037S476
037S47Z
037S4D6
037S4DZ
037S4E6
037S4EZ
037S4F6
037S4FZ
037S4G6
037S4GZ
037S4Z6
037S4ZZ
037T046
037T04Z
037T056
037T05Z
037T066
037T06Z
037T076
037T07Z
037T0D6
037T0DZ
037T0E6
037T0EZ
037T0F6
037T0FZ
037T0G6
037T0GZ
037T0Z6
037T0ZZ
037T346
037T34Z
037T356
037T35Z
037T366
037T36Z
037T376
037T37Z
037T3D6
037T3DZ
037T3E6
037T3EZ
037T3F6
037T3FZ
037T3G6
037T3GZ
037T3Z6
037T3ZZ
037T446
037T44Z
037T456
037T45Z
037T466
037T46Z
037T476
037T47Z
037T4D6
037T4DZ
037T4E6
037T4EZ
037T4F6
037T4FZ
037T4G6
037T4GZ
037T4Z6
037T4ZZ
037U046
037U04Z
037U056
037U05Z
037U066
037U06Z
037U076
037U07Z
037U0D6
037U0DZ
037U0E6
037U0EZ
037U0F6
037U0FZ
037U0G6
037U0GZ
037U0Z6
037U0ZZ
037U346
037U34Z
037U356
037U35Z
037U366
037U36Z
037U376
037U37Z
037U3D6
037U3DZ
037U3E6
037U3EZ
037U3F6
037U3FZ
037U3G6
037U3GZ
037U3Z6
037U3ZZ
037U446
037U44Z
037U456
037U45Z
037U466
037U46Z
037U476
037U47Z
037U4D6
037U4DZ
037U4E6
037U4EZ
037U4F6
037U4FZ
037U4G6
037U4GZ
037U4Z6
037U4ZZ
037V046
037V04Z
037V056
037V05Z
037V066
037V06Z
037V076
037V07Z
037V0D6
037V0DZ
037V0E6
037V0EZ
037V0F6
037V0FZ
037V0G6
037V0GZ
037V0Z6
037V0ZZ
037V346
037V34Z
037V356
037V35Z
037V366
037V36Z
037V376
039000Z
03900ZZ
039030Z
03903ZX
03903ZZ
039040Z
03904ZZ
039100Z
03910ZZ
039130Z
03913ZX
03913ZZ
039140Z
03914ZZ
039200Z
03920ZZ
039230Z
03923ZX
03923ZZ
039240Z
03924ZZ
039300Z
03930ZZ
039330Z
03933ZX
03933ZZ
039340Z
03934ZZ
039400Z
03940ZZ
039430Z
03943ZX
03943ZZ
039440Z
03944ZZ
039500Z
03950ZZ
039530Z
03953ZX
03953ZZ
039540Z
03954ZZ
039600Z
03960ZZ
039630Z
03963ZX
03963ZZ
039640Z
03964ZZ
039700Z
03970ZZ
039730Z
03973ZX
03973ZZ
039740Z
03974ZZ
039800Z
03980ZZ
039830Z
03983ZX
03983ZZ
039840Z
03984ZZ
039900Z
03990ZZ
039930Z
03993ZX
03993ZZ
039940Z
03994ZZ
039A00Z
039A0ZZ
039A30Z
039A3ZX
039A3ZZ
039A40Z
039A4ZZ
039B00Z
039B0ZZ
039B30Z
039B3ZX
039B3ZZ
039B40Z
039B4ZZ
039C00Z
039C0ZZ
039C30Z
039C3ZX
039C3ZZ
039C40Z
039C4ZZ
039D00Z
039D0ZZ
039D30Z
039D3ZX
039D3ZZ
039D40Z
039D4ZZ
039F00Z
039F0ZZ
039F30Z
039F3ZX
039F3ZZ
039F40Z
039F4ZZ
039G00Z
039G0ZZ
039G30Z
039G3ZX
039G3ZZ
039G40Z
039G4ZZ
039H00Z
039H0ZZ
039H30Z
039H3ZX
039H3ZZ
039H40Z
039H4ZZ
039J00Z
039J0ZZ
039J30Z
039J3ZX
039J3ZZ
039J40Z
039J4ZZ
039K00Z
039K0ZZ
039K30Z
039K3ZX
039K3ZZ
039K40Z
039K4ZZ
039L00Z
039L0ZZ
039L30Z
039L3ZX
039L3ZZ
039L40Z
039L4ZZ
039M00Z
039M0ZZ
039M30Z
039M3ZX
039M3ZZ
039M40Z
039M4ZZ
039N00Z
039N0ZZ
039N30Z
039N3ZX
039N3ZZ
039N40Z
039N4ZZ
039P00Z
039P0ZZ
039P30Z
039P3ZX
039P3ZZ
039P40Z
039P4ZZ
039Q00Z
039Q0ZZ
039Q30Z
039Q3ZX
039Q3ZZ
039Q40Z
039Q4ZZ
039R00Z
039R0ZZ
039R30Z
039R3ZX
039R3ZZ
039R40Z
039R4ZZ
039S00Z
039S0ZZ
039S30Z
039S3ZX
039S3ZZ
039S40Z
039S4ZZ
039T00Z
039T0ZZ
039T30Z
039T3ZX
039T3ZZ
039T40Z
039T4ZZ
039U00Z
039U0ZZ
039U30Z
039U3ZX
039U3ZZ
039U40Z
039U4ZZ
039V00Z
039V0ZZ
039V30Z
039V3ZX
039V3ZZ
039V40Z
039V4ZZ
039Y00Z
039Y0ZZ
039Y30Z
039Y3ZX
039Y3ZZ
039Y40Z
039Y4ZZ
03B40ZX
03B40ZZ
03B43ZX
03B43ZZ
03B44ZX
03B44ZZ
03B50ZX
03B50ZZ
03B53ZX
03B53ZZ
03B54ZX
03B54ZZ
03B60ZX
03B60ZZ
03B63ZX
03B63ZZ
03B64ZX
03B64ZZ
03B70ZX
03B70ZZ
03B73ZX
03B73ZZ
03B74ZX
03B74ZZ
03B80ZX
03B80ZZ
03B83ZX
03B83ZZ
03B84ZX
03B84ZZ
03B90ZX
03B90ZZ
03B93ZX
03B93ZZ
03B94ZX
03B94ZZ
03BA0ZX
03BA0ZZ
03BA3ZX
03BA3ZZ
03BA4ZX
03BA4ZZ
03BB0ZX
03BB0ZZ
03BB3ZX
03BB3ZZ
03BB4ZX
03BB4ZZ
03BC0ZX
03BC0ZZ
03BC3ZX
03BC3ZZ
03BC4ZX
03BC4ZZ
03BD0ZX
03BD0ZZ
03BD3ZX
03BD3ZZ
03BD4ZX
03BD4ZZ
03BF0ZX
03BF0ZZ
03BF3ZX
03BF3ZZ
03BF4ZX
03BF4ZZ
03BG0ZX
03BG0ZZ
03BG3ZX
03BG3ZZ
03BG4ZX
03BG4ZZ
03BH0ZX
03BH0ZZ
03BH3ZX
03BH3ZZ
03BH4ZX
03BH4ZZ
03BJ0ZX
03BJ0ZZ
03BJ3ZX
03BJ3ZZ
03BJ4ZX
03BJ4ZZ
03BK0ZX
03BK0ZZ
03BK3ZX
03BK3ZZ
03BK4ZX
03BK4ZZ
03BL0ZX
03BL0ZZ
03BL3ZX
03BL3ZZ
03BL4ZX
03BL4ZZ
03BM0ZX
03BM0ZZ
03BM3ZX
03BM3ZZ
03BM4ZX
03BM4ZZ
03BN0ZX
03BN0ZZ
03BN3ZX
03BN3ZZ
03BN4ZX
03BN4ZZ
03BP0ZX
03BP0ZZ
03BP3ZX
03BP3ZZ
03BP4ZX
03BP4ZZ
03BQ0ZX
03BQ0ZZ
03BQ3ZX
03BQ3ZZ
03BQ4ZX
03BQ4ZZ
03BR0ZX
03BR0ZZ
03BR3ZX
03BR3ZZ
03BR4ZX
03BR4ZZ
03BS0ZX
03BS0ZZ
03BS3ZX
03BS3ZZ
03BS4ZX
03BS4ZZ
03BT0ZX
03BT0ZZ
03BT3ZX
03BT3ZZ
03BT4ZX
03BT4ZZ
03BU0ZX
03BU0ZZ
03BU3ZX
03BU3ZZ
03BU4ZX
03BU4ZZ
03BV0ZX
03BV0ZZ
03BV3ZX
03BV3ZZ
03BV4ZX
03BV4ZZ
03BY0ZX
03BY0ZZ
03BY3ZX
03BY3ZZ
03BY4ZX
03BY4ZZ
03C00Z6
03C00ZZ
03C03Z6
03C03ZZ
03C04Z6
03C04ZZ
03C10Z6
03C10ZZ
03C13Z6
03C13ZZ
03C14Z6
03C14ZZ
03C20Z6
03C20ZZ
03C23Z6
03C23ZZ
03C24Z6
03C24ZZ
03C30Z6
03C30ZZ
03C33Z6
03C33ZZ
03C34Z6
03C34ZZ
03C40Z6
03C40ZZ
03C43Z6
03C43ZZ
03C44Z6
03C44ZZ
03C50Z6
03C50ZZ
03C53Z6
03C53ZZ
03C54Z6
03C54ZZ
03C60Z6
03C60ZZ
03C63Z6
03C63ZZ
03C64Z6
03C64ZZ
03C70Z6
03C70ZZ
03C73Z6
03C73ZZ
03C74Z6
03C74ZZ
03C80Z6
03C80ZZ
03C83Z6
03C83ZZ
03C84Z6
03C84ZZ
03C90Z6
03C90ZZ
03C93Z6
03C93ZZ
03C94Z6
03C94ZZ
03CA0Z6
03CA0ZZ
03CA3Z6
03CA3ZZ
03CA4Z6
03CA4ZZ
03CB0Z6
03CB0ZZ
03CB3Z6
03CB3ZZ
03CB4Z6
03CB4ZZ
03CC0Z6
03CC0ZZ
03CC3Z6
03CC3ZZ
03CC4Z6
03CC4ZZ
03CD0Z6
03CD0ZZ
03CD3Z6
03CD3ZZ
03CD4Z6
03CD4ZZ
03CF0Z6
03CG3Z7
03CH3Z7
03CJ3Z7
03CK3Z7
03CL3Z7
03CM3Z7
03CN3Z7
03CP3Z7
03CQ3Z7
03H003Z
03H00DZ
03H033Z
03H03DZ
03H043Z
03H04DZ
03H103Z
03H10DZ
03H133Z
03H13DZ
03H143Z
03H14DZ
03H203Z
03H20DZ
03H233Z
03H23DZ
03H243Z
03H24DZ
03H303Z
03H30DZ
03H333Z
03H33DZ
03H343Z
03H34DZ
03H403Z
03H40DZ
03H433Z
03H43DZ
03H443Z
03H44DZ
03H503Z
03H50DZ
03H533Z
03H53DZ
03H543Z
03H54DZ
03H603Z
03H60DZ
03H633Z
03H63DZ
03H643Z
03H64DZ
03H703Z
03H70DZ
03H733Z

03H73DZ
03H743Z
03H74DZ
03H803Z
03H80DZ
03H833Z
03H83DZ
03H843Z
03H84DZ
03H903Z
03H90DZ
03H933Z
03H93DZ
03H943Z
03H94DZ
03HA03Z
03HA0DZ
03HA33Z
03HA3DZ
03HA43Z
03HA4DZ
03HB03Z
03HB0DZ
03HB33Z
03HB3DZ
03HB43Z
03HB4DZ
03HC03Z
03HC0DZ
03HC33Z
03HC3DZ
03HC43Z
03HC4DZ
03HD03Z
03HD0DZ
03HD33Z
03HD3DZ
03HD43Z
03HD4DZ
03HF03Z
03HF0DZ
03HF33Z
03HF3DZ
03HF43Z
03HF4DZ
03HG03Z
03HG0DZ
03HG33Z
03HG3DZ
03HG43Z
03HG4DZ
03HH03Z
03HH0DZ
03HH33Z
03HH3DZ
03HH43Z
03HH4DZ
03HJ03Z
03HJ0DZ
03HJ33Z
03HJ3DZ
03HJ43Z
03HJ4DZ
03HK03Z
03HK0DZ
03HK0MZ
03HK33Z
03HK3DZ
03HK3MZ
03HK43Z
03HK4DZ
03HK4MZ
03HL03Z
03HL0DZ
03HL0MZ
03HL33Z
03HL3DZ
03HL3MZ
03HL43Z
03HL4DZ
03HL4MZ
03HM03Z
03HM0DZ
03HM33Z
03HM3DZ
03HM43Z
03HM4DZ
03HN03Z
03HN0DZ
03HN33Z
03HN3DZ
03HN43Z
03HN4DZ
03HP03Z
03HP0DZ
03HP33Z
03HP3DZ
03HP43Z
03HP4DZ
03HQ03Z
03HQ0DZ
03HQ33Z
03HQ3DZ
03HQ43Z
03HQ4DZ
03HR03Z
03HR0DZ
03HR33Z
03HR3DZ
03HR43Z
03HR4DZ
03HS03Z
03HS0DZ
03HS33Z
03HS3DZ
03HS43Z
03HS4DZ
03HT03Z
03HT0DZ
03HT33Z
03HT3DZ
03HT43Z
03HT4DZ
03HU03Z
03HU0DZ
03HU33Z
03HU3DZ
03HU43Z
03HU4DZ
03HV03Z
03HV0DZ
03HV33Z
03HV3DZ
03HV43Z
03HV4DZ
03HY02Z
03HY03Z
03HY0DZ
03HY0YZ
03HY32Z
03HY33Z
03HY3DZ
03HY3YZ
03HY42Z
03HY43Z
03HY4DZ
03HY4YZ
03JY0ZZ
03JY3ZZ
03JY4ZZ
03JYXZZ
03L00CZ
03L00DZ
03L00ZZ
03L03CZ
03L03DZ
03L03ZZ
03L04CZ
03L04DZ
03L04ZZ
03L10CZ
03L10DZ
03L10ZZ
03L13CZ
03L13DZ
03L13ZZ
03L14CZ
03L14DZ
03L14ZZ
03L20CZ
03L20DZ
03L20ZZ
03L23CZ
03L23DZ
03L23ZZ
03L24CZ
03L24DZ
03L24ZZ
03L30CZ
03L30DZ
03L30ZZ
03L33CZ
03L33DZ
03L33ZZ
03L34CZ
03L34DZ
03L34ZZ
03L40CZ
03L40DZ
03L40ZZ
03L43CZ
03L43DZ
03L43ZZ
03L44CZ
03L44DZ
03L44ZZ
03L50CZ
03L50DZ
03L50ZZ
03L53CZ
03L53DZ
03L53ZZ
03L54CZ
03L54DZ
03L54ZZ
03L60CZ
03L60DZ
03L60ZZ
03L63CZ
03L63DZ
03L63ZZ
03L64CZ
03L64DZ
03L64ZZ
03L70CZ
03L70DZ
03L70ZZ
03L73CZ
03L73DZ
03L73ZZ
03L74CZ
03L74DZ
03L74ZZ
03L80CZ
03L80DZ
03L80ZZ
03L83CZ
03L83DZ
03L83ZZ
03L84CZ
03L84DZ
03L84ZZ
03L90CZ
03L90DZ
03L90ZZ
03L93CZ
03LK3DZ
03LK3ZZ
03LK4BZ
03LK4CZ
03LK4DZ
03LK4ZZ
03LL0BZ
03LL0CZ
03LL0DZ
03LL0ZZ
03LL3BZ
03LL3CZ
03LL3DZ
03LL3ZZ
03LL4BZ
03LL4CZ
03LL4DZ
03LL4ZZ
03LM0BZ
03LM0CZ
03LM0DZ
03LM0ZZ
03LM3BZ
03LM3CZ
03LM3DZ
03LM3ZZ
03LM4BZ
03LM4CZ
03LM4DZ
03LM4ZZ
03LN0BZ
03LN0CZ
03LN0DZ
03LN0ZZ
03LN3BZ
03LN3CZ
03LN3DZ
03LN3ZZ
03LN4BZ
03LN4CZ
03LN4DZ
03LN4ZZ
03LP0BZ
03LP0CZ
03LP0DZ
03LP0ZZ
03LP3BZ
03LP3CZ
03LP3DZ
03LP3ZZ
03LP4BZ
03LP4CZ
03LP4DZ
03LP4ZZ
03LQ0BZ
03LQ0CZ
03LQ0DZ
03LQ0ZZ
03LQ3BZ
03LQ3CZ
03LQ3DZ
03LQ3ZZ
03LQ4BZ
03LQ4CZ
03LQ4DZ
03LQ4ZZ
03LR0CZ
03LR0DZ
03LR0ZZ
03LR3CZ
03LR3DZ
03LR3ZZ
03LR4CZ
03LR4DZ
03LR4ZZ
03LS0CZ
03LS0DZ
03LS0ZZ
03LS3CZ
03LS3DZ
03LS3ZZ
03LS4CZ
03LS4DZ
03LS4ZZ
03LT0CZ
03LT0DZ
03LT0ZZ
03LT3CZ
03LT3DZ
03LT3ZZ
03LT4CZ
03LT4DZ
03LT4ZZ
03LU0CZ
03LU0DZ
03LU0ZZ
03LU3CZ
03LU3DZ
03LU3ZZ
03LU4CZ
03LU4DZ
03LU4ZZ
03LV0CZ
03LV0DZ
03LV0ZZ
03LV3CZ
03LV3DZ
03LV3ZZ
03LV4CZ
03LV4DZ
03LV4ZZ
03LY0CZ
03LY0DZ
03LY0ZZ
03LY3CZ
03LY3DZ
03LY3ZZ
03LY4CZ
03LY4DZ
03LY4ZZ
03N00ZZ
03N03ZZ
03N04ZZ
03N10ZZ
03N13ZZ
03N14ZZ
03N20ZZ
03N23ZZ
03N24ZZ
03N30ZZ
03N33ZZ
03N34ZZ
03N40ZZ
03N43ZZ
03N44ZZ
03N50ZZ
03N53ZZ
03N54ZZ
03N60ZZ
03N63ZZ
03N64ZZ
03N70ZZ
03N73ZZ
03N74ZZ
03N80ZZ
03N83ZZ
03N84ZZ
03N90ZZ
03N93ZZ
03N94ZZ
03NA0ZZ
03NA3ZZ
03NA4ZZ
03NB0ZZ
03NB3ZZ
03NB4ZZ
03NC0ZZ
03NC3ZZ
03NC4ZZ
03ND0ZZ
03ND3ZZ
03ND4ZZ
03NF0ZZ
03NF3ZZ
03NF4ZZ
03NG0ZZ
03NG3ZZ
03NG4ZZ
03NH0ZZ
03NH3ZZ
03NH4ZZ
03NJ0ZZ
03NJ3ZZ
03NJ4ZZ
03NK0ZZ
03NK3ZZ
03NK4ZZ
03NL0ZZ
03NL3ZZ
03NL4ZZ
03NM0ZZ
03NM3ZZ
03NM4ZZ
03NN0ZZ
03NN3ZZ
03NN4ZZ
03NP0ZZ
03NP3ZZ
03NP4ZZ
03NQ0ZZ
03NQ3ZZ
03NQ4ZZ
03NR0ZZ
03NR3ZZ
03NR4ZZ
03NS0ZZ
03NS3ZZ
03NS4ZZ
03NT0ZZ
03NT3ZZ
03NT4ZZ
03NU0ZZ
03NU3ZZ
03NU4ZZ
03NV0ZZ
03NV3ZZ
03NV4ZZ
03NY0ZZ
03NY3ZZ
03NY4ZZ
03PY00Z
03PY02Z
03PY03Z
03PY07Z
03PY0CZ
03PY0DZ
03PY0JZ
03PY0KZ
03PY0MZ
03PY0YZ
03PY30Z
03PY32Z
03PY33Z
03PY37Z
03PY3CZ
03PY3DZ
03PY3JZ
03PY3KZ
03PY3MZ
03PY3YZ
03PY40Z
03PY42Z
03PY43Z
03PY47Z
03PY4CZ
03PY4DZ
03PY4JZ
03PY4KZ
03PY4MZ
03PY4YZ
03PYX0Z
03PYX2Z
03PYX3Z
03PYXDZ
03PYXMZ
03Q00ZZ
03Q03ZZ
03Q04ZZ
03Q10ZZ
03Q13ZZ
03Q14ZZ
03Q20ZZ
03Q23ZZ
03Q24ZZ
03Q30ZZ
03Q33ZZ
03Q34ZZ
03Q40ZZ
03Q43ZZ
03Q44ZZ
03Q50ZZ
03Q53ZZ
03Q54ZZ
03Q60ZZ
03Q63ZZ
03Q64ZZ
03Q70ZZ
03R447Z
03R44JZ
03R44KZ
03R507Z
03R50JZ
03R50KZ
03R547Z
03R54JZ
03R54KZ
03R607Z
03R60JZ
03R60KZ
03R647Z
03R64JZ
03R64KZ
03R707Z
03R70JZ
03R70KZ
03R747Z
03R74JZ
03R74KZ
03R807Z
03R80JZ
03R80KZ
03R847Z
03R84JZ
03R84KZ
03R907Z
03R90JZ
03R90KZ
03R947Z
03R94JZ
03R94KZ
03RA07Z
03RA0JZ
03RA0KZ
03RA47Z
03RA4JZ
03RA4KZ
03RB07Z
03RB0JZ
03RB0KZ
03RB47Z
03RB4JZ
03RB4KZ
03RC07Z
03RC0JZ
03RC0KZ
03RC47Z
03RC4JZ
03RC4KZ
03RD07Z
03RD0JZ
03RD0KZ
03RD47Z
03RD4JZ
03RD4KZ
03RF07Z
03RF0JZ
03RF0KZ
03RF47Z
03RF4JZ
03RF4KZ
03RG07Z
03RG0JZ
03RG0KZ
03RG47Z
03RG4JZ
03RG4KZ
03RH07Z
03RH0JZ
03RH0KZ
03RH47Z
03RH4JZ
03RH4KZ
03RJ07Z
03RJ0JZ
03RJ0KZ
03RJ47Z
03RJ4JZ
03RJ4KZ
03RK07Z
03RK0JZ
03RK0KZ
03RK47Z
03RK4JZ
03RK4KZ
03RL07Z
03RL0JZ
03RL0KZ
03RL47Z
03RL4JZ
03RL4KZ
03RM07Z
03RM0JZ
03RM0KZ
03RM47Z
03RM4JZ
03RM4KZ
03RN07Z
03RN0JZ
03RN0KZ
03RN47Z
03RN4JZ
03RN4KZ
03RP07Z
03RP0JZ
03RP0KZ
03RP47Z
03RP4JZ
03RP4KZ
03RQ07Z
03RQ0JZ
03RQ0KZ
03RQ47Z
03RQ4JZ
03RQ4KZ
03RR07Z
03RR0JZ
03RR0KZ
03RR47Z
03RR4JZ
03RR4KZ
03RS07Z
03RS0JZ
03RS0KZ
03RS47Z
03RS4JZ
03RS4KZ
03RT07Z
03RT0JZ
03RT0KZ
03RT47Z
03RT4JZ
03RT4KZ
03RU07Z
03RU0JZ
03RU0KZ
03RU47Z
03RU4JZ
03RU4KZ
03RV07Z
03RV0JZ
03RV0KZ
03RV47Z
03RV4JZ
03RV4KZ
03RY07Z
03RY0JZ
03RY0KZ
03RY47Z
03RY4JZ
03RY4KZ
03S00ZZ
03S03ZZ
03S04ZZ
03S10ZZ
03S13ZZ
03S14ZZ
03S20ZZ
03S23ZZ
03S24ZZ
03S30ZZ
03S33ZZ
03S34ZZ
03S40ZZ
03S43ZZ
03S44ZZ
03S50ZZ
03S53ZZ
03S54ZZ
03S60ZZ
03S63ZZ
03S64ZZ
03S70ZZ
03S73ZZ
03S74ZZ
03S80ZZ
03S83ZZ
03S84ZZ
03S90ZZ
03S93ZZ
03S94ZZ
03SA0ZZ
03SA3ZZ
03SA4ZZ
03SB0ZZ
03SB3ZZ
03SB4ZZ
03SC0ZZ
03SC3ZZ
03SC4ZZ
03SD0ZZ
03SD3ZZ
03SD4ZZ
03SF0ZZ
03SF3ZZ
03SF4ZZ
03SG0ZZ
03SG3ZZ
03SG4ZZ
03SH0ZZ
03SH3ZZ
03SH4ZZ
03SJ0ZZ
03SJ3ZZ
03SJ4ZZ
03SK0ZZ
03SK3ZZ
03SK4ZZ
03SL0ZZ
03SL3ZZ
03SL4ZZ
03SM0ZZ
03SM3ZZ
03SM4ZZ
03SN0ZZ
03SN3ZZ
03SN4ZZ
03SP0ZZ
03SP3ZZ
03SP4ZZ
03SQ0ZZ

03SQ3ZZ
03SQ4ZZ
03SR0ZZ
03SR3ZZ
03SR4ZZ
03SS0ZZ
03SS3ZZ
03SS4ZZ
03ST0ZZ
03ST3ZZ
03ST4ZZ
03SU0ZZ
03SU3ZZ
03SU4ZZ
03SV0ZZ
03SV3ZZ
03SV4ZZ
03SY0ZZ
03SY3ZZ
03SY4ZZ
03U007Z
03U00JZ
03U00KZ
03U037Z
03U03JZ
03U03KZ
03U047Z
03U04JZ
03U04KZ
03U107Z
03U10JZ
03U10KZ
03U137Z
03U13JZ
03U13KZ
03U147Z
03U14JZ
03U14KZ
03U207Z
03U20JZ
03U20KZ
03U237Z
03U23JZ
03U23KZ
03U247Z
03U24JZ
03U24KZ
03U307Z
03U30JZ
03U30KZ
03U337Z
03U33JZ
03U33KZ
03U347Z
03U34JZ
03U34KZ
03U407Z
03U40JZ
03U40KZ
03U437Z
03U43JZ
03U43KZ
03U447Z
03U44JZ
03U44KZ
03U507Z
03U50JZ
03U50KZ
03U537Z
03U53JZ
03U53KZ
03U547Z
03U54JZ
03U54KZ
03U607Z
03U60JZ
03U60KZ
03U637Z
03U63JZ
03U63KZ
03U647Z
03U64JZ
03U64KZ
03U707Z
03U70JZ
03U70KZ
03U737Z
03U73JZ
03U73KZ
03U747Z
03U74JZ
03U74KZ
03U807Z
03UU4JZ
03UU4KZ
03UV07Z
03UV0JZ
03UV0KZ
03UV37Z
03UV3JZ
03UV3KZ
03UV47Z
03UV4JZ
03UV4KZ
03UY07Z
03UY0JZ
03UY0KZ
03UY37Z
03UY3JZ
03UY3KZ
03UY47Z
03UY4JZ
03UY4KZ
03V00CZ
03V00DZ
03V00ZZ
03V03CZ
03V03DZ
03V03ZZ
03V04CZ
03V04DZ
03V04ZZ
03V10CZ
03V10DZ
03V10ZZ
03V13CZ
03V13DZ
03V13ZZ
03V14CZ
03V14DZ
03V14ZZ
03V20CZ
03V20DZ
03V20ZZ
03V23CZ
03V23DZ
03V23ZZ
03V24CZ
03V24DZ
03V24ZZ
03V30CZ
03V30DZ
03V30ZZ
03V33CZ
03V33DZ
03V33ZZ
03V34CZ
03V34DZ
03V34ZZ
03V40CZ
03V40DZ
03V40ZZ
03V43CZ
03V43DZ
03V43ZZ
03V44CZ
03V44DZ
03V44ZZ
03V50CZ
03V50DZ
03V50ZZ
03V53CZ
03V53DZ
03V53ZZ
03V54CZ
03V54DZ
03V54ZZ
03V60CZ
03V60DZ
03V60ZZ
03V63CZ
03V63DZ
03V63ZZ
03V64CZ
03V64DZ
03V64ZZ
03V70CZ
03V70DZ
03V70ZZ
03V73CZ
03V73DZ
03V73ZZ
03V74CZ
03V74DZ
03V74ZZ
03V80CZ
03V80DZ
03V80ZZ
03V83CZ
03V83DZ
03V83ZZ
03V84CZ
03V84DZ
03V84ZZ
03V90CZ
03V90DZ
03V90ZZ
03V93CZ
03V93DZ
03V93ZZ
03V94CZ
03V94DZ
03V94ZZ
03VA0CZ
03VA0DZ
03VA0ZZ
03VA3CZ
03VA3DZ
03VA3ZZ
03VA4CZ
03VA4DZ
03VA4ZZ
03VB0CZ
03VB0DZ
03VB0ZZ
03VB3CZ
03VB3DZ
03VB3ZZ
03VB4CZ
03VB4DZ
03VB4ZZ
03VC0CZ
03VC0DZ
03VC0ZZ
03VC3CZ
03VC3DZ
03VC3ZZ
03VC4CZ
03VC4DZ
03VC4ZZ
03VD0CZ
03VD0DZ
03VD0ZZ
03VD3CZ
03VD3DZ
03VD3ZZ
03VD4CZ
03VD4DZ
03VD4ZZ
03VF0CZ
03VF0DZ
03VF0ZZ
03VF3CZ
03VF3DZ
03VF3ZZ
03VF4CZ
03VF4DZ
03VF4ZZ
03VG0BZ
03VG0CZ
03VG0DZ
03VG0ZZ
03VG3BZ
03VG3CZ
03VG3DZ
03VG3ZZ
03VG4BZ
03VG4CZ
03VG4DZ
03VG4ZZ
03VH0BZ
03VH0CZ
03VH0DZ
03VH0ZZ
03VH3BZ
03VH3CZ
03VH3DZ
03VH3ZZ
03VH4BZ
03VH4CZ
03VH4DZ
03VH4ZZ
03VJ0BZ
03VJ0CZ
03VJ0DZ
03VJ0ZZ
03VJ3BZ
03VJ3CZ
03VJ3DZ
03VJ3ZZ
03VJ4BZ
03VJ4CZ
03VJ4DZ
03VJ4ZZ
03VK0BZ
03VK0CZ
03VK0DZ
03VK0ZZ
03VK3BZ
03VK3CZ
03VK3DZ
03VK3ZZ
03VK4BZ
03VK4CZ
03VK4DZ
03VK4ZZ
03VL0BZ
03VL0CZ
03VL0DZ
03VL0ZZ
03VL3BZ
03VL3CZ
03VL3DZ
03VL3ZZ
03VL4BZ
03VL4CZ
03VL4DZ
03VL4ZZ
03VM0BZ
03VM0CZ
03VM0DZ
03VM0ZZ
03VM3BZ
03VM3CZ
03VM3DZ
03VM3ZZ
03VM4BZ
03VM4CZ
03VM4DZ
03VM4ZZ
03VN0BZ
03VN0CZ
03VN0DZ
03VN0ZZ
03VN3BZ
03VN3CZ
03VN3DZ
03VN3ZZ
03VN4BZ
03VN4CZ
03VN4DZ
03VN4ZZ
03VP0BZ
03VP0CZ
03VP0DZ
03VP0ZZ
03VP3BZ
03VP3CZ
03VP3DZ
03VP3ZZ
03VP4BZ
03VP4CZ
03VP4DZ
03VP4ZZ
03VQ0BZ
03VQ0CZ
03VQ0DZ
03VQ0ZZ
03VQ3BZ
03VQ3CZ
03VQ3DZ
03VQ3ZZ
03VQ4BZ
03VQ4CZ
03VQ4DZ
03VQ4ZZ
03VR0CZ
03VR0DZ
03VR0ZZ
03VR3CZ
03VR3DZ
03VR3ZZ
03VR4CZ
03VR4DZ
03VR4ZZ
03VS0CZ
03VS0DZ
03VS0ZZ
03VS3CZ
03VS3DZ
03VS3ZZ
03VS4CZ
03VS4DZ
03VS4ZZ
03VT0CZ
03VT0DZ
03VT0ZZ
03VT3CZ
03VT3DZ
03WY30Z
03WY32Z
03WY33Z
03WY3DZ
03WY3YZ
03WY4YZ
03WYX0Z
03WYX2Z
03WYX3Z
03WYX7Z
03WYXCZ
03WYXDZ
03WYXJZ
03WYXKZ
03WYXMZ
0410490
0410491
0410492
0410493
0410494
0410495
0410496
0410497
0410498
0410499
041049B
041049C
041049D
041049F
041049G
041049H
041049J
041049K
041049Q
041049R
04104A0
04104A1
04104A2
04104A3
04104A4
04104A5
04104A6
04104A7
04104A8
04104A9
04104AB
04104AC
04104AD
04104AF
04104AG
04104AH
04104AJ
04104AK
04104AQ
04104AR
04104J0
04104J1
04104J2
04104J3
04104J4
04104J5
04104J6
04104J7
04104J8
04104J9
04104JB
04104JC
04104JD
04104JF
04104JG
04104JH
04104JJ
04104JK
04104JQ
04104JR
04104K0
04104K1
04104K2
04104K3
04104K4
04104K5
04104K6
04104K7
04104K8
04104K9
04104KB
04104KC
04104KD
04104KF
04104KG
04104KH
04104KJ
04104KK
04104KQ
04104KR
04104Z0
04104Z1
04104Z2
04104Z3
04104Z4
04104Z5
04104Z6
04104Z7
04104Z8
04104Z9
04104ZB
04104ZC
04104ZD
04104ZF
04104ZG
04104ZH
04104ZJ
04104ZK
04104ZQ
04104ZR
0413093
0413094
0413095
04130A3
04130A4
04130A5
04130J3
04130J4
04130J5
04130K3
04130K4
04130K5
04130Z3
04130Z4
04130Z5
0413493
0413494
0413495
04134A3
04134A4
04134A5
04134J3
04134J4
04134J5
04134K3
04134K4
04134K5
04134Z3
04134Z4
04134Z5
0414093
0414094
0414095
04140A3
04140A4
04140A5
04140J3
04140J4
04140J5
04140K3
04140K4
04140K5
04140Z3
04140Z4
04140Z5
0414493
0414494
0414495
04144A3
04144A4
04144A5
04144J3
04144J4
04144J5
04144K3
04144K4
04144K5
04144Z3
04144Z4
04144Z5
041C090
041C091
041C092
041C093
041C094
041C095
041C096
041C097
041C098
041C099
041C09B
041C09C
041C09D
041C09F
041C09G
041C09H
041C09J
041C09K
041C09Q
041C09R
041C0A0
041C0A1
041C0A2
041C0A3
041C0A4
041C0A5
041C0A6
041C0A7
041C0A8
041C0A9
041C0AB
041C0AC
041C0AD
041C0AF
041C0AG
041C0AH
041C0AJ
041C0AK
041C0AQ
041C0AR
041C0J0
041C0J1
041C0J2
041C0J3
041C0J4
041C0J5
041C0J6
041C0J7
041C0J8
041C0J9
041C0JB
041C0JC
041C0JD
041C0JF
041C0JG
041C0JH
041C0JJ
041C0JK
041C0JQ
041C0JR
041C0K0
041C0K1
041C0K2
041C0K3
041C0K4
041C0K5
041C0K6
041C0K7
041C0K8
041C0K9
041C0KB
041C0KC
041C0KD
041C0KF
041C0KG
041C0KH
041C0KJ
041C0KK
041C0KQ
041C0KR
041C0Z0
041C0Z1
041C0Z2
041C0Z3
041C0Z4
041C0Z5
041C0Z6
041C0Z7
041C0Z8
041C0Z9
041C0ZB
041C0ZC
041C0ZD
041C0ZF
041C0ZG
041C0ZH
041C0ZJ
041C0ZK
041C0ZQ
041C0ZR
041C490
041C491
041C492
041C493
041C494
041C495
041C496
041C497
041C498
041C499
041C49B
041C49C
041C49D
041C49F
041C49G
041C49H
041C49J
041C49K
041C49Q
041C49R
041C4A0
041C4A1
041C4A2
041C4A3
041C4A4
041C4A5
041C4A6
041C4A7
041C4A8
041C4A9
041C4AB
041C4AC
041C4AD
041C4AF
041C4AG
041C4AH
041C4AJ
041C4AK
041C4AQ
041C4AR
041C4J0
041C4J1
041C4J2
041C4J3
041C4J4
041C4J5
041C4J6
041C4J7
041C4J8
041C4J9
041C4JB
041C4JC
041C4JD
041C4JF
041C4JG
041C4JH
041C4JJ
041C4JK
041C4JQ
041C4JR
041C4K0
041C4K1
041C4K2
041C4K3
041C4K4
041C4K5
041C4K6
041C4K7
041C4K8
041C4K9
041C4KB
041C4KC

041C4KD	041D0AQ	041F49Q	041H0AQ	041H4JQ	041J0KQ	041J4ZQ	041K4JH	041P4JQ	041U0ZS	041W3JS
041C4KF	041D0AR	041F4A9	041H0J9	041H4K9	041J0Z9	041K09H	041K4JJ	041P4JS	041U3JQ	041W49P
041C4KG	041D0J0	041F4AB	041H0JB	041H4KB	041J0ZB	041K09J	041K4JK	041Q0JQ	041U3JS	041W49Q
041C4KH	041D0J1	041F4AC	041H0JC	041H4KC	041J0ZC	041K09K	041K4JL	041Q0JS	041U49P	041W49S
041C4KJ	041D0J2	041F4AD	041H0JD	041H4KD	041J0ZD	041K09L	041K4JM	041Q3JQ	041U49Q	041W4AP
041C4KK	041D0J3	041F4AF	041H0JF	041H4KF	041J0ZF	041K09M	041K4JN	041Q3JS	041U49S	041W4AQ
041C4KQ	041D0J4	041F4AG	041H0JG	041H4KG	041J0ZG	041K09N	041K4JP	041Q4JQ	041U4AP	041W4AS
041C4KR	041D0J5	041F4AH	041H0JH	041H4KH	041J0ZH	041K09P	041K4JQ	041Q4JS	041U4AQ	041W4JP
041C4Z0	041D0J6	041F4AJ	041H0JJ	041H4KJ	041J0ZJ	041K09Q	041K4JS	041R0JQ	041U4AS	041W4JQ
041C4Z1	041D0J7	041F4AK	041H0JK	041H4KK	041J0ZK	041K09S	041K4KH	041R0JS	041U4JP	041W4JS
041C4Z2	041D0J8	041F4AP	041H0JP	041H4KP	041J0ZP	041K0AH	041K4KJ	041R3JQ	041U4JQ	041W4KP
041C4Z3	041D0J9	041F4AQ	041H0JQ	041H4KQ	041J0ZQ	041K0AJ	041K4KK	041R3JS	041U4JS	041W4KQ
041C4Z4	041D0JB	041F4J9	041H0K9	041H4Z9	041J499	041K0AK	041K4KL	041R4JQ	041U4KP	041W4KS
041C4Z5	041D0JC	041F4JB	041H0KB	041H4ZB	041J49B	041K0AL	041K4KM	041R4JS	041U4KQ	041W4ZP
041C4Z6	041D0JD	041F4JC	041H0KC	041H4ZC	041J49C	041K0AM	041K4KN	041S0JQ	041U4KS	041W4ZQ
041C4Z7	041D0JF	041F4JD	041H0KD	041H4ZD	041J49D	041K0AN	041K4KP	041S0JS	041U4ZP	041W4ZS
041C4Z8	041D0JG	041F4JF	041H0KF	041H4ZF	041J49F	041K0AP	041K4KQ	041S3JQ	041U4ZQ	04500ZZ
041C4Z9	041D0JH	041F4JG	041H0KG	041H4ZG	041J49G	041K0AQ	041K4KS	041S3JS	041U4ZS	04503ZZ
041C4ZB	041D0JJ	041F4JH	041H0KH	041H4ZH	041J49H	041K0AS	041K4ZH	041S4JQ	041V09P	04504ZZ
041C4ZC	041D0JK	041F4JJ	041H0KJ	041H4ZJ	041J49J	041K0JH	041K4ZJ	041S4JS	041V09Q	04510ZZ
041C4ZD	041D0JQ	041F4JK	041H0KK	041H4ZK	041J49K	041K0JJ	041K4ZK	041T09P	041V09S	04513ZZ
041C4ZF	041F0AP	041F4JP	041H0KP	041H4ZP	041J49P	041K0JK	041K4ZL	041T09Q	041V0AP	04514ZZ
041C4ZG	041F0AQ	041F4JQ	041H0KQ	041H4ZQ	041J49Q	041K0JL	041L3JQ	041T09S	041V0AQ	04520ZZ
041C4ZH	041F0J9	041F4K9	041H0Z9	041J099	041J4A9	041K0JM	041L3JS	041T0AP	041V0AS	04523ZZ
041C4ZJ	041F0JB	041F4KB	041H0ZB	041J09B	041J4AB	041K0JN	041M3JQ	041T0AQ	041V0JP	04524ZZ
041C4ZK	041F0JC	041F4KC	041H0ZC	041J09C	041J4AC	041K0JP	041M3JS	041T0AS	041V0JQ	04530ZZ
041C4ZQ	041F0JD	041F4KD	041H0ZD	041J09D	041J4AD	041K0JQ	041N0KM	041T0JP	041V0JS	04533ZZ
041C4ZR	041F0JF	041F4KF	041H0ZF	041J09F	041J4AF	041K0JS	041N0KP	041T0JQ	041V0KP	04534ZZ
041D090	041F0JG	041F4KG	041H0ZG	041J09G	041J4AG	041K0KH	041N0KQ	041T0JS	041V0KQ	04540ZZ
041D091	041F0JH	041F4KH	041H0ZH	041J09H	041J4AH	041K0KJ	041N0KS	041T0KP	041V0KS	04543ZZ
041D092	041F0JJ	041F4KJ	041H0ZJ	041J09J	041J4AJ	041K0KK	041N0ZL	041T0KQ	041V0ZP	04544ZZ
041D093	041F0JK	041F4KK	041H0ZK	041J09K	041J4AK	041K0KL	041N0ZM	041T0KS	041V0ZQ	04550ZZ
041D094	041F0JP	041F4KP	041H0ZP	041J09P	041J4AP	041K0KM	041N0ZP	041T0ZP	041V0ZS	04553ZZ
041D095	041F0JQ	041F4KQ	041H0ZQ	041J09Q	041J4AQ	041K0KN	041N0ZQ	041T0ZQ	041V3JQ	04554ZZ
041D096	041F0K9	041F4Z9	041H499	041J0A9	041J4J9	041K0KP	041N0ZS	041T0ZS	041V3JS	04560ZZ
041D097	041F0KB	041F4ZB	041H49B	041J0AB	041J4JB	041K0KQ	041N3JQ	041T3JQ	041V49P	04563ZZ
041D098	041F0KC	041F4ZC	041H49C	041J0AC	041J4JC	041K0KS	041N3JS	041T3JS	041V49Q	04564ZZ
041D099	041F0KD	041F4ZD	041H49D	041J0AD	041J4JD	041K0ZH	041N49L	041T49P	041V49S	04570ZZ
041D09B	041F0KF	041F4ZF	041H49F	041J0AF	041J4JF	041K0ZJ	041N49M	041T49Q	041V4AP	04573ZZ
041D09C	041F0KG	041F4ZG	041H49G	041J0AG	041J4JG	041K0ZK	041N49P	041T49S	041V4AQ	04574ZZ
041D09D	041F0KH	041F4ZH	041H49H	041J0AH	041J4JH	041K0ZL	041N49Q	041T4AP	041V4AS	04580ZZ
041D09F	041F0KJ	041F4ZJ	041H49J	041J0AJ	041J4JJ	041K0ZM	041N49S	041T4AQ	041V4JP	04583ZZ
041D09G	041F0KK	041F4ZK	041H49K	041J0AK	041J4JK	041K0ZN	041N4AL	041T4AS	041V4JQ	04584ZZ
041D09H	041F0KP	041F4ZP	041H49P	041J0AP	041J4JP	041K0ZP	041N4AM	041T4JP	041V4JS	04590ZZ
041D09J	041F0KQ	041F4ZQ	041H49Q	041J0AQ	041J4JQ	041K0ZQ	041N4AP	041T4JQ	041V4KP	04593ZZ
041D09K	041F0Z9	041H099	041H4A9	041J0J9	041J4K9	041K0ZS	041N4AQ	041T4JS	041V4KQ	04594ZZ
041D09Q	041F0ZB	041H09B	041H4AB	041J0JB	041J4KB	041K3JQ	041N4AS	041T4KP	041V4KS	045A0ZZ
041D09R	041F0ZC	041H09C	041H4AC	041J0JC	041J4KC	041K3JS	041N4JL	041T4KQ	041V4ZP	045A3ZZ
041D0A0	041F0ZD	041H09D	041H4AD	041J0JD	041J4KD	041K49H	041N4JM	041T4KS	041V4ZQ	045A4ZZ
041D0A1	041F0ZF	041H09F	041H4AF	041J0JF	041J4KF	041K49J	041N4JP	041T4ZP	041V4ZS	045B0ZZ
041D0A2	041F0ZG	041H09G	041H4AG	041J0JG	041J4KG	041K49K	041N4JQ	041T4ZQ	041W09P	045B3ZZ
041D0A3	041F0ZH	041H09H	041H4AH	041J0JH	041J4KH	041K49L	041N4JS	041T4ZS	041W09Q	045B4ZZ
041D0A4	041F0ZJ	041H09J	041H4AJ	041J0JJ	041J4KJ	041K49M	041N4KL	041U09P	041W09S	045C0ZZ
041D0A5	041F0ZK	041H09K	041H4AK	041J0JK	041J4KK	041K49N	041N4KM	041U09Q	041W0AP	045C3ZZ
041D0A6	041F0ZP	041H09P	041H4AP	041J0JP	041J4KP	041K49P	041N4KP	041U09S	041W0AQ	045C4ZZ
041D0A7	041F0ZQ	041H09Q	041H4AQ	041J0JQ	041J4KQ	041K49Q	041N4KQ	041U0AP	041W0AS	045D0ZZ
041D0A8	041F499	041H0A9	041H4J9	041J0K9	041J4Z9	041K49S	041N4KS	041U0AQ	041W0JP	045D3ZZ
041D0A9	041F49B	041H0AB	041H4JB	041J0KB	041J4ZB	041K4AH	041N4ZL	041U0AS	041W0JQ	045D4ZZ
041D0AB	041F49C	041H0AC	041H4JC	041J0KC	041J4ZC	041K4AJ	041N4ZM	041U0JP	041W0JS	045E0ZZ
041D0AC	041F49D	041H0AD	041H4JD	041J0KD	041J4ZD	041K4AK	041N4ZP	041U0JQ	041W0KP	045E3ZZ
041D0AD	041F49F	041H0AF	041H4JF	041J0KF	041J4ZF	041K4AL	041N4ZQ	041U0JS	041W0KQ	045E4ZZ
041D0AF	041F49G	041H0AG	041H4JG	041J0KG	041J4ZG	041K4AM	041N4ZS	041U0KP	041W0KS	045F0ZZ
041D0AG	041F49H	041H0AH	041H4JH	041J0KH	041J4ZH	041K4AN	041P0JQ	041U0KQ	041W0ZP	045F3ZZ
041D0AH	041F49J	041H0AJ	041H4JJ	041J0KJ	041J4ZJ	041K4AP	041P0JS	041U0KS	041W0ZQ	045F4ZZ
041D0AJ	041F49K	041H0AK	041H4JK	041J0KK	041J4ZK	041K4AQ	041P3JQ	041U0ZP	041W0ZS	045H0ZZ
041D0AK	041F49P	041H0AP	041H4JP	041J0KP	041J4ZP	041K4AS	041P3JS	041U0ZQ	041W3JQ	045H3ZZ

045H4ZZ
045J0ZZ
045J3ZZ
045J4ZZ
045K0ZZ
045K3ZZ
045K4ZZ
045L0ZZ
045L3ZZ
045L4ZZ
045M0ZZ
045M3ZZ
045M4ZZ
045N0ZZ
045N3ZZ
045N4ZZ
045P0ZZ
045P3ZZ
045P4ZZ
045Q0ZZ
045Q3ZZ
045Q4ZZ
045R0ZZ
045R3ZZ
045R4ZZ
045S0ZZ
045S3ZZ
045S4ZZ
045T0ZZ
045T3ZZ
045T4ZZ
045U0ZZ
045U3ZZ
045U4ZZ
045V0ZZ
045V3ZZ
045V4ZZ
045W0ZZ
045W3ZZ
045W4ZZ
045Y0ZZ
045Y3ZZ
045Y4ZZ
0470041
0470046
047004Z
0470056
047005Z
0470066
047006Z
0470076
047007Z
04700D1
04700D6
04700DZ
04700E6
04700EZ
04700F6
04700FZ
04700G6
04700GZ
04700Z1
04700Z6
04700ZZ
0470341
0470346
047034Z
0470356
047035Z
0470366
047036Z
0470376
047037Z
04703D1
04703D6
04703DZ
04703E6
04703EZ
04703F6
04703FZ
04703G6
04703GZ
04703Z1
04703Z6
04703ZZ
0470441
0470446
047044Z
0470456
047045Z
0470466
047046Z
0470476
047047Z
04704D1
04704D6
04704DZ
04704E6
04704EZ
04704F6
04704FZ
04704G6
04704GZ
04704Z1
04704Z6
04704ZZ
0471041
0471046
047104Z
0471056
047105Z
0471066
047106Z
0471076
047107Z
04710D1
04710D6
04710DZ
04710E6
04710EZ
04710F6
04710FZ
04710G6
04710GZ
04710Z1
04710Z6
04710ZZ
0471341
0471346
047134Z
0471356
047135Z
0471366
047136Z
0471376
047137Z
04713D1
04713D6
04713DZ
04713E6
04730Z6
04730ZZ
0473341
0473346
047334Z
0473356
047335Z
0473366
047336Z
0473376
047337Z
04733D1
04733D6
04733DZ
04733E6
04733EZ
04733F6
04733FZ
04733G6
04733GZ
04733Z1
04733Z6
04733ZZ
0473441
0473446
047344Z
0473456
047345Z
0473466
047346Z
0473476
047347Z
04734D1
04734D6
04734DZ
04734E6
04734EZ
04734F6
04734FZ
04734G6
04734GZ
04734Z1
04734Z6
04734ZZ
0474041
0474046
047404Z
0474056
047405Z
0474066
047406Z
0474076
047407Z
04740D1
04740D6
04740DZ
04740E6
04740EZ
04740F6
04740FZ
04740G6
04740GZ
04740Z1
04740Z6
04740ZZ
0474341
0474346
047434Z
0474356
047435Z
0474366
047436Z
0474376
047437Z
04743D1
04743D6
04743DZ
04743E6
04743EZ
04743F6
04743FZ
04743G6
04743GZ
04743Z1
04743Z6
04743ZZ
0474441
0474446
047444Z
0474456
047445Z
0474466
047446Z
0474476
047447Z
04744D1
04744D6
04744DZ
04744E6
04744EZ
04744F6
04744FZ
04744G6
04744GZ
04744Z1
04744Z6
04744ZZ
0475041
0475046
047504Z
0475056
047505Z
0475066
047506Z
0475076
047507Z
04750D1
04750D6
04750DZ
04750E6
04750EZ
04750F6
04750FZ
04750G6
04750GZ
04750Z1
04750Z6
04750ZZ
0475341
0475346
047534Z
0475356
047535Z
0475366
047536Z
0475376
047537Z
04753D1
04753D6
04753DZ
04753E6
04753EZ
04753F6
04753FZ
04753G6
04753GZ
04753Z1
04753Z6
04753ZZ
0475441
0475446
047544Z
0475456
047545Z
0475466
047546Z
0475476
047547Z
04754D1
04754D6
04754DZ
04754E6
04754EZ
04754F6
04754FZ
04754G6
04754GZ
04754Z1
04754Z6
04754ZZ
0476041
0476046
047604Z
0476056
047605Z
0476066
047606Z
0476076
04773DZ
04773E6
04773EZ
04773F6
04773FZ
04773G6
04773GZ
04773Z1
04773Z6
04773ZZ
0477441
0477446
047744Z
0477456
047745Z
0477466
047746Z
0477476
047747Z
04774D1
04774D6
04774DZ
04774E6
04774EZ
04774F6
04774FZ
04774G6
04774GZ
04774Z1
04774Z6
04774ZZ
0478041
0478046
047804Z
0478056
047805Z
0478066
047806Z
0478076
047807Z
04780D1
04780D6
04780DZ
04780E6
04780EZ
04780F6
04780FZ
04780G6
04780GZ
04780Z1
04780Z6
04780ZZ
0478341
0478346
047834Z
0478356
047835Z
0478366
047836Z
0478376
047837Z
04783D1
04783D6
04783DZ
04783E6
04783EZ
04783F6
04783FZ
04783G6
04783GZ
04783Z1
04783Z6
04783ZZ
0478441
0478446
047844Z
0478456
047845Z
0478466
047846Z
0478476
047847Z
04784D1
04784D6
04784DZ
04784E6
04784EZ
04784F6
04784FZ
04784G6
04784GZ
04784Z1
04784Z6
04784ZZ
0479041
0479046
047904Z
0479056
047905Z
0479066
047906Z
0479076
047907Z
04790D1
04790D6
04790DZ
04790E6
04790EZ
04790F6
04790FZ
04790G6
04790GZ
04790Z1
04790Z6
04790ZZ
0479341
0479346
047934Z
0479356
047935Z
0479366
047936Z
0479376
047937Z
04793D1
04793D6
04793DZ
04793E6
04793EZ
04793F6
04793FZ
04793G6
04793GZ
04793Z1
04793Z6
04793ZZ
0479441
0479446
047944Z
0479456
047945Z
0479466
047946Z
0479476
047947Z
04794D1
04794D6
04794DZ
04794E6
04794EZ
04794F6
04794FZ
04794G6
04794GZ
04794Z1
04794Z6
04794ZZ
047A041
047A046
047A04Z
047A056
047A05Z
047A066
047A06Z
047A076
047A07Z
047A0D1
047A0D6
047A0DZ
047A0E6
047A0EZ
047A0F6
047A0FZ
047A0G6
047A0GZ
047A0Z1
047A0Z6
047A0ZZ
047A341
047A346
047A34Z
047A356
047A35Z
047A366
047A36Z
047A376
047A37Z
047A3D1
047B476
047B47Z
047B4D1
047B4D6
047B4DZ
047B4E6
047B4EZ
047B4F6
047B4FZ
047B4G6
047B4GZ
047B4Z1
047B4Z6
047B4ZZ
047C041
047C046
047C04Z
047C056
047C05Z
047C066
047C06Z
047C076
047C07Z
047C0D1
047C0D6
047C0DZ
047C0E6
047C0EZ
047C0F6
047C0FZ
047C0G6
047C0GZ
047C0Z1
047C0Z6
047C0ZZ
047C341
047C346
047C34Z
047C356
047C35Z
047C366
047C36Z
047C376
047C37Z
047C3D1
047C3D6
047C3DZ
047C3E6
047C3EZ
047C3F6
047C3FZ
047C3G6
047C3GZ
047C3Z1
047C3Z6
047C3ZZ
047C441
047C446
047C44Z
047C456
047C45Z
047C466
047C46Z
047C476
047C47Z
047C4D1
047C4D6
047C4DZ
047C4E6
047C4EZ
047C4F6
047C4FZ
047C4G6
047C4GZ
047C4Z1
047C4Z6
047C4ZZ
047D041
047D046
047D04Z
047D056
047D05Z
047D066
047D06Z
047D076
047D07Z
047D0D1
047D0D6
047D0DZ
047D0E6
047D0EZ
047D0F6
047D0FZ
047D0G6
047D0GZ
047D0Z1
047D0Z6
047D0ZZ
047D341
047D346
047D34Z
047D356
047D35Z
047D366
047D36Z
047D376
047D37Z
047D3D1
047D3D6
047D3DZ
047D3E6
047D3EZ
047D3F6
047D3FZ
047D3G6
047D3GZ
047D3Z1
047D3Z6
047D3ZZ
047D441
047D446
047D44Z
047D456
047D45Z
047D466
047D46Z
047D476
047D47Z
047D4D1
047D4D6
047D4DZ
047D4E6
047D4EZ
047D4F6
047D4FZ
047D4G6
047D4GZ
047D4Z1
047D4Z6
047D4ZZ
047E041
047E046
047E04Z
047E056
047E05Z
047E066
047E06Z
047E076
047E07Z
047E0D1
047E0D6
047E0DZ
047E0E6
047E0EZ
047E0F6
047E0FZ
047E0G6
047E0GZ
047E0Z1
047E0Z6
047E0ZZ
047E341
047E346
047E34Z
047E356
047E35Z
047E366
047E36Z
047E376
047E37Z
047E3D1
047E3D6
047E3DZ
047E3E6
047E3EZ
047E3F6
047E3FZ
047E3G6
047E3GZ
047E3Z1
047E3Z6
047E3ZZ
047H37Z
047H3D1
047H3D6
047H3DZ
047H3E6
047H3EZ
047H3F6
047H3FZ
047H3G6
047H3GZ
047H3Z1
047H3Z6
047H3ZZ
047H441
047H446
047H44Z
047H456
047H45Z
047H466
047H46Z
047H476
047H47Z
047H4D1
047H4D6
047H4DZ
047H4E6
047H4EZ
047H4F6
047H4FZ
047H4G6
047H4GZ
047H4Z1
047H4Z6
047H4ZZ
047J041
047J046
047J04Z
047J056

047J05Z
047J066
047J06Z
047J076
047J07Z
047J0D1
047J0D6
047J0DZ
047J0E6
047J0EZ
047J0F6
047J0FZ
047J0G6
047J0GZ
047J0Z1
047J0Z6
047J0ZZ
047J341
047J346
047J34Z
047J356
047J35Z
047J366
047J36Z
047J376
047J37Z
047J3D1
047J3D6
047J3DZ
047J3E6
047J3EZ
047J3F6
047J3FZ
047J3G6
047J3GZ
047J3Z1
047J3Z6
047J3ZZ
047J441
047J446
047J44Z
047J456
047J45Z
047J466
047J46Z
047J476
047J47Z
047J4D1
047J4D6
047J4DZ
047J4E6
047J4EZ
047J4F6
047J4FZ
047J4G6
047J4GZ
047J4Z1
047J4Z6
047J4ZZ
047K041
047K046
047K04Z
047K056
047K05Z
047K066
047K06Z
047K076
047K07Z
047K0D1
047K0D6
047K0DZ
047K0E6
047K0EZ
047K0F6
047K0FZ
047K0G6
047K0GZ
047K0Z1
047K0Z6
047K0ZZ
047K341
047K346
047K34Z
047K356
047K35Z
047K366
047K36Z
047K376
047K37Z
047K3D1
047K3D6
047K3DZ
047K3E6
047K3EZ
047K3F6
047K3FZ
047K3G6
047K3GZ
047K3Z1
047K3Z6
047K3ZZ
047K441
047K446
047K44Z
047K456
047K45Z
047K466
047K46Z
047K476
047K47Z
047K4D1
047K4D6
047K4DZ
047K4E6
047K4EZ
047K4F6
047K4FZ
047K4G6
047K4GZ
047K4Z1
047K4Z6
047K4ZZ
047L041
047L046
047L04Z
047L056
047L05Z
047L066
047L06Z
047L076
047L07Z
047L0D1
047L0D6
047L0DZ
047L0E6
047L0EZ
047L0F6
047L0FZ
047M446
047M44Z
047M456
047M45Z
047M466
047M46Z
047M476
047M47Z
047M4D1
047M4D6
047M4DZ
047M4E6
047M4EZ
047M4F6
047M4FZ
047M4G6
047M4GZ
047M4Z1
047M4Z6
047M4ZZ
047N041
047N046
047N04Z
047N056
047N05Z
047N066
047N06Z
047N076
047N07Z
047N0D1
047N0D6
047N0DZ
047N0E6
047N0EZ
047N0F6
047N0FZ
047N0G6
047N0GZ
047N0Z1
047N0Z6
047N0ZZ
047N341
047N346
047N34Z
047N356
047N35Z
047N366
047N36Z
047N376
047N37Z
047N3D1
047N3D6
047N3DZ
047N3E6
047N3EZ
047N3F6
047N3FZ
047N3G6
047N3GZ
047N3Z1
047N3Z6
047N3ZZ
047N441
047N446
047N44Z
047N456
047N45Z
047N466
047N46Z
047N476
047N47Z
047N4D1
047N4D6
047N4DZ
047N4E6
047N4EZ
047N4F6
047N4FZ
047N4G6
047N4GZ
047N4Z1
047N4Z6
047N4ZZ
047P041
047P046
047P04Z
047P056
047P05Z
047P066
047P06Z
047P076
047P07Z
047P0D1
047P0D6
047P0DZ
047P0E6
047P0EZ
047P0F6
047P0FZ
047P0G6
047P0GZ
047P0Z1
047P0Z6
047P0ZZ
047P341
047P346
047P34Z
047P356
047P35Z
047P366
047P36Z
047P376
047P37Z
047P3D1
047P3D6
047P3DZ
047P3E6
047P3EZ
047P3F6
047P3FZ
047P3G6
047P3GZ
047P3Z1
047P3Z6
047P3ZZ
047P441
047P446
047P44Z
047P456
047P45Z
047P466
047P46Z
047P476
047P47Z
047P4D1
047P4D6
047P4DZ
047P4E6
047P4EZ
047P4F6
047P4FZ
047P4G6
047P4GZ
047P4Z1
047P4Z6
047P4ZZ
047Q041
047Q046
047Q04Z
047Q056
047Q05Z
047Q066
047Q06Z
047Q076
047Q07Z
047Q0D1
047Q0D6
047Q0DZ
047Q0E6
047Q0EZ
047Q0F6
047Q0FZ
047Q0G6
047Q0GZ
047Q0Z1
047Q0Z6
047Q0ZZ
047Q341
047Q346
047Q34Z
047Q356
047Q35Z
047Q366
047Q36Z
047Q376
047Q37Z
047Q3D1
047Q3D6
047Q3DZ
047Q3E6
047Q3EZ
047Q3F6
047Q3FZ
047Q3G6
047Q3GZ
047Q3Z1
047Q3Z6
047Q3ZZ
047Q441
047Q446
047Q44Z
047Q456
047Q45Z
047Q466
047Q46Z
047Q476
047Q47Z
047Q4D1
047Q4D6
047Q4DZ
047Q4E6
047Q4EZ
047Q4F6
047Q4FZ
047Q4G6
047Q4GZ
047Q4Z1
047Q4Z6
047Q4ZZ
047R041
047R046
047R04Z
047R056
047R05Z
047R066
047R06Z
047R076
047R07Z
047R0D1
047R0D6
047R0DZ
047R0E6
047R0EZ
047R0F6
047R0FZ
047R0G6
047R0GZ
047R0Z1
047R0Z6
047R0ZZ
047R341
047R346
047R34Z
047R356
047R35Z
047R366
047R36Z
047R376
047R37Z
047R3D1
047R3D6
047R3DZ
047R3E6
047R3EZ
047R3F6
047R3FZ
047R3G6
047R3GZ
047R3Z1
047R3Z6
047R3ZZ
047R441
047R446
047R44Z
047R456
047R45Z
047R466
047R46Z
047R476
047R47Z
047R4D1
047R4D6
047R4DZ
047R4E6
047R4EZ
047R4F6
047R4FZ
047R4G6
047R4GZ
047R4Z1
047R4Z6
047R4ZZ
047S041
047S046
047S04Z
047S056
047S05Z
047S066
047S06Z
047S076
047S07Z
047S0D1
047S0D6
047S0DZ
047S0E6
047S0EZ
047S0F6
047S0FZ
047S0G6
047S0GZ
047S0Z1
047S0Z6
047S0ZZ
047S341
047S346
047S34Z
047S356
047S35Z
047S366
047S36Z
047S376
047S37Z
047S3D1
047S3D6
047S3DZ
047S3E6
047S3EZ
047S3F6
047S3FZ
047S3G6
047S3GZ
047S3Z1
047S3Z6
047S3ZZ
047S441
047S446
047S44Z
047S456
047S45Z
047S466
047S46Z
047S476
047S47Z
047S4D1
047S4D6
047S4DZ
047S4E6
047S4EZ
047S4F6
047S4FZ
047S4G6
047S4GZ
047S4Z1
047S4Z6
047S4ZZ
047T041
047T046
047T04Z
047T056
047T05Z
047T066
047T06Z
047T076
047T07Z
047T0D1
047T0D6
047T0DZ
047T0E6
047T0EZ
047T0F6
047T0FZ
047T0G6
047T0GZ
047T0Z1
047T0Z6
047T0ZZ
047T341
047T346
047T34Z
047T356
047T35Z
047T366
047T36Z
047T376
047T37Z
047T3D1
047T3D6
047T3DZ
047T3E6
047T3EZ
047T3F6
047T3FZ
047T3G6
047T3GZ
047T3Z1
047T3Z6
047T3ZZ
047T441
047T446
047T44Z
047T456
047T45Z
047T466
047T46Z
047T476
047T47Z
047T4D1
047T4D6
047T4DZ
047T4E6
047T4EZ
047T4F6
047T4FZ
047T4G6
047T4GZ
047T4Z1
047T4Z6
047T4ZZ
047U041
047U046
047U04Z
047U056
047U05Z
047U066
047U06Z
047U076
047U07Z
047U0D1
047U0D6
047U0DZ
047U0E6
047U0EZ
047U0F6
047U0FZ
047U0G6
047U0GZ
047U0Z1
047U0Z6
047U0ZZ
047U341
047U346
047U34Z
047U356
047U35Z
047U366
047U36Z
047U376
047U37Z
047U3D1
047U3D6
047U3DZ
047U3E6
047U3EZ
047U3F6
047U3FZ
047U3G6
047U3GZ
047U3Z1
047U3Z6
047U3ZZ
047U441
047U446
047U44Z
047U456
047U45Z
047U466
047U46Z
047U476
047U47Z
047U4D1
047U4D6
047U4DZ
047U4E6
047U4EZ
047U4F6
047U4FZ
047U4G6
047U4GZ
047U4Z1
047U4Z6
047U4ZZ
047V041
047V046
047V04Z
047V056
047V05Z
047V066
047V06Z
047V076
047V07Z
047V0D1
047V0D6
047V0DZ
047V0E6
047V0EZ
047V0F6
047V0FZ
047V0G6
047V0GZ
047V0Z1
047V0Z6
047V0ZZ
047V341
047V346
047V34Z
047V356
047V35Z
047V366
047V36Z
047V376
047V37Z
047V3D1
047V3D6
047V3DZ
047V3E6
047V3EZ
047V3F6
047V3FZ
047V3G6
047V3GZ
047V3Z1
047V3Z6
047V3ZZ
047V441
047V446
047V44Z
047V456
047V45Z
047V466
047V46Z
047V476
047V47Z
047V4D1
047V4D6
047V4DZ
047V4E6
047V4EZ
047V4F6
047V4FZ
047V4G6
047V4GZ
047V4Z1
047V4Z6
047V4ZZ
047W041
047W046
047W04Z
047W056
047W05Z
047W066
047W06Z
047W076
047W07Z
047W0D1
047W0D6
047W0DZ
047W0E6
047W0EZ
047W0F6
047W0FZ
047W0G6
047W0GZ
047W0Z1
047W0Z6
047W0ZZ
047W341
047W346
047W34Z
047W356
047W35Z
047W366
047W36Z
047W376
047W37Z
047W3D1
047W3D6
047W3DZ
047W3E6
047W3EZ
047W3F6
047W3FZ
047W3G6
047W3GZ
047W3Z1
047W3Z6
047W3ZZ
047W441
047W446
047W44Z
047W456
047W45Z
047W466
047W46Z
047W476
047W47Z
047W4D1
047W4D6
047W4DZ
047W4E6
047W4EZ
047W4F6
047W4FZ
047W4G6
047W4GZ
047W4Z1
047W4Z6
047W4ZZ
047Y041

047Y046
047Y04Z
047Y056
047Y05Z
047Y066
047Y06Z
047Y076
047Y07Z
047Y0D1
047Y0D6
047Y0DZ
047Y0E6
047Y0EZ
047Y0F6
047Y0FZ
047Y0G6
047Y0GZ
047Y0Z1
047Y0Z6
047Y0ZZ
047Y341
047Y346
047Y34Z
047Y356
047Y35Z
047Y366
047Y36Z
047Y376
049000Z
04900ZZ
049030Z
04903ZX
04903ZZ
049040Z
04904ZZ
049100Z
04910ZZ
049130Z
04913ZX
04913ZZ
049140Z
04914ZZ
049200Z
04920ZZ
049230Z
04923ZX
04923ZZ
049240Z
04924ZZ
049300Z
04930ZZ
049330Z
04933ZX
04933ZZ
049340Z
04934ZZ
049400Z
04940ZZ
049430Z
04943ZX
04943ZZ
049440Z
04944ZZ
049500Z
04950ZZ
049530Z
04953ZX
04953ZZ
049540Z
04954ZZ
049600Z
04960ZZ
049630Z
04963ZX
04963ZZ
049640Z
04964ZZ
049700Z
04970ZZ
049730Z
04973ZX
04973ZZ
049740Z
04974ZZ
049800Z
04980ZZ
049830Z
04983ZX
04983ZZ
049840Z
04984ZZ
049900Z
04990ZZ
049930Z
04993ZX
04993ZZ
049940Z
04994ZZ
049A00Z
049A0ZZ
049A30Z
049A3ZX
049A3ZZ
049A40Z
049A4ZZ
049B00Z
049B0ZZ
049B30Z
049B3ZX
049B3ZZ
049B40Z
049B4ZZ
049C00Z
049C0ZZ
049C30Z
049C3ZX
049C3ZZ
049C40Z
049C4ZZ
049D00Z
049D0ZZ
049D30Z
049D3ZX
049D3ZZ
049D40Z
049D4ZZ
049E00Z
049E0ZZ
049E30Z
049E3ZX
049E3ZZ
049E40Z
049E4ZZ
049F00Z
049F0ZZ
049F30Z
049F3ZX
049F3ZZ
049F40Z
049F4ZZ
049H00Z
049H0ZZ
049H30Z
049H3ZX
049H3ZZ
049H40Z
049H4ZZ
049J00Z
049J0ZZ
049J30Z
049J3ZX
049J3ZZ
049J40Z
049J4ZZ
049K00Z
049K0ZZ
049K30Z
049K3ZX
049K3ZZ
049K40Z
049K4ZZ
049L00Z
049L0ZZ
049L30Z
049L3ZX
049L3ZZ
049L40Z
049L4ZZ
049M00Z
049M0ZZ
049M30Z
049M3ZX
049M3ZZ
049M40Z
049M4ZZ
049N00Z
049N0ZZ
049N30Z
049N3ZX
049N3ZZ
049N40Z
049N4ZZ
049P00Z
049P0ZZ
049P30Z
049P3ZX
049P3ZZ
049P40Z
049P4ZZ
049Q00Z
049Q0ZZ
049Q30Z
049Q3ZX
049Q3ZZ
049Q40Z
049Q4ZZ
049R00Z
049R0ZZ
049R30Z
049R3ZX
049R3ZZ
049R40Z
049R4ZZ
049S00Z
049S0ZZ
049S30Z
049S3ZX
049S3ZZ
049S40Z
049S4ZZ
049T00Z
049T0ZZ
049T30Z
049T3ZX
049T3ZZ
049T40Z
049T4ZZ
049U00Z
049U0ZZ
049U30Z
049U3ZX
049U3ZZ
049U40Z
049U4ZZ
049V00Z
049V0ZZ
049V30Z
049V3ZX
049V3ZZ
049V40Z
049V4ZZ
049W00Z
049W0ZZ
049W30Z
049W3ZX
049W3ZZ
049W40Z
049W4ZZ
049Y00Z
049Y0ZZ
049Y30Z
049Y3ZX
049Y3ZZ
049Y40Z
049Y4ZZ
04BC3ZX
04BC3ZZ
04BC4ZX
04BC4ZZ
04BD0ZX
04BD0ZZ
04BD3ZX
04BD3ZZ
04BD4ZX
04BD4ZZ
04BE0ZX
04BE0ZZ
04BE3ZX
04BE3ZZ
04BE4ZX
04BE4ZZ
04BF0ZX
04BF0ZZ
04BF3ZX
04BF3ZZ
04BF4ZX
04BF4ZZ
04BH0ZX
04BH0ZZ
04BH3ZX
04BH3ZZ
04BH4ZX
04BH4ZZ
04BJ0ZX
04BJ0ZZ
04BJ3ZX
04BJ3ZZ
04BJ4ZX
04BJ4ZZ
04BK0ZX
04BK0ZZ
04BK3ZX
04BK3ZZ
04BK4ZX
04BK4ZZ
04BL0ZX
04BL0ZZ
04BL3ZX
04BL3ZZ
04BL4ZX
04BL4ZZ
04BM0ZX
04BM0ZZ
04BM3ZX
04BM3ZZ
04BM4ZX
04BM4ZZ
04BN0ZX
04BN0ZZ
04BN3ZX
04BN3ZZ
04BN4ZX
04BN4ZZ
04BP0ZX
04BP0ZZ
04BP3ZX
04BP3ZZ
04BP4ZX
04BP4ZZ
04BQ0ZX
04BQ0ZZ
04BQ3ZX
04BQ3ZZ
04BQ4ZX
04BQ4ZZ
04BR0ZX
04BR0ZZ
04BR3ZX
04BR3ZZ
04BR4ZX
04BR4ZZ
04BS0ZX
04BS0ZZ
04BS3ZX
04BS3ZZ
04BS4ZX
04BS4ZZ
04BT0ZX
04BT0ZZ
04BT3ZX
04BT3ZZ
04BT4ZX
04BT4ZZ
04BU0ZX
04BU0ZZ
04BU3ZX
04BU3ZZ
04BU4ZX
04BU4ZZ
04BV0ZX
04BV0ZZ
04BV3ZX
04BV3ZZ
04BV4ZX
04BV4ZZ
04BW0ZX
04BW0ZZ
04BW3ZX
04BW3ZZ
04BW4ZX
04BW4ZZ
04BY0ZX
04BY0ZZ
04BY3ZX
04BY3ZZ
04BY4ZX
04BY4ZZ
04C00Z6
04C00ZZ
04C03Z6
04C03ZZ
04C04Z6
04C04ZZ
04C10Z6
04C10ZZ
04C13Z6
04C13ZZ
04C14Z6
04C14ZZ
04C20Z6
04C20ZZ
04C23Z6
04C23ZZ
04C24Z6
04C24ZZ
04C30Z6
04C30ZZ
04C33Z6
04C33ZZ
04C34Z6
04C34ZZ
04C40Z6
04C40ZZ
04C43Z6
04C43ZZ
04C44Z6
04C44ZZ
04C50Z6
04C50ZZ
04C53Z6
04C53ZZ
04C54Z6
04C54ZZ
04C60Z6
04C60ZZ
04C63Z6
04C63ZZ
04C64Z6
04C64ZZ
04C70Z6
04C70ZZ
04C73Z6
04C73ZZ
04C74Z6
04C74ZZ
04C80Z6
04C80ZZ
04C83Z6
04C83ZZ
04C84Z6
04C84ZZ
04C90Z6
04C90ZZ
04C93Z6
04C93ZZ
04C94Z6
04C94ZZ
04CA0Z6
04CA0ZZ
04CA3Z6
04CA3ZZ
04CA4Z6
04CA4ZZ
04CB0Z6
04CB0ZZ
04CB3Z6
04CB3ZZ
04CB4Z6
04CB4ZZ
04CC0Z6
04CC0ZZ
04CC3Z6
04CC3ZZ
04CC4Z6
04CC4ZZ
04CD0Z6
04CD0ZZ
04CD3Z6
04CD3ZZ
04CD4Z6
04CD4ZZ
04CE0Z6
04CE0ZZ
04CE3Z6
04CE3ZZ
04CE4Z6
04CE4ZZ
04CF0Z6
04CF0ZZ
04CF3Z6
04CF3ZZ
04CF4Z6
04CF4ZZ
04CH0Z6
04CH0ZZ
04CH3Z6
04CH3ZZ
04CH4Z6
04CH4ZZ
04CJ0Z6
04CJ0ZZ
04CJ3Z6
04CJ3ZZ
04CJ4Z6
04CJ4ZZ
04CW0ZZ
04CW3Z6
04CW3ZZ
04CW4Z6
04CW4ZZ
04CY0Z6
04CY0ZZ
04CY3Z6
04CY3ZZ
04CY4Z6
04CY4ZZ
04H002Z
04H003Z
04H00DZ
04H032Z
04H033Z
04H03DZ
04H042Z
04H043Z
04H04DZ
04H103Z
04H10DZ
04H133Z
04H13DZ
04H143Z
04H14DZ
04H203Z
04H20DZ
04H233Z
04H23DZ
04H243Z
04H24DZ
04H303Z
04H30DZ
04H333Z
04H33DZ
04H343Z
04H34DZ
04H403Z
04H40DZ
04H433Z
04H43DZ
04H443Z
04H44DZ
04H503Z
04H50DZ
04H533Z
04H53DZ
04H543Z
04H54DZ
04H603Z
04H60DZ
04H633Z
04H63DZ
04H643Z
04H64DZ
04H703Z
04H70DZ
04H733Z
04H73DZ
04H743Z
04H74DZ
04H803Z
04H80DZ
04H833Z
04H83DZ
04H843Z
04H84DZ
04H903Z
04H90DZ
04H933Z
04H93DZ
04H943Z
04H94DZ
04HA03Z
04HA0DZ
04HA33Z
04HA3DZ
04HA43Z
04HA4DZ
04HB03Z
04HB0DZ
04HB33Z
04HB3DZ
04HB43Z
04HB4DZ
04HC03Z
04HC0DZ
04HC33Z
04HC3DZ
04HC43Z
04HC4DZ
04HD03Z
04HD0DZ
04HD33Z
04HD3DZ
04HD43Z
04HD4DZ
04HE03Z
04HE0DZ
04HE33Z
04HE3DZ
04HE43Z
04HE4DZ
04HF03Z
04HF0DZ
04HF33Z
04HF3DZ
04HF43Z
04HF4DZ
04HH03Z
04HH0DZ
04HH33Z
04HH3DZ
04HH43Z
04HH4DZ
04HJ03Z
04HJ0DZ
04HJ33Z
04HJ3DZ
04HJ43Z
04HJ4DZ
04HK03Z
04HK0DZ
04HK33Z
04HK3DZ
04HK43Z
04HK4DZ
04HL03Z
04HL0DZ
04HL33Z
04HL3DZ
04HL43Z
04HL4DZ
04HM03Z
04HM0DZ
04HM33Z
04HM3DZ
04HM43Z
04HM4DZ
04HN03Z
04HN0DZ
04HN33Z
04HN3DZ
04HN43Z
04HN4DZ
04HP03Z
04HP0DZ
04HP33Z
04HP3DZ
04HP43Z
04HP4DZ
04HQ03Z
04HQ0DZ
04HQ33Z
04HQ3DZ
04HQ43Z
04HQ4DZ
04HR03Z
04HR0DZ
04HR33Z
04HR3DZ
04HR43Z
04HR4DZ
04HS03Z
04HS0DZ
04HS33Z
04HS3DZ
04HS43Z
04HS4DZ
04HT03Z
04HT0DZ
04HT33Z
04HT3DZ
04HT43Z
04HT4DZ
04HU03Z
04HU0DZ
04HU33Z
04HU3DZ
04HU43Z
04HU4DZ
04HV03Z
04HV0DZ
04HV33Z
04HV3DZ
04HV43Z
04HV4DZ
04HW03Z
04HW0DZ
04HW33Z
04HW3DZ
04HW43Z
04HW4DZ
04HY02Z
04HY03Z
04HY0DZ
04HY0YZ
04HY32Z
04HY33Z
04HY3DZ
04HY3YZ
04HY42Z
04HY43Z
04HY4DZ
04HY4YZ
04JY0ZZ
04JY3ZZ
04JY4ZZ
04JYXZZ
04L00CZ
04L00DZ
04L00ZZ
04L03CZ
04L03DJ
04L03DZ
04L03ZZ
04L04CZ
04L04DZ
04L04ZZ
04L10CZ
04L10DZ
04L10ZZ
04L13CZ
04L13DZ
04L13ZZ
04L14CZ
04L14DZ
04L14ZZ
04L20CZ
04L20DZ
04L20ZZ
04L23CZ
04L23DZ
04L23ZZ
04L24CZ
04L24DZ
04L24ZZ
04L30CZ
04L30DZ
04L30ZZ
04L33CZ
04L33DZ
04L33ZZ
04L34CZ
04L34DZ
04L34ZZ
04L40CZ
04L40DZ
04L40ZZ
04L43CZ
04L43DZ
04L43ZZ
04L44CZ
04L44DZ
04L44ZZ
04L50CZ
04L50DZ
04L50ZZ
04L53CZ
04L53DZ

04L53ZZ
04L54CZ
04L54DZ
04L54ZZ
04L60CZ
04L60DZ
04L60ZZ
04LH4ZZ
04LJ0CZ
04LJ0DZ
04LJ0ZZ
04LJ3CZ
04LJ3DZ
04LJ3ZZ
04LJ4CZ
04LJ4DZ
04LJ4ZZ
04LK0CZ
04LK0DZ
04LK0ZZ
04LK3CZ
04LK3DZ
04LK3ZZ
04LK4CZ
04LK4DZ
04LK4ZZ
04LL0CZ
04LL0DZ
04LL0ZZ
04LL3CZ
04LL3DZ
04LL3ZZ
04LL4CZ
04LL4DZ
04LL4ZZ
04LM0CZ
04LM0DZ
04LM0ZZ
04LM3CZ
04LM3DZ
04LM3ZZ
04LM4CZ
04LM4DZ
04LM4ZZ
04LN0CZ
04LN0DZ
04LN0ZZ
04LN3CZ
04LN3DZ
04LN3ZZ
04LN4CZ
04LN4DZ
04LN4ZZ
04LP0CZ
04LP0DZ
04LP0ZZ
04LP3CZ
04LP3DZ
04LP3ZZ
04LP4CZ
04LP4DZ
04LP4ZZ
04LQ0CZ
04LQ0DZ
04LQ0ZZ
04LQ3CZ
04LQ3DZ
04LQ3ZZ
04LQ4CZ
04LQ4DZ
04LQ4ZZ
04LR0CZ
04LR0DZ
04LR0ZZ
04LR3CZ
04LR3DZ
04LR3ZZ
04LR4CZ
04LR4DZ
04LR4ZZ
04LS0CZ
04LS0DZ
04LS0ZZ
04LS3CZ
04LS3DZ
04LS3ZZ
04LS4CZ
04LS4DZ
04LS4ZZ
04LT0CZ
04LT0DZ
04LT0ZZ
04LT3CZ
04LT3DZ
04LT3ZZ
04LT4CZ
04LT4DZ
04LT4ZZ
04LU0CZ
04LU0DZ
04LU0ZZ
04LU3CZ
04LU3DZ
04LU3ZZ
04LU4CZ
04LU4DZ
04LU4ZZ
04LV0CZ
04LV0DZ
04LV0ZZ
04LV3CZ
04LV3DZ
04LV3ZZ
04LV4CZ
04LV4DZ
04LV4ZZ
04LW0CZ
04LW0DZ
04LW0ZZ
04LW3CZ
04LW3DZ
04LW3ZZ
04LW4CZ
04LW4DZ
04LW4ZZ
04LY0CZ
04LY0DZ
04LY0ZZ
04LY3CZ
04LY3DZ
04LY3ZZ
04LY4CZ
04LY4DZ
04LY4ZZ
04N00ZZ
04N03ZZ
04N04ZZ
04N10ZZ
04N13ZZ
04N14ZZ
04N20ZZ
04N23ZZ
04N24ZZ
04N30ZZ
04N33ZZ
04N34ZZ
04N40ZZ
04N43ZZ
04N44ZZ
04N50ZZ
04N53ZZ
04N54ZZ
04N60ZZ
04N63ZZ
04N64ZZ
04N70ZZ
04N73ZZ
04N74ZZ
04N80ZZ
04N83ZZ
04N84ZZ
04N90ZZ
04N93ZZ
04N94ZZ
04NA0ZZ
04NA3ZZ
04NA4ZZ
04NB0ZZ
04NB3ZZ
04NB4ZZ
04NC0ZZ
04NC3ZZ
04NC4ZZ
04ND0ZZ
04ND3ZZ
04ND4ZZ
04NE0ZZ
04NE3ZZ
04NE4ZZ
04NF0ZZ
04NF3ZZ
04NF4ZZ
04NH0ZZ
04NH3ZZ
04NH4ZZ
04NJ0ZZ
04NJ3ZZ
04NJ4ZZ
04NK0ZZ
04NK3ZZ
04NK4ZZ
04NL0ZZ
04NL3ZZ
04NL4ZZ
04NM0ZZ
04NM3ZZ
04NM4ZZ
04NN0ZZ
04NN3ZZ
04NN4ZZ
04NP0ZZ
04NP3ZZ
04NP4ZZ
04NQ0ZZ
04NQ3ZZ
04NQ4ZZ
04NR0ZZ
04NR3ZZ
04NR4ZZ
04NS0ZZ
04NS3ZZ
04NS4ZZ
04NT0ZZ
04NT3ZZ
04NT4ZZ
04NU0ZZ
04NU3ZZ
04NU4ZZ
04NV0ZZ
04NV3ZZ
04NV4ZZ
04NW0ZZ
04NW3ZZ
04NW4ZZ
04NY0ZZ
04NY3ZZ
04NY4ZZ
04PY00Z
04PY02Z
04PY03Z
04PY07Z
04PY0CZ
04PY0DZ
04PY0JZ
04PY0KZ
04PY0YZ
04PY30Z
04PY32Z
04PY33Z
04PY37Z
04PY3CZ
04PY3DZ
04PY3JZ
04PY3KZ
04PY3YZ
04PY40Z
04PY42Z
04PY43Z
04PY47Z
04PY4CZ
04PY4DZ
04PY4JZ
04PY4KZ
04PY4YZ
04PYX0Z
04PYX1Z
04PYX2Z
04PYX3Z
04PYXDZ
04Q00ZZ
04Q03ZZ
04Q04ZZ
04Q10ZZ
04Q13ZZ
04Q14ZZ
04Q20ZZ
04Q23ZZ
04Q24ZZ
04Q30ZZ
04Q33ZZ
04Q34ZZ
04Q40ZZ
04Q43ZZ
04Q44ZZ
04Q50ZZ
04Q53ZZ
04Q54ZZ
04Q60ZZ
04Q63ZZ
04Q64ZZ
04Q70ZZ
04Q73ZZ
04Q74ZZ
04Q80ZZ
04Q83ZZ
04Q84ZZ
04Q90ZZ
04Q93ZZ
04Q94ZZ
04QA0ZZ
04QA3ZZ
04QA4ZZ
04QB0ZZ
04QB3ZZ
04QB4ZZ
04QC0ZZ
04QC3ZZ
04QC4ZZ
04QD0ZZ
04QD3ZZ
04QD4ZZ
04QE0ZZ
04QE3ZZ
04QE4ZZ
04QF0ZZ
04QF3ZZ
04QF4ZZ
04QH0ZZ
04QH3ZZ
04QH4ZZ
04QJ0ZZ
04QJ3ZZ
04QJ4ZZ
04QK0ZZ
04QK3ZZ
04RC0KZ
04RC47Z
04RC4JZ
04RC4KZ
04RD07Z
04RD0JZ
04RD0KZ
04RD47Z
04RD4JZ
04RD4KZ
04RE07Z
04RE0JZ
04RE0KZ
04RE47Z
04RE4JZ
04RE4KZ
04RF07Z
04RF0JZ
04RF0KZ
04RF47Z
04RF4JZ
04RF4KZ
04RH07Z
04RH0JZ
04RH0KZ
04RH47Z
04RH4JZ
04RH4KZ
04RJ07Z
04RJ0JZ
04RJ0KZ
04RJ47Z
04RJ4JZ
04RJ4KZ
04RK07Z
04RK0JZ
04RK0KZ
04RK47Z
04RK4JZ
04RK4KZ
04RL07Z
04RL0JZ
04RL0KZ
04RL47Z
04RL4JZ
04RL4KZ
04RM07Z
04RM0JZ
04RM0KZ
04RM47Z
04RM4JZ
04RM4KZ
04RN07Z
04RN0JZ
04RN0KZ
04RN47Z
04RN4JZ
04RN4KZ
04RP07Z
04RP0JZ
04RP0KZ
04RP47Z
04RP4JZ
04RP4KZ
04RQ07Z
04RQ0JZ
04RQ0KZ
04RQ47Z
04RQ4JZ
04RQ4KZ
04RR07Z
04RR0JZ
04RR0KZ
04RR47Z
04RR4JZ
04RR4KZ
04RS07Z
04RS0JZ
04RS0KZ
04RS47Z
04RS4JZ
04RS4KZ
04RT07Z
04RT0JZ
04RT0KZ
04RT47Z
04RT4JZ
04RT4KZ
04RU07Z
04RU0JZ
04RU0KZ
04RU47Z
04RU4JZ
04RU4KZ
04RV07Z
04RV0JZ
04RV0KZ
04RV47Z
04RV4JZ
04RV4KZ
04RW07Z
04RW0JZ
04RW0KZ
04RW47Z
04RW4JZ
04RW4KZ
04RY07Z
04RY0JZ
04RY0KZ
04RY47Z
04RY4JZ
04RY4KZ
04S00ZZ
04S03ZZ
04S04ZZ
04S10ZZ
04S13ZZ
04S14ZZ
04S20ZZ
04S23ZZ
04S24ZZ
04S30ZZ
04S33ZZ
04S34ZZ
04S40ZZ
04S43ZZ
04S44ZZ
04S50ZZ
04S53ZZ
04S54ZZ
04S60ZZ
04S63ZZ
04S64ZZ
04S70ZZ
04S73ZZ
04S74ZZ
04S80ZZ
04S83ZZ
04S84ZZ
04S90ZZ
04S93ZZ
04S94ZZ
04SA0ZZ
04SA3ZZ
04SA4ZZ
04SB0ZZ
04SB3ZZ
04SB4ZZ
04SC0ZZ
04SC3ZZ
04SC4ZZ
04SD0ZZ
04SD3ZZ
04SD4ZZ
04SE0ZZ
04SE3ZZ
04SE4ZZ
04SF0ZZ
04SF3ZZ
04SF4ZZ
04SH0ZZ
04SH3ZZ
04SH4ZZ
04SJ0ZZ
04SJ3ZZ
04SJ4ZZ
04SK0ZZ
04SK3ZZ
04SK4ZZ
04SL0ZZ
04SL3ZZ
04SL4ZZ
04SM0ZZ
04SM3ZZ
04SM4ZZ
04SN0ZZ
04SN3ZZ
04SN4ZZ
04SP0ZZ
04SP3ZZ
04SP4ZZ
04SQ0ZZ
04SQ3ZZ
04SQ4ZZ
04SR0ZZ
04SR3ZZ
04SR4ZZ
04SS0ZZ
04SS3ZZ
04SS4ZZ
04ST0ZZ
04ST3ZZ
04ST4ZZ
04SU0ZZ
04SU3ZZ
04SU4ZZ
04SV0ZZ
04SV3ZZ
04SV4ZZ
04SW0ZZ
04SW3ZZ
04SW4ZZ
04SY0ZZ
04SY3ZZ
04SY4ZZ
04U007Z
04U00JZ
04U00KZ
04U037Z
04U03JZ
04U03KZ
04U047Z
04UP37Z
04UP3JZ
04UP3KZ
04UP47Z
04UP4JZ
04UP4KZ
04UQ07Z
04UQ0JZ
04UQ0KZ
04UQ37Z
04UQ3JZ
04UQ3KZ
04UQ47Z
04UQ4JZ
04UQ4KZ
04UR07Z
04UR0JZ
04UR0KZ
04UR37Z
04UR3JZ
04UR3KZ
04UR47Z
04UR4JZ
04UR4KZ
04US07Z
04US0JZ
04US0KZ
04US37Z
04US3JZ
04US3KZ
04US47Z
04US4JZ
04US4KZ
04UT07Z
04UT0JZ
04UT0KZ
04UT37Z
04UT3JZ
04UT3KZ
04UT47Z
04UT4JZ
04UT4KZ
04UU07Z
04UU0JZ
04UU0KZ
04UU37Z
04UU3JZ
04UU3KZ
04UU47Z
04UU4JZ
04UU4KZ
04UV07Z
04UV0JZ
04UV0KZ
04UV37Z
04UV3JZ
04UV3KZ
04UV47Z
04UV4JZ
04UV4KZ
04UW07Z
04UW0JZ
04UW0KZ
04UW37Z
04UW3JZ
04UW3KZ
04UW47Z
04UW4JZ
04UW4KZ
04UY07Z
04UY0JZ
04UY0KZ
04UY37Z
04UY3JZ
04UY3KZ
04UY47Z
04UY4JZ
04UY4KZ
04V00C6
04V00CZ
04V00D6
04V00DJ
04V00DZ
04V00E6
04V00EZ
04V00F6
04V00FZ
04V00Z6
04V00ZZ
04V03C6
04V03CZ
04V03D6
04V03DJ
04V03DZ
04V03E6
04V03EZ
04V03F6
04V03FZ
04V03Z6
04V03ZZ
04V04C6
04V04CZ
04V04D6
04V04DJ
04V04DZ
04V04E6
04V04EZ
04V04F6
04V04FZ
04V04Z6
04V04ZZ
04V10CZ
04V10DZ
04V10ZZ
04V13CZ
04V13DZ
04V13ZZ
04V14CZ
04V14DZ
04V14ZZ
04V20CZ
04V20DZ
04V20ZZ
04V23CZ
04V23DZ
04V23ZZ
04V24CZ
04V24DZ
04V24ZZ
04V30CZ
04V30DZ
04V30ZZ
04V33CZ
04V33DZ
04V33ZZ
04V34CZ
04V34DZ
04V34ZZ
04V40CZ
04V40DZ
04V40ZZ
04V43CZ
04V43DZ
04V43ZZ
04V44CZ
04V44DZ
04V44ZZ
04V50CZ
04V50DZ
04V50ZZ
04V53CZ
04V53DZ
04V53ZZ
04V54CZ
04V54DZ
04V54ZZ
04V60CZ
04V60DZ
04V60ZZ
04V63CZ
04V63DZ
04V63ZZ
04V64CZ
04V64DZ
04V64ZZ
04V70CZ
04V70DZ
04V70ZZ
04V73CZ
04V73DZ
04V73ZZ
04V74CZ
04V74DZ
04V74ZZ
04V80CZ
04V80DZ
04V80ZZ
04V83CZ
04V83DZ
04V83ZZ
04V84CZ
04V84DZ
04V84ZZ
04V90CZ
04V90DZ
04V90ZZ
04V93CZ
04V93DZ
04V93ZZ
04V94CZ
04V94DZ
04V94ZZ
04VA0CZ
04VA0DZ
04VA0ZZ
04VA3CZ
04VA3DZ
04VA3ZZ
04VA4CZ

04VA4DZ
04VA4ZZ
04VB0CZ
04VB0DZ
04VB0ZZ
04VB3CZ
04VB3DZ
04VB3ZZ
04VB4CZ
04VB4DZ
04VB4ZZ
04VC0CZ
04VC0DZ
04VC0EZ
04VC0ZZ
04VC3CZ
04VC3DZ
04VC3EZ
04VC3ZZ
04VC4CZ
04VC4DZ
04VC4EZ
04VC4ZZ
04VD0CZ
04VD0DZ
04VD0EZ
04VD0ZZ
04VD3CZ
04VD3DZ
04VD3EZ
04VD3ZZ
04VD4CZ
04VD4DZ
04VD4EZ
04VD4ZZ
04VE0CZ
04VE0DZ
04VE0ZZ
04VE3CZ
04VE3DZ
04VE3ZZ
04VE4CZ
04VE4DZ
04VE4ZZ
04VF0CZ
04VF0DZ
04VF0ZZ
04VF3CZ
04VF3DZ
04VF3ZZ
04VF4CZ
04VF4DZ
04VF4ZZ
04VH0CZ
04VH0DZ
04VH0ZZ
04VH3CZ
04VH3DZ
04VH3ZZ
04VH4CZ
04VH4DZ
04VH4ZZ
04VJ0CZ
04VJ0DZ
04VJ0ZZ
04VJ3CZ
04VJ3DZ
04VJ3ZZ
04VJ4CZ
04VJ4DZ
04VJ4ZZ
04VK0CZ
04VK0DZ
04VK0ZZ
04VK3CZ
04VK3DZ
04VK3ZZ
04VK4CZ
04VK4DZ
04VK4ZZ
04VL0CZ
04VL0DZ
04VL0ZZ
04VL3CZ
04VL3DZ
04VL3ZZ
04VL4CZ
04VL4DZ
04VL4ZZ
04VM0CZ
04VM0DZ
04VM0ZZ
04VM3CZ
04VM3DZ
04VM3ZZ
04VM4CZ
04VM4DZ
04VM4ZZ
04VN0CZ
04VN0DZ
04VN0ZZ
04VN3CZ
04VN3DZ
04VN3ZZ
04VN4CZ
04VN4DZ
04VN4ZZ
04VP0CZ
04VP0DZ
04VP0ZZ
04VP3CZ
04VP3DZ
04VP3ZZ
04VP4CZ
04VP4DZ
04VP4ZZ
04VQ0CZ
04VQ0DZ
04VQ0ZZ
04VQ3CZ
04VQ3DZ
04VQ3ZZ
04VQ4CZ
04VQ4DZ
04VQ4ZZ
04VR0CZ
04VR0DZ
04VR0ZZ
04VR3CZ
04VR3DZ
04VR3ZZ
04VR4CZ
04VR4DZ
04VR4ZZ
04VS0CZ
04VS0DZ
04VS0ZZ
04VS3CZ
04VS3DZ
04VS3ZZ
04VS4CZ
04VS4DZ
04VS4ZZ
04VT0CZ
04VT0DZ
04VT0ZZ
04VT3CZ
04VT3DZ
04VT3ZZ
04VT4CZ
04VT4DZ
04VT4ZZ
04VU0CZ
04VU0DZ
04VU0ZZ
04VU3CZ
04VU3DZ
04VU3ZZ
04VU4CZ
04WY30Z
04WY32Z
04WY33Z
04WY3DZ
04WY3YZ
04WY4YZ
04WYX0Z
04WYX2Z
04WYX3Z
04WYX7Z
04WYXCZ
04WYXDZ
04WYXJZ
04WYXKZ
051A4JY
051A4KY
051A4ZY
051B07Y
051B09Y
051B0AY
051B0JY
051B0KY
051B0ZY
051B47Y
051B49Y
051B4AY
051B4JY
051B4KY
051B4ZY
051C07Y
051C09Y
051C0AY
051C0JY
051C0KY
051C0ZY
051C47Y
051C49Y
051C4AY
051C4JY
051C4KY
051C4ZY
051D07Y
051D09Y
051D0AY
051D0JY
051D0KY
051D0ZY
051D47Y
051D49Y
051D4AY
051D4JY
051D4KY
051D4ZY
051F07Y
051F09Y
051F0AY
051F0JY
051F0KY
051F0ZY
051F47Y
051F49Y
051F4AY
051F4JY
051F4KY
051F4ZY
051G07Y
051G09Y
051G0AY
051G0JY
051G0KY
051G0ZY
051G47Y
051G49Y
051G4AY
051G4JY
051G4KY
051G4ZY
051H07Y
051H09Y
051H0AY
051H0JY
051H0KY
051H0ZY
051H47Y
051H49Y
051H4AY
051H4JY
051H4KY
051H4ZY
051L07Y
051L09Y
051L0AY
051L0JY
051L0KY
051L0ZY
051L47Y
051L49Y
051L4AY
051L4JY
051L4KY
051L4ZY
051M07Y
051M09Y
051M0AY
051M0JY
051M0KY
051M0ZY
051M47Y
051M49Y
051M4AY
051M4JY
051M4KY
051M4ZY
051N07Y
051N09Y
051N0AY
051N0JY
051N0KY
051N0ZY
051N47Y
051N49Y
051N4AY
051N4JY
051N4KY
051N4ZY
051P07Y
051P09Y
051P0AY
051P0JY
051P0KY
051P0ZY
051P47Y
051P49Y
051P4AY
051P4JY
051P4KY
051P4ZY
051Q07Y
051Q09Y
051Q0AY
051Q0JY
051Q0KY
051Q0ZY
051Q47Y
051Q49Y
051Q4AY
051Q4JY
051Q4KY
051Q4ZY
051R07Y
051R09Y
051R0AY
051R0JY
051R0KY
051R0ZY
051R47Y
051R49Y
051R4AY
051R4JY
051R4KY
051R4ZY
051S07Y
051S09Y
051S0AY
051S0JY
051S0KY
051S0ZY
051S47Y
051S49Y
051S4AY
051S4JY
051S4KY
051S4ZY
051T07Y
051T09Y
051T0AY
051T0JY
051T0KY
051T0ZY
051T47Y
051T49Y
051T4AY
051T4JY
051T4KY
051T4ZY
051V07Y
051V09Y
051V0AY
051V0JY
051V0KY
051V0ZY
051V47Y
051V49Y
051V4AY
051V4JY
051V4KY
051V4ZY
05500ZZ
05503ZZ
05504ZZ
05510ZZ
05513ZZ
05514ZZ
05530ZZ
05533ZZ
05534ZZ
05540ZZ
05543ZZ
05544ZZ
05550ZZ
05553ZZ
05554ZZ
05560ZZ
05563ZZ
05564ZZ
05570ZZ
05573ZZ
05574ZZ
05580ZZ
05583ZZ
05584ZZ
05590ZZ
05593ZZ
05594ZZ
055A0ZZ
055A3ZZ
055A4ZZ
055B0ZZ
055B3ZZ
055B4ZZ
055C0ZZ
055C3ZZ
055C4ZZ
055D0ZZ
055D3ZZ
055D4ZZ
055F0ZZ
055F3ZZ
055F4ZZ
055G0ZZ
055G3ZZ
055G4ZZ
055H0ZZ
055H3ZZ
055H4ZZ
055L0ZZ
055L3ZZ
055L4ZZ
055M0ZZ
055M3ZZ
055M4ZZ
055N0ZZ
055N3ZZ
055N4ZZ
055P0ZZ
055P3ZZ
055P4ZZ
055Q0ZZ
055Q3ZZ
055Q4ZZ
055R0ZZ
055R3ZZ
055R4ZZ
055S0ZZ
055S3ZZ
055S4ZZ
055T0ZZ
055T3ZZ
055T4ZZ
055V0ZZ
055V3ZZ
055V4ZZ
055Y0ZZ
055Y3ZZ
055Y4ZZ
05700DZ
05700ZZ
05703DZ
05703ZZ
05704DZ
05704ZZ
05710DZ
05710ZZ
05713DZ
05713ZZ
05714DZ
05714ZZ
05730D1
05730DZ
05730Z1
05730ZZ
05733D1
05733DZ
05733Z1
05733ZZ
05734D1
05734DZ
05734Z1
05734ZZ
05740D1
05740DZ
05740Z1
05740ZZ
05743D1
05743DZ
05743Z1
05743ZZ
05744D1
05744DZ
05744Z1
05744ZZ
05750D1
05750DZ
05750Z1
05750ZZ
05753D1
05753DZ
05753Z1
05753ZZ
05754D1
05754DZ
05754Z1
05754ZZ
05760D1
05760DZ
05760Z1
05760ZZ
05763D1
05763DZ
05763Z1
05763ZZ
05764D1
05764DZ
05764Z1
05764ZZ
05770D1
05770DZ
05770Z1
05770ZZ
05773D1
05773DZ
05773Z1
05773ZZ
05774D1
05774DZ
05774Z1
05774ZZ
05780D1
05780DZ
05780Z1
05780ZZ
05783D1
05783DZ
05783Z1
05783ZZ
05784D1
05784DZ
05784Z1
05784ZZ
05790D1
05790DZ
05790Z1
05790ZZ
05793D1
05793DZ
05793Z1
05793ZZ
05794D1
05794DZ
05794Z1
05794ZZ
057A0D1
057A0DZ
057A0Z1
057A0ZZ
057A3D1
057A3DZ
057A3Z1
057A3ZZ
057A4D1
057A4DZ
057A4Z1
057A4ZZ
057B0D1
057B0DZ
057B0Z1
057B0ZZ
057B3D1
057B3DZ
057B3Z1
057B3ZZ
057B4D1
057B4DZ
057B4Z1
057B4ZZ
057C0D1
057C0DZ
057C0Z1
057C0ZZ
057C3D1
057C3DZ
057C3Z1
057C3ZZ
057C4D1
057C4DZ
057C4Z1
057C4ZZ
057D0D1
057D0DZ
057D0Z1
057D0ZZ
057D3D1
057D3DZ
057D3Z1
057D3ZZ
057D4D1
057D4DZ
057D4Z1
057D4ZZ
057F0D1
057F0DZ
057F0Z1
057F0ZZ
057F3D1
057F3DZ
057F3Z1
057F3ZZ
057F4D1
057F4DZ
057F4Z1
057F4ZZ
057G0DZ
057G0ZZ
057G3DZ
057G3ZZ
057G4DZ
057G4ZZ
057H0DZ
057H0ZZ
057H3DZ
057H3ZZ
057H4DZ
057H4ZZ
057L0DZ
057L0ZZ
057L3DZ
057L3ZZ
057L4DZ
057L4ZZ
057M0DZ
057M0ZZ
057M3DZ
057M3ZZ
057M4DZ
057M4ZZ
057N0DZ
057N0ZZ
057N3DZ
057N3ZZ
057N4DZ
057N4ZZ
057P0DZ
057P0ZZ
057P3DZ
057P3ZZ
057P4DZ
057P4ZZ
057Q0DZ
057Q0ZZ
057Q3DZ
057Q3ZZ
057Q4DZ
057Q4ZZ
057R0DZ
057R0ZZ
057R3DZ
057R3ZZ
057R4DZ
057R4ZZ
057S0DZ
057S0ZZ
057S3DZ
057S3ZZ
057S4DZ
057S4ZZ
057T0DZ
057T0ZZ
057T3DZ
057T3ZZ
057T4DZ
057T4ZZ
057V0DZ
057V0ZZ
057V3DZ
057V3ZZ
057V4DZ
057V4ZZ
057Y0DZ
057Y0ZZ
057Y3DZ
057Y3ZZ
057Y4DZ
057Y4ZZ
059000Z
05900ZX
05900ZZ
059030Z
05903ZX
05903ZZ
059040Z
05904ZX
05904ZZ
059100Z
05910ZX
05910ZZ
059130Z
05913ZX
05913ZZ
059140Z
05914ZX
05914ZZ
059300Z
05930ZX
05930ZZ
059330Z
05933ZX
05933ZZ
059340Z
05934ZX
05934ZZ
059400Z
05940ZX
05940ZZ
059430Z
05943ZX
05943ZZ
059440Z
05944ZX
05944ZZ
059500Z
05950ZX
05950ZZ
059530Z
05953ZX
05953ZZ
059540Z
05954ZX
05954ZZ
059600Z
05960ZX
05960ZZ
059630Z
05963ZX
05963ZZ
059640Z
05964ZX
05964ZZ
059700Z
05970ZX
05970ZZ
059730Z
05973ZX
05973ZZ
059740Z
05974ZX
05974ZZ
059800Z

05980ZX
05980ZZ
059830Z
05983ZX
05983ZZ
059840Z
05984ZX
05984ZZ
059900Z
05990ZX
05990ZZ
059930Z
05993ZX
05993ZZ
059940Z
05994ZX
05994ZZ
059A00Z
059A0ZX
059A0ZZ
059A30Z
059A3ZX
059A3ZZ
059A40Z
059A4ZX
059A4ZZ
059B00Z
059B0ZX
059B0ZZ
059B30Z
059B3ZX
059B3ZZ
059B40Z
059B4ZX
059B4ZZ
059C00Z
059C0ZX
059C0ZZ
059C30Z
059C3ZX
059C3ZZ
059C40Z
059C4ZX
059C4ZZ
059D00Z
059D0ZX
059D0ZZ
059D30Z
059D3ZX
059D3ZZ
059D40Z
059D4ZX
059D4ZZ
059F00Z
059F0ZX
059F0ZZ
059F30Z
059F3ZX
059F3ZZ
059F40Z
059F4ZX
059F4ZZ
059G00Z
059G0ZX
059G0ZZ
059G30Z
059G3ZX
059G3ZZ
059G40Z
059G4ZX
059G4ZZ
059H00Z
059H0ZX
059H0ZZ
059H30Z
059H3ZX
059H3ZZ
059H40Z
059H4ZX
059H4ZZ
059L00Z
059L0ZX
059L0ZZ
059L30Z
059L3ZX
059L3ZZ
059L40Z
059L4ZX
059L4ZZ
059M00Z
059M0ZX
059M0ZZ
059M30Z
059M3ZX
059M3ZZ
059M40Z
059M4ZX
059M4ZZ
059N00Z
059N0ZX
059N0ZZ
059N30Z
059N3ZX
059N3ZZ
059N40Z
059N4ZX
059N4ZZ
059P00Z
059P0ZX
059P0ZZ
059P30Z
059P3ZX
059P3ZZ
059P40Z
059P4ZX
059P4ZZ
059Q00Z
059Q0ZX
059Q0ZZ
059Q30Z
059Q3ZX
059Q3ZZ
059Q40Z
059Q4ZX
059Q4ZZ
059R00Z
059R0ZX
059R0ZZ
059R30Z
059R3ZX
059R3ZZ
059R40Z
059R4ZX
059R4ZZ
059S00Z
059S0ZX
059S0ZZ
059S30Z
059S3ZX
059S3ZZ
059S40Z
059S4ZX
059S4ZZ
059T00Z
059T0ZX
059T0ZZ
059T30Z
059T3ZX
059T3ZZ
059T40Z
059T4ZX
059T4ZZ
059V00Z
059V0ZX
059V0ZZ
059V30Z
059V3ZX
059V3ZZ
059V40Z
059V4ZZ
059Y00Z
059Y0ZZ
059Y30Z
059Y3ZX
059Y3ZZ
059Y40Z
059Y4ZZ
05C83ZZ
05C84ZZ
05C90ZZ
05C93ZZ
05C94ZZ
05CA0ZZ
05CA3ZZ
05CA4ZZ
05CB0ZZ
05CB3ZZ
05CB4ZZ
05CC0ZZ
05CC3ZZ
05CC4ZZ
05CD0ZZ
05CD3ZZ
05CD4ZZ
05CF0ZZ
05CF3ZZ
05CF4ZZ
05CG0ZZ
05CG3ZZ
05CG4ZZ
05CH0ZZ
05CH3ZZ
05CH4ZZ
05CL0ZZ
05CL3ZZ
05CL4ZZ
05CM0ZZ
05CM3ZZ
05CM4ZZ
05CN0ZZ
05CN3ZZ
05CN4ZZ
05CP0ZZ
05CP3ZZ
05CP4ZZ
05CQ0ZZ
05CQ3ZZ
05CQ4ZZ
05CR0ZZ
05CR3ZZ
05CR4ZZ
05CS0ZZ
05CS3ZZ
05CS4ZZ
05CT0ZZ
05CT3ZZ
05CT4ZZ
05CV0ZZ
05CV3ZZ
05CV4ZZ
05CY0ZZ
05CY3ZZ
05CY4ZZ
05D90ZZ
05D93ZZ
05DA0ZZ
05DA3ZZ
05DB0ZZ
05DB3ZZ
05DC0ZZ
05DC3ZZ
05DD0ZZ
05DD3ZZ
05DF0ZZ
05DF3ZZ
05DG0ZZ
05DG3ZZ
05DH0ZZ
05DH3ZZ
05DY0ZZ
05DY3ZZ
05H002Z
05H003Z
05H00DZ
05H00MZ
05H032Z
05H033Z
05H03DZ
05H03MZ
05H042Z
05H043Z
05H04DZ
05H04MZ
05H103Z
05H10DZ
05H133Z
05H13DZ
05H143Z
05H14DZ
05H303Z
05H30DZ
05H30MZ
05H333Z
05H33DZ
05H33MZ
05H343Z
05H34DZ
05H34MZ
05H403Z
05H40DZ
05H40MZ
05H433Z
05H43DZ
05H43MZ
05H443Z
05H44DZ
05H44MZ
05H503Z
05H50DZ
05H533Z
05H53DZ
05H543Z
05H54DZ
05H603Z
05H60DZ
05H633Z
05H63DZ
05H643Z
05H64DZ
05H703Z
05H70DZ
05H733Z
05H73DZ
05H743Z
05H74DZ
05H803Z
05H80DZ
05H833Z
05H83DZ
05H843Z
05H84DZ
05H903Z
05H90DZ
05H933Z
05H93DZ
05H943Z
05H94DZ
05HA03Z
05HA0DZ
05HA33Z
05HA3DZ
05HA43Z
05HA4DZ
05HB03Z
05HB0DZ
05HB33Z
05HB3DZ
05HB43Z
05HB4DZ
05HC03Z
05HC0DZ
05HC33Z
05HC3DZ
05HC43Z
05HC4DZ
05HD03Z
05HD0DZ
05HD33Z
05HD3DZ
05HD43Z
05HD4DZ
05HF03Z
05HF0DZ
05HF33Z
05HF3DZ
05HF43Z
05HF4DZ
05HG03Z
05HG0DZ
05HG33Z
05HG3DZ
05HG43Z
05HG4DZ
05HH03Z
05HH0DZ
05HH33Z
05HH3DZ
05HH43Z
05HH4DZ
05HL03Z
05HL0DZ
05HL33Z
05HL3DZ
05HL43Z
05HL4DZ
05HM03Z
05HM0DZ
05HM33Z
05HM3DZ
05HM43Z
05HM4DZ
05HN03Z
05HN0DZ
05HN33Z
05HN3DZ
05HN43Z
05HN4DZ
05HP03Z
05HP0DZ
05HP33Z
05HP3DZ
05HP43Z
05HP4DZ
05HQ03Z
05HQ0DZ
05HQ33Z
05HQ3DZ
05HQ43Z
05HQ4DZ
05HR03Z
05HR0DZ
05HR33Z
05HR3DZ
05HR43Z
05HR4DZ
05HS03Z
05HS0DZ
05HS33Z
05HS3DZ
05HS43Z
05HS4DZ
05HT03Z
05HT0DZ
05HT33Z
05HT3DZ
05HT43Z
05HT4DZ
05HV03Z
05HV0DZ
05HV33Z
05HV3DZ
05HV43Z
05HV4DZ
05HY02Z
05HY03Z
05HY0DZ
05HY0YZ
05HY32Z
05HY33Z
05HY3DZ
05HY3YZ
05HY43Z
05HY4YZ
05JY3ZZ
05JYXZZ
05LD0ZZ
05LD3CZ
05LD3DZ
05LD3ZZ
05LD4CZ
05LD4DZ
05LD4ZZ
05LF0CZ
05LF0DZ
05LF0ZZ
05LF3CZ
05LF3DZ
05LF3ZZ
05LF4CZ
05LF4DZ
05LF4ZZ
05LG0CZ
05LG0DZ
05LG0ZZ
05LG3CZ
05LG3DZ
05LG3ZZ
05LG4CZ
05LG4DZ
05LG4ZZ
05LH0CZ
05LH0DZ
05LH0ZZ
05LH3CZ
05LH3DZ
05LH3ZZ
05LH4CZ
05LH4DZ
05LH4ZZ
05LL0CZ
05LL0DZ
05LL0ZZ
05LL3CZ
05LL3DZ
05LL3ZZ
05LL4CZ
05LL4DZ
05LL4ZZ
05LM0CZ
05LM0DZ
05LM0ZZ
05LM3CZ
05LM3DZ
05LM3ZZ
05LM4CZ
05LM4DZ
05LM4ZZ
05LN0CZ
05LN0DZ
05LN0ZZ
05LN3CZ
05LN3DZ
05LN3ZZ
05LN4CZ
05LN4DZ
05LN4ZZ
05LP0CZ
05LP0DZ
05LP0ZZ
05LP3CZ
05LP3DZ
05LP3ZZ
05LP4CZ
05LP4DZ
05LP4ZZ
05LQ0CZ
05LQ0DZ
05LQ0ZZ
05LQ3CZ
05LQ3DZ
05LQ3ZZ
05LQ4CZ
05LQ4DZ
05LQ4ZZ
05LR0CZ
05LR0DZ
05LR0ZZ
05LR3CZ
05LR3DZ
05LR3ZZ
05LR4CZ
05LR4DZ
05LR4ZZ
05LS0CZ
05LS0DZ
05LS0ZZ
05LS3CZ
05LS3DZ
05LS3ZZ
05LS4CZ
05LS4DZ
05LS4ZZ
05LT0CZ
05LT0DZ
05LT0ZZ
05LT3CZ
05LT3DZ
05LT3ZZ
05LT4CZ
05LT4DZ
05LT4ZZ
05LV0CZ
05LV0DZ
05LV0ZZ
05LV3CZ
05LV3DZ
05LV3ZZ
05LV4CZ
05LV4DZ
05LV4ZZ
05LY0CZ
05LY0DZ
05LY0ZZ
05LY3CZ
05LY3DZ
05LY3ZZ
05LY4CZ
05LY4DZ
05LY4ZZ
05N00ZZ
05N03ZZ
05N04ZZ
05N10ZZ
05N13ZZ
05N14ZZ
05N30ZZ
05N33ZZ
05N34ZZ
05N40ZZ
05N43ZZ
05N44ZZ
05N50ZZ
05N53ZZ
05N54ZZ
05N60ZZ
05N63ZZ
05N64ZZ
05N70ZZ
05N73ZZ
05N74ZZ
05N80ZZ
05N83ZZ
05N84ZZ
05N90ZZ
05N93ZZ
05N94ZZ
05NA0ZZ
05NA3ZZ
05NA4ZZ
05NB0ZZ
05NB3ZZ
05NB4ZZ
05NC0ZZ
05NC3ZZ
05NC4ZZ
05ND0ZZ
05ND3ZZ
05ND4ZZ
05NF0ZZ
05NF3ZZ
05NF4ZZ
05NG0ZZ
05NG3ZZ
05NG4ZZ
05NH0ZZ
05NH3ZZ
05NH4ZZ
05NL0ZZ
05NL3ZZ
05NL4ZZ
05NM0ZZ
05NM3ZZ
05NM4ZZ
05NN0ZZ
05NN3ZZ
05NN4ZZ
05NP0ZZ
05NP3ZZ
05NP4ZZ
05NQ0ZZ
05NQ3ZZ
05NQ4ZZ
05NR0ZZ
05NR3ZZ
05NR4ZZ
05NS0ZZ
05NS3ZZ
05NS4ZZ
05NT0ZZ
05NT3ZZ
05NT4ZZ
05NV0ZZ
05NV3ZZ
05NV4ZZ
05NY0ZZ
05NY3ZZ
05NY4ZZ
05P002Z
05P00MZ
05P032Z
05P03MZ
05P042Z
05P04MZ
05P0X2Z
05P0XMZ
05P30MZ
05P33MZ
05P34MZ
05P3XMZ
05P40MZ
05P43MZ
05P44MZ
05P4XMZ
05PY00Z
05PY02Z
05PY03Z
05PY07Z
05PY0CZ
05PY0DZ
05PY0JZ
05PY0KZ
05PY0YZ
05PY30Z
05PY32Z
05PY33Z
05PY37Z
05PY3CZ
05PY3DZ
05PY3JZ
05PY3KZ
05PY3YZ
05PY40Z
05PY42Z
05PY43Z
05PY47Z
05PY4CZ
05PY4DZ
05PY4JZ
05PY4KZ
05PY4YZ
05PYX0Z
05PYX2Z
05PYX3Z
05PYXDZ
05Q00ZZ
05Q03ZZ
05Q04ZZ
05Q10ZZ
05Q13ZZ
05Q14ZZ
05Q30ZZ
05Q33ZZ
05Q34ZZ
05Q40ZZ
05Q43ZZ
05Q44ZZ
05Q50ZZ
05Q53ZZ
05Q54ZZ
05Q60ZZ
05Q63ZZ
05Q64ZZ
05Q70ZZ
05Q73ZZ
05Q74ZZ
05Q80ZZ
05Q83ZZ
05Q84ZZ
05RD47Z
05RD4JZ
05RD4KZ
05RF07Z
05RF0JZ
05RF0KZ
05RF47Z
05RF4JZ
05RF4KZ
05RG07Z
05RG0JZ
05RG0KZ
05RG47Z
05RG4JZ
05RG4KZ
05RH07Z
05RH0JZ
05RH0KZ
05RH47Z
05RH4JZ
05RH4KZ
05RL07Z
05RL0JZ
05RL0KZ
05RL47Z
05RL4JZ
05RL4KZ
05RM07Z
05RM0JZ
05RM0KZ
05RM47Z
05RM4JZ
05RM4KZ
05RN07Z
05RN0JZ
05RN0KZ
05RN47Z
05RN4JZ

05RN4KZ
05RP07Z
05RP0JZ
05RP0KZ
05RP47Z
05RP4JZ
05RP4KZ
05RQ07Z
05RQ0JZ
05RQ0KZ
05RQ47Z
05RQ4JZ
05RQ4KZ
05RR07Z
05RR0JZ
05RR0KZ
05RR47Z
05RR4JZ
05RR4KZ
05RS07Z
05RS0JZ
05RS0KZ
05RS47Z
05RS4JZ
05RS4KZ
05RT07Z
05RT0JZ
05RT0KZ
05RT47Z
05RT4JZ
05RT4KZ
05RV07Z
05RV0JZ
05RV0KZ
05RV47Z
05RV4JZ
05RV4KZ
05RY07Z
05RY0JZ
05RY0KZ
05RY47Z
05RY4JZ
05RY4KZ
05S00ZZ
05S03ZZ
05S04ZZ
05S10ZZ
05S13ZZ
05S14ZZ
05S30ZZ
05S33ZZ
05S34ZZ
05S40ZZ
05S43ZZ
05S44ZZ
05S50ZZ
05S53ZZ
05S54ZZ
05S60ZZ
05S63ZZ
05S64ZZ
05S70ZZ
05S73ZZ
05S74ZZ
05S80ZZ
05S83ZZ
05S84ZZ
05S90ZZ
05S93ZZ
05S94ZZ
05SA0ZZ
05SA3ZZ
05SA4ZZ
05SB0ZZ
05SB3ZZ
05SB4ZZ
05SC0ZZ
05SC3ZZ
05SC4ZZ
05SD0ZZ
05SD3ZZ
05SD4ZZ
05SF0ZZ
05SF3ZZ
05SF4ZZ
05SG0ZZ
05SG3ZZ
05SG4ZZ
05SH0ZZ
05SH3ZZ
05SH4ZZ
05SL0ZZ
05SL3ZZ
05SL4ZZ
05SM0ZZ
05SM3ZZ
05SM4ZZ
05SN0ZZ
05SN3ZZ
05SN4ZZ
05SP0ZZ
05SP3ZZ
05SP4ZZ
05SQ0ZZ
05SQ3ZZ
05SQ4ZZ
05SR0ZZ
05SR3ZZ
05SR4ZZ
05SS0ZZ
05SS3ZZ
05SS4ZZ
05ST0ZZ
05ST3ZZ
05ST4ZZ
05SV0ZZ
05SV3ZZ
05SV4ZZ
05SY0ZZ
05SY3ZZ
05SY4ZZ
05U007Z
05U00JZ
05U00KZ
05U037Z
05U03JZ
05U03KZ
05U047Z
05U04JZ
05U04KZ
05U107Z
05U10JZ
05U10KZ
05U137Z
05U13JZ
05U13KZ
05U147Z
05U14JZ
05U14KZ
05U307Z
05U30JZ
05U30KZ
05U337Z
05U33JZ
05U33KZ
05U347Z
05U34JZ
05U34KZ
05U407Z
05U40JZ
05U40KZ
05U437Z
05U43JZ
05U43KZ
05U447Z
05U44JZ
05U44KZ
05U507Z
05U50JZ
05U50KZ
05U537Z
05U53JZ
05U53KZ
05U547Z
05U54JZ
05U54KZ
05U607Z
05U60JZ
05U60KZ
05U637Z
05U63JZ
05U63KZ
05U647Z
05U64JZ
05U64KZ
05U707Z
05U70JZ
05U70KZ
05U737Z
05U73JZ
05U73KZ
05U747Z
05U74JZ
05U74KZ
05U807Z
05U80JZ
05U80KZ
05U837Z
05U83JZ
05U83KZ
05U847Z
05U84JZ
05U84KZ
05U907Z
05U90JZ
05U90KZ
05U937Z
05U93JZ
05U93KZ
05U947Z
05U94JZ
05U94KZ
05UA07Z
05UA0JZ
05UA0KZ
05UA37Z
05UA3JZ
05UA3KZ
05UA47Z
05UA4JZ
05UA4KZ
05UB07Z
05UB0JZ
05UB0KZ
05UB37Z
05UB3JZ
05UB3KZ
05UB47Z
05UB4JZ
05UB4KZ
05UC07Z
05UC0JZ
05UC0KZ
05UC37Z
05UC3JZ
05UC3KZ
05UC47Z
05UC4JZ
05UC4KZ
05UD07Z
05UD0JZ
05UD0KZ
05UD37Z
05UD3JZ
05UD3KZ
05UD47Z
05UD4JZ
05UD4KZ
05UF07Z
05UF0JZ
05UF0KZ
05UF37Z
05UF3JZ
05UF3KZ
05UF47Z
05UF4JZ
05UF4KZ
05UG07Z
05UG0JZ
05UG0KZ
05UG37Z
05UG3JZ
05UG3KZ
05UG47Z
05UG4JZ
05UG4KZ
05UH07Z
05UH0JZ
05UH0KZ
05UH37Z
05UH3JZ
05UH3KZ
05UH47Z
05UH4JZ
05UH4KZ
05UL07Z
05UL0JZ
05UL0KZ
05UL37Z
05UL3JZ
05UL3KZ
05UL47Z
05UL4JZ
05UL4KZ
05UM07Z
05UM0JZ
05UM0KZ
05UM37Z
05UM3JZ
05UM3KZ
05UM47Z
05UM4JZ
05UM4KZ
05UN07Z
05UN0JZ
05UN0KZ
05UN37Z
05UN3JZ
05UN3KZ
05UN47Z
05UN4JZ
05UN4KZ
05UP07Z
05UP0JZ
05UP0KZ
05UP37Z
05UP3JZ
05UP3KZ
05UP47Z
05UP4JZ
05UP4KZ
05UQ07Z
05UQ0JZ
05VH4ZZ
05VL0CZ
05VL0DZ
05VL0ZZ
05VL3CZ
05VL3DZ
05VL3ZZ
05VL4CZ
05VL4DZ
05VL4ZZ
05VM0CZ
05VM0DZ
05VM0ZZ
05VM3CZ
05VM3DZ
05VM3ZZ
05VM4CZ
05VM4DZ
05VM4ZZ
05VN0CZ
05VN0DZ
05VN0ZZ
05VN3CZ
05VN3DZ
05VN3ZZ
05VN4CZ
05VN4DZ
05VN4ZZ
05VP0CZ
05VP0DZ
05VP0ZZ
05VP3CZ
05VP3DZ
05VP3ZZ
05VP4CZ
05VP4DZ
05VP4ZZ
05VQ0CZ
05VQ0DZ
05VQ0ZZ
05VQ3CZ
05VQ3DZ
05VQ3ZZ
05VQ4CZ
05VQ4DZ
05VQ4ZZ
05VR0CZ
05VR0DZ
05VR0ZZ
05VR3CZ
05VR3DZ
05VR3ZZ
05VR4CZ
05VR4DZ
05VR4ZZ
05VS0CZ
05VS0DZ
05VS0ZZ
05VS3CZ
05VS3DZ
05VS3ZZ
05VS4CZ
05VS4DZ
05VS4ZZ
05VT0CZ
05VT0DZ
05VT0ZZ
05VT3CZ
05VT3DZ
05VT3ZZ
05VT4CZ
05VT4DZ
05VT4ZZ
05VV0CZ
05VV0DZ
05VV0ZZ
05VV3CZ
05VV3DZ
05VV3ZZ
05VV4CZ
05VV4DZ
05VV4ZZ
05VY0CZ
05VY0DZ
05VY0ZZ
05VY3CZ
05VY3DZ
05VY3ZZ
05VY4CZ
05VY4DZ
05VY4ZZ
05W002Z
05W00MZ
05W032Z
05W03MZ
05W042Z
05W04MZ
05W0X2Z
05W0XMZ
05W30MZ
05W33MZ
05W34MZ
05W3XMZ
05W40MZ
05W43MZ
05W44MZ
05W4XMZ
05WY00Z
05WY02Z
05WY03Z
05WY07Z
05WY0CZ
05WY0DZ
05WY0JZ
05WY0KZ
05WY0YZ
05WY30Z
05WY32Z
05WY33Z
05WY37Z
05WY3CZ
05WY3DZ
05WY3JZ
05WY3KZ
05WY3YZ
05WY40Z
05WY42Z
05WY43Z
05WY47Z
05WY4CZ
05WY4DZ
05WY4JZ
05WY4KZ
05WY4YZ
05WYX0Z
05WYX2Z
05WYX3Z
05WYX7Z
05WYXCZ
05WYXDZ
05WYXJZ
05WYXKZ
0610075
0610076
061007P
061007Q
061007R
061007Y
0610095
0610096
061009P
061009Q
061009R
061009Y
06100A5
06100A6
06100AP
06100AQ
06100AR
06100AY
06100J5
06100J6
06100JP
06100JQ
06100JR
06100JY
06100K5
06100K6
06100KP
06100KQ
06100KR
06100KY
06100Z5
06100Z6
06100ZP
06100ZQ
06100ZR
06100ZY
0610475
0610476
061047P
061047Q
061047R
061047Y
0610495
0610496
061049P
061049Q
061049R
061049Y
06104A5
06104A6
06104AP
06104AQ
06104AR
06104AY
06104J5
06104J6
06104JP
06104JQ
06104JR
06104JY
06104K5
06104K6
06104KP
06104KQ
06104KR
06104KY
06104Z5
06104Z6
06104ZP
06104ZQ
06104ZR
06104ZY
0611079
061107B
061107Y
0611099
061109B
061109Y
06110A9
06110AB
06110AY
06110J9
06110JB
06110JY
06110K9
06110KB
06110KY
06110Z9
06110ZB
06110ZY
0611479
061147B
061147Y
0611499
061149B
061149Y
06114A9
06114AB
06114AY
06114J9
06114JB
06114JY
06114K9
06114KB
06114KY
06114Z9
06114ZB
06114ZY
061207Y
061209Y
06120AY
06120JY
06120KY
06120ZY
061247Y
061249Y
06124AY
06124JY
06124KY
06124ZY
061307Y
061309Y
06130AY
06130JY
06130KY
06130ZY
061347Y
061349Y
06134AY
06134JY
06134KY
06134ZY
061407Y
061409Y
06140AY
06140JY
06140KY
06140ZY
061447Y
061449Y
06144AY
06144JY
06144KY
06144ZY
061507Y
061509Y
06150AY
06150JY
06150KY
06150ZY
061547Y
061549Y
06154AY
06154JY
06154KY
06154ZY
061607Y
061609Y
06160AY
06160JY
06160KY
06160ZY
061647Y
061649Y
06164AY
06164JY
06164KY
06164ZY
061707Y
061709Y
06170AY
06170JY
06170KY
06170ZY
061747Y
061749Y
06174AY
06174JY
06174KY
06174ZY
0618079
061807B
061807Y
0618099
061809B
061809Y
06180A9
06180AB
06180AY
06180J9
06180JB
06180JY
06180K9
06180KB
06180KY
06180Z9
06180ZB
06180ZY
06183J4
06183JY
0618479
061847B
061847Y
0618499
061849B
061849Y
06184A9
06184AB
06184AY
06184J4
06184J9
06184JB
06184JY
06184K9
06184KB
06184KY
06184Z9
06184ZB
06184ZY
061907Y
061909Y
06190AY
06190JY
06190KY
06190ZY
061947Y
061949Y
06194AY
06194JY
06194KY
06194ZY
061B07Y
061B09Y
061B0AY
061B0JY
061B0KY
061B0ZY
061B47Y
061B49Y
061B4AY
061B4JY
061B4KY
061B4ZY
061C07Y
061C09Y
061C0AY
061C0JY
061C0KY
061C0ZY
061C47Y
061C49Y
061C4AY
061C4JY
061C4KY
061C4ZY
061D07Y
061D09Y
061D0AY
061D0JY
061D0KY
061D0ZY
061D47Y
061D49Y
061D4AY
061D4JY
061D4KY
061D4ZY
061F07Y
061F09Y
061F0AY
061F0JY
061F0KY
061F0ZY
061F47Y
061F49Y
061F4AY
061F4JY
061F4KY
061F4ZY
061G07Y
061G09Y

05RN4KZ-061G09Y
APPENDIX H: NON-OR NOT AFFECTING MS-DRG ASSIGNMENT

061G0AY
061G0JY
061G0KY
061G0ZY
061G47Y
061G49Y
061G4AY
061G4JY
061G4KY
061G4ZY
061H07Y
061H09Y
061H0AY
061H0JY
061H0KY
061H0ZY
061H47Y
061H49Y
061H4AY
061H4JY
061H4KY
061H4ZY
061J07Y
061J09Y
061J0AY
061J0JY
061J0KY
061J0ZY
061J47Y
061J49Y
061J4AY
061J4JY
061J4KY
061J4ZY
061M07Y
061M09Y
061M0AY
061M0JY
061M0KY
061M0ZY
061M47Y
061M49Y
061M4AY
061M4JY
061M4KY
061M4ZY
061N07Y
061N09Y
061N0AY
061N0JY
061N0KY
061N0ZY
061N47Y
061N49Y
061N4AY
061N4JY
061N4KY
061N4ZY
061P07Y
061P09Y
061P0AY
061P0JY
061P0KY
061P0ZY
061P47Y
061P49Y
061P4AY
061P4JY
061P4KY
061P4ZY
061Q07Y
061Q09Y
061Q0AY
061Q0JY
061Q0KY
061Q0ZY
061Q47Y
061Q49Y
061Q4AY
061Q4JY
061Q4KY
061Q4ZY
061T07Y
061T09Y
061T0AY
061T0JY
061T0KY
061T0ZY
061T47Y
061T49Y
061T4AY
061T4JY
061T4KY
061T4ZY
061V07Y
061V09Y
061V0AY
061V0JY
061V0KY
061V0ZY
061V47Y
061V49Y
061V4AY
061V4JY
061V4KY
061V4ZY
06500ZZ
06503ZZ
06504ZZ
06510ZZ
06513ZZ
06514ZZ
06520ZZ
06523ZZ
06524ZZ
06530ZZ
06533ZZ
06534ZZ
06540ZZ
06543ZZ
06544ZZ
06550ZZ
06553ZZ
06554ZZ
06560ZZ
06563ZZ
06564ZZ
06570ZZ
06573ZZ
06574ZZ
06580ZZ
06583ZZ
06584ZZ
06590ZZ
06593ZZ
06594ZZ
065B0ZZ
065B3ZZ
065B4ZZ
065C0ZZ
065C3ZZ
065C4ZZ
065D0ZZ
065D3ZZ
065D4ZZ
065F0ZZ
065F3ZZ
065F4ZZ
065G0ZZ
065G3ZZ
065G4ZZ
065H0ZZ
065H3ZZ
065H4ZZ
065J0ZZ
065J3ZZ
065J4ZZ
065M0ZZ
065M3ZZ
065M4ZZ
065N0ZZ
065N3ZZ
065N4ZZ
065P0ZZ
065P3ZZ
065P4ZZ
065Q0ZZ
065Q3ZZ
065Q4ZZ
065T0ZZ
065T3ZZ
065T4ZZ
065V0ZZ
065V3ZZ
069000Z
06900ZZ
069030Z
06903ZX
06903ZZ
069040Z
06904ZZ
069100Z
06910ZZ
069130Z
06913ZX
06913ZZ
069140Z
06914ZZ
069200Z
06920ZZ
069230Z
06923ZX
06923ZZ
069240Z
06924ZZ
069330Z
06933ZX
06933ZZ
069400Z
06940ZZ
069430Z
06943ZX
06943ZZ
069440Z
06944ZZ
069500Z
06950ZZ
069530Z
06953ZX
06953ZZ
069540Z
06954ZZ
069600Z
06960ZZ
069630Z
06963ZX
06963ZZ
069640Z
06964ZZ
069700Z
06970ZZ
069730Z
06973ZX
06973ZZ
069740Z
06974ZZ
069800Z
06980ZZ
069830Z
06983ZX
06983ZZ
069840Z
06984ZZ
069900Z
06990ZZ
069930Z
06993ZX
06993ZZ
069940Z
06994ZZ
069B00Z
069B0ZZ
069B30Z
069B3ZX
069B3ZZ
069B40Z
069B4ZZ
069C00Z
069C0ZZ
069C30Z
069C3ZX
069C3ZZ
069C40Z
069C4ZZ
069D00Z
069D0ZZ
069D30Z
069D3ZX
069D3ZZ
069D40Z
069D4ZZ
069F00Z
069F0ZZ
069F30Z
069F3ZX
069F3ZZ
069F40Z
069F4ZZ
069G00Z
069G0ZZ
069G30Z
069G3ZX
069G3ZZ
069G40Z
069G4ZZ
069H00Z
069H0ZZ
069H30Z
069H3ZX
069H3ZZ
069H40Z
069H4ZZ
069J00Z
069J0ZZ
069J30Z
069J3ZX
069J3ZZ
069J40Z
069J4ZZ
069M00Z
069M0ZZ
069M30Z
069M3ZX
069M3ZZ
069M40Z
069M4ZZ
069N00Z
069N0ZZ
069N30Z
069N3ZX
069N3ZZ
069N40Z
069N4ZZ
069P00Z
069P0ZZ
069P30Z
069P3ZX
069P3ZZ
069P40Z
069P4ZZ
069Q00Z
069Q0ZZ
069Q30Z
069Q3ZX
069Q3ZZ
069Q40Z
069Q4ZZ
069T00Z
069T0ZZ
069T30Z
069T3ZX
069T3ZZ
069T40Z
069T4ZZ
069V00Z
069V0ZZ
069V30Z
069V3ZX
069V3ZZ
069V40Z
069V4ZZ
069Y00Z
069Y0ZZ
069Y30Z
069Y3ZX
069Y3ZZ
069Y40Z
069Y4ZZ
06BQ4ZX
06BQ4ZZ
06BT0ZX
06BT0ZZ
06BT3ZX
06BT3ZZ
06BT4ZX
06BT4ZZ
06BV0ZX
06BV0ZZ
06BV3ZX
06BV3ZZ
06BV4ZX
06BV4ZZ
06BY0ZC
06BY0ZX
06BY0ZZ
06BY3ZC
06BY3ZX
06BY3ZZ
06BY4ZC
06BY4ZX
06BY4ZZ
06C00ZZ
06C03ZZ
06C04ZZ
06C10ZZ
06C13ZZ
06C14ZZ
06C20ZZ
06C23ZZ
06C24ZZ
06C30ZZ
06C33ZZ
06C34ZZ
06C40ZZ
06C43ZZ
06C44ZZ
06C50ZZ
06C53ZZ
06C54ZZ
06C60ZZ
06C63ZZ
06C64ZZ
06C70ZZ
06C73ZZ
06C74ZZ
06C80ZZ
06C83ZZ
06C84ZZ
06C90ZZ
06C93ZZ
06C94ZZ
06CB0ZZ
06CB3ZZ
06CB4ZZ
06CC0ZZ
06CC3ZZ
06CC4ZZ
06CD0ZZ
06CD3ZZ
06CD4ZZ
06CF0ZZ
06CF3ZZ
06CF4ZZ
06CG0ZZ
06CG3ZZ
06CG4ZZ
06CH0ZZ
06CH3ZZ
06CH4ZZ
06CJ0ZZ
06CJ3ZZ
06CJ4ZZ
06CM0ZZ
06CM3ZZ
06CM4ZZ
06CN0ZZ
06CN3ZZ
06CN4ZZ
06CP0ZZ
06CP3ZZ
06CP4ZZ
06CQ0ZZ
06CQ3ZZ
06CQ4ZZ
06CT0ZZ
06CT3ZZ
06CT4ZZ
06CV0ZZ
06CV3ZZ
06CV4ZZ
06CY0ZZ
06CY3ZZ
06CY4ZZ
06DM0ZZ
06DM3ZZ
06DM4ZZ
06DN0ZZ
06DN3ZZ
06DN4ZZ
06DP0ZZ
06DP3ZZ
06DP4ZZ
06DQ0ZZ
06DQ3ZZ
06DQ4ZZ
06DT0ZZ
06DT3ZZ
06DT4ZZ
06DV0ZZ
06DV3ZZ
06DV4ZZ
06DY0ZZ
06DY3ZZ
06DY4ZZ
06H003T
06H003Z
06H00DZ
06H033T
06H033Z
06H03DZ
06H043Z
06H04DZ
06H103Z
06H10DZ
06H133Z
06H13DZ
06H143Z
06H14DZ
06H203Z
06H20DZ
06H233Z
06H23DZ
06H243Z
06H24DZ
06H303Z
06H30DZ
06H333Z
06H33DZ
06H343Z
06H34DZ
06H403Z
06H40DZ
06H433Z
06H43DZ
06H443Z
06H44DZ
06H503Z
06H50DZ
06H533Z
06H53DZ
06H543Z
06H54DZ
06H603Z
06H60DZ
06H633Z
06H63DZ
06H643Z
06H64DZ
06H703Z
06H70DZ
06H733Z
06H73DZ
06H743Z
06H74DZ
06H803Z
06H80DZ
06H833Z
06H83DZ
06H843Z
06H84DZ
06H903Z
06H90DZ
06H933Z
06H93DZ
06H943Z
06H94DZ
06HB03Z
06HB0DZ
06HB33Z
06HB3DZ
06HB43Z
06HB4DZ
06HC03Z
06HC0DZ
06HC33Z
06HC3DZ
06HC43Z
06HC4DZ
06HD03Z
06HD0DZ
06HD33Z
06HD3DZ
06HD43Z
06HD4DZ
06HF03Z
06HF0DZ
06HF33Z
06HF3DZ
06HF43Z
06HF4DZ
06HG03Z
06HG0DZ
06HG33Z
06HG3DZ
06HG43Z
06HG4DZ
06HH03Z
06HH0DZ
06HH33Z
06HH3DZ
06HH43Z
06HH4DZ
06HJ03Z
06HJ0DZ
06HJ33Z
06HJ3DZ
06HJ43Z
06HJ4DZ
06HM03Z
06HM0DZ
06HM33Z
06HM3DZ
06HM43Z
06HM4DZ
06HN03Z
06HN0DZ
06HN33Z
06HN3DZ
06HN43Z
06HN4DZ
06HP03Z
06HP0DZ
06HP33Z
06HP3DZ
06HP43Z
06HP4DZ
06HQ03Z
06HQ0DZ
06HQ33Z
06HQ3DZ
06HQ43Z
06HQ4DZ
06HT03Z
06HT0DZ
06HT33Z
06HT3DZ
06HT43Z
06HT4DZ
06HV03Z
06HV0DZ
06HV33Z
06HV3DZ
06HV43Z
06HV4DZ
06HY02Z
06HY03Z
06HY0DZ
06HY0YZ
06HY32Z
06HY33Z
06HY3DZ
06HY3YZ
06HY42Z
06HY43Z
06HY4DZ
06HY4YZ
06JY0ZZ
06JY3ZZ
06JY4ZZ
06JYXZZ
06L00CZ
06L00DZ
06L00ZZ
06L03CZ
06L03DZ
06L03ZZ
06L04CZ
06L04DZ
06L04ZZ
06L10CZ
06L10DZ
06L10ZZ
06L33CZ
06L33DZ
06L33ZZ
06L34CZ
06L34DZ
06L34ZZ
06L37CZ
06L37DZ
06L37ZZ
06L38CZ
06L38DZ
06L38ZZ
06LD4CZ
06LD4DZ
06LD4ZZ
06LF0CZ
06LF0DZ
06LF0ZZ
06LF3CZ
06LF3DZ
06LF3ZZ
06LF4CZ
06LF4DZ
06LF4ZZ
06LG0CZ
06LG0DZ
06LG0ZZ
06LG3CZ
06LG3DZ
06LG3ZZ
06LG4CZ
06LG4DZ
06LG4ZZ
06LH0CZ
06LH0DZ
06LH0ZZ
06LH3CZ
06LH3DZ
06LH3ZZ
06LH4CZ
06LH4DZ
06LH4ZZ
06LJ0CZ
06LJ0DZ
06LJ0ZZ
06LJ3CZ
06LJ3DZ
06LJ3ZZ
06LJ4CZ
06LJ4DZ
06LJ4ZZ
06LM0CZ
06LM0DZ
06LM0ZZ
06LM3CZ
06LM3DZ
06LM3ZZ
06LM4CZ
06LM4DZ
06LM4ZZ
06LN0CZ
06LN0DZ
06LN0ZZ
06LN3CZ
06LN3DZ
06LN3ZZ
06LN4CZ
06LN4DZ
06LN4ZZ
06LP0CZ
06LP0DZ
06LP0ZZ
06LP3CZ
06LP3DZ
06LP3ZZ
06LP4CZ
06LP4DZ
06LP4ZZ
06LQ0CZ
06LQ0DZ
06LQ0ZZ
06LQ3CZ
06LQ3DZ
06LQ3ZZ
06LQ4CZ
06LQ4DZ
06LQ4ZZ
06LT0CZ
06LT0DZ
06LT0ZZ
06LT3CZ
06LT3DZ
06LT3ZZ
06LT4CZ
06LT4DZ
06LT4ZZ
06LV0CZ
06LV0DZ
06LV0ZZ
06LV3CZ
06LV3DZ
06LV3ZZ
06LV4CZ
06LV4DZ

06LV4ZZ
06LY0CC
06LY0CZ
06LY0DC
06LY0DZ
06LY0ZC
06LY0ZZ
06LY3CC
06LY3CZ
06LY3DC
06LY3DZ
06LY3ZC
06LY3ZZ
06LY4CC
06LY4CZ
06LY4DC
06LY4DZ
06LY4ZC
06LY4ZZ
06N00ZZ
06N03ZZ
06N04ZZ
06N10ZZ
06N13ZZ
06N14ZZ
06N20ZZ
06N23ZZ
06N24ZZ
06N30ZZ
06N33ZZ
06N34ZZ
06N40ZZ
06N43ZZ
06N44ZZ
06N50ZZ
06N53ZZ
06N54ZZ
06N60ZZ
06N63ZZ
06N64ZZ
06N70ZZ
06N73ZZ
06N74ZZ
06N80ZZ
06N83ZZ
06N84ZZ
06N90ZZ
06N93ZZ
06N94ZZ
06NB0ZZ
06NB3ZZ
06NB4ZZ
06NC0ZZ
06NC3ZZ
06NC4ZZ
06ND0ZZ
06ND3ZZ
06ND4ZZ
06NF0ZZ
06NF3ZZ
06NF4ZZ
06NG0ZZ
06NG3ZZ
06NG4ZZ
06NH0ZZ
06NH3ZZ
06NH4ZZ
06NJ0ZZ
06NJ3ZZ
06NJ4ZZ
06NM0ZZ
06NM3ZZ
06NM4ZZ
06NN0ZZ
06NN3ZZ
06NN4ZZ
06NP0ZZ
06NP3ZZ
06NP4ZZ
06NQ0ZZ
06NQ3ZZ
06NQ4ZZ
06NT0ZZ
06NT3ZZ
06NT4ZZ
06NV0ZZ
06NV3ZZ
06NV4ZZ
06NY0ZZ
06NY3ZZ
06NY4ZZ
06PY00Z
06PY02Z
06PY03Z
06PY07Z
06PY0CZ
06PY0DZ
06PY0JZ
06PY0KZ
06PY0YZ
06PY30Z
06PY32Z
06PY33Z
06PY37Z
06PY3CZ
06PY3DZ
06PY3JZ
06PY3KZ
06PY3YZ
06PY40Z
06PY42Z
06PY43Z
06PY47Z
06PY4CZ
06PY4DZ
06PY4JZ
06PY4KZ
06PY4YZ
06PYX0Z
06PYX2Z
06PYX3Z
06PYXDZ
06Q00ZZ
06Q03ZZ
06Q04ZZ
06Q10ZZ
06Q13ZZ
06Q14ZZ
06Q20ZZ
06Q23ZZ
06Q24ZZ
06Q30ZZ
06Q33ZZ
06Q34ZZ
06Q40ZZ
06Q43ZZ
06Q44ZZ
06Q50ZZ
06Q53ZZ
06Q54ZZ
06Q60ZZ
06Q63ZZ
06Q64ZZ
06Q70ZZ
06Q73ZZ
06Q74ZZ
06Q80ZZ
06Q83ZZ
06Q84ZZ
06Q90ZZ
06Q93ZZ
06Q94ZZ
06QB0ZZ
06QB3ZZ
06QB4ZZ
06QC0ZZ
06QC3ZZ
06QC4ZZ
06QD0ZZ
06QD3ZZ
06QD4ZZ
06QF0ZZ
06QF3ZZ
06QF4ZZ
06QG0ZZ
06QG3ZZ
06QG4ZZ
06QH0ZZ
06QH3ZZ
06QH4ZZ
06QJ0ZZ
06QJ3ZZ
06QJ4ZZ
06QM0ZZ
06QM3ZZ
06QM4ZZ
06QN0ZZ
06QN3ZZ
06QN4ZZ
06QP0ZZ
06QP3ZZ
06QP4ZZ
06QQ0ZZ
06QQ3ZZ
06QQ4ZZ
06QT0ZZ
06QT3ZZ
06QT4ZZ
06QV0ZZ
06QV3ZZ
06QV4ZZ
06QY0ZZ
06QY3ZZ
06QY4ZZ
06R007Z
06R00JZ
06R00KZ
06R047Z
06R04JZ
06R04KZ
06R107Z
06R10JZ
06R10KZ
06R147Z
06R14JZ
06R14KZ
06R207Z
06R20JZ
06R20KZ
06R247Z
06R24JZ
06R24KZ
06R307Z
06R30JZ
06R30KZ
06R347Z
06R34JZ
06R34KZ
06R407Z
06R40JZ
06R40KZ
06R447Z
06R44JZ
06R44KZ
06R507Z
06R50JZ
06R50KZ
06R547Z
06R54JZ
06R54KZ
06R607Z
06R60JZ
06R60KZ
06R647Z
06R64JZ
06R64KZ
06R707Z
06R70JZ
06R70KZ
06R747Z
06R74JZ
06R74KZ
06R807Z
06R80JZ
06R80KZ
06R847Z
06R84JZ
06R84KZ
06R907Z
06R90JZ
06R90KZ
06R947Z
06R94JZ
06R94KZ
06RB07Z
06RB0JZ
06RB0KZ
06RB47Z
06RB4JZ
06RB4KZ
06RC07Z
06RC0JZ
06RC0KZ
06RC47Z
06RC4JZ
06SQ4ZZ
06ST0ZZ
06ST3ZZ
06ST4ZZ
06SV0ZZ
06SV3ZZ
06SV4ZZ
06SY0ZZ
06SY3ZZ
06SY4ZZ
06U007Z
06U00JZ
06U00KZ
06U037Z
06U03JZ
06U03KZ
06U047Z
06U04JZ
06U04KZ
06U107Z
06U10JZ
06U10KZ
06U137Z
06U13JZ
06U13KZ
06U147Z
06U14JZ
06U14KZ
06U207Z
06U20JZ
06U20KZ
06U237Z
06U23JZ
06U23KZ
06U247Z
06U24JZ
06U24KZ
06U307Z
06U30JZ
06U30KZ
06U337Z
06U33JZ
06U33KZ
06U347Z
06U34JZ
06U34KZ
06U407Z
06U40JZ
06U40KZ
06U437Z
06U43JZ
06U43KZ
06U447Z
06U44JZ
06U44KZ
06U507Z
06U50JZ
06U50KZ
06U537Z
06U53JZ
06U53KZ
06U547Z
06U54JZ
06U54KZ
06U607Z
06U60JZ
06U60KZ
06U637Z
06U63JZ
06U63KZ
06U647Z
06U64JZ
06U64KZ
06U707Z
06U70JZ
06U70KZ
06U737Z
06U73JZ
06U73KZ
06U747Z
06U74JZ
06U74KZ
06U807Z
06U80JZ
06U80KZ
06U837Z
06U83JZ
06U83KZ
06U847Z
06U84JZ
06U84KZ
06U907Z
06U90JZ
06U90KZ
06U937Z
06U93JZ
06U93KZ
06U947Z
06U94JZ
06U94KZ
06UB07Z
06UB0JZ
06UB0KZ
06UB37Z
06UB3JZ
06UB3KZ
06UB47Z
06UB4JZ
06UB4KZ
06UC07Z
06UC0JZ
06UC0KZ
06UC37Z
06UC3JZ
06UC3KZ
06UC47Z
06UC4JZ
06UC4KZ
06UD07Z
06UD0JZ
06UD0KZ
06UD37Z
06UD3JZ
06UD3KZ
06UD47Z
06UD4JZ
06UD4KZ
06UF07Z
06UF0JZ
06UF0KZ
06UF37Z
06UF3JZ
06UF3KZ
06UF47Z
06UF4JZ
06UF4KZ
06UG07Z
06UG0JZ
06UG0KZ
06UG37Z
06UG3JZ
06UG3KZ
06UG47Z
06UG4JZ
06UG4KZ
06UH07Z
06UH0JZ
06UH0KZ
06UH37Z
06UH3JZ
06UH3KZ
06UH47Z
06UH4JZ
06UH4KZ
06UJ07Z
06UJ0JZ
06UJ0KZ
06UJ37Z
06UJ3JZ
06UJ3KZ
06UJ47Z
06UJ4JZ
06UJ4KZ
06UM07Z
06UM0JZ
06UM0KZ
06UM37Z
06UM3JZ
06UM3KZ
06UM47Z
06UM4JZ
06UM4KZ
06UN07Z
06UN0JZ
06UN0KZ
06UN37Z
06UN3JZ
06UN3KZ
06UN47Z
06UN4JZ
06UN4KZ
06UP07Z
06UP0JZ
06UP0KZ
06UP37Z
06UP3JZ
06UP3KZ
06UP47Z
06UP4JZ
06UP4KZ
06UQ07Z
06UQ0JZ
06UQ0KZ
06UQ37Z
06UQ3JZ
06UQ3KZ
06UQ47Z
06UQ4JZ
06UQ4KZ
06UT07Z
06UT0JZ
06UT0KZ
06UT37Z
06UT3JZ
06UT3KZ
06UT47Z
06UT4JZ
06UT4KZ
06UV07Z
06UV0JZ
06UV0KZ
06UV37Z
06UV3JZ
06UV3KZ
06UV47Z
06UV4JZ
06UV4KZ
06UY07Z
06UY0JZ
06UY0KZ
06UY37Z
06UY3JZ
06UY3KZ
06UY47Z
06UY4JZ
06UY4KZ
06V00CZ
06V00DZ
06V00ZZ
06V03CZ
06V03DZ
06V03ZZ
06V04CZ
06V04DZ
06V04ZZ
06V10CZ
06V10DZ
06V10ZZ
06V13CZ
06V13DZ
06V13ZZ
06V14CZ
06V14DZ
06V14ZZ
06V20CZ
06V20DZ
06V20ZZ
06V23CZ
06V23DZ
06V23ZZ
06V24CZ
06V24DZ
06V24ZZ
06V30CZ
06V30DZ
06V30ZZ
06V33CZ
06V33DZ
06V33ZZ
06V34CZ
06V34DZ
06V34ZZ
06V40CZ
06V40DZ
06V40ZZ
06V43CZ
06V43DZ
06V43ZZ
06V44CZ
06V44DZ
06V44ZZ
06V50CZ
06V50DZ
06V50ZZ
06V53CZ
06V53DZ
06V53ZZ
06V54CZ
06V54DZ
06V54ZZ
06V60CZ
06V60DZ
06V60ZZ
06V63CZ
06V63DZ
06V63ZZ
06V64CZ
06V64DZ
06V64ZZ
06V70CZ
06V70DZ
06V70ZZ
06V73CZ
06V73DZ
06V73ZZ
06V74CZ
06V74DZ
06V74ZZ
06V80CZ
06V80DZ
06V80ZZ
06V83CZ
06V83DZ
06V83ZZ
06V84CZ
06V84DZ
06V84ZZ
06V90CZ
06V90DZ
06V90ZZ
06V93CZ
06V93DZ
06V93ZZ
06V94CZ
06V94DZ
06V94ZZ
06VB0CZ
06VB0DZ
06WY30Z
06WY32Z
06WY33Z
06WY3DZ
06WY3YZ
06WY4YZ
06WYX0Z
06WYX2Z
06WYX3Z
06WYX7Z
06WYXCZ
06WYXDZ
06WYXJZ
06WYXKZ
072KX0Z
072KXYZ
072LX0Z
072LXYZ
072MX0Z
072MXYZ
072NX0Z
072NXYZ
072PX0Z
072PXYZ
072TX0Z
072TXYZ
07590ZZ
07593ZZ
07594ZZ
075B0ZZ
075B3ZZ
075B4ZZ
075C0ZZ
075C3ZZ
075C4ZZ
075D0ZZ
075D3ZZ
075D4ZZ
075F0ZZ
075F3ZZ
075F4ZZ
075G0ZZ
075G3ZZ
075G4ZZ
075H0ZZ
075H3ZZ
075H4ZZ
075J0ZZ
075J3ZZ
075J4ZZ
075K0ZZ
075K3ZZ
075K4ZZ
075L0ZZ
075L3ZZ
075L4ZZ
075M0ZZ
075M3ZZ
075M4ZZ
075P0ZZ
075P3ZZ
075P4ZZ
079000Z
07900ZX
07900ZZ
079030Z
07903ZX
07903ZZ
079040Z
07904ZX
07904ZZ
079080Z
07908ZX
07908ZZ
079100Z
07910ZX
07910ZZ
079130Z
07913ZX
07913ZZ
079140Z
07914ZX
07914ZZ
079180Z
07918ZX
07918ZZ
079200Z
07920ZX
07920ZZ
079230Z
07923ZX
07923ZZ
079240Z
07924ZX
07924ZZ
079280Z
07928ZX
07928ZZ
079300Z
07930ZX
07930ZZ
079330Z
07933ZX
07933ZZ
079340Z
07934ZX
07934ZZ
079380Z
07938ZX
07938ZZ
079400Z
07940ZX
07940ZZ
079430Z
07943ZX
07943ZZ
079440Z
07944ZX
07944ZZ
079480Z
07948ZX
07948ZZ
079500Z
07950ZX
07950ZZ
079530Z
07953ZX
07953ZZ
079540Z
07954ZX
07954ZZ
079580Z
07958ZX
07958ZZ
079600Z
07960ZX
07960ZZ
079630Z
07963ZX
07963ZZ
079640Z
07964ZX
07964ZZ

079680Z
07968ZX
07968ZZ
079700Z
07970ZX
07970ZZ
079730Z
07973ZX
07973ZZ
079740Z
07974ZX
07974ZZ
079780Z
07978ZX
07978ZZ
079800Z
07980ZX
07980ZZ
079830Z
07983ZX
07983ZZ
079840Z
07984ZX
07984ZZ
079880Z
07988ZX
07988ZZ
079900Z
07990ZX
07990ZZ
079930Z
07993ZX
07993ZZ
079940Z
07994ZX
07994ZZ
079980Z
07998ZX
07998ZZ
079B00Z
079B0ZX
079B0ZZ
079B30Z
079B3ZX
079B3ZZ
079B40Z
079B4ZX
079B4ZZ
079B80Z
079B8ZX
079B8ZZ
079C00Z
079C0ZX
079C0ZZ
079C30Z
079C3ZX
079C3ZZ
079C40Z
079C4ZX
079C4ZZ
079C80Z
079C8ZX
079C8ZZ
079D00Z
079D0ZX
079D0ZZ
079D30Z
079D3ZX
079D3ZZ
079D40Z
079D4ZX
079D4ZZ
079D80Z
079D8ZX
079D8ZZ
079F00Z
079F0ZX
079F0ZZ
079F30Z
079F3ZX
079F3ZZ
079F40Z
079F4ZX
079F4ZZ
079F80Z
079F8ZX
079F8ZZ
079G00Z
079G0ZX
079G0ZZ
079G30Z
079G3ZX
079G3ZZ
079G40Z
079G4ZX
079G4ZZ
079G80Z
079G8ZX
079G8ZZ
079H00Z
079H0ZX
079H0ZZ
079H30Z
079H3ZX
079H3ZZ
079H40Z
079H4ZX
079H4ZZ
079H80Z
079H8ZX
079H8ZZ
079J00Z
079J0ZX
079J0ZZ
079J30Z
079J3ZX
079J3ZZ
079J40Z
079J4ZX
079J4ZZ
079J80Z
079J8ZX
079J8ZZ
079K00Z
079K0ZX
079K0ZZ
079K30Z
079K3ZX
079K3ZZ
079K40Z
079K4ZX
079K4ZZ
079K80Z
079K8ZX
079K8ZZ
079L00Z
079L0ZX
079L0ZZ
079L30Z
079L3ZX
079L3ZZ
079L40Z
079L4ZX
079L4ZZ
079L80Z
079L8ZX
079L8ZZ
079M00Z
079M0ZX
079M0ZZ
079M30Z
079M3ZX
079M3ZZ
079M40Z
079M4ZX
079M4ZZ
079P00Z
079P0ZX
079P0ZZ
079P30Z
079P3ZX
079P3ZZ
079P40Z
079P4ZX
079P4ZZ
079T00Z
079T0ZX
079T0ZZ
079T30Z
079T3ZX
079T3ZZ
079T40Z
079T4ZX
079T4ZZ
07B00ZX
07B00ZZ
07B03ZX
07B03ZZ
07B04ZX
07B04ZZ
07B10ZX
07BD0ZX
07BD0ZZ
07BD3ZX
07BD3ZZ
07BD4ZX
07BD4ZZ
07BF0ZX
07BF0ZZ
07BF3ZX
07BF3ZZ
07BF4ZX
07BF4ZZ
07BG0ZX
07BG0ZZ
07BG3ZX
07BG3ZZ
07BG4ZX
07BG4ZZ
07BH0ZX
07BH0ZZ
07BH3ZX
07BH3ZZ
07BH4ZX
07BH4ZZ
07BJ0ZX
07BJ0ZZ
07BJ3ZX
07BJ3ZZ
07BJ4ZX
07BJ4ZZ
07BK0ZX
07BK0ZZ
07BK3ZX
07BK3ZZ
07BK4ZX
07BK4ZZ
07BL0ZX
07BL0ZZ
07BL3ZX
07BL3ZZ
07BL4ZX
07BL4ZZ
07BM0ZX
07BM0ZZ
07BM3ZX
07BM3ZZ
07BM4ZX
07BM4ZZ
07BP0ZX
07BP0ZZ
07BP3ZX
07BP3ZZ
07BP4ZX
07BP4ZZ
07C00ZZ
07C03ZZ
07C04ZZ
07C10ZZ
07C13ZZ
07C14ZZ
07C20ZZ
07C23ZZ
07C24ZZ
07C30ZZ
07C33ZZ
07C34ZZ
07C40ZZ
07C43ZZ
07C44ZZ
07C50ZZ
07C53ZZ
07C54ZZ
07C60ZZ
07C63ZZ
07C64ZZ
07C70ZZ
07C73ZZ
07C74ZZ
07C80ZZ
07C83ZZ
07C84ZZ
07C90ZZ
07C93ZZ
07C94ZZ
07CB0ZZ
07CB3ZZ
07CB4ZZ
07CC0ZZ
07CC3ZZ
07CC4ZZ
07CD0ZZ
07CD3ZZ
07CD4ZZ
07CF0ZZ
07CF3ZZ
07CF4ZZ
07CG0ZZ
07CG3ZZ
07CG4ZZ
07CH0ZZ
07CH3ZZ
07CH4ZZ
07CJ0ZZ
07CJ3ZZ
07CJ4ZZ
07CK0ZZ
07CK3ZZ
07CK4ZZ
07CL0ZZ
07CL3ZZ
07CL4ZZ
07CM0ZZ
07CM3ZZ
07CM4ZZ
07CP0ZZ
07CP3ZZ
07CP4ZZ
07D03ZX
07D04ZX
07D08ZX
07D13ZX
07D14ZX
07D18ZX
07D23ZX
07D24ZX
07D28ZX
07D33ZX
07D34ZX
07D38ZX
07D43ZX
07D44ZX
07D48ZX
07D53ZX
07D54ZX
07D58ZX
07D63ZX
07D64ZX
07D68ZX
07D73ZX
07D74ZX
07D78ZX
07D83ZX
07D84ZX
07D88ZX
07D93ZX
07D94ZX
07D98ZX
07DB3ZX
07DB4ZX
07DB8ZX
07DC3ZX
07DC4ZX
07DC8ZX
07DD3ZX
07DD4ZX
07DD8ZX
07DF3ZX
07DF4ZX
07DF8ZX
07DG3ZX
07DG4ZX
07DG8ZX
07DH3ZX
07DH4ZX
07DH8ZX
07DJ3ZX
07DJ4ZX
07DJ8ZX
07DK3ZX
07DK4ZX
07DK8ZX
07DL3ZX
07DL4ZX
07DL8ZX
07DM3ZX
07DM4ZX
07DP3ZX
07DP4ZX
07DQ0ZX
07DQ0ZZ
07DQ3ZX
07DQ3ZZ
07DR0ZX
07DR0ZZ
07DR3ZX
07DR3ZZ
07DS0ZX
07DS0ZZ
07DS3ZX
07DS3ZZ
07HK03Z
07HK0YZ
07HK33Z
07HK3YZ
07HK43Z
07HK4YZ
07HL03Z
07HL0YZ
07HL33Z
07HL3YZ
07HL43Z
07HL4YZ
07HM03Z
07HM0YZ
07HM33Z
07HM3YZ
07HM43Z
07HM4YZ
07HN03Z
07HN0YZ
07HN33Z
07HN3YZ
07HN43Z
07HN4YZ
07HP03Z
07HP0YZ
07HP33Z
07HP3YZ
07HP43Z
07HP4YZ
07JK0ZZ
07JK3ZZ
07JK4ZZ
07JL0ZZ
07JL3ZZ
07JL4ZZ
07JM0ZZ
07JM3ZZ
07JM4ZZ
07JN0ZZ
07JN3ZZ
07JN4ZZ
07JN8ZZ
07JNXZZ
07JP0ZZ
07JP3ZZ
07JP4ZZ
07JPXZZ
07JT0ZZ
07JT3ZZ
07JT4ZZ
07L00CZ
07L00DZ
07L00ZZ
07L03CZ
07L03DZ
07L03ZZ
07L04CZ
07L04DZ
07L04ZZ
07L10CZ
07L10DZ
07L10ZZ
07L13CZ
07L13DZ
07L13ZZ
07L14CZ
07L14DZ
07L14ZZ
07L20CZ
07L20DZ
07L20ZZ
07L23CZ
07L23DZ
07L23ZZ
07L24CZ
07L24DZ
07L24ZZ
07L30CZ
07L30DZ
07L30ZZ
07L33CZ
07L33DZ
07L33ZZ
07L34CZ
07L34DZ
07L34ZZ
07L40CZ
07L40DZ
07L40ZZ
07L43CZ
07L43DZ
07L43ZZ
07L44CZ
07L44DZ
07L44ZZ
07L50CZ
07L50DZ
07L50ZZ
07L53CZ
07L53DZ
07L53ZZ
07L54CZ
07L54DZ
07L54ZZ
07L60CZ
07L60DZ
07L60ZZ
07L63CZ
07L63DZ
07L63ZZ
07L64CZ
07L64DZ
07L64ZZ
07L70CZ
07L70DZ
07LL4ZZ
07N00ZZ
07N03ZZ
07N04ZZ
07N10ZZ
07N13ZZ
07N14ZZ
07N20ZZ
07N23ZZ
07N24ZZ
07N30ZZ
07N33ZZ
07N34ZZ
07N40ZZ
07N43ZZ
07N44ZZ
07N50ZZ
07N53ZZ
07N54ZZ
07N60ZZ
07N63ZZ
07N64ZZ
07N70ZZ
07N73ZZ
07N74ZZ
07N80ZZ
07N83ZZ
07N84ZZ
07N90ZZ
07N93ZZ
07N94ZZ
07NB0ZZ
07NB3ZZ
07NB4ZZ
07NC0ZZ
07NC3ZZ
07NC4ZZ
07ND0ZZ
07ND3ZZ
07ND4ZZ
07NF0ZZ
07NF3ZZ
07NF4ZZ
07NG0ZZ
07NG3ZZ
07NG4ZZ
07NH0ZZ
07NH3ZZ
07NH4ZZ
07NJ0ZZ
07NJ3ZZ
07NJ4ZZ
07NK0ZZ
07NK3ZZ
07NK4ZZ
07NL0ZZ
07NL3ZZ
07NL4ZZ
07NM0ZZ
07NM3ZZ
07NM4ZZ
07NP0ZZ
07NP3ZZ
07NP4ZZ
07PK00Z
07PK03Z
07PK07Z
07PK0CZ
07PK0DZ
07PK0JZ
07PK0KZ
07PK0YZ
07PK30Z
07PK33Z
07PK37Z
07PK3CZ
07PK3DZ
07PK3JZ
07PK3KZ
07PK3YZ
07PK40Z
07PK43Z
07PK47Z
07PK4CZ
07PK4DZ
07PK4JZ
07PK4KZ
07PK4YZ
07PKX0Z
07PKX3Z
07PKXDZ
07PL00Z
07PL03Z
07PL07Z
07PL0CZ
07PL0DZ
07PL0JZ
07PL0KZ
07PL0YZ
07PL30Z
07PL33Z
07PL37Z
07PL3CZ
07PL3DZ
07PL3JZ
07PL3KZ
07PL3YZ
07PL40Z
07PL43Z
07PL47Z
07PL4CZ
07PL4DZ
07PL4JZ
07PL4KZ
07PL4YZ
07PLX0Z
07PLX3Z
07PLXDZ
07PM00Z
07PM03Z
07PM0YZ
07PM30Z
07PM33Z
07PM3YZ
07PM40Z
07PM43Z
07PM4YZ
07PMX0Z
07PMX3Z
07PN00Z
07PN03Z
07PN07Z
07PN0CZ
07PN0DZ
07PN0JZ
07PN0KZ
07PN0YZ
07PN30Z
07PN33Z
07PN37Z
07PN3CZ
07PN3DZ
07PN3JZ
07PN3KZ
07PN3YZ
07PN40Z
07PN43Z
07PN47Z
07PN4CZ
07PN4DZ
07PN4JZ
07PN4KZ
07PN4YZ
07PNX0Z
07PNX3Z
07PNXDZ
07PP00Z
07PP03Z
07PP0YZ
07PP30Z
07PP33Z
07PP3YZ
07PP40Z
07PP43Z
07PP4YZ
07PPX0Z
07PPX3Z
07PT00Z
07PT30Z
07PT40Z
07PTX0Z
07Q00ZZ
07Q03ZZ
07Q04ZZ
07Q08ZZ
07Q10ZZ
07Q13ZZ
07Q14ZZ
07Q18ZZ
07Q20ZZ
07Q23ZZ
07Q24ZZ
07Q28ZZ
07Q30ZZ
07Q33ZZ
07Q34ZZ
07Q38ZZ
07Q40ZZ
07Q43ZZ
07Q44ZZ
07Q48ZZ
07Q50ZZ
07Q53ZZ
07Q54ZZ
07Q58ZZ
07Q60ZZ
07Q63ZZ
07Q64ZZ
07Q68ZZ
07Q70ZZ
07Q73ZZ
07Q74ZZ
07Q78ZZ
07Q80ZZ
07Q83ZZ
07Q84ZZ
07Q88ZZ
07Q90ZZ
07Q93ZZ
07Q94ZZ
07Q98ZZ
07QB0ZZ
07QB3ZZ
07QB4ZZ
07QB8ZZ
07QC0ZZ
07QC3ZZ
07QC4ZZ
07QC8ZZ
07QD0ZZ
07QD3ZZ
07QD4ZZ
07QD8ZZ
07QF0ZZ
07QF3ZZ
07QF4ZZ
07QF8ZZ
07QG0ZZ
07QG3ZZ
07QG4ZZ
07QG8ZZ
07QH0ZZ
07QH3ZZ
07QH4ZZ
07QH8ZZ
07QJ0ZZ
07QJ3ZZ
07QJ4ZZ
07QJ8ZZ

07QK0ZZ
07QK3ZZ
07QK4ZZ
07QK8ZZ
07QL0ZZ
07QL3ZZ
07QL4ZZ
07QL8ZZ
07QM0ZZ
07QM3ZZ
07QM4ZZ
07T50ZZ
07T60ZZ
07T70ZZ
07T80ZZ
07T90ZZ
07U107Z
07U10JZ
07U10KZ
07U147Z
07U14JZ
07U14KZ
07U207Z
07U20JZ
07U20KZ
07U247Z
07U24JZ
07U24KZ
07U307Z
07U30JZ
07U30KZ
07U347Z
07U34JZ
07U34KZ
07U407Z
07U40JZ
07U40KZ
07U447Z
07U44JZ
07U44KZ
07U507Z
07U50JZ
07U50KZ
07U547Z
07U54JZ
07U54KZ
07U607Z
07U60JZ
07U60KZ
07U647Z
07U64JZ
07U64KZ
07U707Z
07U70JZ
07U70KZ
07U747Z
07U74JZ
07U74KZ
07U807Z
07U80JZ
07U80KZ
07U847Z
07U84JZ
07U84KZ
07U907Z
07U90JZ

07U90KZ
07U947Z
07U94JZ
07U94KZ
07UB07Z
07UB0JZ
07UB0KZ
07UB47Z
07UB4JZ
07UB4KZ
07UC07Z
07UC0JZ
07UC0KZ
07UC47Z
07UC4JZ
07UC4KZ
07UD07Z
07UD0JZ
07UD0KZ
07UD47Z
07UD4JZ
07UD4KZ
07UF07Z
07UF0JZ
07UF0KZ
07UF47Z
07UF4JZ
07UF4KZ
07UG07Z
07UG0JZ
07UG0KZ
07UG47Z
07UG4JZ
07UG4KZ
07UH07Z
07UH0JZ
07UH0KZ
07UH47Z
07UH4JZ
07UH4KZ
07UJ07Z
07UJ0JZ
07UJ0KZ
07UJ47Z
07UJ4JZ
07UJ4KZ
07UK07Z
07UK0JZ
07UK0KZ
07UK47Z
07UK4JZ
07UK4KZ
07UL07Z
07UL0JZ
07UL0KZ
07UL47Z
07UL4JZ
07UL4KZ
07V00CZ
07V00DZ
07V00ZZ
07V03CZ
07V03DZ
07V03ZZ
07V04CZ
07V04DZ

07V04ZZ
07V10CZ
07V10DZ
07V10ZZ
07V13CZ
07V13DZ
07V13ZZ
07V14CZ
07V14DZ
07V14ZZ
07V20CZ
07V20DZ
07V20ZZ
07V23CZ
07V23DZ
07V23ZZ
07V24CZ
07V24DZ
07V24ZZ
07V30CZ
07V30DZ
07V30ZZ
07V33CZ
07V33DZ
07V33ZZ
07V34CZ
07V34DZ
07V34ZZ
07V40CZ
07V40DZ
07V40ZZ
07V43CZ
07V43DZ
07V43ZZ
07V44CZ
07V44DZ
07V44ZZ
07V50CZ
07V50DZ
07V50ZZ
07V53CZ
07V53DZ
07V53ZZ
07V54CZ
07V54DZ
07V54ZZ
07V60CZ
07V60DZ
07V60ZZ
07V63CZ
07V63DZ
07V63ZZ
07V64CZ
07V64DZ
07V64ZZ
07V70CZ
07V70DZ
07V70ZZ
07V73CZ
07V73DZ
07V73ZZ
07V74CZ
07V74DZ
07V74ZZ
07V80CZ
07V80DZ

07V80ZZ
07V83CZ
07V83DZ
07V83ZZ
07V84CZ
07V84DZ
07V84ZZ
07V90CZ
07V90DZ
07V90ZZ
07V93CZ
07V93DZ
07V93ZZ
07V94CZ
07V94DZ
07V94ZZ
07VB0CZ
07VB0DZ
07VB0ZZ
07VB3CZ
07VB3DZ
07VB3ZZ
07VB4CZ
07VB4DZ
07VB4ZZ
07VC0CZ
07VC0DZ
07VC0ZZ
07VC3CZ
07WK3YZ
07WK4YZ
07WKX0Z
07WKX3Z
07WKX7Z
07WKXCZ
07WKXDZ
07WKXJZ
07WKXKZ
07WL3YZ
07WL4YZ
07WLX0Z
07WLX3Z
07WLX7Z
07WLXCZ
07WLXDZ
07WLXJZ
07WLXKZ
07WM3YZ
07WM4YZ
07WMX0Z
07WMX3Z
07WN3KZ
07WN3YZ
07WN40Z
07WN43Z
07WN47Z
07WN4CZ
07WN4DZ
07WN4JZ
07WN4KZ
07WN4YZ
07WNX0Z
07WNX3Z
07WNX7Z
07WNXCZ
07WNXDZ

07WNXJZ
07WNXKZ
07WP00Z
07WP03Z
07WP0YZ
07WP30Z
07WP33Z
07WP3YZ
07WP40Z
07WP43Z
07WP4YZ
07WPX0Z
07WPX3Z
07WT00Z
07WT30Z
07WT40Z
07WTX0Z
07YM0Z0
07YM0Z1
07YM0Z2
07YP0Z0
07YP0Z1
07YP0Z2
080N07Z
080N0JZ
080N0KZ
080N0ZZ
080N37Z
080N3JZ
080N3KZ
080N3ZZ
080NX7Z
080NXJZ
080NXKZ
080NXZZ
080P07Z
080P0JZ
080P0KZ
080P0ZZ
080P37Z
080P3JZ
080P3KZ
080P3ZZ
080PX7Z
080PXJZ
080PXKZ
080PXZZ
080Q07Z
080Q0JZ
080Q0KZ
080Q0ZZ
080Q37Z
080Q3JZ
080Q3KZ
080Q3ZZ
080QX7Z
080QXJZ
080QXKZ
080QXZZ
080R07Z
080R0JZ
080R0KZ
080R0ZZ
080R37Z
080R3JZ
080R3KZ

080R3ZZ
080RX7Z
080RXJZ
080RXKZ
080RXZZ
08123J4
08123K4
08123Z4
08133J4
08133K4
08133Z4
081X0J3
081X0K3
081X0Z3
081X3J3
081X3K3
081X3Z3
081Y0J3
081Y0K3
081Y0Z3
081Y3J3
081Y3K3
081Y3Z3
0820X0Z
0820XYZ
0821X0Z
0821XYZ
0850XZZ
0851XZZ
08523ZZ
08533ZZ
08543ZZ
08553ZZ
0856XZZ
0857XZZ
0858XZZ
0859XZZ
085A0ZZ
085A3ZZ
085B0ZZ
085B3ZZ
085C3ZZ
085D3ZZ
085E3ZZ
085F3ZZ
085G3ZZ
085H3ZZ
085J3ZZ
085K3ZZ
085L0ZZ
085L3ZZ
085M0ZZ
085M3ZZ
085N0ZZ
085N3ZZ
085NXZZ
085P0ZZ
085P3ZZ
085PXZZ
085Q0ZZ
085Q3ZZ
085QXZZ
085R0ZZ
085R3ZZ
085RXZZ
085SXZZ

085TXZZ
085V0ZZ
085V3ZZ
085W0ZZ
085W3ZZ
085X0ZZ
085X3ZZ
085X7ZZ
085X8ZZ
085Y0ZZ
085Y3ZZ
085Y7ZZ
085Y8ZZ
087X0DZ
087X0ZZ
087X3DZ
087X3ZZ
087X7DZ
087X7ZZ
087X8DZ
087X8ZZ
087Y0DZ
087Y0ZZ
087Y3DZ
087Y3ZZ
087Y7DZ
087Y7ZZ
087Y8DZ
087Y8ZZ
0890X0Z
0890XZX
0890XZZ
0891X0Z
0891XZX
0891XZZ
089230Z
08923ZX
08923ZZ
089330Z
08933ZX
08933ZZ
089430Z
08943ZX
08943ZZ
089530Z
08953ZX
08953ZZ
0896X0Z
0896XZX
0896XZZ
0897X0Z
0897XZX
0897XZZ
0898X0Z
0898XZX
0898XZZ
0899X0Z
0899XZX
0899XZZ
089A00Z
089A0ZX
089A0ZZ
089A30Z
089A3ZX
089A3ZZ
089B00Z

089B0ZX
089B0ZZ
089B30Z
089B3ZX
089B3ZZ
089C30Z
089C3ZX
089C3ZZ
089D30Z
089D3ZX
089D3ZZ
089E30Z
089E3ZX
089E3ZZ
089F30Z
089F3ZX
089F3ZZ
089G30Z
089G3ZX
089G3ZZ
089H30Z
089H3ZX
089H3ZZ
089J30Z
089J3ZX
089J3ZZ
089K30Z
089K3ZX
089K3ZZ
089L00Z
089L0ZX
089L0ZZ
089L30Z
089L3ZX
089L3ZZ
089M00Z
089M0ZX
089M0ZZ
089M30Z
089M3ZX
089M3ZZ
089N00Z
089N0ZX
089N0ZZ
089N30Z
089N3ZX
089N3ZZ
089NX0Z
089NXZX
089NXZZ
089P00Z
089P0ZX
089P0ZZ
089P30Z
089P3ZX
089P3ZZ
089PX0Z
089PXZX
089PXZZ
089Q00Z
089Q0ZX
089Q0ZZ
089Q30Z
089Q3ZX
089Q3ZZ
089QX0Z

089QXZX
089QXZZ
089R00Z
089R0ZX
089R0ZZ
089R30Z
089R3ZX
089R3ZZ
089RX0Z
089RXZX
089RXZZ
089SX0Z
089SXZX
089SXZZ
089TX0Z
089TXZX
089TXZZ
089V00Z
089V0ZX
089V0ZZ
089V30Z
089V3ZX
089V3ZZ
089W00Z
089W0ZX
089W0ZZ
089W30Z
089W3ZX
089W3ZZ
089X00Z
089X0ZX
089X0ZZ
089X30Z
089X3ZX
089X3ZZ
089X70Z
089X7ZX
089X7ZZ
089X80Z
089X8ZX
089X8ZZ
089Y00Z
089Y0ZX
089Y0ZZ
089Y30Z
089Y3ZX
089Y3ZZ
089Y70Z
089Y7ZX
089Y7ZZ
089Y80Z
089Y8ZX
089Y8ZZ
08B00ZX
08B00ZZ
08B03ZX
08B03ZZ
08B0XZX
08B0XZZ
08B10ZX
08B10ZZ
08B13ZX
08B13ZZ
08B1XZX
08B1XZZ
08B43ZX

08B43ZZ
08B53ZX
08B53ZZ
08B6XZX
08B6XZZ
08B7XZX
08B7XZZ
08B8XZX
08B8XZZ
08B9XZX
08B9XZZ
08BA0ZX
08BA0ZZ
08BA3ZX
08BA3ZZ
08BB0ZX
08BB0ZZ
08BB3ZX
08BB3ZZ
08BC3ZX
08BC3ZZ
08BD3ZX
08BD3ZZ
08BE3ZX
08BE3ZZ
08BF3ZX
08BF3ZZ
08BJ3ZX
08BJ3ZZ
08BK3ZX
08BK3ZZ
08BL0ZX
08BL0ZZ
08BL3ZX
08BL3ZZ
08BM0ZX
08BM0ZZ
08BM3ZX
08BM3ZZ
08BN0ZX
08BN0ZZ
08BN3ZX
08BN3ZZ
08BNXZX
08BNXZZ
08BP0ZX
08BP0ZZ
08BP3ZX
08BP3ZZ
08BPXZX
08BPXZZ
08BQ0ZX
08BQ0ZZ
08BQ3ZX
08BQ3ZZ
08BQXZX
08BQXZZ
08BR0ZX
08BR0ZZ
08BR3ZX
08BR3ZZ
08C0XZZ
08C1XZZ
08C2XZZ
08C3XZZ
08C6XZZ

08C7XZZ
08CN0ZZ
08CN3ZZ
08CNXZZ
08CP0ZZ
08CP3ZZ
08CPXZZ
08CQ0ZZ
08CQ3ZZ
08CQXZZ
08CR0ZZ
08CR3ZZ
08CRXZZ
08CSXZZ
08CTXZZ
08F4XZZ
08F5XZZ
08H03YZ
08H07YZ
08H08YZ
08H13YZ
08H17YZ
08H18YZ
08J0XZZ
08J1XZZ
08JJXZZ
08JKXZZ
08JLXZZ
08JMXZZ
08NM3ZZ
08NN0ZZ
08NN3ZZ
08NNXZZ
08NP0ZZ
08NP3ZZ
08NPXZZ
08NQ0ZZ
08NQ3ZZ
08NQXZZ
08NR0ZZ
08NR3ZZ
08NRXZZ
08NSXZZ
08NTXZZ
08NV0ZZ
08NV3ZZ
08NW0ZZ
08NW3ZZ
08NX0ZZ
08NX3ZZ
08NX7ZZ
08NX8ZZ
08NY0ZZ
08NY3ZZ
08NY7ZZ
08NY8ZZ
08P000Z
08P001Z
08P003Z
08P007Z
08P00CZ
08P00DZ
08P00JZ
08P00KZ
08P00YZ
08P030Z

08P031Z
08P033Z
08P037Z
08P03CZ
08P03DZ
08P03JZ
08P03KZ
08P03YZ
08P070Z
08P071Z
08P073Z
08P077Z
08P07CZ
08P07DZ
08P07JZ
08P07KZ
08P07YZ
08P080Z
08P081Z
08P083Z
08P087Z
08P08CZ
08P08DZ
08P08JZ
08P08KZ
08P08YZ
08P0X0Z
08P0X1Z
08P0X3Z
08P0X7Z
08P0XCZ
08P0XDZ
08P0XJZ
08P0XKZ
08P100Z
08P101Z
08P103Z
08P107Z
08P10CZ
08P10DZ
08P10JZ
08P10KZ
08P10YZ
08P130Z
08P131Z
08P133Z
08P137Z
08P13CZ
08P13DZ
08P13JZ
08P13KZ
08P13YZ
08P170Z
08P171Z
08P173Z
08P177Z
08P17CZ
08P17DZ
08P17JZ
08P17KZ
08P17YZ
08P180Z
08P181Z
08P183Z
08P187Z
08P18CZ
08P18DZ
08P18JZ
08P18KZ
08P18YZ
08P1X0Z
08P1X1Z
08P1X3Z
08P1X7Z
08P1XCZ
08P1XDZ
08P1XJZ
08P1XKZ
08PJ3JZ
08PJ3YZ
08PK3JZ
08PK3YZ
08PL00Z
08PL07Z
08PL0JZ
08PL0KZ
08PL0YZ
08PL30Z
08PL37Z
08PL3JZ
08PL3KZ
08PL3YZ
08PM00Z
08PM07Z
08PM0JZ
08PM0KZ
08PM0YZ
08PM30Z
08PM37Z
08PM3JZ
08PM3KZ
08PM3YZ
08Q0XZZ
08Q1XZZ
08Q23ZZ
08Q33ZZ
08Q43ZZ
08Q53ZZ
08Q6XZZ
08Q7XZZ
08Q8XZZ
08Q9XZZ
08QA0ZZ
08QA3ZZ
08QB0ZZ
08QB3ZZ
08QC3ZZ
08QD3ZZ
08QE3ZZ
08QF3ZZ
08QG3ZZ
08QH3ZZ
08QJ3ZZ
08QK3ZZ
08QL0ZZ
08QL3ZZ
08QM0ZZ
08QM3ZZ
08QN0ZZ
08QN3ZZ
08QNXZZ
08QP0ZZ
08QP3ZZ
08QPXZZ
08QQ0ZZ
08QQ3ZZ
08QQXZZ
08QR0ZZ
08QR3ZZ
08QRXZZ
08QSXZZ
08QTXZZ
08QV0ZZ
08QV3ZZ
08QW0ZZ
08QW3ZZ
08QX0ZZ
08QX3ZZ
08QX7ZZ
08QX8ZZ
08QY0ZZ
08QY3ZZ
08QY7ZZ
08QY8ZZ
08R007Z
08R00JZ
08R00KZ
08R037Z
08R03JZ
08R03KZ
08R107Z
08R10JZ
08R10KZ
08R137Z
08R13JZ
08R13KZ
08R437Z
08R43JZ
08R43KZ
08R537Z
08R53JZ
08R53KZ
08R6X7Z
08R6XJZ
08R6XKZ
08R7X7Z
08R7XJZ
08R7XKZ
08R837Z
08R83JZ
08R83KZ
08R8X7Z
08R8XJZ
08R8XKZ
08R937Z
08R93JZ
08R93KZ
08R9X7Z
08R9XJZ
08R9XKZ
08RA07Z
08RA0JZ
08RA0KZ
08RA37Z
08RA3JZ
08RA3KZ
08RB07Z
08RB0JZ
08RB0KZ
08RB37Z
08RB3JZ
08RB3KZ
08RC37Z
08RC3JZ
08RC3KZ
08RD37Z
08RD3JZ
08RD3KZ
08RG37Z
08RG3JZ
08RG3KZ
08RH37Z
08RH3JZ
08RH3KZ
08RJ30Z
08RJ37Z
08RJ3JZ
08RJ3KZ
08RK30Z
08RK37Z
08RK3JZ
08RK3KZ
08RN07Z
08RN0JZ
08RN0KZ
08RN37Z
08RN3JZ
08RN3KZ
08RNX7Z
08RNXJZ
08RNXKZ
08RP07Z
08RP0JZ
08RP0KZ
08RP37Z
08RP3JZ
08RP3KZ
08RPX7Z
08RPXJZ
08RPXKZ
08RQ07Z
08RQ0JZ
08RQ0KZ
08RQ37Z
08RQ3JZ
08RQ3KZ
08RQX7Z
08RQXJZ
08RQXKZ
08RR07Z
08RR0JZ
08RR0KZ
08RR37Z
08RR3JZ
08RR3KZ
08RRX7Z
08RRXJZ
08RRXKZ
08RSX7Z
08RSXJZ
08RSXKZ
08RTX7Z
08RTXJZ
08RTXKZ
08RX07Z
08RX0JZ
08RX0KZ
08RX37Z
08RX3JZ
08RX3KZ
08RX77Z
08RX7JZ
08RX7KZ
08RX87Z
08RX8JZ
08RX8KZ
08RY07Z
08RY0JZ
08RY0KZ
08RY37Z
08RY3JZ
08RY3KZ
08UD0KZ
08UD37Z
08UD3JZ
08UD3KZ
08UE07Z
08UE0JZ
08UE0KZ
08UE37Z
08UE3JZ
08UE3KZ
08UF07Z
08UF0JZ
08UF0KZ
08UF37Z
08UF3JZ
08UF3KZ
08UG07Z
08UG0JZ
08UG0KZ
08UG37Z
08UG3JZ
08UG3KZ
08UH07Z
08UH0JZ
08UH0KZ
08UH37Z
08UH3JZ
08UH3KZ
08UL07Z
08UL0JZ
08UL0KZ
08UL37Z
08UL3JZ
08UL3KZ
08UM07Z
08UM0JZ
08UM0KZ
08UM37Z
08UM3JZ
08UM3KZ
08UN07Z
08UN0JZ
08UN0KZ
08UN37Z
08UN3JZ
08UN3KZ
08UNX7Z
08UNXJZ
08UNXKZ
08UP07Z
08UP0JZ
08UP0KZ
08UP37Z
08UP3JZ
08UP3KZ
08UPX7Z
08UPXJZ
08UPXKZ
08UQ07Z
08UQ0JZ
08UQ0KZ
08UQ37Z
08UQ3JZ
08UQ3KZ
08UQX7Z
08UQXJZ
08UQXKZ
08UR07Z
08UR0JZ
08UR0KZ
08UR37Z
08UR3JZ
08UR3KZ
08URX7Z
08URXJZ
08URXKZ
08UX07Z
08UX0JZ
08UX0KZ
08UX37Z
08UX3JZ
08UX3KZ
08UX77Z
08UX7JZ
08UX7KZ
08UX87Z
08UX8JZ
08UX8KZ
08UY07Z
08UY0JZ
08UY0KZ
08UY37Z
08UY3JZ
08UY3KZ
08UY77Z
08UY7JZ
08UY7KZ
08UY87Z
08UY8JZ
08UY8KZ
08VX0CZ
08VX0DZ
08VX0ZZ
08VX3CZ
08VX3DZ
08VX3ZZ
08VX7DZ
08VX7ZZ
08VX8DZ
08VX8ZZ
08VY0CZ
08VY0DZ
08VY0ZZ
08VY3CZ
08VY3DZ
08VY3ZZ
08VY7DZ
08VY7ZZ
08VY8DZ
08VY8ZZ
08W000Z
08W003Z
08W007Z
08W00CZ
08W00DZ
08W00JZ
08W00KZ
08W00YZ
08W030Z
08W033Z
08W037Z
08W03CZ
08W03DZ
08W03JZ
08W03KZ
08W03YZ
08W070Z
08W073Z
08W077Z
08W07CZ
08W07DZ
08W07JZ
08W07KZ
08W07YZ
08W080Z
08W083Z
08W087Z
08W08CZ
08W08DZ
08W08JZ
08W08KZ
08W08YZ
08W0X0Z
08W0X3Z
08W0X7Z
08W0XCZ
08W0XDZ
08W0XJZ
08W0XKZ
08W100Z
08W103Z
08W107Z
08W10CZ
08W10DZ
08W10JZ
08W10KZ
08W10YZ
08W130Z
08W133Z
08W137Z
08W13CZ
08W13DZ
08W13JZ
08W13KZ
08W13YZ
08W170Z
08W173Z
08W177Z
08W17CZ
08W17DZ
08W17JZ
08W17KZ
08W17YZ
08W180Z
08W183Z
08W187Z
08W18CZ
08W18DZ
08W18JZ
08W18KZ
08W18YZ
08W1X0Z
08W1X3Z
08W1X7Z
08W1XCZ
08W1XDZ
08W1XJZ
08W1XKZ
08WJ3JZ
08WJ3YZ
08WJXJZ
08WK3JZ
08WK3YZ
08WKXJZ
08WL00Z
08WL07Z
08WL0JZ
08WL0KZ
08WL0YZ
08WL30Z
08WL37Z
08WL3JZ
08WL3KZ
08WL3YZ
08WM00Z
08WM07Z
08WM0JZ
08WM0KZ
08WM0YZ
08WM30Z
08WM37Z
08WM3JZ
08WM3KZ
08WM3YZ
08XL0ZZ
08XL3ZZ
08XM0ZZ
08XM3ZZ
090007Z
09000JZ
09000KZ
09000ZZ
090037Z
09003JZ
09003KZ
09003ZZ
090047Z
09004JZ
09004KZ
09004ZZ
0900X7Z
0900XJZ
0900XKZ
0900XZZ
090107Z
09010JZ
09010KZ
09010ZZ
090137Z
09013JZ
09013KZ
09013ZZ
090147Z
09014JZ
09014KZ
09014ZZ
0901X7Z
0901XJZ
0901XKZ
0901XZZ
090207Z
09020JZ
09020KZ
09020ZZ
090237Z
09023JZ
09023KZ
09023ZZ
090247Z
09024JZ
09024KZ
09024ZZ
0902X7Z
0902XJZ
0902XKZ
0902XZZ
090K07Z
090K0JZ
090K0KZ
090K0ZZ
090K37Z
090K3JZ
090K3KZ
090K3ZZ
090K47Z
090K4JZ
090K4KZ
090K4ZZ
090KX7Z
090KXJZ
090KXKZ
092HX0Z
092HXYZ
092JX0Z
092JXYZ
092KX0Z
092KXYZ
092YX0Z
092YXYZ
093K7ZZ
093K8ZZ
09500ZZ
09503ZZ
09504ZZ
0950XZZ
09510ZZ
09513ZZ
09514ZZ
0951XZZ
09530ZZ
09533ZZ
09534ZZ
09537ZZ
09538ZZ
0953XZZ
09540ZZ
09543ZZ
09544ZZ
09547ZZ
09548ZZ
0954XZZ
095F0ZZ
095F3ZZ
095F4ZZ
095F7ZZ
095F8ZZ
095G0ZZ
095G3ZZ
095G4ZZ
095G7ZZ
095G8ZZ
095K0ZZ
095K3ZZ
095K4ZZ
095K8ZZ
095KXZZ
095M0ZZ
095M3ZZ
095M4ZZ
095M8ZZ
097F0DZ
097F0ZZ
097F3ZZ
097F4ZZ
097F7DZ
097F7ZZ
097F8DZ
097F8ZZ
097G0DZ
097G0ZZ
097G3ZZ
097G4ZZ
097G7DZ
097G7ZZ
097G8DZ
097G8ZZ
099000Z
09900ZX
09900ZZ
099030Z
09903ZX
09903ZZ
099040Z
09904ZX
09904ZZ
0990X0Z
0990XZX
0990XZZ
099100Z
09910ZX
09910ZZ
099130Z
09913ZX
09913ZZ
099140Z
09914ZX
09914ZZ
0991X0Z
0991XZX
0991XZZ
099300Z
09930ZX
09930ZZ
099330Z
09933ZX
09933ZZ
099340Z
09934ZX
09934ZZ
099370Z
09937ZX
09937ZZ
099380Z
09938ZX
09938ZZ
0993X0Z
0993XZX
0993XZZ
099400Z
09940ZX
09940ZZ
099430Z
09943ZX
09943ZZ
099440Z
09944ZX
09944ZZ
099470Z
09947ZX
09947ZZ
099480Z
09948ZX
09948ZZ
0994X0Z
0994XZX
0994XZZ
09950ZZ
09957ZX
09957ZZ
099580Z
09958ZX
09958ZZ
09960ZZ
099670Z
09967ZX
09967ZZ
099680Z
09968ZX
09968ZZ
09970ZZ
09973ZZ
09974ZZ
09977ZX
09977ZZ
09978ZX
09978ZZ
09980ZZ
09983ZZ
09984ZZ
09987ZX
09987ZZ
09988ZX
09988ZZ
099970Z

09997ZX
09997ZZ
099980Z
09998ZX
09998ZZ
099A70Z
099A7ZX
099A7ZZ
099A80Z
099A8ZX
099A8ZZ
099B30Z
099B3ZZ
099B70Z
099B7ZX
099B7ZZ
099B80Z
099B8ZX
099B8ZZ
099C30Z
099C3ZZ
099C70Z
099C7ZX
099C7ZZ
099C80Z
099C8ZX
099C8ZZ
099D70Z
099D7ZX
099D7ZZ
099D80Z
099D8ZX
099D8ZZ
099E70Z
099E7ZX
099E7ZZ
099E80Z
099E8ZX
099E8ZZ
099F00Z
099F0ZZ
099F30Z
099F3ZZ
099F40Z
099F4ZZ
099F70Z
099F7ZX
099F7ZZ
099F80Z
099F8ZX
099F8ZZ
099G00Z
099G0ZZ
099G30Z
099G3ZZ
099G40Z
099G4ZZ
099G70Z
099G7ZX
099G7ZZ
099G80Z
099G8ZX
099G8ZZ
099K00Z
099K0ZX
099K0ZZ
099K30Z
099K3ZX
099K3ZZ
099K40Z
099K4ZX
099K4ZZ
099K70Z
099K7ZX
099K7ZZ
099K80Z
099K8ZX
099K8ZZ
099KX0Z
099KXZX
099KXZZ
099L00Z
099L0ZX
099L0ZZ
099L30Z
099L3ZX
099L3ZZ
099L40Z
099L4ZX
099L4ZZ
099L70Z
099L7ZX
099L7ZZ
099L80Z
099L8ZX
099L8ZZ
099M00Z
099M0ZX
099M0ZZ
099M30Z
099M3ZX
099M3ZZ
099M40Z
099M4ZX
099M4ZZ
099M70Z
099M7ZX
099M7ZZ
099M80Z
099M8ZX
099M8ZZ
099N0ZX
099N30Z
099N3ZX
099N3ZZ
099N4ZX
099N7ZX
099N8ZX
099P30Z
099P3ZX
099P3ZZ
099P40Z
099P4ZX
099P4ZZ
099P70Z
099P7ZX
099P7ZZ
099P80Z
099P8ZX
099P8ZZ
099Q30Z
099Q3ZX
099Q3ZZ
099Q40Z
099Q4ZX
099Q4ZZ
099Q70Z
099Q7ZX
099Q7ZZ
099Q80Z
099Q8ZX
099Q8ZZ
099R30Z
099R3ZX
099R3ZZ
099R40Z
099R4ZX
099R4ZZ
099R70Z
099R7ZX
099R7ZZ
099R80Z
099R8ZX
099R8ZZ
099S30Z
099S3ZX
099S3ZZ
099S40Z
099S4ZX
099S4ZZ
099S70Z
099S7ZX
099S7ZZ
099S80Z
099S8ZX
099S8ZZ
099T30Z
099T3ZX
099T3ZZ
099T40Z
099T4ZX
099T4ZZ
099T70Z
099T7ZX
099T7ZZ
099T80Z
099T8ZX
099T8ZZ
099U30Z
099U3ZX
099U3ZZ
099U40Z
099U4ZX
099U4ZZ
099U70Z
099U7ZX
099U7ZZ
099U80Z
099U8ZX
099U8ZZ
099V30Z
099V3ZX
099V3ZZ
099V40Z
099V4ZX
099V4ZZ
099V70Z
099V7ZX
099V7ZZ
099V80Z
099V8ZX
099V8ZZ
099W30Z
099W3ZX
099W3ZZ
099W40Z
099W4ZX
099W4ZZ
099W70Z
099W7ZX
099W7ZZ
099W80Z
099W8ZX
099W8ZZ
099X30Z
099X3ZX
099X3ZZ
099X40Z
099X4ZX
099X4ZZ
099X70Z
099X7ZX
099X7ZZ
099X80Z
099X8ZX
099X8ZZ
09B00ZX
09B00ZZ
09B03ZX
09B03ZZ
09B04ZX
09B04ZZ
09B0XZX
09B0XZZ
09B10ZX
09B10ZZ
09B13ZX
09B13ZZ
09B14ZX
09B14ZZ
09B1XZX
09B1XZZ
09B30ZX
09B30ZZ
09B33ZX
09B33ZZ
09B34ZX
09B34ZZ
09B37ZX
09B37ZZ
09B38ZX
09B38ZZ
09B3XZX
09B3XZZ
09B40ZX
09B40ZZ
09B43ZX
09B43ZZ
09B44ZX
09B44ZZ
09B47ZX
09B47ZZ
09B48ZX
09B48ZZ
09B4XZX
09B4XZZ
09BF0ZX
09BF0ZZ
09BF3ZX
09BF3ZZ
09BF4ZX
09BF4ZZ
09BF7ZX
09BF7ZZ
09BF8ZX
09BF8ZZ
09BG0ZX
09BG0ZZ
09BG3ZX
09BG3ZZ
09BG4ZX
09BG4ZZ
09BG7ZX
09BG7ZZ
09BG8ZX
09BG8ZZ
09BK0ZX
09BK0ZZ
09BK3ZX
09BK3ZZ
09BK4ZX
09BK4ZZ
09BK8ZX
09BK8ZZ
09BKXZX
09BKXZZ
09BL0ZX
09BL3ZX
09BL4ZX
09BL7ZX
09BL8ZX
09BM0ZX
09BM3ZX
09BM4ZX
09BM8ZX
09BN0ZX
09BN3ZX
09BN4ZX
09BN7ZX
09BN8ZX
09BP3ZX
09BP4ZX
09BP8ZX
09BQ3ZX
09BQ4ZX
09BQ8ZX
09BR3ZX
09BR4ZX
09BR8ZX
09BS3ZX
09BS4ZX
09BS8ZX
09BT3ZX
09BT4ZX
09BT8ZX
09BU3ZX
09BU4ZX
09BU8ZX
09BV3ZX
09BV4ZX
09BV8ZX
09BW3ZX
09BW4ZX
09BW8ZX
09BX3ZX
09BX4ZX
09BX8ZX
09C00ZZ
09C03ZZ
09C04ZZ
09C0XZZ
09C10ZZ
09C13ZZ
09C14ZZ
09C1XZZ
09C30ZZ
09C33ZZ
09C34ZZ
09C37ZZ
09C38ZZ
09C3XZZ
09C40ZZ
09C43ZZ
09C44ZZ
09C47ZZ
09C48ZZ
09C4XZZ
09C70ZZ
09C73ZZ
09C74ZZ
09C77ZZ
09C78ZZ
09C80ZZ
09C83ZZ
09C84ZZ
09C87ZZ
09C88ZZ
09CF0ZZ
09CF3ZZ
09CF4ZZ
09CF7ZZ
09CF8ZZ
09CG0ZZ
09CG3ZZ
09CG4ZZ
09CG7ZZ
09CG8ZZ
09CK0ZZ
09CK3ZZ
09CK4ZZ
09CK8ZZ
09CKXZZ
09CL0ZZ
09CL3ZZ
09CL4ZZ
09CL7ZZ
09CL8ZZ
09CM0ZZ
09CM3ZZ
09CM4ZZ
09CM8ZZ
09CP8ZZ
09CQ0ZZ
09CQ3ZZ
09CQ4ZZ
09CQ8ZZ
09CR0ZZ
09CR3ZZ
09CR4ZZ
09CR8ZZ
09CS0ZZ
09CS3ZZ
09CS4ZZ
09CS8ZZ
09CT0ZZ
09CT3ZZ
09CT4ZZ
09CT8ZZ
09CU0ZZ
09CU3ZZ
09CU4ZZ
09CU8ZZ
09CV0ZZ
09CV3ZZ
09CV4ZZ
09CV8ZZ
09CW0ZZ
09CW3ZZ
09CW4ZZ
09CW8ZZ
09CX0ZZ
09CX3ZZ
09CX4ZZ
09CX8ZZ
09D70ZZ
09D73ZZ
09D74ZZ
09D77ZZ
09D78ZZ
09D80ZZ
09D83ZZ
09D84ZZ
09D87ZZ
09D88ZZ
09D90ZZ
09DA0ZZ
09DB0ZZ
09DB3ZZ
09DB4ZZ
09DC0ZZ
09DC3ZZ
09DC4ZZ
09DL0ZZ
09DL3ZZ
09DL4ZZ
09DL7ZZ
09DL8ZZ
09DM0ZZ
09DM3ZZ
09DM4ZZ
09DP0ZZ
09DP3ZZ
09DP4ZZ
09DQ0ZZ
09DQ3ZZ
09DQ4ZZ
09DR0ZZ
09DR3ZZ
09DR4ZZ
09DS0ZZ
09DS3ZZ
09DS4ZZ
09DT0ZZ
09DT3ZZ
09DT4ZZ
09DU0ZZ
09DU3ZZ
09DU4ZZ
09DV0ZZ
09DV3ZZ
09DV4ZZ
09DW0ZZ
09DW3ZZ
09DW4ZZ
09DX0ZZ
09DX3ZZ
09DX4ZZ
09HD04Z
09HD05Z
09HD06Z
09HD0SZ
09HD34Z
09HD35Z
09HD36Z
09HD3SZ
09HD44Z
09HD45Z
09HD46Z
09HD4SZ
09HE04Z
09HE05Z
09HE06Z
09HE0SZ
09HE34Z
09HE35Z
09HE36Z
09HE3SZ
09HE44Z
09HE45Z
09HE46Z
09HE4SZ
09HH0YZ
09HH3YZ
09HH4YZ
09HH7YZ
09HH8YZ
09HJ0YZ
09HJ3YZ
09HJ4YZ
09HJ7YZ
09HJ8YZ
09HK0YZ
09HK3YZ
09HK4YZ
09HK7YZ
09HK8YZ
09HN7BZ
09HN8BZ
09HY0YZ
09HY3YZ
09HY4YZ
09HY7YZ
09HY8YZ
09J70ZZ
09J73ZZ
09J74ZZ
09J77ZZ
09J78ZZ
09J7XZZ
09J80ZZ
09J83ZZ
09J84ZZ
09J87ZZ
09J88ZZ
09J8XZZ
09JD0ZZ
09JD3ZZ
09JD4ZZ
09JD8ZZ
09JDXZZ
09JE0ZZ
09JE3ZZ
09JE4ZZ
09JE8ZZ
09JEXZZ
09JH0ZZ
09JH3ZZ
09JH4ZZ
09JH7ZZ
09JH8ZZ
09JHXZZ
09JJ0ZZ
09JJ3ZZ
09JJ4ZZ
09JJ7ZZ
09JJ8ZZ
09JJXZZ
09JK0ZZ
09JK3ZZ
09JK4ZZ
09JK8ZZ
09JKXZZ
09JY0ZZ
09JY3ZZ
09JY4ZZ
09JY8ZZ
09JYXZZ
09M0XZZ
09M1XZZ
09MKXZZ
09N00ZZ
09N03ZZ
09N04ZZ
09N0XZZ
09N10ZZ
09N13ZZ
09N14ZZ
09N1XZZ
09N30ZZ
09N33ZZ
09N34ZZ
09N37ZZ
09N38ZZ
09N3XZZ
09N40ZZ
09N43ZZ
09N44ZZ
09N47ZZ
09N48ZZ
09N4XZZ
09N50ZZ
09N58ZZ
09N60ZZ
09N68ZZ
09N70ZZ
09N73ZZ
09N74ZZ
09N77ZZ
09N78ZZ
09N80ZZ
09N83ZZ
09N84ZZ
09N87ZZ
09N88ZZ
09N90ZZ
09N98ZZ
09NA0ZZ
09NA8ZZ
09NB0ZZ
09NB3ZZ
09NB4ZZ
09NB8ZZ
09NC0ZZ
09NC3ZZ
09NC4ZZ
09NC8ZZ
09ND0ZZ
09ND8ZZ
09NE0ZZ
09NE8ZZ
09NF0ZZ
09NF3ZZ
09NF4ZZ
09NF7ZZ
09NF8ZZ
09NG0ZZ
09NG3ZZ
09NG4ZZ
09NG7ZZ
09NG8ZZ
09NK0ZZ
09NK3ZZ
09NK4ZZ
09NK8ZZ
09NKXZZ
09NL0ZZ
09NL3ZZ
09NL4ZZ
09NL7ZZ
09NL8ZZ
09NM0ZZ
09NM3ZZ
09NM4ZZ
09NM8ZZ
09NN0ZZ
09NN3ZZ
09NN4ZZ
09NN7ZZ
09NN8ZZ
09NP0ZZ
09NP3ZZ
09NP4ZZ
09NP8ZZ
09NQ0ZZ
09NQ3ZZ
09NQ4ZZ
09NQ8ZZ
09NR0ZZ
09NR3ZZ
09NR4ZZ
09NR8ZZ
09NS0ZZ
09NS3ZZ
09NS4ZZ
09NS8ZZ
09NT0ZZ
09NT3ZZ
09NT4ZZ
09NT8ZZ
09NU0ZZ
09NU3ZZ
09NU4ZZ
09NU8ZZ
09NV0ZZ
09NV3ZZ
09NV4ZZ
09NV8ZZ
09NW0ZZ
09NW3ZZ
09NW4ZZ
09NW8ZZ
09NX0ZZ
09NX3ZZ
09NX4ZZ
09NX8ZZ
09P700Z
09P770Z
09P780Z
09P7X0Z
09P800Z
09P870Z
09P880Z
09P8X0Z
09PD0SZ
09PD7SZ
09PD8SZ
09PE0SZ
09PE7SZ
09PE8SZ
09PH00Z
09PH07Z
09PH0DZ
09PH0JZ
09PH0KZ
09PH0YZ
09PH30Z
09PH37Z
09PH3DZ
09PH3JZ
09PH3KZ
09PH3YZ
09PH40Z
09PH47Z
09PH4DZ
09PH4JZ
09PH4KZ
09PH4YZ
09PH70Z
09PH77Z
09PH7DZ
09PH7JZ
09PH7KZ
09PH7YZ
09PH80Z
09PH87Z
09PH8DZ

09PH8JZ
09PH8KZ
09PH8YZ
09PHX0Z
09PHX7Z
09PHXDZ
09PHXJZ
09PHXKZ
09PJ00Z
09PJ07Z
09PJ0DZ
09PJ0JZ
09PJ0KZ
09PJ0YZ
09PJ30Z
09PJ37Z
09PJ3DZ
09PJ3JZ
09PJ3KZ
09PJ3YZ
09PJ40Z
09PJ47Z
09PJ4DZ
09PJ4JZ
09PJ4KZ
09PJ4YZ
09PJ70Z
09PJ77Z
09PJ7DZ
09PJ7JZ
09PJ7KZ
09PJ7YZ
09PJ80Z
09PJ87Z
09PJ8DZ
09PJ8JZ
09PJ8KZ
09PJ8YZ
09PJX0Z
09PJX7Z
09PJXDZ
09PJXJZ
09PJXKZ
09PK00Z
09PK07Z
09PK0DZ
09PK0JZ
09PK0KZ
09PK0YZ
09PK30Z
09PK37Z
09PK3DZ
09PK3JZ
09PK3KZ
09PK3YZ
09PK40Z
09PK47Z
09PK4DZ
09PK4JZ
09PK4KZ
09PK4YZ
09PK70Z
09PK77Z
09PK7DZ
09PK7JZ
09PK7KZ
09PK7YZ
09PK80Z
09PK87Z
09PK8DZ
09PK8JZ
09PK8KZ
09PK8YZ
09PKX0Z
09PKX7Z
09PKXDZ
09PKXJZ
09PKXKZ
09PY00Z
09PY0YZ
09PY30Z
09PY3YZ
09PY40Z
09PY4YZ
09PY7YZ
09PY8YZ
09PYX0Z
09Q00ZZ
09Q03ZZ
09Q04ZZ
09Q0XZZ
09Q10ZZ
09Q13ZZ
09Q14ZZ
09Q1XZZ
09Q20ZZ
09Q23ZZ
09Q24ZZ
09Q2XZZ
09Q30ZZ
09Q33ZZ
09Q34ZZ
09Q37ZZ
09Q38ZZ
09Q3XZZ
09Q40ZZ
09Q43ZZ
09Q44ZZ
09Q47ZZ
09Q48ZZ
09Q4XZZ
09Q50ZZ
09Q58ZZ
09Q60ZZ
09Q68ZZ
09Q70ZZ
09Q73ZZ
09Q74ZZ
09Q77ZZ
09Q78ZZ
09Q80ZZ
09Q83ZZ
09Q84ZZ
09Q87ZZ
09Q88ZZ
09Q90ZZ
09Q98ZZ
09QA0ZZ
09QA8ZZ
09QB0ZZ
09QB3ZZ
09QB4ZZ
09QB8ZZ
09QC0ZZ
09QC3ZZ
09QC4ZZ
09QC8ZZ
09QD0ZZ
09QD8ZZ
09QE0ZZ
09QE8ZZ
09QF0ZZ
09QF3ZZ
09QF4ZZ
09QF7ZZ
09QF8ZZ
09QFXZZ
09QG0ZZ
09QG3ZZ
09QG4ZZ
09QG7ZZ
09QG8ZZ
09QGXZZ
09QK0ZZ
09QK3ZZ
09QK4ZZ
09QK8ZZ
09QKXZZ
09QL0ZZ
09QL3ZZ
09QL4ZZ
09QL7ZZ
09QL8ZZ
09QM0ZZ
09QM3ZZ
09QM4ZZ
09QM8ZZ
09QN0ZZ
09QN3ZZ
09QN4ZZ
09QN7ZZ
09QN8ZZ
09QP0ZZ
09QP3ZZ
09QP4ZZ
09QP8ZZ
09QQ0ZZ
09QQ3ZZ
09QQ4ZZ
09QQ8ZZ
09QR0ZZ
09QR3ZZ
09QR4ZZ
09QR8ZZ
09QS0ZZ
09QS3ZZ
09QS4ZZ
09QS8ZZ
09QT0ZZ
09QT3ZZ
09QT4ZZ
09QT8ZZ
09QU0ZZ
09QU3ZZ
09QU4ZZ
09QU8ZZ
09QV0ZZ
09QV3ZZ
09QV4ZZ
09QV8ZZ
09QW0ZZ
09QW3ZZ
09QW4ZZ
09QW8ZZ
09QX0ZZ
09QX3ZZ
09QX4ZZ
09QX8ZZ
09R007Z
09R00JZ
09R00KZ
09R0X7Z
09R0XJZ
09R0XKZ
09R107Z
09R10JZ
09R10KZ
09R1X7Z
09R1XJZ
09R1XKZ
09R207Z
09R20JZ
09R20KZ
09R2X7Z
09R2XJZ
09R2XKZ
09R507Z
09R50JZ
09R50KZ
09R607Z
09R60JZ
09R60KZ
09R707Z
09R70JZ
09R70KZ
09R777Z
09R77JZ
09R77KZ
09R787Z
09R78JZ
09R78KZ
09R807Z
09R80JZ
09R80KZ
09R877Z
09R87JZ
09R87KZ
09R887Z
09R88JZ
09R88KZ
09R907Z
09R90JZ
09R90KZ
09RA07Z
09RA0JZ
09RA0KZ
09RD07Z
09RD0JZ
09RD0KZ
09RE07Z
09RE0JZ
09RE0KZ
09RK07Z
09RK0JZ
09RK0KZ
09RKX7Z
09RKXJZ
09RKXKZ
09RL07Z
09RL0JZ
09RL0KZ
09RL37Z
09RL3JZ
09RL3KZ
09RL47Z
09RL4JZ
09RL4KZ
09RL77Z
09RL7JZ
09RL7KZ
09RL87Z
09RL8JZ
09RL8KZ
09RM07Z
09RM0JZ
09RM0KZ
09RM37Z
09RM3JZ
09RM3KZ
09RM47Z
09RM4JZ
09RM4KZ
09RN07Z
09RN0JZ
09RN0KZ
09SF0ZZ
09SF4ZZ
09SF7ZZ
09SF8ZZ
09SG0ZZ
09SG4ZZ
09SG7ZZ
09SG8ZZ
09TF0ZZ
09TF4ZZ
09TF7ZZ
09TF8ZZ
09TG0ZZ
09TG4ZZ
09TG7ZZ
09TG8ZZ
09UKXKZ
09UL07Z
09UL0JZ
09UL0KZ
09UL37Z
09UL3JZ
09UL3KZ
09UL47Z
09UL4JZ
09UL4KZ
09UL77Z
09UL7JZ
09UL7KZ
09UL87Z
09UL8JZ
09UL8KZ
09UM07Z
09UM0JZ
09UM0KZ
09UM37Z
09UM3JZ
09UM3KZ
09UM47Z
09UM4JZ
09UM4KZ
09UM87Z
09UM8JZ
09UM8KZ
09UN07Z
09UN0JZ
09UN0KZ
09UN77Z
09UN7JZ
09UN7KZ
09UN87Z
09UN8JZ
09UN8KZ
09W707Z
09W70JZ
09W70KZ
09W777Z
09W77JZ
09W77KZ
09W787Z
09W78JZ
09W78KZ
09W807Z
09W80JZ
09W80KZ
09W877Z
09W87JZ
09W87KZ
09W887Z
09W88JZ
09W88KZ
09W907Z
09W90JZ
09W90KZ
09W977Z
09W97JZ
09W97KZ
09W987Z
09W98JZ
09W98KZ
09WA07Z
09WA0JZ
09WA0KZ
09WA77Z
09WA7JZ
09WA7KZ
09WA87Z
09WA8JZ
09WA8KZ
09WD0SZ
09WD7SZ
09WD8SZ
09WE0SZ
09WE7SZ
09WE8SZ
09WH00Z
09WH07Z
09WH0DZ
09WH0JZ
09WH0KZ
09WH0YZ
09WH30Z
09WH37Z
09WH3DZ
09WH3JZ
09WH3KZ
09WH3YZ
09WH40Z
09WH47Z
09WH4DZ
09WH4JZ
09WH4KZ
09WH4YZ
09WH70Z
09WH77Z
09WH7DZ
09WH7JZ
09WH7KZ
09WH7YZ
09WH80Z
09WH87Z
09WH8DZ
09WH8JZ
09WH8KZ
09WH8YZ
09WHX0Z
09WHX7Z
09WHXDZ
09WHXJZ
09WHXKZ
09WJ00Z
09WJ07Z
09WJ0DZ
09WJ0JZ
09WJ0KZ
09WJ0YZ
09WJ30Z
09WJ37Z
09WJ3DZ
09WJ3JZ
09WJ3KZ
09WJ3YZ
09WJ40Z
09WJ47Z
09WJ4DZ
09WJ4JZ
09WJ4KZ
09WJ4YZ
09WJ70Z
09WJ77Z
09WJ7DZ
09WJ7JZ
09WJ7KZ
09WJ7YZ
09WJ80Z
09WJ87Z
09WJ8DZ
09WJ8JZ
09WJ8KZ
09WJ8YZ
09WJX0Z
09WJX7Z
09WJXDZ
09WJXJZ
09WJXKZ
09WK00Z
09WK07Z
09WK0DZ
09WK0JZ
09WK0KZ
09WK0YZ
09WK30Z
09WK37Z
09WK3DZ
09WK3JZ
09WK3KZ
09WK3YZ
09WK40Z
09WK47Z
09WK4DZ
09WK4JZ
09WK4KZ
09WK4YZ
09WK70Z
09WK77Z
09WK7DZ
09WK7JZ
09WK7KZ
09WK7YZ
09WK80Z
09WK87Z
09WK8DZ
09WK8JZ
09WK8KZ
09WK8YZ
09WKX0Z
09WKX7Z
09WKXDZ
09WKXJZ
09WKXKZ
09WY00Z
09WY0YZ
09WY30Z
09WY3YZ
09WY40Z
09WY4YZ
09WY7YZ
09WY8YZ
09WYX0Z
0B110D6
0B110F4
0B110Z4
0B113F4
0B113Z4
0B114F4
0B114Z4
0B20X0Z
0B20XYZ
0B21X0Z
0B21XEZ
0B21XFZ
0B21XYZ
0B2KX0Z
0B2KXYZ
0B2LX0Z
0B2LXYZ
0B2QX0Z
0B2QXYZ
0B2TX0Z
0B2TXYZ
0B510ZZ
0B513ZZ
0B514ZZ
0B517ZZ
0B518ZZ
0B520ZZ
0B523ZZ
0B524ZZ
0B527ZZ
0B528ZZ
0B530ZZ
0B533ZZ
0B534ZZ
0B537ZZ
0B538ZZ
0B540ZZ
0B543ZZ
0B544ZZ
0B547ZZ
0B548ZZ
0B550ZZ
0B553ZZ
0B554ZZ
0B557ZZ
0B558ZZ
0B560ZZ
0B563ZZ
0B564ZZ
0B567ZZ
0B568ZZ
0B570ZZ
0B573ZZ
0B574ZZ
0B577ZZ
0B578ZZ
0B580ZZ
0B583ZZ
0B584ZZ
0B587ZZ
0B588ZZ
0B590ZZ
0B593ZZ
0B594ZZ
0B597ZZ
0B598ZZ
0B5B0ZZ
0B5B3ZZ
0B5B4ZZ
0B5B7ZZ
0B5B8ZZ
0B5C0ZZ
0B5C3ZZ
0B5C4ZZ
0B5C7ZZ
0B5C8ZZ
0B5D0ZZ
0B5D3ZZ
0B5D4ZZ
0B5D7ZZ
0B5D8ZZ
0B5F0ZZ
0B5F3ZZ
0B5F4ZZ
0B5F7ZZ
0B5F8ZZ
0B5G0ZZ
0B5G3ZZ
0B5G4ZZ
0B5G7ZZ
0B5G8ZZ
0B5H0ZZ
0B5H3ZZ
0B5H4ZZ
0B5H7ZZ
0B5H8ZZ
0B5J0ZZ
0B5J3ZZ
0B5J4ZZ
0B5J7ZZ
0B5J8ZZ
0B5K0ZZ
0B5K3ZZ
0B5K4ZZ
0B5K7ZZ
0B5K8ZZ
0B5L0ZZ
0B5L3ZZ
0B5L4ZZ
0B5L7ZZ
0B5L8ZZ
0B5M0ZZ
0B5M3ZZ
0B5M4ZZ
0B5M7ZZ
0B5M8ZZ
0B5N0ZZ
0B5N3ZZ
0B5N4ZZ
0B5P0ZZ
0B5P3ZZ
0B5P4ZZ
0B5T0ZZ
0B5T3ZZ
0B5T4ZZ
0B710DZ
0B710ZZ
0B713DZ
0B713ZZ
0B714DZ
0B714ZZ
0B717DZ
0B717ZZ
0B718DZ
0B718ZZ
0B720DZ
0B720ZZ
0B723DZ
0B723ZZ
0B724DZ
0B724ZZ
0B727DZ
0B727ZZ
0B728DZ
0B728ZZ
0B730DZ
0B730ZZ
0B733DZ
0B733ZZ
0B734DZ
0B734ZZ
0B737DZ
0B737ZZ
0B738DZ
0B738ZZ
0B740DZ
0B740ZZ
0B743DZ
0B743ZZ
0B744DZ
0B744ZZ
0B747DZ
0B747ZZ
0B748DZ
0B748ZZ
0B750DZ
0B750ZZ
0B753DZ
0B753ZZ
0B754DZ
0B754ZZ
0B757DZ
0B757ZZ
0B758DZ
0B758ZZ
0B760DZ
0B760ZZ
0B763DZ
0B763ZZ
0B764DZ
0B764ZZ
0B767DZ
0B767ZZ
0B768DZ
0B768ZZ
0B770DZ
0B770ZZ
0B773DZ
0B773ZZ
0B774DZ
0B774ZZ
0B777DZ
0B777ZZ
0B778DZ
0B778ZZ
0B780DZ
0B780ZZ
0B783DZ
0B783ZZ
0B784DZ
0B784ZZ
0B787DZ
0B787ZZ
0B788DZ
0B788ZZ
0B790DZ
0B790ZZ
0B793DZ
0B793ZZ
0B794DZ
0B794ZZ
0B797DZ
0B797ZZ
0B798DZ
0B798ZZ
0B7B0DZ
0B7B0ZZ
0B7B3DZ
0B7B3ZZ
0B7B4DZ
0B7B4ZZ
0B7B7DZ

0B7B7ZZ
0B7B8DZ
0B7B8ZZ
0B9100Z
0B910ZX
0B910ZZ
0B9130Z
0B913ZX
0B913ZZ
0B9140Z
0B914ZX
0B914ZZ
0B9170Z
0B917ZX
0B917ZZ
0B9180Z
0B918ZX
0B918ZZ
0B9200Z
0B920ZX
0B920ZZ
0B9230Z
0B923ZX
0B923ZZ
0B9240Z
0B924ZX
0B924ZZ
0B9270Z
0B927ZX
0B927ZZ
0B9280Z
0B928ZX
0B928ZZ
0B9300Z
0B930ZX
0B930ZZ
0B9330Z
0B933ZX
0B933ZZ
0B9340Z
0B934ZX
0B934ZZ
0B9370Z
0B937ZX
0B937ZZ
0B9380Z
0B938ZX
0B938ZZ
0B9400Z
0B940ZX
0B940ZZ
0B9430Z
0B943ZX
0B943ZZ
0B9440Z
0B944ZX
0B944ZZ
0B9470Z
0B947ZX
0B947ZZ
0B9480Z
0B948ZX
0B948ZZ
0B9500Z
0B950ZX
0B950ZZ
0B9530Z
0B953ZX
0B953ZZ
0B9540Z
0B954ZX
0B954ZZ
0B9570Z
0B957ZX
0B957ZZ
0B9580Z
0B958ZX
0B958ZZ
0B9600Z
0B960ZX
0B960ZZ
0B9630Z
0B963ZX
0B963ZZ
0B9640Z
0B964ZX
0B964ZZ
0B9670Z
0B967ZX
0B967ZZ
0B9680Z
0B968ZX
0B968ZZ
0B9700Z
0B970ZX
0B970ZZ
0B9730Z
0B973ZX
0B973ZZ
0B9740Z
0B974ZX
0B974ZZ
0B9770Z
0B977ZX
0B977ZZ
0B9780Z
0B978ZX
0B978ZZ
0B9800Z
0B980ZX
0B980ZZ
0B9830Z
0B983ZX
0B983ZZ
0B9840Z
0B984ZX
0B984ZZ
0B9870Z
0B987ZX
0B987ZZ
0B9880Z
0B988ZX
0B988ZZ
0B9900Z
0B990ZX
0B990ZZ
0B9930Z
0B993ZX
0B993ZZ
0B9940Z
0B994ZX
0B994ZZ
0B9970Z
0B997ZX
0B997ZZ
0B9980Z
0B998ZX
0B998ZZ
0B9B00Z
0B9B0ZX
0B9B0ZZ
0B9B30Z
0B9B3ZX
0B9B3ZZ
0B9B40Z
0B9B4ZX
0B9B4ZZ
0B9B70Z
0B9B7ZX
0B9B7ZZ
0B9B80Z
0B9B8ZX
0B9B8ZZ
0B9C00Z
0B9C0ZX
0B9C0ZZ
0B9C30Z
0B9C3ZX
0B9C3ZZ
0B9C40Z
0B9C4ZX
0B9C4ZZ
0B9C70Z
0B9C7ZX
0B9C7ZZ
0B9C80Z
0B9C8ZX
0B9C8ZZ
0B9D00Z
0B9D0ZX
0B9D0ZZ
0B9D30Z
0B9D3ZX
0B9D3ZZ
0B9D40Z
0B9D4ZX
0B9D4ZZ
0B9D70Z
0B9D7ZX
0B9D7ZZ
0B9D80Z
0B9D8ZX
0B9D8ZZ
0B9F00Z
0B9F0ZX
0B9F0ZZ
0B9F30Z
0B9F3ZX
0B9F3ZZ
0B9F40Z
0B9F4ZX
0B9F4ZZ
0B9F70Z
0B9F7ZX
0B9F7ZZ
0B9F80Z
0B9F8ZX
0B9F8ZZ
0B9G00Z
0B9G0ZX
0B9G0ZZ
0B9G30Z
0B9G3ZX
0B9G3ZZ
0B9G40Z
0B9G4ZX
0B9G4ZZ
0B9G70Z
0B9G7ZX
0B9G7ZZ
0B9G80Z
0B9G8ZX
0B9G8ZZ
0B9H00Z
0B9H0ZX
0B9H0ZZ
0B9H30Z
0B9H3ZX
0B9H3ZZ
0B9H40Z
0B9H4ZX
0B9H4ZZ
0B9H70Z
0B9H7ZX
0B9H7ZZ
0B9H80Z
0B9H8ZX
0B9H8ZZ
0B9J00Z
0B9J0ZX
0B9J0ZZ
0B9J30Z
0B9J3ZX
0B9J3ZZ
0B9J40Z
0B9J4ZX
0B9J4ZZ
0B9J70Z
0B9J7ZX
0B9J7ZZ
0B9J80Z
0B9J8ZX
0B9J8ZZ
0B9K00Z
0B9K0ZX
0B9K0ZZ
0B9K30Z
0B9K3ZX
0B9K3ZZ
0B9K40Z
0B9K4ZX
0B9K4ZZ
0B9K70Z
0B9K7ZX
0B9K7ZZ
0B9K80Z
0B9K8ZX
0B9K8ZZ
0B9L00Z
0B9L0ZX
0B9L0ZZ
0B9L30Z
0B9L3ZX
0B9L3ZZ
0B9L40Z
0B9L4ZX
0B9L4ZZ
0B9L70Z
0B9L7ZX
0B9L7ZZ
0B9L80Z
0B9L8ZX
0B9L8ZZ
0B9M00Z
0B9M0ZX
0B9M0ZZ
0B9M30Z
0B9M3ZX
0B9M3ZZ
0B9M40Z
0B9M4ZX
0B9M4ZZ
0B9M70Z
0B9M7ZX
0B9M7ZZ
0B9M80Z
0B9M8ZX
0B9M8ZZ
0B9N00Z
0B9N0ZX
0B9N0ZZ
0B9N30Z
0B9N3ZX
0B9N3ZZ
0B9N40Z
0B9N4ZX
0B9N4ZZ
0B9N80Z
0B9N8ZX
0B9N8ZZ
0B9P00Z
0B9P0ZX
0B9P0ZZ
0B9P30Z
0B9P3ZX
0B9P3ZZ
0B9P40Z
0B9P4ZX
0B9P4ZZ
0B9P80Z
0B9P8ZX
0B9P8ZZ
0B9T00Z
0B9T0ZX
0B9T0ZZ
0B9T30Z
0B9T3ZX
0B9T3ZZ
0B9T40Z
0B9T4ZX
0B9T4ZZ
0BB10ZX
0BB10ZZ
0BB13ZX
0BB13ZZ
0BB14ZX
0BB14ZZ
0BB17ZX
0BB17ZZ
0BB18ZX
0BB18ZZ
0BB20ZX
0BB20ZZ
0BB23ZX
0BB23ZZ
0BB24ZX
0BB24ZZ
0BB27ZX
0BB27ZZ
0BB28ZX
0BB28ZZ
0BB30ZX
0BB30ZZ
0BB33ZX
0BB33ZZ
0BB34ZX
0BB34ZZ
0BB37ZX
0BB37ZZ
0BB38ZX
0BB38ZZ
0BB40ZX
0BB40ZZ
0BB43ZX
0BB43ZZ
0BB44ZX
0BB44ZZ
0BB47ZX
0BB47ZZ
0BB48ZX
0BB48ZZ
0BB50ZX
0BB50ZZ
0BB53ZX
0BB53ZZ
0BB54ZX
0BB54ZZ
0BB57ZX
0BB57ZZ
0BB58ZX
0BB58ZZ
0BB63ZX
0BB64ZX
0BB64ZZ
0BB67ZX
0BB68ZX
0BB68ZZ
0BB73ZX
0BB74ZX
0BB74ZZ
0BB77ZX
0BB78ZX
0BB78ZZ
0BB83ZX
0BB84ZX
0BB84ZZ
0BB87ZX
0BB88ZX
0BB88ZZ
0BB93ZX
0BB94ZX
0BB94ZZ
0BB97ZX
0BB98ZX
0BB98ZZ
0BBB3ZX
0BBB4ZX
0BBB4ZZ
0BBB7ZX
0BBB8ZX
0BBB8ZZ
0BBC3ZX
0BBC8ZZ
0BBD3ZX
0BBD8ZZ
0BBF3ZX
0BBF8ZZ
0BBG3ZX
0BBG8ZZ
0BBH3ZX
0BBH8ZZ
0BBJ3ZX
0BBJ8ZZ
0BBK3ZX
0BBK8ZZ
0BBL3ZX
0BBL8ZZ
0BBM3ZX
0BBM4ZZ
0BBM8ZZ
0BBN0ZX
0BBN3ZX
0BBP0ZX
0BBP3ZX
0BC17ZZ
0BC18ZZ
0BC27ZZ
0BC28ZZ
0BC37ZZ
0BC38ZZ
0BC47ZZ
0BC48ZZ
0BC57ZZ
0BC58ZZ
0BC67ZZ
0BC68ZZ
0BC77ZZ
0BC78ZZ
0BC87ZZ
0BC88ZZ
0BC97ZZ
0BC98ZZ
0BCB7ZZ
0BCB8ZZ
0BCC8ZZ
0BCK7ZZ
0BCK8ZZ
0BCL0ZZ
0BCL3ZZ
0BCL4ZZ
0BCL7ZZ
0BCL8ZZ
0BCM0ZZ
0BCM3ZZ
0BCM4ZZ
0BCM7ZZ
0BCM8ZZ
0BCN0ZZ
0BCN3ZZ
0BCN4ZZ
0BCP0ZZ
0BCP3ZZ
0BCP4ZZ
0BCT0ZZ
0BCT3ZZ
0BCT4ZZ
0BD14ZX
0BD18ZX
0BD24ZX
0BD28ZX
0BD34ZX
0BD38ZX
0BD44ZX
0BD48ZX
0BD54ZX
0BD58ZX
0BD64ZX
0BD68ZX
0BD74ZX
0BD78ZX
0BD84ZX
0BD88ZX
0BD94ZX
0BD98ZX
0BDB4ZX
0BDB8ZX
0BDC4ZX
0BDC8ZX
0BDD4ZX
0BDD8ZX
0BDF4ZX
0BDF8ZX
0BDG4ZX
0BDG8ZX
0BDH4ZX
0BDH8ZX
0BDJ4ZX
0BDJ8ZX
0BDK4ZX
0BDK8ZX
0BDL4ZX
0BDL8ZX
0BDM4ZX
0BDM8ZX
0BDN0ZX
0BDN0ZZ
0BDN3ZX
0BDN3ZZ
0BDN4ZX
0BDN4ZZ
0BDP0ZX
0BDP0ZZ
0BDP3ZX
0BDP3ZZ
0BDP4ZX
0BDP4ZZ
0BF10ZZ
0BF13ZZ
0BF14ZZ
0BF17ZZ
0BF18ZZ
0BF1XZZ
0BF20ZZ
0BF23ZZ
0BF24ZZ
0BF27ZZ
0BF28ZZ
0BF2XZZ
0BF30ZZ
0BF33ZZ
0BF34ZZ
0BF37ZZ
0BF38ZZ
0BF3XZZ
0BF40ZZ
0BF43ZZ
0BF44ZZ
0BF47ZZ
0BF48ZZ
0BF4XZZ
0BF50ZZ
0BF53ZZ
0BF54ZZ
0BF57ZZ
0BF58ZZ
0BF5XZZ
0BF60ZZ
0BF63ZZ
0BF64ZZ
0BF67ZZ
0BF68ZZ
0BF6XZZ
0BF70ZZ
0BF73ZZ
0BF74ZZ
0BF77ZZ
0BF78ZZ
0BF7XZZ
0BF80ZZ
0BF83ZZ
0BF84ZZ
0BF87ZZ
0BF88ZZ
0BF8XZZ
0BF90ZZ
0BF93ZZ
0BF94ZZ
0BF97ZZ
0BF98ZZ
0BF9XZZ
0BFB0ZZ
0BFB3ZZ
0BFB4ZZ
0BFB7ZZ
0BFB8ZZ
0BFBXZZ
0BH001Z
0BH002Z
0BH003Z
0BH00DZ
0BH00YZ
0BH031Z
0BH032Z
0BH033Z
0BH03DZ
0BH03YZ
0BH041Z
0BH042Z
0BH043Z
0BH04DZ
0BH04YZ
0BH071Z
0BH072Z
0BH073Z
0BH07DZ
0BH07YZ
0BH081Z
0BH082Z
0BH083Z
0BH08DZ
0BH08YZ
0BH102Z
0BH10DZ
0BH10YZ
0BH13DZ
0BH13EZ
0BH13YZ
0BH14DZ
0BH14YZ
0BH172Z
0BH17DZ
0BH17EZ
0BH17YZ
0BH182Z
0BH18DZ
0BH18EZ
0BH18YZ
0BH30GZ
0BH33GZ
0BH34GZ
0BH37GZ
0BH38GZ
0BH40GZ
0BH43GZ
0BH44GZ
0BH47GZ
0BH48GZ
0BH50GZ
0BH53GZ
0BH54GZ
0BH57GZ
0BH58GZ
0BH60GZ
0BH63GZ
0BH64GZ
0BH67GZ
0BH68GZ
0BH70GZ
0BH73GZ
0BH74GZ
0BH77GZ
0BH78GZ
0BH80GZ
0BH83GZ
0BH84GZ
0BH87GZ
0BH88GZ
0BH90GZ
0BH93GZ
0BH94GZ
0BH97GZ
0BH98GZ
0BHB0GZ
0BHB3GZ
0BHB4GZ
0BHB7GZ
0BHB8GZ
0BHK01Z
0BHK02Z
0BHK03Z
0BHK0YZ
0BHK31Z
0BHK32Z
0BHK33Z
0BHK3YZ
0BHK41Z
0BHK42Z
0BHK43Z
0BHK4YZ
0BHK71Z
0BHK72Z
0BHK73Z
0BHK7YZ
0BHK81Z
0BHK82Z
0BHK83Z
0BHK8YZ
0BHL01Z
0BHL02Z
0BHL03Z
0BHL0YZ
0BHL31Z
0BHL32Z
0BHL33Z
0BHL3YZ
0BHL41Z
0BHL42Z
0BHL43Z
0BHL4YZ
0BHL71Z
0BHL72Z
0BHL73Z
0BHL7YZ
0BHL81Z
0BHL82Z
0BHL83Z
0BHL8YZ
0BHQ0YZ
0BHQ3YZ
0BHQ4YZ
0BHQ7YZ
0BHQ8YZ
0BHT02Z
0BHT0MZ
0BHT0YZ
0BHT32Z
0BHT3MZ
0BHT3YZ
0BHT42Z
0BHT4MZ
0BHT4YZ
0BHT7YZ
0BHT8YZ
0BJ00ZZ
0BJ03ZZ
0BJ04ZZ
0BJ07ZZ
0BJ08ZZ
0BJ0XZZ
0BJ10ZZ
0BJ13ZZ
0BJ14ZZ
0BJ17ZZ
0BJ18ZZ
0BJ1XZZ
0BJK0ZZ

0B7B7ZZ-0BJK0ZZ
APPENDIX H: NON-OR NOT AFFECTING MS-DRG ASSIGNMENT

0BJK3ZZ-0BV60DZ
APPENDIX H: NON-OR NOT AFFECTING MS-DRG ASSIGNMENT

0BJK3ZZ
0BJK4ZZ
0BJK7ZZ
0BJK8ZZ
0BJKXZZ
0BJL0ZZ
0BJL3ZZ
0BJL4ZZ
0BJL7ZZ
0BJL8ZZ
0BJLXZZ
0BJQ0ZZ
0BJQ3ZZ
0BJQ4ZZ
0BJQ7ZZ
0BJQ8ZZ
0BJQXZZ
0BJT0ZZ
0BJT3ZZ
0BJT4ZZ
0BJT7ZZ
0BJT8ZZ
0BJTXZZ
0BL10CZ
0BL10DZ
0BL10ZZ
0BL13CZ
0BL13DZ
0BL13ZZ
0BL14CZ
0BL14DZ
0BL14ZZ
0BL17DZ
0BL17ZZ
0BL18DZ
0BL18ZZ
0BL20CZ
0BL20DZ
0BL20ZZ
0BL23CZ
0BL23DZ
0BL23ZZ
0BL24CZ
0BL24DZ
0BL24ZZ
0BL27DZ
0BL27ZZ
0BL28DZ
0BL28ZZ
0BL30CZ
0BL30DZ
0BL30ZZ
0BL33CZ
0BL33DZ
0BL33ZZ
0BL34CZ
0BL34DZ
0BL34ZZ
0BL37DZ
0BL37ZZ
0BL38DZ
0BL38ZZ
0BL40CZ
0BL40DZ
0BL40ZZ
0BL43CZ
0BL43DZ
0BL43ZZ
0BL44CZ
0BL44DZ
0BL44ZZ
0BL47DZ
0BL47ZZ
0BL48DZ
0BL48ZZ
0BL50CZ
0BL50DZ
0BL50ZZ
0BL53CZ
0BL53DZ
0BL53ZZ
0BL54CZ
0BL54DZ
0BL54ZZ
0BL57DZ
0BL57ZZ
0BL58DZ
0BL58ZZ
0BL60CZ
0BL60DZ
0BL60ZZ
0BL63CZ
0BL63DZ
0BL63ZZ
0BL64CZ
0BL64DZ
0BL64ZZ
0BL67DZ
0BL67ZZ
0BL68DZ
0BL68ZZ
0BL70CZ
0BL70DZ
0BL70ZZ
0BL73CZ
0BL73DZ
0BL73ZZ
0BL74CZ
0BL74DZ
0BL74ZZ
0BL77DZ
0BL77ZZ
0BL78DZ
0BL78ZZ
0BL80CZ
0BL80DZ
0BL80ZZ
0BL83CZ
0BL83DZ
0BL83ZZ
0BL84CZ
0BL84DZ
0BL84ZZ
0BL87DZ
0BL87ZZ
0BL88DZ
0BL88ZZ
0BL90CZ
0BL90DZ
0BL90ZZ
0BL93CZ
0BL93DZ
0BL93ZZ
0BL94CZ
0BL94DZ
0BL94ZZ
0BL97DZ
0BL97ZZ
0BL98DZ
0BL98ZZ
0BLB0CZ
0BLB0DZ
0BLB0ZZ
0BLB3CZ
0BLB3DZ
0BLB3ZZ
0BLB4CZ
0BLB4DZ
0BLB4ZZ
0BLB7DZ
0BLB7ZZ
0BLB8DZ
0BLB8ZZ
0BM10ZZ
0BM20ZZ
0BM30ZZ
0BM40ZZ
0BM50ZZ
0BM60ZZ
0BM70ZZ
0BM80ZZ
0BM90ZZ
0BMB0ZZ
0BMC0ZZ
0BMD0ZZ
0BMF0ZZ
0BMG0ZZ
0BMH0ZZ
0BMJ0ZZ
0BMK0ZZ
0BML0ZZ
0BMT0ZZ
0BN10ZZ
0BN13ZZ
0BN14ZZ
0BN17ZZ
0BN18ZZ
0BN20ZZ
0BN23ZZ
0BN24ZZ
0BN27ZZ
0BN28ZZ
0BN30ZZ
0BN33ZZ
0BN34ZZ
0BN37ZZ
0BN38ZZ
0BN40ZZ
0BN43ZZ
0BN44ZZ
0BN47ZZ
0BN48ZZ
0BN50ZZ
0BN53ZZ
0BN54ZZ
0BN57ZZ
0BN58ZZ
0BN60ZZ
0BN63ZZ
0BN64ZZ
0BN67ZZ
0BN68ZZ
0BN70ZZ
0BN73ZZ
0BN74ZZ
0BN77ZZ
0BN78ZZ
0BN80ZZ
0BN83ZZ
0BN84ZZ
0BN87ZZ
0BN88ZZ
0BN90ZZ
0BN93ZZ
0BN94ZZ
0BN97ZZ
0BN98ZZ
0BNB0ZZ
0BNB3ZZ
0BNB4ZZ
0BNB7ZZ
0BNB8ZZ
0BNC0ZZ
0BNC3ZZ
0BNC4ZZ
0BNC7ZZ
0BNC8ZZ
0BND0ZZ
0BND3ZZ
0BND4ZZ
0BND7ZZ
0BND8ZZ
0BNF0ZZ
0BNF3ZZ
0BNF4ZZ
0BNF7ZZ
0BNF8ZZ
0BNG0ZZ
0BNG3ZZ
0BNG4ZZ
0BNG7ZZ
0BNG8ZZ
0BNH0ZZ
0BNH3ZZ
0BNH4ZZ
0BNH7ZZ
0BNH8ZZ
0BNJ0ZZ
0BNJ3ZZ
0BNJ4ZZ
0BNJ7ZZ
0BNJ8ZZ
0BNK0ZZ
0BNK3ZZ
0BNK4ZZ
0BNK7ZZ
0BNK8ZZ
0BNL0ZZ
0BNL3ZZ
0BNL4ZZ
0BNL7ZZ
0BNL8ZZ
0BNM0ZZ
0BNM3ZZ
0BNM4ZZ
0BNM7ZZ
0BNM8ZZ
0BNN0ZZ
0BNN3ZZ
0BNN4ZZ
0BNP0ZZ
0BNP3ZZ
0BNP4ZZ
0BNT0ZZ
0BNT3ZZ
0BNT4ZZ
0BP000Z
0BP001Z
0BP002Z
0BP003Z
0BP007Z
0BP00CZ
0BP00DZ
0BP00JZ
0BP00KZ
0BP00YZ
0BP030Z
0BP031Z
0BP032Z
0BP033Z
0BP037Z
0BP03CZ
0BP03DZ
0BP03JZ
0BP03KZ
0BP03YZ
0BP040Z
0BP041Z
0BP042Z
0BP043Z
0BP047Z
0BP04CZ
0BP04DZ
0BP04JZ
0BP04KZ
0BP04YZ
0BP070Z
0BP071Z
0BP072Z
0BP073Z
0BP077Z
0BP07CZ
0BP07DZ
0BP07JZ
0BP07KZ
0BP07YZ
0BP080Z
0BP081Z
0BP082Z
0BP083Z
0BP087Z
0BP08CZ
0BP08DZ
0BP08JZ
0BP08KZ
0BP08YZ
0BP0X0Z
0BP0X1Z
0BP0X2Z
0BP0X3Z
0BP0XDZ
0BP100Z
0BP102Z
0BP107Z
0BP10CZ
0BP10DZ
0BP10FZ
0BP10JZ
0BP10KZ
0BP130Z
0BP132Z
0BP137Z
0BP13CZ
0BP13DZ
0BP13FZ
0BP13JZ
0BP13KZ
0BP140Z
0BP142Z
0BP147Z
0BP14CZ
0BP14DZ
0BP14FZ
0BP14JZ
0BP14KZ
0BP170Z
0BP172Z
0BP177Z
0BP17CZ
0BP17DZ
0BP17FZ
0BP17JZ
0BP17KZ
0BP180Z
0BP182Z
0BP187Z
0BP18CZ
0BP18DZ
0BP18FZ
0BP18JZ
0BP18KZ
0BP1X0Z
0BP1X2Z
0BP1XDZ
0BP1XFZ
0BPK00Z
0BPK01Z
0BPK02Z
0BPK03Z
0BPK0YZ
0BPK30Z
0BPK31Z
0BPK32Z
0BPK33Z
0BPK3YZ
0BPK40Z
0BPK41Z
0BPK42Z
0BPK43Z
0BPK4YZ
0BPK70Z
0BPK71Z
0BPK72Z
0BPK73Z
0BPK7YZ
0BPK80Z
0BPK81Z
0BPK82Z
0BPK83Z
0BPK8YZ
0BPKX0Z
0BPKX1Z
0BPKX2Z
0BPKX3Z
0BPL00Z
0BPL01Z
0BPL02Z
0BPL03Z
0BPL0YZ
0BPL30Z
0BPL31Z
0BPL32Z
0BPL33Z
0BPL3YZ
0BPL70Z
0BPL72Z
0BPL73Z
0BPL7YZ
0BPL80Z
0BPL82Z
0BPL83Z
0BPLX0Z
0BPLX1Z
0BPLX2Z
0BPLX3Z
0BPQ00Z
0BPQ01Z
0BPQ02Z
0BPQ30Z
0BPQ31Z
0BPQ32Z
0BPQ3YZ
0BPQ40Z
0BPQ41Z
0BPQ42Z
0BPQ70Z
0BPQ71Z
0BPQ72Z
0BPQ7YZ
0BPQ80Z
0BPQ81Z
0BPQ82Z
0BPQX0Z
0BPQX1Z
0BPQX2Z
0BPT3YZ
0BPT70Z
0BPT72Z
0BPT7YZ
0BPT80Z
0BPT82Z
0BPT8YZ
0BPTX0Z
0BPTX2Z
0BPTXMZ
0BR34KZ
0BR407Z
0BR40JZ
0BR40KZ
0BR447Z
0BR44JZ
0BR44KZ
0BR507Z
0BR50JZ
0BR50KZ
0BR547Z
0BR54JZ
0BR54KZ
0BR607Z
0BR60JZ
0BR60KZ
0BR647Z
0BR64JZ
0BR64KZ
0BR707Z
0BR70JZ
0BR70KZ
0BR747Z
0BR74JZ
0BR74KZ
0BR807Z
0BR80JZ
0BR80KZ
0BR847Z
0BR84JZ
0BR84KZ
0BR907Z
0BR90JZ
0BR90KZ
0BR947Z
0BR94JZ
0BR94KZ
0BRB07Z
0BRB0JZ
0BRB0KZ
0BRB47Z
0BRB4JZ
0BRB4KZ
0BRT07Z
0BRT0JZ
0BRT0KZ
0BRT47Z
0BRT4JZ
0BRT4KZ
0BS10ZZ
0BS20ZZ
0BS30ZZ
0BS40ZZ
0BS50ZZ
0BS60ZZ
0BS70ZZ
0BS80ZZ
0BS90ZZ
0BSB0ZZ
0BSC0ZZ
0BSD0ZZ
0BSF0ZZ
0BSG0ZZ
0BSH0ZZ
0BSJ0ZZ
0BSK0ZZ
0BSL0ZZ
0BST0ZZ
0BT10ZZ
0BT14ZZ
0BT20ZZ
0BT24ZZ
0BT30ZZ
0BT34ZZ
0BT40ZZ
0BT44ZZ
0BT50ZZ
0BT54ZZ
0BT60ZZ
0BT64ZZ
0BT70ZZ
0BT74ZZ
0BT80ZZ
0BT84ZZ
0BT90ZZ
0BT94ZZ
0BTB0ZZ
0BTB4ZZ
0BTC0ZZ
0BTC4ZZ
0BTD0ZZ
0BTD4ZZ
0BTF0ZZ
0BTF4ZZ
0BTG0ZZ
0BTG4ZZ
0BTH0ZZ
0BTH4ZZ
0BTJ0ZZ
0BTJ4ZZ
0BTK0ZZ
0BTK4ZZ
0BTL0ZZ
0BTL4ZZ
0BTM0ZZ
0BTM4ZZ
0BTT0ZZ
0BTT4ZZ
0BU107Z
0BU10JZ
0BU10KZ
0BU147Z
0BU14JZ
0BU14KZ
0BU187Z
0BU18JZ
0BU18KZ
0BU207Z
0BU20JZ
0BU20KZ
0BU247Z
0BU24JZ
0BU24KZ
0BU287Z
0BU28JZ
0BU28KZ
0BU307Z
0BU30JZ
0BU30KZ
0BU347Z
0BU34JZ
0BU34KZ
0BU387Z
0BU38JZ
0BU38KZ
0BU407Z
0BU40JZ
0BU40KZ
0BU447Z
0BU44JZ
0BU44KZ
0BU487Z
0BU48JZ
0BU48KZ
0BU507Z
0BU50JZ
0BU50KZ
0BU547Z
0BU54JZ
0BU54KZ
0BU587Z
0BU58JZ
0BU58KZ
0BU607Z
0BU60JZ
0BU60KZ
0BU647Z
0BU64JZ
0BU64KZ
0BU687Z
0BU68JZ
0BU68KZ
0BU707Z
0BU70JZ
0BU70KZ
0BU747Z
0BU74JZ
0BU74KZ
0BU787Z
0BU78JZ
0BU78KZ
0BU807Z
0BU80JZ
0BU80KZ
0BU847Z
0BU84JZ
0BU84KZ
0BU887Z
0BU88JZ
0BU88KZ
0BU907Z
0BU90JZ
0BU90KZ
0BU947Z
0BU94JZ
0BU94KZ
0BU987Z
0BU98JZ
0BU98KZ
0BUB07Z
0BUB0JZ
0BUB0KZ
0BUB47Z
0BUB4JZ
0BUB4KZ
0BUB87Z
0BUB8JZ
0BUB8KZ
0BUT07Z
0BUT0JZ
0BUT0KZ
0BUT47Z
0BUT4JZ
0BUT4KZ
0BV10CZ
0BV10DZ
0BV10ZZ
0BV13CZ
0BV13DZ
0BV13ZZ
0BV14CZ
0BV14DZ
0BV14ZZ
0BV17DZ
0BV17ZZ
0BV18DZ
0BV18ZZ
0BV20CZ
0BV20DZ
0BV20ZZ
0BV23CZ
0BV23DZ
0BV23ZZ
0BV24CZ
0BV24DZ
0BV24ZZ
0BV27DZ
0BV27ZZ
0BV28DZ
0BV28ZZ
0BV30CZ
0BV30DZ
0BV30ZZ
0BV33CZ
0BV33DZ
0BV33ZZ
0BV34CZ
0BV34DZ
0BV34ZZ
0BV37DZ
0BV37ZZ
0BV38DZ
0BV38ZZ
0BV40CZ
0BV40DZ
0BV40ZZ
0BV43CZ
0BV43DZ
0BV43ZZ
0BV44CZ
0BV44DZ
0BV44ZZ
0BV47DZ
0BV47ZZ
0BV48DZ
0BV48ZZ
0BV50CZ
0BV50DZ
0BV50ZZ
0BV53CZ
0BV53DZ
0BV53ZZ
0BV54CZ
0BV54DZ
0BV54ZZ
0BV57DZ
0BV57ZZ
0BV58DZ
0BV58ZZ
0BV60CZ
0BV60DZ

0BV60ZZ
0BV63CZ
0BV63DZ
0BV63ZZ
0BV64CZ
0BV64DZ
0BV64ZZ
0BV67DZ
0BV67ZZ
0BV68DZ
0BV68ZZ
0BV70CZ
0BV70DZ
0BV70ZZ
0BV73CZ
0BV73DZ
0BV73ZZ
0BV74CZ
0BV74DZ
0BV74ZZ
0BV77DZ
0BV77ZZ
0BV78DZ
0BV78ZZ
0BV80CZ
0BV80DZ
0BV80ZZ
0BV83CZ
0BV83DZ
0BV83ZZ
0BV84CZ
0BV84DZ
0BV84ZZ
0BV87DZ
0BV87ZZ
0BV88DZ
0BV88ZZ
0BV90CZ
0BV90DZ
0BV90ZZ
0BV93CZ
0BV93DZ
0BV93ZZ
0BV94CZ
0BV94DZ
0BV94ZZ
0BV97DZ
0BV97ZZ
0BV98DZ
0BV98ZZ
0BVB0CZ
0BVB0DZ
0BVB0ZZ
0BVB3CZ
0BVB3DZ
0BVB3ZZ
0BVB4CZ
0BVB4DZ
0BVB4ZZ
0BVB7DZ
0BVB7ZZ
0BVB8DZ
0BVB8ZZ
0BW000Z
0BW002Z
0BW003Z
0BW007Z
0BW00CZ
0BW00DZ
0BW00JZ
0BW00KZ
0BW00YZ
0BW030Z
0BW032Z
0BW033Z
0BW037Z
0BW03CZ
0BW03DZ
0BW03JZ
0BW03KZ
0BW03YZ
0BW040Z
0BW042Z
0BW043Z
0BW047Z
0BW04CZ
0BW04DZ
0BW04JZ
0BW04KZ
0BW04YZ
0BW070Z
0BW072Z
0BW073Z
0BW077Z
0BW07CZ
0BW07DZ
0BW07JZ
0BW07KZ
0BW07YZ
0BW080Z
0BW082Z
0BW083Z
0BW087Z
0BW08CZ
0BW08DZ
0BW08JZ
0BW08KZ
0BW08YZ
0BW0X0Z
0BW0X2Z
0BW0X3Z
0BW0X7Z
0BW0XCZ
0BW0XDZ
0BW0XJZ
0BW0XKZ
0BW100Z
0BW102Z
0BW107Z
0BW10CZ
0BW10DZ
0BW10FZ
0BW10JZ
0BW10KZ
0BW130Z
0BW132Z
0BW137Z
0BW13CZ
0BW13DZ
0BW13FZ
0BW13JZ
0BW13KZ
0BW140Z
0BW142Z
0BW147Z
0BW14CZ
0BW14DZ
0BW14FZ
0BW14JZ
0BW14KZ
0BW170Z
0BW172Z
0BW177Z
0BW17CZ
0BW17DZ
0BW17FZ
0BW17JZ
0BW17KZ
0BW180Z
0BW182Z
0BW187Z
0BW18CZ
0BW18DZ
0BW18FZ
0BW18JZ
0BW18KZ
0BW1X0Z
0BW1X2Z
0BW1X7Z
0BW1XCZ
0BW1XDZ
0BW1XFZ
0BW1XJZ
0BW1XKZ
0BWK00Z
0BWK02Z
0BWK03Z
0BWK0YZ
0BWK30Z
0BWK32Z
0BWK33Z
0BWK3YZ
0BWK40Z
0BWK42Z
0BWK43Z
0BWK4YZ
0BWK70Z
0BWK72Z
0BWK73Z
0BWK7YZ
0BWK80Z
0BWK82Z
0BWK83Z
0BWK8YZ
0BWKX0Z
0BWKX2Z
0BWKX3Z
0BWL00Z
0BWL02Z
0BWL03Z
0BWL3YZ
0BWL70Z
0BWL72Z
0BWL73Z
0BWL7YZ
0BWL80Z
0BWL82Z
0BWL83Z
0BWLX0Z
0BWLX2Z
0BWLX3Z
0BWQ00Z
0BWQ02Z
0BWQ0YZ
0BWQ30Z
0BWQ32Z
0BWQ3YZ
0BWQ40Z
0BWQ42Z
0BWQ70Z
0BWQ72Z
0BWQ7YZ
0BWQ80Z
0BWQ82Z
0BWQX0Z
0BWQX2Z
0BWT3YZ
0BWT7YZ
0BWT8YZ
0BWTX0Z
0BWTX2Z
0BWTX7Z
0BWTXJZ
0BWTXKZ
0BWTXMZ
0C2AX0Z
0C2AXYZ
0C2SX0Z
0C2SXYZ
0C2YX0Z
0C2YXYZ
0C550ZZ
0C553ZZ
0C55XZZ
0C560ZZ
0C563ZZ
0C56XZZ
0C5W0Z0
0C5W0Z1
0C5W0Z2
0C5WXZ0
0C5WXZ1
0C5WXZ2
0C5X0Z0
0C5X0Z1
0C5X0Z2
0C5XXZ0
0C5XXZ1
0C5XXZ2
0C7B0DZ
0C7B0ZZ
0C7B3DZ
0C7B3ZZ
0C7B7DZ
0C7B7ZZ
0C7C0DZ
0C7C0ZZ
0C7C3DZ
0C7C3ZZ
0C7C7DZ
0C7C7ZZ
0C7M7DZ
0C7M7ZZ
0C7M8DZ
0C7M8ZZ
0C900ZX
0C9030Z
0C903ZX
0C903ZZ
0C90XZX
0C910ZX
0C9130Z
0C913ZX
0C913ZZ
0C91XZX
0C9230Z
0C923ZZ
0C9330Z
0C933ZZ
0C940ZX
0C9430Z
0C943ZX
0C943ZZ
0C94XZX
0C9500Z
0C950ZX
0C950ZZ
0C9530Z
0C953ZX
0C953ZZ
0C95X0Z
0C95XZX
0C95XZZ
0C9600Z
0C960ZX
0C960ZZ
0C9630Z
0C963ZX
0C963ZZ
0C96X0Z
0C96XZX
0C96XZZ
0C9730Z
0C973ZX
0C973ZZ
0C97XZX
0C9800Z
0C980ZZ
0C9830Z
0C983ZX
0C983ZZ
0C9900Z
0C990ZZ
0C9930Z
0C993ZX
0C993ZZ
0C9B00Z
0C9B0ZZ
0C9B30Z
0C9B3ZX
0C9B3ZZ
0C9C00Z
0C9C0ZZ
0C9C30Z
0C9C3ZX
0C9C3ZZ
0C9D00Z
0C9D0ZZ
0C9D30Z
0C9D3ZX
0C9D3ZZ
0C9F00Z
0C9F0ZZ
0C9F30Z
0C9F3ZX
0C9F3ZZ
0C9G00Z
0C9G0ZZ
0C9G30Z
0C9G3ZX
0C9G3ZZ
0C9H00Z
0C9H0ZZ
0C9H30Z
0C9H3ZX
0C9H3ZZ
0C9J00Z
0C9J0ZZ
0C9J30Z
0C9J3ZX
0C9J3ZZ
0C9M0ZX
0C9M30Z
0C9M3ZX
0C9M3ZZ
0C9M4ZX
0C9M7ZX
0C9M8ZX
0C9N30Z
0C9N3ZZ
0C9P30Z
0C9P3ZZ
0C9Q30Z
0C9Q3ZZ
0C9R30Z
0C9R3ZX
0C9R3ZZ
0C9R4ZX
0C9R7ZX
0C9R8ZX
0C9S30Z
0C9S3ZX
0C9S3ZZ
0C9S4ZX
0C9S7ZX
0C9S8ZX
0C9T0ZX
0C9T0ZZ
0C9T30Z
0C9T3ZX
0C9T3ZZ
0C9T40Z
0C9T4ZX
0C9T4ZZ
0C9T70Z
0C9T7ZX
0C9T7ZZ
0C9T80Z
0C9T8ZX
0C9T8ZZ
0C9V00Z
0C9V0ZX
0C9V0ZZ
0C9V30Z
0C9V3ZX
0C9V3ZZ
0C9V40Z
0C9V4ZX
0C9V4ZZ
0C9V70Z
0C9V7ZX
0C9V7ZZ
0C9V80Z
0C9V8ZX
0C9V8ZZ
0C9W000
0C9W001
0C9W002
0C9W0Z0
0C9W0Z1
0C9W0Z2
0C9WX00
0C9WX01
0C9WX02
0C9WXZ0
0C9WXZ1
0C9WXZ2
0C9X000
0C9X001
0C9X002
0C9X0Z0
0C9X0Z1
0C9X0Z2
0C9XX00
0C9XX01
0C9XX02
0C9XXZ0
0C9XXZ1
0C9XXZ2
0CB00ZX
0CB00ZZ
0CB03ZX
0CB03ZZ
0CB0XZX
0CB0XZZ
0CB10ZX
0CB10ZZ
0CB13ZX
0CB13ZZ
0CB1XZX
0CB1XZZ
0CB20ZX
0CB20ZZ
0CB23ZX
0CB23ZZ
0CB2XZX
0CB2XZZ
0CB30ZX
0CB30ZZ
0CB33ZX
0CB33ZZ
0CB3XZX
0CB3XZZ
0CB40ZX
0CB40ZZ
0CB43ZX
0CB43ZZ
0CB4XZX
0CB4XZZ
0CB50ZX
0CB50ZZ
0CB53ZX
0CB53ZZ
0CB5XZX
0CB5XZZ
0CB60ZX
0CB60ZZ
0CB63ZX
0CB63ZZ
0CB6XZX
0CB6XZZ
0CB70ZX
0CB70ZZ
0CB73ZX
0CB73ZZ
0CB7XZX
0CB7XZZ
0CB80ZX
0CB80ZZ
0CB83ZX
0CB83ZZ
0CB90ZX
0CB90ZZ
0CB93ZX
0CB93ZZ
0CBB0ZX
0CBB0ZZ
0CBB3ZX
0CBB3ZZ
0CBC0ZX
0CBC0ZZ
0CBC3ZX
0CBC3ZZ
0CBD0ZX
0CBD0ZZ
0CBD3ZX
0CBD3ZZ
0CBF0ZX
0CBF0ZZ
0CBF3ZX
0CBF3ZZ
0CBG0ZX
0CBG0ZZ
0CBG3ZX
0CBG3ZZ
0CBH0ZX
0CBH0ZZ
0CBH3ZX
0CBH3ZZ
0CBJ0ZX
0CBJ0ZZ
0CBJ3ZX
0CBJ3ZZ
0CBM0ZX
0CBM0ZZ
0CBM3ZX
0CBM3ZZ
0CBM4ZX
0CBM4ZZ
0CBM7ZX
0CBM7ZZ
0CBM8ZX
0CBM8ZZ
0CBN0ZX
0CBN0ZZ
0CBN3ZX
0CBN3ZZ
0CBNXZX
0CBNXZZ
0CBP0ZX
0CBP0ZZ
0CBP3ZX
0CBP3ZZ
0CBPXZX
0CBPXZZ
0CBQ0ZX
0CBQ0ZZ
0CBQ3ZX
0CBQ3ZZ
0CBQXZX
0CBQXZZ
0CBR0ZX
0CBR0ZZ
0CBR3ZX
0CBR3ZZ
0CBR4ZX
0CBR4ZZ
0CBR7ZX
0CBR7ZZ
0CBR8ZX
0CBR8ZZ
0CBS0ZX
0CBS0ZZ
0CBS3ZX
0CBS3ZZ
0CBS4ZX
0CBS4ZZ
0CBS7ZX
0CBS7ZZ
0CBS8ZX
0CBS8ZZ
0CBT0ZX
0CBT0ZZ
0CBT3ZX
0CBT3ZZ
0CBT4ZX
0CBT4ZZ
0CBT7ZX
0CBT7ZZ
0CBT8ZX
0CBT8ZZ
0CBV0ZX
0CBV0ZZ
0CBV3ZX
0CBV3ZZ
0CBV4ZX
0CBV4ZZ
0CBV7ZX
0CBV7ZZ
0CBV8ZX
0CBV8ZZ
0CBW0Z0
0CBW0Z1
0CBW0Z2
0CBWXZ0
0CBWXZ1
0CBWXZ2
0CBX0Z0
0CBX0Z1
0CBX0Z2
0CBXXZ0
0CBXXZ1
0CBXXZ2
0CC00ZZ
0CC03ZZ
0CC0XZZ
0CC10ZZ
0CC13ZZ
0CC1XZZ
0CC20ZZ
0CC23ZZ
0CC2XZZ
0CC30ZZ
0CC33ZZ
0CC3XZZ
0CC40ZZ
0CC43ZZ
0CC4XZZ
0CC50ZZ
0CC53ZZ
0CC5XZZ
0CC60ZZ
0CC63ZZ
0CC6XZZ
0CC70ZZ
0CC73ZZ
0CC7XZZ
0CC80ZZ
0CC83ZZ
0CC90ZZ
0CC93ZZ
0CCB0ZZ
0CCB3ZZ
0CCC0ZZ
0CCC3ZZ
0CCD0ZZ
0CCD3ZZ
0CCF0ZZ
0CCF3ZZ
0CCG0ZZ
0CCG3ZZ
0CCH0ZZ
0CCH3ZZ
0CCJ0ZZ
0CCJ3ZZ
0CCM0ZZ
0CCM3ZZ
0CCM4ZZ
0CCM7ZZ
0CCM8ZZ
0CCN0ZZ
0CCN3ZZ
0CCNXZZ
0CCP0ZZ
0CCP3ZZ
0CCPXZZ
0CCQ0ZZ
0CCQ3ZZ
0CCQXZZ
0CCR0ZZ
0CCR3ZZ
0CCR4ZZ
0CCR7ZZ
0CCR8ZZ
0CCS0ZZ
0CCS3ZZ
0CCS4ZZ
0CCS7ZZ
0CCS8ZZ
0CCT0ZZ
0CCT3ZZ
0CCT4ZZ
0CCT7ZZ
0CCT8ZZ
0CCV0ZZ
0CCV3ZZ
0CCV4ZZ
0CCV7ZZ
0CCV8ZZ
0CCW0Z0
0CCW0Z1
0CCW0Z2
0CCWXZ0
0CCWXZ1
0CCWXZ2
0CCX0Z0
0CCX0Z1
0CCX0Z2
0CCXXZ0
0CCXXZ1
0CCXXZ2
0CDT0ZZ
0CDT3ZZ
0CDT4ZZ
0CDT7ZZ
0CDT8ZZ
0CDV0ZZ
0CDV3ZZ
0CDV4ZZ
0CDV7ZZ
0CDV8ZZ
0CDWXZ0
0CDWXZ1
0CDWXZ2
0CDXXZ0
0CDXXZ1
0CDXXZ2
0CFB0ZZ
0CFB3ZZ
0CFB7ZZ
0CFBXZZ
0CFC0ZZ
0CFC3ZZ
0CFC7ZZ
0CFCXZZ
0CH701Z
0CH731Z
0CH7X1Z
0CHA0YZ
0CHA3YZ
0CHA7YZ
0CHA8YZ
0CHS0YZ
0CHS3YZ
0CHS7YZ
0CHS8YZ
0CHY0YZ
0CHY3YZ
0CHY7BZ
0CHY7YZ
0CHY8BZ
0CHY8YZ
0CJA0ZZ
0CJA3ZZ
0CJAXZZ
0CJS0ZZ

0CJS3ZZ
0CJS4ZZ
0CJS7ZZ
0CJS8ZZ
0CJSXZZ
0CJY0ZZ
0CJY3ZZ
0CJY4ZZ
0CJY7ZZ
0CJY8ZZ
0CJYXZZ
0CLB0CZ
0CLB0DZ
0CLB0ZZ
0CLB3CZ
0CLB3DZ
0CLB3ZZ
0CLB4CZ
0CLB4DZ
0CLB4ZZ
0CLB7DZ
0CLB7ZZ
0CLB8DZ
0CLB8ZZ
0CLC0CZ
0CLC0DZ
0CLC0ZZ
0CLC3CZ
0CLC3DZ
0CLC3ZZ
0CLC4CZ
0CLC4DZ
0CLC4ZZ
0CLC7DZ
0CLC7ZZ
0CLC8DZ
0CLC8ZZ
0CM00ZZ
0CM10ZZ
0CM30ZZ
0CM70ZZ
0CMN0ZZ
0CMW0Z0
0CMW0Z1
0CMW0Z2
0CMWXZ0
0CMWXZ1
0CMWXZ2
0CMX0Z0
0CMX0Z1
0CMX0Z2
0CMXXZ0
0CMXXZ1
0CMXXZ2
0CN00ZZ
0CN03ZZ
0CN0XZZ
0CN10ZZ
0CN13ZZ
0CN1XZZ
0CN20ZZ
0CN23ZZ
0CN2XZZ
0CN30ZZ
0CN33ZZ
0CN3XZZ
0CN40ZZ
0CN43ZZ
0CN4XZZ
0CN50ZZ
0CN53ZZ
0CN5XZZ
0CN60ZZ
0CN63ZZ
0CN6XZZ
0CN70ZZ
0CN73ZZ
0CN7XZZ
0CN80ZZ
0CN83ZZ
0CN90ZZ
0CN93ZZ
0CNB0ZZ
0CNB3ZZ
0CNC0ZZ
0CNC3ZZ
0CND0ZZ
0CND3ZZ
0CNF0ZZ
0CNF3ZZ
0CNG0ZZ
0CNG3ZZ
0CNH0ZZ
0CNH3ZZ
0CNJ0ZZ
0CNJ3ZZ
0CNM0ZZ
0CNM3ZZ
0CNM4ZZ
0CNM7ZZ
0CNM8ZZ
0CNN0ZZ
0CNN3ZZ
0CNNXZZ
0CNP0ZZ
0CNP3ZZ
0CNPXZZ
0CNQ0ZZ
0CNQ3ZZ
0CNQXZZ
0CNR0ZZ
0CNR3ZZ
0CNR4ZZ
0CNR7ZZ
0CNR8ZZ
0CNS0ZZ
0CNS3ZZ
0CNS4ZZ
0CNS7ZZ
0CNS8ZZ
0CNT0ZZ
0CNT3ZZ
0CNT4ZZ
0CNT7ZZ
0CNT8ZZ
0CNV0ZZ
0CNV3ZZ
0CNV4ZZ
0CNV7ZZ
0CNV8ZZ
0CNW0Z0
0CNW0Z1
0CNW0Z2
0CNWXZ0
0CNWXZ1
0CNWXZ2
0CNX0Z0
0CNX0Z1
0CNX0Z2
0CNXXZ0
0CNXXZ1
0CNXXZ2
0CPA00Z
0CPA0CZ
0CPA0YZ
0CPA30Z
0CPA3CZ
0CPA3YZ
0CPA7YZ
0CPA8YZ
0CPS00Z
0CPS07Z
0CPS0DZ
0CPS0JZ
0CPS0KZ
0CPS0YZ
0CPS30Z
0CPS37Z
0CPS3DZ
0CPS3JZ
0CPS3KZ
0CPS3YZ
0CPS70Z
0CPS77Z
0CPS7DZ
0CPS7JZ
0CPS7KZ
0CPS7YZ
0CPS80Z
0CPS87Z
0CPS8DZ
0CPS8JZ
0CPS8KZ
0CPS8YZ
0CPSX0Z
0CPSX7Z
0CPSXDZ
0CPSXJZ
0CPSXKZ
0CPY00Z
0CPY01Z
0CPY07Z
0CPY0DZ
0CPY0JZ
0CPY0KZ
0CPY0YZ
0CPY30Z
0CPY31Z
0CPY37Z
0CPY3DZ
0CPY3JZ
0CPY3KZ
0CPY3YZ
0CPY70Z
0CPY71Z
0CPY77Z
0CPY7DZ
0CPY7JZ
0CPY7KZ
0CPY7YZ
0CPY80Z
0CPY81Z
0CPY87Z
0CPY8DZ
0CPY8JZ
0CPY8KZ
0CPY8YZ
0CPYX0Z
0CPYX1Z
0CPYX7Z
0CPYXDZ
0CPYXJZ
0CPYXKZ
0CQ00ZZ
0CQ03ZZ
0CQ0XZZ
0CQ10ZZ
0CQ13ZZ
0CQ1XZZ
0CQ20ZZ
0CQ23ZZ
0CQ2XZZ
0CQ30ZZ
0CQ33ZZ
0CQ3XZZ
0CQ40ZZ
0CQ43ZZ
0CQ4XZZ
0CQ50ZZ
0CQ53ZZ
0CQ5XZZ
0CQ60ZZ
0CQ63ZZ
0CQ6XZZ
0CQ70ZZ
0CQ73ZZ
0CQ7XZZ
0CQ80ZZ
0CQ83ZZ
0CQ90ZZ
0CQ93ZZ
0CQB0ZZ
0CQB3ZZ
0CQC0ZZ
0CQC3ZZ
0CQD0ZZ
0CQD3ZZ
0CQF0ZZ
0CQF3ZZ
0CQG0ZZ
0CQG3ZZ
0CQH0ZZ
0CQH3ZZ
0CQJ0ZZ
0CQJ3ZZ
0CQM0ZZ
0CQM3ZZ
0CQM4ZZ
0CQM7ZZ
0CQM8ZZ
0CQN0ZZ
0CQN3ZZ
0CQNXZZ
0CQP0ZZ
0CQP3ZZ
0CQPXZZ
0CQQ0ZZ
0CQQ3ZZ
0CQQXZZ
0CQR0ZZ
0CQR3ZZ
0CQR4ZZ
0CQR7ZZ
0CQR8ZZ
0CQS0ZZ
0CQS3ZZ
0CQS4ZZ
0CQS7ZZ
0CQS8ZZ
0CQT0ZZ
0CQT3ZZ
0CQW0Z0
0CQW0Z1
0CQW0Z2
0CQWXZ0
0CQWXZ1
0CQWXZ2
0CQX0Z0
0CQX0Z1
0CQX0Z2
0CQXXZ0
0CQXXZ1
0CQXXZ2
0CRT07Z
0CRT0JZ
0CRT0KZ
0CRT77Z
0CRT7JZ
0CRT7KZ
0CRT87Z
0CRT8JZ
0CRT8KZ
0CRV07Z
0CRV0JZ
0CRV0KZ
0CRV77Z
0CRV7JZ
0CRV7KZ
0CRV87Z
0CRV8JZ
0CRV8KZ
0CRW070
0CRW071
0CRW072
0CRW0J0
0CRW0J1
0CRW0J2
0CRW0K0
0CRW0K1
0CRW0K2
0CRWX70
0CRWX71
0CRWX72
0CRWXJ0
0CRWXJ1
0CRWXJ2
0CRWXK0
0CRWXK1
0CRWXK2
0CRX070
0CRX071
0CRX072
0CRX0J0
0CRX0J1
0CRX0J2
0CRX0K0
0CRX0K1
0CRX0K2
0CRXX70
0CRXX71
0CRXX72
0CRXXJ0
0CRXXJ1
0CRXXJ2
0CRXXK0
0CRXXK1
0CRXXK2
0CS00ZZ
0CS0XZZ
0CS10ZZ
0CS1XZZ
0CS20ZZ
0CS2XZZ
0CS30ZZ
0CS3XZZ
0CS70ZZ
0CS7XZZ
0CSB0ZZ
0CSB3ZZ
0CSC0ZZ
0CSC3ZZ
0CSN0ZZ
0CSNXZZ
0CSR0ZZ
0CSR7ZZ
0CSR8ZZ
0CST0ZZ
0CST7ZZ
0CST8ZZ
0CSV0ZZ
0CSV7ZZ
0CSV8ZZ
0CSW050
0CSW051
0CSW052
0CSW0Z0
0CSW0Z1
0CSW0Z2
0CSWX50
0CSWX51
0CSWX52
0CSWXZ0
0CSWXZ1
0CSWXZ2
0CSX050
0CSX051
0CSX052
0CSX0Z0
0CSX0Z1
0CSX0Z2
0CSXX50
0CSXX51
0CSXX52
0CSXXZ0
0CSXXZ1
0CSXXZ2
0CT00ZZ
0CT0XZZ
0CT10ZZ
0CT1XZZ
0CT20ZZ
0CT2XZZ
0CT30ZZ
0CT3XZZ
0CT70ZZ
0CT7XZZ
0CT80ZZ
0CT90ZZ
0CTB0ZZ
0CTC0ZZ
0CTD0ZZ
0CTF0ZZ
0CTG0ZZ
0CTH0ZZ
0CTJ0ZZ
0CTM0ZZ
0CTM4ZZ
0CTM7ZZ
0CTM8ZZ
0CTN0ZZ
0CTNXZZ
0CTP0ZZ
0CTPXZZ
0CTQ0ZZ
0CTQXZZ
0CTR0ZZ
0CTR4ZZ
0CTR7ZZ
0CTR8ZZ
0CTS0ZZ
0CTS4ZZ
0CTS7ZZ
0CTS8ZZ
0CTT0ZZ
0CTT4ZZ
0CTT7ZZ
0CTT8ZZ
0CTV0ZZ
0CTV4ZZ
0CTV7ZZ
0CTV8ZZ
0CTW0Z0
0CTW0Z1
0CTW0Z2
0CTX0Z0
0CTX0Z1
0CTX0Z2
0CU007Z
0CU00JZ
0CU00KZ
0CU037Z
0CU03JZ
0CU03KZ
0CU0X7Z
0CU0XJZ
0CU0XKZ
0CU107Z
0CU10JZ
0CU10KZ
0CU137Z
0CU13JZ
0CU13KZ
0CU1X7Z
0CU1XJZ
0CU1XKZ
0CU207Z
0CU20JZ
0CU20KZ
0CU237Z
0CU23JZ
0CU23KZ
0CU2X7Z
0CU2XJZ
0CU2XKZ
0CU307Z
0CU30JZ
0CU30KZ
0CU337Z
0CU33JZ
0CU33KZ
0CU3X7Z
0CU3XJZ
0CU3XKZ
0CU407Z
0CU40JZ
0CU40KZ
0CU437Z
0CU43JZ
0CU43KZ
0CU4X7Z
0CU4XJZ
0CU4XKZ
0CU507Z
0CU50JZ
0CU50KZ
0CU537Z
0CU53JZ
0CU53KZ
0CU5X7Z
0CU5XJZ
0CU5XKZ
0CU607Z
0CU60JZ
0CU60KZ
0CU637Z
0CU63JZ
0CU63KZ
0CU6X7Z
0CU6XJZ
0CU6XKZ
0CU707Z
0CU70JZ
0CU70KZ
0CU737Z
0CU73JZ
0CU73KZ
0CU7X7Z
0CU7XJZ
0CU7XKZ
0CUM07Z
0CUM0JZ
0CUM0KZ
0CUM77Z
0CUM7JZ
0CUM7KZ
0CUM87Z
0CUM8JZ
0CUM8KZ
0CUN07Z
0CUN0JZ
0CUN0KZ
0CUN37Z
0CUN3JZ
0CUN3KZ
0CUNX7Z
0CUNXJZ
0CUNXKZ
0CUR07Z
0CUR0JZ
0CUR0KZ
0CUR77Z
0CUR7JZ
0CUR7KZ
0CUR87Z
0CUR8JZ
0CUR8KZ
0CUS07Z
0CUS0JZ
0CUS0KZ
0CUS77Z
0CUS7JZ
0CUS7KZ
0CUS87Z
0CUS8JZ
0CUS8KZ
0CUT07Z
0CUT0JZ
0CUT0KZ
0CUT77Z
0CUT7JZ
0CUT7KZ
0CUT87Z
0CUT8JZ
0CUT8KZ
0CUV07Z
0CUV0JZ
0CUV0KZ
0CUV77Z
0CUV7JZ
0CUV7KZ
0CUV87Z
0CUV8JZ
0CUV8KZ
0CVB0CZ
0CVB0DZ
0CVB0ZZ
0CVB3CZ
0CVB3DZ
0CVB3ZZ
0CVB7DZ
0CVB7ZZ
0CVB8DZ
0CVB8ZZ
0CVC0CZ
0CVC0DZ
0CVC0ZZ
0CVC3CZ
0CVC3DZ
0CVC3ZZ
0CVC7DZ
0CVC7ZZ
0CVC8DZ
0CVC8ZZ
0CWA00Z
0CWA0CZ
0CWA0YZ
0CWA30Z
0CWA3CZ
0CWA3YZ
0CWA7YZ
0CWA8YZ
0CWAX0Z
0CWAXCZ
0CWS00Z
0CWS07Z
0CWS0DZ
0CWS0JZ
0CWS0KZ
0CWS0YZ
0CWS30Z
0CWS37Z
0CWS3DZ
0CWS3JZ
0CWS3KZ
0CWS3YZ
0CWS70Z
0CWS77Z
0CWS7DZ
0CWS7JZ
0CWS7KZ
0CWS7YZ
0CWS80Z
0CWS87Z
0CWS8DZ
0CWS8JZ
0CWS8KZ
0CWS8YZ
0CWSX0Z
0CWSX7Z
0CWSXDZ
0CWSXJZ
0CWSXKZ
0CWY00Z
0CWY01Z
0CWY07Z
0CWY0DZ
0CWY0JZ
0CWY0KZ
0CWY0YZ
0CWY30Z
0CWY31Z
0CWY37Z
0CWY3DZ
0CWY3JZ
0CWY3KZ
0CWY3YZ
0CWY70Z
0CWY71Z
0CWY77Z
0CWY7DZ
0CWY7JZ
0CWY7KZ
0CWY7YZ
0CWY80Z
0CWY81Z
0CWY87Z
0CWY8DZ
0CWY8JZ
0CWY8KZ
0CWY8YZ
0CWYX0Z
0CWYX1Z
0CWYX7Z
0CWYXDZ
0CWYXJZ
0CWYXKZ
0CX00ZZ
0CX0XZZ
0CX10ZZ
0CX1XZZ
0CX30ZZ
0CX3XZZ
0CX40ZZ
0CX4XZZ
0CX50ZZ
0CX5XZZ
0CX60ZZ
0CX6XZZ
0D130J9
0D130JA
0D130JB
0D130K4
0D130K6
0D130K9
0D130KA
0D130KB
0D130Z4
0D130Z6
0D130Z9
0D130ZA
0D130ZB
0D133J4
0D13474
0D13476
0D13479
0D1347A
0D1347B
0D134J4
0D134J6
0D134J9
0D134JA
0D134JB
0D134K4
0D134K6
0D134K9
0D134KA
0D134KB
0D134Z4
0D134Z6
0D134Z9
0D134ZA
0D134ZB
0D13874
0D13876
0D13879
0D1387A
0D1387B
0D138J4
0D138J6
0D138J9
0D138JA
0D138JB
0D138K4
0D138K6
0D138K9
0D138KA

0D138KB
0D138Z4
0D138Z6
0D138Z9
0D138ZA
0D138ZB
0D15074
0D15076
0D15079
0D1507A
0D1507B
0D150J4
0D150J6
0D150J9
0D150JA
0D150JB
0D150K4
0D150K6
0D150K9
0D150KA
0D150KB
0D150Z4
0D150Z6
0D150Z9
0D150ZA
0D150ZB
0D153J4
0D15474
0D15476
0D15479
0D1547A
0D1547B
0D154J4
0D154J6
0D154J9
0D154JA
0D154JB
0D154K4
0D154K6
0D154K9
0D154KA
0D154KB
0D154Z4
0D154Z6
0D154Z9
0D154ZA
0D154ZB
0D15874
0D15876
0D15879
0D1587A
0D1587B
0D158J4
0D158J6
0D158J9
0D158JA
0D158JB
0D158K4
0D158K6
0D158K9
0D158KA
0D158KB
0D158Z4
0D158Z6
0D158Z9
0D158ZA
0D158ZB
0D16074
0D16079
0D1607A
0D1607B
0D1607L
0D160J4
0D160J9
0D160JA
0D160JB
0D160JL
0D160K4
0D160K9
0D160KA
0D160KB
0D160KL
0D160Z4
0D160Z9
0D160ZA
0D160ZB
0D160ZL
0D163J4
0D16474
0D16479
0D1647A
0D1647B
0D1647L
0D164J4
0D164J9
0D164JA
0D164JB
0D164JL
0D164K4
0D164K9
0D164KA
0D164KB
0D164KL
0D164Z4
0D164Z9
0D164ZA
0D164ZB
0D164ZL
0D16874
0D16879
0D1687A
0D1687B
0D1687L
0D168J4
0D168J9
0D168JA
0D168JB
0D168JL
0D168K4
0D168K9
0D168KA
0D168KB
0D168KL
0D168Z4
0D168Z9
0D168ZA
0D168ZB
0D1A0JA
0D1A0JB
0D1A0JH
0D1A0JK
0D1A0JL
0D1A0JM
0D1A0JN
0D1A0JP
0D1A0JQ
0D1A0K4
0D1A0KA
0D1A0KB
0D1A0KH
0D1A0KK
0D1A0KL
0D1A0KM
0D1A0KN
0D1A0KP
0D1A0KQ
0D1A0Z4
0D1A0ZA
0D1A0ZB
0D1A0ZH
0D1A0ZK
0D1A0ZL
0D1A0ZM
0D1A0ZN
0D1A0ZP
0D1A0ZQ
0D1A3J4
0D1A474
0D1A47A
0D1A47B
0D1A47H
0D1A47K
0D1A47L
0D1A47M
0D1A47N
0D1A47P
0D1A47Q
0D1A4J4
0D1A4JA
0D1A4JB
0D1A4JH
0D1A4JK
0D1A4JL
0D1A4JM
0D1A4JN
0D1A4JP
0D1A4JQ
0D1A4K4
0D1A4KA
0D1A4KB
0D1A4KH
0D1A4KK
0D1A4KL
0D1A4KM
0D1A4KN
0D1A4KP
0D1A4KQ
0D1A4Z4
0D1A4ZA
0D1A4ZB
0D1A4ZH
0D1A4ZK
0D1A4ZL
0D1A4ZM
0D1A4ZN
0D1A4ZP
0D1A4ZQ
0D1A874
0D1A87A
0D1A87B
0D1A87H
0D1A87K
0D1A87L
0D1A87M
0D1A87N
0D1A87P
0D1A87Q
0D1A8J4
0D1A8JA
0D1A8JB
0D1A8JH
0D1A8JK
0D1A8JL
0D1A8JM
0D1A8JN
0D1A8JP
0D1A8JQ
0D1A8K4
0D1A8KA
0D1A8KB
0D1A8KH
0D1A8KK
0D1A8KL
0D1A8KM
0D1A8KN
0D1A8KP
0D1A8KQ
0D1A8Z4
0D1A8ZA
0D1A8ZB
0D1A8ZH
0D1A8ZK
0D1A8ZL
0D1A8ZM
0D1A8ZN
0D1A8ZP
0D1A8ZQ
0D1B074
0D1B07B
0D1B07H
0D1B07K
0D1B07L
0D1B07M
0D1B07N
0D1B07P
0D1B07Q
0D1B0J4
0D1B0JB
0D1B0JH
0D1B0JK
0D1B0JL
0D1B0JM
0D1B0JN
0D1B0JP
0D1B0JQ
0D1B0K4
0D1B0KB
0D1B0KH
0D1B0KK
0D1B0KL
0D1B0KM
0D1B0KN
0D1B0KP
0D1B0KQ
0D1B0Z4
0D1B0ZB
0D1B0ZH
0D1B0ZK
0D1B0ZL
0D1B0ZM
0D1B0ZN
0D1B0ZP
0D1B0ZQ
0D1B3J4
0D1B474
0D1B47B
0D1B47H
0D1B47K
0D1B47L
0D1B47M
0D1B47N
0D1H0KN
0D1H0KP
0D1H0Z4
0D1H0ZH
0D1H0ZK
0D1H0ZL
0D1H0ZM
0D1H0ZN
0D1H0ZP
0D1H3J4
0D1H474
0D1H47H
0D1H47K
0D1H47L
0D1H47M
0D1H47N
0D1H47P
0D1H4J4
0D1H4JH
0D1H4JK
0D1H4JL
0D1H4JM
0D1H4JN
0D1H4JP
0D1H4K4
0D1H4KH
0D1H4KK
0D1H4KL
0D1H4KM
0D1H4KN
0D1H4KP
0D1H4Z4
0D1H4ZH
0D1H4ZK
0D1H4ZL
0D1H4ZM
0D1H4ZN
0D1H4ZP
0D1H874
0D1H87H
0D1H87K
0D1H87L
0D1H87M
0D1H87N
0D1H87P
0D1H8J4
0D1H8JH
0D1H8JK
0D1H8JL
0D1H8JM
0D1H8JN
0D1H8JP
0D1H8K4
0D1H8KH
0D1H8KK
0D1H8KL
0D1H8KM
0D1H8KN
0D1H8KP
0D1H8Z4
0D1H8ZH
0D1H8ZK
0D1H8ZL
0D1H8ZM
0D1H8ZN
0D1H8ZP
0D1K074
0D1K07K
0D1K07L
0D1K07M
0D1K07N
0D1K07P
0D1K0J4
0D1K0JK
0D1K0JL
0D1K0JM
0D1K0JN
0D1K0JP
0D1K0K4
0D1K0KK
0D1K0KL
0D1K0KM
0D1K0KN
0D1K0KP
0D1K0Z4
0D1K0ZK
0D1K0ZL
0D1K0ZM
0D1K0ZN
0D1K0ZP
0D1K3J4
0D1K474
0D1K47K
0D1K47L
0D1K47M
0D1K47N
0D1K47P
0D1K4J4
0D1K4JK
0D1K4JL
0D1K4JM
0D1K4JN
0D1K4JP
0D1K4K4
0D1K4KK
0D1K4KL
0D1K4KM
0D1K4KN
0D1K4KP
0D1K4Z4
0D1K4ZK
0D1K4ZL
0D1K4ZM
0D1K4ZN
0D1K4ZP
0D1K874
0D1K87K
0D1K87L
0D1K87M
0D1K87N
0D1K87P
0D1K8J4
0D1K8JK
0D1K8JL
0D1K8JM
0D1K8JN
0D1K8JP
0D1K8K4
0D1K8KK
0D1K8KL
0D1K8KM
0D1K8KN
0D1K8KP
0D1K8Z4
0D1K8ZK
0D1K8ZL
0D1K8ZM
0D1K8ZN
0D1K8ZP
0D1L074
0D1L07L
0D1L07M
0D1L07N
0D1L07P
0D1L0J4
0D1L0JL
0D1L0JM
0D1L0JN
0D1L0JP
0D1L0K4
0D1L0KL
0D1L0KM
0D1L0KN
0D1L0KP
0D1L0Z4
0D1L0ZL
0D1L0ZM
0D1L0ZN
0D1L0ZP
0D1L3J4
0D1L474
0D1L47L
0D1L47M
0D1L47N
0D1L47P
0D1L4J4
0D1L4JL
0D1L4JM
0D1L4JN
0D1L4JP
0D1L4K4
0D1L4KL
0D1L4KM
0D1L4KN
0D1L4KP
0D1L4Z4
0D1L4ZL
0D1L4ZM
0D1L4ZN
0D1L4ZP
0D1L874
0D1L87L
0D1L87M
0D1L87N
0D1L87P
0D1L8J4
0D1L8JL
0D1L8JM
0D1L8JN
0D1L8JP
0D1L8K4
0D1L8KL
0D1L8KM
0D1L8KN
0D1L8KP
0D1L8Z4
0D1L8ZL
0D1L8ZM
0D1L8ZN
0D1L8ZP
0D1M074
0D1M07M
0D1M07N
0D1M07P
0D1M0J4
0D1M0JM
0D1M0JN
0D1M0JP
0D1M0K4
0D1M0KM
0D1M0KN
0D1M0KP
0D1M0Z4
0D1M0ZM
0D1M0ZN
0D1M0ZP
0D1M3J4
0D1M474
0D1M47M
0D1M47N
0D1M47P
0D1M4J4
0D1M4JM
0D1M4JN
0D1M4JP
0D1M4K4
0D1M4KM
0D1M4KN
0D1M4KP
0D1M4Z4
0D1M4ZM
0D1M4ZN
0D1M4ZP
0D20X0Z
0D20XUZ
0D20XYZ
0D2DX0Z
0D2DXUZ
0D2DXYZ
0D2UX0Z
0D2UXYZ
0D2VX0Z
0D2VXYZ
0D2WX0Z
0D2WXYZ
0D514ZZ
0D518ZZ
0D524ZZ
0D528ZZ
0D534ZZ
0D538ZZ
0D544ZZ
0D548ZZ
0D554ZZ
0D558ZZ
0D564ZZ
0D568ZZ
0D574ZZ
0D578ZZ
0D594ZZ
0D598ZZ
0D5E4ZZ
0D5E8ZZ
0D5F4ZZ
0D5F8ZZ
0D5G4ZZ
0D5G8ZZ
0D5H4ZZ
0D5H8ZZ
0D5K4ZZ
0D5K8ZZ
0D5L4ZZ
0D5L8ZZ
0D5M4ZZ
0D5M8ZZ
0D5N4ZZ
0D5N7ZZ
0D5N8ZZ
0D5P0ZZ
0D5P3ZZ
0D5P4ZZ
0D5P7ZZ
0D5P8ZZ
0D5Q0ZZ
0D5Q3ZZ
0D5Q4ZZ
0D5Q7ZZ
0D5Q8ZZ
0D5QXZZ
0D5R0ZZ
0D5R3ZZ
0D5R4ZZ
0D5U0ZZ
0D5U3ZZ
0D5U4ZZ
0D5V0ZZ
0D5V3ZZ
0D5V4ZZ
0D5W0ZZ
0D5W3ZZ
0D5W4ZZ
0D710DZ
0D710ZZ
0D713DZ
0D713ZZ
0D714DZ
0D714ZZ
0D717DZ
0D717ZZ
0D718DZ
0D718ZZ
0D720DZ
0D720ZZ
0D723DZ
0D723ZZ
0D724DZ
0D724ZZ
0D727DZ
0D727ZZ
0D728DZ
0D728ZZ
0D730DZ
0D730ZZ
0D733DZ
0D733ZZ
0D734DZ
0D734ZZ
0D737DZ
0D737ZZ
0D738DZ
0D738ZZ
0D740DZ
0D740ZZ
0D743DZ
0D743ZZ
0D744DZ
0D744ZZ
0D747DZ
0D747ZZ
0D748DZ
0D748ZZ
0D750DZ
0D750ZZ
0D753DZ
0D753ZZ
0D754DZ
0D754ZZ
0D757DZ
0D757ZZ
0D758DZ
0D758ZZ
0D760DZ
0D760ZZ
0D763DZ
0D763ZZ
0D764DZ
0D764ZZ
0D767DZ
0D767ZZ
0D768DZ
0D768ZZ
0D770DZ
0D770ZZ
0D773DZ
0D773ZZ
0D774DZ
0D774ZZ
0D777DZ
0D777ZZ
0D778DZ
0D778ZZ
0D780DZ
0D780ZZ
0D783DZ
0D783ZZ
0D784DZ
0D784ZZ
0D787DZ
0D787ZZ
0D788DZ
0D788ZZ
0D790DZ
0D790ZZ
0D793DZ
0D793ZZ
0D794DZ
0D794ZZ
0D797DZ
0D797ZZ
0D798DZ
0D798ZZ
0D7A0DZ
0D7A0ZZ
0D7A3DZ
0D7A3ZZ
0D7A4DZ
0D7A4ZZ
0D7A7DZ
0D7A7ZZ
0D7A8DZ
0D7A8ZZ
0D7B0DZ
0D7B0ZZ
0D7B3DZ
0D7B3ZZ
0D7B4DZ
0D7B4ZZ
0D7B7DZ
0D7B7ZZ
0D7B8DZ
0D7B8ZZ
0D7C0DZ
0D7C0ZZ
0D7C3DZ
0D7C3ZZ
0D7C4DZ
0D7C4ZZ
0D7C7DZ
0D7C7ZZ
0D7C8DZ
0D7C8ZZ
0D7E0DZ
0D7E0ZZ
0D7E3DZ
0D7E3ZZ
0D7E4DZ
0D7E4ZZ
0D7E7DZ
0D7E7ZZ
0D7E8DZ
0D7E8ZZ
0D7F0DZ
0D7F0ZZ
0D7F3DZ
0D7F3ZZ
0D7F4DZ
0D7F4ZZ
0D7F7DZ
0D7F7ZZ
0D7F8DZ
0D7F8ZZ
0D7G0DZ
0D7G0ZZ
0D7G3DZ
0D7G3ZZ

0D138KB-0D7G3ZZ
APPENDIX H: NON-OR NOT AFFECTING MS-DRG ASSIGNMENT

0D7G4DZ
0D7G4ZZ
0D7G7DZ
0D7G7ZZ
0D7G8DZ
0D7G8ZZ
0D7H0DZ
0D7H0ZZ
0D7H3DZ
0D7H3ZZ
0D7H4DZ
0D7H4ZZ
0D7H7DZ
0D7H7ZZ
0D7H8DZ
0D7H8ZZ
0D7K0DZ
0D7K0ZZ
0D7K3DZ
0D7K3ZZ
0D7K4DZ
0D7K4ZZ
0D7K7DZ
0D7K7ZZ
0D7K8DZ
0D7K8ZZ
0D7L0DZ
0D7L0ZZ
0D7L3DZ
0D7L3ZZ
0D7L4DZ
0D7L4ZZ
0D7L7DZ
0D7L7ZZ
0D7L8DZ
0D7L8ZZ
0D7M0DZ
0D7M0ZZ
0D7M3DZ
0D7M3ZZ
0D7M4DZ
0D7M4ZZ
0D7M7DZ
0D7M7ZZ
0D7M8DZ
0D7M8ZZ
0D7N0DZ
0D7N0ZZ
0D7N3DZ
0D7N3ZZ
0D7N4DZ
0D7N4ZZ
0D7N7DZ
0D7N7ZZ
0D7N8DZ
0D7N8ZZ
0D7P0DZ
0D7P0ZZ
0D7P3DZ
0D7P3ZZ
0D7P4DZ
0D7P4ZZ
0D7P7DZ
0D7P7ZZ
0D7P8DZ
0D7P8ZZ
0D7Q0DZ
0D7Q0ZZ
0D7Q3DZ
0D7Q3ZZ
0D7Q4DZ
0D7Q4ZZ
0D7Q7DZ
0D7Q7ZZ
0D7Q8DZ
0D7Q8ZZ
0D840ZZ
0D843ZZ
0D844ZZ
0D847ZZ
0D848ZZ
0D870ZZ
0D873ZZ
0D874ZZ
0D877ZZ
0D878ZZ
0D8R0ZZ
0D8R3ZZ
0D9100Z
0D910ZX
0D910ZZ
0D9130Z
0D913ZX
0D913ZZ
0D9140Z
0D914ZX
0D914ZZ
0D9170Z
0D917ZX
0D917ZZ
0D9180Z
0D918ZX
0D918ZZ
0D9200Z
0D920ZX
0D920ZZ
0D9230Z
0D923ZX
0D923ZZ
0D9240Z
0D924ZX
0D924ZZ
0D9270Z
0D927ZX
0D927ZZ
0D9280Z
0D928ZX
0D928ZZ
0D9300Z
0D930ZX
0D930ZZ
0D9330Z
0D933ZX
0D933ZZ
0D9340Z
0D934ZX
0D934ZZ
0D9370Z
0D937ZX
0D937ZZ
0D9380Z
0D938ZX
0D938ZZ
0D9400Z
0D940ZX
0D940ZZ
0D9430Z
0D943ZX
0D943ZZ
0D9440Z
0D944ZX
0D944ZZ
0D9470Z
0D947ZX
0D947ZZ
0D9480Z
0D948ZX
0D948ZZ
0D9500Z
0D950ZX
0D950ZZ
0D9530Z
0D953ZX
0D953ZZ
0D9540Z
0D954ZX
0D954ZZ
0D9570Z
0D957ZX
0D957ZZ
0D9580Z
0D958ZX
0D958ZZ
0D9600Z
0D960ZX
0D960ZZ
0D9630Z
0D963ZX
0D963ZZ
0D9640Z
0D964ZX
0D964ZZ
0D9670Z
0D967ZX
0D967ZZ
0D9680Z
0D968ZX
0D968ZZ
0D9700Z
0D970ZX
0D970ZZ
0D9730Z
0D973ZX
0D973ZZ
0D9740Z
0D974ZX
0D974ZZ
0D9770Z
0D977ZX
0D977ZZ
0D9780Z
0D978ZX
0D978ZZ
0D9800Z
0D980ZX
0D980ZZ
0D9830Z
0D983ZX
0D983ZZ
0D9840Z
0D984ZX
0D984ZZ
0D9870Z
0D987ZX
0D987ZZ
0D9880Z
0D988ZX
0D988ZZ
0D9900Z
0D990ZX
0D990ZZ
0D9930Z
0D993ZX
0D993ZZ
0D9940Z
0D994ZX
0D994ZZ
0D9970Z
0D997ZX
0D997ZZ
0D9980Z
0D998ZX
0D998ZZ
0D9A00Z
0D9A0ZX
0D9A0ZZ
0D9A30Z
0D9A3ZX
0D9A3ZZ
0D9A40Z
0D9A4ZX
0D9A4ZZ
0D9A70Z
0D9A7ZX
0D9A7ZZ
0D9A80Z
0D9A8ZX
0D9A8ZZ
0D9B00Z
0D9B0ZX
0D9B0ZZ
0D9B30Z
0D9B3ZX
0D9B3ZZ
0D9B40Z
0D9B4ZX
0D9B4ZZ
0D9B70Z
0D9B7ZX
0D9B7ZZ
0D9B80Z
0D9B8ZX
0D9B8ZZ
0D9C00Z
0D9C0ZX
0D9C0ZZ
0D9C30Z
0D9C3ZX
0D9C3ZZ
0D9C40Z
0D9C4ZX
0D9C4ZZ
0D9C70Z
0D9C7ZX
0D9C7ZZ
0D9C80Z
0D9C8ZX
0D9C8ZZ
0D9E00Z
0D9E0ZX
0D9E0ZZ
0D9E30Z
0D9E3ZX
0D9E3ZZ
0D9E40Z
0D9E4ZX
0D9E4ZZ
0D9E70Z
0D9E7ZX
0D9E7ZZ
0D9E80Z
0D9E8ZX
0D9E8ZZ
0D9F00Z
0D9F0ZX
0D9F0ZZ
0D9F30Z
0D9F3ZX
0D9F3ZZ
0D9F40Z
0D9F4ZX
0D9F4ZZ
0D9F70Z
0D9F7ZX
0D9F7ZZ
0D9F80Z
0D9F8ZX
0D9F8ZZ
0D9G00Z
0D9G0ZX
0D9G0ZZ
0D9G30Z
0D9G3ZX
0D9G3ZZ
0D9G40Z
0D9G4ZX
0D9G4ZZ
0D9G70Z
0D9G7ZX
0D9G7ZZ
0D9G80Z
0D9G8ZX
0D9G8ZZ
0D9H00Z
0D9H0ZX
0D9H0ZZ
0D9H30Z
0D9H3ZX
0D9H3ZZ
0D9H40Z
0D9H4ZX
0D9H4ZZ
0D9H70Z
0D9H7ZX
0D9H7ZZ
0D9H80Z
0D9H8ZX
0D9H8ZZ
0D9J00Z
0D9J0ZX
0D9J0ZZ
0D9J30Z
0D9J3ZX
0D9J3ZZ
0D9J40Z
0D9J4ZX
0D9J4ZZ
0D9J70Z
0D9J7ZX
0D9J7ZZ
0D9J80Z
0D9J8ZX
0D9J8ZZ
0D9K00Z
0D9K0ZX
0D9K0ZZ
0D9K30Z
0D9K3ZX
0D9K3ZZ
0D9K40Z
0D9K4ZX
0D9K4ZZ
0D9K70Z
0D9K7ZX
0D9K7ZZ
0D9K80Z
0D9K8ZX
0D9K8ZZ
0D9L00Z
0D9L0ZX
0D9L0ZZ
0D9L30Z
0D9L3ZX
0D9L3ZZ
0D9L40Z
0D9L4ZX
0D9L4ZZ
0D9L70Z
0D9L7ZX
0D9L7ZZ
0D9L80Z
0D9L8ZX
0D9L8ZZ
0D9M00Z
0D9M0ZX
0D9M0ZZ
0D9M30Z
0D9M3ZX
0D9M3ZZ
0D9M40Z
0D9M4ZX
0D9M4ZZ
0D9M70Z
0D9M7ZX
0D9M7ZZ
0D9M80Z
0D9M8ZX
0D9M8ZZ
0D9N00Z
0D9N0ZX
0D9N0ZZ
0D9N30Z
0D9N3ZX
0D9N3ZZ
0D9N40Z
0D9N4ZX
0D9N4ZZ
0D9N70Z
0D9N7ZX
0D9N7ZZ
0D9N80Z
0D9N8ZX
0D9N8ZZ
0D9P00Z
0D9P0ZX
0D9P0ZZ
0D9P30Z
0D9P3ZX
0D9P3ZZ
0D9P40Z
0D9P4ZX
0D9P4ZZ
0D9P70Z
0D9P7ZX
0D9P7ZZ
0D9P80Z
0D9P8ZX
0D9P8ZZ
0D9Q00Z
0D9Q0ZX
0D9Q0ZZ
0D9Q30Z
0D9Q3ZX
0D9Q3ZZ
0D9Q40Z
0D9Q4ZX
0D9Q4ZZ
0D9Q70Z
0D9Q7ZX
0D9Q7ZZ
0D9Q80Z
0D9Q8ZX
0D9Q8ZZ
0D9QX0Z
0D9QXZX
0D9QXZZ
0D9R00Z
0D9R0ZX
0D9R0ZZ
0D9R30Z
0D9R3ZX
0D9R3ZZ
0D9R40Z
0D9R4ZX
0D9R4ZZ
0D9U00Z
0D9U0ZX
0D9U0ZZ
0D9U30Z
0D9U3ZX
0D9U3ZZ
0D9U40Z
0D9U4ZX
0D9U4ZZ
0D9V00Z
0D9V0ZX
0D9V0ZZ
0D9V30Z
0D9V3ZX
0D9V3ZZ
0D9V40Z
0D9V4ZX
0D9V4ZZ
0D9W00Z
0D9W0ZX
0D9W30Z
0D9W3ZX
0D9W3ZZ
0D9W40Z
0D9W4ZZ
0DB13ZX
0DB14ZX
0DB14ZZ
0DB17ZX
0DB18ZX
0DB18ZZ
0DB23ZX
0DB24ZX
0DB24ZZ
0DB27ZX
0DB28ZX
0DB28ZZ
0DB33ZX
0DB34ZX
0DB34ZZ
0DB37ZX
0DB38ZX
0DB38ZZ
0DB43ZX
0DB44ZX
0DB47ZX
0DB48ZX
0DB48ZZ
0DB53ZX
0DB54ZX
0DB54ZZ
0DB57ZX
0DB58ZX
0DB58ZZ
0DB63ZX
0DB64ZX
0DB64ZZ
0DB67ZX
0DB68ZX
0DB68ZZ
0DB73ZX
0DB74ZX
0DB74ZZ
0DB77ZX
0DB78ZX
0DB78ZZ
0DB83ZX
0DB84ZX
0DB87ZX
0DB88ZX
0DB93ZX
0DB94ZX
0DB94ZZ
0DB97ZX
0DB98ZX
0DB98ZZ
0DBA3ZX
0DBA4ZX
0DBA7ZX
0DBA8ZX
0DBB3ZX
0DBB4ZX
0DBB7ZX
0DBB8ZX
0DBC3ZX
0DBC4ZX
0DBC7ZX
0DBC8ZX
0DBE3ZX
0DBE4ZX
0DBE7ZX
0DBE8ZX
0DBE8ZZ
0DBF3ZX
0DBF4ZX
0DBF7ZX
0DBF8ZX
0DBF8ZZ
0DBG3ZX
0DBG4ZX
0DBG7ZX
0DBG8ZX
0DBG8ZZ
0DBH3ZX
0DBH4ZX
0DBH7ZX
0DBH8ZX
0DBH8ZZ
0DBK3ZX
0DBK4ZX
0DBK7ZX
0DBK8ZX
0DBK8ZZ
0DBL3ZX
0DBL4ZX
0DBL7ZX
0DBL8ZX
0DBL8ZZ
0DBM0ZX
0DBM0ZZ
0DBM3ZX
0DBM3ZZ
0DBM4ZX
0DBM4ZZ
0DBM7ZX
0DBM7ZZ
0DBM8ZX
0DBM8ZZ
0DBMFZZ
0DBN0ZX
0DBN0ZZ
0DBN3ZX
0DBN3ZZ
0DBN4ZX
0DBN4ZZ
0DBN7ZX
0DBN7ZZ
0DBN8ZX
0DBN8ZZ
0DBNFZZ
0DBP0ZX
0DBP0ZZ
0DBP3ZX
0DBP3ZZ
0DBP4ZX
0DBP4ZZ
0DBP7ZX
0DBP7ZZ
0DBP8ZX
0DBP8ZZ
0DBQ0ZX
0DBQ0ZZ
0DBQ3ZX
0DBQ3ZZ
0DBQ4ZX
0DBQ4ZZ
0DBQ7ZX
0DBQ7ZZ
0DBQ8ZX
0DBQ8ZZ
0DBQXZX
0DBQXZZ
0DBR0ZX
0DBR0ZZ
0DBR3ZX
0DBR3ZZ
0DBR4ZX
0DBR4ZZ
0DBU0ZX
0DBU0ZZ
0DBU3ZX
0DBU3ZZ
0DBU4ZX
0DBU4ZZ
0DBV0ZX
0DBV0ZZ
0DBV3ZX
0DBV3ZZ
0DBV4ZX
0DBV4ZZ
0DBW0ZX
0DBW0ZZ
0DBW3ZX
0DBW3ZZ
0DBW4ZX
0DBW4ZZ
0DC10ZZ
0DC13ZZ
0DC14ZZ
0DC17ZZ
0DC18ZZ
0DC20ZZ
0DC23ZZ
0DC24ZZ
0DC27ZZ
0DC28ZZ
0DC30ZZ
0DC33ZZ
0DC34ZZ
0DC37ZZ
0DC38ZZ
0DC40ZZ
0DC43ZZ
0DC44ZZ
0DC47ZZ
0DC48ZZ
0DC50ZZ
0DC53ZZ
0DC54ZZ
0DC57ZZ
0DC58ZZ
0DC60ZZ
0DC63ZZ
0DC64ZZ
0DC67ZZ
0DC68ZZ
0DC70ZZ
0DC73ZZ
0DC74ZZ
0DC77ZZ
0DC78ZZ
0DC80ZZ
0DC83ZZ
0DC84ZZ
0DC87ZZ
0DC88ZZ
0DC90ZZ
0DC93ZZ
0DC94ZZ
0DC97ZZ
0DC98ZZ
0DCA0ZZ
0DCA3ZZ
0DCA4ZZ
0DCA7ZZ
0DCA8ZZ
0DCB0ZZ
0DCB3ZZ
0DCB4ZZ
0DCB7ZZ
0DCB8ZZ
0DCC0ZZ
0DCC3ZZ
0DCC4ZZ
0DCC7ZZ
0DCC8ZZ
0DCE0ZZ
0DCE3ZZ
0DCE4ZZ
0DCE7ZZ
0DCE8ZZ
0DCF0ZZ
0DCF3ZZ
0DCF4ZZ
0DCF7ZZ
0DCF8ZZ
0DCG0ZZ
0DCG3ZZ
0DCG4ZZ
0DCG7ZZ
0DCG8ZZ
0DCH0ZZ
0DCH3ZZ
0DCH4ZZ
0DCH7ZZ
0DCH8ZZ
0DCJ0ZZ
0DCJ3ZZ
0DCJ4ZZ
0DCJ7ZZ
0DCJ8ZZ
0DCK0ZZ
0DCK3ZZ
0DCK4ZZ
0DCK7ZZ
0DCK8ZZ
0DCL0ZZ
0DCL3ZZ
0DCL4ZZ
0DCL7ZZ
0DCL8ZZ

0DCM0ZZ
0DCM3ZZ
0DCM4ZZ
0DCM7ZZ
0DCM8ZZ
0DCN0ZZ
0DCN3ZZ
0DCN4ZZ
0DCN7ZZ
0DCN8ZZ
0DCP0ZZ
0DCP3ZZ
0DCP4ZZ
0DCP7ZZ
0DCP8ZZ
0DCQ0ZZ
0DCQ3ZZ
0DCQ4ZZ
0DCQ7ZZ
0DCQ8ZZ
0DCQXZZ
0DCR0ZZ
0DCR3ZZ
0DCR4ZZ
0DCU0ZZ
0DCU3ZZ
0DCU4ZZ
0DCV0ZZ
0DCV3ZZ
0DCV4ZZ
0DCW0ZZ
0DCW3ZZ
0DCW4ZZ
0DD13ZX
0DD14ZX
0DD18ZX
0DD23ZX
0DD24ZX
0DD28ZX
0DD33ZX
0DD34ZX
0DD38ZX
0DD43ZX
0DD44ZX
0DD48ZX
0DD53ZX
0DD54ZX
0DD58ZX
0DD63ZX
0DD64ZX
0DD68ZX
0DD73ZX
0DD74ZX
0DD78ZX
0DD83ZX
0DD84ZX
0DD88ZX
0DD93ZX
0DD94ZX
0DD98ZX
0DDA3ZX
0DDA4ZX
0DDA8ZX
0DDB3ZX
0DDB4ZX
0DDB8ZX
0DDC3ZX
0DDC4ZX
0DDC8ZX
0DDE3ZX
0DDE4ZX
0DDE8ZX
0DDF3ZX
0DDF4ZX
0DDF8ZX
0DDG3ZX
0DDG4ZX
0DDG8ZX
0DDH3ZX
0DDH4ZX
0DDH8ZX
0DDJ3ZX
0DDJ4ZX
0DDJ8ZX
0DDK3ZX
0DDK4ZX
0DDK8ZX
0DDL3ZX
0DDL4ZX
0DDL8ZX
0DDM3ZX
0DDM4ZX
0DDM8ZX
0DDN3ZX
0DDN4ZX
0DDN8ZX
0DDP3ZX
0DDP4ZX
0DDP8ZX
0DDQ3ZX
0DDQ4ZX
0DDQ8ZX
0DDQXZX
0DF50ZZ
0DF53ZZ
0DF54ZZ
0DF57ZZ
0DF58ZZ
0DF5XZZ
0DF60ZZ
0DF63ZZ
0DF64ZZ
0DF67ZZ
0DF68ZZ
0DF6XZZ
0DF80ZZ
0DF83ZZ
0DF84ZZ
0DF87ZZ
0DF88ZZ
0DF8XZZ
0DF90ZZ
0DF93ZZ
0DF94ZZ
0DF97ZZ
0DF98ZZ
0DF9XZZ
0DFA0ZZ
0DFA3ZZ
0DFA4ZZ
0DFA7ZZ
0DFA8ZZ
0DFAXZZ
0DFB0ZZ
0DFB3ZZ
0DFB4ZZ
0DFB7ZZ
0DFB8ZZ
0DFBXZZ
0DFE0ZZ
0DFE3ZZ
0DFE4ZZ
0DFE7ZZ
0DFE8ZZ
0DFEXZZ
0DFF0ZZ
0DFF3ZZ
0DFF4ZZ
0DFF7ZZ
0DFF8ZZ
0DFFXZZ
0DFG0ZZ
0DFG3ZZ
0DFG4ZZ
0DFG7ZZ
0DFG8ZZ
0DFGXZZ
0DFH0ZZ
0DFH3ZZ
0DFH4ZZ
0DFH7ZZ
0DFH8ZZ
0DFHXZZ
0DFJ0ZZ
0DFJ3ZZ
0DFJ4ZZ
0DFJ7ZZ
0DFJ8ZZ
0DFJXZZ
0DFK0ZZ
0DFK3ZZ
0DFK4ZZ
0DFK7ZZ
0DFK8ZZ
0DFKXZZ
0DFL0ZZ
0DFL3ZZ
0DFL4ZZ
0DFL7ZZ
0DFL8ZZ
0DFLXZZ
0DFM0ZZ
0DFM3ZZ
0DFM4ZZ
0DFM7ZZ
0DFM8ZZ
0DFMXZZ
0DFN0ZZ
0DFN3ZZ
0DFN4ZZ
0DFN7ZZ
0DFN8ZZ
0DFNXZZ
0DFP0ZZ
0DFP3ZZ
0DFP4ZZ
0DFP7ZZ
0DFP8ZZ
0DFPXZZ
0DFQ0ZZ
0DFQ3ZZ
0DFQ4ZZ
0DFQ7ZZ
0DFQ8ZZ
0DFQXZZ
0DH00YZ
0DH03YZ
0DH04YZ
0DH07YZ
0DH08YZ
0DH501Z
0DH502Z
0DH503Z
0DH50DZ
0DH50UZ
0DH50YZ
0DH531Z
0DH532Z
0DH533Z
0DH53DZ
0DH53UZ
0DH53YZ
0DH541Z
0DH542Z
0DH543Z
0DH54DZ
0DH54UZ
0DH54YZ
0DH571Z
0DH572Z
0DH573Z
0DH57BZ
0DH57DZ
0DH57UZ
0DH57YZ
0DH581Z
0DH582Z
0DH583Z
0DH58BZ
0DH58DZ
0DH58UZ
0DH58YZ
0DH602Z
0DH603Z
0DH60DZ
0DH60MZ
0DH60UZ
0DH60YZ
0DH632Z
0DH633Z
0DH63DZ
0DH63MZ
0DH63UZ
0DH63YZ
0DH642Z
0DH643Z
0DH64DZ
0DH64MZ
0DH64UZ
0DH64YZ
0DH672Z
0DH673Z
0DH67DZ
0DH67UZ
0DH67YZ
0DH682Z
0DH683Z
0DH68DZ
0DH68UZ
0DH68YZ
0DH802Z
0DH803Z
0DH80DZ
0DH80UZ
0DH832Z
0DH833Z
0DH83DZ
0DH83UZ
0DH842Z
0DH843Z
0DH84DZ
0DH84UZ
0DH872Z
0DH873Z
0DH87DZ
0DH87UZ
0DH882Z
0DH883Z
0DH88DZ
0DH88UZ
0DH902Z
0DH903Z
0DH90DZ
0DH90UZ
0DH932Z
0DH933Z
0DH93DZ
0DH93UZ
0DH942Z
0DH943Z
0DH94DZ
0DH94UZ
0DH972Z
0DH973Z
0DH97DZ
0DH97UZ
0DH982Z
0DH983Z
0DH98DZ
0DH98UZ
0DHA02Z
0DHA03Z
0DHA0DZ
0DHA0UZ
0DHA32Z
0DHA33Z
0DHA3DZ
0DHA3UZ
0DHA42Z
0DHA43Z
0DHA4DZ
0DHA4UZ
0DHA72Z
0DHA73Z
0DHA7DZ
0DHA7UZ
0DHA82Z
0DHA83Z
0DHA8DZ
0DHA8UZ
0DHB02Z
0DHB03Z
0DHB0DZ
0DHB0UZ
0DHB32Z
0DHB33Z
0DHB3DZ
0DHB3UZ
0DHB42Z
0DHB43Z
0DHB4DZ
0DHB4UZ
0DHB72Z
0DHB73Z
0DHB7DZ
0DHB7UZ
0DHB82Z
0DHB83Z
0DHB8DZ
0DHB8UZ
0DHD0YZ
0DHD3YZ
0DHD4YZ
0DHD7YZ
0DHD8YZ
0DHE0DZ
0DHE3DZ
0DHE4DZ
0DHE7DZ
0DHE8DZ
0DHP01Z
0DHP0DZ
0DHP31Z
0DHP3DZ
0DHP41Z
0DHP4DZ
0DHP71Z
0DHP7DZ
0DHP81Z
0DHP8DZ
0DHQ0DZ
0DHQ0LZ
0DHQ3DZ
0DHQ3LZ
0DHQ4DZ
0DHQ4LZ
0DHQ7DZ
0DHQ8DZ
0DHR0MZ
0DHR3MZ
0DHR4MZ
0DJ00ZZ
0DJ03ZZ
0DJ04ZZ
0DJ07ZZ
0DJ08ZZ
0DJ0XZZ
0DJ60ZZ
0DJ63ZZ
0DJ64ZZ
0DJ67ZZ
0DJ68ZZ
0DJ6XZZ
0DJD0ZZ
0DJD3ZZ
0DJD4ZZ
0DJD7ZZ
0DJD8ZZ
0DJDXZZ
0DJU3ZZ
0DJUXZZ
0DJV3ZZ
0DJVXZZ
0DJW3ZZ
0DJWXZZ
0DL10CZ
0DL10DZ
0DL10ZZ
0DL13CZ
0DL13DZ
0DL13ZZ
0DL14CZ
0DL14DZ
0DL14ZZ
0DL17DZ
0DL17ZZ
0DL18DZ
0DL18ZZ
0DL20CZ
0DL20DZ
0DL20ZZ
0DL23CZ
0DL23DZ
0DL23ZZ
0DL24CZ
0DL24DZ
0DL24ZZ
0DL27DZ
0DL27ZZ
0DL28DZ
0DL28ZZ
0DL30CZ
0DL30DZ
0DL30ZZ
0DL33CZ
0DL33DZ
0DL33ZZ
0DL34CZ
0DL34DZ
0DL34ZZ
0DL37DZ
0DL37ZZ
0DL38DZ
0DL38ZZ
0DL40CZ
0DL40DZ
0DL40ZZ
0DL43CZ
0DL43DZ
0DL43ZZ
0DL44CZ
0DL44DZ
0DL44ZZ
0DL47DZ
0DL47ZZ
0DL48DZ
0DL48ZZ
0DL50CZ
0DL50DZ
0DL50ZZ
0DL53CZ
0DL53DZ
0DL53ZZ
0DL54CZ
0DL54DZ
0DL54ZZ
0DL57DZ
0DL57ZZ
0DL58DZ
0DL58ZZ
0DLQ4CZ
0DLQ4DZ
0DLQ4ZZ
0DLQ7DZ
0DLQ7ZZ
0DLQ8DZ
0DLQ8ZZ
0DLQXCZ
0DLQXDZ
0DLQXZZ
0DM50ZZ
0DM54ZZ
0DM60ZZ
0DM64ZZ
0DM80ZZ
0DM84ZZ
0DM90ZZ
0DM94ZZ
0DMA0ZZ
0DMA4ZZ
0DMB0ZZ
0DMB4ZZ
0DME0ZZ
0DME4ZZ
0DMF0ZZ
0DMF4ZZ
0DMG0ZZ
0DMG4ZZ
0DMH0ZZ
0DMH4ZZ
0DMK0ZZ
0DMK4ZZ
0DML0ZZ
0DML4ZZ
0DMM0ZZ
0DMM4ZZ
0DMN0ZZ
0DMN4ZZ
0DMP0ZZ
0DMP4ZZ
0DN10ZZ
0DN13ZZ
0DN14ZZ
0DN17ZZ
0DN18ZZ
0DN20ZZ
0DN23ZZ
0DN24ZZ
0DN27ZZ
0DN28ZZ
0DN30ZZ
0DN33ZZ
0DN34ZZ
0DN37ZZ
0DN38ZZ
0DN40ZZ
0DN43ZZ
0DN44ZZ
0DN47ZZ
0DN48ZZ
0DN50ZZ
0DN53ZZ
0DN54ZZ
0DN57ZZ
0DN58ZZ
0DN60ZZ
0DN63ZZ
0DN64ZZ
0DN67ZZ
0DN68ZZ
0DN70ZZ
0DN73ZZ
0DN74ZZ
0DN77ZZ
0DN78ZZ
0DN80ZZ
0DN83ZZ
0DN84ZZ
0DN87ZZ
0DN88ZZ
0DN90ZZ
0DN93ZZ
0DN94ZZ
0DN97ZZ
0DN98ZZ
0DNA0ZZ
0DNA3ZZ
0DNA4ZZ
0DNA7ZZ
0DNA8ZZ
0DNB0ZZ
0DNB3ZZ
0DNB4ZZ
0DNB7ZZ
0DNB8ZZ
0DNC0ZZ
0DNC3ZZ
0DNC4ZZ
0DNC7ZZ
0DNC8ZZ
0DNE0ZZ
0DNE3ZZ
0DNE4ZZ
0DNE7ZZ
0DNE8ZZ
0DNF0ZZ
0DNF3ZZ
0DNF4ZZ
0DNF7ZZ
0DNF8ZZ
0DNG0ZZ
0DNG3ZZ
0DNG4ZZ
0DNG7ZZ
0DNG8ZZ
0DNH0ZZ
0DNH3ZZ
0DNH4ZZ
0DNH7ZZ
0DNH8ZZ
0DNJ0ZZ
0DNJ3ZZ
0DNJ4ZZ
0DNJ7ZZ
0DNJ8ZZ
0DNK0ZZ
0DNK3ZZ
0DNK4ZZ
0DNK7ZZ
0DNK8ZZ
0DNL0ZZ
0DNL3ZZ
0DNL4ZZ
0DNL7ZZ
0DNL8ZZ
0DNM0ZZ
0DNM3ZZ
0DNM4ZZ
0DNM7ZZ
0DNM8ZZ
0DNN0ZZ
0DNN3ZZ
0DNN4ZZ
0DNN7ZZ
0DNN8ZZ
0DNP0ZZ
0DNP3ZZ
0DNP4ZZ
0DNP7ZZ
0DNP8ZZ
0DNQ0ZZ
0DNQ3ZZ
0DNQ4ZZ
0DNQ7ZZ
0DNQ8ZZ
0DNQXZZ
0DNR0ZZ
0DNR3ZZ
0DNR4ZZ
0DNU0ZZ
0DNU3ZZ
0DNU4ZZ
0DNV0ZZ
0DNV3ZZ
0DNV4ZZ
0DNW0ZZ
0DNW3ZZ
0DNW4ZZ
0DP000Z
0DP002Z
0DP003Z
0DP007Z
0DP00CZ
0DP00DZ
0DP00JZ
0DP00KZ
0DP00UZ
0DP00YZ
0DP030Z
0DP032Z
0DP033Z
0DP037Z
0DP03CZ
0DP03DZ
0DP03JZ
0DP03KZ
0DP03UZ
0DP03YZ
0DP040Z
0DP042Z
0DP043Z
0DP047Z
0DP04CZ
0DP04DZ
0DP04JZ
0DP04KZ
0DP04UZ
0DP04YZ
0DP070Z
0DP072Z
0DP073Z
0DP077Z
0DP07CZ
0DP07DZ
0DP07JZ
0DP07KZ
0DP07UZ
0DP07YZ
0DP080Z
0DP082Z
0DP083Z
0DP087Z
0DP08CZ
0DP08DZ
0DP08JZ
0DP08KZ
0DP08UZ
0DP08YZ
0DP0X0Z
0DP0X2Z
0DP0X3Z
0DP0XDZ
0DP0XUZ
0DP501Z
0DP502Z
0DP503Z
0DP50UZ
0DP50YZ
0DP531Z
0DP532Z
0DP533Z
0DP53UZ
0DP53YZ
0DP541Z
0DP542Z
0DP543Z
0DP54UZ
0DP54YZ
0DP571Z
0DP57DZ
0DP57YZ
0DP581Z
0DP58DZ
0DP58YZ
0DP5X1Z
0DP5X2Z
0DP5X3Z
0DP5XDZ
0DP5XUZ
0DP600Z
0DP602Z
0DP603Z
0DP607Z
0DP60CZ
0DP60DZ
0DP60JZ

0DP60KZ
0DP60MZ
0DP60UZ
0DP60YZ
0DP630Z
0DP632Z
0DP633Z
0DP637Z
0DP63CZ
0DP63DZ
0DP63JZ
0DP63KZ
0DP63MZ
0DP63UZ
0DP63YZ
0DP640Z
0DP642Z
0DP643Z
0DP647Z
0DP64CZ
0DP64DZ
0DP64JZ
0DP64KZ
0DP64MZ
0DP64UZ
0DP64YZ
0DP670Z
0DP672Z
0DP673Z
0DP677Z
0DP67CZ
0DP67DZ
0DP67JZ
0DP67KZ
0DP67UZ
0DP67YZ
0DP680Z
0DP682Z
0DP683Z
0DP687Z
0DP68CZ
0DP68DZ
0DP68JZ
0DP68KZ
0DP68UZ
0DP68YZ
0DP6X0Z
0DP6X2Z
0DP6X3Z
0DP6XDZ
0DP6XUZ
0DPD00Z
0DPD02Z
0DPD03Z
0DPD07Z
0DPD0CZ
0DPD0DZ
0DPD0JZ
0DPD0KZ
0DPD0UZ
0DPD0YZ
0DPD30Z
0DPD32Z
0DPD33Z
0DPD37Z
0DPD3CZ
0DPD3DZ
0DPD3JZ
0DPD3KZ
0DPD3UZ
0DPD3YZ
0DPD40Z
0DPD42Z
0DPD43Z
0DPD47Z
0DPD4CZ
0DPD4DZ
0DPD4JZ
0DPD4KZ
0DPD4UZ
0DPD4YZ
0DPD70Z
0DPD72Z
0DPD73Z
0DPD77Z
0DPD7CZ
0DPD7DZ
0DPD7JZ
0DPD7UZ
0DPD7YZ
0DPD80Z
0DPD82Z
0DPD83Z
0DPD8DZ
0DPD8UZ
0DPD8YZ
0DPDX0Z
0DPDX2Z
0DPDX3Z
0DPDXDZ
0DPDXUZ
0DPP71Z
0DPP81Z
0DPPX1Z
0DQ80ZZ
0DQ90ZZ
0DQA0ZZ
0DQB0ZZ
0DQE0ZZ
0DQF0ZZ
0DQG0ZZ
0DQH0ZZ
0DQK0ZZ
0DQL0ZZ
0DQM0ZZ
0DQN0ZZ
0DQP0ZZ
0DQP3ZZ
0DQP4ZZ
0DQP7ZZ
0DQP8ZZ
0DQQ0ZZ
0DQQ3ZZ
0DQQ4ZZ
0DQQ7ZZ
0DQQ8ZZ
0DQQXZZ
0DQR0ZZ
0DQR3ZZ
0DQR4ZZ
0DQU0ZZ
0DQU3ZZ
0DQU4ZZ
0DQV0ZZ
0DQV3ZZ
0DQV4ZZ
0DQW0ZZ
0DQW3ZZ
0DQW4ZZ
0DR507Z
0DR50JZ
0DR50KZ
0DR547Z
0DR54JZ
0DR54KZ
0DR577Z
0DR57JZ
0DR57KZ
0DR587Z
0DR58JZ
0DR58KZ
0DRR07Z
0DRR0JZ
0DRR0KZ
0DRR47Z
0DRR4JZ
0DRR4KZ
0DRU07Z
0DRU0JZ
0DRU0KZ
0DRU47Z
0DRU4JZ
0DRU4KZ
0DRV07Z
0DRV0JZ
0DRV0KZ
0DRV47Z
0DRV4JZ
0DRV4KZ
0DRW07Z
0DRW0JZ
0DRW0KZ
0DRW47Z
0DRW4JZ
0DRW4KZ
0DS50ZZ
0DS54ZZ
0DS57ZZ
0DS58ZZ
0DS5XZZ
0DS60ZZ
0DS64ZZ
0DS67ZZ
0DS68ZZ
0DS6XZZ
0DS80ZZ
0DS84ZZ
0DS87ZZ
0DS88ZZ
0DS90ZZ
0DS94ZZ
0DS97ZZ
0DS98ZZ
0DS9XZZ
0DSA0ZZ
0DSA4ZZ
0DSA7ZZ
0DSA8ZZ
0DSAXZZ
0DSB0ZZ
0DSB4ZZ
0DSB7ZZ
0DSB8ZZ
0DSBXZZ
0DSE0ZZ
0DSE4ZZ
0DSE7ZZ
0DSE8ZZ
0DSH0ZZ
0DSH4ZZ
0DSH7ZZ
0DSH8ZZ
0DSHXZZ
0DSK0ZZ
0DSK4ZZ
0DSK7ZZ
0DSK8ZZ
0DSKXZZ
0DSL0ZZ
0DSL4ZZ
0DSL7ZZ
0DSL8ZZ
0DSLXZZ
0DSM0ZZ
0DSM4ZZ
0DSM7ZZ
0DSM8ZZ
0DSMXZZ
0DSN0ZZ
0DSN4ZZ
0DSN7ZZ
0DSN8ZZ
0DSNXZZ
0DSP0ZZ
0DSP4ZZ
0DSP7ZZ
0DSP8ZZ
0DSPXZZ
0DSQ0ZZ
0DSQ4ZZ
0DSQ7ZZ
0DSQ8ZZ
0DSQXZZ
0DT10ZZ
0DT14ZZ
0DT17ZZ
0DT18ZZ
0DT20ZZ
0DT24ZZ
0DT27ZZ
0DT28ZZ
0DT30ZZ
0DT34ZZ
0DT37ZZ
0DT38ZZ
0DT40ZZ
0DT44ZZ
0DT47ZZ
0DT48ZZ
0DT50ZZ
0DT54ZZ
0DT57ZZ
0DT58ZZ
0DT60ZZ
0DT64ZZ
0DT67ZZ
0DT68ZZ
0DT70ZZ
0DT74ZZ
0DT77ZZ
0DT78ZZ
0DT80ZZ
0DT84ZZ
0DT87ZZ
0DT88ZZ
0DT90ZZ
0DT94ZZ
0DT97ZZ
0DT98ZZ
0DTA0ZZ
0DTA4ZZ
0DTA7ZZ
0DTA8ZZ
0DTB0ZZ
0DTB4ZZ
0DTB7ZZ
0DTB8ZZ
0DTC0ZZ
0DTC4ZZ
0DTC7ZZ
0DTC8ZZ
0DTE0ZZ
0DTE4ZZ
0DTE7ZZ
0DTE8ZZ
0DTF0ZZ
0DTF4ZZ
0DTF7ZZ
0DU377Z
0DU37JZ
0DU37KZ
0DU387Z
0DU38JZ
0DU38KZ
0DU407Z
0DU40JZ
0DU40KZ
0DU447Z
0DU44JZ
0DU44KZ
0DU477Z
0DU47JZ
0DU47KZ
0DU487Z
0DU48JZ
0DU48KZ
0DU507Z
0DU50JZ
0DU50KZ
0DU547Z
0DU54JZ
0DU54KZ
0DU577Z
0DU57JZ
0DU57KZ
0DU587Z
0DU58JZ
0DU58KZ
0DU607Z
0DU60JZ
0DU60KZ
0DU647Z
0DU64JZ
0DU64KZ
0DU677Z
0DU67JZ
0DU67KZ
0DU687Z
0DU68JZ
0DU68KZ
0DU707Z
0DU70JZ
0DU70KZ
0DU747Z
0DU74JZ
0DU74KZ
0DU777Z
0DU77JZ
0DU77KZ
0DU787Z
0DU78JZ
0DU78KZ
0DU807Z
0DU80JZ
0DU80KZ
0DU847Z
0DU84JZ
0DU84KZ
0DU877Z
0DU87JZ
0DU87KZ
0DU887Z
0DU88JZ
0DU88KZ
0DU907Z
0DU90JZ
0DU90KZ
0DU947Z
0DU94JZ
0DU94KZ
0DU977Z
0DU97JZ
0DU97KZ
0DU987Z
0DU98JZ
0DU98KZ
0DUA07Z
0DUA0JZ
0DUA0KZ
0DUA47Z
0DUA4JZ
0DUA4KZ
0DUA77Z
0DUA7JZ
0DUA7KZ
0DUA87Z
0DUA8JZ
0DUA8KZ
0DUB07Z
0DUB0JZ
0DUB0KZ
0DUB47Z
0DUB4JZ
0DUB4KZ
0DUB77Z
0DUB7JZ
0DUB7KZ
0DUB87Z
0DUB8JZ
0DUB8KZ
0DUC07Z
0DUC0JZ
0DUC0KZ
0DUC47Z
0DUC4JZ
0DUC4KZ
0DUC77Z
0DUC7JZ
0DUC7KZ
0DUC87Z
0DUC8JZ
0DUC8KZ
0DUE07Z
0DUE0JZ
0DUE0KZ
0DUE47Z
0DUE4JZ
0DUE4KZ
0DUE77Z
0DUE7JZ
0DUE7KZ
0DUE87Z
0DUE8JZ
0DUE8KZ
0DUF07Z
0DUF0JZ
0DUF0KZ
0DUF47Z
0DUF4JZ
0DUF4KZ
0DUF77Z
0DUF7JZ
0DUF7KZ
0DUF87Z
0DUF8JZ
0DUF8KZ
0DUG07Z
0DUG0JZ
0DUG0KZ
0DUG47Z
0DUG4JZ
0DUG4KZ
0DUG77Z
0DUG7JZ
0DUG7KZ
0DUG87Z
0DUG8JZ
0DUG8KZ
0DUH07Z
0DUH0JZ
0DUH0KZ
0DUH47Z
0DUH4JZ
0DUH4KZ
0DUH77Z
0DUH7JZ
0DUH7KZ
0DUH87Z
0DUH8JZ
0DUH8KZ
0DUK07Z
0DUK0JZ
0DUK0KZ
0DUK47Z
0DUK4JZ
0DUK4KZ
0DUK77Z
0DUK7JZ
0DUK7KZ
0DUK87Z
0DUK8JZ
0DUK8KZ
0DUL07Z
0DUL0JZ
0DUL0KZ
0DUL47Z
0DUL4JZ
0DUL4KZ
0DUL77Z
0DUL7JZ
0DUL7KZ
0DUL87Z
0DUL8JZ
0DUL8KZ
0DUM07Z
0DUM0JZ
0DUM0KZ
0DUM47Z
0DUM4JZ
0DUM4KZ
0DUM77Z
0DUM7JZ
0DUM7KZ
0DUM87Z
0DUM8JZ
0DUM8KZ
0DUN07Z
0DUN0JZ
0DUN0KZ
0DUN47Z
0DUN4JZ
0DUN4KZ
0DUN77Z
0DUN7JZ
0DUN7KZ
0DUN87Z
0DUN8JZ
0DUN8KZ
0DUP07Z
0DUP0JZ
0DUP0KZ
0DUP47Z
0DUP4JZ
0DUP4KZ
0DUP77Z
0DUP7JZ
0DUP7KZ
0DUP87Z
0DUP8JZ
0DUP8KZ
0DUQ07Z
0DUQ0JZ
0DUQ0KZ
0DUQ47Z
0DUQ4JZ
0DUQ4KZ
0DUQ77Z
0DUQ7JZ
0DUQ7KZ
0DUQ87Z
0DUQ8JZ
0DUQ8KZ
0DUQX7Z
0DUQXJZ
0DUQXKZ
0DUR07Z
0DUR0JZ
0DUR0KZ
0DUR47Z
0DUR4JZ
0DUR4KZ
0DUU07Z
0DUU0JZ
0DUU0KZ
0DUU47Z
0DUU4JZ
0DUU4KZ
0DUV07Z
0DUV0JZ
0DUV0KZ
0DUV47Z
0DUV4JZ
0DUV4KZ
0DUW07Z
0DUW0JZ
0DUW0KZ
0DUW47Z
0DUW4JZ
0DUW4KZ
0DV10CZ
0DV10DZ
0DV10ZZ
0DV13CZ
0DV13DZ
0DV13ZZ
0DV14CZ
0DV14DZ
0DV14ZZ
0DV17DZ
0DV17ZZ
0DV18DZ
0DV18ZZ
0DV20CZ
0DV20DZ
0DV20ZZ
0DV23CZ
0DV23DZ
0DV23ZZ
0DV24CZ
0DV24DZ
0DV24ZZ
0DV27DZ
0DV27ZZ
0DV28DZ
0DV28ZZ
0DV30CZ
0DV30DZ
0DV30ZZ
0DV33CZ
0DV33DZ
0DV67DZ
0DV68DZ
0DVL0ZZ
0DVL3CZ
0DVL3DZ
0DVL3ZZ
0DVL4CZ
0DVL4DZ
0DVL4ZZ
0DVL7DZ
0DVL7ZZ
0DVL8DZ
0DVL8ZZ
0DVM0CZ
0DVM0DZ
0DVM0ZZ
0DVM3CZ
0DVM3DZ
0DVM3ZZ
0DVM4CZ
0DVM4DZ
0DVM4ZZ
0DVM7DZ
0DVM7ZZ
0DVM8DZ
0DVM8ZZ
0DVN0CZ
0DVN0DZ
0DVN0ZZ
0DVN3CZ
0DVN3DZ
0DVN3ZZ
0DVN4CZ
0DVN4DZ
0DVN4ZZ
0DVN7DZ
0DVN7ZZ
0DVN8DZ
0DVN8ZZ
0DVP0CZ
0DVP0DZ
0DVP0ZZ
0DVP3CZ
0DVP3DZ
0DVP3ZZ
0DVP4CZ
0DVP4DZ
0DVP4ZZ
0DVP7DZ
0DVP7ZZ
0DVP8DZ
0DVP8ZZ
0DVQ0CZ
0DVQ0DZ
0DVQ0ZZ
0DVQ3CZ
0DVQ3DZ
0DVQ3ZZ
0DVQ4CZ
0DVQ4DZ
0DVQ4ZZ
0DVQ7DZ
0DVQ7ZZ
0DVQ8DZ
0DVQ8ZZ
0DVQXCZ
0DVQXDZ
0DVQXZZ
0DW000Z
0DW002Z
0DW003Z
0DW007Z
0DW00CZ
0DW00DZ
0DW00JZ
0DW00KZ
0DW00UZ
0DW00YZ
0DW030Z
0DW032Z
0DW033Z
0DW037Z
0DW03CZ
0DW03DZ
0DW03JZ
0DW03KZ
0DW03UZ
0DW03YZ
0DW040Z
0DW042Z
0DW043Z
0DW047Z
0DW04CZ
0DW04DZ
0DW04JZ
0DW04KZ
0DW04UZ
0DW04YZ
0DW070Z
0DW072Z
0DW073Z
0DW077Z
0DW07CZ
0DW07DZ
0DW07JZ
0DW07KZ
0DW07UZ
0DW07YZ
0DW080Z
0DW082Z
0DW083Z
0DW087Z
0DW08CZ
0DW08DZ
0DW08JZ
0DW08KZ
0DW08UZ
0DW08YZ
0DW0X0Z
0DW0X2Z
0DW0X3Z
0DW0X7Z
0DW0XCZ
0DW0XDZ
0DW0XJZ
0DW0XKZ
0DW0XUZ
0DW50YZ
0DW53YZ
0DW54YZ
0DW57DZ
0DW57YZ
0DW58DZ
0DW58YZ
0DW5XDZ
0DW600Z

0DW602Z
0DW603Z
0DW607Z
0DW60CZ
0DW60DZ
0DW60JZ
0DW60KZ
0DW60MZ
0DW60UZ
0DW60YZ
0DW630Z
0DW632Z
0DW633Z
0DW637Z
0DW63CZ
0DW63DZ
0DW63JZ
0DW63KZ
0DW63MZ
0DW63UZ
0DW63YZ
0DW640Z
0DW642Z
0DW643Z
0DW647Z
0DW64CZ
0DW64DZ
0DW64JZ
0DW64KZ
0DW64MZ
0DW64UZ
0DW64YZ
0DW670Z
0DW672Z
0DW673Z
0DW677Z
0DW67CZ
0DW67DZ
0DW67JZ
0DW67KZ
0DW67UZ
0DW67YZ
0DW680Z
0DW682Z
0DW683Z
0DW687Z
0DW68CZ
0DW68DZ
0DW68JZ
0DW68KZ
0DW68UZ
0DW68YZ
0DW6X0Z
0DW6X2Z
0DW6X3Z
0DW6X7Z
0DW6XCZ
0DW6XDZ
0DW6XJZ
0DW6XKZ
0DW6XUZ
0DW807Z
0DW80JZ
0DW80KZ
0DW847Z
0DW84JZ
0DW84KZ
0DW877Z
0DW87JZ
0DW87KZ
0DW887Z
0DW88JZ
0DW88KZ
0DWD00Z
0DWD02Z
0DWD03Z
0DWD07Z
0DWD0CZ
0DWD0DZ
0DWD0JZ
0DWD0KZ
0DWD0UZ
0DWD0YZ
0DWD30Z
0DWD32Z
0DWD33Z
0DWD37Z
0DWD3CZ
0DWD3DZ
0DWD3JZ
0DWD3KZ
0DWD3UZ
0DWD3YZ
0DWD40Z
0DWD42Z
0DWD43Z
0DWD47Z
0DWD4CZ
0DWD4DZ
0DWD4JZ
0DWD4KZ
0DWD4UZ
0DWD4YZ
0DWD70Z
0DWD72Z
0DWD73Z
0DWD77Z
0DWD7CZ
0DWD7DZ
0DWD7JZ
0DWD7KZ
0DWD7UZ
0DWD7YZ
0DWD80Z
0DWD82Z
0DWD83Z
0DWD87Z
0DWD8CZ
0DWD8DZ
0DWD8JZ
0DWD8KZ
0DWD8UZ
0DWD8YZ
0DWDX0Z
0DWDX2Z
0DWDX3Z
0DWDX7Z
0DWDXCZ
0DWDXDZ
0DWDXJZ
0DWDXKZ
0DWDXUZ
0DWE07Z
0DWE0JZ
0DWE0KZ
0DWE47Z
0DWE4JZ
0DWE4KZ
0DWE77Z
0DWE7JZ
0DWE7KZ
0DWE87Z
0DWE8JZ
0DWE8KZ
0DWQ0LZ
0DWQ3LZ
0DWQ4LZ
0DWQ7LZ
0DWQ8LZ
0DWR0MZ
0DWR3MZ
0DWR4MZ
0DWU00Z
0DWU07Z
0DWU0JZ
0DWU0KZ
0DWU30Z
0DWU37Z
0DWU3JZ
0DWU3KZ
0DWU40Z
0DWU47Z
0DWU4JZ
0DWU4KZ
0DWV00Z
0DWV07Z
0DWV0JZ
0DWV0KZ
0DWV30Z
0DWV37Z
0DWV3JZ
0DWV3KZ
0DWV40Z
0DWV47Z
0DWV4JZ
0DWV4KZ
0DWW00Z
0DWW07Z
0DWW0JZ
0DWW0KZ
0DWW30Z
0DWW37Z
0DWW3JZ
0DWW3KZ
0DWW40Z
0DWW47Z
0DWW4JZ
0DWW4KZ
0DX60Z5
0DX64Z5
0DX80Z5
0DX84Z5
0DXE0Z5
0DXE4Z5
0DY50Z0
0DY50Z1
0DY50Z2
0DY60Z0
0DY60Z1
0DY60Z2
0DY80Z0
0DY80Z1
0DY80Z2
0DYE0Z0
0DYE0Z1
0DYE0Z2
0F140D3
0F140D4
0F140D5
0F140D6
0F140D7
0F140D8
0F140D9
0F140DB
0F140Z3
0F140Z4
0F140Z5
0F140Z6
0F140Z7
0F140Z8
0F140Z9
0F140ZB
0F144D3
0F144D4
0F144D5
0F144D6
0F144D7
0F144D8
0F144D9
0F144DB
0F144Z3
0F144Z4
0F144Z5
0F144Z6
0F144Z7
0F144Z8
0F144Z9
0F144ZB
0F170Z6
0F170Z7
0F170Z8
0F170Z9
0F170ZB
0F174D3
0F174D4
0F174D5
0F174D6
0F174D7
0F174D8
0F174D9
0F174DB
0F174Z3
0F174Z4
0F174Z5
0F174Z6
0F174Z7
0F174Z8
0F174Z9
0F174ZB
0F180D3
0F180D4
0F180D5
0F180D6
0F180D7
0F180D8
0F180D9
0F180DB
0F180Z3
0F180Z4
0F180Z5
0F180Z6
0F180Z7
0F180Z8
0F180Z9
0F180ZB
0F184D3
0F184D4
0F184D5
0F184D6
0F184D7
0F184D8
0F184D9
0F184DB
0F184Z3
0F184Z4
0F184Z5
0F184Z6
0F184Z7
0F184Z8
0F184Z9
0F184ZB
0F190D3
0F190D4
0F190D5
0F190D6
0F190D7
0F190D8
0F190D9
0F190DB
0F190Z3
0F190Z4
0F190Z5
0F190Z6
0F190Z7
0F190Z8
0F190Z9
0F190ZB
0F194D3
0F194D4
0F194D5
0F194D6
0F194D7
0F194D8
0F194D9
0F194DB
0F194Z3
0F194Z4
0F194Z5
0F194Z6
0F194Z7
0F194Z8
0F194Z9
0F194ZB
0F1D0D3
0F1D0DB
0F1D0DC
0F1D0Z3
0F1D0ZB
0F1D0ZC
0F1D4D3
0F1D4DB
0F1D4DC
0F1D4Z3
0F1D4ZB
0F1D4ZC
0F1F0D3
0F1F0DB
0F1F0DC
0F1F0Z3
0F1F0ZB
0F1F0ZC
0F1F4D3
0F1F4DB
0F1F4DC
0F1F4Z3
0F1F4ZB
0F1F4ZC
0F1G0D3
0F1G0DB
0F1G0DC
0F1G0Z3
0F1G0ZB
0F1G0ZC
0F1G4D3
0F1G4DB
0F1G4DC
0F1G4Z3
0F1G4ZB
0F1G4ZC
0F20X0Z
0F20XYZ
0F24X0Z
0F24XYZ
0F2BX0Z
0F2BXYZ
0F2DX0Z
0F2DXYZ
0F2GX0Z
0F2GXYZ
0F500ZF
0F500ZZ
0F503ZF
0F503ZZ
0F504ZF
0F504ZZ
0F510ZF
0F510ZZ
0F513ZF
0F513ZZ
0F514ZF
0F514ZZ
0F520ZF
0F520ZZ
0F523ZF
0F523ZZ
0F524ZF
0F524ZZ
0F540ZZ
0F543ZZ
0F544ZZ
0F548ZZ
0F550ZZ
0F553ZZ
0F554ZZ
0F557ZZ
0F558ZZ
0F560ZZ
0F563ZZ
0F564ZZ
0F567ZZ
0F568ZZ
0F570ZZ
0F573ZZ
0F574ZZ
0F577ZZ
0F578ZZ
0F580ZZ
0F583ZZ
0F584ZZ
0F587ZZ
0F588ZZ
0F590ZZ
0F593ZZ
0F594ZZ
0F597ZZ
0F598ZZ
0F5C0ZZ
0F5C3ZZ
0F5C4ZZ
0F5C7ZZ
0F5C8ZZ
0F5D0ZZ
0F5D3ZZ
0F5D4ZZ
0F5D7ZZ
0F5D8ZZ
0F5F0ZZ
0F5F3ZZ
0F5F4ZZ
0F5F7ZZ
0F5F8ZZ
0F5G0ZF
0F5G0ZZ
0F5G3ZF
0F5G3ZZ
0F5G4ZF
0F5G4ZZ
0F5G8ZZ
0F750DZ
0F750ZZ
0F753DZ
0F753ZZ
0F754DZ
0F754ZZ
0F757DZ
0F757ZZ
0F758DZ
0F758ZZ
0F760DZ
0F760ZZ
0F763DZ
0F763ZZ
0F764DZ
0F764ZZ
0F767DZ
0F767ZZ
0F768DZ
0F768ZZ
0F770DZ
0F770ZZ
0F773DZ
0F773ZZ
0F774DZ
0F774ZZ
0F777DZ
0F777ZZ
0F778DZ
0F778ZZ
0F780DZ
0F780ZZ
0F783DZ
0F783ZZ
0F784DZ
0F784ZZ
0F787DZ
0F787ZZ
0F788DZ
0F788ZZ
0F790DZ
0F790ZZ
0F793DZ
0F793ZZ
0F794DZ
0F794ZZ
0F797DZ
0F797ZZ
0F798DZ
0F798ZZ
0F7C0DZ
0F7C0ZZ
0F7C3DZ
0F7C3ZZ
0F7C4DZ
0F7C4ZZ
0F7C7DZ
0F7C7ZZ
0F7C8DZ
0F7C8ZZ
0F7D0DZ
0F7D0ZZ
0F7D3DZ
0F7D3ZZ
0F7D4DZ
0F7D4ZZ
0F7D7DZ
0F7D7ZZ
0F7D8DZ
0F7D8ZZ
0F7F0DZ
0F7F0ZZ
0F7F3DZ
0F7F3ZZ
0F7F4DZ
0F7F4ZZ
0F7F7DZ
0F7F7ZZ
0F7F8DZ
0F7F8ZZ
0F8G0ZZ
0F8G3ZZ
0F8G4ZZ
0F9000Z
0F900ZX
0F9030Z
0F903ZX
0F903ZZ
0F9040Z
0F904ZX
0F904ZZ
0F9130Z
0F913ZX
0F913ZZ
0F9140Z
0F914ZX
0F914ZZ
0F9230Z
0F923ZX
0F923ZZ
0F9240Z
0F924ZX
0F924ZZ
0F9430Z
0F943ZX
0F943ZZ
0F9440Z
0F944ZX
0F944ZZ
0F9480Z
0F948ZX
0F948ZZ
0F9530Z
0F953ZX
0F953ZZ
0F954ZX
0F957ZX
0F9580Z
0F958ZX
0F958ZZ
0F9630Z
0F963ZX
0F963ZZ
0F964ZX
0F967ZX
0F9680Z
0F968ZX
0F968ZZ
0F9730Z
0F973ZX
0F973ZZ
0F9740Z
0F974ZX
0F974ZZ
0F9770Z
0F977ZX
0F977ZZ
0F9780Z
0F978ZX
0F978ZZ
0F9830Z
0F983ZX
0F983ZZ
0F984ZX
0F987ZX
0F9880Z
0F988ZX
0F988ZZ
0F9930Z
0F993ZX
0F993ZZ
0F994ZX
0F994ZZ
0F997ZX
0F997ZZ
0F9980Z
0F998ZX
0F998ZZ
0F9C30Z
0F9C3ZX
0F9C3ZZ
0F9C40Z
0F9C4ZX
0F9C4ZZ
0F9C7ZX
0F9C80Z
0F9C8ZX
0F9C8ZZ
0F9D30Z
0F9D3ZX
0F9D3ZZ
0F9D4ZX
0F9D7ZX
0F9D80Z
0F9D8ZX
0F9D8ZZ
0F9F30Z
0F9F3ZX
0F9F3ZZ
0F9F4ZX
0F9F7ZX
0F9F80Z
0F9F8ZX
0F9F8ZZ
0F9G30Z
0F9G3ZX
0F9G3ZZ
0F9G4ZX
0F9G80Z
0F9G8ZX
0F9G8ZZ
0FB03ZX
0FB13ZX
0FB23ZX
0FB43ZX
0FB44ZX
0FB48ZX
0FB53ZX
0FB54ZX
0FB54ZZ
0FB57ZX
0FB58ZX
0FB58ZZ
0FB63ZX
0FB64ZX
0FB64ZZ
0FB67ZX
0FB68ZX
0FB68ZZ
0FB73ZX
0FB74ZX
0FB74ZZ
0FB77ZX
0FB78ZX
0FB78ZZ
0FB83ZX
0FB84ZX
0FB84ZZ
0FB87ZX
0FB88ZX
0FB88ZZ
0FB93ZX
0FB94ZX
0FB94ZZ
0FB97ZX
0FB98ZX
0FB98ZZ
0FBC3ZX
0FBC4ZX
0FBC4ZZ
0FBC7ZX
0FBC8ZX
0FBC8ZZ
0FBD3ZX
0FBD4ZX
0FBD4ZZ
0FBD7ZX
0FBD8ZX
0FBD8ZZ
0FBF3ZX
0FBF4ZX
0FBF4ZZ
0FBF7ZX
0FBF8ZX
0FBF8ZZ
0FBG3ZX
0FBG4ZX
0FBG8ZX
0FBG8ZZ
0FC00ZZ
0FC03ZZ
0FC04ZZ
0FC10ZZ
0FC13ZZ
0FC14ZZ
0FC20ZZ
0FC23ZZ
0FC24ZZ
0FC40ZZ
0FC43ZZ
0FC44ZZ
0FC48ZZ
0FC50ZZ
0FC53ZZ
0FC54ZZ
0FC57ZZ
0FC58ZZ
0FC60ZZ
0FC63ZZ
0FC64ZZ
0FC67ZZ
0FC68ZZ
0FC70ZZ
0FC73ZZ
0FC74ZZ
0FC77ZZ
0FC78ZZ
0FC80ZZ
0FC83ZZ
0FC84ZZ
0FC87ZZ
0FC88ZZ
0FC90ZZ
0FC93ZZ
0FC94ZZ
0FC97ZZ
0FC98ZZ
0FCC0ZZ

0DW602Z-0FCC0ZZ
APPENDIX H: NON-OR NOT AFFECTING MS-DRG ASSIGNMENT

0FCC3ZZ
0FCC4ZZ
0FCC7ZZ
0FCC8ZZ
0FCD0ZZ
0FCD3ZZ
0FCD4ZZ
0FCD7ZZ
0FCD8ZZ
0FCF0ZZ
0FCF3ZZ
0FCF4ZZ
0FCF7ZZ
0FCF8ZZ
0FCG0ZZ
0FCG3ZZ
0FCG4ZZ
0FCG8ZZ
0FD03ZX
0FD04ZX
0FD13ZX
0FD14ZX
0FD23ZX
0FD24ZX
0FD43ZX
0FD44ZX
0FD48ZX
0FD53ZX
0FD54ZX
0FD58ZX
0FD63ZX
0FD64ZX
0FD68ZX
0FD73ZX
0FD74ZX
0FD78ZX
0FD83ZX
0FD84ZX
0FD88ZX
0FD93ZX
0FD94ZX
0FD98ZX
0FDC3ZX
0FDC4ZX
0FDC8ZX
0FDD3ZX
0FDD4ZX
0FDD8ZX
0FDF3ZX
0FDF4ZX
0FDF8ZX
0FDG3ZX
0FDG4ZX
0FDG8ZX
0FF40ZZ
0FF43ZZ
0FF44ZZ
0FF47ZZ
0FF48ZZ
0FF4XZZ
0FF50ZZ
0FF53ZZ
0FF54ZZ
0FF57ZZ
0FF58ZZ
0FF5XZZ
0FF60ZZ
0FF63ZZ
0FF64ZZ
0FF67ZZ
0FF68ZZ
0FF6XZZ
0FF70ZZ
0FF73ZZ
0FF74ZZ
0FF77ZZ
0FF78ZZ
0FF7XZZ
0FF80ZZ
0FF83ZZ
0FF84ZZ
0FF87ZZ
0FF88ZZ
0FF8XZZ
0FF90ZZ
0FF93ZZ
0FF94ZZ
0FF97ZZ
0FF98ZZ
0FF9XZZ
0FFC0ZZ
0FFC3ZZ
0FFC4ZZ
0FFC7ZZ
0FFC8ZZ
0FFCXZZ
0FFD0ZZ
0FFD3ZZ
0FFD4ZZ
0FFD7ZZ
0FFD8ZZ
0FFDXZZ
0FFF0ZZ
0FFF3ZZ
0FFF4ZZ
0FFF7ZZ
0FFF8ZZ
0FFFXZZ
0FH002Z
0FH003Z
0FH00YZ
0FH032Z
0FH033Z
0FH03YZ
0FH042Z
0FH043Z
0FH04YZ
0FH102Z
0FH103Z
0FH132Z
0FH133Z
0FH142Z
0FH143Z
0FH202Z
0FH203Z
0FH232Z
0FH233Z
0FH242Z
0FH243Z
0FH402Z
0FH403Z
0FH40YZ
0FH432Z
0FH433Z
0FH43YZ
0FH442Z
0FH443Z
0FH44YZ
0FHB01Z
0FHB02Z
0FHB03Z
0FHB0DZ
0FHB0YZ
0FHB31Z
0FHB32Z
0FHB33Z
0FHB3DZ
0FHB3YZ
0FHB41Z
0FHB42Z
0FHB43Z
0FHB4DZ
0FHB4YZ
0FHB71Z
0FHB72Z
0FHB73Z
0FHB7DZ
0FHB7YZ
0FHB81Z
0FHB82Z
0FHB83Z
0FHB8DZ
0FHB8YZ
0FHD01Z
0FHD02Z
0FHD03Z
0FHD0DZ
0FHD0YZ
0FHD31Z
0FHD32Z
0FHD33Z
0FHD3DZ
0FHD3YZ
0FHD41Z
0FHD42Z
0FHD43Z
0FHD4DZ
0FHD4YZ
0FHD71Z
0FHD72Z
0FHD73Z
0FHD7DZ
0FHD7YZ
0FHD81Z
0FHD82Z
0FHD83Z
0FHD8DZ
0FHD8YZ
0FHG02Z
0FHG03Z
0FHG0YZ
0FHG32Z
0FHG33Z
0FHG3YZ
0FHG42Z
0FHG43Z
0FHG4YZ
0FJ00ZZ
0FJ03ZZ
0FJ04ZZ
0FJ0XZZ
0FJ40ZZ
0FJ43ZZ
0FJ44ZZ
0FJ48ZZ
0FJ4XZZ
0FJB0ZZ
0FJB3ZZ
0FJB4ZZ
0FJB7ZZ
0FJB8ZZ
0FJD0ZZ
0FJD3ZZ
0FJD4ZZ
0FJD7ZZ
0FJD8ZZ
0FJG0ZZ
0FJG3ZZ
0FJG4ZZ
0FJG8ZZ
0FJGXZZ
0FL50CZ
0FL50DZ
0FL50ZZ
0FL53CZ
0FL53DZ
0FL53ZZ
0FL54CZ
0FL54DZ
0FL54ZZ
0FL57DZ
0FL57ZZ
0FL58DZ
0FL58ZZ
0FL60CZ
0FL60DZ
0FL60ZZ
0FL63CZ
0FL63DZ
0FL63ZZ
0FL64CZ
0FL64DZ
0FL64ZZ
0FL67DZ
0FL67ZZ
0FL68DZ
0FL68ZZ
0FL70CZ
0FL70DZ
0FL70ZZ
0FL73CZ
0FL73DZ
0FL73ZZ
0FL74CZ
0FL74DZ
0FL74ZZ
0FL77DZ
0FL77ZZ
0FL78DZ
0FL78ZZ
0FL80CZ
0FL80DZ
0FL80ZZ
0FL83CZ
0FL83DZ
0FL83ZZ
0FL84CZ
0FL84DZ
0FL84ZZ
0FL87DZ
0FL87ZZ
0FL88DZ
0FL88ZZ
0FL90CZ
0FL90DZ
0FL90ZZ
0FL93CZ
0FL93DZ
0FL93ZZ
0FL94CZ
0FL94DZ
0FL94ZZ
0FL97DZ
0FL97ZZ
0FL98DZ
0FL98ZZ
0FLC0CZ
0FLC0DZ
0FLC0ZZ
0FLC3CZ
0FLC3DZ
0FLC3ZZ
0FLC4CZ
0FLC4DZ
0FLC4ZZ
0FLC7DZ
0FLC7ZZ
0FLC8DZ
0FLC8ZZ
0FLD0CZ
0FLD0DZ
0FLD0ZZ
0FLD3CZ
0FLD3DZ
0FLD3ZZ
0FLD4CZ
0FLD4DZ
0FLD4ZZ
0FLD7DZ
0FLD7ZZ
0FLD8DZ
0FLD8ZZ
0FLF0CZ
0FLF0DZ
0FLF0ZZ
0FLF3CZ
0FLF3DZ
0FLF3ZZ
0FLF4CZ
0FLF4DZ
0FLF4ZZ
0FLF7DZ
0FLF7ZZ
0FLF8DZ
0FLF8ZZ
0FM00ZZ
0FM04ZZ
0FM10ZZ
0FM14ZZ
0FM20ZZ
0FM24ZZ
0FM40ZZ
0FM44ZZ
0FM50ZZ
0FM54ZZ
0FM60ZZ
0FM64ZZ
0FM70ZZ
0FM74ZZ
0FM80ZZ
0FM84ZZ
0FM90ZZ
0FM94ZZ
0FMC0ZZ
0FMC4ZZ
0FMD0ZZ
0FMD4ZZ
0FMF0ZZ
0FMF4ZZ
0FMG0ZZ
0FMG4ZZ
0FN00ZZ
0FN03ZZ
0FN04ZZ
0FN10ZZ
0FN13ZZ
0FN14ZZ
0FN20ZZ
0FN23ZZ
0FN24ZZ
0FN40ZZ
0FN43ZZ
0FN44ZZ
0FN48ZZ
0FN50ZZ
0FN53ZZ
0FN54ZZ
0FN57ZZ
0FN58ZZ
0FN60ZZ
0FN63ZZ
0FN64ZZ
0FN67ZZ
0FN68ZZ
0FN70ZZ
0FN73ZZ
0FN74ZZ
0FN77ZZ
0FN78ZZ
0FN80ZZ
0FN83ZZ
0FP03YZ
0FP04YZ
0FP0X0Z
0FP0X2Z
0FP0X3Z
0FP43YZ
0FP44YZ
0FP4X0Z
0FP4X2Z
0FP4X3Z
0FP4XDZ
0FPB3YZ
0FPB4YZ
0FPB70Z
0FPB72Z
0FPB73Z
0FPB7DZ
0FPB7YZ
0FPB80Z
0FPB82Z
0FPB83Z
0FPB8DZ
0FPB8YZ
0FPBX0Z
0FPBX1Z
0FPBX2Z
0FPBX3Z
0FPBXDZ
0FPD3YZ
0FPD4YZ
0FPD70Z
0FPD72Z
0FPD73Z
0FPD7DZ
0FPD7YZ
0FPD80Z
0FPD82Z
0FPD83Z
0FPD8DZ
0FPD8YZ
0FPDX0Z
0FPDX1Z
0FPDX2Z
0FPDX3Z
0FPDXDZ
0FPG3YZ
0FPG4YZ
0FPGX0Z
0FPGX2Z
0FPGX3Z
0FQ44ZZ
0FQ48ZZ
0FQ50ZZ
0FQ53ZZ
0FQ54ZZ
0FQ57ZZ
0FQ58ZZ
0FQ60ZZ
0FQ63ZZ
0FQ64ZZ
0FQ67ZZ
0FQ68ZZ
0FQ70ZZ
0FQ73ZZ
0FQ74ZZ
0FQ77ZZ
0FQ78ZZ
0FQ80ZZ
0FQ83ZZ
0FQ84ZZ
0FQ87ZZ
0FQ88ZZ
0FQ90ZZ
0FQ93ZZ
0FQ94ZZ
0FQ97ZZ
0FQ98ZZ
0FQC0ZZ
0FQC3ZZ
0FQC4ZZ
0FQC7ZZ
0FQC8ZZ
0FQD0ZZ
0FQD3ZZ
0FQD4ZZ
0FQD7ZZ
0FQD8ZZ
0FQF0ZZ
0FQF3ZZ
0FQF4ZZ
0FQF7ZZ
0FQF8ZZ
0FQG0ZZ
0FQG3ZZ
0FQG4ZZ
0FQG8ZZ
0FR507Z
0FR50JZ
0FR50KZ
0FR547Z
0FR54JZ
0FR54KZ
0FR587Z
0FR58JZ
0FR58KZ
0FR607Z
0FR60JZ
0FR60KZ
0FR647Z
0FR64JZ
0FR64KZ
0FR687Z
0FR68JZ
0FR68KZ
0FR707Z
0FR70JZ
0FR70KZ
0FR747Z
0FR74JZ
0FR74KZ
0FR787Z
0FR78JZ
0FR78KZ
0FR807Z
0FR80JZ
0FR80KZ
0FR847Z
0FR84JZ
0FR84KZ
0FR887Z
0FR88JZ
0FR88KZ
0FR907Z
0FR90JZ
0FR90KZ
0FR947Z
0FR94JZ
0FR94KZ
0FR987Z
0FR98JZ
0FR98KZ
0FRC07Z
0FRC0JZ
0FRC0KZ
0FRC47Z
0FRC4JZ
0FRC4KZ
0FRC87Z
0FRC8JZ
0FRC8KZ
0FRD07Z
0FRD0JZ
0FRD0KZ
0FRD47Z
0FRD4JZ
0FRD4KZ
0FRD87Z
0FRD8JZ
0FRD8KZ
0FRF07Z
0FRF0JZ
0FRF0KZ
0FRF47Z
0FRF4JZ
0FRF4KZ
0FRF87Z
0FRF8JZ
0FRF8KZ
0FS00ZZ
0FS04ZZ
0FS40ZZ
0FS44ZZ
0FS50ZZ
0FS54ZZ
0FS60ZZ
0FS64ZZ
0FS70ZZ
0FS74ZZ
0FS80ZZ
0FS84ZZ
0FS90ZZ
0FS94ZZ
0FSC0ZZ
0FSC4ZZ
0FSD0ZZ
0FSD4ZZ
0FSF0ZZ
0FSF4ZZ
0FSG0ZZ
0FSG4ZZ
0FT00ZZ
0FT04ZZ
0FT10ZZ
0FT14ZZ
0FT20ZZ
0FT24ZZ
0FT40ZZ
0FT44ZZ
0FT50ZZ
0FT54ZZ
0FT57ZZ
0FT58ZZ
0FT60ZZ
0FT64ZZ
0FT67ZZ
0FT68ZZ
0FT70ZZ
0FT74ZZ
0FT77ZZ
0FT78ZZ
0FT80ZZ
0FT84ZZ
0FT87ZZ
0FT88ZZ
0FT90ZZ
0FT94ZZ
0FT97ZZ
0FT98ZZ
0FTC0ZZ
0FTC4ZZ
0FTC7ZZ
0FTC8ZZ
0FTD0ZZ
0FTD4ZZ
0FTD7ZZ
0FTD8ZZ
0FTF0ZZ
0FTF4ZZ
0FTF7ZZ
0FTF8ZZ
0FTG0ZZ
0FTG4ZZ
0FU507Z
0FU50JZ
0FU50KZ
0FU537Z
0FU53JZ
0FU53KZ
0FU547Z
0FU54JZ
0FU54KZ
0FU587Z
0FU58JZ
0FU58KZ
0FU607Z
0FU60JZ
0FU60KZ
0FU637Z
0FU63JZ
0FU63KZ
0FU647Z
0FU64JZ
0FU64KZ
0FU687Z
0FU68JZ
0FU68KZ
0FU707Z
0FU70JZ
0FU70KZ
0FU737Z
0FU73JZ
0FU73KZ
0FU747Z
0FU74JZ
0FU74KZ
0FU787Z
0FU78JZ
0FU78KZ
0FU807Z
0FU80JZ
0FU80KZ
0FU837Z
0FU83JZ
0FU83KZ
0FU847Z
0FU84JZ
0FU84KZ
0FU887Z
0FU88JZ
0FU88KZ
0FU907Z
0FU90JZ
0FU90KZ
0FU937Z
0FU93JZ
0FU93KZ
0FU947Z
0FU94JZ
0FU94KZ
0FU987Z
0FU98JZ
0FU98KZ
0FUC07Z
0FUC0JZ
0FUC0KZ
0FUC37Z
0FUC3JZ
0FUC3KZ
0FUC47Z
0FV53CZ
0FV53DZ
0FV53ZZ
0FV54CZ
0FV54DZ
0FV54ZZ
0FV57DZ
0FV57ZZ
0FV58DZ
0FV58ZZ
0FV63CZ
0FV63DZ
0FV63ZZ
0FV64CZ
0FV64DZ
0FV64ZZ
0FV67DZ
0FV67ZZ
0FV68DZ
0FV68ZZ
0FV73CZ
0FV73DZ
0FV73ZZ
0FV74CZ
0FV74DZ
0FV74ZZ
0FV77DZ
0FV77ZZ
0FV78DZ
0FV78ZZ
0FV83CZ
0FV83DZ
0FV83ZZ
0FV84CZ
0FV84DZ
0FV84ZZ
0FV87DZ
0FV87ZZ
0FV88DZ
0FV88ZZ
0FV93CZ
0FV93DZ
0FV93ZZ
0FV94CZ
0FV94DZ
0FV94ZZ

0FV97DZ
0FV97ZZ
0FV98DZ
0FV98ZZ
0FW03YZ
0FW04YZ
0FW0X0Z
0FW0X2Z
0FW0X3Z
0FW43YZ
0FW44YZ
0FW4X0Z
0FW4X2Z
0FW4X3Z
0FW4XDZ
0FWB3YZ
0FWB4YZ
0FWB7YZ
0FWB80Z
0FWB82Z
0FWB8CZ
0FWB8DZ
0FWB8JZ
0FWB8KZ
0FWB8YZ
0FWBX0Z
0FWBX2Z
0FWBX3Z
0FWBX7Z
0FWBXCZ
0FWBXDZ
0FWBXJZ
0FWBXKZ
0FWD00Z
0FWD02Z
0FWD03Z
0FWD07Z
0FWD0CZ
0FWD0DZ
0FWD0JZ
0FWD0KZ
0FWD0YZ
0FWD30Z
0FWD32Z
0FWD33Z
0FWD37Z
0FWD3CZ
0FWD3DZ
0FWD3JZ
0FWD3KZ
0FWD3YZ
0FWD40Z
0FWD42Z
0FWD43Z
0FWD47Z
0FWD4CZ
0FWD4DZ
0FWD4JZ
0FWD4KZ
0FWD4YZ
0FWD70Z
0FWD72Z
0FWD73Z
0FWD77Z
0FWD7CZ
0FWD7DZ
0FWD7JZ
0FWD7KZ
0FWD7YZ
0FWD80Z
0FWD82Z
0FWD83Z
0FWD87Z
0FWD8CZ
0FWD8DZ
0FWD8JZ
0FWD8KZ
0FWD8YZ
0FWDX0Z
0FWDX2Z
0FWDX3Z
0FWDX7Z
0FWDXCZ
0FWDXDZ
0FWDXJZ
0FWDXKZ
0FWG00Z
0FWG02Z
0FWG03Z
0FWG0DZ
0FWG0YZ
0FWG30Z
0FWG32Z
0FWG33Z
0FWG3DZ
0FWG3YZ
0FWG40Z
0FWG42Z
0FWG43Z
0FWG4DZ
0FWG4YZ
0FWGX0Z
0FWGX2Z
0FWGX3Z
0FWGXDZ
0FY00Z0
0FY00Z1
0FY00Z2
0FYG0Z0
0FYG0Z1
0FYG0Z2
0G20X0Z
0G20XYZ
0G21X0Z
0G21XYZ
0G25X0Z
0G25XYZ
0G2KX0Z
0G2KXYZ
0G2RX0Z
0G2RXYZ
0G2SX0Z
0G2SXYZ
0G500ZZ
0G503ZZ
0G504ZZ
0G510ZZ
0G513ZZ
0G514ZZ
0G520ZZ
0G523ZZ
0G524ZZ
0G530ZZ
0G533ZZ
0G534ZZ
0G540ZZ
0G543ZZ
0G544ZZ
0G560ZZ
0G563ZZ
0G564ZZ
0G570ZZ
0G573ZZ
0G574ZZ
0G580ZZ
0G583ZZ
0G584ZZ
0G590ZZ
0G593ZZ
0G594ZZ
0G5B0ZZ
0G5B3ZZ
0G5B4ZZ
0G5C0ZZ
0G5C3ZZ
0G5C4ZZ
0G5D0ZZ
0G5D3ZZ
0G5D4ZZ
0G5F0ZZ
0G5F3ZZ
0G5F4ZZ
0G5G0ZZ
0G5G3ZZ
0G5G4ZZ
0G5H0ZZ
0G5H3ZZ
0G5H4ZZ
0G5K0ZZ
0G5K3ZZ
0G5K4ZZ
0G5L0ZZ
0G5L3ZZ
0G5L4ZZ
0G5M0ZZ
0G5M3ZZ
0G5M4ZZ
0G5N0ZZ
0G5N3ZZ
0G5N4ZZ
0G5P0ZZ
0G5P3ZZ
0G5P4ZZ
0G5Q0ZZ
0G5Q3ZZ
0G5Q4ZZ
0G5R0ZZ
0G5R3ZZ
0G5R4ZZ
0G800ZZ
0G803ZZ
0G804ZZ
0G8J0ZZ
0G8J3ZZ
0G8J4ZZ
0G9000Z
0G900ZX
0G900ZZ
0G9030Z
0G903ZX
0G903ZZ
0G9040Z
0G904ZX
0G904ZZ
0G9100Z
0G910ZX
0G910ZZ
0G9130Z
0G913ZX
0G913ZZ
0G9140Z
0G914ZX
0G914ZZ
0G9200Z
0G920ZX
0G920ZZ
0G9230Z
0G923ZX
0G923ZZ
0G9240Z
0G924ZX
0G924ZZ
0G9300Z
0G930ZX
0G930ZZ
0G9330Z
0G933ZX
0G933ZZ
0G9340Z
0G934ZX
0G934ZZ
0G9400Z
0G940ZX
0G940ZZ
0G9430Z
0G943ZX
0G943ZZ
0G9440Z
0G944ZX
0G944ZZ
0G9600Z
0G960ZX
0G960ZZ
0G9630Z
0G963ZX
0G963ZZ
0G9640Z
0G964ZX
0G964ZZ
0G9700Z
0G970ZX
0G970ZZ
0G9730Z
0G973ZX
0G973ZZ
0G9740Z
0G974ZX
0G974ZZ
0G9800Z
0G980ZX
0G980ZZ
0G9830Z
0G983ZX
0G983ZZ
0G9840Z
0G984ZX
0G984ZZ
0G9900Z
0G990ZX
0G990ZZ
0G9930Z
0G993ZX
0G993ZZ
0G9940Z
0G994ZX
0G994ZZ
0G9B00Z
0G9B0ZX
0G9B0ZZ
0G9B30Z
0G9B3ZX
0G9B3ZZ
0G9B40Z
0G9B4ZX
0G9B4ZZ
0G9C00Z
0G9C0ZX
0G9C0ZZ
0G9C30Z
0G9C3ZX
0G9C3ZZ
0G9C40Z
0G9C4ZX
0G9C4ZZ
0G9D00Z
0G9D0ZX
0G9D0ZZ
0G9D30Z
0G9D3ZX
0G9D3ZZ
0G9D40Z
0G9D4ZX
0G9D4ZZ
0G9F00Z
0G9F0ZX
0G9F0ZZ
0G9F30Z
0G9F3ZX
0G9F3ZZ
0G9F40Z
0G9F4ZX
0G9F4ZZ
0G9G00Z
0G9G0ZX
0G9G0ZZ
0G9G30Z
0G9G3ZX
0G9G3ZZ
0G9G40Z
0G9G4ZX
0G9G4ZZ
0G9H00Z
0G9H0ZX
0G9H0ZZ
0G9H30Z
0G9H3ZX
0G9H3ZZ
0G9H40Z
0G9H4ZX
0G9H4ZZ
0G9K00Z
0G9K0ZX
0G9K0ZZ
0G9K30Z
0G9K3ZX
0G9K3ZZ
0G9K40Z
0G9K4ZX
0G9K4ZZ
0G9L00Z
0G9L0ZX
0G9L0ZZ
0G9L30Z
0G9L3ZX
0G9L3ZZ
0G9L40Z
0G9L4ZX
0G9L4ZZ
0G9M00Z
0G9M0ZX
0G9M0ZZ
0G9M30Z
0G9M3ZX
0G9M3ZZ
0G9M40Z
0G9M4ZX
0G9M4ZZ
0G9N00Z
0G9N0ZX
0G9N0ZZ
0G9N30Z
0G9N3ZX
0G9N3ZZ
0G9N40Z
0G9N4ZX
0G9N4ZZ
0G9P00Z
0G9P0ZX
0G9P0ZZ
0G9P30Z
0G9P3ZX
0G9P3ZZ
0G9P40Z
0G9P4ZX
0G9P4ZZ
0G9Q00Z
0G9Q0ZX
0G9Q0ZZ
0G9Q30Z
0G9Q3ZX
0G9Q3ZZ
0G9Q40Z
0G9Q4ZX
0G9Q4ZZ
0G9R00Z
0G9R0ZX
0G9R0ZZ
0G9R30Z
0G9R3ZX
0G9R3ZZ
0G9R40Z
0G9R4ZX
0G9R4ZZ
0GB00ZX
0GB00ZZ
0GB03ZX
0GB03ZZ
0GB04ZX
0GB04ZZ
0GB10ZX
0GB10ZZ
0GB13ZX
0GB13ZZ
0GB14ZX
0GB14ZZ
0GB20ZX
0GB20ZZ
0GB23ZX
0GB23ZZ
0GB24ZX
0GB24ZZ
0GB30ZX
0GB30ZZ
0GB33ZX
0GB33ZZ
0GB34ZX
0GB34ZZ
0GB40ZX
0GB40ZZ
0GB43ZX
0GB43ZZ
0GB44ZX
0GB44ZZ
0GB60ZX
0GB60ZZ
0GB63ZX
0GB63ZZ
0GB64ZX
0GB64ZZ
0GB70ZX
0GB70ZZ
0GB73ZX
0GB73ZZ
0GB74ZX
0GB74ZZ
0GB80ZX
0GB80ZZ
0GB83ZX
0GB83ZZ
0GB84ZX
0GB84ZZ
0GB90ZX
0GB90ZZ
0GB93ZX
0GB93ZZ
0GB94ZX
0GB94ZZ
0GBB0ZX
0GBB0ZZ
0GBB3ZX
0GBB3ZZ
0GBB4ZX
0GBB4ZZ
0GBC0ZX
0GBC0ZZ
0GBC3ZX
0GBC3ZZ
0GBC4ZX
0GBC4ZZ
0GBD0ZX
0GBD0ZZ
0GBD3ZX
0GBD3ZZ
0GBD4ZX
0GBD4ZZ
0GBF0ZX
0GBF0ZZ
0GBF3ZX
0GBF3ZZ
0GBF4ZX
0GBF4ZZ
0GBG0ZX
0GBG0ZZ
0GBG3ZX
0GBG3ZZ
0GBG4ZX
0GBG4ZZ
0GBH0ZX
0GBH0ZZ
0GBH3ZX
0GBH3ZZ
0GBH4ZX
0GBH4ZZ
0GBJ0ZX
0GBJ0ZZ
0GBJ3ZX
0GBJ3ZZ
0GBJ4ZX
0GBJ4ZZ
0GBL0ZX
0GBL0ZZ
0GBL3ZX
0GBL3ZZ
0GBL4ZX
0GBL4ZZ
0GBM0ZX
0GBM0ZZ
0GBM3ZX
0GBM3ZZ
0GBM4ZX
0GBM4ZZ
0GBN0ZX
0GBN0ZZ
0GBN3ZX
0GBN3ZZ
0GBN4ZX
0GBN4ZZ
0GBP0ZX
0GBP0ZZ
0GBP3ZX
0GBP3ZZ
0GBP4ZX
0GBP4ZZ
0GBQ0ZX
0GBQ0ZZ
0GBQ3ZX
0GBQ3ZZ
0GBQ4ZX
0GBQ4ZZ
0GBR0ZX
0GBR0ZZ
0GBR3ZX
0GBR3ZZ
0GBR4ZX
0GBR4ZZ
0GC00ZZ
0GC03ZZ
0GC04ZZ
0GC10ZZ
0GC13ZZ
0GC14ZZ
0GC20ZZ
0GC23ZZ
0GC24ZZ
0GC30ZZ
0GC33ZZ
0GC34ZZ
0GC40ZZ
0GC43ZZ
0GC44ZZ
0GC60ZZ
0GC63ZZ
0GC64ZZ
0GC70ZZ
0GC73ZZ
0GC74ZZ
0GC80ZZ
0GC83ZZ
0GC84ZZ
0GC90ZZ
0GC93ZZ
0GC94ZZ
0GCB0ZZ
0GCB3ZZ
0GCB4ZZ
0GCC0ZZ
0GCC3ZZ
0GCC4ZZ
0GCD0ZZ
0GCD3ZZ
0GCD4ZZ
0GCF0ZZ
0GCF3ZZ
0GCF4ZZ
0GCG0ZZ
0GCG3ZZ
0GCG4ZZ
0GCH0ZZ
0GCH3ZZ
0GCH4ZZ
0GCK0ZZ
0GCK3ZZ
0GCK4ZZ
0GCL0ZZ
0GCL3ZZ
0GCL4ZZ
0GCM0ZZ
0GCM3ZZ
0GCM4ZZ
0GCN0ZZ
0GCN3ZZ
0GCN4ZZ
0GCP0ZZ
0GCP3ZZ
0GCP4ZZ
0GCQ0ZZ
0GCQ3ZZ
0GCQ4ZZ
0GCR0ZZ
0GCR3ZZ
0GCR4ZZ
0GHS02Z
0GHS03Z
0GHS0YZ
0GHS32Z
0GHS33Z
0GHS3YZ
0GHS42Z
0GHS43Z
0GHS4YZ
0GJ00ZZ
0GJ03ZZ
0GJ04ZZ
0GJ10ZZ
0GJ13ZZ
0GJ14ZZ
0GJ50ZZ
0GJ53ZZ
0GJ54ZZ
0GJK3ZZ
0GJR3ZZ
0GJS3ZZ
0GP0X0Z
0GP1X0Z
0GP5X0Z
0GPKX0Z
0GPRX0Z
0GPS3YZ
0GPS4YZ
0GPSX0Z
0GPSX2Z
0GPSX3Z
0GTN0ZZ
0GTN4ZZ
0GTP0ZZ
0GTP4ZZ
0GTQ0ZZ
0GTQ4ZZ
0GTR0ZZ
0GTR4ZZ
0GW000Z
0GW030Z
0GW040Z
0GW0X0Z
0GW100Z
0GW130Z
0GW140Z
0GW1X0Z
0GW500Z
0GW530Z
0GW540Z
0GW5X0Z
0GWK00Z
0GWK30Z
0GWK40Z
0GWKX0Z
0GWR00Z
0GWR30Z
0GWR40Z
0GWRX0Z
0GWS00Z
0GWS02Z
0GWS03Z
0GWS0YZ
0GWS30Z
0GWS32Z
0GWS33Z
0GWS3YZ
0GWS40Z
0GWS42Z
0GWS43Z
0GWS4YZ
0GWSX0Z
0GWSX2Z
0GWSX3Z
0H0T07Z
0H0T0JZ
0H0T0KZ
0H0T0ZZ
0H0T37Z
0H0T3JZ
0H0T3KZ
0H0T3ZZ
0H0TX7Z
0H0TXJZ
0H0TXKZ
0H0TXZZ
0H0U07Z
0H0U0JZ
0H0U0KZ
0H0U0ZZ
0H0U37Z
0H0U3JZ
0H0U3KZ
0H0U3ZZ
0H0UX7Z
0H0UXJZ
0H0UXKZ
0H0UXZZ
0H0V07Z
0H0V0JZ
0H0V0KZ
0H0V0ZZ
0H0V37Z
0H0V3JZ
0H0V3KZ
0H0V3ZZ
0H0VX7Z
0H0VXJZ
0H0VXKZ
0H0VXZZ
0H2PX0Z
0H2PXYZ
0H2TX0Z
0H2TXYZ
0H2UX0Z
0H2UXYZ
0H50XZD
0H50XZZ
0H51XZD
0H51XZZ
0H52XZD
0H52XZZ
0H53XZD
0H53XZZ
0H54XZD
0H54XZZ
0H55XZD
0H55XZZ
0H56XZD
0H56XZZ
0H57XZD
0H57XZZ
0H58XZD
0H58XZZ
0H59XZD

0H59XZZ
0H5AXZD
0H5AXZZ
0H5BXZD
0H5BXZZ
0H5CXZD
0H5CXZZ
0H5DXZD
0H5DXZZ
0H5EXZD
0H5EXZZ
0H5FXZD
0H5FXZZ
0H5GXZD
0H5GXZZ
0H5HXZD
0H5HXZZ
0H5JXZD
0H5JXZZ
0H5KXZD
0H5KXZZ
0H5LXZD
0H5LXZZ
0H5MXZD
0H5MXZZ
0H5NXZD
0H5NXZZ
0H5QXZZ
0H5RXZZ
0H5T0ZZ
0H5T3ZZ
0H5T7ZZ
0H5T8ZZ
0H5TXZZ
0H5U0ZZ
0H5U3ZZ
0H5U7ZZ
0H5U8ZZ
0H5UXZZ
0H5V0ZZ
0H5V3ZZ
0H5V7ZZ
0H5V8ZZ
0H5VXZZ
0H5W0ZZ
0H5W3ZZ
0H5W7ZZ
0H5W8ZZ
0H5WXZZ
0H5X0ZZ
0H5X3ZZ
0H5X7ZZ
0H5X8ZZ
0H5XXZZ
0H80XZZ
0H81XZZ
0H82XZZ
0H83XZZ
0H84XZZ
0H85XZZ
0H86XZZ
0H87XZZ
0H88XZZ
0H89XZZ
0H8AXZZ
0H8BXZZ
0H8CXZZ
0H8DXZZ
0H8EXZZ
0H8FXZZ
0H8GXZZ
0H8HXZZ
0H8JXZZ
0H8KXZZ
0H8LXZZ
0H8MXZZ
0H8NXZZ
0H90X0Z
0H90XZX
0H90XZZ
0H91X0Z
0H91XZX
0H91XZZ
0H92X0Z
0H92XZX
0H92XZZ
0H93X0Z
0H93XZX
0H93XZZ
0H94X0Z
0H94XZX
0H94XZZ
0H95X0Z
0H95XZX
0H95XZZ
0H96X0Z
0H96XZX
0H96XZZ
0H97X0Z
0H97XZX
0H97XZZ
0H98X0Z
0H98XZX
0H98XZZ
0H99X0Z
0H99XZX
0H99XZZ
0H9AX0Z
0H9AXZX
0H9AXZZ
0H9BX0Z
0H9BXZX
0H9BXZZ
0H9CX0Z
0H9CXZX
0H9CXZZ
0H9DX0Z
0H9DXZX
0H9DXZZ
0H9EX0Z
0H9EXZX
0H9EXZZ
0H9FX0Z
0H9FXZX
0H9FXZZ
0H9GX0Z
0H9GXZX
0H9GXZZ
0H9HX0Z
0H9HXZX
0H9HXZZ
0H9JX0Z
0H9JXZX
0H9JXZZ
0H9KX0Z
0H9KXZX
0H9KXZZ
0H9LX0Z
0H9LXZX
0H9LXZZ
0H9MX0Z
0H9MXZX
0H9MXZZ
0H9NX0Z
0H9NXZX
0H9NXZZ
0H9QX0Z
0H9QXZX
0H9QXZZ
0H9RX0Z
0H9RXZX
0H9RXZZ
0H9T00Z
0H9T0ZX
0H9T0ZZ
0H9T30Z
0H9T3ZX
0H9T3ZZ
0H9T70Z
0H9T7ZX
0H9T7ZZ
0H9T80Z
0H9T8ZX
0H9T8ZZ
0H9TX0Z
0H9TXZX
0H9TXZZ
0H9U00Z
0H9U0ZX
0H9U0ZZ
0H9U30Z
0H9U3ZX
0H9U3ZZ
0H9U70Z
0H9U7ZX
0H9U7ZZ
0H9U80Z
0H9U8ZX
0H9U8ZZ
0H9UX0Z
0H9UXZX
0H9UXZZ
0H9V00Z
0H9V0ZX
0H9V0ZZ
0H9V30Z
0H9V3ZX
0H9V3ZZ
0H9V70Z
0H9V7ZX
0H9V7ZZ
0H9V80Z
0H9V8ZX
0H9V8ZZ
0H9VX0Z
0H9VXZX
0H9VXZZ
0H9W00Z
0H9W0ZX
0H9W0ZZ
0H9W30Z
0H9W3ZX
0H9W3ZZ
0H9W70Z
0H9W7ZX
0H9W7ZZ
0H9W80Z
0H9W8ZX
0H9W8ZZ
0H9WX0Z
0H9WXZX
0H9WXZZ
0H9X00Z
0H9X0ZX
0H9X0ZZ
0H9X30Z
0H9X3ZX
0H9X3ZZ
0H9X70Z
0H9X7ZX
0H9X7ZZ
0H9X80Z
0H9X8ZX
0H9X8ZZ
0H9XX0Z
0H9XXZX
0H9XXZZ
0HB0XZX
0HB0XZZ
0HB1XZX
0HB1XZZ
0HB2XZX
0HB2XZZ
0HB3XZX
0HB3XZZ
0HB4XZX
0HB4XZZ
0HB5XZX
0HB5XZZ
0HB6XZX
0HB6XZZ
0HB7XZX
0HB7XZZ
0HB8XZX
0HB8XZZ
0HB9XZX
0HB9XZZ
0HBAXZX
0HBAXZZ
0HBBXZX
0HBBXZZ
0HBCXZX
0HBCXZZ
0HBDXZX
0HBDXZZ
0HBEXZX
0HBEXZZ
0HBFXZX
0HBFXZZ
0HBGXZX
0HBGXZZ
0HBHXZX
0HBHXZZ
0HBJXZX
0HBJXZZ
0HBKXZX
0HBKXZZ
0HBLXZX
0HBLXZZ
0HBMXZX
0HBMXZZ
0HBNXZX
0HBNXZZ
0HBQXZX
0HBQXZZ
0HBRXZX
0HBRXZZ
0HBT0ZX
0HBT0ZZ
0HBT3ZX
0HBT3ZZ
0HBT7ZX
0HBT7ZZ
0HBT8ZX
0HBT8ZZ
0HBTXZX
0HBTXZZ
0HBU0ZX
0HBU0ZZ
0HBU3ZX
0HBU3ZZ
0HBU7ZX
0HBU7ZZ
0HBU8ZX
0HBU8ZZ
0HBUXZX
0HBUXZZ
0HBV0ZX
0HBV0ZZ
0HBV3ZX
0HBV3ZZ
0HBV7ZX
0HBV7ZZ
0HBV8ZX
0HBV8ZZ
0HBVXZX
0HBVXZZ
0HBW0ZX
0HBW0ZZ
0HBW3ZX
0HBW3ZZ
0HBW7ZX
0HBW7ZZ
0HBW8ZX
0HBW8ZZ
0HBWXZX
0HBWXZZ
0HBX0ZX
0HBX0ZZ
0HBX3ZX
0HBX3ZZ
0HBX7ZX
0HBX7ZZ
0HBX8ZX
0HBX8ZZ
0HBXXZX
0HBXXZZ
0HBY0ZX
0HBY0ZZ
0HBY3ZX
0HBY3ZZ
0HBY7ZX
0HBY7ZZ
0HBY8ZX
0HBY8ZZ
0HBYXZX
0HBYXZZ
0HC0XZZ
0HC1XZZ
0HC2XZZ
0HC3XZZ
0HC4XZZ
0HC5XZZ
0HC6XZZ
0HC7XZZ
0HC8XZZ
0HC9XZZ
0HCAXZZ
0HCBXZZ
0HCCXZZ
0HCDXZZ
0HCEXZZ
0HCFXZZ
0HCGXZZ
0HCHXZZ
0HCJXZZ
0HCKXZZ
0HCLXZZ
0HCMXZZ
0HCNXZZ
0HCQXZZ
0HCRXZZ
0HCT0ZZ
0HCT3ZZ
0HCT7ZZ
0HCT8ZZ
0HCTXZZ
0HCU0ZZ
0HCU3ZZ
0HCU7ZZ
0HCU8ZZ
0HCUXZZ
0HCV0ZZ
0HCV3ZZ
0HCV7ZZ
0HCV8ZZ
0HCVXZZ
0HCW0ZZ
0HCW3ZZ
0HCW7ZZ
0HCW8ZZ
0HCWXZZ
0HCX0ZZ
0HCX3ZZ
0HCX7ZZ
0HCX8ZZ
0HCXXZZ
0HD0XZZ
0HD1XZZ
0HD2XZZ
0HD3XZZ
0HD4XZZ
0HD5XZZ
0HD6XZZ
0HD7XZZ
0HD8XZZ
0HD9XZZ
0HDAXZZ
0HDBXZZ
0HDCXZZ
0HDDXZZ
0HDEXZZ
0HDFXZZ
0HDGXZZ
0HDHXZZ
0HDJXZZ
0HDKXZZ
0HDLXZZ
0HDMXZZ
0HDNXZZ
0HDQXZZ
0HDRXZZ
0HDSXZZ
0HHPXYZ
0HHT01Z
0HHT0NZ
0HHT0YZ
0HHT31Z
0HHT3NZ
0HHT3YZ
0HHT71Z
0HHT7NZ
0HHT7YZ
0HHT81Z
0HHT8NZ
0HHT8YZ
0HHTX1Z
0HHU01Z
0HHU0NZ
0HHU0YZ
0HHU31Z
0HHU3NZ
0HHU3YZ
0HHU71Z
0HHU7NZ
0HHU7YZ
0HHU81Z
0HHU8NZ
0HHU8YZ
0HHUX1Z
0HHV01Z
0HHV0NZ
0HHV31Z
0HHV3NZ
0HHV71Z
0HHV7NZ
0HHV81Z
0HHV8NZ
0HHVX1Z
0HHW01Z
0HHW0NZ
0HHW31Z
0HHW3NZ
0HHW71Z
0HHW7NZ
0HHW81Z
0HHW8NZ
0HHWX1Z
0HHX01Z
0HHX0NZ
0HHX31Z
0HHX3NZ
0HHX71Z
0HHX7NZ
0HHX81Z
0HHX8NZ
0HHXX1Z
0HJPXZZ
0HJQXZZ
0HJRXZZ
0HJT0ZZ
0HJT3ZZ
0HJT7ZZ
0HJT8ZZ
0HJTXZZ
0HJU0ZZ
0HJU3ZZ
0HJU7ZZ
0HJU8ZZ
0HJUXZZ
0HM0XZZ
0HM1XZZ
0HM2XZZ
0HM3XZZ
0HM4XZZ
0HM5XZZ
0HM6XZZ
0HM7XZZ
0HM8XZZ
0HM9XZZ
0HMAXZZ
0HMBXZZ
0HMCXZZ
0HMDXZZ
0HMEXZZ
0HMFXZZ
0HMGXZZ
0HMHXZZ
0HMJXZZ
0HMKXZZ
0HMLXZZ
0HMMXZZ
0HMNXZZ
0HMTXZZ
0HMUXZZ
0HMVXZZ
0HMWXZZ
0HMXXZZ
0HN0XZZ
0HN1XZZ
0HN2XZZ
0HN3XZZ
0HN4XZZ
0HN5XZZ
0HN6XZZ
0HN7XZZ
0HN8XZZ
0HN9XZZ
0HNAXZZ
0HNBXZZ
0HNCXZZ
0HNDXZZ
0HNEXZZ
0HNFXZZ
0HNGXZZ
0HNHXZZ
0HNJXZZ
0HNKXZZ
0HNLXZZ
0HNMXZZ
0HNNXZZ
0HNQXZZ
0HNRXZZ
0HNT0ZZ
0HNT3ZZ
0HNT7ZZ
0HNT8ZZ
0HNTXZZ
0HNU0ZZ
0HNU3ZZ
0HNU7ZZ
0HNU8ZZ
0HNUXZZ
0HNV0ZZ
0HNV3ZZ
0HNV7ZZ
0HNV8ZZ
0HNVXZZ
0HNW0ZZ
0HNW3ZZ
0HNW7ZZ
0HNW8ZZ
0HNWXZZ
0HNX0ZZ
0HNX3ZZ
0HNX7ZZ
0HNX8ZZ
0HNXXZZ
0HPPX0Z
0HPPX7Z
0HPPXJZ
0HPPXKZ
0HPPXYZ
0HPQX0Z
0HPQX7Z
0HPQXJZ
0HPQXKZ
0HPRX0Z
0HPRX7Z
0HPRXJZ
0HPRXKZ
0HPSX7Z
0HPSXJZ
0HPSXKZ
0HPT00Z
0HPT01Z
0HPT07Z
0HPT0JZ
0HPT0KZ
0HPT0NZ
0HPT0YZ
0HPT30Z
0HPT31Z
0HPT37Z
0HPT3JZ
0HPT3KZ
0HPT3NZ
0HPT3YZ
0HPT70Z
0HPT71Z
0HPT77Z
0HPT7JZ
0HPT7KZ
0HPT7NZ
0HPT7YZ
0HPT80Z
0HPT81Z
0HPT87Z
0HPT8JZ
0HPT8KZ
0HPT8NZ
0HPT8YZ
0HPTX0Z
0HPTX1Z
0HPTX7Z
0HPTXJZ
0HPTXKZ
0HPU00Z
0HPU01Z
0HPU07Z
0HPU0JZ
0HPU0KZ
0HPU0NZ
0HPU0YZ
0HPU30Z
0HPU31Z
0HPU37Z
0HPU3JZ
0HPU3KZ
0HPU3NZ
0HPU3YZ
0HPU70Z
0HPU71Z
0HPU77Z
0HPU7JZ
0HPU7KZ
0HPU7NZ
0HPU7YZ
0HPU80Z
0HPU81Z
0HPU87Z
0HPU8JZ
0HPU8KZ
0HPU8NZ
0HPU8YZ
0HPUX0Z
0HPUX1Z
0HPUX7Z
0HPUXJZ
0HPUXKZ
0HQ0XZZ
0HQ1XZZ
0HQ2XZZ
0HQ3XZZ
0HQ4XZZ
0HQ5XZZ
0HQ6XZZ
0HQ7XZZ
0HQ8XZZ
0HQ9XZZ
0HQAXZZ
0HQBXZZ
0HQCXZZ
0HQDXZZ
0HQEXZZ
0HQFXZZ
0HQGXZZ
0HQHXZZ
0HQJXZZ
0HQKXZZ
0HQLXZZ
0HQMXZZ
0HQNXZZ
0HQQXZZ
0HQRXZZ
0HQT0ZZ
0HQT3ZZ
0HQT7ZZ
0HQT8ZZ
0HQTXZZ
0HQU0ZZ
0HQU3ZZ
0HQU7ZZ
0HQU8ZZ
0HQUXZZ
0HQV0ZZ
0HQV3ZZ
0HQV7ZZ
0HQV8ZZ
0HQVXZZ
0HQW0ZZ
0HQW3ZZ
0HQW7ZZ
0HQW8ZZ
0HQWXZZ
0HQX0ZZ
0HQX3ZZ
0HQX7ZZ
0HQX8ZZ
0HQXXZZ
0HQYXZZ
0HR7X74
0HR7XJ3
0HR7XJ4
0HR7XJZ
0HR7XK3
0HR7XK4
0HR8X73
0HR8X74
0HR8XJ3
0HR8XJ4
0HR8XJZ
0HR8XK3
0HR8XK4
0HR9X73
0HR9X74
0HR9XJ3
0HR9XJ4
0HR9XJZ
0HR9XK3
0HR9XK4
0HRAX73
0HRAX74
0HRAXJ3
0HRAXJ4
0HRAXJZ
0HRAXK3
0HRAXK4
0HRBX73
0HRBX74
0HRBXJ3
0HRBXJ4
0HRBXJZ
0HRBXK3
0HRBXK4
0HRCX73

0HRCX74
0HRCXJ3
0HRCXJ4
0HRCXJZ
0HRCXK3
0HRCXK4
0HRDX73
0HRDX74
0HRDXJ3
0HRDXJ4
0HRDXJZ
0HRDXK3
0HRDXK4
0HREX73
0HREX74
0HREXJ3
0HREXJ4
0HREXJZ
0HREXK3
0HREXK4
0HRFX73
0HRFX74
0HRFXJ3
0HRFXJ4
0HRFXJZ
0HRFXK3
0HRFXK4
0HRGX73
0HRGX74
0HRGXJ3
0HRGXJ4
0HRGXJZ
0HRGXK3
0HRGXK4
0HRHX73
0HRHX74
0HRHXJ3
0HRHXJ4
0HRHXJZ
0HRHXK3
0HRHXK4
0HRJX73
0HRJX74
0HRJXJ3
0HRJXJ4
0HRJXJZ
0HRJXK3
0HRJXK4
0HRKX73
0HRKX74
0HRKXJ3
0HRKXJ4
0HRKXJZ
0HRKXK3
0HRKXK4
0HRLX73
0HRLX74
0HRLXJ3
0HRLXJ4
0HRLXJZ
0HRSX7Z
0HRT37Z
0HRU37Z
0HRV37Z
0HSSXZZ
0HTQXZZ
0HTRXZZ
0HTT0ZZ
0HTU0ZZ
0HTV0ZZ
0HUT3JZ
0HUT8KZ
0HUTX7Z
0HUTXJZ
0HUTXKZ
0HUU07Z
0HUU0JZ
0HUU0KZ
0HUU37Z
0HUU3JZ
0HUU3KZ
0HUU77Z
0HUU7JZ
0HUU7KZ
0HUU87Z
0HUU8JZ
0HUU8KZ
0HUUX7Z
0HUUXJZ
0HUUXKZ
0HUV07Z
0HUV0JZ
0HUV0KZ
0HUV37Z
0HUV3JZ
0HUV3KZ
0HUV77Z
0HUV7JZ
0HUV7KZ
0HUV87Z
0HUV8JZ
0HUV8KZ
0HUVX7Z
0HUVXJZ
0HUVXKZ
0HUW07Z
0HUW0JZ
0HUW0KZ
0HUW37Z
0HUW3JZ
0HUW3KZ
0HUW77Z
0HUW7JZ
0HUW7KZ
0HUW87Z
0HUW8JZ
0HUW8KZ
0HUWX7Z
0HUWXJZ
0HUWXKZ
0HUX07Z
0HUX0JZ
0HUX0KZ
0HUX37Z
0HUX3JZ
0HUX3KZ
0HUX77Z
0HUX7JZ
0HUX7KZ
0HUX87Z
0HUX8JZ
0HUX8KZ
0HUXX7Z
0HUXXJZ
0HUXXKZ
0HWPX0Z
0HWPX7Z
0HWPXJZ
0HWPXKZ
0HWPXYZ
0HWQX0Z
0HWQX7Z
0HWQXJZ
0HWQXKZ
0HWRX0Z
0HWRX7Z
0HWRXJZ
0HWRXKZ
0HWSX7Z
0HWSXJZ
0HWSXKZ
0HWT00Z
0HWT07Z
0HWT0JZ
0HWT0KZ
0HWT0NZ
0HWT0YZ
0HWT30Z
0HWT37Z
0HWT3JZ
0HWT3KZ
0HWT3NZ
0HWT3YZ
0HWT70Z
0HWT77Z
0HWT7JZ
0HWT7KZ
0HWT7NZ
0HWT7YZ
0HWT80Z
0HWT87Z
0HWT8JZ
0HWT8KZ
0HWT8NZ
0HWT8YZ
0HWTX0Z
0HWTX7Z
0HWTXJZ
0HWTXKZ
0HWU00Z
0HWU07Z
0HWU0JZ
0HWU0KZ
0HWU0NZ
0HWU0YZ
0HWU30Z
0HWU37Z
0HWU3JZ
0HWU3KZ
0HWU3NZ
0HWU3YZ
0HWU70Z
0HWU77Z
0HWU7JZ
0HWU7KZ
0HWU7NZ
0HWU7YZ
0HWU80Z
0HWU87Z
0HWU8JZ
0HWU8KZ
0HWU8NZ
0HWU8YZ
0HWUX0Z
0HWUX7Z
0HWUXJZ
0HWUXKZ
0HX0XZZ
0HX1XZZ
0HX2XZZ
0HX3XZZ
0HX4XZZ
0HX5XZZ
0HX6XZZ
0HX7XZZ
0HX8XZZ
0HX9XZZ
0HXAXZZ
0HXBXZZ
0HXCXZZ
0HXDXZZ
0HXEXZZ
0HXFXZZ
0HXGXZZ
0HXHXZZ
0HXJXZZ
0HXKXZZ
0HXLXZZ
0HXMXZZ
0HXNXZZ
0J010ZZ
0J013ZZ
0J040ZZ
0J043ZZ
0J050ZZ
0J053ZZ
0J060ZZ
0J063ZZ
0J070ZZ
0J073ZZ
0J080ZZ
0J083ZZ
0J090ZZ
0J093ZZ
0J0D0ZZ
0J0D3ZZ
0J0F0ZZ
0J0F3ZZ
0J0G0ZZ
0J0G3ZZ
0J0H0ZZ
0J0H3ZZ
0J0L0ZZ
0J0L3ZZ
0J0M0ZZ
0J0M3ZZ
0J0N0ZZ
0J0N3ZZ
0J0P0ZZ
0J0P3ZZ
0J2SX0Z
0J2SXYZ
0J2TX0Z
0J2TXYZ
0J2VX0Z
0J2VXYZ
0J2WX0Z
0J2WXYZ
0J500ZZ
0J503ZZ
0J510ZZ
0J513ZZ
0J540ZZ
0J543ZZ
0J550ZZ
0J553ZZ
0J560ZZ
0J563ZZ
0J570ZZ
0J573ZZ
0J580ZZ
0J583ZZ
0J590ZZ
0J593ZZ
0J5B0ZZ
0J5B3ZZ
0J5C0ZZ
0J5C3ZZ
0J5D0ZZ
0J5D3ZZ
0J5F0ZZ
0J5F3ZZ
0J5G0ZZ
0J5G3ZZ
0J5H0ZZ
0J5H3ZZ
0J5J0ZZ
0J5J3ZZ
0J5K0ZZ
0J5K3ZZ
0J5L0ZZ
0J5L3ZZ
0J5M0ZZ
0J5M3ZZ
0J5N0ZZ
0J5N3ZZ
0J5P0ZZ
0J5P3ZZ
0J5Q0ZZ
0J5Q3ZZ
0J5R0ZZ
0J5R3ZZ
0J800ZZ
0J803ZZ
0J810ZZ
0J813ZZ
0J840ZZ
0J843ZZ
0J850ZZ
0J853ZZ
0J860ZZ
0J863ZZ
0J870ZZ
0J873ZZ
0J880ZZ
0J883ZZ
0J890ZZ
0J893ZZ
0J8B0ZZ
0J8B3ZZ
0J8C0ZZ
0J8C3ZZ
0J8D0ZZ
0J8D3ZZ
0J8F0ZZ
0J8F3ZZ
0J8G0ZZ
0J8G3ZZ
0J8H0ZZ
0J8H3ZZ
0J8J0ZZ
0J8J3ZZ
0J8K0ZZ
0J8K3ZZ
0J8L0ZZ
0J8L3ZZ
0J8M0ZZ
0J8M3ZZ
0J8N0ZZ
0J8N3ZZ
0J8P0ZZ
0J8P3ZZ
0J8Q0ZZ
0J8Q3ZZ
0J8R0ZZ
0J8R3ZZ
0J8S0ZZ
0J8S3ZZ
0J8T0ZZ
0J8T3ZZ
0J8V0ZZ
0J8V3ZZ
0J8W0ZZ
0J8W3ZZ
0J9000Z
0J900ZX
0J900ZZ
0J9030Z
0J903ZX
0J903ZZ
0J9100Z
0J910ZX
0J910ZZ
0J9130Z
0J913ZX
0J913ZZ
0J9400Z
0J940ZX
0J940ZZ
0J9430Z
0J943ZX
0J943ZZ
0J9500Z
0J950ZX
0J950ZZ
0J9530Z
0J953ZX
0J953ZZ
0J9600Z
0J960ZX
0J960ZZ
0J9630Z
0J963ZX
0J963ZZ
0J9700Z
0J970ZX
0J970ZZ
0J9730Z
0J973ZX
0J973ZZ
0J9800Z
0J980ZX
0J980ZZ
0J9830Z
0J983ZX
0J983ZZ
0J9900Z
0J990ZX
0J990ZZ
0J9930Z
0J993ZX
0J993ZZ
0J9B00Z
0J9B0ZX
0J9B0ZZ
0J9B30Z
0J9B3ZX
0J9B3ZZ
0J9C00Z
0J9C0ZX
0J9C30Z
0J9C3ZX
0J9C3ZZ
0J9D00Z
0J9D0ZX
0J9D30Z
0J9D3ZX
0J9D3ZZ
0J9F00Z
0J9F0ZX
0J9F30Z
0J9F3ZX
0J9F3ZZ
0J9G00Z
0J9G0ZX
0J9G30Z
0J9G3ZX
0J9G3ZZ
0J9H00Z
0J9H0ZX
0J9H30Z
0J9H3ZX
0J9H3ZZ
0J9J00Z
0J9J0ZX
0J9J30Z
0J9J3ZX
0J9J3ZZ
0J9K00Z
0J9K0ZX
0J9K30Z
0J9K3ZX
0J9K3ZZ
0J9L00Z
0J9L0ZX
0J9L30Z
0J9L3ZX
0J9L3ZZ
0J9M00Z
0J9M0ZX
0J9M30Z
0J9M3ZX
0J9M3ZZ
0J9N00Z
0J9N0ZX
0J9N30Z
0J9N3ZX
0J9N3ZZ
0J9P00Z
0J9P0ZX
0J9P30Z
0J9P3ZX
0J9P3ZZ
0J9Q00Z
0J9Q0ZX
0J9Q30Z
0J9Q3ZX
0J9Q3ZZ
0J9R00Z
0J9R0ZX
0J9R30Z
0J9R3ZX
0J9R3ZZ
0JB00ZX
0JB03ZX
0JB10ZX
0JB13ZX
0JB40ZX
0JB43ZX
0JB50ZX
0JB53ZX
0JB60ZX
0JB63ZX
0JB70ZX
0JB73ZX
0JB80ZX
0JB83ZX
0JB90ZX
0JB93ZX
0JBB0ZX
0JBB3ZX
0JBC0ZX
0JBC3ZX
0JBD0ZX
0JBD3ZX
0JBF0ZX
0JBF3ZX
0JBG0ZX
0JBG3ZX
0JBH0ZX
0JBH3ZX
0JBJ0ZX
0JBJ3ZX
0JBK0ZX
0JBK3ZX
0JBL0ZX
0JBL3ZX
0JBM0ZX
0JBM3ZX
0JBN0ZX
0JBN3ZX
0JBP0ZX
0JBP3ZX
0JBQ0ZX
0JBQ3ZX
0JBR0ZX
0JBR3ZX
0JBR3ZZ
0JC00ZZ
0JC03ZZ
0JC10ZZ
0JC13ZZ
0JC40ZZ
0JC43ZZ
0JC50ZZ
0JC53ZZ
0JC60ZZ
0JC63ZZ
0JC70ZZ
0JC73ZZ
0JC80ZZ
0JC83ZZ
0JC90ZZ
0JC93ZZ
0JCB0ZZ
0JCB3ZZ
0JCC0ZZ
0JCC3ZZ
0JCD0ZZ
0JCD3ZZ
0JCF0ZZ
0JCF3ZZ
0JCG0ZZ
0JCG3ZZ
0JCH0ZZ
0JCH3ZZ
0JCJ0ZZ
0JCJ3ZZ
0JCK0ZZ
0JCK3ZZ
0JCL0ZZ
0JCL3ZZ
0JCM0ZZ
0JCM3ZZ
0JCN0ZZ
0JCN3ZZ
0JCP0ZZ
0JCP3ZZ
0JCQ0ZZ
0JCQ3ZZ
0JCR0ZZ
0JCR3ZZ
0JD00ZZ
0JD03ZZ
0JD10ZZ
0JD13ZZ
0JD40ZZ
0JD43ZZ
0JD50ZZ
0JD53ZZ
0JD60ZZ
0JD63ZZ
0JD70ZZ
0JD73ZZ
0JD80ZZ
0JD83ZZ
0JD90ZZ
0JD93ZZ
0JDB0ZZ
0JDB3ZZ
0JDC0ZZ
0JDC3ZZ
0JDD0ZZ
0JDD3ZZ
0JDF0ZZ
0JDF3ZZ
0JDG0ZZ
0JDG3ZZ
0JDH0ZZ
0JDH3ZZ
0JDJ0ZZ
0JDJ3ZZ
0JDK0ZZ
0JDK3ZZ
0JDL0ZZ
0JDL3ZZ
0JDM0ZZ
0JDM3ZZ
0JDN0ZZ
0JDN3ZZ
0JDP0ZZ
0JDP3ZZ
0JDQ0ZZ
0JDQ3ZZ
0JDR0ZZ
0JDR3ZZ
0JH00NZ
0JH03NZ
0JH10NZ
0JH13NZ
0JH40NZ
0JH43NZ
0JH50NZ
0JH53NZ
0JH600Z
0JH602Z
0JH604Z
0JH605Z
0JH606Z
0JH607Z
0JH608Z
0JH609Z
0JH60AZ
0JH60BZ
0JH60CZ
0JH60DZ
0JH60EZ
0JH60HZ
0JH60MZ
0JH60NZ
0JH60PZ
0JH60VZ
0JH60WZ
0JH60XZ
0JH630Z
0JH632Z
0JH634Z
0JH635Z
0JH636Z
0JH637Z
0JH638Z
0JH639Z
0JH63AZ
0JH63BZ
0JH63CZ
0JH63DZ
0JH63EZ
0JH63HZ
0JH63MZ
0JH63NZ
0JH63PZ
0JH63VZ
0JH63WZ
0JH63XZ
0JH70BZ
0JH70CZ
0JH70DZ
0JH70EZ
0JH70MZ
0JH70NZ
0JH70VZ
0JH73BZ
0JH73CZ
0JH73DZ
0JH73EZ
0JH73MZ
0JH73NZ
0JH73VZ
0JH800Z
0JH802Z
0JH804Z
0JH805Z
0JH806Z
0JH807Z
0JH808Z
0JH809Z
0JH80AZ
0JH80BZ
0JH80CZ
0JH80DZ
0JH80EZ
0JH80HZ
0JH80MZ
0JH80NZ
0JH80PZ
0JH80VZ
0JH80WZ
0JH80XZ
0JH830Z
0JH832Z
0JH834Z
0JH835Z
0JH836Z
0JH837Z
0JH838Z
0JH839Z
0JH83AZ
0JH83BZ
0JH83CZ
0JH83DZ
0JH83EZ
0JH83HZ
0JH83MZ
0JH83NZ
0JH83PZ
0JH83VZ
0JH83WZ
0JH83XZ
0JH90NZ
0JH93NZ
0JHB0NZ
0JHB3NZ
0JHC0NZ
0JHC3NZ
0JHD0HZ
0JHD0NZ

0JHD0VZ
0JHD0WZ
0JHD0XZ
0JHD3HZ
0JHD3NZ
0JHD3VZ
0JHD3WZ
0JHD3XZ
0JHF0HZ
0JHF0NZ
0JHF0VZ
0JHF0WZ
0JHF0XZ
0JHF3HZ
0JHF3NZ
0JHF3VZ
0JHF3WZ
0JHF3XZ
0JHG0HZ
0JHG0NZ
0JHG0VZ
0JHG0WZ
0JHG0XZ
0JHG3HZ
0JHG3NZ
0JHG3VZ
0JHG3WZ
0JHG3XZ
0JHH0HZ
0JHH0NZ
0JHH0VZ
0JHH0WZ
0JHH0XZ
0JHH3HZ
0JHH3NZ
0JHH3VZ
0JHH3WZ
0JHH3XZ
0JHJ0NZ
0JHJ3NZ
0JHK0NZ
0JHK3NZ
0JHL0HZ
0JHL0NZ
0JHL0VZ
0JHL3HZ
0JHM0HZ
0JHM3HZ
0JHN0HZ
0JHS03Z
0JHS33Z
0JHS3YZ
0JHT03Z
0JHT33Z
0JHT3YZ
0JHV03Z
0JHV33Z
0JHV3YZ
0JHW03Z
0JHW33Z
0JHW3YZ
0JJS0ZZ
0JJS3ZZ
0JJSXZZ
0JJT0ZZ
0JJT3ZZ
0JJTXZZ
0JJV0ZZ
0JJV3ZZ
0JJVXZZ
0JJW0ZZ
0JJW3ZZ
0JJWXZZ
0JN0XZZ
0JN1XZZ
0JN4XZZ
0JN5XZZ
0JN6XZZ
0JN7XZZ
0JN8XZZ
0JN9XZZ
0JNBXZZ
0JNCXZZ
0JNDXZZ
0JNFXZZ
0JNGXZZ
0JNHXZZ
0JNJXZZ
0JNKXZZ
0JNLXZZ
0JNMXZZ
0JNNXZZ
0JNPXZZ
0JNQXZZ
0JNRXZZ
0JPS00Z
0JPS01Z
0JPS03Z
0JPS07Z
0JPS0JZ
0JPS0KZ
0JPS0NZ
0JPS0YZ
0JPS30Z
0JPS31Z
0JPS33Z
0JPS37Z
0JPS3JZ
0JPS3KZ
0JPS3NZ
0JPS3YZ
0JPSX0Z
0JPSX1Z
0JPSX3Z
0JPT00Z
0JPT01Z
0JPT02Z
0JPT03Z
0JPT07Z
0JPT0HZ
0JPT0JZ
0JPT0KZ
0JPT0MZ
0JPT0NZ
0JPT0VZ
0JPT0WZ
0JPT0XZ
0JPT0YZ
0JPT30Z
0JPT31Z
0JPT32Z
0JPT33Z
0JPT37Z
0JPT3HZ
0JPT3JZ
0JPT3KZ
0JPT3MZ
0JPT3NZ
0JPT3VZ
0JPT3WZ
0JPT3XZ
0JPT3YZ
0JPTX0Z
0JPTX1Z
0JPTX2Z
0JPTX3Z
0JPTXHZ
0JPTXVZ
0JPTXXZ
0JPV00Z
0JPV01Z
0JPV03Z
0JPV07Z
0JPV0HZ
0JPV0JZ
0JPV0KZ
0JPV0NZ
0JPV0VZ
0JPV0WZ
0JPV0XZ
0JPV0YZ
0JPV30Z
0JPV31Z
0JPV33Z
0JPV37Z
0JPV3HZ
0JPV3JZ
0JPV3KZ
0JPV3NZ
0JPV3VZ
0JPV3WZ
0JPV3XZ
0JPV3YZ
0JPVX0Z
0JPVX1Z
0JPVX3Z
0JPVXHZ
0JPVXVZ
0JPVXXZ
0JPW00Z
0JPW01Z
0JPW03Z
0JPW07Z
0JPW0HZ
0JPW0JZ
0JPW0KZ
0JPW0NZ
0JPW0VZ
0JPW0WZ
0JPW0XZ
0JPW0YZ
0JPW30Z
0JPW31Z
0JPW33Z
0JPW37Z
0JPW3HZ
0JPW3JZ
0JPW3KZ
0JPW3NZ
0JPW3VZ
0JPW3WZ
0JPW3XZ
0JPW3YZ
0JPWX0Z
0JPWX1Z
0JPWX3Z
0JPWXHZ
0JPWXVZ
0JPWXXZ
0JQ03ZZ
0JQ13ZZ
0JQ43ZZ
0JQ53ZZ
0JQ63ZZ
0JQ73ZZ
0JQ83ZZ
0JQ93ZZ
0JQB3ZZ
0JQC3ZZ
0JQD3ZZ
0JQF3ZZ
0JQG0ZZ
0JQG3ZZ
0JQH0ZZ
0JQH3ZZ
0JQJ0ZZ
0JQJ3ZZ
0JQK0ZZ
0JQK3ZZ
0JQL0ZZ
0JQL3ZZ
0JQM0ZZ
0JQM3ZZ
0JQN0ZZ
0JQN3ZZ
0JQP0ZZ
0JQP3ZZ
0JQQ0ZZ
0JQQ3ZZ
0JQR0ZZ
0JQR3ZZ
0JR007Z
0JR00JZ
0JR00KZ
0JR037Z
0JR03JZ
0JR03KZ
0JR107Z
0JR10JZ
0JR10KZ
0JR137Z
0JR13JZ
0JR13KZ
0JR407Z
0JR40JZ
0JR40KZ
0JR437Z
0JR43JZ
0JR43KZ
0JR507Z
0JR50JZ
0JR50KZ
0JR537Z
0JR53JZ
0JR53KZ
0JR607Z
0JR60JZ
0JR60KZ
0JR637Z
0JR63JZ
0JR63KZ
0JR707Z
0JR70JZ
0JR70KZ
0JR737Z
0JR73JZ
0JR73KZ
0JR807Z
0JR80JZ
0JR80KZ
0JR837Z
0JR83JZ
0JR83KZ
0JR907Z
0JR90JZ
0JR90KZ
0JR937Z
0JR93JZ
0JR93KZ
0JRB07Z
0JRB0JZ
0JRB0KZ
0JRB37Z
0JRB3JZ
0JRB3KZ
0JRC07Z
0JRC0JZ
0JRC0KZ
0JRC37Z
0JRC3JZ
0JRC3KZ
0JRD07Z
0JRD0JZ
0JRD0KZ
0JRD37Z
0JRD3JZ
0JRD3KZ
0JRF07Z
0JRF0JZ
0JRF0KZ
0JRF37Z
0JRF3JZ
0JRF3KZ
0JRG07Z
0JRG0JZ
0JRG0KZ
0JRG37Z
0JRG3JZ
0JRG3KZ
0JRH07Z
0JRH0JZ
0JRH0KZ
0JRH37Z
0JRH3JZ
0JRH3KZ
0JRJ07Z
0JRJ0JZ
0JRJ0KZ
0JRJ37Z
0JRJ3JZ
0JRJ3KZ
0JRK07Z
0JRK0JZ
0JRK0KZ
0JRK37Z
0JRK3JZ
0JRK3KZ
0JRL07Z
0JRL0JZ
0JRL0KZ
0JRL37Z
0JRL3JZ
0JRL3KZ
0JRM07Z
0JRM0JZ
0JRM0KZ
0JRM37Z
0JRM3JZ
0JRM3KZ
0JRN07Z
0JRN0JZ
0JRN0KZ
0JRN37Z
0JRN3JZ
0JRN3KZ
0JRP07Z
0JRP0JZ
0JRP0KZ
0JRP37Z
0JRP3JZ
0JRP3KZ
0JRQ07Z
0JRQ0JZ
0JRQ0KZ
0JRQ37Z
0JRQ3JZ
0JRQ3KZ
0JRR07Z
0JRR0JZ
0JRR0KZ
0JRR37Z
0JRR3JZ
0JRR3KZ
0JU007Z
0JU00JZ
0JU00KZ
0JU037Z
0JU03JZ
0JU03KZ
0JU107Z
0JU10JZ
0JU10KZ
0JU137Z
0JU13JZ
0JU13KZ
0JU407Z
0JU40JZ
0JU40KZ
0JU437Z
0JU43JZ
0JU43KZ
0JU507Z
0JU50JZ
0JU50KZ
0JU537Z
0JU53JZ
0JU53KZ
0JU607Z
0JU60JZ
0JU60KZ
0JU637Z
0JU63JZ
0JU63KZ
0JU707Z
0JU70JZ
0JU70KZ
0JU737Z
0JU73JZ
0JU73KZ
0JU807Z
0JU80JZ
0JU80KZ
0JU837Z
0JU83JZ
0JU83KZ
0JU907Z
0JU90JZ
0JU90KZ
0JU937Z
0JU93JZ
0JU93KZ
0JUB07Z
0JUB0JZ
0JUB0KZ
0JUB37Z
0JUB3JZ
0JUB3KZ
0JUC07Z
0JUC0JZ
0JUC0KZ
0JUC37Z
0JUC3JZ
0JUC3KZ
0JUD07Z
0JUD0JZ
0JUD0KZ
0JUD37Z
0JUD3JZ
0JUD3KZ
0JUF07Z
0JUF0JZ
0JUF0KZ
0JUF37Z
0JUF3JZ
0JUF3KZ
0JUG07Z
0JUG0JZ
0JUG0KZ
0JUG37Z
0JUG3JZ
0JUG3KZ
0JUH07Z
0JUH0JZ
0JUH0KZ
0JUH37Z
0JUH3JZ
0JUH3KZ
0JWSX0Z
0JWSX3Z
0JWSX7Z
0JWSXJZ
0JWSXKZ
0JWSXNZ
0JWT3YZ
0JWTX0Z
0JWTX2Z
0JWTX3Z
0JWTX7Z
0JWTXHZ
0JWTXJZ
0JWTXKZ
0JWTXNZ
0JWTXPZ
0JWTXVZ
0JWTXWZ
0JWTXXZ
0JWVX0Z
0JWVX3Z
0JWVX7Z
0JWVXHZ
0JWVXJZ
0JWVXKZ
0JWVXNZ
0JWVXVZ
0JWVXWZ
0JWVXXZ
0JWWX0Z
0JWWX3Z
0JWWX7Z
0JWWXHZ
0JWWXJZ
0JWWXKZ
0JWWXNZ
0JWWXVZ
0JWWXWZ
0JWWXXZ
0JX43ZC
0JX43ZZ
0JX50ZB
0JX50ZC
0JX50ZZ
0JX53ZB
0JX53ZC
0JX53ZZ
0JX60ZB
0JX60ZC
0JX60ZZ
0JX63ZB
0JX63ZC
0JX63ZZ
0JX70ZB
0JX70ZC
0JX70ZZ
0JX73ZB
0JX73ZC
0JX73ZZ
0JX80ZB
0JX80ZC
0JX80ZZ
0JX83ZB
0JX83ZC
0JX83ZZ
0JX90ZB
0JX90ZC
0JX90ZZ
0JX93ZB
0JX93ZC
0JX93ZZ
0JXB0ZB
0JXB0ZC
0JXB0ZZ
0JXB3ZB
0JXB3ZC
0JXB3ZZ
0JXC0ZB
0JXC0ZC
0JXC0ZZ
0JXC3ZB
0JXC3ZC
0JXC3ZZ
0JXD0ZB
0JXD0ZC
0JXD0ZZ
0JXD3ZB
0JXD3ZC
0JXD3ZZ
0JXF0ZB
0JXF0ZC
0JXF0ZZ
0JXF3ZB
0JXF3ZC
0JXF3ZZ
0JXG0ZB
0JXG0ZC
0JXG0ZZ
0JXG3ZB
0JXG3ZC
0JXG3ZZ
0JXH0ZB
0JXH0ZC
0JXH0ZZ
0JXH3ZB
0JXH3ZC
0JXH3ZZ
0JXJ0ZB
0JXJ0ZC
0JXJ0ZZ
0JXJ3ZB
0JXJ3ZC
0JXJ3ZZ
0JXK0ZB
0JXK0ZC
0JXK0ZZ
0JXK3ZB
0JXK3ZC
0JXK3ZZ
0JXL0ZB
0JXL0ZC
0JXL0ZZ
0JXL3ZB
0JXL3ZC
0JXL3ZZ
0JXM0ZB
0JXM0ZC
0JXM0ZZ
0JXM3ZB
0JXM3ZC
0JXM3ZZ
0JXN0ZB
0JXN0ZC
0JXN0ZZ
0JXN3ZB
0JXN3ZC
0JXN3ZZ
0JXP0ZB
0JXP0ZC
0JXP0ZZ
0JXP3ZB
0JXP3ZC
0JXP3ZZ
0JXQ0ZB
0JXQ0ZC
0JXQ0ZZ
0JXQ3ZB
0JXQ3ZC
0K2XX0Z
0K2XXYZ
0K2YX0Z
0K2YXYZ
0K820ZZ
0K823ZZ
0K824ZZ
0K830ZZ
0K833ZZ
0K834ZZ
0K840ZZ
0K843ZZ
0K844ZZ
0K850ZZ
0K853ZZ
0K854ZZ
0K860ZZ
0K863ZZ
0K864ZZ
0K870ZZ
0K873ZZ
0K874ZZ
0K880ZZ
0K883ZZ
0K884ZZ
0K890ZZ
0K893ZZ
0K894ZZ
0K8B0ZZ
0K8B3ZZ
0K8B4ZZ
0K8C0ZZ
0K8C3ZZ
0K8C4ZZ
0K8D0ZZ
0K8D3ZZ
0K8D4ZZ
0K8F0ZZ
0K8F3ZZ
0K8F4ZZ
0K8G0ZZ
0K8G3ZZ
0K8G4ZZ
0K8H0ZZ
0K8H3ZZ
0K8H4ZZ
0K8J0ZZ
0K8J3ZZ
0K8J4ZZ
0K8K0ZZ
0K8K3ZZ
0K8K4ZZ
0K8L0ZZ
0K8L3ZZ
0K8L4ZZ
0K8M0ZZ
0K8M3ZZ
0K8M4ZZ
0K8N0ZZ
0K8N3ZZ
0K8N4ZZ
0K8P0ZZ
0K8P3ZZ
0K8P4ZZ
0K8Q0ZZ
0K8Q3ZZ
0K8Q4ZZ
0K8R0ZZ
0K8R3ZZ
0K8R4ZZ
0K8S0ZZ
0K8S3ZZ
0K8S4ZZ
0K8T0ZZ
0K8T3ZZ
0K8T4ZZ
0K8V0ZZ
0K8V3ZZ
0K8V4ZZ
0K8W0ZZ
0K8W3ZZ
0K8W4ZZ
0K9000Z
0K900ZX
0K900ZZ
0K9030Z
0K903ZX
0K903ZZ
0K9040Z
0K904ZX
0K904ZZ
0K9100Z
0K910ZX
0K910ZZ
0K9130Z
0K913ZX
0K913ZZ
0K9140Z
0K914ZX
0K914ZZ
0K9200Z
0K920ZX
0K920ZZ
0K9230Z
0K923ZX
0K923ZZ
0K9240Z
0K924ZX
0K924ZZ
0K9300Z
0K930ZX
0K930ZZ
0K9330Z
0K933ZX
0K933ZZ
0K9340Z
0K934ZX
0K934ZZ
0K9400Z
0K940ZX
0K940ZZ

0K9430Z
0K943ZX
0K943ZZ
0K9440Z
0K944ZX
0K944ZZ
0K9500Z
0K950ZX
0K950ZZ
0K9530Z
0K953ZX
0K953ZZ
0K9540Z
0K954ZX
0K954ZZ
0K9600Z
0K960ZX
0K960ZZ
0K9630Z
0K963ZX
0K963ZZ
0K9640Z
0K964ZX
0K964ZZ
0K9700Z
0K970ZX
0K970ZZ
0K9730Z
0K973ZX
0K973ZZ
0K9740Z
0K974ZX
0K974ZZ
0K9800Z
0K980ZX
0K980ZZ
0K9830Z
0K983ZX
0K983ZZ
0K9840Z
0K984ZX
0K984ZZ
0K9900Z
0K990ZX
0K990ZZ
0K9930Z
0K993ZX
0K993ZZ
0K9940Z
0K994ZX
0K994ZZ
0K9B00Z
0K9B0ZX
0K9B0ZZ
0K9B30Z
0K9B3ZX
0K9B3ZZ
0K9B40Z
0K9B4ZX
0K9B4ZZ
0K9C00Z
0K9C0ZX
0K9C0ZZ
0K9C30Z
0K9C3ZX
0K9C3ZZ
0K9C40Z
0K9C4ZX
0K9C4ZZ
0K9D00Z
0K9D0ZX
0K9D0ZZ
0K9D30Z
0K9D3ZX
0K9D3ZZ
0K9D40Z
0K9D4ZX
0K9D4ZZ
0K9F00Z
0K9F0ZX
0K9F0ZZ
0K9F30Z
0K9F3ZX
0K9F3ZZ
0K9F40Z
0K9F4ZX
0K9F4ZZ
0K9G00Z
0K9G0ZX
0K9G0ZZ
0K9G30Z
0K9G3ZX
0K9G3ZZ
0K9G40Z
0K9G4ZX
0K9G4ZZ
0K9H00Z
0K9H0ZX
0K9H0ZZ
0K9H30Z
0K9H3ZX
0K9H3ZZ
0K9H40Z
0K9H4ZX
0K9H4ZZ
0K9J00Z
0K9J0ZX
0K9J0ZZ
0K9J30Z
0K9J3ZX
0K9J3ZZ
0K9J40Z
0K9J4ZX
0K9J4ZZ
0K9K00Z
0K9K0ZX
0K9K0ZZ
0K9K30Z
0K9K3ZX
0K9K3ZZ
0K9K40Z
0K9K4ZX
0K9K4ZZ
0K9L00Z
0K9L0ZX
0K9L0ZZ
0K9L30Z
0K9L3ZX
0K9L3ZZ
0K9L40Z
0K9L4ZX
0K9L4ZZ
0K9M00Z
0K9M0ZX
0K9M0ZZ
0K9M30Z
0K9M3ZX
0K9M3ZZ
0K9M40Z
0K9M4ZX
0K9M4ZZ
0K9N00Z
0K9N0ZX
0K9N0ZZ
0K9N30Z
0K9N3ZX
0K9N3ZZ
0K9N40Z
0K9N4ZX
0K9N4ZZ
0K9P00Z
0K9P0ZX
0K9P0ZZ
0K9P30Z
0K9P3ZX
0K9P3ZZ
0K9P40Z
0K9P4ZX
0K9P4ZZ
0K9Q00Z
0K9Q0ZX
0K9Q0ZZ
0K9Q30Z
0K9Q3ZX
0K9Q3ZZ
0K9Q40Z
0K9Q4ZX
0K9Q4ZZ
0K9R00Z
0K9R0ZX
0K9R0ZZ
0K9R30Z
0K9R3ZX
0K9R3ZZ
0K9R40Z
0K9R4ZX
0K9R4ZZ
0K9S00Z
0K9S0ZX
0K9S0ZZ
0K9S30Z
0K9S3ZX
0K9S3ZZ
0K9S40Z
0K9S4ZX
0K9S4ZZ
0K9T00Z
0K9T0ZX
0K9T0ZZ
0K9T30Z
0K9T3ZX
0K9T3ZZ
0K9T40Z
0K9T4ZX
0K9T4ZZ
0K9V00Z
0K9V0ZX
0K9V0ZZ
0K9V30Z
0K9V3ZX
0K9V3ZZ
0K9V40Z
0K9V4ZX
0K9V4ZZ
0K9W00Z
0K9W0ZX
0K9W30Z
0K9W3ZZ
0KBM0ZZ
0KBM3ZX
0KBM3ZZ
0KBM4ZX
0KBM4ZZ
0KBN0ZX
0KBN0ZZ
0KBN3ZX
0KBN3ZZ
0KBN4ZX
0KBN4ZZ
0KBP0ZX
0KBP0ZZ
0KBP3ZX
0KBP3ZZ
0KBP4ZX
0KBP4ZZ
0KBQ0ZX
0KBQ0ZZ
0KBQ3ZX
0KBQ3ZZ
0KBQ4ZX
0KBQ4ZZ
0KBR0ZX
0KBR0ZZ
0KBR3ZX
0KBR3ZZ
0KBR4ZX
0KBR4ZZ
0KBS0ZX
0KBS0ZZ
0KBS3ZX
0KBS3ZZ
0KBS4ZX
0KBS4ZZ
0KBT0ZX
0KBT0ZZ
0KBT3ZX
0KBT3ZZ
0KBT4ZX
0KBT4ZZ
0KBV0ZX
0KBV0ZZ
0KBV3ZX
0KBV3ZZ
0KBV4ZX
0KBV4ZZ
0KBW0ZX
0KBW0ZZ
0KBW3ZX
0KBW3ZZ
0KBW4ZX
0KBW4ZZ
0KC00ZZ
0KC03ZZ
0KC04ZZ
0KC10ZZ
0KC13ZZ
0KC14ZZ
0KC20ZZ
0KC23ZZ
0KC24ZZ
0KC30ZZ
0KC33ZZ
0KC34ZZ
0KC40ZZ
0KC43ZZ
0KC44ZZ
0KC50ZZ
0KC53ZZ
0KC54ZZ
0KC60ZZ
0KC63ZZ
0KC64ZZ
0KC70ZZ
0KC73ZZ
0KC74ZZ
0KC80ZZ
0KC83ZZ
0KC84ZZ
0KC90ZZ
0KC93ZZ
0KC94ZZ
0KCB0ZZ
0KCB3ZZ
0KCB4ZZ
0KCC0ZZ
0KCC3ZZ
0KCC4ZZ
0KCD0ZZ
0KCD3ZZ
0KCD4ZZ
0KCF0ZZ
0KCF3ZZ
0KCF4ZZ
0KCG0ZZ
0KCG3ZZ
0KCG4ZZ
0KCH0ZZ
0KCH3ZZ
0KCH4ZZ
0KCJ0ZZ
0KCJ3ZZ
0KCJ4ZZ
0KCK0ZZ
0KCK3ZZ
0KCK4ZZ
0KCL0ZZ
0KCL3ZZ
0KCL4ZZ
0KCM0ZZ
0KCM3ZZ
0KCM4ZZ
0KCN0ZZ
0KCN3ZZ
0KCN4ZZ
0KCP0ZZ
0KCP3ZZ
0KCP4ZZ
0KCQ0ZZ
0KCQ3ZZ
0KCQ4ZZ
0KCR0ZZ
0KCR3ZZ
0KCR4ZZ
0KCS0ZZ
0KCS3ZZ
0KCS4ZZ
0KCT0ZZ
0KCT3ZZ
0KCT4ZZ
0KCV0ZZ
0KCV3ZZ
0KCV4ZZ
0KCW0ZZ
0KCW3ZZ
0KCW4ZZ
0KD00ZZ
0KD10ZZ
0KD20ZZ
0KD30ZZ
0KD40ZZ
0KD50ZZ
0KD60ZZ
0KD70ZZ
0KD80ZZ
0KD90ZZ
0KDB0ZZ
0KDC0ZZ
0KDD0ZZ
0KDF0ZZ
0KDG0ZZ
0KDH0ZZ
0KDJ0ZZ
0KDK0ZZ
0KDL0ZZ
0KDM0ZZ
0KDN0ZZ
0KDP0ZZ
0KDQ0ZZ
0KDR0ZZ
0KDS0ZZ
0KDT0ZZ
0KDV0ZZ
0KDW0ZZ
0KHX0MZ
0KHX0YZ
0KHX3MZ
0KHX3YZ
0KHX4MZ
0KHX4YZ
0KHY0MZ
0KHY0YZ
0KHY3MZ
0KHY3YZ
0KHY4MZ
0KHY4YZ
0KJX0ZZ
0KJX3ZZ
0KJX4ZZ
0KJXXZZ
0KJY0ZZ
0KJY3ZZ
0KJY4ZZ
0KJYXZZ
0KM00ZZ
0KM04ZZ
0KM10ZZ
0KM14ZZ
0KM20ZZ
0KM24ZZ
0KM30ZZ
0KM34ZZ
0KM40ZZ
0KM44ZZ
0KM50ZZ
0KM54ZZ
0KM60ZZ
0KM64ZZ
0KM70ZZ
0KM74ZZ
0KM80ZZ
0KM84ZZ
0KM90ZZ
0KM94ZZ
0KMB0ZZ
0KMB4ZZ
0KMC0ZZ
0KMC4ZZ
0KMD0ZZ
0KMD4ZZ
0KMF0ZZ
0KMF4ZZ
0KMG0ZZ
0KMG4ZZ
0KMH0ZZ
0KMH4ZZ
0KMJ0ZZ
0KMJ4ZZ
0KMK0ZZ
0KMK4ZZ
0KML0ZZ
0KML4ZZ
0KMM0ZZ
0KMM4ZZ
0KMN0ZZ
0KMN4ZZ
0KMP0ZZ
0KMP4ZZ
0KMQ0ZZ
0KMQ4ZZ
0KN0XZZ
0KN1XZZ
0KN2XZZ
0KN3XZZ
0KN4XZZ
0KN5XZZ
0KN6XZZ
0KN7XZZ
0KN8XZZ
0KN9XZZ
0KNBXZZ
0KNCXZZ
0KNDXZZ
0KNFXZZ
0KNGXZZ
0KNHXZZ
0KNJXZZ
0KNKXZZ
0KNLXZZ
0KNMXZZ
0KNNXZZ
0KNPXZZ
0KNQXZZ
0KNRXZZ
0KNSXZZ
0KNTXZZ
0KNVXZZ
0KNWXZZ
0KPX3YZ
0KPX4YZ
0KPXX0Z
0KPXXMZ
0KPY3YZ
0KPY4YZ
0KPYX0Z
0KPYXMZ
0KQ93ZZ
0KQ94ZZ
0KQB0ZZ
0KQB3ZZ
0KQB4ZZ
0KQC0ZZ
0KQC3ZZ
0KQC4ZZ
0KQD0ZZ
0KQD3ZZ
0KQD4ZZ
0KQF0ZZ
0KQF3ZZ
0KQF4ZZ
0KQG0ZZ
0KQG3ZZ
0KQG4ZZ
0KQH0ZZ
0KQH3ZZ
0KQH4ZZ
0KQJ0ZZ
0KQJ3ZZ
0KQJ4ZZ
0KQK0ZZ
0KQK3ZZ
0KQK4ZZ
0KQL0ZZ
0KQL3ZZ
0KQL4ZZ
0KQM0ZZ
0KQM3ZZ
0KQM4ZZ
0KQN0ZZ
0KQN3ZZ
0KQN4ZZ
0KQP0ZZ
0KQP3ZZ
0KQP4ZZ
0KQQ0ZZ
0KQQ3ZZ
0KQQ4ZZ
0KQR0ZZ
0KQR3ZZ
0KQR4ZZ
0KQS0ZZ
0KQS3ZZ
0KQS4ZZ
0KQT0ZZ
0KQT3ZZ
0KQT4ZZ
0KQV0ZZ
0KQV3ZZ
0KQV4ZZ
0KQW0ZZ
0KQW3ZZ
0KQW4ZZ
0KR007Z
0KR00JZ
0KR00KZ
0KR047Z
0KR04JZ
0KR04KZ
0KR107Z
0KR10JZ
0KR10KZ
0KR147Z
0KR14JZ
0KR14KZ
0KR207Z
0KR20JZ
0KR20KZ
0KR247Z
0KR24JZ
0KR24KZ
0KR307Z
0KR30JZ
0KR30KZ
0KR347Z
0KR34JZ
0KR34KZ
0KR407Z
0KR40JZ
0KR40KZ
0KR447Z
0KR44JZ
0KR44KZ
0KR507Z
0KR50JZ
0KR50KZ
0KR547Z
0KR54JZ
0KR54KZ
0KR607Z
0KR60JZ
0KR60KZ
0KR647Z
0KR64JZ
0KR64KZ
0KR707Z
0KR70JZ
0KR70KZ
0KR747Z
0KR74JZ
0KR74KZ
0KR807Z
0KR80JZ
0KR80KZ
0KR847Z
0KR84JZ
0KR84KZ
0KR907Z
0KR90JZ
0KR90KZ
0KR947Z
0KR94JZ
0KR94KZ
0KRB07Z
0KRB0JZ
0KRB0KZ
0KRB47Z
0KRB4JZ
0KRB4KZ
0KRC07Z
0KRC0JZ
0KRC0KZ
0KRC47Z
0KRC4JZ
0KRC4KZ
0KRD07Z
0KRD0JZ
0KRD0KZ
0KRD47Z
0KRD4JZ
0KRD4KZ
0KRF07Z
0KRF0JZ
0KRF0KZ
0KRF47Z
0KRF4JZ
0KRF4KZ
0KRG07Z
0KRG0JZ
0KRG0KZ
0KRG47Z
0KRG4JZ
0KRG4KZ
0KRH07Z
0KRH0JZ
0KRH0KZ
0KRH47Z
0KRH4JZ
0KRH4KZ
0KRJ07Z
0KRJ0JZ
0KRJ0KZ
0KRJ47Z
0KRJ4JZ
0KRJ4KZ
0KRK07Z
0KS64ZZ
0KS70ZZ
0KS74ZZ
0KS80ZZ
0KS84ZZ
0KS90ZZ
0KS94ZZ
0KSB0ZZ
0KSB4ZZ
0KSC0ZZ
0KSC4ZZ
0KSD0ZZ
0KSD4ZZ
0KSF0ZZ
0KSF4ZZ
0KSG0ZZ
0KSG4ZZ
0KSH0ZZ
0KSH4ZZ
0KSJ0ZZ
0KSJ4ZZ
0KSK0ZZ
0KSK4ZZ
0KSL0ZZ
0KSL4ZZ
0KSM0ZZ
0KSM4ZZ
0KSN0ZZ
0KSN4ZZ
0KSP0ZZ
0KSP4ZZ
0KSQ0ZZ
0KSQ4ZZ
0KSR0ZZ
0KSR4ZZ
0KSS0ZZ
0KSS4ZZ
0KST0ZZ
0KST4ZZ
0KSV0ZZ
0KSV4ZZ
0KSW0ZZ
0KSW4ZZ
0KT00ZZ
0KT04ZZ
0KT10ZZ
0KT14ZZ
0KT20ZZ
0KT24ZZ
0KT30ZZ
0KT34ZZ
0KT40ZZ
0KT44ZZ
0KT50ZZ
0KT54ZZ
0KT60ZZ
0KT64ZZ
0KT70ZZ
0KT74ZZ
0KT80ZZ
0KT84ZZ
0KT90ZZ
0KT94ZZ
0KTB0ZZ
0KTB4ZZ
0KTC0ZZ
0KTC4ZZ
0KTD0ZZ
0KTD4ZZ
0KTF0ZZ
0KTF4ZZ
0KTG0ZZ
0KTG4ZZ
0KTH0ZZ
0KTH4ZZ
0KTJ0ZZ
0KTJ4ZZ
0KTK0ZZ
0KTK4ZZ
0KTL0ZZ
0KTL4ZZ
0KTM0ZZ
0KTM4ZZ
0KTN0ZZ
0KTN4ZZ
0KTP0ZZ
0KTP4ZZ
0KTQ0ZZ
0KTQ4ZZ
0KTR0ZZ
0KTR4ZZ
0KTS0ZZ

0KTS4ZZ
0KTT0ZZ
0KTT4ZZ
0KTV0ZZ
0KTV4ZZ
0KTW0ZZ
0KTW4ZZ
0KU007Z
0KU00JZ
0KU00KZ
0KU047Z
0KU04JZ
0KU04KZ
0KU107Z
0KU10JZ
0KU10KZ
0KU147Z
0KU14JZ
0KU14KZ
0KU207Z
0KU20JZ
0KU20KZ
0KU247Z
0KU24JZ
0KU24KZ
0KU307Z
0KU30JZ
0KU30KZ
0KU347Z
0KU34JZ
0KU34KZ
0KU407Z
0KU40JZ
0KU40KZ
0KU447Z
0KU44JZ
0KU44KZ
0KU507Z
0KU50JZ
0KU50KZ
0KU547Z
0KU54JZ
0KU54KZ
0KU607Z
0KU60JZ
0KU60KZ
0KU647Z
0KU64JZ
0KU64KZ
0KU707Z
0KU70JZ
0KU70KZ
0KU747Z
0KU74JZ
0KU74KZ
0KU807Z
0KU80JZ
0KU80KZ
0KU847Z
0KU84JZ
0KU84KZ
0KU907Z
0KU90JZ
0KU90KZ
0KU947Z
0KU94JZ
0KU94KZ
0KUB07Z
0KUB0JZ
0KUB0KZ
0KUB47Z
0KUB4JZ
0KUB4KZ
0KUC07Z
0KUC0JZ
0KUC0KZ
0KUC47Z
0KUC4JZ
0KUC4KZ
0KUD07Z
0KUD0JZ
0KUD0KZ
0KUD47Z
0KUD4JZ
0KUD4KZ
0KUF07Z
0KUF0JZ
0KUF0KZ
0KUF47Z
0KUF4JZ
0KUF4KZ
0KUG07Z
0KUG0JZ
0KUG0KZ
0KUG47Z
0KUG4JZ
0KUG4KZ
0KUH07Z
0KWX3YZ
0KWX4YZ
0KWXX0Z
0KWXX7Z
0KWXXJZ
0KWXXKZ
0KWXXMZ
0KWY3YZ
0KWY4JZ
0KWY4KZ
0KWY4MZ
0KWY4YZ
0KWYX0Z
0KWYX7Z
0KWYXJZ
0KWYXKZ
0KWYXMZ
0KX00Z0
0KX00Z1
0KX00Z2
0KX00ZZ
0KX04Z0
0KX04Z1
0KX04Z2
0KX04ZZ
0KX10Z0
0KX10Z1
0KX10Z2
0KX10ZZ
0KX14Z0
0KX14Z1
0KX14Z2
0KX14ZZ
0KX20Z0
0KX20Z1
0KX20Z2
0KX20ZZ
0KX24Z0
0KX24Z1
0KX24Z2
0KX24ZZ
0KX30Z0
0KX30Z1
0KX30Z2
0KX30ZZ
0KX34Z0
0KX34Z1
0KX34Z2
0KX34ZZ
0KX40Z0
0KX40Z1
0KX40Z2
0KX40ZZ
0KX44Z0
0KX44Z1
0KX44Z2
0KX44ZZ
0KX50Z0
0KX50Z1
0KX50Z2
0KX50ZZ
0KX54Z0
0KX54Z1
0KX54Z2
0KX54ZZ
0KX60Z0
0KX60Z1
0KX60Z2
0KX60ZZ
0KX64Z0
0KX64Z1
0KX64Z2
0KX64ZZ
0KX70Z0
0KX70Z1
0KX70Z2
0KX70ZZ
0KX74Z0
0KX74Z1
0KX74Z2
0KX74ZZ
0KX80Z0
0KX80Z1
0KX80Z2
0KX80ZZ
0KX84Z0
0KX84Z1
0KX84Z2
0KX84ZZ
0KX90Z0
0KX90Z1
0KX90Z2
0KX90ZZ
0KX94Z0
0KX94Z1
0KX94Z2
0KX94ZZ
0KXB0Z0
0KXB0Z1
0KXB0Z2
0KXB0ZZ
0KXB4Z0
0KXB4Z1
0KXB4Z2
0KXB4ZZ
0KXC0Z0
0KXC0Z1
0KXC0Z2
0KXC0ZZ
0KXC4Z0
0KXC4Z1
0KXC4Z2
0KXC4ZZ
0KXD0Z0
0KXD0Z1
0KXD0Z2
0KXD0ZZ
0KXD4Z0
0KXD4Z1
0KXD4Z2
0KXD4ZZ
0KXF0Z0
0KXF0Z1
0KXF0Z2
0KXF0Z5
0KXF0Z7
0KXF0Z8
0KXF0Z9
0KXF0ZZ
0KXF4Z0
0KXF4Z1
0KXF4Z2
0KXF4Z5
0KXF4Z7
0KXF4Z8
0KXF4Z9
0KXF4ZZ
0KXG0Z0
0KXG0Z1
0KXG0Z2
0KXG0Z5
0KXG0Z7
0KXG0Z8
0KXG0Z9
0KXG0ZZ
0KXG4Z0
0KXG4Z1
0KXG4Z2
0KXG4Z5
0KXG4Z7
0KXG4Z8
0KXG4Z9
0KXG4ZZ
0KXH0Z0
0KXH0Z1
0KXH0Z2
0KXH0ZZ
0KXH4Z0
0KXH4Z1
0KXH4Z2
0KXH4ZZ
0KXJ0Z0
0KXJ0Z1
0KXJ0Z2
0KXJ0ZZ
0KXJ4Z0
0KXJ4Z1
0KXJ4Z2
0KXJ4ZZ
0KXK0Z0
0KXK0Z1
0KXK0Z2
0KXK0Z6
0KXK0ZZ
0KXK4Z0
0KXK4Z1
0KXK4Z2
0KXK4Z6
0KXK4ZZ
0KXL0Z0
0KXL0Z1
0KXL0Z2
0KXL0Z6
0KXL0ZZ
0KXL4Z0
0KXL4Z1
0KXL4Z2
0KXL4Z6
0KXL4ZZ
0KXM0Z0
0KXM0Z1
0KXM0Z2
0KXM0ZZ
0KXM4Z0
0KXM4Z1
0KXM4Z2
0KXM4ZZ
0KXN0Z0
0KXN0Z1
0KXN0Z2
0KXN0ZZ
0KXN4Z0
0KXN4Z1
0KXN4Z2
0KXN4ZZ
0KXP0Z0
0KXP0Z1
0KXP0Z2
0KXP0ZZ
0KXP4Z0
0KXP4Z1
0KXP4Z2
0KXP4ZZ
0KXQ0Z0
0KXQ0Z1
0KXQ0Z2
0KXQ0ZZ
0KXQ4Z0
0KXQ4Z1
0KXQ4Z2
0KXQ4ZZ
0KXR0Z0
0KXR0Z1
0KXR0Z2
0KXR0ZZ
0KXR4Z0
0KXR4Z1
0KXR4Z2
0KXR4ZZ
0KXS0Z0
0KXS0Z1
0KXS0Z2
0KXS0ZZ
0KXS4Z0
0KXS4Z1
0KXS4Z2
0KXS4ZZ
0KXT0Z0
0KXT0Z1
0KXT0Z2
0KXT0ZZ
0KXT4Z0
0KXT4Z1
0KXT4Z2
0KXT4ZZ
0KXV0Z0
0KXV0Z1
0KXV0Z2
0KXV0ZZ
0KXV4Z0
0KXV4Z1
0KXV4Z2
0KXV4ZZ
0KXW0Z0
0KXW0Z1
0KXW0Z2
0KXW0ZZ
0KXW4Z0
0KXW4Z1
0KXW4Z2
0KXW4ZZ
0L2XX0Z
0L2XXYZ
0L2YX0Z
0L2YXYZ
0L500ZZ
0L503ZZ
0L504ZZ
0L510ZZ
0L513ZZ
0L514ZZ
0L520ZZ
0L523ZZ
0L524ZZ
0L530ZZ
0L533ZZ
0L534ZZ
0L540ZZ
0L543ZZ
0L544ZZ
0L550ZZ
0L553ZZ
0L554ZZ
0L560ZZ
0L563ZZ
0L564ZZ
0L570ZZ
0L573ZZ
0L574ZZ
0L580ZZ
0L583ZZ
0L584ZZ
0L590ZZ
0L593ZZ
0L594ZZ
0L5B0ZZ
0L5B3ZZ
0L5B4ZZ
0L5C0ZZ
0L5C3ZZ
0L5C4ZZ
0L5D0ZZ
0L5D3ZZ
0L5D4ZZ
0L5F0ZZ
0L5F3ZZ
0L5F4ZZ
0L5G0ZZ
0L5G3ZZ
0L5G4ZZ
0L5H0ZZ
0L5H3ZZ
0L5H4ZZ
0L5J0ZZ
0L5J3ZZ
0L5J4ZZ
0L5K0ZZ
0L5K3ZZ
0L5K4ZZ
0L5L0ZZ
0L5L3ZZ
0L8T4ZZ
0L8V0ZZ
0L8V3ZZ
0L8V4ZZ
0L8W0ZZ
0L8W3ZZ
0L8W4ZZ
0L9000Z
0L900ZX
0L900ZZ
0L9030Z
0L903ZX
0L903ZZ
0L9040Z
0L904ZX
0L904ZZ
0L9100Z
0L910ZX
0L910ZZ
0L9130Z
0L913ZX
0L913ZZ
0L9140Z
0L914ZX
0L914ZZ
0L9200Z
0L920ZX
0L920ZZ
0L9230Z
0L923ZX
0L923ZZ
0L9240Z
0L924ZX
0L924ZZ
0L9300Z
0L930ZX
0L930ZZ
0L9330Z
0L933ZX
0L933ZZ
0L9340Z
0L934ZX
0L934ZZ
0L9400Z
0L940ZX
0L940ZZ
0L9430Z
0L943ZX
0L943ZZ
0L9440Z
0L944ZX
0L944ZZ
0L9500Z
0L950ZX
0L950ZZ
0L9530Z
0L953ZX
0L953ZZ
0L9540Z
0L954ZX
0L954ZZ
0L9600Z
0L960ZX
0L960ZZ
0L9630Z
0L963ZX
0L963ZZ
0L9640Z
0L964ZX
0L964ZZ
0L9700Z
0L970ZX
0L970ZZ
0L9730Z
0L973ZX
0L973ZZ
0L9740Z
0L974ZX
0L974ZZ
0L9800Z
0L980ZX
0L980ZZ
0L9830Z
0L983ZX
0L983ZZ
0L9840Z
0L984ZX
0L984ZZ
0L9900Z
0L990ZX
0L990ZZ
0L9930Z
0L993ZX
0L993ZZ
0L9940Z
0L994ZX
0L994ZZ
0L9B00Z
0L9B0ZX
0L9B0ZZ
0L9B30Z
0L9B3ZX
0L9B3ZZ
0L9B40Z
0L9B4ZX
0L9B4ZZ
0L9C00Z
0L9C0ZX
0L9C0ZZ
0L9C30Z
0L9C3ZX
0L9C3ZZ
0L9C40Z
0L9C4ZX
0L9C4ZZ
0L9D00Z
0L9D0ZX
0L9D0ZZ
0L9D30Z
0L9D3ZX
0L9D3ZZ
0L9D40Z
0L9D4ZX
0L9D4ZZ
0L9F00Z
0L9F0ZX
0L9F0ZZ
0L9F30Z
0L9F3ZX
0L9F3ZZ
0L9F40Z
0L9F4ZX
0L9F4ZZ
0L9G00Z
0L9G0ZX
0L9G0ZZ
0L9G30Z
0L9G3ZX
0L9G3ZZ
0L9G40Z
0L9G4ZX
0L9G4ZZ
0L9H00Z
0L9H0ZX
0L9H0ZZ
0L9H30Z
0L9H3ZX
0L9H3ZZ
0L9H40Z
0L9H4ZX
0L9H4ZZ
0L9J00Z
0L9J0ZX
0L9J0ZZ
0L9J30Z
0L9J3ZX
0L9J3ZZ
0L9J40Z
0L9J4ZX
0L9J4ZZ
0L9K00Z
0L9K0ZX
0L9K0ZZ
0L9K30Z
0L9K3ZX
0L9K3ZZ
0L9K40Z
0L9K4ZX
0L9K4ZZ
0L9L00Z
0L9L0ZX
0L9L0ZZ
0L9L30Z
0L9L3ZX
0L9L3ZZ
0L9L40Z
0L9L4ZX
0L9L4ZZ
0L9M00Z
0L9M0ZX
0L9M0ZZ
0L9M30Z
0L9M3ZX
0L9M3ZZ
0L9M40Z
0L9M4ZX
0L9M4ZZ
0L9N00Z
0L9N0ZX
0L9N0ZZ
0L9N30Z
0L9N3ZX
0L9N3ZZ
0L9N40Z
0L9N4ZX
0L9N4ZZ
0L9P00Z
0L9P0ZX
0L9P0ZZ
0L9P30Z
0L9P3ZX
0L9P3ZZ
0L9P40Z
0L9P4ZX
0L9P4ZZ
0L9Q00Z
0L9Q0ZX
0L9Q0ZZ
0L9Q30Z
0L9Q3ZX
0L9Q3ZZ
0L9Q40Z
0L9Q4ZX
0L9Q4ZZ
0L9R00Z
0L9R0ZX
0L9R0ZZ
0L9R30Z
0L9R3ZX
0L9R3ZZ
0L9R40Z
0L9R4ZX
0L9R4ZZ
0L9S00Z
0L9S0ZX
0L9S0ZZ
0L9S30Z
0L9S3ZX
0L9S3ZZ
0L9S40Z
0L9S4ZX
0L9S4ZZ
0L9T00Z
0L9T0ZX
0L9T0ZZ
0L9T30Z
0L9T3ZX
0L9T3ZZ
0L9T40Z
0L9T4ZX
0L9T4ZZ
0L9V00Z
0L9V0ZX
0L9V0ZZ
0L9V30Z
0L9V3ZX
0L9V3ZZ
0L9V40Z
0L9V4ZX
0L9V4ZZ
0L9W00Z
0L9W0ZX
0L9W0ZZ
0L9W30Z
0L9W3ZX
0L9W3ZZ
0L9W40Z
0L9W4ZX
0L9W4ZZ
0LB00ZX
0LB00ZZ
0LB03ZX
0LB03ZZ
0LB04ZX
0LB04ZZ
0LB10ZX
0LB10ZZ
0LB13ZX
0LB13ZZ
0LB14ZX
0LB14ZZ
0LB20ZX
0LB20ZZ
0LB23ZX
0LB23ZZ
0LB24ZX
0LB24ZZ
0LB30ZX
0LB30ZZ
0LB33ZX
0LB33ZZ
0LB34ZX
0LB34ZZ
0LB40ZX
0LB40ZZ
0LB43ZX
0LB43ZZ
0LB44ZX
0LB44ZZ
0LB50ZX
0LB50ZZ
0LB53ZX
0LB53ZZ
0LB54ZX
0LB54ZZ
0LB60ZX
0LB60ZZ
0LB63ZX
0LB63ZZ
0LB64ZX
0LB64ZZ
0LB70ZX
0LB70ZZ
0LB73ZX
0LB73ZZ
0LB74ZX
0LB74ZZ

0LB80ZX
0LB80ZZ
0LB83ZX
0LB83ZZ
0LB84ZX
0LB84ZZ
0LB90ZX
0LB90ZZ
0LB93ZX
0LB93ZZ
0LB94ZX
0LB94ZZ
0LBB0ZX
0LBB0ZZ
0LBB3ZX
0LBB3ZZ
0LBB4ZX
0LBB4ZZ
0LBC0ZX
0LBC0ZZ
0LBC3ZX
0LBC3ZZ
0LBC4ZX
0LBC4ZZ
0LBD0ZX
0LBD0ZZ
0LBD3ZX
0LBD3ZZ
0LBD4ZX
0LBD4ZZ
0LBF0ZX
0LBF0ZZ
0LBF3ZX
0LBF3ZZ
0LBF4ZX
0LBF4ZZ
0LBG0ZX
0LBG0ZZ
0LBG3ZX
0LBG3ZZ
0LBG4ZX
0LBG4ZZ
0LBH0ZX
0LBH0ZZ
0LBH3ZX
0LBH3ZZ
0LBH4ZX
0LBH4ZZ
0LBJ0ZX
0LBJ0ZZ
0LBJ3ZX
0LBJ3ZZ
0LBJ4ZX
0LBJ4ZZ
0LBK0ZX
0LBK0ZZ
0LBK3ZX
0LBK3ZZ
0LBK4ZX
0LBK4ZZ
0LBL0ZX
0LBL0ZZ
0LBL3ZX
0LBL3ZZ
0LBL4ZX
0LBL4ZZ
0LBM0ZX
0LBM0ZZ
0LBM3ZX
0LBM3ZZ
0LBM4ZX
0LBM4ZZ
0LBN0ZX
0LBN0ZZ
0LBN3ZX
0LBN3ZZ
0LBN4ZX
0LBN4ZZ
0LBP0ZX
0LBP0ZZ
0LBP3ZX
0LBP3ZZ
0LBP4ZX
0LBP4ZZ
0LBQ0ZX
0LBQ0ZZ
0LBQ3ZX
0LBQ3ZZ
0LBQ4ZX
0LBQ4ZZ
0LBR0ZX
0LBR0ZZ
0LBR3ZX
0LBR3ZZ
0LBR4ZX
0LBR4ZZ
0LBS0ZX
0LBS0ZZ
0LBS3ZX
0LBS3ZZ
0LBS4ZX
0LBS4ZZ
0LBT0ZX
0LBT0ZZ
0LBT3ZX
0LBT3ZZ
0LBT4ZX
0LBT4ZZ
0LBV0ZX
0LBV0ZZ
0LBV3ZX
0LBV3ZZ
0LBV4ZX
0LBV4ZZ
0LBW0ZX
0LBW0ZZ
0LHX3YZ
0LHX4YZ
0LHY3YZ
0LHY4YZ
0LJX3ZZ
0LJXXZZ
0LJY3ZZ
0LJYXZZ
0LM84ZZ
0LM90ZZ
0LM94ZZ
0LMB0ZZ
0LMB4ZZ
0LMC0ZZ
0LMC4ZZ
0LMD0ZZ
0LMD4ZZ
0LMF0ZZ
0LMF4ZZ
0LMG0ZZ
0LMG4ZZ
0LMH0ZZ
0LMH4ZZ
0LMJ0ZZ
0LMJ4ZZ
0LMK0ZZ
0LMK4ZZ
0LML0ZZ
0LML4ZZ
0LMM0ZZ
0LMM4ZZ
0LMN0ZZ
0LMN4ZZ
0LMP0ZZ
0LMP4ZZ
0LMQ0ZZ
0LMQ4ZZ
0LMR0ZZ
0LMR4ZZ
0LMS0ZZ
0LMS4ZZ
0LMT0ZZ
0LMT4ZZ
0LMV0ZZ
0LMV4ZZ
0LMW0ZZ
0LMW4ZZ
0LN00ZZ
0LN03ZZ
0LN04ZZ
0LN0XZZ
0LN10ZZ
0LN13ZZ
0LN14ZZ
0LN1XZZ
0LN20ZZ
0LN23ZZ
0LN24ZZ
0LN2XZZ
0LN30ZZ
0LN33ZZ
0LN34ZZ
0LN3XZZ
0LN40ZZ
0LN43ZZ
0LN44ZZ
0LN4XZZ
0LN50ZZ
0LN53ZZ
0LN54ZZ
0LN5XZZ
0LN60ZZ
0LN63ZZ
0LN64ZZ
0LN6XZZ
0LN70ZZ
0LN73ZZ
0LN74ZZ
0LN7XZZ
0LN80ZZ
0LN83ZZ
0LN84ZZ
0LN8XZZ
0LN90ZZ
0LN93ZZ
0LN94ZZ
0LN9XZZ
0LNB0ZZ
0LNB3ZZ
0LNB4ZZ
0LNBXZZ
0LNC0ZZ
0LNC3ZZ
0LNC4ZZ
0LNCXZZ
0LND0ZZ
0LND3ZZ
0LND4ZZ
0LNDXZZ
0LNF0ZZ
0LNF3ZZ
0LNF4ZZ
0LNFXZZ
0LNG0ZZ
0LNG3ZZ
0LNG4ZZ
0LNGXZZ
0LNH0ZZ
0LNH3ZZ
0LNH4ZZ
0LNHXZZ
0LNJ0ZZ
0LNJ3ZZ
0LNJ4ZZ
0LNJXZZ
0LNK0ZZ
0LNK3ZZ
0LNK4ZZ
0LNKXZZ
0LNL0ZZ
0LNL3ZZ
0LNL4ZZ
0LNLXZZ
0LNM0ZZ
0LNM3ZZ
0LNM4ZZ
0LNMXZZ
0LNN0ZZ
0LNN3ZZ
0LNN4ZZ
0LNNXZZ
0LNP0ZZ
0LNP3ZZ
0LNP4ZZ
0LNPXZZ
0LNQ0ZZ
0LNQ3ZZ
0LNQ4ZZ
0LNQXZZ
0LNR0ZZ
0LNR3ZZ
0LNR4ZZ
0LNRXZZ
0LNS0ZZ
0LNS3ZZ
0LNS4ZZ
0LNSXZZ
0LNT0ZZ
0LNT3ZZ
0LNT4ZZ
0LNTXZZ
0LNV0ZZ
0LNV3ZZ
0LNV4ZZ
0LNVXZZ
0LNW0ZZ
0LNW3ZZ
0LNW4ZZ
0LNWXZZ
0LPX00Z
0LPX07Z
0LPX0JZ
0LPX0KZ
0LPX0YZ
0LPX30Z
0LPX37Z
0LPX3JZ
0LPX3KZ
0LPX3YZ
0LPX40Z
0LPX47Z
0LPX4JZ
0LPX4KZ
0LPX4YZ
0LPXX0Z
0LPY00Z
0LPY07Z
0LPY0JZ
0LPY0KZ
0LPY0YZ
0LPY30Z
0LPY37Z
0LPY3JZ
0LPY3KZ
0LPY3YZ
0LPY40Z
0LPY47Z
0LPY4JZ
0LPY4KZ
0LPY4YZ
0LPYX0Z
0LQ00ZZ
0LQ03ZZ
0LQ04ZZ
0LQ10ZZ
0LQ13ZZ
0LQ14ZZ
0LQ20ZZ
0LQ23ZZ
0LQ24ZZ
0LQ30ZZ
0LQ33ZZ
0LQ34ZZ
0LQ40ZZ
0LQ43ZZ
0LQ44ZZ
0LQ50ZZ
0LQ53ZZ
0LQ54ZZ
0LQ60ZZ
0LQ63ZZ
0LQ64ZZ
0LQ70ZZ
0LQ73ZZ
0LQ74ZZ
0LQ80ZZ
0LQ83ZZ
0LQ84ZZ
0LQ90ZZ
0LQ93ZZ
0LQ94ZZ
0LQB0ZZ
0LQB3ZZ
0LQB4ZZ
0LQC0ZZ
0LQC3ZZ
0LQC4ZZ
0LQD0ZZ
0LQD3ZZ
0LQD4ZZ
0LQF0ZZ
0LQF3ZZ
0LQF4ZZ
0LQG0ZZ
0LQG3ZZ
0LQG4ZZ
0LQH0ZZ
0LQH3ZZ
0LQH4ZZ
0LQJ0ZZ
0LQJ3ZZ
0LQJ4ZZ
0LQK0ZZ
0LQK3ZZ
0LQK4ZZ
0LQL0ZZ
0LQL3ZZ
0LQL4ZZ
0LQM0ZZ
0LQM3ZZ
0LQM4ZZ
0LQN0ZZ
0LQN3ZZ
0LQN4ZZ
0LQP0ZZ
0LQP3ZZ
0LQP4ZZ
0LQQ0ZZ
0LQQ3ZZ
0LQQ4ZZ
0LQR0ZZ
0LQR3ZZ
0LQR4ZZ
0LQS0ZZ
0LQS3ZZ
0LQS4ZZ
0LQT0ZZ
0LQT3ZZ
0LQT4ZZ
0LQV0ZZ
0LQV3ZZ
0LQV4ZZ
0LQW0ZZ
0LQW3ZZ
0LQW4ZZ
0LR007Z
0LR00JZ
0LR00KZ
0LR047Z
0LR04JZ
0LR04KZ
0LR107Z
0LR10JZ
0LR10KZ
0LR147Z
0LR14JZ
0LR14KZ
0LR207Z
0LR20JZ
0LR20KZ
0LR247Z
0LR24JZ
0LR24KZ
0LR307Z
0LR30JZ
0LR30KZ
0LR347Z
0LR34JZ
0LR34KZ
0LR407Z
0LR40JZ
0LR40KZ
0LR447Z
0LR44JZ
0LR44KZ
0LR507Z
0LR50JZ
0LR50KZ
0LR547Z
0LR54JZ
0LR54KZ
0LR607Z
0LR60JZ
0LR60KZ
0LR647Z
0LR64JZ
0LR64KZ
0LR707Z
0LR70JZ
0LR70KZ
0LR747Z
0LR74JZ
0LR74KZ
0LR807Z
0LSH4ZZ
0LSJ0ZZ
0LSJ4ZZ
0LSK0ZZ
0LSK4ZZ
0LSL0ZZ
0LSL4ZZ
0LSM0ZZ
0LSM4ZZ
0LSN0ZZ
0LSN4ZZ
0LSP0ZZ
0LSP4ZZ
0LSQ0ZZ
0LSQ4ZZ
0LSR0ZZ
0LSR4ZZ
0LSS0ZZ
0LSS4ZZ
0LST0ZZ
0LST4ZZ
0LSV0ZZ
0LSV4ZZ
0LSW0ZZ
0LSW4ZZ
0LT00ZZ
0LT04ZZ
0LT10ZZ
0LT14ZZ
0LT20ZZ
0LT24ZZ
0LT30ZZ
0LT34ZZ
0LT40ZZ
0LT44ZZ
0LT50ZZ
0LT54ZZ
0LT60ZZ
0LT64ZZ
0LT70ZZ
0LT74ZZ
0LT80ZZ
0LT84ZZ
0LT90ZZ
0LT94ZZ
0LTB0ZZ
0LTB4ZZ
0LTC0ZZ
0LTC4ZZ
0LTD0ZZ
0LTD4ZZ
0LTF0ZZ
0LTF4ZZ
0LTG0ZZ
0LTG4ZZ
0LTH0ZZ
0LTH4ZZ
0LTJ0ZZ
0LTJ4ZZ
0LTK0ZZ
0LTK4ZZ
0LTL0ZZ
0LTL4ZZ
0LTM0ZZ
0LTM4ZZ
0LTN0ZZ
0LTN4ZZ
0LTP0ZZ
0LTP4ZZ
0LTQ0ZZ
0LTQ4ZZ
0LTR0ZZ
0LTR4ZZ
0LTS0ZZ
0LTS4ZZ
0LTT0ZZ
0LTT4ZZ
0LTV0ZZ
0LTV4ZZ
0LTW0ZZ
0LTW4ZZ
0LU007Z
0LU00JZ
0LU00KZ
0LU047Z
0LU04JZ
0LU04KZ
0LU107Z
0LU10JZ
0LU10KZ
0LU147Z
0LU14JZ
0LU14KZ
0LU207Z
0LU20JZ
0LU20KZ
0LU247Z
0LU24JZ
0LU24KZ
0LU307Z
0LU30JZ
0LU30KZ
0LU347Z
0LU34JZ
0LU34KZ
0LU407Z
0LU40JZ
0LU40KZ
0LU447Z
0LU44JZ
0LU44KZ
0LU507Z
0LU50JZ
0LU50KZ
0LU547Z
0LU54JZ
0LU54KZ
0LU607Z
0LU60JZ
0LU60KZ
0LU647Z
0LU64JZ
0LU64KZ
0LU707Z
0LU70JZ
0LU70KZ
0LU747Z
0LU74JZ
0LU74KZ
0LU807Z
0LU80JZ
0LU80KZ
0LU847Z
0LU84JZ
0LU84KZ
0LU907Z
0LU90JZ
0LU90KZ
0LU947Z
0LU94JZ
0LU94KZ
0LUB07Z
0LUB0JZ
0LUB0KZ
0LUB47Z
0LUB4JZ
0LUB4KZ
0LUC07Z
0LUC0JZ
0LUC0KZ
0LUC47Z
0LUC4JZ
0LUC4KZ
0LUD07Z
0LUD0JZ
0LUD0KZ
0LUD47Z
0LUD4JZ
0LUD4KZ
0LUF07Z
0LUF0JZ
0LUF0KZ
0LUF47Z
0LUF4JZ
0LUF4KZ
0LUG07Z
0LUG0JZ
0LUG0KZ
0LUG47Z
0LUG4JZ
0LUG4KZ
0LUH07Z
0LUH0JZ
0LUH0KZ
0LUH47Z
0LUH4JZ
0LUH4KZ
0LUJ07Z
0LUJ0JZ
0LUJ0KZ
0LUJ47Z
0LUJ4JZ
0LUJ4KZ
0LUK07Z
0LUK0JZ
0LUK0KZ
0LUK47Z
0LUK4JZ
0LUK4KZ
0LUL07Z
0LUL0JZ
0LUL0KZ
0LUL47Z
0LUL4JZ
0LUL4KZ
0LUM07Z
0LUM0JZ
0LUM0KZ
0LUM47Z
0LUM4JZ
0LUM4KZ
0LUN07Z
0LUN0JZ
0LUN0KZ
0LUN47Z
0LUN4JZ
0LUN4KZ
0LUP07Z
0LUP0JZ
0LUP0KZ
0LUP47Z
0LUP4JZ
0LUP4KZ
0LUQ07Z
0LUQ0JZ
0LUQ0KZ
0LUQ47Z
0LUQ4JZ
0LUQ4KZ
0LUR07Z
0LUR0JZ
0LUR0KZ
0LUR47Z
0LUR4JZ
0LUR4KZ
0LUS07Z
0LUS0JZ
0LUS0KZ
0LUS47Z
0LUS4JZ
0LUS4KZ
0LUT07Z
0LUT0JZ
0LUT0KZ
0LUT47Z
0LUT4JZ
0LUT4KZ
0LUV07Z
0LUV0JZ
0LUV0KZ
0LUV47Z
0LUV4JZ
0LUV4KZ
0LUW07Z
0LUW0JZ
0LUW0KZ
0LUW47Z
0LUW4JZ
0LUW4KZ
0LWX00Z
0LWX07Z
0LWX0JZ
0LWX0KZ
0LWX0YZ
0LWX30Z
0LWX37Z
0LWX3JZ
0LWX3KZ
0LWX3YZ
0LWX40Z
0LWX47Z
0LWX4JZ
0LWX4KZ
0LWX4YZ
0LWXX0Z
0LWXX7Z
0LWXXJZ
0LWXXKZ
0LWY00Z
0LWY07Z
0LWY0JZ
0LWY0KZ
0LWY0YZ
0LWY30Z
0LWY37Z
0LWY3JZ
0LWY3KZ
0LWY3YZ
0LWY40Z
0LWY47Z
0LWY4JZ
0LWY4KZ
0LWY4YZ
0LWYX0Z
0LWYX7Z
0LWYXJZ

0LWYXKZ
0LX00ZZ
0LX04ZZ
0LX10ZZ
0LX14ZZ
0LX20ZZ
0LX24ZZ
0LX30ZZ
0LX34ZZ
0LX40ZZ
0LX44ZZ
0LX50ZZ
0LX54ZZ
0LX60ZZ
0LX64ZZ
0LX70ZZ
0LX74ZZ
0LX80ZZ
0LX84ZZ
0LX90ZZ
0LX94ZZ
0LXB0ZZ
0LXB4ZZ
0LXC0ZZ
0LXC4ZZ
0LXD0ZZ
0LXD4ZZ
0LXF0ZZ
0LXF4ZZ
0M2XX0Z
0M2XXYZ
0M2YX0Z
0M2YXYZ
0M803ZZ
0M804ZZ
0M810ZZ
0M813ZZ
0M814ZZ
0M820ZZ
0M823ZZ
0M824ZZ
0M830ZZ
0M833ZZ
0M834ZZ
0M840ZZ
0M843ZZ
0M844ZZ
0M850ZZ
0M853ZZ
0M854ZZ
0M860ZZ
0M863ZZ
0M864ZZ
0M870ZZ
0M873ZZ
0M874ZZ
0M880ZZ
0M883ZZ
0M884ZZ
0M890ZZ
0M893ZZ
0M894ZZ
0M8B0ZZ
0M8B3ZZ
0M8B4ZZ
0M8C0ZZ
0M8C3ZZ
0M8C4ZZ
0M8D0ZZ
0M8D3ZZ
0M8D4ZZ
0M8F0ZZ
0M8F3ZZ
0M8F4ZZ
0M8G0ZZ
0M8G3ZZ
0M8G4ZZ
0M8H0ZZ
0M8H3ZZ
0M8H4ZZ
0M8J0ZZ
0M8J3ZZ
0M8J4ZZ
0M8K0ZZ
0M8K3ZZ
0M8K4ZZ
0M8L0ZZ
0M8L3ZZ
0M8L4ZZ
0M8M0ZZ
0M8M3ZZ
0M8M4ZZ
0M8N0ZZ
0M8N3ZZ
0M8N4ZZ
0M8P0ZZ
0M8P3ZZ
0M8P4ZZ
0M8Q0ZZ
0M8Q3ZZ
0M8Q4ZZ
0M8R0ZZ
0M8R3ZZ
0M8R4ZZ
0M8S0ZZ
0M8S3ZZ
0M8S4ZZ
0M8T0ZZ
0M8T3ZZ
0M8T4ZZ
0M8V0ZZ
0M8V3ZZ
0M8V4ZZ
0M8W0ZZ
0M8W3ZZ
0M8W4ZZ
0M9000Z
0M900ZX
0M900ZZ
0M9030Z
0M903ZX
0M903ZZ
0M9040Z
0M904ZX
0M904ZZ
0M9100Z
0M910ZX
0M910ZZ
0M9130Z
0M913ZX
0M913ZZ
0M9140Z
0M914ZX
0M914ZZ
0M9200Z
0M920ZX
0M920ZZ
0M9230Z
0M923ZX
0M923ZZ
0M9240Z
0M924ZX
0M924ZZ
0M9300Z
0M930ZX
0M930ZZ
0M9330Z
0M933ZX
0M933ZZ
0M9340Z
0M934ZX
0M934ZZ
0M9400Z
0M940ZX
0M940ZZ
0M9430Z
0M943ZX
0M943ZZ
0M9440Z
0M944ZX
0M944ZZ
0M9500Z
0M950ZX
0M950ZZ
0M9530Z
0M953ZX
0M953ZZ
0M9540Z
0M954ZX
0M954ZZ
0M9600Z
0M960ZX
0M960ZZ
0M9630Z
0M963ZX
0M963ZZ
0M9640Z
0M964ZX
0M964ZZ
0M9700Z
0M970ZX
0M970ZZ
0M9730Z
0M973ZX
0M973ZZ
0M9740Z
0M974ZX
0M974ZZ
0M9800Z
0M980ZX
0M980ZZ
0M9830Z
0M983ZX
0M983ZZ
0M9840Z
0M984ZX
0M984ZZ
0M9900Z
0M990ZX
0M990ZZ
0M9930Z
0M993ZX
0M993ZZ
0M9940Z
0M994ZX
0M994ZZ
0M9B00Z
0M9B0ZX
0M9B0ZZ
0M9B30Z
0M9B3ZX
0M9B3ZZ
0M9B40Z
0M9B4ZX
0M9B4ZZ
0M9C00Z
0M9C0ZX
0M9C0ZZ
0M9C30Z
0M9C3ZX
0M9C3ZZ
0M9C40Z
0M9C4ZX
0M9C4ZZ
0M9D00Z
0M9D0ZX
0M9D0ZZ
0M9D30Z
0M9D3ZX
0M9D3ZZ
0M9D40Z
0M9D4ZX
0M9D4ZZ
0M9F00Z
0M9F0ZX
0M9F0ZZ
0M9F30Z
0M9F3ZX
0M9F3ZZ
0M9F40Z
0M9F4ZX
0M9F4ZZ
0M9G00Z
0M9G0ZX
0M9G0ZZ
0M9G30Z
0M9G3ZX
0M9G3ZZ
0M9G40Z
0M9G4ZX
0M9G4ZZ
0M9H00Z
0M9H0ZX
0M9H0ZZ
0M9H30Z
0M9H3ZX
0M9H3ZZ
0M9H40Z
0M9H4ZX
0M9H4ZZ
0M9J00Z
0M9J0ZX
0M9J0ZZ
0M9J30Z
0M9J3ZX
0M9J3ZZ
0M9J40Z
0M9J4ZX
0M9J4ZZ
0M9K00Z
0M9K0ZX
0M9K0ZZ
0M9K30Z
0M9K3ZX
0M9K3ZZ
0M9K40Z
0M9K4ZX
0M9K4ZZ
0M9L00Z
0M9L0ZX
0M9L0ZZ
0M9L30Z
0M9L3ZX
0M9L3ZZ
0M9L40Z
0M9L4ZX
0M9L4ZZ
0M9M00Z
0M9M0ZX
0M9M0ZZ
0M9M30Z
0M9M3ZX
0M9M3ZZ
0M9M40Z
0M9M4ZX
0M9M4ZZ
0M9N00Z
0M9N0ZX
0M9N0ZZ
0M9N30Z
0M9N3ZX
0M9N3ZZ
0M9N40Z
0M9N4ZX
0M9N4ZZ
0M9P00Z
0M9P0ZX
0M9P0ZZ
0M9P30Z
0M9P3ZX
0M9P3ZZ
0M9P40Z
0M9P4ZX
0M9P4ZZ
0M9Q00Z
0M9Q0ZX
0M9Q0ZZ
0M9Q30Z
0M9Q3ZX
0M9Q3ZZ
0M9Q40Z
0M9Q4ZX
0M9Q4ZZ
0M9R00Z
0M9R0ZX
0M9R0ZZ
0M9R30Z
0M9R3ZX
0M9R3ZZ
0M9R40Z
0M9R4ZX
0M9R4ZZ
0M9S00Z
0M9S0ZX
0M9S0ZZ
0M9S30Z
0M9S3ZX
0M9S3ZZ
0M9S40Z
0M9S4ZX
0M9S4ZZ
0M9T00Z
0M9T0ZX
0M9T0ZZ
0M9T30Z
0M9T3ZX
0M9T3ZZ
0M9T40Z
0M9T4ZX
0M9T4ZZ
0M9V00Z
0M9V0ZX
0M9V0ZZ
0M9V30Z
0M9V3ZX
0M9V3ZZ
0M9V40Z
0M9V4ZX
0M9V4ZZ
0M9W00Z
0M9W0ZX
0M9W0ZZ
0M9W30Z
0M9W3ZX
0M9W3ZZ
0M9W40Z
0M9W4ZX
0M9W4ZZ
0MB00ZX
0MB00ZZ
0MB03ZX
0MB03ZZ
0MB04ZX
0MB04ZZ
0MB10ZX
0MB10ZZ
0MB13ZX
0MB13ZZ
0MB14ZX
0MB14ZZ
0MB20ZX
0MB20ZZ
0MB23ZX
0MB23ZZ
0MB24ZX
0MB24ZZ
0MB30ZX
0MB30ZZ
0MB33ZX
0MB33ZZ
0MB34ZX
0MB34ZZ
0MB40ZX
0MB40ZZ
0MB43ZX
0MB43ZZ
0MB44ZX
0MB44ZZ
0MB50ZX
0MB50ZZ
0MB53ZX
0MB53ZZ
0MB54ZX
0MB54ZZ
0MB60ZX
0MB60ZZ
0MB63ZX
0MB63ZZ
0MB64ZX
0MB64ZZ
0MB70ZX
0MB70ZZ
0MB73ZX
0MB73ZZ
0MB74ZX
0MB74ZZ
0MB80ZX
0MB80ZZ
0MB83ZX
0MB83ZZ
0MB84ZX
0MB84ZZ
0MB90ZX
0MB90ZZ
0MB93ZX
0MB93ZZ
0MB94ZX
0MB94ZZ
0MBB0ZX
0MBB0ZZ
0MBB3ZX
0MBB3ZZ
0MBB4ZX
0MBB4ZZ
0MBC0ZX
0MBC0ZZ
0MBC3ZX
0MBC3ZZ
0MBC4ZX
0MBC4ZZ
0MBD0ZX
0MBD0ZZ
0MBD3ZX
0MBD3ZZ
0MBD4ZX
0MBD4ZZ
0MBF0ZX
0MBF0ZZ
0MBF3ZX
0MBF3ZZ
0MBF4ZX
0MBF4ZZ
0MBG0ZX
0MBG0ZZ
0MBG3ZX
0MBG3ZZ
0MBG4ZX
0MBG4ZZ
0MBH0ZX
0MBH0ZZ
0MBH3ZX
0MBH3ZZ
0MBH4ZX
0MBH4ZZ
0MBJ0ZX
0MBJ0ZZ
0MBJ3ZX
0MBJ3ZZ
0MBJ4ZX
0MBJ4ZZ
0MBK0ZX
0MBK0ZZ
0MBK3ZX
0MBK3ZZ
0MBK4ZX
0MBK4ZZ
0MBL0ZX
0MBL0ZZ
0MBL3ZX
0MBL3ZZ
0MBL4ZX
0MBL4ZZ
0MBM0ZX
0MBM0ZZ
0MBM3ZX
0MBM3ZZ
0MBM4ZX
0MBM4ZZ
0MBN0ZX
0MBN0ZZ
0MBN3ZX
0MBN3ZZ
0MBN4ZX
0MBN4ZZ
0MBP0ZX
0MBP0ZZ
0MBP3ZX
0MBP3ZZ
0MBP4ZX
0MBP4ZZ
0MBQ0ZX
0MBQ0ZZ
0MBQ3ZX
0MBQ3ZZ
0MBQ4ZX
0MBQ4ZZ
0MBR0ZX
0MBR0ZZ
0MBR3ZX
0MBR3ZZ
0MBR4ZX
0MBR4ZZ
0MBS0ZX
0MBS0ZZ
0MBS3ZX
0MBS3ZZ
0MBS4ZX
0MBS4ZZ
0MBT0ZX
0MBT0ZZ
0MBT3ZX
0MBT3ZZ
0MBT4ZX
0MBT4ZZ
0MBV0ZX
0MBV0ZZ
0MBV3ZX
0MBV3ZZ
0MBV4ZX
0MBV4ZZ
0MBW0ZX
0MBW0ZZ
0MBW3ZX
0MBW3ZZ
0MBW4ZX
0MBW4ZZ
0MC00ZZ
0MC03ZZ
0MC04ZZ
0MC10ZZ
0MC13ZZ
0MC14ZZ
0MC20ZZ
0MC23ZZ
0MC24ZZ
0MC30ZZ
0MC33ZZ
0MC34ZZ
0MC40ZZ
0MC43ZZ
0MC44ZZ
0MC50ZZ
0MC53ZZ
0MC54ZZ
0MC60ZZ
0MC63ZZ
0MC64ZZ
0MC70ZZ
0MC73ZZ
0MC74ZZ
0MC80ZZ
0MC83ZZ
0MC84ZZ
0MC90ZZ
0MC93ZZ
0MC94ZZ
0MCB0ZZ
0MCB3ZZ
0MCB4ZZ
0MCC0ZZ
0MCC3ZZ
0MCC4ZZ
0MCD0ZZ
0MCD3ZZ
0MCD4ZZ
0MCF0ZZ
0MCF3ZZ
0MHX3YZ
0MHX4YZ
0MHY3YZ
0MHY4YZ
0MJX3ZZ
0MJXXZZ
0MJY3ZZ
0MJYXZZ
0MN0XZZ
0MN1XZZ
0MN2XZZ
0MN3XZZ
0MN4XZZ
0MN5XZZ
0MN6XZZ
0MN7XZZ
0MN80ZZ
0MN83ZZ
0MN84ZZ
0MN8XZZ
0MN90ZZ
0MN93ZZ
0MN94ZZ
0MN9XZZ
0MNB0ZZ
0MNB3ZZ
0MNB4ZZ
0MNBXZZ
0MNC0ZZ
0MNC3ZZ
0MNC4ZZ
0MNCXZZ
0MND0ZZ
0MND3ZZ
0MND4ZZ
0MNDXZZ
0MNF0ZZ
0MNF3ZZ
0MNF4ZZ
0MNFXZZ
0MNG0ZZ
0MNG3ZZ
0MNG4ZZ
0MNGXZZ
0MNH0ZZ
0MNH3ZZ
0MNH4ZZ
0MNHXZZ
0MNJ0ZZ
0MNJ3ZZ
0MNJ4ZZ
0MNJXZZ
0MNK0ZZ
0MNK3ZZ
0MNK4ZZ
0MNKXZZ
0MNL0ZZ
0MNL3ZZ
0MNL4ZZ
0MNLXZZ
0MNM0ZZ
0MNM3ZZ
0MNM4ZZ
0MNMXZZ
0MNN0ZZ
0MNN3ZZ
0MNN4ZZ
0MNNXZZ
0MNP0ZZ
0MNP3ZZ
0MNP4ZZ
0MNPXZZ
0MNQ0ZZ
0MNQ3ZZ
0MNQ4ZZ
0MNQXZZ
0MNR0ZZ
0MNR3ZZ
0MNR4ZZ
0MNRXZZ
0MNS0ZZ
0MNS3ZZ
0MNS4ZZ
0MNSXZZ
0MNT0ZZ
0MNT3ZZ
0MNT4ZZ
0MNTXZZ
0MNV0ZZ
0MNV3ZZ
0MNV4ZZ
0MNVXZZ
0MNW0ZZ
0MNW3ZZ
0MNW4ZZ
0MNWXZZ
0MPX00Z
0MPX07Z
0MPX0JZ
0MPX0KZ
0MPX0YZ
0MPX30Z
0MPX37Z
0MPX3JZ
0MPX3KZ
0MPX3YZ
0MPX40Z
0MPX47Z
0MPX4JZ
0MPX4KZ
0MPX4YZ
0MPXX0Z
0MPY00Z
0MPY07Z
0MPY0JZ
0MPY0KZ
0MPY0YZ
0MPY30Z
0MPY37Z
0MPY3JZ
0MPY3KZ
0MPY3YZ
0MPY40Z
0MPY47Z
0MPY4JZ
0MPY4KZ
0MPY4YZ
0MPYX0Z
0MQ00ZZ
0MQ03ZZ
0MQ04ZZ
0MQ10ZZ
0MQ13ZZ
0MQ14ZZ
0MQ20ZZ
0MQ23ZZ
0MQ24ZZ
0MQ30ZZ
0MQ33ZZ
0MQ34ZZ
0MQ40ZZ
0MQ43ZZ
0MQ44ZZ
0MQ50ZZ
0MQ53ZZ
0MQ54ZZ
0MQ60ZZ
0MQ63ZZ
0MQ64ZZ

0MQ70ZZ
0MQ73ZZ
0MQ74ZZ
0MQ80ZZ
0MQ83ZZ
0MQ84ZZ
0MQ90ZZ
0MQ93ZZ
0MQ94ZZ
0MQB0ZZ
0MQB3ZZ
0MQB4ZZ
0MQC0ZZ
0MQC3ZZ
0MQC4ZZ
0MQD0ZZ
0MQD3ZZ
0MQD4ZZ
0MQF0ZZ
0MQF3ZZ
0MQF4ZZ
0MQG0ZZ
0MQG3ZZ
0MQG4ZZ
0MQH0ZZ
0MQH3ZZ
0MQH4ZZ
0MQJ0ZZ
0MQJ3ZZ
0MQJ4ZZ
0MQK0ZZ
0MQK3ZZ
0MQK4ZZ
0MQL0ZZ
0MQL3ZZ
0MQL4ZZ
0MQM0ZZ
0MQM3ZZ
0MQM4ZZ
0MQN0ZZ
0MQN3ZZ
0MQN4ZZ
0MQP0ZZ
0MQP3ZZ
0MQP4ZZ
0MQQ0ZZ
0MQQ3ZZ
0MQQ4ZZ
0MQR0ZZ
0MQR3ZZ
0MQR4ZZ
0MQS0ZZ
0MQS3ZZ
0MQS4ZZ
0MQT0ZZ
0MQT3ZZ
0MQT4ZZ
0MQV0ZZ
0MQV3ZZ
0MQV4ZZ
0MQW0ZZ
0MQW3ZZ
0MQW4ZZ
0MR007Z
0MR00JZ
0MR00KZ
0MR047Z
0MR04JZ
0MR04KZ
0MR107Z
0MR10JZ
0MR10KZ
0MR147Z
0MR14JZ
0MR14KZ
0MR207Z
0MR20JZ
0MR20KZ
0MR247Z
0MR24JZ
0MR24KZ
0MR307Z
0MR30JZ
0MR30KZ
0MR347Z
0MR34JZ
0MR34KZ
0MR407Z
0MR40JZ
0MR40KZ
0MR447Z
0MR44JZ
0MR44KZ
0MR507Z
0MR50JZ
0MR50KZ
0MR547Z
0MR54JZ
0MR54KZ
0MR607Z
0MR60JZ
0MR60KZ
0MR647Z
0MR64JZ
0MR64KZ
0MR707Z
0MR70JZ
0MR70KZ
0MR747Z
0MR74JZ
0MR74KZ
0MR807Z
0MR80JZ
0MR80KZ
0MR847Z
0MR84JZ
0MR84KZ
0MR907Z
0MR90JZ
0MR90KZ
0MR947Z
0MR94JZ
0MR94KZ
0MRB07Z
0MRB0JZ
0MRB0KZ
0MRB47Z
0MRB4JZ
0MRB4KZ
0MRC07Z
0MRC0JZ
0MRC0KZ
0MRC47Z
0MRC4JZ
0MRC4KZ
0MRD07Z
0MRD0JZ
0MRD0KZ
0MRD47Z
0MRD4JZ
0MRD4KZ
0MRF07Z
0MRF0JZ
0MRF0KZ
0MRF47Z
0MRF4JZ
0MRF4KZ
0MRG07Z
0MRG0JZ
0MRG0KZ
0MRG47Z
0MRG4JZ
0MRG4KZ
0MRH07Z
0MRH0JZ
0MRH0KZ
0MRH47Z
0MRH4JZ
0MRH4KZ
0MRJ07Z
0MRJ0JZ
0MRJ0KZ
0MRJ47Z
0MRJ4JZ
0MRJ4KZ
0MRK07Z
0MRK0JZ
0MRK0KZ
0MRK47Z
0MRK4JZ
0MRK4KZ
0MRL07Z
0MRL0JZ
0MRL0KZ
0MRL47Z
0MRL4JZ
0MRL4KZ
0MRM07Z
0MRM0JZ
0MRM0KZ
0MRM47Z
0MRM4JZ
0MRM4KZ
0MRN07Z
0MRN0JZ
0MRN0KZ
0MRN47Z
0MRN4JZ
0MRN4KZ
0MRP07Z
0MRP0JZ
0MRP0KZ
0MRP47Z
0MRP4JZ
0MRP4KZ
0MRQ07Z
0MRQ0JZ
0MRQ0KZ
0MRQ47Z
0MRQ4JZ
0MRQ4KZ
0MRR07Z
0MRR0JZ
0MRR0KZ
0MRR47Z
0MRR4JZ
0MRR4KZ
0MRS07Z
0MRS0JZ
0MRS0KZ
0MRS47Z
0MRS4JZ
0MRS4KZ
0MRT07Z
0MRT0JZ
0MRT0KZ
0MRT47Z
0MRT4JZ
0MRT4KZ
0MRV07Z
0MRV0JZ
0MRV0KZ
0MRV47Z
0MRV4JZ
0MRV4KZ
0MRW07Z
0MRW0JZ
0MRW0KZ
0MRW47Z
0MRW4JZ
0MRW4KZ
0MS00ZZ
0MS04ZZ
0MS10ZZ
0MS14ZZ
0MS20ZZ
0MS24ZZ
0MS30ZZ
0MS34ZZ
0MS40ZZ
0MS44ZZ
0MS50ZZ
0MS54ZZ
0MS60ZZ
0MS64ZZ
0MS70ZZ
0MS74ZZ
0MS80ZZ
0MS84ZZ
0MS90ZZ
0MS94ZZ
0MSB0ZZ
0MSB4ZZ
0MSC0ZZ
0MSC4ZZ
0MSD0ZZ
0MSD4ZZ
0MSF0ZZ
0MSF4ZZ
0MSG0ZZ
0MSG4ZZ
0MSH0ZZ
0MSH4ZZ
0MSJ0ZZ
0MSJ4ZZ
0MSK0ZZ
0MSK4ZZ
0MSL0ZZ
0MSL4ZZ
0MSM0ZZ
0MSM4ZZ
0MSN0ZZ
0MSN4ZZ
0MSP0ZZ
0MSP4ZZ
0MSQ0ZZ
0MSQ4ZZ
0MSR0ZZ
0MSR4ZZ
0MSS0ZZ
0MSS4ZZ
0MST0ZZ
0MST4ZZ
0MSV0ZZ
0MSV4ZZ
0MSW0ZZ
0MSW4ZZ
0MT00ZZ
0MT04ZZ
0MT10ZZ
0MT14ZZ
0MT20ZZ
0MT24ZZ
0MT30ZZ
0MT34ZZ
0MT40ZZ
0MT44ZZ
0MT50ZZ
0MT54ZZ
0MT60ZZ
0MT64ZZ
0MT70ZZ
0MT74ZZ
0MT80ZZ
0MT84ZZ
0MT90ZZ
0MT94ZZ
0MTB0ZZ
0MTB4ZZ
0MTC0ZZ
0MTC4ZZ
0MTD0ZZ
0MTD4ZZ
0MTF0ZZ
0MTF4ZZ
0MTG0ZZ
0MTG4ZZ
0MTH0ZZ
0MTH4ZZ
0MTJ0ZZ
0MTJ4ZZ
0MTK0ZZ
0MTK4ZZ
0MTL0ZZ
0MTL4ZZ
0MTM0ZZ
0MTM4ZZ
0MTN0ZZ
0MTN4ZZ
0MTP0ZZ
0MTP4ZZ
0MTQ0ZZ
0MTQ4ZZ
0MTR0ZZ
0MTR4ZZ
0MTS0ZZ
0MTS4ZZ
0MTT0ZZ
0MTT4ZZ
0MTV0ZZ
0MTV4ZZ
0MWX3YZ
0MWX4YZ
0MWXX0Z
0MWXX7Z
0MWXXJZ
0MWXXKZ
0MWY3YZ
0MWY4YZ
0MWYX0Z
0MWYX7Z
0MWYXJZ
0MWYXKZ
0N20X0Z
0N20XYZ
0N2BX0Z
0N2BXYZ
0N2WX0Z
0N2WXYZ
0N554ZZ
0N560ZZ
0N563ZZ
0N564ZZ
0N570ZZ
0N573ZZ
0N574ZZ
0N5B0ZZ
0N5B3ZZ
0N5B4ZZ
0N5C0ZZ
0N5C3ZZ
0N5C4ZZ
0N5F0ZZ
0N5F3ZZ
0N5F4ZZ
0N5G0ZZ
0N5G3ZZ
0N5G4ZZ
0N5H0ZZ
0N5H3ZZ
0N5H4ZZ
0N5J0ZZ
0N5J3ZZ
0N5J4ZZ
0N5K0ZZ
0N5K3ZZ
0N5K4ZZ
0N5L0ZZ
0N5L3ZZ
0N5L4ZZ
0N5M0ZZ
0N5M3ZZ
0N5M4ZZ
0N5N0ZZ
0N5N3ZZ
0N5N4ZZ
0N5P0ZZ
0N5P3ZZ
0N5P4ZZ
0N5Q0ZZ
0N5Q3ZZ
0N5Q4ZZ
0N5R0ZZ
0N5R3ZZ
0N5R4ZZ
0N5T0ZZ
0N5T3ZZ
0N5T4ZZ
0N5V0ZZ
0N5V3ZZ
0N5V4ZZ
0N5X0ZZ
0N5X3ZZ
0N5X4ZZ
0N800ZZ
0N803ZZ
0N804ZZ
0N810ZZ
0N813ZZ
0N814ZZ
0N830ZZ
0N833ZZ
0N834ZZ
0N840ZZ
0N843ZZ
0N844ZZ
0N850ZZ
0N853ZZ
0N854ZZ
0N860ZZ
0N863ZZ
0N864ZZ
0N870ZZ
0N873ZZ
0N874ZZ
0N8B0ZZ
0N8B3ZZ
0N8B4ZZ
0N8C0ZZ
0N8C3ZZ
0N8C4ZZ
0N8F0ZZ
0N8F3ZZ
0N8F4ZZ
0N8G0ZZ
0N8G3ZZ
0N8G4ZZ
0N8H0ZZ
0N8H3ZZ
0N8H4ZZ
0N8J0ZZ
0N8J3ZZ
0N8J4ZZ
0N8K0ZZ
0N8K3ZZ
0N8K4ZZ
0N8L0ZZ
0N8L3ZZ
0N8L4ZZ
0N8M0ZZ
0N8M3ZZ
0N8M4ZZ
0N8N0ZZ
0N8N3ZZ
0N8N4ZZ
0N8P0ZZ
0N8P3ZZ
0N8P4ZZ
0N8Q0ZZ
0N8Q3ZZ
0N8Q4ZZ
0N8R0ZZ
0N8R3ZZ
0N8R4ZZ
0N8T0ZZ
0N8T3ZZ
0N8T4ZZ
0N8V0ZZ
0N8V3ZZ
0N8V4ZZ
0N8X0ZZ
0N8X3ZZ
0N8X4ZZ
0N9000Z
0N900ZX
0N900ZZ
0N9030Z
0N903ZX
0N903ZZ
0N9040Z
0N904ZX
0N904ZZ
0N9100Z
0N910ZX
0N910ZZ
0N9130Z
0N913ZX
0N913ZZ
0N9140Z
0N914ZX
0N914ZZ
0N9300Z
0N930ZX
0N930ZZ
0N9330Z
0N933ZX
0N933ZZ
0N9340Z
0N934ZX
0N934ZZ
0N9400Z
0N940ZX
0N940ZZ
0N9430Z
0N943ZX
0N943ZZ
0N9440Z
0N944ZX
0N944ZZ
0N9500Z
0N950ZX
0N950ZZ
0N9530Z
0N953ZX
0N953ZZ
0N9540Z
0N954ZX
0N954ZZ
0N9600Z
0N960ZX
0N960ZZ
0N9630Z
0N963ZX
0N963ZZ
0N9640Z
0N964ZX
0N964ZZ
0N9700Z
0N970ZX
0N970ZZ
0N9730Z
0N973ZX
0N973ZZ
0N9740Z
0N974ZX
0N974ZZ
0N9B00Z
0N9B0ZX
0N9B0ZZ
0N9B30Z
0N9B3ZX
0N9B3ZZ
0N9B40Z
0N9B4ZX
0N9B4ZZ
0N9C00Z
0N9C0ZX
0N9C0ZZ
0N9C30Z
0N9C3ZX
0N9C3ZZ
0N9C40Z
0N9C4ZX
0N9C4ZZ
0N9F00Z
0N9F0ZX
0N9F0ZZ
0N9F30Z
0N9F3ZX
0N9F3ZZ
0N9F40Z
0N9F4ZX
0N9F4ZZ
0N9G00Z
0N9G0ZX
0N9G0ZZ
0N9G30Z
0N9G3ZX
0N9G3ZZ
0N9G40Z
0N9G4ZX
0N9G4ZZ
0N9H00Z
0N9H0ZX
0N9H0ZZ
0N9H30Z
0N9H3ZX
0N9H3ZZ
0N9H40Z
0N9H4ZX
0N9H4ZZ
0N9J00Z
0N9J0ZX
0N9J0ZZ
0N9J30Z
0N9J3ZX
0N9J3ZZ
0N9J40Z
0N9J4ZX
0N9J4ZZ
0N9K00Z
0N9K0ZX
0N9K0ZZ
0N9K30Z
0N9K3ZX
0N9K3ZZ
0N9K40Z
0N9K4ZX
0N9K4ZZ
0N9L00Z
0N9L0ZX
0N9L0ZZ
0N9L30Z
0N9L3ZX
0N9L3ZZ
0N9L40Z
0N9L4ZX
0N9L4ZZ
0N9M00Z
0N9M0ZX
0N9M0ZZ
0N9M30Z
0N9M3ZX
0N9M3ZZ
0N9M40Z
0N9M4ZX
0N9M4ZZ
0N9N00Z
0N9N0ZX
0N9N0ZZ
0N9N30Z
0N9N3ZX
0N9N3ZZ
0N9N40Z
0N9N4ZX
0N9N4ZZ
0N9P00Z
0N9P0ZX
0N9P0ZZ
0N9P30Z
0N9P3ZX
0N9P3ZZ
0N9P40Z
0N9P4ZX
0N9P4ZZ
0N9Q00Z
0N9Q0ZX
0N9Q0ZZ
0N9Q30Z
0N9Q3ZX
0N9Q3ZZ
0N9Q40Z
0N9Q4ZX
0N9Q4ZZ
0N9R00Z
0N9R0ZX
0N9R0ZZ
0N9R30Z
0N9R3ZX
0N9R3ZZ
0N9R40Z
0N9R4ZX
0N9R4ZZ
0N9T00Z
0N9T0ZX
0N9T0ZZ
0N9T30Z
0N9T3ZX
0N9T3ZZ
0N9T40Z
0N9T4ZX
0N9T4ZZ
0N9V00Z
0N9V0ZX
0N9V0ZZ
0N9V30Z
0N9V3ZX
0N9V3ZZ
0N9V40Z
0N9V4ZX
0N9V4ZZ
0N9X00Z
0N9X0ZX
0N9X0ZZ
0N9X30Z
0N9X3ZX
0N9X3ZZ
0N9X40Z
0N9X4ZX
0N9X4ZZ
0NB00ZX
0NB00ZZ
0NB03ZX
0NB03ZZ
0NB04ZX
0NB04ZZ
0NB10ZX
0NB10ZZ
0NB13ZX
0NB13ZZ
0NB14ZX
0NB14ZZ
0NB30ZX
0NB30ZZ
0NB33ZX
0NB33ZZ
0NB34ZX
0NB34ZZ
0NB40ZX
0NB40ZZ
0NB43ZX
0NB43ZZ
0NB44ZX
0NB44ZZ
0NB50ZX
0NB50ZZ
0NB53ZX
0NB53ZZ
0NB54ZX
0NB54ZZ
0NB60ZX
0NB60ZZ
0NB63ZX
0NB63ZZ
0NB64ZX
0NB64ZZ

0MQ70ZZ-0NB64ZZ

APPENDIX H: NON-OR NOT AFFECTING MS-DRG ASSIGNMENT

0NB70ZX
0NB70ZZ
0NB73ZX
0NB73ZZ
0NB74ZX
0NB74ZZ
0NBB0ZX
0NBB3ZX
0NBB4ZX
0NBR0ZX
0NBR3ZX
0NBR4ZX
0NBT0ZX
0NBT3ZX
0NBT4ZX
0NBV0ZX
0NBV3ZX
0NBV4ZX
0NCB0ZZ
0NCB3ZZ
0NCB4ZZ
0NCR0ZZ
0NCR3ZZ
0NCR4ZZ
0NCT0ZZ
0NCT3ZZ
0NCT4ZZ
0NCV0ZZ
0NCV3ZZ
0NCV4ZZ
0NCX4ZZ
0ND00ZZ
0ND10ZZ
0ND30ZZ
0ND40ZZ
0ND50ZZ
0ND60ZZ
0ND70ZZ
0NDB0ZZ
0NDC0ZZ
0NDF0ZZ
0NDG0ZZ
0NDH0ZZ
0NDJ0ZZ
0NDK0ZZ
0NDL0ZZ
0NDM0ZZ
0NDN0ZZ
0NDP0ZZ
0NDQ0ZZ
0NDR0ZZ
0NDT0ZZ
0NDV0ZZ
0NDX0ZZ
0NH004Z
0NH005Z
0NH00MZ
0NH00NZ
0NH034Z
0NH035Z
0NH03MZ
0NH044Z
0NH045Z
0NH04MZ
0NH104Z
0NH134Z
0NH144Z
0NH304Z
0NH334Z
0NH344Z
0NH404Z
0NH434Z
0NH444Z
0NH504Z
0NH50SZ
0NH534Z
0NH53SZ
0NH544Z
0NH54SZ
0NH604Z
0NH60SZ
0NH634Z
0NH63SZ
0NH644Z
0NH64SZ
0NH704Z
0NH734Z
0NH744Z
0NHB04Z
0NHB0MZ
0NHB34Z
0NHB3MZ
0NHB44Z
0NHB4MZ
0NHC04Z
0NHC34Z
0NHC44Z
0NHF04Z
0NHF34Z
0NHF44Z
0NHG04Z
0NHG34Z
0NHG44Z
0NHH04Z
0NHH34Z
0NHH44Z
0NHJ04Z
0NHJ34Z
0NHJ44Z
0NHK04Z
0NHK34Z
0NHK44Z
0NHL04Z
0NHL34Z
0NHL44Z
0NHM04Z
0NHM34Z
0NHM44Z
0NHN04Z
0NHN34Z
0NHN44Z
0NHP04Z
0NHP34Z
0NHP44Z
0NHQ04Z
0NHQ34Z
0NHQ44Z
0NHR04Z
0NHR05Z
0NHR34Z
0NHR35Z
0NHR44Z
0NHR45Z
0NHT04Z
0NHT05Z
0NHT34Z
0NHT35Z
0NHT44Z
0NHT45Z
0NHV04Z
0NHV05Z
0NHV34Z
0NHV35Z
0NHV44Z
0NHV45Z
0NHW0MZ
0NHW3MZ
0NHW4MZ
0NHX04Z
0NHX34Z
0NHX44Z
0NJ00ZZ
0NJ03ZZ
0NJ04ZZ
0NJ0XZZ
0NJB0ZZ
0NJB3ZZ
0NJB4ZZ
0NJBXZZ
0NJW0ZZ
0NJW3ZZ
0NJW4ZZ
0NJWXZZ
0NN10ZZ
0NN13ZZ
0NN14ZZ
0NN30ZZ
0NN33ZZ
0NN34ZZ
0NN40ZZ
0NN43ZZ
0NN44ZZ
0NN50ZZ
0NN53ZZ
0NN54ZZ
0NN60ZZ
0NN63ZZ
0NN64ZZ
0NN70ZZ
0NN73ZZ
0NN74ZZ
0NNB0ZZ
0NNB3ZZ
0NNB4ZZ
0NNC0ZZ
0NNC3ZZ
0NNC4ZZ
0NNF0ZZ
0NNF3ZZ
0NNF4ZZ
0NNG0ZZ
0NNG3ZZ
0NNG4ZZ
0NNH0ZZ
0NNH3ZZ
0NNH4ZZ
0NNJ0ZZ
0NNJ3ZZ
0NNJ4ZZ
0NNK0ZZ
0NNK3ZZ
0NNK4ZZ
0NNL0ZZ
0NNL3ZZ
0NNL4ZZ
0NNM0ZZ
0NNM3ZZ
0NNM4ZZ
0NNN0ZZ
0NNN3ZZ
0NNN4ZZ
0NNP0ZZ
0NNP3ZZ
0NNP4ZZ
0NNQ0ZZ
0NNQ3ZZ
0NNQ4ZZ
0NNR0ZZ
0NNR3ZZ
0NNR4ZZ
0NNT0ZZ
0NNT3ZZ
0NNT4ZZ
0NNV0ZZ
0NNV3ZZ
0NNV4ZZ
0NNX0ZZ
0NNX3ZZ
0NNX4ZZ
0NP000Z
0NP004Z
0NP005Z
0NP007Z
0NP00JZ
0NP00KZ
0NP00MZ
0NP00NZ
0NP00SZ
0NP030Z
0NP034Z
0NP035Z
0NP037Z
0NP03JZ
0NP03KZ
0NP03MZ
0NP03SZ
0NP040Z
0NP044Z
0NP045Z
0NP047Z
0NP04JZ
0NP04KZ
0NP04MZ
0NP04SZ
0NP0X0Z
0NP0X4Z
0NP0X5Z
0NP0XMZ
0NP0XSZ
0NPB00Z
0NPB04Z
0NPB07Z
0NPB0JZ
0NPB0KZ
0NPB0MZ
0NPB30Z
0NPB34Z
0NPB37Z
0NPB3JZ
0NPB3KZ
0NPB3MZ
0NPB40Z
0NPB44Z
0NPB47Z
0NPB4JZ
0NPB4KZ
0NPB4MZ
0NPBX0Z
0NPBX4Z
0NPBXMZ
0NPW00Z
0NPW04Z
0NPW07Z
0NPW0JZ
0NPW0KZ
0NPW0MZ
0NPW30Z
0NPW34Z
0NPW37Z
0NPW3JZ
0NPW3KZ
0NPW3MZ
0NPW40Z
0NPW44Z
0NPW47Z
0NPW4JZ
0NPW4KZ
0NPW4MZ
0NPWX0Z
0NPWX4Z
0NPWXMZ
0NQ00ZZ
0NQ03ZZ
0NQ04ZZ
0NQ0XZZ
0NQ10ZZ
0NQ13ZZ
0NQ14ZZ
0NQ1XZZ
0NQ30ZZ
0NQ33ZZ
0NQ34ZZ
0NQ3XZZ
0NQ40ZZ
0NQ43ZZ
0NQ44ZZ
0NQ4XZZ
0NQ50ZZ
0NQ53ZZ
0NQ54ZZ
0NQ5XZZ
0NQ60ZZ
0NQ63ZZ
0NQ64ZZ
0NQ6XZZ
0NQ70ZZ
0NQ73ZZ
0NQ74ZZ
0NQ7XZZ
0NQB0ZZ
0NQB3ZZ
0NQB4ZZ
0NQBXZZ
0NQC0ZZ
0NQC3ZZ
0NQC4ZZ
0NQCXZZ
0NQF0ZZ
0NQF3ZZ
0NQF4ZZ
0NQFXZZ
0NQG0ZZ
0NQG3ZZ
0NQG4ZZ
0NQGXZZ
0NQH0ZZ
0NQH3ZZ
0NQH4ZZ
0NQHXZZ
0NQJ0ZZ
0NQJ3ZZ
0NQJ4ZZ
0NQJXZZ
0NQK0ZZ
0NQK3ZZ
0NQKXZZ
0NQLXZZ
0NQMXZZ
0NQNXZZ
0NQPXZZ
0NQQXZZ
0NQRXZZ
0NQTXZZ
0NQVXZZ
0NQXXZZ
0NRC47Z
0NRC4JZ
0NRC4KZ
0NRF07Z
0NRF0JZ
0NRF0KZ
0NRF37Z
0NRF3JZ
0NRF3KZ
0NRF47Z
0NRF4JZ
0NRF4KZ
0NRG07Z
0NRG0JZ
0NRG0KZ
0NRG37Z
0NRG3JZ
0NRG3KZ
0NRG47Z
0NRG4JZ
0NRG4KZ
0NRH07Z
0NRH0JZ
0NRH0KZ
0NRH37Z
0NRH3JZ
0NRH3KZ
0NRH47Z
0NRH4JZ
0NRH4KZ
0NRJ07Z
0NRJ0JZ
0NRJ0KZ
0NRJ37Z
0NRJ3JZ
0NRJ3KZ
0NRJ47Z
0NRJ4JZ
0NRJ4KZ
0NRK07Z
0NRK0JZ
0NRK0KZ
0NRK37Z
0NRK3JZ
0NRK3KZ
0NRK47Z
0NRK4JZ
0NRK4KZ
0NRL07Z
0NRL0JZ
0NRL0KZ
0NRL37Z
0NRL3JZ
0NRL3KZ
0NRL47Z
0NRL4JZ
0NRL4KZ
0NRM07Z
0NRM0JZ
0NRM0KZ
0NRM37Z
0NRM3JZ
0NRM3KZ
0NRM47Z
0NRM4JZ
0NRM4KZ
0NRN07Z
0NRN0JZ
0NRN0KZ
0NRN37Z
0NRN3JZ
0NRN3KZ
0NRN47Z
0NRN4JZ
0NRN4KZ
0NRP07Z
0NRP0JZ
0NRP0KZ
0NRP37Z
0NRP3JZ
0NRP3KZ
0NRP47Z
0NRP4JZ
0NRP4KZ
0NRQ07Z
0NRQ0JZ
0NRQ0KZ
0NRQ37Z
0NRQ3JZ
0NRQ3KZ
0NRQ47Z
0NRQ4JZ
0NRQ4KZ
0NRR07Z
0NRR0JZ
0NRR0KZ
0NRR37Z
0NRR3JZ
0NRR3KZ
0NRR47Z
0NRR4JZ
0NRR4KZ
0NRT07Z
0NRT0JZ
0NRT0KZ
0NRT37Z
0NRT3JZ
0NRT3KZ
0NRT47Z
0NRT4JZ
0NRT4KZ
0NRV07Z
0NRV0JZ
0NRV0KZ
0NRV37Z
0NRV3JZ
0NRV3KZ
0NRV47Z
0NRV4JZ
0NRV4KZ
0NRX07Z
0NRX0JZ
0NRX0KZ
0NRX37Z
0NRX3JZ
0NRX3KZ
0NRX47Z
0NRX4JZ
0NRX4KZ
0NS004Z
0NS005Z
0NS00ZZ
0NS034Z
0NS035Z
0NS03ZZ
0NS044Z
0NS045Z
0NS04ZZ
0NS0XZZ
0NS104Z
0NS10ZZ
0NS134Z
0NS13ZZ
0NS144Z
0NS14ZZ
0NS1XZZ
0NS304Z
0NS30ZZ
0NS334Z
0NS33ZZ
0NS344Z
0NS34ZZ
0NS3XZZ
0NS404Z
0NS40ZZ
0NS434Z
0NS43ZZ
0NS444Z
0NS44ZZ
0NS4XZZ
0NS504Z
0NS50ZZ
0NS534Z
0NS53ZZ
0NS544Z
0NS54ZZ
0NS5XZZ
0NS604Z
0NS60ZZ
0NS634Z
0NS63ZZ
0NS644Z
0NS64ZZ
0NS6XZZ
0NS704Z
0NS70ZZ
0NS734Z
0NS73ZZ
0NS744Z
0NS74ZZ
0NS7XZZ
0NSB04Z
0NSB0ZZ
0NSB34Z
0NSB3ZZ
0NSB44Z
0NSB4ZZ
0NSBXZZ
0NSC04Z
0NSC0ZZ
0NSC34Z
0NSC3ZZ
0NSC44Z
0NSC4ZZ
0NSCXZZ
0NSF04Z
0NSF0ZZ
0NSF34Z
0NSF3ZZ
0NSF44Z
0NSF4ZZ
0NSFXZZ
0NSG04Z
0NSG0ZZ
0NSG34Z
0NSG3ZZ
0NSG44Z
0NSG4ZZ
0NSGXZZ
0NSH04Z
0NSH0ZZ
0NSH34Z
0NSH3ZZ
0NSH44Z
0NSH4ZZ
0NSHXZZ
0NSJ04Z
0NSJ0ZZ
0NSJ34Z
0NSJ3ZZ
0NSJ44Z
0NSJ4ZZ
0NSJXZZ
0NSK04Z
0NSK0ZZ
0NSK34Z
0NSK3ZZ
0NSK44Z
0NSK4ZZ
0NSKXZZ
0NSL04Z
0NSL0ZZ
0NSL34Z
0NSL3ZZ
0NSL44Z
0NSL4ZZ
0NSLXZZ
0NSM04Z
0NSM0ZZ
0NSM34Z
0NSM3ZZ
0NSM44Z
0NSM4ZZ
0NSMXZZ
0NSN04Z
0NSN0ZZ
0NSN34Z
0NSN3ZZ
0NSN44Z
0NSN4ZZ
0NSNXZZ
0NSP04Z
0NSP0ZZ
0NSP34Z
0NSP3ZZ
0NSP44Z
0NSP4ZZ
0NSPXZZ
0NSQ04Z
0NSQ0ZZ
0NSQ34Z
0NSQ3ZZ
0NSQ44Z
0NSQ4ZZ
0NSQXZZ
0NSR04Z
0NSR05Z
0NSR0ZZ
0NSR34Z
0NSR35Z
0NSR3ZZ
0NSR44Z
0NSR45Z
0NSR4ZZ
0NSRXZZ
0NST04Z
0NST05Z
0NST0ZZ
0NST34Z
0NST35Z
0NST3ZZ
0NST44Z
0NST45Z
0NST4ZZ
0NSTXZZ
0NSV04Z
0NSV05Z
0NSV0ZZ
0NSV34Z
0NSV35Z
0NSV3ZZ
0NSV44Z
0NSV45Z
0NSV4ZZ
0NSVXZZ
0NSX04Z
0NSX0ZZ
0NSX34Z
0NSX3ZZ
0NSX44Z
0NSX4ZZ
0NSXXZZ
0NT10ZZ
0NT30ZZ
0NT40ZZ
0NT50ZZ
0NT60ZZ
0NT70ZZ
0NTB0ZZ
0NTC0ZZ
0NTF0ZZ
0NTG0ZZ
0NTH0ZZ
0NTJ0ZZ
0NTK0ZZ
0NUJ0KZ
0NUJ37Z
0NUJ3JZ
0NUJ3KZ
0NUJ47Z
0NUJ4JZ
0NUJ4KZ
0NUK07Z
0NUK0JZ
0NUK0KZ
0NUK37Z
0NUK3JZ
0NUK3KZ
0NUK47Z
0NUK4JZ
0NUK4KZ
0NUL07Z
0NUL0JZ
0NUL0KZ
0NUL37Z
0NUL3JZ
0NUL3KZ
0NUL47Z
0NUL4JZ
0NUL4KZ
0NUM07Z
0NUM0JZ
0NUM0KZ
0NUM37Z
0NUM3JZ
0NUM3KZ
0NUM47Z
0NUM4JZ
0NUM4KZ
0NUN07Z
0NUN0JZ
0NUN0KZ
0NUN37Z
0NUN3JZ
0NUN3KZ
0NUN47Z
0NUN4JZ
0NUN4KZ
0NUP07Z
0NUP0JZ
0NUP0KZ

0NUP37Z
0NUP3JZ
0NUP3KZ
0NUP47Z
0NUP4JZ
0NUP4KZ
0NUQ07Z
0NUQ0JZ
0NUQ0KZ
0NUQ37Z
0NUQ3JZ
0NUQ3KZ
0NUQ47Z
0NUQ4JZ
0NUQ4KZ
0NUR07Z
0NUR0JZ
0NUR0KZ
0NUR37Z
0NUR3JZ
0NUR3KZ
0NUR47Z
0NUR4JZ
0NUR4KZ
0NUT07Z
0NUT0JZ
0NUT0KZ
0NUT37Z
0NUT3JZ
0NUT3KZ
0NUT47Z
0NUT4JZ
0NUT4KZ
0NUV07Z
0NUV0JZ
0NUV0KZ
0NUV37Z
0NUV3JZ
0NUV3KZ
0NUV47Z
0NUV4JZ
0NUV4KZ
0NUX07Z
0NUX0JZ
0NUX0KZ
0NUX37Z
0NUX3JZ
0NUX3KZ
0NUX47Z
0NUX4JZ
0NUX4KZ
0NW000Z
0NW004Z
0NW005Z
0NW007Z
0NW00JZ
0NW00KZ
0NW00MZ
0NW00NZ
0NW00SZ
0NW030Z
0NW034Z
0NW035Z
0NW037Z
0NW03JZ
0NW03KZ
0NW03MZ
0NW03SZ
0NW040Z
0NW044Z
0NW045Z
0NW047Z
0NW04JZ
0NW04KZ
0NW04MZ
0NW04SZ
0NW0X0Z
0NW0X4Z
0NW0X5Z
0NW0X7Z
0NW0XJZ
0NW0XKZ
0NW0XMZ
0NW0XSZ
0NWB00Z
0NWB04Z
0NWB07Z
0NWB0JZ
0NWB0KZ
0NWB0MZ
0NWB30Z
0NWB34Z
0NWB37Z
0NWB3JZ
0NWB3KZ
0NWB3MZ
0NWB40Z
0NWB44Z
0NWB47Z
0NWB4JZ
0NWB4KZ
0NWB4MZ
0NWBX0Z
0NWBX4Z
0NWBX7Z
0NWBXJZ
0NWBXKZ
0NWBXMZ
0NWW00Z
0NWW04Z
0NWW07Z
0NWW0JZ
0NWW0KZ
0NWW0MZ
0NWW30Z
0NWW34Z
0NWW37Z
0NWW3JZ
0NWW3KZ
0NWW3MZ
0NWW40Z
0NWW44Z
0NWW47Z
0NWW4JZ
0NWW4KZ
0NWW4MZ
0NWWX0Z
0NWWX4Z
0NWWX7Z
0NWWXJZ
0NWWXKZ
0NWWXMZ
0P2YX0Z
0P2YXYZ
0P500ZZ
0P503ZZ
0P504ZZ
0P510ZZ
0P513ZZ
0P514ZZ
0P520ZZ
0P523ZZ
0P524ZZ
0P530ZZ
0P533ZZ
0P534ZZ
0P540ZZ
0P543ZZ
0P544ZZ
0P550ZZ
0P553ZZ
0P554ZZ
0P560ZZ
0P563ZZ
0P564ZZ
0P570ZZ
0P573ZZ
0P574ZZ
0P580ZZ
0P583ZZ
0P584ZZ
0P590ZZ
0P593ZZ
0P594ZZ
0P5B0ZZ
0P5B3ZZ
0P5B4ZZ
0P5C0ZZ
0P5C3ZZ
0P5C4ZZ
0P5D0ZZ
0P5D3ZZ
0P5D4ZZ
0P5F0ZZ
0P5F3ZZ
0P5F4ZZ
0P5G0ZZ
0P5G3ZZ
0P5G4ZZ
0P5H0ZZ
0P5H3ZZ
0P5H4ZZ
0P5J0ZZ
0P5J3ZZ
0P5J4ZZ
0P5K0ZZ
0P5K3ZZ
0P5K4ZZ
0P5L0ZZ
0P5L3ZZ
0P5L4ZZ
0P5M0ZZ
0P5M3ZZ
0P5M4ZZ
0P5N0ZZ
0P5N3ZZ
0P5N4ZZ
0P5P0ZZ
0P5P3ZZ
0P5P4ZZ
0P5Q0ZZ
0P5Q3ZZ
0P5Q4ZZ
0P5R0ZZ
0P5R3ZZ
0P5R4ZZ
0P5S0ZZ
0P5S3ZZ
0P5S4ZZ
0P5T0ZZ
0P5T3ZZ
0P5T4ZZ
0P5V0ZZ
0P5V3ZZ
0P5V4ZZ
0P800ZZ
0P803ZZ
0P804ZZ
0P810ZZ
0P813ZZ
0P814ZZ
0P820ZZ
0P823ZZ
0P824ZZ
0P830ZZ
0P833ZZ
0P834ZZ
0P840ZZ
0P843ZZ
0P844ZZ
0P850ZZ
0P853ZZ
0P854ZZ
0P860ZZ
0P863ZZ
0P864ZZ
0P870ZZ
0P873ZZ
0P874ZZ
0P880ZZ
0P883ZZ
0P884ZZ
0P890ZZ
0P893ZZ
0P894ZZ
0P8B0ZZ
0P8B3ZZ
0P8B4ZZ
0P8C0ZZ
0P8C3ZZ
0P8C4ZZ
0P8D0ZZ
0P8D3ZZ
0P8D4ZZ
0P8F0ZZ
0P8F3ZZ
0P8F4ZZ
0P8G0ZZ
0P8G3ZZ
0P8G4ZZ
0P8H0ZZ
0P8H3ZZ
0P8H4ZZ
0P8J0ZZ
0P8J3ZZ
0P8J4ZZ
0P8K0ZZ
0P8K3ZZ
0P8K4ZZ
0P8L0ZZ
0P9030Z
0P903ZZ
0P9130Z
0P913ZZ
0P9230Z
0P923ZZ
0P9330Z
0P933ZZ
0P9430Z
0P943ZZ
0P9530Z
0P953ZZ
0P9630Z
0P963ZZ
0P9730Z
0P973ZZ
0P9830Z
0P983ZZ
0P9930Z
0P993ZZ
0P9B30Z
0P9B3ZZ
0P9C30Z
0P9C3ZZ
0P9D30Z
0P9D3ZZ
0P9F30Z
0P9F3ZZ
0P9G30Z
0P9G3ZZ
0P9H30Z
0P9H3ZZ
0P9J0ZZ
0P9J30Z
0P9J3ZX
0P9J3ZZ
0P9J40Z
0P9J4ZX
0P9J4ZZ
0P9K00Z
0P9K0ZX
0P9K0ZZ
0P9K30Z
0P9K3ZX
0P9K3ZZ
0P9K40Z
0P9K4ZX
0P9K4ZZ
0P9L00Z
0P9L0ZX
0P9L0ZZ
0P9L30Z
0P9L3ZX
0P9L3ZZ
0P9L40Z
0P9L4ZX
0P9L4ZZ
0P9M00Z
0P9M0ZX
0P9M0ZZ
0P9M30Z
0P9M3ZX
0P9M3ZZ
0P9M40Z
0P9M4ZX
0P9M4ZZ
0P9N00Z
0P9N0ZX
0P9N0ZZ
0P9N30Z
0P9N3ZX
0P9N3ZZ
0P9N40Z
0P9N4ZX
0P9N4ZZ
0P9P00Z
0P9P0ZX
0P9P0ZZ
0P9P30Z
0P9P3ZX
0P9P3ZZ
0P9P40Z
0P9P4ZX
0P9P4ZZ
0P9Q00Z
0P9Q0ZX
0P9Q0ZZ
0P9Q30Z
0P9Q3ZX
0P9Q3ZZ
0P9Q40Z
0P9Q4ZX
0P9Q4ZZ
0P9R00Z
0P9R0ZX
0P9R0ZZ
0P9R30Z
0P9R3ZX
0P9R3ZZ
0P9R40Z
0P9R4ZX
0P9R4ZZ
0P9S00Z
0P9S0ZX
0P9S0ZZ
0P9S30Z
0P9S3ZX
0P9S3ZZ
0P9S40Z
0P9S4ZX
0P9S4ZZ
0P9T00Z
0P9T0ZX
0P9T0ZZ
0P9T30Z
0P9T3ZX
0P9T3ZZ
0P9T40Z
0P9T4ZX
0P9T4ZZ
0P9V00Z
0P9V0ZX
0P9V0ZZ
0P9V30Z
0P9V3ZX
0P9V3ZZ
0P9V40Z
0P9V4ZX
0P9V4ZZ
0PB00ZX
0PB00ZZ
0PB03ZX
0PB03ZZ
0PB04ZX
0PB04ZZ
0PB10ZX
0PB10ZZ
0PB13ZX
0PB13ZZ
0PB14ZX
0PB14ZZ
0PB20ZX
0PB20ZZ
0PB23ZX
0PB23ZZ
0PB24ZX
0PB24ZZ
0PB30ZX
0PB30ZZ
0PB33ZX
0PB33ZZ
0PB34ZX
0PB34ZZ
0PB40ZX
0PB40ZZ
0PB43ZX
0PB43ZZ
0PB44ZX
0PB44ZZ
0PB50ZX
0PB50ZZ
0PB53ZX
0PB53ZZ
0PB54ZX
0PB54ZZ
0PB60ZX
0PB60ZZ
0PB63ZX
0PB63ZZ
0PB64ZX
0PB64ZZ
0PB70ZX
0PB70ZZ
0PB73ZX
0PB73ZZ
0PB74ZX
0PB74ZZ
0PB80ZX
0PB80ZZ
0PB83ZX
0PB83ZZ
0PB84ZX
0PB84ZZ
0PB90ZX
0PB90ZZ
0PB93ZX
0PB93ZZ
0PB94ZX
0PB94ZZ
0PBB0ZX
0PBB0ZZ
0PBB3ZX
0PBB3ZZ
0PBB4ZX
0PBB4ZZ
0PBC0ZX
0PBC0ZZ
0PBC3ZX
0PBC3ZZ
0PBC4ZX
0PBC4ZZ
0PBD0ZX
0PBD0ZZ
0PBD3ZX
0PBD3ZZ
0PBD4ZX
0PBD4ZZ
0PBF0ZX
0PBF0ZZ
0PBF3ZX
0PBF3ZZ
0PBF4ZX
0PBF4ZZ
0PBG0ZX
0PBG0ZZ
0PBG3ZX
0PBG3ZZ
0PBG4ZX
0PBG4ZZ
0PBH0ZX
0PBH0ZZ
0PBH3ZX
0PBH3ZZ
0PBH4ZX
0PBH4ZZ
0PBJ0ZX
0PBJ0ZZ
0PBJ3ZX
0PBJ3ZZ
0PBJ4ZX
0PBJ4ZZ
0PBK0ZX
0PBK0ZZ
0PBK3ZX
0PBK3ZZ
0PBK4ZX
0PBK4ZZ
0PBL0ZX
0PBL0ZZ
0PBL3ZX
0PBL3ZZ
0PBL4ZX
0PBL4ZZ
0PBM0ZX
0PBM0ZZ
0PBM3ZX
0PBM3ZZ
0PBM4ZX
0PBM4ZZ
0PBN0ZX
0PBN0ZZ
0PBN3ZX
0PBN3ZZ
0PBN4ZX
0PBN4ZZ
0PBP0ZX
0PCT0ZZ
0PCT3ZZ
0PCT4ZZ
0PCV0ZZ
0PCV3ZZ
0PCV4ZZ
0PD00ZZ
0PD10ZZ
0PD20ZZ
0PD30ZZ
0PD40ZZ
0PD50ZZ
0PD60ZZ
0PD70ZZ
0PD80ZZ
0PD90ZZ
0PDB0ZZ
0PDC0ZZ
0PDD0ZZ
0PDF0ZZ
0PDG0ZZ
0PDH0ZZ
0PDJ0ZZ
0PDK0ZZ
0PDL0ZZ
0PDM0ZZ
0PDN0ZZ
0PDP0ZZ
0PDQ0ZZ
0PDR0ZZ
0PDS0ZZ
0PDT0ZZ
0PDV0ZZ
0PH000Z
0PH004Z
0PH030Z
0PH034Z
0PH040Z
0PH044Z
0PH104Z
0PH134Z
0PH144Z
0PH204Z
0PH234Z
0PH244Z
0PH304Z
0PH334Z
0PH344Z
0PH404Z
0PH434Z
0PH444Z
0PH504Z
0PH534Z
0PH544Z
0PH604Z
0PH634Z
0PH644Z
0PH704Z
0PH734Z
0PH744Z
0PH804Z
0PH834Z
0PH844Z
0PH904Z
0PH934Z
0PH944Z
0PHB04Z
0PHB34Z
0PHB44Z
0PHC04Z
0PHC05Z
0PHC06Z
0PHC08Z
0PHC0BZ
0PHC0CZ
0PHC0DZ
0PHC34Z
0PHC35Z
0PHC36Z
0PHC38Z
0PHC3BZ
0PHC3CZ
0PHC3DZ
0PHC44Z
0PHC45Z
0PHC46Z
0PHC48Z
0PHC4BZ
0PHC4CZ
0PHC4DZ
0PHD04Z
0PHD05Z
0PHD06Z
0PHD08Z
0PHD0BZ
0PHD0CZ
0PHD0DZ
0PHD34Z
0PHD35Z
0PHD36Z
0PHD38Z
0PHD3BZ
0PHD3CZ
0PHD3DZ
0PHD44Z
0PHD45Z
0PHD46Z
0PHD48Z
0PHD4BZ
0PHD4CZ
0PHD4DZ
0PHF04Z
0PHF05Z
0PHF06Z
0PHF08Z
0PHF0BZ
0PHF0CZ
0PHF0DZ
0PHF34Z
0PHF35Z
0PHF36Z
0PHF38Z
0PHF3BZ
0PHF3CZ
0PHF3DZ
0PHF44Z
0PHF45Z
0PHF46Z
0PHF48Z
0PHF4BZ
0PHF4CZ
0PHF4DZ
0PHG04Z
0PHG05Z
0PHG06Z
0PHG08Z
0PHG0BZ
0PHG0CZ
0PHG0DZ
0PHG34Z
0PHG35Z
0PHG36Z
0PHG38Z
0PHG3BZ
0PHG3CZ
0PHG3DZ
0PHG44Z
0PHG45Z
0PHG46Z
0PHG48Z
0PHG4BZ
0PHG4CZ
0PHG4DZ
0PHH04Z
0PHH05Z
0PHH06Z
0PHH08Z
0PHH0BZ
0PHH0CZ
0PHH0DZ
0PHH34Z
0PHH35Z
0PHH36Z
0PHH38Z
0PHH3BZ
0PHH3CZ
0PHH3DZ
0PHH44Z
0PHH45Z
0PHH46Z
0PHH48Z
0PHH4BZ
0PHH4CZ
0PHH4DZ
0PHJ04Z
0PHJ05Z
0PHJ06Z
0PHJ08Z
0PHJ0BZ
0PHJ0CZ
0PHJ0DZ
0PHJ34Z
0PHJ35Z
0PHJ36Z
0PHJ38Z
0PHJ3BZ
0PHJ3CZ
0PHJ3DZ
0PHJ44Z
0PHJ45Z
0PHJ46Z
0PHJ48Z
0PHJ4BZ
0PHJ4CZ
0PHJ4DZ
0PHK04Z
0PHK05Z
0PHK06Z
0PHK08Z
0PHK0BZ

0PHK0CZ-0PSF3DZ

APPENDIX H: NON-OR NOT AFFECTING MS-DRG ASSIGNMENT

0PHK0CZ
0PHK0DZ
0PHK34Z
0PHK35Z
0PHK36Z
0PHK38Z
0PHK3BZ
0PHK3CZ
0PHK3DZ
0PHK44Z
0PHK45Z
0PHK46Z
0PHK48Z
0PHK4BZ
0PHK4CZ
0PHK4DZ
0PHL04Z
0PHL05Z
0PHL06Z
0PHL08Z
0PHL0BZ
0PHL0CZ
0PHL0DZ
0PHL34Z
0PHL35Z
0PHL36Z
0PHL38Z
0PHL3BZ
0PHL3CZ
0PHL3DZ
0PHL44Z
0PHL45Z
0PHL46Z
0PHL48Z
0PHL4BZ
0PHL4CZ
0PHL4DZ
0PHM04Z
0PHM05Z
0PHM34Z
0PHM35Z
0PHM44Z
0PHM45Z
0PHN04Z
0PHN05Z
0PHN34Z
0PHN35Z
0PHN44Z
0PHN45Z
0PHP04Z
0PHP05Z
0PHP34Z
0PHP35Z
0PHP44Z
0PHP45Z
0PHQ04Z
0PHQ05Z
0PHQ34Z
0PHQ35Z
0PHQ44Z
0PHQ45Z
0PHR04Z
0PHR05Z
0PHR34Z
0PHR35Z
0PHR44Z
0PHR45Z
0PHS04Z
0PJY3ZZ
0PJYXZZ
0PP0X4Z
0PP1X4Z
0PP2X4Z
0PP3X4Z
0PP4X4Z
0PP534Z
0PP537Z
0PP53JZ
0PP53KZ
0PP544Z
0PP547Z
0PP54JZ
0PP54KZ
0PP5X4Z
0PP604Z
0PP607Z
0PP60JZ
0PP60KZ
0PP634Z
0PP637Z
0PP63JZ
0PP63KZ
0PP644Z
0PP647Z
0PP64JZ
0PP64KZ
0PP6X4Z
0PP704Z
0PP707Z
0PP70JZ
0PP70KZ
0PP734Z
0PP737Z
0PP73JZ
0PP73KZ
0PP744Z
0PP747Z
0PP74JZ
0PP74KZ
0PP7X4Z
0PP804Z
0PP807Z
0PP80JZ
0PP80KZ
0PP834Z
0PP837Z
0PP83JZ
0PP83KZ
0PP844Z
0PP847Z
0PP84JZ
0PP84KZ
0PP8X4Z
0PP904Z
0PP907Z
0PP90JZ
0PP90KZ
0PP934Z
0PP937Z
0PP93JZ
0PP93KZ
0PP944Z
0PP947Z
0PP94JZ
0PP94KZ
0PP9X4Z
0PPB04Z
0PPB07Z
0PPB0JZ
0PPB0KZ
0PPB34Z
0PPB37Z
0PPB3JZ
0PPB3KZ
0PPB44Z
0PPB47Z
0PPB4JZ
0PPB4KZ
0PPBX4Z
0PPC04Z
0PPC05Z
0PPC07Z
0PPC0JZ
0PPC0KZ
0PPC34Z
0PPC35Z
0PPC37Z
0PPC3JZ
0PPC3KZ
0PPC44Z
0PPC45Z
0PPC47Z
0PPC4JZ
0PPC4KZ
0PPCX4Z
0PPCX5Z
0PPD04Z
0PPD05Z
0PPD07Z
0PPD0JZ
0PPD0KZ
0PPD34Z
0PPD35Z
0PPD37Z
0PPD3JZ
0PPD3KZ
0PPD44Z
0PPD45Z
0PPD47Z
0PPD4JZ
0PPD4KZ
0PPDX4Z
0PPDX5Z
0PPF04Z
0PPF05Z
0PPF07Z
0PPF0JZ
0PPF0KZ
0PPF34Z
0PPF35Z
0PPF37Z
0PPF3JZ
0PPF3KZ
0PPF44Z
0PPF45Z
0PPF47Z
0PPF4JZ
0PPF4KZ
0PPFX4Z
0PPFX5Z
0PPG04Z
0PPG05Z
0PPG07Z
0PPG0JZ
0PPG0KZ
0PPG34Z
0PPG35Z
0PPG37Z
0PPG3JZ
0PPG3KZ
0PPG44Z
0PPG45Z
0PPG47Z
0PPG4JZ
0PPG4KZ
0PPGX4Z
0PPGX5Z
0PPH04Z
0PPH05Z
0PPH07Z
0PPH0JZ
0PPH0KZ
0PPH34Z
0PPH35Z
0PPH37Z
0PPH3JZ
0PPH3KZ
0PPH44Z
0PPH45Z
0PPH47Z
0PPH4JZ
0PPH4KZ
0PPHX4Z
0PPHX5Z
0PPJ04Z
0PPJ05Z
0PPJ07Z
0PPJ0JZ
0PPJ0KZ
0PPJ34Z
0PPJ35Z
0PPJ37Z
0PPJ3JZ
0PPJ3KZ
0PPJ44Z
0PPJ45Z
0PPJ47Z
0PPJ4JZ
0PPJ4KZ
0PPJX4Z
0PPJX5Z
0PPK04Z
0PPK05Z
0PPK07Z
0PPK0JZ
0PPK0KZ
0PPK34Z
0PPK35Z
0PPK37Z
0PPK3JZ
0PPK3KZ
0PPK44Z
0PPK45Z
0PPK47Z
0PPK4JZ
0PPK4KZ
0PPKX4Z
0PPKX5Z
0PPL04Z
0PPL05Z
0PPL07Z
0PPL0JZ
0PPL0KZ
0PPL34Z
0PPL35Z
0PPL37Z
0PPL3JZ
0PPL3KZ
0PPL44Z
0PPL45Z
0PPL47Z
0PPL4JZ
0PPL4KZ
0PPLX4Z
0PPLX5Z
0PPM04Z
0PPM05Z
0PPM07Z
0PPM0JZ
0PPM0KZ
0PPM34Z
0PPM35Z
0PPM37Z
0PPM3JZ
0PPM3KZ
0PPM44Z
0PPM45Z
0PPM47Z
0PPM4JZ
0PPM4KZ
0PPMX4Z
0PPMX5Z
0PPN04Z
0PPN05Z
0PPN07Z
0PPN0JZ
0PPN0KZ
0PPN34Z
0PPN35Z
0PPN37Z
0PPN3JZ
0PPN3KZ
0PPN44Z
0PPN45Z
0PPN47Z
0PPN4JZ
0PPN4KZ
0PPNX4Z
0PPNX5Z
0PPP04Z
0PPP05Z
0PPP07Z
0PPP0JZ
0PPP0KZ
0PPP34Z
0PPP35Z
0PPP37Z
0PPP3JZ
0PPP3KZ
0PPP44Z
0PPP45Z
0PPP47Z
0PPP4JZ
0PPP4KZ
0PPPX4Z
0PPPX5Z
0PPQ04Z
0PPQ05Z
0PPQ07Z
0PPQ0JZ
0PPQ0KZ
0PPQ34Z
0PPQ35Z
0PPQ37Z
0PPQ3JZ
0PPQ3KZ
0PPQ44Z
0PPQ45Z
0PPQ47Z
0PPQ4JZ
0PPQ4KZ
0PPQX4Z
0PPQX5Z
0PPR04Z
0PPR05Z
0PPR07Z
0PPR0JZ
0PPR0KZ
0PPR34Z
0PPR35Z
0PPR37Z
0PPR3JZ
0PPR3KZ
0PPR44Z
0PPR45Z
0PPR47Z
0PPR4JZ
0PPR4KZ
0PPRX4Z
0PPRX5Z
0PPS04Z
0PPS05Z
0PPS07Z
0PPS0JZ
0PPS0KZ
0PPS34Z
0PPS35Z
0PPS37Z
0PPS3JZ
0PPS3KZ
0PPS44Z
0PPS45Z
0PPS47Z
0PPS4JZ
0PPS4KZ
0PPSX4Z
0PPSX5Z
0PPT04Z
0PPT05Z
0PPT07Z
0PPT0JZ
0PPT0KZ
0PPT34Z
0PPT35Z
0PPT37Z
0PPT3JZ
0PPT3KZ
0PPT44Z
0PPT45Z
0PPT47Z
0PPT4JZ
0PPT4KZ
0PPTX4Z
0PPTX5Z
0PPV04Z
0PPV05Z
0PPV07Z
0PPV0JZ
0PPV0KZ
0PPV34Z
0PPV35Z
0PPV37Z
0PPV3JZ
0PPV3KZ
0PPV44Z
0PPV45Z
0PPV47Z
0PPV4JZ
0PPV4KZ
0PPVX4Z
0PPVX5Z
0PPY00Z
0PPY0MZ
0PPY30Z
0PPY3MZ
0PPY40Z
0PPY4MZ
0PPYX0Z
0PPYXMZ
0PQ0XZZ
0PQ1XZZ
0PQ2XZZ
0PQ3XZZ
0PQ4XZZ
0PQ5XZZ
0PQ6XZZ
0PQ7XZZ
0PQ8XZZ
0PQ9XZZ
0PQBXZZ
0PQCXZZ
0PQDXZZ
0PQFXZZ
0PQGXZZ
0PQHXZZ
0PQJXZZ
0PQKXZZ
0PQLXZZ
0PQMXZZ
0PQNXZZ
0PQPXZZ
0PQQXZZ
0PQRXZZ
0PQSXZZ
0PQTXZZ
0PQVXZZ
0PRD0KZ
0PRD37Z
0PRD3JZ
0PRD3KZ
0PRD47Z
0PRD4JZ
0PRD4KZ
0PRF07Z
0PRF0JZ
0PRF0KZ
0PRF37Z
0PRF3JZ
0PRF3KZ
0PRF47Z
0PRF4JZ
0PRF4KZ
0PRG07Z
0PRG0JZ
0PRG0KZ
0PRG37Z
0PRG3JZ
0PRG3KZ
0PRG47Z
0PRG4JZ
0PRG4KZ
0PRH07Z
0PRH0JZ
0PRH0KZ
0PRH37Z
0PRH3JZ
0PRH3KZ
0PRH47Z
0PRH4JZ
0PRH4KZ
0PRJ07Z
0PRJ0JZ
0PRJ0KZ
0PRJ37Z
0PRJ3JZ
0PRJ3KZ
0PRJ47Z
0PRJ4JZ
0PRJ4KZ
0PRK07Z
0PRK0JZ
0PRK0KZ
0PRK37Z
0PRK3JZ
0PRK3KZ
0PRK47Z
0PRK4JZ
0PRK4KZ
0PRL07Z
0PRL0JZ
0PRL0KZ
0PRL37Z
0PRL3JZ
0PRL3KZ
0PRL47Z
0PRL4JZ
0PRL4KZ
0PRM07Z
0PRM0JZ
0PRM0KZ
0PRM37Z
0PRM3JZ
0PRM3KZ
0PRM47Z
0PRM4JZ
0PRM4KZ
0PRN07Z
0PRN0JZ
0PRN0KZ
0PRN37Z
0PRN3JZ
0PRN3KZ
0PRN47Z
0PRN4JZ
0PRN4KZ
0PRP07Z
0PRP0JZ
0PRP0KZ
0PRP37Z
0PRP3JZ
0PRP3KZ
0PRP47Z
0PRP4JZ
0PRP4KZ
0PRQ07Z
0PRQ0JZ
0PRQ0KZ
0PRQ37Z
0PRQ3JZ
0PRQ3KZ
0PRQ47Z
0PRQ4JZ
0PRQ4KZ
0PRR07Z
0PRR0JZ
0PRR0KZ
0PRR37Z
0PRR3JZ
0PRR3KZ
0PRR47Z
0PRR4JZ
0PRR4KZ
0PRS07Z
0PRS0JZ
0PRS0KZ
0PRS37Z
0PRS3JZ
0PRS3KZ
0PRS47Z
0PRS4JZ
0PRS4KZ
0PRT07Z
0PRT0JZ
0PRT0KZ
0PRT37Z
0PRT3JZ
0PRT3KZ
0PRT47Z
0PRT4JZ
0PRT4KZ
0PRV07Z
0PRV0JZ
0PRV0KZ
0PRV37Z
0PRV3JZ
0PRV3KZ
0PRV47Z
0PRV4JZ
0PRV4KZ
0PS000Z
0PS004Z
0PS00ZZ
0PS030Z
0PS034Z
0PS03ZZ
0PS040Z
0PS044Z
0PS04ZZ
0PS0XZZ
0PS104Z
0PS10ZZ
0PS134Z
0PS13ZZ
0PS144Z
0PS14ZZ
0PS1XZZ
0PS204Z
0PS20ZZ
0PS234Z
0PS23ZZ
0PS244Z
0PS24ZZ
0PS2XZZ
0PS304Z
0PS30ZZ
0PS334Z
0PS33ZZ
0PS344Z
0PS34ZZ
0PS3XZZ
0PS404Z
0PS40ZZ
0PS434Z
0PS43ZZ
0PS444Z
0PS44ZZ
0PS4XZZ
0PS504Z
0PS50ZZ
0PS534Z
0PS53ZZ
0PS544Z
0PS54ZZ
0PS5XZZ
0PS604Z
0PS60ZZ
0PS634Z
0PS63ZZ
0PS644Z
0PS64ZZ
0PS6XZZ
0PS704Z
0PS70ZZ
0PS734Z
0PS73ZZ
0PS744Z
0PS74ZZ
0PS7XZZ
0PS804Z
0PS80ZZ
0PS834Z
0PS83ZZ
0PS844Z
0PS84ZZ
0PS8XZZ
0PS904Z
0PS90ZZ
0PS934Z
0PS93ZZ
0PS944Z
0PS94ZZ
0PS9XZZ
0PSB04Z
0PSB0ZZ
0PSB34Z
0PSB3ZZ
0PSB44Z
0PSB4ZZ
0PSBXZZ
0PSC04Z
0PSC05Z
0PSC06Z
0PSC0BZ
0PSC0CZ
0PSC0DZ
0PSC0ZZ
0PSC34Z
0PSC35Z
0PSC36Z
0PSC3BZ
0PSC3CZ
0PSC3DZ
0PSC3ZZ
0PSC44Z
0PSC45Z
0PSC46Z
0PSC4BZ
0PSC4CZ
0PSC4DZ
0PSC4ZZ
0PSCXZZ
0PSD04Z
0PSD05Z
0PSD06Z
0PSD0BZ
0PSD0CZ
0PSD0DZ
0PSD0ZZ
0PSD34Z
0PSD35Z
0PSD36Z
0PSD3BZ
0PSD3CZ
0PSD3DZ
0PSD3ZZ
0PSD44Z
0PSD45Z
0PSD46Z
0PSD4BZ
0PSD4CZ
0PSD4DZ
0PSD4ZZ
0PSDXZZ
0PSF04Z
0PSF05Z
0PSF06Z
0PSF0BZ
0PSF0CZ
0PSF0DZ
0PSF0ZZ
0PSF34Z
0PSF35Z
0PSF36Z
0PSF3BZ
0PSF3CZ
0PSF3DZ

0PSF3ZZ-0Q8S4ZZ

0PSF3ZZ
0PSF44Z
0PSF45Z
0PSF46Z
0PSF4BZ
0PSF4CZ
0PSF4DZ
0PSF4ZZ
0PSFXZZ
0PSG04Z
0PSG05Z
0PSG06Z
0PSG0BZ
0PSG0CZ
0PSG0DZ
0PSG0ZZ
0PSG34Z
0PSG35Z
0PSG36Z
0PSG3BZ
0PSG3CZ
0PSG3DZ
0PSG3ZZ
0PSG44Z
0PSG45Z
0PSG46Z
0PSG4BZ
0PSG4CZ
0PSG4DZ
0PSG4ZZ
0PSGXZZ
0PSH04Z
0PSH05Z
0PSH06Z
0PSH0BZ
0PSH0CZ
0PSH0DZ
0PSH0ZZ
0PSH3ZZ
0PSH4ZZ
0PSHXZZ
0PSJ3ZZ
0PSJ4ZZ
0PSJXZZ
0PSK3ZZ
0PSK4ZZ
0PSKXZZ
0PSL3ZZ
0PSL4ZZ
0PSLXZZ
0PSM3ZZ
0PSM4ZZ
0PSMXZZ
0PSN3ZZ
0PSN4ZZ
0PSNXZZ
0PSP3ZZ
0PSP4ZZ
0PSPXZZ
0PSQ3ZZ
0PSQ4ZZ
0PSQXZZ
0PSR3ZZ
0PSR4ZZ
0PSRXZZ
0PSS3ZZ
0PSS4ZZ
0PSSXZZ
0PST3ZZ
0PST4ZZ
0PSTXZZ
0PSV3ZZ
0PSV4ZZ
0PSVXZZ
0PT80ZZ
0PT90ZZ
0PTB0ZZ
0PTC0ZZ
0PTD0ZZ
0PTF0ZZ
0PTG0ZZ
0PTH0ZZ
0PTJ0ZZ
0PTK0ZZ
0PTL0ZZ
0PTM0ZZ
0PTN0ZZ
0PTP0ZZ
0PTQ0ZZ
0PTR0ZZ
0PTS0ZZ
0PTT0ZZ
0PTV0ZZ
0PU007Z
0PU00JZ
0PU00KZ
0PU037Z
0PU03JZ
0PU03KZ
0PU047Z
0PU04JZ
0PU04KZ
0PU107Z
0PU10JZ
0PU10KZ
0PU137Z
0PU13JZ
0PU13KZ
0PU147Z
0PU14JZ
0PU14KZ
0PU207Z
0PU20JZ
0PU20KZ
0PU237Z
0PU23JZ
0PU23KZ
0PU247Z
0PU24JZ
0PU24KZ
0PU307Z
0PU30JZ
0PU30KZ
0PU337Z
0PU33JZ
0PU33KZ
0PU347Z
0PU34JZ
0PU34KZ
0PU407Z
0PU40JZ
0PU40KZ
0PU437Z
0PU43JZ
0PU43KZ
0PU447Z
0PU44JZ
0PU44KZ
0PU507Z
0PU50JZ
0PU50KZ
0PU537Z
0PU53JZ
0PU53KZ
0PU547Z
0PU54JZ
0PU54KZ
0PU607Z
0PU60JZ
0PU60KZ
0PU637Z
0PU63JZ
0PU63KZ
0PU647Z
0PU64JZ
0PU64KZ
0PU707Z
0PU70JZ
0PU70KZ
0PU737Z
0PU73JZ
0PU73KZ
0PU747Z
0PU74JZ
0PU74KZ
0PU807Z
0PU80JZ
0PU80KZ
0PU837Z
0PU83JZ
0PU83KZ
0PU847Z
0PU84JZ
0PU84KZ
0PU907Z
0PU90JZ
0PU90KZ
0PU937Z
0PU93JZ
0PU93KZ
0PU947Z
0PU94JZ
0PU94KZ
0PUB07Z
0PUB0JZ
0PUB0KZ
0PUB37Z
0PUB3JZ
0PUB3KZ
0PUB47Z
0PUB4JZ
0PUB4KZ
0PUC07Z
0PUC0JZ
0PUC0KZ
0PUC37Z
0PUC3JZ
0PUC3KZ
0PUC47Z
0PUC4JZ
0PUC4KZ
0PUD07Z
0PUD0JZ
0PUD0KZ
0PUD37Z
0PUD3JZ
0PUD3KZ
0PUD47Z
0PUD4JZ
0PUD4KZ
0PUF07Z
0PUF0JZ
0PUF0KZ
0PUF37Z
0PUF3JZ
0PUF3KZ
0PUF47Z
0PUF4JZ
0PUF4KZ
0PUG07Z
0PUG0JZ
0PUG0KZ
0PUG37Z
0PUG3JZ
0PUG3KZ
0PUG47Z
0PUG4JZ
0PUG4KZ
0PUH07Z
0PUH0JZ
0PUH0KZ
0PUH37Z
0PUH3JZ
0PUH3KZ
0PUH47Z
0PUH4JZ
0PUH4KZ
0PUJ07Z
0PUJ0JZ
0PUJ0KZ
0PUJ37Z
0PUJ3JZ
0PUJ3KZ
0PUJ47Z
0PUJ4JZ
0PUJ4KZ
0PUK07Z
0PUK0JZ
0PUK0KZ
0PUK37Z
0PUK3JZ
0PUK3KZ
0PUK47Z
0PUK4JZ
0PUK4KZ
0PUL07Z
0PUL0JZ
0PUL0KZ
0PUL37Z
0PUL3JZ
0PUL3KZ
0PUL47Z
0PUL4JZ
0PUL4KZ
0PUM07Z
0PUM0JZ
0PUM0KZ
0PUM37Z
0PUM3JZ
0PUM3KZ
0PUM47Z
0PUM4JZ
0PUM4KZ
0PUN07Z
0PUN0JZ
0PUN0KZ
0PUN37Z
0PUN3JZ
0PUN3KZ
0PUN47Z
0PUN4JZ
0PUN4KZ
0PUP07Z
0PUP0JZ
0PUP0KZ
0PUP37Z
0PUP3JZ
0PUP3KZ
0PUP47Z
0PUP4JZ
0PUP4KZ
0PUQ07Z
0PUQ0JZ
0PUQ0KZ
0PUQ37Z
0PUQ3JZ
0PUQ3KZ
0PUQ47Z
0PUQ4JZ
0PUQ4KZ
0PUR07Z
0PUR0JZ
0PUR0KZ
0PUR37Z
0PUR3JZ
0PUR3KZ
0PUR47Z
0PUR4JZ
0PUR4KZ
0PUS07Z
0PUS0JZ
0PUS0KZ
0PUS37Z
0PUS3JZ
0PUS3KZ
0PUS47Z
0PUS4JZ
0PUS4KZ
0PUT07Z
0PUT0JZ
0PUT0KZ
0PUT37Z
0PUT3JZ
0PUT3KZ
0PUT47Z
0PUT4JZ
0PUT4KZ
0PUV07Z
0PUV0JZ
0PUV0KZ
0PUV37Z
0PUV3JZ
0PUV3KZ
0PUV47Z
0PUV4JZ
0PUV4KZ
0PW004Z
0PW007Z
0PW00JZ
0PW00KZ
0PW034Z
0PW037Z
0PW03JZ
0PW03KZ
0PW044Z
0PW047Z
0PW04JZ
0PW04KZ
0PW0X4Z
0PW0X7Z
0PW0XJZ
0PW0XKZ
0PW104Z
0PW107Z
0PW10JZ
0PW10KZ
0PW134Z
0PW137Z
0PW13JZ
0PW13KZ
0PW144Z
0PW147Z
0PW14JZ
0PW14KZ
0PW1X4Z
0PW1X7Z
0PW1XJZ
0PW1XKZ
0PW204Z
0PW207Z
0PW20JZ
0PW20KZ
0PW234Z
0PW237Z
0PW23JZ
0PW23KZ
0PW244Z
0PW247Z
0PW24JZ
0PW24KZ
0PW2X4Z
0PW2X7Z
0PW2XJZ
0PW2XKZ
0PW304Z
0PW307Z
0PW30JZ
0PW30KZ
0PW334Z
0PW337Z
0PW33JZ
0PW33KZ
0PW344Z
0PW347Z
0PW34JZ
0PW34KZ
0PW3X4Z
0PW3X7Z
0PW3XJZ
0PW3XKZ
0PW404Z
0PW407Z
0PW40JZ
0PW40KZ
0PW434Z
0PW437Z
0PW43JZ
0PW43KZ
0PW444Z
0PW447Z
0PW44JZ
0PW44KZ
0PW4X4Z
0PW4X7Z
0PW4XJZ
0PW4XKZ
0PW504Z
0PW507Z
0PW50JZ
0PW50KZ
0PW534Z
0PW537Z
0PW53JZ
0PW53KZ
0PW544Z
0PW547Z
0PW54JZ
0PW54KZ
0PW5X4Z
0PW5X7Z
0PW5XJZ
0PW5XKZ
0PW604Z
0PW607Z
0PW60JZ
0PW60KZ
0PW634Z
0PW637Z
0PW63JZ
0PW63KZ
0PW644Z
0PW647Z
0PW64JZ
0PW64KZ
0PW6X4Z
0PW6X7Z
0PW6XJZ
0PW6XKZ
0PW704Z
0PW707Z
0PW70JZ
0PW70KZ
0PW734Z
0PW737Z
0PW73JZ
0PW73KZ
0PW744Z
0PW747Z
0PW74JZ
0PW74KZ
0PW7X4Z
0PW7X7Z
0PW7XJZ
0PW7XKZ
0PW804Z
0PW807Z
0PW80JZ
0PW80KZ
0PW834Z
0PW837Z
0PW83JZ
0PW83KZ
0PW844Z
0PW847Z
0PW84JZ
0PW84KZ
0PW8X4Z
0PW8X7Z
0PW8XJZ
0PW8XKZ
0PW904Z
0PW907Z
0PW90JZ
0PW90KZ
0PW934Z
0PW937Z
0PW93JZ
0PW93KZ
0PW944Z
0PW947Z
0PW94JZ
0PW94KZ
0PW9X4Z
0PW9X7Z
0PW9XJZ
0PW9XKZ
0PWB04Z
0PWB07Z
0PWB0JZ
0PWB0KZ
0PWB34Z
0PWB37Z
0PWB3JZ
0PWB3KZ
0PWB44Z
0PWB47Z
0PWB4JZ
0PWB4KZ
0PWBX4Z
0PWBX7Z
0PWBXJZ
0PWBXKZ
0PWC04Z
0PWC05Z
0PWC07Z
0PWC0JZ
0PWC0KZ
0PWC34Z
0PWC35Z
0PWC37Z
0PWC3JZ
0PWC3KZ
0PWC44Z
0PWC45Z
0PWC47Z
0PWC4JZ
0PWC4KZ
0PWCX4Z
0PWCX5Z
0PWCX7Z
0PWCXJZ
0PWCXKZ
0PWD04Z
0PWD05Z
0PWD07Z
0PWD0JZ
0PWD0KZ
0PWD34Z
0PWD35Z
0PWD37Z
0PWD3JZ
0PWD3KZ
0PWD44Z
0PWD45Z
0PWD47Z
0PWD4JZ
0PWD4KZ
0PWDX4Z
0PWDX5Z
0PWDX7Z
0PWDXJZ
0PWDXKZ
0PWF04Z
0PWF05Z
0PWF07Z
0PWF0JZ
0PWF0KZ
0PWF34Z
0PWF35Z
0PWF37Z
0PWF3JZ
0PWF3KZ
0PWF44Z
0PWF45Z
0PWF47Z
0PWF4JZ
0PWFX4Z
0PWFX5Z
0PWFX7Z
0PWFXJZ
0PWFXKZ
0PWGX4Z
0PWGX5Z
0PWGX7Z
0PWGXJZ
0PWGXKZ
0PWHX4Z
0PWHX5Z
0PWHX7Z
0PWHXJZ
0PWHXKZ
0PWJX4Z
0PWJX5Z
0PWJX7Z
0PWJXJZ
0PWJXKZ
0PWKX4Z
0PWKX5Z
0PWKX7Z
0PWKXJZ
0PWKXKZ
0PWLX4Z
0PWLX5Z
0PWLX7Z
0PWLXJZ
0PWLXKZ
0PWMX4Z
0PWMX5Z
0PWMX7Z
0PWMXJZ
0PWMXKZ
0PWNX4Z
0PWNX5Z
0PWNX7Z
0PWNXJZ
0PWNXKZ
0PWPX4Z
0PWPX5Z
0PWPX7Z
0PWPXJZ
0PWPXKZ
0PWQX4Z
0PWQX5Z
0PWQX7Z
0PWQXJZ
0PWQXKZ
0PWRX4Z
0PWRX5Z
0PWRX7Z
0PWRXJZ
0PWRXKZ
0PWSX4Z
0PWSX5Z
0PWSX7Z
0PWSXJZ
0PWSXKZ
0PWTX4Z
0PWTX5Z
0PWTX7Z
0PWTXJZ
0PWTXKZ
0PWVX4Z
0PWVX5Z
0PWVX7Z
0PWVXJZ
0PWVXKZ
0PWYX0Z
0PWYXMZ
0Q2YX0Z
0Q2YXYZ
0Q5P3ZZ
0Q5P4ZZ
0Q5Q0ZZ
0Q5Q3ZZ
0Q5Q4ZZ
0Q5R0ZZ
0Q5R3ZZ
0Q5R4ZZ
0Q5S0ZZ
0Q5S3ZZ
0Q5S4ZZ
0Q800ZZ
0Q803ZZ
0Q804ZZ
0Q810ZZ
0Q813ZZ
0Q814ZZ
0Q820ZZ
0Q823ZZ
0Q824ZZ
0Q830ZZ
0Q833ZZ
0Q834ZZ
0Q840ZZ
0Q843ZZ
0Q844ZZ
0Q850ZZ
0Q853ZZ
0Q854ZZ
0Q860ZZ
0Q863ZZ
0Q864ZZ
0Q870ZZ
0Q873ZZ
0Q874ZZ
0Q880ZZ
0Q883ZZ
0Q884ZZ
0Q890ZZ
0Q893ZZ
0Q894ZZ
0Q8B0ZZ
0Q8B3ZZ
0Q8B4ZZ
0Q8C0ZZ
0Q8C3ZZ
0Q8C4ZZ
0Q8D0ZZ
0Q8D3ZZ
0Q8D4ZZ
0Q8F0ZZ
0Q8F3ZZ
0Q8F4ZZ
0Q8G0ZZ
0Q8G3ZZ
0Q8G4ZZ
0Q8H0ZZ
0Q8H3ZZ
0Q8H4ZZ
0Q8J0ZZ
0Q8J3ZZ
0Q8J4ZZ
0Q8K0ZZ
0Q8K3ZZ
0Q8K4ZZ
0Q8L0ZZ
0Q8L3ZZ
0Q8L4ZZ
0Q8M0ZZ
0Q8M3ZZ
0Q8M4ZZ
0Q8N0ZZ
0Q8N3ZZ
0Q8N4ZZ
0Q8P0ZZ
0Q8P3ZZ
0Q8P4ZZ
0Q8Q0ZZ
0Q8Q3ZZ
0Q8Q4ZZ
0Q8R0ZZ
0Q8R3ZZ
0Q8R4ZZ
0Q8S0ZZ
0Q8S3ZZ
0Q8S4ZZ

0Q9000Z
0Q900ZX
0Q900ZZ
0Q9030Z
0Q903ZX
0Q903ZZ
0Q9040Z
0Q904ZX
0Q904ZZ
0Q9100Z
0Q910ZX
0Q910ZZ
0Q9130Z
0Q913ZX
0Q913ZZ
0Q9140Z
0Q914ZX
0Q914ZZ
0Q9200Z
0Q920ZX
0Q920ZZ
0Q9230Z
0Q923ZX
0Q923ZZ
0Q9240Z
0Q924ZX
0Q924ZZ
0Q9300Z
0Q930ZX
0Q930ZZ
0Q9330Z
0Q933ZX
0Q933ZZ
0Q9340Z
0Q934ZX
0Q934ZZ
0Q9400Z
0Q940ZX
0Q940ZZ
0Q9430Z
0Q943ZX
0Q943ZZ
0Q9440Z
0Q944ZX
0Q944ZZ
0Q9500Z
0Q950ZX
0Q950ZZ
0Q9530Z
0Q953ZX
0Q953ZZ
0Q9540Z
0Q954ZX
0Q954ZZ
0Q9600Z
0Q960ZX
0Q960ZZ
0Q9630Z
0Q963ZX
0Q963ZZ
0Q9640Z
0Q964ZX
0Q964ZZ
0Q9700Z
0Q970ZX
0Q970ZZ
0Q9730Z
0Q973ZX
0Q973ZZ
0Q9740Z
0Q974ZX
0Q974ZZ
0Q9800Z
0Q980ZX
0Q980ZZ
0Q9830Z
0Q983ZX
0Q983ZZ
0Q9840Z
0Q984ZX
0Q984ZZ
0Q9900Z
0Q990ZX
0Q990ZZ
0Q9930Z
0Q993ZX
0Q993ZZ
0Q9940Z
0Q994ZX
0Q994ZZ
0Q9B00Z
0Q9B0ZX
0Q9B0ZZ
0Q9B30Z
0Q9B3ZX
0Q9B3ZZ
0Q9B40Z
0Q9B4ZX
0Q9B4ZZ
0Q9C00Z
0Q9C0ZX
0Q9C0ZZ
0Q9C30Z
0Q9C3ZX
0Q9C3ZZ
0Q9C40Z
0Q9C4ZX
0Q9C4ZZ
0Q9D00Z
0Q9D0ZX
0Q9D0ZZ
0Q9D30Z
0Q9D3ZX
0Q9D3ZZ
0Q9D40Z
0Q9D4ZX
0Q9D4ZZ
0Q9F00Z
0Q9F0ZX
0Q9F0ZZ
0Q9F30Z
0Q9F3ZX
0Q9F3ZZ
0Q9F40Z
0Q9F4ZX
0Q9F4ZZ
0Q9G00Z
0Q9G0ZX
0Q9G0ZZ
0Q9G30Z
0Q9G3ZX
0Q9G3ZZ
0Q9G40Z
0Q9G4ZX
0Q9G4ZZ
0Q9H00Z
0Q9H0ZX
0Q9H0ZZ
0Q9H30Z
0Q9H3ZX
0Q9H3ZZ
0Q9H40Z
0Q9H4ZX
0Q9H4ZZ
0Q9J00Z
0Q9J0ZX
0Q9J0ZZ
0Q9J30Z
0Q9J3ZX
0Q9J3ZZ
0Q9J40Z
0Q9J4ZX
0Q9J4ZZ
0Q9K00Z
0Q9K0ZX
0Q9K0ZZ
0Q9K30Z
0Q9K3ZX
0Q9K3ZZ
0Q9K40Z
0Q9K4ZX
0Q9K4ZZ
0Q9L00Z
0Q9L0ZX
0Q9L0ZZ
0Q9L30Z
0Q9L3ZX
0Q9L3ZZ
0Q9L40Z
0Q9L4ZX
0Q9L4ZZ
0Q9M00Z
0Q9M0ZX
0Q9M0ZZ
0Q9M30Z
0Q9M3ZX
0Q9M3ZZ
0Q9M40Z
0Q9M4ZX
0Q9M4ZZ
0Q9N00Z
0Q9N0ZX
0Q9N0ZZ
0Q9N30Z
0Q9N3ZX
0Q9N3ZZ
0Q9N40Z
0Q9N4ZX
0Q9N4ZZ
0Q9P00Z
0Q9P0ZX
0Q9P0ZZ
0Q9P30Z
0Q9P3ZX
0Q9P3ZZ
0Q9P40Z
0Q9P4ZX
0Q9P4ZZ
0Q9Q00Z
0Q9Q0ZX
0Q9Q0ZZ
0Q9Q30Z
0Q9Q3ZX
0Q9Q3ZZ
0Q9Q40Z
0Q9Q4ZX
0Q9Q4ZZ
0Q9R00Z
0Q9R0ZX
0Q9R0ZZ
0Q9R30Z
0Q9R3ZX
0Q9R3ZZ
0Q9R40Z
0Q9R4ZX
0Q9R4ZZ
0Q9S00Z
0Q9S0ZX
0Q9S0ZZ
0Q9S30Z
0Q9S3ZX
0Q9S3ZZ
0Q9S40Z
0Q9S4ZX
0Q9S4ZZ
0QB00ZX
0QB00ZZ
0QB03ZX
0QB03ZZ
0QB04ZX
0QB04ZZ
0QB10ZX
0QBJ4ZX
0QBJ4ZZ
0QBK0ZX
0QBK0ZZ
0QBK3ZX
0QBK3ZZ
0QBK4ZX
0QBK4ZZ
0QBL0ZX
0QBL0ZZ
0QBL3ZX
0QBL3ZZ
0QBL4ZX
0QBL4ZZ
0QBM0ZX
0QBM0ZZ
0QBM3ZX
0QBM3ZZ
0QBM4ZX
0QBM4ZZ
0QBN0ZX
0QBN0ZZ
0QBN3ZX
0QBN3ZZ
0QBN4ZX
0QBN4ZZ
0QBP0ZX
0QBP0ZZ
0QBP3ZX
0QBP3ZZ
0QBP4ZX
0QBP4ZZ
0QBQ0ZX
0QBQ0ZZ
0QBQ3ZX
0QBQ3ZZ
0QBQ4ZX
0QBQ4ZZ
0QBR0ZX
0QBR0ZZ
0QBR3ZX
0QBR3ZZ
0QBR4ZX
0QBR4ZZ
0QBS0ZX
0QBS0ZZ
0QBS3ZX
0QBS3ZZ
0QBS4ZX
0QBS4ZZ
0QC00ZZ
0QC03ZZ
0QC04ZZ
0QC10ZZ
0QC13ZZ
0QC14ZZ
0QC20ZZ
0QC23ZZ
0QC24ZZ
0QC30ZZ
0QC33ZZ
0QC34ZZ
0QC40ZZ
0QC43ZZ
0QC44ZZ
0QC50ZZ
0QC53ZZ
0QC54ZZ
0QC60ZZ
0QC63ZZ
0QC64ZZ
0QC70ZZ
0QC73ZZ
0QC74ZZ
0QC80ZZ
0QC83ZZ
0QC84ZZ
0QC90ZZ
0QC93ZZ
0QC94ZZ
0QCB0ZZ
0QCB3ZZ
0QCB4ZZ
0QCC0ZZ
0QCC3ZZ
0QCC4ZZ
0QCD0ZZ
0QCD3ZZ
0QCD4ZZ
0QCF0ZZ
0QCF3ZZ
0QCF4ZZ
0QCG0ZZ
0QCG3ZZ
0QCG4ZZ
0QCH0ZZ
0QCH3ZZ
0QCH4ZZ
0QCJ0ZZ
0QCJ3ZZ
0QCJ4ZZ
0QCK0ZZ
0QCK3ZZ
0QCK4ZZ
0QCL0ZZ
0QCL3ZZ
0QCL4ZZ
0QCM0ZZ
0QCM3ZZ
0QCM4ZZ
0QCN0ZZ
0QCN3ZZ
0QCN4ZZ
0QCP0ZZ
0QCP3ZZ
0QCP4ZZ
0QCQ0ZZ
0QCQ3ZZ
0QCQ4ZZ
0QCR0ZZ
0QCR3ZZ
0QCR4ZZ
0QCS0ZZ
0QCS3ZZ
0QCS4ZZ
0QD00ZZ
0QD10ZZ
0QD20ZZ
0QD30ZZ
0QD40ZZ
0QD50ZZ
0QD60ZZ
0QD70ZZ
0QD80ZZ
0QD90ZZ
0QDB0ZZ
0QDC0ZZ
0QDD0ZZ
0QDF0ZZ
0QDG0ZZ
0QDH0ZZ
0QDJ0ZZ
0QDK0ZZ
0QDL0ZZ
0QDM0ZZ
0QDN0ZZ
0QDP0ZZ
0QDQ0ZZ
0QDR0ZZ
0QDS0ZZ
0QH004Z
0QH005Z
0QH034Z
0QH035Z
0QH044Z
0QH045Z
0QH104Z
0QH105Z
0QH134Z
0QH135Z
0QH144Z
0QH145Z
0QH204Z
0QH205Z
0QH234Z
0QH235Z
0QH244Z
0QH245Z
0QH304Z
0QH305Z
0QH334Z
0QH335Z
0QH344Z
0QH345Z
0QH404Z
0QH405Z
0QH434Z
0QH435Z
0QH444Z
0QH445Z
0QH504Z
0QH505Z
0QH534Z
0QH535Z
0QH544Z
0QH545Z
0QH604Z
0QH605Z
0QH606Z
0QH608Z
0QH60BZ
0QH60CZ
0QH60DZ
0QH634Z
0QH635Z
0QH636Z
0QH638Z
0QH63BZ
0QH63CZ
0QH63DZ
0QH644Z
0QH645Z
0QH646Z
0QH648Z
0QH64BZ
0QH64CZ
0QH64DZ
0QH704Z
0QH705Z
0QH706Z
0QH708Z
0QH70BZ
0QH70CZ
0QH70DZ
0QH734Z
0QH735Z
0QH736Z
0QH738Z
0QH73BZ
0QH73CZ
0QH73DZ
0QH744Z
0QH745Z
0QH746Z
0QH748Z
0QH74BZ
0QH74CZ
0QH74DZ
0QH804Z
0QH805Z
0QH806Z
0QH808Z
0QH80BZ
0QH80CZ
0QH80DZ
0QH838Z
0QH848Z
0QH908Z
0QH938Z
0QH948Z
0QHB08Z
0QHB38Z
0QHB48Z
0QHC08Z
0QHC38Z
0QHC48Z
0QHG08Z
0QHG38Z
0QHG48Z
0QHH08Z
0QHH38Z
0QHH48Z
0QHJ08Z
0QHJ38Z
0QHJ48Z
0QHK06Z
0QHK08Z
0QHK0BZ
0QHK0CZ
0QHK0DZ
0QHK34Z
0QHK35Z
0QHK36Z
0QHK38Z
0QHK3BZ
0QHK3CZ
0QHK3DZ
0QHK44Z
0QHK45Z
0QHK46Z
0QHK48Z
0QHK4BZ
0QHK4CZ
0QHK4DZ
0QHL04Z
0QHL05Z
0QHL34Z
0QHL35Z
0QHL44Z
0QHL45Z
0QHM04Z
0QHM05Z
0QHM34Z
0QHM35Z
0QHM44Z
0QHM45Z
0QHN04Z
0QHN05Z
0QHN34Z
0QHN35Z
0QHN44Z
0QHN45Z
0QHP04Z
0QHP05Z
0QHP34Z
0QHP35Z
0QHP44Z
0QHP45Z
0QHQ04Z
0QHQ05Z
0QHQ34Z
0QHQ35Z
0QHQ44Z
0QHQ45Z
0QHR04Z
0QHR05Z
0QHR34Z
0QHR35Z
0QHR44Z
0QHR45Z
0QHS04Z
0QHS05Z
0QHS34Z
0QHS35Z
0QHS44Z
0QHS45Z
0QHY0MZ
0QHY3MZ
0QHY4MZ
0QJY0ZZ
0QJY3ZZ
0QJY4ZZ
0QJYXZZ
0QN00ZZ
0QN03ZZ
0QN04ZZ
0QN10ZZ
0QN13ZZ
0QN14ZZ
0QN20ZZ
0QN23ZZ
0QN24ZZ
0QN30ZZ
0QN33ZZ
0QN34ZZ
0QN40ZZ
0QN43ZZ
0QN44ZZ
0QN50ZZ
0QN53ZZ
0QN54ZZ
0QN60ZZ
0QN63ZZ
0QN64ZZ
0QN70ZZ
0QN73ZZ
0QN74ZZ
0QN80ZZ
0QN83ZZ
0QN84ZZ
0QN90ZZ
0QN93ZZ
0QN94ZZ
0QNB0ZZ
0QNB3ZZ
0QNB4ZZ
0QNC0ZZ
0QNC3ZZ
0QNC4ZZ
0QND0ZZ
0QND3ZZ
0QND4ZZ
0QNF0ZZ
0QNF3ZZ
0QNF4ZZ
0QNG0ZZ
0QNG3ZZ
0QNG4ZZ
0QNH0ZZ
0QNH3ZZ
0QNH4ZZ
0QNJ0ZZ
0QNJ3ZZ
0QNJ4ZZ
0QNK0ZZ
0QNK3ZZ
0QNK4ZZ
0QNL0ZZ
0QNL3ZZ
0QNL4ZZ
0QNM0ZZ
0QNM3ZZ
0QNM4ZZ
0QNN0ZZ
0QNN3ZZ
0QNN4ZZ
0QNP0ZZ
0QNP3ZZ
0QNP4ZZ
0QNQ0ZZ
0QNQ3ZZ
0QNQ4ZZ
0QNR0ZZ
0QNR3ZZ
0QNR4ZZ
0QNS0ZZ
0QNS3ZZ
0QNS4ZZ
0QP004Z
0QP007Z
0QP00JZ
0QP00KZ
0QP034Z
0QP037Z
0QP03JZ
0QP03KZ
0QP044Z
0QP047Z
0QP04JZ
0QP04KZ
0QP0X4Z
0QP104Z
0QP107Z
0QP10JZ
0QP10KZ
0QP134Z
0QP137Z
0QP13JZ
0QP13KZ
0QP144Z
0QP147Z
0QP14JZ
0QP14KZ
0QP1X4Z
0QP204Z
0QP205Z
0QP207Z
0QP20JZ
0QP20KZ
0QP234Z
0QP235Z
0QP237Z
0QP23JZ
0QP23KZ
0QP244Z
0QP245Z
0QP247Z
0QP24JZ
0QP24KZ
0QP2X4Z
0QP2X5Z
0QP304Z
0QP305Z
0QP307Z
0QP30JZ
0QP30KZ
0QP334Z
0QP335Z
0QP337Z
0QP33JZ
0QP33KZ
0QP344Z
0QP345Z
0QP347Z
0QP34JZ
0QP34KZ
0QP3X4Z
0QP3X5Z
0QP404Z
0QP407Z
0QP40JZ
0QP40KZ
0QP434Z
0QP437Z
0QP43JZ
0QP43KZ
0QP444Z
0QP447Z
0QP44JZ
0QP44KZ
0QP4X4Z
0QP504Z
0QP507Z
0QP50JZ
0QP50KZ
0QP534Z
0QP537Z
0QP53JZ
0QP53KZ
0QP544Z
0QP547Z
0QP54JZ
0QP54KZ
0QP5X4Z
0QP604Z
0QP605Z
0QP607Z
0QP60JZ
0QP60KZ
0QP634Z
0QP635Z
0QP637Z
0QP63JZ
0QP63KZ

0QP644Z
0QP645Z
0QP647Z
0QP64JZ
0QP64KZ
0QP6X4Z
0QP6X5Z
0QP704Z
0QP705Z
0QP707Z
0QP70JZ
0QP70KZ
0QP734Z
0QP735Z
0QP737Z
0QP73JZ
0QP73KZ
0QP744Z
0QP745Z
0QP747Z
0QP74JZ
0QP74KZ
0QP7X4Z
0QP7X5Z
0QP804Z
0QP805Z
0QP807Z
0QP80JZ
0QP80KZ
0QP834Z
0QP835Z
0QP837Z
0QP83JZ
0QP83KZ
0QP844Z
0QP845Z
0QP847Z
0QP84JZ
0QP84KZ
0QP8X4Z
0QP8X5Z
0QP904Z
0QP905Z
0QP907Z
0QP90JZ
0QP90KZ
0QP934Z
0QP935Z
0QP937Z
0QP93JZ
0QP93KZ
0QP944Z
0QP945Z
0QP947Z
0QP94JZ
0QP94KZ
0QP9X4Z
0QP9X5Z
0QPB04Z
0QPB05Z
0QPB07Z
0QPB0JZ
0QPB0KZ
0QPB34Z
0QPB35Z
0QPB37Z
0QPB3JZ
0QPB3KZ
0QPB44Z
0QPB45Z
0QPB47Z
0QPB4JZ
0QPB4KZ
0QPBX4Z
0QPBX5Z
0QPC04Z
0QPC05Z
0QPC07Z
0QPC0JZ
0QPC0KZ
0QPC34Z
0QPC35Z
0QPC37Z
0QPC3JZ
0QPC3KZ
0QPC44Z
0QPC45Z
0QPC47Z
0QPC4JZ
0QPC4KZ
0QPCX4Z
0QPCX5Z
0QPD04Z
0QPD05Z
0QPD07Z
0QPD0JZ
0QPD0KZ
0QPD34Z
0QPD35Z
0QPDX4Z
0QPDX5Z
0QPFX4Z
0QPFX5Z
0QPGX4Z
0QPGX5Z
0QPHX4Z
0QPHX5Z
0QPJX4Z
0QPJX5Z
0QPKX4Z
0QPKX5Z
0QPLX4Z
0QPLX5Z
0QPMX4Z
0QPMX5Z
0QPNX4Z
0QPNX5Z
0QPP35Z
0QPP37Z
0QPP3JZ
0QPP3KZ
0QPP44Z
0QPP45Z
0QPP47Z
0QPP4JZ
0QPP4KZ
0QPPX4Z
0QPPX5Z
0QPQ04Z
0QPQ05Z
0QPQ07Z
0QPQ0JZ
0QPQ0KZ
0QPQ34Z
0QPQ35Z
0QPQ37Z
0QPQ3JZ
0QPQ3KZ
0QPQ44Z
0QPQ45Z
0QPQ47Z
0QPQ4JZ
0QPQ4KZ
0QPQX4Z
0QPQX5Z
0QPR04Z
0QPR05Z
0QPR07Z
0QPR0JZ
0QPR0KZ
0QPR34Z
0QPR35Z
0QPR37Z
0QPR3JZ
0QPR3KZ
0QPR44Z
0QPR45Z
0QPR47Z
0QPR4JZ
0QPR4KZ
0QPRX4Z
0QPRX5Z
0QPS04Z
0QPS07Z
0QPS0JZ
0QPS0KZ
0QPS34Z
0QPS37Z
0QPS3JZ
0QPS3KZ
0QPS44Z
0QPS47Z
0QPS4JZ
0QPS4KZ
0QPSX4Z
0QPY00Z
0QPY0MZ
0QPY30Z
0QPY3MZ
0QPY40Z
0QPY4MZ
0QPYX0Z
0QPYXMZ
0QQ00ZZ
0QQ03ZZ
0QQ04ZZ
0QQ0XZZ
0QQ10ZZ
0QQ13ZZ
0QQ14ZZ
0QQ1XZZ
0QQ20ZZ
0QQ23ZZ
0QQ24ZZ
0QQ2XZZ
0QQ30ZZ
0QQ33ZZ
0QQ34ZZ
0QQ3XZZ
0QQ40ZZ
0QQ43ZZ
0QQ44ZZ
0QQ4XZZ
0QQ50ZZ
0QQ53ZZ
0QQ54ZZ
0QQ5XZZ
0QQ60ZZ
0QQ63ZZ
0QQ64ZZ
0QQ6XZZ
0QQ70ZZ
0QQ73ZZ
0QQ74ZZ
0QQ7XZZ
0QQ80ZZ
0QQ83ZZ
0QQ84ZZ
0QQ8XZZ
0QQ90ZZ
0QQ93ZZ
0QQ94ZZ
0QQ9XZZ
0QQB0ZZ
0QQB3ZZ
0QQB4ZZ
0QQBXZZ
0QQC0ZZ
0QQC3ZZ
0QQC4ZZ
0QQCXZZ
0QQD0ZZ
0QQD3ZZ
0QQD4ZZ
0QQDXZZ
0QQF0ZZ
0QQF3ZZ
0QQF4ZZ
0QQFXZZ
0QQG0ZZ
0QQG3ZZ
0QQG4ZZ
0QQGXZZ
0QQH0ZZ
0QQH3ZZ
0QQH4ZZ
0QQHXZZ
0QQJ0ZZ
0QQJ3ZZ
0QQJ4ZZ
0QQJXZZ
0QQK0ZZ
0QQK3ZZ
0QQK4ZZ
0QQKXZZ
0QQL0ZZ
0QQL3ZZ
0QQL4ZZ
0QQLXZZ
0QQM0ZZ
0QQM3ZZ
0QQM4ZZ
0QQMXZZ
0QQN0ZZ
0QQN3ZZ
0QQN4ZZ
0QQNXZZ
0QQP0ZZ
0QQP3ZZ
0QQP4ZZ
0QQPXZZ
0QQQ0ZZ
0QQQ3ZZ
0QQQ4ZZ
0QQQXZZ
0QQR0ZZ
0QQR3ZZ
0QQR4ZZ
0QQRXZZ
0QQS0ZZ
0QQS3ZZ
0QQS4ZZ
0QQSXZZ
0QR007Z
0QR00JZ
0QR00KZ
0QR037Z
0QR03JZ
0QR03KZ
0QR047Z
0QR04JZ
0QR04KZ
0QR107Z
0QR10JZ
0QR10KZ
0QR137Z
0QR13JZ
0QR13KZ
0QR147Z
0QR14JZ
0QR14KZ
0QR207Z
0QR20JZ
0QR20KZ
0QR237Z
0QR23JZ
0QR23KZ
0QR247Z
0QR24JZ
0QR24KZ
0QR307Z
0QR30JZ
0QR30KZ
0QR337Z
0QR33JZ
0QR33KZ
0QR347Z
0QR34JZ
0QR34KZ
0QR407Z
0QR40JZ
0QR40KZ
0QR437Z
0QR43JZ
0QR43KZ
0QR447Z
0QR44JZ
0QR44KZ
0QR507Z
0QR50JZ
0QR50KZ
0QR537Z
0QR53JZ
0QR53KZ
0QR547Z
0QR54JZ
0QR54KZ
0QR607Z
0QR60JZ
0QR60KZ
0QR637Z
0QR63JZ
0QR63KZ
0QR647Z
0QR64JZ
0QR64KZ
0QR707Z
0QR70JZ
0QR70KZ
0QR737Z
0QR73JZ
0QR73KZ
0QR747Z
0QR74JZ
0QR74KZ
0QR807Z
0QR80JZ
0QR80KZ
0QR837Z
0QR83JZ
0QR83KZ
0QR847Z
0QR84JZ
0QR84KZ
0QR907Z
0QR90JZ
0QR90KZ
0QR937Z
0QR93JZ
0QR93KZ
0QR947Z
0QR94JZ
0QR94KZ
0QRB07Z
0QRB0JZ
0QRB0KZ
0QRB37Z
0QRB3JZ
0QRB3KZ
0QRB47Z
0QRB4JZ
0QRB4KZ
0QRC07Z
0QRC0JZ
0QRC0KZ
0QRC37Z
0QRC3JZ
0QRC3KZ
0QRC47Z
0QRC4JZ
0QRC4KZ
0QRD07Z
0QRD0JZ
0QRD0KZ
0QRD37Z
0QRD3JZ
0QRD3KZ
0QRD47Z
0QRD4JZ
0QRD4KZ
0QRF07Z
0QRF0JZ
0QRF0KZ
0QRF37Z
0QRF3JZ
0QRF3KZ
0QRF47Z
0QRF4JZ
0QRF4KZ
0QRG07Z
0QRG0JZ
0QRG0KZ
0QRG37Z
0QRG3JZ
0QRG3KZ
0QRG47Z
0QRG4JZ
0QRG4KZ
0QRH07Z
0QRH0JZ
0QRH0KZ
0QRH37Z
0QRH3JZ
0QRH3KZ
0QRH47Z
0QRH4JZ
0QRH4KZ
0QRJ07Z
0QRJ0JZ
0QRJ0KZ
0QRJ37Z
0QRJ3JZ
0QRJ3KZ
0QRJ47Z
0QRJ4JZ
0QRJ4KZ
0QRK07Z
0QRK0JZ
0QRK0KZ
0QRK37Z
0QRK3JZ
0QRK3KZ
0QRK47Z
0QRK4JZ
0QRK4KZ
0QRL07Z
0QRL0JZ
0QRL0KZ
0QRL37Z
0QRL3JZ
0QRL3KZ
0QRL47Z
0QRL4JZ
0QRL4KZ
0QRM07Z
0QRM0JZ
0QRM0KZ
0QRM37Z
0QRM3JZ
0QRM3KZ
0QRM47Z
0QRM4JZ
0QRM4KZ
0QRN07Z
0QRN0JZ
0QRN0KZ
0QRN37Z
0QRN3JZ
0QRN3KZ
0QRN47Z
0QRN4JZ
0QRN4KZ
0QS03ZZ
0QS0XZZ
0QS13ZZ
0QS1XZZ
0QS23ZZ
0QS24ZZ
0QS2XZZ
0QS33ZZ
0QS34ZZ
0QS3XZZ
0QS43ZZ
0QS44ZZ
0QS4XZZ
0QS53ZZ
0QS54ZZ
0QS5XZZ
0QS63ZZ
0QS64ZZ
0QS6XZZ
0QS73ZZ
0QS74ZZ
0QS7XZZ
0QS83ZZ
0QS84ZZ
0QS8XZZ
0QS90DZ
0QS90ZZ
0QS934Z
0QS935Z
0QS936Z
0QS93BZ
0QS93CZ
0QS93DZ
0QS93ZZ
0QS944Z
0QS945Z
0QS946Z
0QS94BZ
0QS94CZ
0QS94DZ
0QS94ZZ
0QS9XZZ
0QSB04Z
0QSB05Z
0QSB06Z
0QSB0BZ
0QSB0CZ
0QSB0DZ
0QSB0ZZ
0QSB34Z
0QSB35Z
0QSB36Z
0QSB3BZ
0QSB3CZ
0QSB3DZ
0QSB3ZZ
0QSB44Z
0QSB45Z
0QSB46Z
0QSB4BZ
0QSB4CZ
0QSB4DZ
0QSB4ZZ
0QSBXZZ
0QSC04Z
0QSC05Z
0QSC06Z
0QSC0BZ
0QSC0CZ
0QSC0DZ
0QSC0ZZ
0QSC34Z
0QSC35Z
0QSC36Z
0QSC3BZ
0QSC3CZ
0QSC3DZ
0QSC3ZZ
0QSC44Z
0QSC45Z
0QSC46Z
0QSC4BZ
0QSC4CZ
0QSC4DZ
0QSC4ZZ
0QSCXZZ
0QSD04Z
0QSD05Z
0QSD0ZZ
0QSD34Z
0QSD35Z
0QSD3ZZ
0QSD44Z
0QSD45Z
0QSD4ZZ
0QSDXZZ
0QSF04Z
0QSF05Z
0QSF0ZZ
0QSF34Z
0QSF35Z
0QSF3ZZ
0QSF44Z
0QSF45Z
0QSF4ZZ
0QSFXZZ
0QSG04Z
0QSG05Z
0QSG06Z
0QSG0BZ
0QSG0CZ
0QSG0DZ
0QSG0ZZ
0QSG34Z
0QSG35Z
0QSG36Z
0QSG3BZ
0QSG3CZ
0QSG3DZ
0QSG3ZZ
0QSG44Z
0QSG45Z
0QSG46Z
0QSG4BZ
0QSG4CZ
0QSG4DZ
0QSG4ZZ
0QSGXZZ
0QSH04Z
0QSH05Z
0QSH06Z
0QSH0BZ
0QSH0CZ
0QSH0DZ
0QSH0ZZ
0QSH34Z
0QSH35Z
0QSH36Z
0QSH3BZ
0QSH3CZ
0QSH3DZ
0QSH3ZZ
0QSH44Z
0QSH45Z
0QSH46Z
0QSH4BZ
0QSH4CZ
0QSH4DZ
0QSH4ZZ
0QSHXZZ
0QSJ04Z
0QSJ05Z
0QSJ06Z
0QSJ0BZ
0QSJ0CZ
0QSJ0DZ
0QSJ0ZZ
0QSJ34Z
0QSJ35Z
0QSJ36Z
0QSJ3BZ
0QSJ3CZ
0QSJ3DZ
0QSJ3ZZ
0QSJ44Z
0QSJ45Z
0QSJ46Z
0QSJ4BZ
0QSJ4CZ
0QSJ4DZ
0QSJ4ZZ
0QSJXZZ
0QSK04Z
0QSK05Z
0QSK06Z
0QSK0BZ
0QSK0CZ
0QSK0DZ
0QSK0ZZ
0QSK34Z
0QSK35Z
0QSK36Z
0QSK3BZ
0QSK3CZ
0QSK3DZ
0QSK3ZZ
0QSK44Z
0QSK45Z
0QSK46Z
0QSK4BZ
0QSK4CZ
0QSK4DZ
0QSK4ZZ
0QSKXZZ
0QSL04Z
0QSL05Z
0QSL0ZZ
0QSL34Z
0QSL35Z
0QSL3ZZ
0QSL44Z
0QSL45Z
0QSL4ZZ
0QSLXZZ
0QSM04Z
0QSM05Z
0QSM0ZZ
0QSM34Z
0QSM35Z
0QSM3ZZ
0QSM44Z
0QSM45Z
0QSM4ZZ
0QSMXZZ
0QSN042
0QSN04Z
0QSN052
0QSN05Z
0QSN0Z2
0QSN0ZZ
0QSN342
0QSN34Z
0QSN352
0QSN35Z
0QSN3Z2
0QSN3ZZ
0QSN442
0QSN44Z
0QSN452
0QSN45Z
0QSN4Z2
0QSN4ZZ
0QSNXZ2
0QSNXZZ
0QSP042
0QSP04Z
0QSP052
0QSP05Z
0QSP0Z2
0QSP0ZZ
0QSP342
0QSP34Z
0QSP352
0QSP35Z
0QSP3Z2
0QSP3ZZ
0QSP442
0QSP44Z
0QSP452
0QSP45Z
0QSP4Z2
0QSP4ZZ
0QSPXZ2
0QSPXZZ

0QSQ04Z
0QSQ05Z
0QSQ0ZZ
0QSQ34Z
0QSQ35Z
0QSQ3ZZ
0QSQ44Z
0QSQ45Z
0QSQ4ZZ
0QSQXZZ
0QSR04Z
0QSR05Z
0QSR0ZZ
0QSR34Z
0QSR35Z
0QSR3ZZ
0QSR44Z
0QSR45Z
0QSR4ZZ
0QSRXZZ
0QSS04Z
0QSS0ZZ
0QSS34Z
0QSS3ZZ
0QSS44Z
0QSS4ZZ
0QSSXZZ
0QT20ZZ
0QT30ZZ
0QT40ZZ
0QT50ZZ
0QT60ZZ
0QT70ZZ
0QT80ZZ
0QT90ZZ
0QTB0ZZ
0QTC0ZZ
0QTD0ZZ
0QTF0ZZ
0QTG0ZZ
0QTH0ZZ
0QTJ0ZZ
0QTK0ZZ
0QTL0ZZ
0QTM0ZZ
0QTN0ZZ
0QTP0ZZ
0QTQ0ZZ
0QTR0ZZ
0QTS0ZZ
0QU007Z
0QU00JZ
0QU00KZ
0QU037Z
0QU03JZ
0QU03KZ
0QU047Z
0QU04JZ
0QU04KZ
0QU107Z
0QU10JZ
0QU10KZ
0QU137Z
0QU13JZ
0QU13KZ
0QU147Z
0QU14JZ
0QU14KZ
0QU207Z
0QU20JZ
0QU20KZ
0QU237Z
0QU23JZ
0QU23KZ
0QU247Z
0QU24JZ
0QU24KZ
0QU307Z
0QU30JZ
0QU30KZ
0QU337Z
0QU33JZ
0QU33KZ
0QU347Z
0QU34JZ
0QU34KZ
0QU407Z
0QU40JZ
0QU40KZ
0QU437Z
0QU43JZ
0QU43KZ
0QUM4KZ
0QUN07Z
0QUN0JZ
0QUN0KZ
0QUN37Z
0QUN3JZ
0QUN3KZ
0QUN47Z
0QUN4JZ
0QUN4KZ
0QUP07Z
0QUP0JZ
0QUP0KZ
0QUP37Z
0QUP3JZ
0QUP3KZ
0QUP47Z
0QUP4JZ
0QUP4KZ
0QUQ07Z
0QUQ0JZ
0QUQ0KZ
0QUQ37Z
0QUQ3JZ
0QUQ3KZ
0QUQ47Z
0QUQ4JZ
0QUQ4KZ
0QUR07Z
0QUR0JZ
0QUR0KZ
0QUR37Z
0QUR3JZ
0QUR3KZ
0QUR47Z
0QUR4JZ
0QUR4KZ
0QUS07Z
0QUS0JZ
0QUS0KZ
0QUS37Z
0QUS3JZ
0QUS3KZ
0QUS47Z
0QUS4JZ
0QUS4KZ
0QW004Z
0QW007Z
0QW00JZ
0QW00KZ
0QW034Z
0QW037Z
0QW03JZ
0QW03KZ
0QW044Z
0QW047Z
0QW04JZ
0QW04KZ
0QW0X4Z
0QW0X7Z
0QW0XJZ
0QW0XKZ
0QW104Z
0QW107Z
0QW10JZ
0QW10KZ
0QW134Z
0QW137Z
0QW13JZ
0QW13KZ
0QW144Z
0QW147Z
0QW14JZ
0QW14KZ
0QW1X4Z
0QW1X7Z
0QW1XJZ
0QW1XKZ
0QW204Z
0QW205Z
0QW207Z
0QW20JZ
0QW20KZ
0QW234Z
0QW235Z
0QW237Z
0QW23JZ
0QW23KZ
0QW244Z
0QW245Z
0QW247Z
0QW24JZ
0QW24KZ
0QW2X4Z
0QW2X5Z
0QW2X7Z
0QW2XJZ
0QW2XKZ
0QW304Z
0QW305Z
0QW307Z
0QW30JZ
0QW30KZ
0QW334Z
0QW335Z
0QW337Z
0QW33JZ
0QW33KZ
0QW344Z
0QW345Z
0QW347Z
0QW34JZ
0QW34KZ
0QW3X4Z
0QW3X5Z
0QW3X7Z
0QW3XJZ
0QW3XKZ
0QW404Z
0QW407Z
0QW40JZ
0QW40KZ
0QW434Z
0QW437Z
0QW43JZ
0QW43KZ
0QW444Z
0QW447Z
0QW44JZ
0QW44KZ
0QW4X4Z
0QW4X7Z
0QW4XJZ
0QW4XKZ
0QW504Z
0QW507Z
0QW50JZ
0QW50KZ
0QW534Z
0QW537Z
0QW53JZ
0QW53KZ
0QW544Z
0QW547Z
0QW54JZ
0QW54KZ
0QW5X4Z
0QW5X7Z
0QW5XJZ
0QW5XKZ
0QW604Z
0QW605Z
0QW607Z
0QW60JZ
0QW60KZ
0QW634Z
0QW635Z
0QW637Z
0QW63JZ
0QW63KZ
0QW644Z
0QW645Z
0QW647Z
0QW64JZ
0QW64KZ
0QW6X4Z
0QW6X5Z
0QW6X7Z
0QW6XJZ
0QW6XKZ
0QW704Z
0QW705Z
0QW707Z
0QW70JZ
0QW70KZ
0QW734Z
0QW735Z
0QW737Z
0QW73JZ
0QW73KZ
0QW744Z
0QW745Z
0QW747Z
0QW74JZ
0QW74KZ
0QW7X4Z
0QW7X5Z
0QW7X7Z
0QW7XJZ
0QW7XKZ
0QW804Z
0QW805Z
0QW807Z
0QW80JZ
0QW80KZ
0QW834Z
0QW835Z
0QW837Z
0QW83JZ
0QW83KZ
0QW844Z
0QW845Z
0QW847Z
0QW84JZ
0QW84KZ
0QW8X4Z
0QW8X5Z
0QW8X7Z
0QW8XJZ
0QW8XKZ
0QW904Z
0QW905Z
0QW907Z
0QW90JZ
0QW90KZ
0QW934Z
0QW935Z
0QW937Z
0QW93JZ
0QW93KZ
0QW944Z
0QW945Z
0QW947Z
0QW94JZ
0QW94KZ
0QW9X4Z
0QW9X5Z
0QW9X7Z
0QW9XJZ
0QW9XKZ
0QWB04Z
0QWB05Z
0QWB07Z
0QWB0JZ
0QWB0KZ
0QWB34Z
0QWB35Z
0QWB37Z
0QWB3JZ
0QWB3KZ
0QWB44Z
0QWB45Z
0QWB47Z
0QWB4JZ
0QWB4KZ
0QWBX4Z
0QWBX5Z
0QWBX7Z
0QWBXJZ
0QWBXKZ
0QWC04Z
0QWC05Z
0QWC07Z
0QWC0JZ
0QWC0KZ
0QWC34Z
0QWC35Z
0QWC37Z
0QWC3JZ
0QWC3KZ
0QWC44Z
0QWC45Z
0QWC47Z
0QWC4JZ
0QWC4KZ
0QWCX4Z
0QWCX5Z
0QWCX7Z
0QWCXJZ
0QWCXKZ
0QWD04Z
0QWD05Z
0QWD07Z
0QWD0JZ
0QWD0KZ
0QWD34Z
0QWD35Z
0QWD37Z
0QWD3JZ
0QWD3KZ
0QWD44Z
0QWD45Z
0QWD47Z
0QWD4JZ
0QWD4KZ
0QWDX4Z
0QWDX5Z
0QWDX7Z
0QWDXJZ
0QWDXKZ
0QWF04Z
0QWF05Z
0QWF07Z
0QWF0JZ
0QWF0KZ
0QWF34Z
0QWF35Z
0QWF37Z
0QWF3JZ
0QWF3KZ
0QWF44Z
0QWF45Z
0QWF47Z
0QWF4JZ
0QWF4KZ
0QWFX4Z
0QWFX5Z
0QWFX7Z
0QWFXJZ
0QWFXKZ
0QWG04Z
0QWG05Z
0QWG07Z
0QWG0JZ
0QWG0KZ
0QWG34Z
0QWG35Z
0QWG37Z
0QWG3JZ
0QWG3KZ
0QWG44Z
0QWG45Z
0QWG47Z
0QWG4JZ
0QWG4KZ
0QWGX4Z
0QWGX5Z
0QWGX7Z
0QWGXJZ
0QWGXKZ
0QWH04Z
0QWH05Z
0QWH07Z
0QWH0JZ
0QWH0KZ
0QWH34Z
0QWH35Z
0QWH37Z
0QWH3JZ
0QWH3KZ
0QWH44Z
0QWH45Z
0QWH47Z
0QWH4JZ
0QWH4KZ
0QWHX4Z
0QWHX5Z
0QWHX7Z
0QWHXJZ
0QWHXKZ
0QWJ04Z
0QWJ05Z
0QWJ07Z
0QWJ0JZ
0QWJ0KZ
0QWJ34Z
0QWJ35Z
0QWJ37Z
0QWJ3JZ
0QWJ3KZ
0QWJ44Z
0QWJ45Z
0QWJ47Z
0QWJ4JZ
0QWJ4KZ
0QWJX4Z
0QWJX5Z
0QWJX7Z
0QWJXJZ
0QWJXKZ
0QWK04Z
0QWK05Z
0QWK07Z
0QWK0JZ
0QWK0KZ
0QWK34Z
0QWK35Z
0QWK37Z
0QWK3JZ
0QWK3KZ
0QWK44Z
0QWK45Z
0QWK47Z
0QWK4JZ
0QWK4KZ
0QWKX4Z
0QWKX5Z
0QWKX7Z
0QWKXJZ
0QWKXKZ
0QWL04Z
0QWL05Z
0QWL07Z
0QWL0JZ
0QWL0KZ
0QWL34Z
0QWL35Z
0QWL37Z
0QWL3JZ
0QWL3KZ
0QWL44Z
0QWL45Z
0QWL47Z
0QWL4JZ
0QWL4KZ
0QWLX4Z
0QWLX5Z
0QWLX7Z
0QWLXJZ
0QWLXKZ
0QWM04Z
0QWM05Z
0QWM07Z
0QWM0JZ
0QWM0KZ
0QWM34Z
0QWM35Z
0QWM37Z
0QWM3JZ
0QWM3KZ
0QWM44Z
0QWM45Z
0QWM47Z
0QWM4JZ
0QWM4KZ
0QWMX4Z
0QWMX5Z
0QWMX7Z
0QWMXJZ
0QWMXKZ
0QWN04Z
0QWN05Z
0QWN07Z
0QWN0JZ
0QWN0KZ
0QWN34Z
0QWN35Z
0QWN37Z
0QWN3JZ
0QWN3KZ
0QWN44Z
0QWN45Z
0QWN47Z
0QWN4JZ
0QWN4KZ
0QWNX4Z
0QWNX5Z
0QWNX7Z
0QWNXJZ
0QWNXKZ
0QWP04Z
0QWP05Z
0QWP07Z
0QWP0JZ
0QWP0KZ
0QWP34Z
0QWP35Z
0QWP37Z
0QWP3JZ
0QWP3KZ
0QWP44Z
0QWP45Z
0QWP47Z
0QWP4JZ
0QWP4KZ
0QWPX4Z
0QWPX5Z
0QWPX7Z
0QWPXJZ
0QWPXKZ
0QWQ04Z
0QWQ05Z
0QWQ07Z
0QWQ0JZ
0QWQ0KZ
0QWQ34Z
0QWQ35Z
0QWQ37Z
0QWQ3JZ
0QWQ3KZ
0QWQ44Z
0QWQ45Z
0QWQ47Z
0QWQ4JZ
0QWQ4KZ
0QWQX4Z
0QWQX5Z
0QWQX7Z
0QWQXJZ
0QWQXKZ
0QWR04Z
0QWR05Z
0QWR07Z
0QWR0JZ
0QWR0KZ
0QWR34Z
0QWR35Z
0QWR37Z
0QWR3JZ
0QWR3KZ
0QWR44Z
0QWR45Z
0QWR47Z
0QWR4JZ
0QWR4KZ
0QWRX4Z
0QWRX5Z
0QWRX7Z
0QWRXJZ
0QWRXKZ
0QWS04Z
0QWS07Z
0QWS0JZ
0QWS0KZ
0QWS34Z
0QWS37Z
0QWS3JZ
0QWS3KZ
0QWS44Z
0QWS47Z
0QWS4JZ
0QWS4KZ
0QWSX4Z
0QWSX7Z
0QWSXJZ
0QWSXKZ
0QWY00Z
0QWY0MZ
0QWY30Z
0QWY3MZ
0QWY40Z
0QWY4MZ
0QWYX0Z
0QWYXMZ
0R2YX0Z
0R2YXYZ
0R500ZZ
0R503ZZ
0R504ZZ
0R510ZZ
0R513ZZ
0R514ZZ
0R530ZZ
0R533ZZ
0R534ZZ
0R540ZZ
0R543ZZ
0R544ZZ
0R550ZZ
0R553ZZ
0R554ZZ
0R560ZZ
0R563ZZ
0R564ZZ
0R590ZZ
0R593ZZ
0R594ZZ
0R5A0ZZ
0R5A3ZZ
0R5A4ZZ
0R5B0ZZ
0R5B3ZZ
0R5B4ZZ
0R5C0ZZ
0R5C3ZZ
0R5C4ZZ
0R5D0ZZ
0R5D3ZZ
0R5D4ZZ
0R5E0ZZ
0R5E3ZZ
0R5E4ZZ
0R5F0ZZ
0R5F3ZZ
0R5F4ZZ
0R5G0ZZ
0R5G3ZZ
0R5G4ZZ
0R5H0ZZ
0R5H3ZZ
0R5H4ZZ
0R5J0ZZ
0R5J3ZZ
0R5J4ZZ
0R5K0ZZ
0R5K3ZZ
0R5K4ZZ
0R5L0ZZ
0R5L3ZZ
0R5L4ZZ
0R5M0ZZ
0R5M3ZZ
0R5M4ZZ
0R5N0ZZ
0R5N3ZZ
0R5N4ZZ
0R5P0ZZ
0R5P3ZZ
0R5P4ZZ
0R5Q0ZZ
0R5Q3ZZ
0R5Q4ZZ
0R5R0ZZ
0R5R3ZZ
0R5R4ZZ
0R5S0ZZ
0R5S3ZZ
0R5S4ZZ
0R5T0ZZ
0R5T3ZZ
0R5T4ZZ
0R5U0ZZ
0R5U3ZZ
0R5U4ZZ
0R5V0ZZ
0R5V3ZZ
0R5V4ZZ
0R5W0ZZ
0R5W3ZZ
0R5W4ZZ
0R5X0ZZ
0R5X3ZZ
0R5X4ZZ
0R9000Z
0R900ZX
0R900ZZ
0R9030Z
0R903ZX
0R903ZZ
0R9040Z
0R904ZX
0R904ZZ
0R9100Z
0R910ZX

0R910ZZ
0R9130Z
0R913ZX
0R913ZZ
0R9140Z
0R914ZX
0R914ZZ
0R9300Z
0R930ZX
0R930ZZ
0R9330Z
0R933ZX
0R933ZZ
0R9340Z
0R934ZX
0R934ZZ
0R9400Z
0R940ZX
0R940ZZ
0R9430Z
0R943ZX
0R943ZZ
0R9440Z
0R944ZX
0R944ZZ
0R9500Z
0R950ZX
0R950ZZ
0R9530Z
0R953ZX
0R953ZZ
0R9540Z
0R954ZX
0R954ZZ
0R9600Z
0R960ZX
0R960ZZ
0R9630Z
0R963ZX
0R963ZZ
0R9640Z
0R964ZX
0R964ZZ
0R9900Z
0R990ZX
0R990ZZ
0R9930Z
0R993ZX
0R993ZZ
0R9940Z
0R994ZX
0R994ZZ
0R9A00Z
0R9A0ZX
0R9A30Z
0R9A3ZX
0R9A3ZZ
0R9A40Z
0R9A4ZX
0R9A4ZZ
0R9B0ZX
0R9B30Z
0R9B3ZX
0R9B3ZZ
0R9B40Z
0R9B4ZX
0R9B4ZZ
0R9C30Z
0R9C3ZZ
0R9D30Z
0R9D3ZZ
0R9E0ZX
0R9E30Z
0R9E3ZX
0R9E3ZZ
0R9E40Z
0R9E4ZX
0R9E4ZZ
0R9F0ZX
0R9F30Z
0R9F3ZX
0R9F3ZZ
0R9F40Z
0R9F4ZX
0R9F4ZZ
0R9G0ZX
0R9G30Z
0R9G3ZX
0R9G3ZZ
0R9G40Z
0R9G4ZX
0R9G4ZZ
0R9H0ZX
0R9H30Z
0R9H3ZX
0R9H3ZZ
0R9H40Z
0R9H4ZX
0R9H4ZZ
0R9J0ZX
0R9J30Z
0R9J3ZX
0R9J3ZZ
0R9J40Z
0R9J4ZX
0R9J4ZZ
0R9K0ZX
0R9K30Z
0R9K3ZX
0R9K3ZZ
0R9K40Z
0R9K4ZX
0R9K4ZZ
0R9L0ZX
0R9L30Z
0R9L3ZX
0R9L3ZZ
0R9L40Z
0R9L4ZX
0R9L4ZZ
0R9M0ZX
0R9M30Z
0R9M3ZX
0R9M3ZZ
0R9M40Z
0R9M4ZX
0R9M4ZZ
0R9N0ZX
0R9N30Z
0R9N3ZX
0R9N3ZZ
0R9N40Z
0R9N4ZX
0R9N4ZZ
0R9P0ZX
0R9P30Z
0R9P3ZX
0R9P3ZZ
0R9P40Z
0R9P4ZX
0R9P4ZZ
0R9Q0ZX
0R9Q30Z
0R9Q3ZX
0R9Q3ZZ
0R9Q40Z
0R9Q4ZX
0R9Q4ZZ
0R9R0ZX
0R9R30Z
0R9R3ZX
0R9R3ZZ
0R9R40Z
0R9R4ZX
0R9R4ZZ
0R9S0ZX
0R9S30Z
0R9S3ZX
0R9S3ZZ
0R9S40Z
0R9S4ZX
0R9S4ZZ
0R9T0ZX
0R9T30Z
0R9T3ZX
0R9T3ZZ
0R9T40Z
0R9T4ZX
0R9T4ZZ
0R9U0ZX
0R9U30Z
0R9U3ZX
0R9U3ZZ
0R9U40Z
0R9U4ZX
0R9U4ZZ
0R9V0ZX
0R9V30Z
0R9V3ZX
0R9V3ZZ
0R9V40Z
0R9V4ZX
0R9V4ZZ
0R9W0ZX
0R9W30Z
0R9W3ZX
0R9W3ZZ
0R9W40Z
0R9W4ZX
0R9W4ZZ
0R9X0ZX
0R9X30Z
0R9X3ZX
0R9X3ZZ
0R9X40Z
0R9X4ZX
0R9X4ZZ
0RB00ZX
0RB03ZX
0RB04ZX
0RB10ZX
0RB13ZX
0RB14ZX
0RB30ZX
0RB33ZX
0RB34ZX
0RB40ZX
0RB43ZX
0RB44ZX
0RB50ZX
0RB53ZX
0RB54ZX
0RB60ZX
0RB63ZX
0RB64ZX
0RB90ZX
0RB93ZX
0RB94ZX
0RBA0ZX
0RBA3ZX
0RBA4ZX
0RBB0ZX
0RBB3ZX
0RBB4ZX
0RBE0ZX
0RBE3ZX
0RBE4ZX
0RBF0ZX
0RBF3ZX
0RBF4ZX
0RBG0ZX
0RBG3ZX
0RBG4ZX
0RBH0ZX
0RBH3ZX
0RBH4ZX
0RBJ0ZX
0RBJ3ZX
0RBJ4ZX
0RBK0ZX
0RBK3ZX
0RBK4ZX
0RBL0ZX
0RBL3ZX
0RBL4ZX
0RBM0ZX
0RBM3ZX
0RBM4ZX
0RBN0ZX
0RBN3ZX
0RBN4ZX
0RBP0ZX
0RBP3ZX
0RBP4ZX
0RBQ0ZX
0RBQ3ZX
0RBQ4ZX
0RBR0ZX
0RBR3ZX
0RBR4ZX
0RBS0ZX
0RBS3ZX
0RBS4ZX
0RBT0ZX
0RBT3ZX
0RBT4ZX
0RBU0ZX
0RBU3ZX
0RBU3ZZ
0RBU4ZX
0RBU4ZZ
0RBV0ZX
0RBV0ZZ
0RBV3ZX
0RBV3ZZ
0RBV4ZX
0RBV4ZZ
0RBW0ZX
0RBW0ZZ
0RBW3ZX
0RBW3ZZ
0RBW4ZX
0RBW4ZZ
0RBX0ZX
0RBX0ZZ
0RBX3ZX
0RBX3ZZ
0RBX4ZX
0RBX4ZZ
0RC00ZZ
0RC03ZZ
0RC04ZZ
0RC10ZZ
0RC13ZZ
0RC14ZZ
0RC30ZZ
0RC33ZZ
0RC34ZZ
0RC40ZZ
0RC43ZZ
0RC44ZZ
0RC50ZZ
0RC53ZZ
0RC54ZZ
0RC60ZZ
0RC63ZZ
0RC64ZZ
0RC90ZZ
0RC93ZZ
0RC94ZZ
0RCA0ZZ
0RCA3ZZ
0RCA4ZZ
0RCB0ZZ
0RCB3ZZ
0RCB4ZZ
0RCC0ZZ
0RCC3ZZ
0RCC4ZZ
0RCD0ZZ
0RCD3ZZ
0RCD4ZZ
0RCE0ZZ
0RCE3ZZ
0RCE4ZZ
0RCF0ZZ
0RCF3ZZ
0RCF4ZZ
0RCG0ZZ
0RCG3ZZ
0RCG4ZZ
0RCH0ZZ
0RCH3ZZ
0RCH4ZZ
0RCJ0ZZ
0RCJ3ZZ
0RCJ4ZZ
0RCK0ZZ
0RCK3ZZ
0RCK4ZZ
0RCL0ZZ
0RCL3ZZ
0RCL4ZZ
0RCM0ZZ
0RCM3ZZ
0RCM4ZZ
0RCN0ZZ
0RCN3ZZ
0RCN4ZZ
0RCP0ZZ
0RCP3ZZ
0RCP4ZZ
0RCQ0ZZ
0RCQ3ZZ
0RCQ4ZZ
0RCR0ZZ
0RCR3ZZ
0RCR4ZZ
0RCS0ZZ
0RCS3ZZ
0RCS4ZZ
0RCT0ZZ
0RCT3ZZ
0RCT4ZZ
0RCU0ZZ
0RCU3ZZ
0RCU4ZZ
0RCV0ZZ
0RCV3ZZ
0RCV4ZZ
0RCW0ZZ
0RCW3ZZ
0RCW4ZZ
0RCX0ZZ
0RCX3ZZ
0RCX4ZZ
0RG0070
0RG0071
0RG007J
0RG00A0
0RG00AJ
0RG00J0
0RG00J1
0RG00JJ
0RG00K0
0RG00K1
0RG00KJ
0RG0370
0RG0371
0RG037J
0RG03A0
0RG03AJ
0RG03J0
0RG03J1
0RG03JJ
0RG03K0
0RG03K1
0RG03KJ
0RG0470
0RG0471
0RG047J
0RG04A0
0RG04AJ
0RG04J0
0RG04J1
0RG04JJ
0RG04K0
0RG04K1
0RG04KJ
0RG1070
0RG1071
0RG107J
0RG10A0
0RG10AJ
0RG10J0
0RG10J1
0RG10JJ
0RG10K0
0RG10K1
0RG10KJ
0RG1370
0RG1371
0RG137J
0RG13A0
0RG13AJ
0RG13J0
0RG13J1
0RG13JJ
0RG13K0
0RG13K1
0RG13KJ
0RG1470
0RG1471
0RG147J
0RG14A0
0RG14AJ
0RG14J0
0RG14J1
0RG14JJ
0RG14K0
0RG14K1
0RG14KJ
0RG2070
0RG2071
0RG207J
0RG20A0
0RG20AJ
0RG20J0
0RG20J1
0RG20JJ
0RG20K0
0RG20K1
0RG20KJ
0RG2370
0RG2371
0RG237J
0RG23A0
0RG23AJ
0RG23J0
0RG23J1
0RG23JJ
0RG23K0
0RG23K1
0RG23KJ
0RG2470
0RG2471
0RG247J
0RG24A0
0RG24AJ
0RG24J0
0RG24J1
0RG24JJ
0RG24K0
0RG24K1
0RG24KJ
0RG4070
0RG4071
0RG407J
0RG40A0
0RG64K0
0RG64K1
0RG64KJ
0RG7070
0RG7071
0RG707J
0RG70A0
0RG70AJ
0RG70J0
0RG70J1
0RG70JJ
0RG70K0
0RG70K1
0RG70KJ
0RG7370
0RG7371
0RG737J
0RG73A0
0RG73AJ
0RG73J0
0RG73J1
0RG73JJ
0RG73K0
0RG73K1
0RG73KJ
0RG7470
0RG7471
0RG747J
0RG74A0
0RG74AJ
0RG74J0
0RG74J1
0RG74JJ
0RG74K0
0RG74K1
0RG74KJ
0RG8070
0RG8071
0RG807J
0RG80A0
0RG80AJ
0RG80J0
0RG80J1
0RG80JJ
0RG80K0
0RG80K1
0RG80KJ
0RG8370
0RG8371
0RG837J
0RG83A0
0RG83AJ
0RG83J0
0RG83J1
0RG83JJ
0RG83K0
0RG83K1
0RG83KJ
0RG8470
0RG8471
0RG847J
0RG84A0
0RG84AJ
0RG84J0
0RG84J1
0RG84JJ
0RG84K0
0RG84K1
0RG84KJ
0RGA070
0RGA071
0RGA07J
0RGA0A0
0RGA0AJ
0RGA0J0
0RGA0J1
0RGA0JJ
0RGA0K0
0RGA0K1
0RGA0KJ
0RGA370
0RGA371
0RGA37J
0RGA3A0
0RGA3AJ
0RGA3J0
0RGA3J1
0RGA3JJ
0RGA3K0
0RGA3K1
0RGA3KJ
0RGA470
0RGA471
0RGA47J
0RGA4A0
0RGA4AJ
0RGA4J0
0RGA4J1
0RGA4JJ
0RGA4K0
0RGA4K1
0RGA4KJ
0RGC04Z
0RGC07Z
0RGC0JZ
0RGP47Z
0RGP4JZ
0RGP4KZ
0RGQ04Z
0RGQ05Z
0RGQ07Z
0RGQ0JZ
0RGQ0KZ
0RGQ34Z
0RGQ35Z
0RGQ37Z
0RGQ3JZ
0RGQ3KZ
0RGQ44Z
0RGQ45Z
0RGQ47Z
0RGQ4JZ
0RGQ4KZ
0RGR04Z
0RGR05Z
0RGR07Z
0RGR0JZ
0RGR0KZ
0RGR34Z
0RGR35Z
0RGR37Z
0RGR3JZ
0RGR3KZ
0RGR44Z
0RGR45Z
0RGR47Z
0RGR4JZ
0RGR4KZ
0RGS04Z
0RGS05Z
0RGS07Z
0RGS0JZ
0RGS0KZ
0RGS34Z
0RGS35Z
0RGS37Z
0RGS3JZ
0RGS3KZ
0RGS44Z
0RGS45Z
0RGS47Z
0RGS4JZ
0RGS4KZ
0RGT04Z
0RGT05Z
0RGT07Z
0RGT0JZ
0RGT0KZ
0RGT34Z
0RGT35Z
0RGT37Z
0RGT3JZ
0RGT3KZ
0RGT44Z
0RGT45Z
0RGT47Z
0RGT4JZ
0RGT4KZ
0RGU04Z
0RGU05Z
0RGU07Z
0RGU0JZ
0RGU0KZ
0RGU34Z
0RGU35Z
0RGU37Z
0RGU3JZ
0RGU3KZ
0RGU44Z
0RGU45Z
0RGU47Z
0RGU4JZ
0RGU4KZ
0RGV04Z
0RGV05Z
0RGV07Z
0RGV0JZ
0RGV0KZ
0RGV34Z
0RGV35Z
0RGV37Z
0RGV3JZ
0RGV3KZ
0RGV44Z
0RGV45Z
0RGV47Z
0RGV4JZ
0RGV4KZ
0RGW04Z
0RGW05Z
0RGW07Z
0RGW0JZ
0RGW0KZ
0RGW34Z
0RGW35Z
0RGW37Z
0RGW3JZ
0RGW3KZ
0RGW44Z
0RGW45Z
0RGW47Z
0RGW4JZ
0RGW4KZ
0RGX04Z
0RGX05Z
0RGX07Z
0RGX0JZ
0RGX0KZ
0RGX34Z
0RGX35Z
0RGX37Z
0RGX3JZ
0RGX3KZ
0RGX44Z
0RGX45Z
0RGX47Z
0RGX4JZ
0RGX4KZ
0RH003Z
0RH004Z
0RH008Z
0RH00BZ
0RH00CZ
0RH00DZ
0RH033Z
0RH034Z
0RH038Z
0RH03BZ
0RH03CZ
0RH03DZ
0RH043Z
0RH044Z
0RH048Z
0RH04BZ
0RH04CZ
0RH04DZ
0RH103Z

0RH104Z
0RH108Z
0RH10BZ
0RH10CZ
0RH10DZ
0RH133Z
0RH134Z
0RH138Z
0RH13BZ
0RH13CZ
0RH13DZ
0RH143Z
0RH144Z
0RH148Z
0RH14BZ
0RH14CZ
0RH14DZ
0RH303Z
0RH333Z
0RH343Z
0RH403Z
0RH404Z
0RH408Z
0RH40BZ
0RH40CZ
0RH40DZ
0RH433Z
0RH434Z
0RH438Z
0RH43BZ
0RH43CZ
0RH43DZ
0RH443Z
0RH444Z
0RH448Z
0RH44BZ
0RH44CZ
0RH44DZ
0RH503Z
0RH533Z
0RH543Z
0RH603Z
0RH604Z
0RH608Z
0RH60BZ
0RH60CZ
0RH60DZ
0RH633Z
0RH634Z
0RH638Z
0RH63BZ
0RH63CZ
0RH63DZ
0RH643Z
0RH644Z
0RH648Z
0RH64BZ
0RH64CZ
0RH64DZ
0RH903Z
0RH933Z
0RH943Z
0RHA03Z
0RHA04Z
0RHA08Z
0RHA0BZ
0RHA0CZ
0RHA0DZ
0RHA33Z
0RHA34Z
0RHA38Z
0RHA3BZ
0RHA3CZ
0RHA3DZ
0RHA43Z
0RHA44Z
0RHA48Z
0RHA4BZ
0RHA4CZ
0RHA4DZ
0RHB03Z
0RHB33Z
0RHB43Z
0RHC03Z
0RHC04Z
0RHC08Z
0RHC33Z
0RHC34Z
0RHC38Z
0RHC43Z
0RHC44Z
0RHC48Z
0RHD03Z
0RHD04Z
0RHD08Z
0RHD33Z
0RHD34Z
0RHD38Z
0RHD43Z
0RHD44Z
0RHD48Z
0RHE03Z
0RHE04Z
0RHE08Z
0RHE33Z
0RHE34Z
0RHE38Z
0RHE43Z
0RHE44Z
0RHE48Z
0RHF03Z
0RHF04Z
0RHF08Z
0RHF33Z
0RHF34Z
0RHF38Z
0RHF43Z
0RHF44Z
0RHF48Z
0RHG03Z
0RHG04Z
0RHG08Z
0RHG33Z
0RHG34Z
0RHG38Z
0RHG43Z
0RHG44Z
0RHG48Z
0RHH03Z
0RHH04Z
0RHH08Z
0RHH33Z
0RHH34Z
0RHH38Z
0RHH43Z
0RHH44Z
0RHH48Z
0RHJ03Z
0RHJ04Z
0RHJ08Z
0RHJ33Z
0RHJ34Z
0RHJ38Z
0RHJ43Z
0RHJ44Z
0RHJ48Z
0RHK03Z
0RHK04Z
0RHK08Z
0RHK33Z
0RHK34Z
0RHK38Z
0RHK43Z
0RHK44Z
0RHK48Z
0RHL03Z
0RHL04Z
0RHL05Z
0RHL08Z
0RHL33Z
0RHL34Z
0RHL35Z
0RHL38Z
0RHL43Z
0RHL44Z
0RHL45Z
0RHL48Z
0RHM03Z
0RHM04Z
0RHM05Z
0RHM08Z
0RHM33Z
0RHM34Z
0RHM35Z
0RHM38Z
0RHM43Z
0RHM44Z
0RHM45Z
0RHM48Z
0RHN03Z
0RHN04Z
0RHN05Z
0RHN08Z
0RHN33Z
0RHN34Z
0RHN35Z
0RHN38Z
0RHN43Z
0RHN44Z
0RHN45Z
0RHN48Z
0RHP03Z
0RHP04Z
0RHP05Z
0RHP08Z
0RHP33Z
0RHP34Z
0RHP35Z
0RHP38Z
0RHP43Z
0RHP44Z
0RHP45Z
0RHP48Z
0RHQ03Z
0RHQ04Z
0RHQ05Z
0RHQ08Z
0RHQ33Z
0RHQ34Z
0RHQ35Z
0RHQ38Z
0RHQ43Z
0RHQ44Z
0RHQ45Z
0RHQ48Z
0RHR03Z
0RHR04Z
0RHR05Z
0RHR08Z
0RHR33Z
0RHR34Z
0RHR35Z
0RHR38Z
0RHR43Z
0RHR44Z
0RHR45Z
0RHR48Z
0RHS03Z
0RHS04Z
0RHS05Z
0RHS08Z
0RHS33Z
0RHS34Z
0RHS35Z
0RHS38Z
0RHS43Z
0RHS44Z
0RHS45Z
0RHS48Z
0RHT03Z
0RHT04Z
0RHT05Z
0RHT08Z
0RHT33Z
0RHT34Z
0RHT35Z
0RHT38Z
0RHT43Z
0RHT44Z
0RHT45Z
0RHT48Z
0RHU03Z
0RHU04Z
0RHU05Z
0RHU08Z
0RHU33Z
0RHU34Z
0RHU35Z
0RHU38Z
0RHU43Z
0RHU44Z
0RHU45Z
0RHU48Z
0RHV03Z
0RHV04Z
0RHV05Z
0RHV08Z
0RHV33Z
0RHV34Z
0RHV35Z
0RHV38Z
0RHV43Z
0RHV44Z
0RHV48Z
0RHW03Z
0RHW08Z
0RHW33Z
0RHW38Z
0RHW43Z
0RHW48Z
0RHX03Z
0RHX08Z
0RHX33Z
0RHX38Z
0RHX43Z
0RHX48Z
0RJ03ZZ
0RJ0XZZ
0RJ13ZZ
0RJ1XZZ
0RJ33ZZ
0RJ3XZZ
0RJ43ZZ
0RJ4XZZ
0RJ53ZZ
0RJ5XZZ
0RJ63ZZ
0RJ6XZZ
0RJ93ZZ
0RJ9XZZ
0RJA3ZZ
0RJAXZZ
0RJB3ZZ
0RJBXZZ
0RJC3ZZ
0RJCXZZ
0RJD3ZZ
0RJDXZZ
0RJE3ZZ
0RJEXZZ
0RJF3ZZ
0RJFXZZ
0RJG3ZZ
0RJGXZZ
0RJH3ZZ
0RJHXZZ
0RJJ3ZZ
0RJJXZZ
0RJK3ZZ
0RJKXZZ
0RJL3ZZ
0RJLXZZ
0RJM3ZZ
0RJMXZZ
0RJN3ZZ
0RJNXZZ
0RJP3ZZ
0RJPXZZ
0RJQ3ZZ
0RJQXZZ
0RJR3ZZ
0RJRXZZ
0RJS3ZZ
0RJSXZZ
0RJT3ZZ
0RJTXZZ
0RJU3ZZ
0RJUXZZ
0RJV3ZZ
0RJVXZZ
0RJW3ZZ
0RJWXZZ
0RJX3ZZ
0RJXXZZ
0RN0XZZ
0RN1XZZ
0RN3XZZ
0RN4XZZ
0RN5XZZ
0RN6XZZ
0RN9XZZ
0RNAXZZ
0RNBXZZ
0RNCXZZ
0RNDXZZ
0RNEXZZ
0RNFXZZ
0RNGXZZ
0RNHXZZ
0RNJXZZ
0RNKXZZ
0RNLXZZ
0RNMXZZ
0RNNXZZ
0RNPXZZ
0RNQXZZ
0RNRXZZ
0RNSXZZ
0RNTXZZ
0RNUXZZ
0RNVXZZ
0RNWXZZ
0RNXXZZ
0RP000Z
0RP003Z
0RP004Z
0RP007Z
0RP008Z
0RP00AZ
0RP00JZ
0RP00KZ
0RP030Z
0RP033Z
0RP034Z
0RP037Z
0RP038Z
0RP03AZ
0RP03JZ
0RP03KZ
0RP040Z
0RP043Z
0RP044Z
0RP047Z
0RP048Z
0RP04AZ
0RP04JZ
0RP04KZ
0RP0X0Z
0RP0X3Z
0RP0X4Z
0RP100Z
0RP103Z
0RP104Z
0RP107Z
0RP108Z
0RP10AZ
0RP10JZ
0RP10KZ
0RP130Z
0RP133Z
0RP134Z
0RP137Z
0RP138Z
0RP13AZ
0RP13JZ
0RP13KZ
0RP140Z
0RP143Z
0RP144Z
0RP147Z
0RP148Z
0RP14AZ
0RP14JZ
0RP14KZ
0RP1X0Z
0RP1X3Z
0RP1X4Z
0RP300Z
0RP303Z
0RP307Z
0RP30JZ
0RP30KZ
0RP330Z
0RP333Z
0RP337Z
0RP33JZ
0RP33KZ
0RP340Z
0RP343Z
0RP347Z
0RP34JZ
0RP34KZ
0RP3X0Z
0RP3X3Z
0RP400Z
0RP403Z
0RP404Z
0RP407Z
0RP408Z
0RP40AZ
0RP40JZ
0RP40KZ
0RP430Z
0RP433Z
0RP434Z
0RP437Z
0RP438Z
0RP43AZ
0RP43JZ
0RP43KZ
0RP440Z
0RP443Z
0RP444Z
0RP447Z
0RP448Z
0RP44AZ
0RP44JZ
0RP44KZ
0RP4X0Z
0RP4X3Z
0RP4X4Z
0RP500Z
0RP503Z
0RP507Z
0RP50JZ
0RP50KZ
0RP530Z
0RP533Z
0RP537Z
0RP53JZ
0RP53KZ
0RP540Z
0RP543Z
0RP547Z
0RP54JZ
0RP54KZ
0RP5X0Z
0RP5X3Z
0RP600Z
0RP603Z
0RP604Z
0RP607Z
0RP608Z
0RP60AZ
0RP60JZ
0RP60KZ
0RP630Z
0RP633Z
0RP634Z
0RP637Z
0RP638Z
0RP63AZ
0RP63JZ
0RP63KZ
0RP640Z
0RP643Z
0RP644Z
0RP647Z
0RP648Z
0RP64AZ
0RP64JZ
0RP64KZ
0RP6X0Z
0RP6X3Z
0RP6X4Z
0RP900Z
0RP903Z
0RP907Z
0RP90JZ
0RP90KZ
0RP930Z
0RP933Z
0RP937Z
0RP93JZ
0RP93KZ
0RP940Z
0RP943Z
0RP947Z
0RP94JZ
0RP94KZ
0RP9X0Z
0RP9X3Z
0RPA00Z
0RPA03Z
0RPA04Z
0RPA07Z
0RPA08Z
0RPA0AZ
0RPA0JZ
0RPA0KZ
0RPA30Z
0RPA33Z
0RPA34Z
0RPA37Z
0RPA38Z
0RPA3AZ
0RPA3JZ
0RPA3KZ
0RPA40Z
0RPA43Z
0RPA44Z
0RPA47Z
0RPA48Z
0RPA4AZ
0RPA4JZ
0RPA4KZ
0RPAX0Z
0RPAX3Z
0RPAX4Z
0RPB00Z
0RPB03Z
0RPB07Z
0RPB0JZ
0RPB0KZ
0RPB30Z
0RPB33Z
0RPB37Z
0RPB3JZ
0RPB3KZ
0RPB40Z
0RPB43Z
0RPB47Z
0RPB4JZ
0RPB4KZ
0RPBX0Z
0RPBX3Z
0RPC00Z
0RPC03Z
0RPC04Z
0RPC07Z
0RPC08Z
0RPC0JZ
0RPC0KZ
0RPC30Z
0RPC33Z
0RPC34Z
0RPC37Z
0RPC38Z
0RPC3JZ
0RPC3KZ
0RPC40Z
0RPC43Z
0RPC44Z
0RPC47Z
0RPC48Z
0RPC4JZ
0RPC4KZ
0RPCX0Z
0RPCX3Z
0RPCX4Z
0RPD00Z
0RPD03Z
0RPD04Z
0RPD07Z
0RPD08Z
0RPD0JZ
0RPD0KZ
0RPD30Z
0RPD33Z
0RPD34Z
0RPD37Z
0RPD38Z
0RPD3JZ
0RPD3KZ
0RPD40Z
0RPD43Z
0RPD44Z
0RPD47Z
0RPD48Z
0RPD4JZ
0RPD4KZ
0RPDX0Z
0RPDX3Z
0RPDX4Z
0RPE00Z
0RPE03Z
0RPE04Z
0RPE07Z
0RPE08Z
0RPE0JZ
0RPE0KZ
0RPE30Z
0RPE33Z
0RPE34Z
0RPE37Z
0RPE38Z
0RPE3JZ
0RPE3KZ
0RPE40Z
0RPE43Z
0RPE44Z
0RPE47Z
0RPE48Z
0RPE4JZ
0RPE4KZ
0RPEX0Z
0RPEX3Z
0RPEX4Z
0RPF00Z
0RPF03Z
0RPF04Z
0RPF07Z
0RPF08Z
0RPF0JZ
0RPF0KZ
0RPF30Z
0RPF33Z
0RPF34Z
0RPF37Z
0RPF38Z
0RPF3JZ
0RPF3KZ
0RPF40Z
0RPF43Z
0RPF44Z
0RPF47Z
0RPF48Z
0RPF4JZ
0RPF4KZ
0RPFX0Z
0RPFX3Z
0RPFX4Z
0RPG00Z
0RPG03Z
0RPG04Z
0RPG07Z
0RPG08Z
0RPG0JZ
0RPG0KZ
0RPG30Z
0RPG33Z
0RPG34Z
0RPG37Z
0RPG38Z
0RPG3JZ
0RPG3KZ
0RPG40Z
0RPG43Z
0RPG44Z
0RPG47Z
0RPG48Z
0RPG4JZ
0RPG4KZ
0RPGX0Z
0RPGX3Z
0RPGX4Z
0RPH00Z
0RPH03Z
0RPH04Z
0RPH07Z
0RPH08Z
0RPH0JZ
0RPH0KZ
0RPH30Z
0RPH33Z
0RPH34Z
0RPH37Z
0RPH38Z
0RPH3JZ
0RPH3KZ
0RPH40Z
0RPH43Z
0RPH44Z
0RPH47Z
0RPH48Z
0RPH4JZ
0RPH4KZ
0RPHX0Z
0RPHX3Z
0RPHX4Z
0RPJ00Z
0RPJ03Z
0RPJ04Z
0RPJ07Z
0RPJ08Z
0RPJ0JZ

0RPJ0KZ
0RPJ30Z
0RPJ33Z
0RPJ34Z
0RPJ37Z
0RPJ38Z
0RPJ3JZ
0RPJ3KZ
0RPJ40Z
0RPJ43Z
0RPJ44Z
0RPJ47Z
0RPJ48Z
0RPJ4JZ
0RPJ4KZ
0RPJX0Z
0RPJX3Z
0RPJX4Z
0RPK00Z
0RPK03Z
0RPK04Z
0RPK07Z
0RPK08Z
0RPK0JZ
0RPK0KZ
0RPK30Z
0RPK33Z
0RPK34Z
0RPK37Z
0RPK38Z
0RPK3JZ
0RPK3KZ
0RPK40Z
0RPK43Z
0RPK44Z
0RPK47Z
0RPK48Z
0RPK4JZ
0RPK4KZ
0RPKX0Z
0RPKX3Z
0RPKX4Z
0RPL00Z
0RPL03Z
0RPL04Z
0RPL05Z
0RPL07Z
0RPL08Z
0RPL0JZ
0RPL0KZ
0RPL30Z
0RPL33Z
0RPL34Z
0RPL35Z
0RPL37Z
0RPL38Z
0RPL3JZ
0RPL3KZ
0RPL40Z
0RPL43Z
0RPL44Z
0RPL45Z
0RPL47Z
0RPL48Z
0RPL4JZ
0RPL4KZ
0RPLX0Z
0RPLX3Z
0RPLX4Z
0RPLX5Z
0RPM00Z
0RPM03Z
0RPM04Z
0RPM05Z
0RPM07Z
0RPM08Z
0RPM0JZ
0RPM0KZ
0RPM30Z
0RPM33Z
0RPM34Z
0RPM35Z
0RPM37Z
0RPM38Z
0RPM3JZ
0RPM3KZ
0RPM40Z
0RPM43Z
0RPM44Z
0RPM45Z
0RPM47Z
0RPM48Z
0RPM4JZ
0RPM4KZ
0RPMX0Z
0RPMX3Z
0RPMX4Z
0RPMX5Z
0RPN00Z
0RPN03Z
0RPN04Z
0RPN05Z
0RPN07Z
0RPN08Z
0RPN0JZ
0RPN0KZ
0RPN30Z
0RPN33Z
0RPN34Z
0RPN35Z
0RPN37Z
0RPN38Z
0RPN3JZ
0RPN3KZ
0RPN40Z
0RPN43Z
0RPN44Z
0RPN45Z
0RPN47Z
0RPN48Z
0RPN4JZ
0RPN4KZ
0RPNX0Z
0RPNX3Z
0RPNX4Z
0RPNX5Z
0RPP00Z
0RPP03Z
0RPP04Z
0RPP05Z
0RPP07Z
0RPP08Z
0RPP0JZ
0RPP0KZ
0RPP30Z
0RPP33Z
0RPP34Z
0RPP35Z
0RPP37Z
0RPP38Z
0RPP3JZ
0RPP3KZ
0RPP40Z
0RPP43Z
0RPP44Z
0RPP45Z
0RPP47Z
0RPP48Z
0RPP4JZ
0RPP4KZ
0RPPX0Z
0RPPX3Z
0RPPX4Z
0RPPX5Z
0RPQ00Z
0RPQ03Z
0RPQ04Z
0RPQ05Z
0RPQ07Z
0RPQ08Z
0RPQ0JZ
0RPQ0KZ
0RPQ30Z
0RPQ33Z
0RPQ34Z
0RPQ35Z
0RPQ37Z
0RPQ38Z
0RPQ3JZ
0RPQ3KZ
0RPQ40Z
0RPQ43Z
0RPQ44Z
0RPQ45Z
0RPQ47Z
0RPQ48Z
0RPQ4JZ
0RPQ4KZ
0RPQX0Z
0RPQX3Z
0RPQX4Z
0RPQX5Z
0RPR00Z
0RPR03Z
0RPR04Z
0RPR05Z
0RPR07Z
0RPR08Z
0RPR0JZ
0RPR0KZ
0RPR30Z
0RPR33Z
0RPR34Z
0RPR35Z
0RPR37Z
0RPR38Z
0RPR3JZ
0RPR3KZ
0RPR40Z
0RPR43Z
0RPR44Z
0RPR45Z
0RPR47Z
0RPR48Z
0RPR4JZ
0RPR4KZ
0RPRX0Z
0RPRX3Z
0RPRX4Z
0RPRX5Z
0RPS00Z
0RPS03Z
0RPS04Z
0RPS05Z
0RPS07Z
0RPS08Z
0RPS0JZ
0RPS0KZ
0RPS30Z
0RPS33Z
0RPS34Z
0RPS35Z
0RPS37Z
0RPS38Z
0RPS3JZ
0RPS3KZ
0RPS40Z
0RPS43Z
0RPS44Z
0RPS45Z
0RPS47Z
0RPS48Z
0RPS4JZ
0RPS4KZ
0RPSX0Z
0RPSX3Z
0RPSX4Z
0RPSX5Z
0RPT00Z
0RPT03Z
0RPT04Z
0RPT05Z
0RPT07Z
0RPT08Z
0RPT0JZ
0RPT0KZ
0RPT30Z
0RPT33Z
0RPT34Z
0RPT35Z
0RPT37Z
0RPT38Z
0RPT48Z
0RPTX0Z
0RPTX3Z
0RPTX4Z
0RPTX5Z
0RPU08Z
0RPU30Z
0RPU33Z
0RPU38Z
0RPU48Z
0RPUX0Z
0RPUX3Z
0RPUX4Z
0RPUX5Z
0RPV08Z
0RPV30Z
0RPV33Z
0RPV38Z
0RPV48Z
0RPVX0Z
0RPVX3Z
0RPVX4Z
0RPVX5Z
0RPW08Z
0RPW30Z
0RPW33Z
0RPW38Z
0RPW48Z
0RPWX0Z
0RPWX3Z
0RPWX4Z
0RPWX5Z
0RPX08Z
0RPX30Z
0RPX33Z
0RPX38Z
0RPX48Z
0RPXX0Z
0RPXX3Z
0RPXX4Z
0RPXX5Z
0RQ0XZZ
0RQ1XZZ
0RQ3XZZ
0RQ4XZZ
0RQ5XZZ
0RQ6XZZ
0RQ9XZZ
0RQAXZZ
0RQBXZZ
0RQCXZZ
0RQDXZZ
0RQEXZZ
0RQFXZZ
0RQGXZZ
0RQHXZZ
0RQJXZZ
0RQKXZZ
0RQLXZZ
0RQMXZZ
0RQNXZZ
0RQPXZZ
0RQQXZZ
0RQRXZZ
0RQSXZZ
0RQTXZZ
0RQU4ZZ
0RQUXZZ
0RQV0ZZ
0RQV3ZZ
0RQV4ZZ
0RQVXZZ
0RQW0ZZ
0RQW3ZZ
0RQW4ZZ
0RQWXZZ
0RQX0ZZ
0RQX3ZZ
0RQX4ZZ
0RQXXZZ
0RR007Z
0RR00JZ
0RR00KZ
0RR107Z
0RR10JZ
0RR10KZ
0RR307Z
0RR30JZ
0RR30KZ
0RR407Z
0RR40JZ
0RR40KZ
0RR507Z
0RR50JZ
0RR50KZ
0RR607Z
0RR60JZ
0RR60KZ
0RR907Z
0RR90JZ
0RR90KZ
0RRA07Z
0RRA0JZ
0RRA0KZ
0RRB07Z
0RRB0JZ
0RRB0KZ
0RRC07Z
0RRC0JZ
0RRC0KZ
0RRD07Z
0RRD0JZ
0RRD0KZ
0RRE07Z
0RRE0JZ
0RRE0KZ
0RRF07Z
0RRF0JZ
0RRF0KZ
0RRG07Z
0RRG0JZ
0RRG0KZ
0RRH07Z
0RRH0JZ
0RRH0KZ
0RRJ00Z
0RRJ07Z
0RRJ0J6
0RRJ0J7
0RRJ0JZ
0RRJ0KZ
0RRK00Z
0RRK07Z
0RRK0J6
0RRK0J7
0RRK0JZ
0RRK0KZ
0RRL07Z
0RRL0JZ
0RRL0KZ
0RRM07Z
0RRM0JZ
0RRM0KZ
0RRN07Z
0RRN0JZ
0RRN0KZ
0RRP07Z
0RRP0JZ
0RRP0KZ
0RRQ07Z
0RRQ0JZ
0RRQ0KZ
0RRR07Z
0RRR0JZ
0RRR0KZ
0RRS07Z
0RRS0JZ
0RRS0KZ
0RRT07Z
0RRT0JZ
0RRT0KZ
0RRU07Z
0RRU0JZ
0RRU0KZ
0RRV07Z
0RRV0JZ
0RRV0KZ
0RRW07Z
0RRW0JZ
0RRW0KZ
0RRX07Z
0RRX0JZ
0RRX0KZ
0RS004Z
0RS00ZZ
0RS034Z
0RS03ZZ
0RS044Z
0RS04ZZ
0RS0X4Z
0RS0XZZ
0RS104Z
0RS10ZZ
0RS134Z
0RS13ZZ
0RS144Z
0RS14ZZ
0RS1X4Z
0RS1XZZ
0RS404Z
0RS40ZZ
0RS434Z
0RS43ZZ
0RS444Z
0RS44ZZ
0RS4X4Z
0RS4XZZ
0RS604Z
0RS60ZZ
0RS634Z
0RS63ZZ
0RS644Z
0RS64ZZ
0RS6X4Z
0RS6XZZ
0RSA04Z
0RSA0ZZ
0RSA34Z
0RSA3ZZ
0RSA44Z
0RSA4ZZ
0RSAX4Z
0RSAXZZ
0RSC04Z
0RSC0ZZ
0RSC34Z
0RSC3ZZ
0RSC44Z
0RSC4ZZ
0RSCX4Z
0RSCXZZ
0RSD04Z
0RSD0ZZ
0RSD34Z
0RSD3ZZ
0RSD44Z
0RSD4ZZ
0RSDX4Z
0RSDXZZ
0RSE04Z
0RSE0ZZ
0RSE34Z
0RSE3ZZ
0RSE44Z
0RSE4ZZ
0RSEX4Z
0RSEXZZ
0RSF04Z
0RSF0ZZ
0RSF34Z
0RSF3ZZ
0RSF44Z
0RSF4ZZ
0RSFX4Z
0RSFXZZ
0RSG04Z
0RSG0ZZ
0RSG34Z
0RSG3ZZ
0RSG44Z
0RSG4ZZ
0RSGX4Z
0RSGXZZ
0RSH04Z
0RSH0ZZ
0RSH34Z
0RSH3ZZ
0RSH44Z
0RSH4ZZ
0RSHX4Z
0RSHXZZ
0RSJ04Z
0RSJ0ZZ
0RSJ34Z
0RSJ3ZZ
0RSJ44Z
0RSJ4ZZ
0RSJX4Z
0RSJXZZ
0RSK04Z
0RSK0ZZ
0RSK34Z
0RSK3ZZ
0RSK44Z
0RSK4ZZ
0RSKX4Z
0RSKXZZ
0RSL04Z
0RSL05Z
0RSL0ZZ
0RSL34Z
0RSL35Z
0RSL3ZZ
0RSL44Z
0RSL45Z
0RSL4ZZ
0RSLX4Z
0RSLX5Z
0RSLXZZ
0RSM04Z
0RSM05Z
0RSM0ZZ
0RSM34Z
0RSM35Z
0RSM3ZZ
0RSM44Z
0RSM45Z
0RSM4ZZ
0RSMX4Z
0RSMX5Z
0RSMXZZ
0RSN04Z
0RSN05Z
0RSN0ZZ
0RSN34Z
0RSN35Z
0RSN3ZZ
0RSN44Z
0RSN45Z
0RSN4ZZ
0RSNX4Z
0RSNX5Z
0RSNXZZ
0RSP04Z
0RSP05Z
0RSP0ZZ
0RSP34Z
0RSP35Z
0RSP3ZZ
0RSP44Z
0RSP45Z
0RSP4ZZ
0RSPX4Z
0RSPX5Z
0RSPXZZ
0RSQ04Z
0RSQ05Z
0RSQ0ZZ
0RSQ34Z
0RSQ35Z
0RSQ3ZZ
0RSQ44Z
0RSQ45Z
0RSQ4ZZ
0RSQX4Z
0RSQX5Z
0RSQXZZ
0RSR04Z
0RSR05Z
0RSR0ZZ
0RSR34Z
0RSR35Z
0RSR3ZZ
0RSR44Z
0RSR45Z
0RSR4ZZ
0RSRX4Z
0RSRX5Z
0RSRXZZ
0RSS04Z
0RSS05Z
0RSS0ZZ
0RSS34Z
0RSS35Z
0RSS3ZZ
0RSS44Z
0RSS45Z
0RSS4ZZ
0RSSX4Z
0RSSX5Z
0RSSXZZ
0RST04Z
0RST05Z
0RST0ZZ
0RST34Z
0RST35Z
0RST3ZZ
0RST44Z
0RST45Z
0RST4ZZ
0RSTX4Z
0RSTX5Z
0RSTXZZ
0RSU04Z
0RSU05Z
0RSU0ZZ
0RSU34Z
0RSU35Z
0RSU3ZZ
0RSU44Z
0RSU45Z
0RSU4ZZ
0RSUX4Z
0RSUX5Z
0RSUXZZ
0RSV04Z
0RSV05Z
0RSV0ZZ
0RSV34Z
0RSV35Z
0RSV3ZZ
0RSV44Z
0RSV45Z
0RSV4ZZ
0RSVX4Z
0RSVX5Z
0RSVXZZ
0RSW04Z
0RSW05Z
0RSW0ZZ
0RSW34Z
0RSW35Z
0RSW3ZZ
0RSW44Z
0RSW45Z
0RSW4ZZ
0RSWX4Z
0RSWX5Z
0RSWXZZ
0RSX04Z
0RSX05Z
0RSX0ZZ
0RSX34Z
0RSX35Z
0RSX3ZZ
0RSX44Z
0RSX45Z
0RSX4ZZ
0RSXX4Z
0RSXX5Z
0RSXXZZ
0RT30ZZ
0RT40ZZ
0RT50ZZ
0RT90ZZ
0RTB0ZZ
0RTC0ZZ
0RTD0ZZ
0RTE0ZZ
0RTF0ZZ
0RTG0ZZ
0RTH0ZZ
0RTJ0ZZ
0RTK0ZZ
0RTL0ZZ
0RTM0ZZ
0RTN0ZZ
0RTP0ZZ
0RTQ0ZZ
0RTR0ZZ
0RTS0ZZ
0RTT0ZZ
0RTU0ZZ
0RTV0ZZ
0RTW0ZZ
0RTX0ZZ
0RU007Z
0RU00JZ
0RU00KZ
0RU037Z
0RU03JZ
0RU03KZ
0RU047Z
0RU04JZ
0RU04KZ
0RU107Z
0RU10JZ
0RU10KZ
0RU137Z
0RU13JZ
0RU13KZ
0RU147Z
0RU14JZ
0RU14KZ
0RU307Z
0RU30JZ
0RU30KZ
0RU337Z
0RU33JZ
0RU33KZ
0RU347Z
0RU34JZ
0RU34KZ
0RU407Z

0RU40JZ
0RU40KZ
0RU437Z
0RU43JZ
0RU43KZ
0RU447Z
0RU44JZ
0RU44KZ
0RU507Z
0RU50JZ
0RU50KZ
0RU537Z
0RU53JZ
0RU53KZ
0RU547Z
0RU54JZ
0RU54KZ
0RU607Z
0RU60JZ
0RU60KZ
0RU637Z
0RU63JZ
0RU63KZ
0RU647Z
0RU64JZ
0RU64KZ
0RU907Z
0RU90JZ
0RU90KZ
0RU937Z
0RU93JZ
0RU93KZ
0RU947Z
0RU94JZ
0RU94KZ
0RUA07Z
0RUA0JZ
0RUA0KZ
0RUA37Z
0RUA3JZ
0RUA3KZ
0RUA47Z
0RUA4JZ
0RUA4KZ
0RUB07Z
0RUB0JZ
0RUQ07Z
0RUQ0JZ
0RUQ0KZ
0RUQ37Z
0RUQ3JZ
0RUQ3KZ
0RUQ47Z
0RUQ4JZ
0RUQ4KZ
0RUR07Z
0RUR0JZ
0RUR0KZ
0RUR37Z
0RUR3JZ
0RUR3KZ
0RUR47Z
0RUR4JZ
0RUR4KZ
0RUS07Z
0RUS0JZ
0RUS0KZ
0RUS37Z
0RUS3JZ
0RUS3KZ
0RUS47Z
0RUS4JZ
0RUS4KZ
0RUT07Z
0RUT0JZ
0RUT0KZ
0RUT37Z
0RUT3JZ
0RUT3KZ
0RUT47Z
0RUT4JZ
0RUT4KZ
0RUU07Z
0RUU0JZ
0RUU0KZ
0RUU37Z
0RUU3JZ
0RUU3KZ
0RUU47Z
0RUU4JZ
0RUU4KZ
0RUV07Z
0RUV0JZ
0RUV0KZ
0RUV37Z
0RUV3JZ
0RUV3KZ
0RUV47Z
0RUV4JZ
0RUV4KZ
0RUW07Z
0RUW0JZ
0RUW0KZ
0RUW37Z
0RUW3JZ
0RUW3KZ
0RUW47Z
0RUW4JZ
0RUW4KZ
0RUX07Z
0RUX0JZ
0RUX0KZ
0RUX37Z
0RUX3JZ
0RUX3KZ
0RUX47Z
0RUX4JZ
0RUX4KZ
0RW000Z
0RW003Z
0RW004Z
0RW007Z
0RW008Z
0RW00AZ
0RW00JZ
0RW00KZ
0RW030Z
0RW033Z
0RW034Z
0RW037Z
0RW038Z
0RW03AZ
0RW03JZ
0RW03KZ
0RW040Z
0RW043Z
0RW044Z
0RW047Z
0RW048Z
0RW04AZ
0RW04JZ
0RW04KZ
0RW0X0Z
0RW0X3Z
0RW0X4Z
0RW0X7Z
0RW0X8Z
0RW0XAZ
0RW0XJZ
0RW0XKZ
0RW100Z
0RW103Z
0RW104Z
0RW107Z
0RW108Z
0RW10AZ
0RW10JZ
0RW10KZ
0RW130Z
0RW133Z
0RW134Z
0RW137Z
0RW138Z
0RW13AZ
0RW13JZ
0RW13KZ
0RW140Z
0RW143Z
0RW144Z
0RW147Z
0RW148Z
0RW14AZ
0RW14JZ
0RW14KZ
0RW1X0Z
0RW1X3Z
0RW1X4Z
0RW1X7Z
0RW1X8Z
0RW1XAZ
0RW1XJZ
0RW1XKZ
0RW300Z
0RW303Z
0RW307Z
0RW30JZ
0RW30KZ
0RW330Z
0RW333Z
0RW337Z
0RW33JZ
0RW33KZ
0RW340Z
0RW343Z
0RW347Z
0RW34JZ
0RW34KZ
0RW3X0Z
0RW3X3Z
0RW3X7Z
0RW3XJZ
0RW3XKZ
0RW400Z
0RW403Z
0RW404Z
0RW407Z
0RW408Z
0RW40AZ
0RW40JZ
0RW40KZ
0RW430Z
0RW433Z
0RW434Z
0RW437Z
0RW438Z
0RW43AZ
0RW43JZ
0RW43KZ
0RW440Z
0RW443Z
0RW444Z
0RW447Z
0RW448Z
0RW44AZ
0RW44JZ
0RW44KZ
0RW4X0Z
0RW4X3Z
0RW4X4Z
0RW4X7Z
0RW4X8Z
0RW4XAZ
0RW4XJZ
0RW4XKZ
0RW500Z
0RW503Z
0RW507Z
0RW50JZ
0RW50KZ
0RW530Z
0RW533Z
0RW537Z
0RW53JZ
0RW53KZ
0RW540Z
0RW543Z
0RW547Z
0RW54JZ
0RW54KZ
0RW5X0Z
0RW5X3Z
0RW5X7Z
0RW5XJZ
0RW5XKZ
0RW600Z
0RW603Z
0RW604Z
0RW607Z
0RW608Z
0RW60AZ
0RW60JZ
0RW60KZ
0RW630Z
0RW633Z
0RW634Z
0RW637Z
0RW638Z
0RW63AZ
0RW63JZ
0RW63KZ
0RW640Z
0RW643Z
0RW644Z
0RW647Z
0RW648Z
0RW64AZ
0RW64JZ
0RW64KZ
0RW6X0Z
0RW6X3Z
0RW6X4Z
0RW6X7Z
0RW6X8Z
0RW6XAZ
0RW6XJZ
0RW6XKZ
0RW900Z
0RW903Z
0RW907Z
0RW90JZ
0RW90KZ
0RW930Z
0RW933Z
0RW937Z
0RW93JZ
0RW93KZ
0RW940Z
0RW943Z
0RW947Z
0RW94JZ
0RW94KZ
0RW9X0Z
0RW9X3Z
0RW9X7Z
0RW9XJZ
0RW9XKZ
0RWA00Z
0RWA03Z
0RWA04Z
0RWA07Z
0RWA08Z
0RWA0AZ
0RWA0JZ
0RWA0KZ
0RWA30Z
0RWA33Z
0RWA34Z
0RWA37Z
0RWA38Z
0RWA3AZ
0RWA3JZ
0RWA3KZ
0RWA40Z
0RWA43Z
0RWA44Z
0RWA47Z
0RWA48Z
0RWA4AZ
0RWA4JZ
0RWA4KZ
0RWAX0Z
0RWAX3Z
0RWAX4Z
0RWAX7Z
0RWAX8Z
0RWAXAZ
0RWAXJZ
0RWAXKZ
0RWB00Z
0RWB03Z
0RWB07Z
0RWB0JZ
0RWB0KZ
0RWB30Z
0RWB33Z
0RWB37Z
0RWB3JZ
0RWB3KZ
0RWB40Z
0RWB43Z
0RWB47Z
0RWB4JZ
0RWB4KZ
0RWBX0Z
0RWBX3Z
0RWBX7Z
0RWBXJZ
0RWBXKZ
0RWC00Z
0RWC03Z
0RWC04Z
0RWC07Z
0RWC08Z
0RWC0JZ
0RWC0KZ
0RWC30Z
0RWC33Z
0RWC34Z
0RWC37Z
0RWC38Z
0RWC3JZ
0RWC3KZ
0RWC40Z
0RWC43Z
0RWC44Z
0RWC47Z
0RWC48Z
0RWC4JZ
0RWC4KZ
0RWCX0Z
0RWCX3Z
0RWCX4Z
0RWCX7Z
0RWCX8Z
0RWCXJZ
0RWCXKZ
0RWD00Z
0RWD03Z
0RWD04Z
0RWD07Z
0RWD08Z
0RWD0JZ
0RWD0KZ
0RWD30Z
0RWD33Z
0RWD34Z
0RWD37Z
0RWD38Z
0RWD3JZ
0RWD3KZ
0RWD40Z
0RWD43Z
0RWD44Z
0RWD47Z
0RWD48Z
0RWD4JZ
0RWD4KZ
0RWDX0Z
0RWDX3Z
0RWDX4Z
0RWDX7Z
0RWDX8Z
0RWDXJZ
0RWDXKZ
0RWE00Z
0RWE03Z
0RWE04Z
0RWE07Z
0RWE08Z
0RWE0JZ
0RWE0KZ
0RWE30Z
0RWE33Z
0RWE34Z
0RWE37Z
0RWE38Z
0RWE3JZ
0RWE3KZ
0RWE40Z
0RWE43Z
0RWE44Z
0RWE47Z
0RWE48Z
0RWE4JZ
0RWE4KZ
0RWEX0Z
0RWEX3Z
0RWEX4Z
0RWEX7Z
0RWEX8Z
0RWEXJZ
0RWEXKZ
0RWF00Z
0RWF03Z
0RWF04Z
0RWF07Z
0RWF08Z
0RWF0JZ
0RWF0KZ
0RWF30Z
0RWF33Z
0RWF34Z
0RWF37Z
0RWF38Z
0RWF3JZ
0RWF3KZ
0RWF40Z
0RWF43Z
0RWF44Z
0RWF47Z
0RWF48Z
0RWF4JZ
0RWF4KZ
0RWFX0Z
0RWFX3Z
0RWFX4Z
0RWFX7Z
0RWFX8Z
0RWFXJZ
0RWFXKZ
0RWG00Z
0RWG03Z
0RWG04Z
0RWG07Z
0RWG08Z
0RWG0JZ
0RWG0KZ
0RWG30Z
0RWG33Z
0RWG34Z
0RWG37Z
0RWG38Z
0RWG3JZ
0RWG3KZ
0RWG40Z
0RWG43Z
0RWG44Z
0RWG47Z
0RWG48Z
0RWG4JZ
0RWG4KZ
0RWGX0Z
0RWGX3Z
0RWGX4Z
0RWGX7Z
0RWGX8Z
0RWGXJZ
0RWGXKZ
0RWH00Z
0RWH03Z
0RWH04Z
0RWH07Z
0RWH08Z
0RWH0JZ
0RWH0KZ
0RWH30Z
0RWH33Z
0RWH34Z
0RWH37Z
0RWH38Z
0RWH3JZ
0RWH3KZ
0RWH40Z
0RWH43Z
0RWH44Z
0RWH47Z
0RWH48Z
0RWH4JZ
0RWH4KZ
0RWHX0Z
0RWHX3Z
0RWHX4Z
0RWHX7Z
0RWHX8Z
0RWHXJZ
0RWHXKZ
0RWJ00Z
0RWJ03Z
0RWJ04Z
0RWJ07Z
0RWJ08Z
0RWJ0JZ
0RWJ0KZ
0RWJ30Z
0RWJ33Z
0RWJ34Z
0RWJ37Z
0RWJX0Z
0RWJX3Z
0RWJX4Z
0RWJX7Z
0RWJX8Z
0RWJXJZ
0RWJXKZ
0RWKX0Z
0RWKX3Z
0RWKX4Z
0RWKX7Z
0RWKX8Z
0RWKXJZ
0RWKXKZ
0RWLX0Z
0RWLX3Z
0RWLX4Z
0RWLX5Z
0RWLX7Z
0RWLX8Z
0RWLXJZ
0RWLXKZ
0RWMX0Z
0RWMX3Z
0RWMX4Z
0RWMX5Z
0RWMX7Z
0RWMX8Z
0RWMXJZ
0RWMXKZ
0RWNX0Z
0RWNX3Z
0RWNX4Z
0RWNX5Z
0RWNX7Z
0RWNX8Z
0RWNXJZ
0RWNXKZ
0RWPX0Z
0RWPX3Z
0RWPX4Z
0RWPX5Z
0RWPX7Z
0RWPX8Z
0RWPXJZ
0RWPXKZ
0RWQX0Z
0RWQX3Z
0RWQX4Z
0RWQX5Z
0RWQX7Z
0RWQX8Z
0RWQXJZ
0RWQXKZ
0RWRX0Z
0RWRX3Z
0RWRX4Z
0RWRX5Z
0RWRX7Z
0RWRX8Z
0RWRXJZ
0RWRXKZ
0RWS3JZ
0RWS3KZ
0RWS40Z
0RWS43Z
0RWS44Z
0RWS45Z
0RWS47Z
0RWS48Z
0RWS4JZ
0RWS4KZ
0RWSX0Z
0RWSX3Z
0RWSX4Z
0RWSX5Z
0RWSX7Z
0RWSX8Z
0RWSXJZ
0RWSXKZ
0RWT00Z
0RWT03Z
0RWT04Z
0RWT05Z
0RWT07Z
0RWT08Z
0RWT0JZ
0RWT0KZ
0RWT30Z
0RWT33Z
0RWT34Z
0RWT35Z
0RWT37Z
0RWT38Z
0RWT3JZ
0RWT3KZ
0RWT40Z
0RWT43Z
0RWT44Z
0RWT45Z
0RWT47Z
0RWT48Z
0RWT4JZ
0RWT4KZ
0RWTX0Z
0RWTX3Z
0RWTX4Z
0RWTX5Z
0RWTX7Z
0RWTX8Z
0RWTXJZ
0RWTXKZ
0RWU00Z
0RWU03Z
0RWU04Z
0RWU05Z
0RWU07Z
0RWU08Z
0RWU0JZ
0RWU0KZ
0RWU30Z
0RWU33Z
0RWU34Z
0RWU35Z
0RWU37Z
0RWU38Z
0RWU3JZ
0RWU3KZ
0RWU40Z
0RWU43Z
0RWU44Z
0RWU45Z
0RWU47Z
0RWU48Z
0RWU4JZ
0RWU4KZ
0RWUX0Z
0RWUX3Z
0RWUX4Z
0RWUX5Z
0RWUX7Z
0RWUX8Z
0RWUXJZ
0RWUXKZ
0RWV00Z
0RWV03Z
0RWV04Z
0RWV05Z
0RWV07Z
0RWV08Z
0RWV0JZ
0RWV0KZ
0RWV30Z
0RWV33Z
0RWV34Z
0RWV35Z
0RWV37Z
0RWV38Z
0RWV3JZ
0RWV3KZ
0RWV40Z
0RWV43Z
0RWV44Z
0RWV45Z
0RWV47Z
0RWV48Z
0RWV4JZ
0RWV4KZ
0RWVX0Z
0RWVX3Z
0RWVX4Z
0RWVX5Z
0RWVX7Z
0RWVX8Z
0RWVXJZ
0RWVXKZ
0RWW00Z
0RWW03Z
0RWW04Z
0RWW05Z
0RWW07Z
0RWW08Z
0RWW0JZ
0RWW0KZ
0RWW30Z
0RWW33Z
0RWW34Z
0RWW35Z
0RWW37Z

0RWW38Z
0RWW3JZ
0RWW3KZ
0RWW40Z
0RWW43Z
0RWW44Z
0RWW45Z
0RWW47Z
0RWW48Z
0RWW4JZ
0RWW4KZ
0RWWX0Z
0RWWX3Z
0RWWX4Z
0RWWX5Z
0RWWX7Z
0RWWX8Z
0RWWXJZ
0RWWXKZ
0RWX00Z
0RWX03Z
0RWX04Z
0RWX05Z
0RWX07Z
0RWX08Z
0RWX0JZ
0RWX0KZ
0RWX30Z
0RWX33Z
0RWX34Z
0RWX35Z
0RWX37Z
0RWX38Z
0RWX3JZ
0RWX3KZ
0RWX40Z
0RWX43Z
0RWX44Z
0RWX45Z
0RWX47Z
0RWX48Z
0RWX4JZ
0RWX4KZ
0RWXX0Z
0RWXX3Z
0RWXX4Z
0RWXX5Z
0RWXX7Z
0RWXX8Z
0RWXXJZ
0RWXXKZ
0S2YX0Z
0S2YXYZ
0S500ZZ
0S503ZZ
0S504ZZ
0S520ZZ
0S523ZZ
0S524ZZ
0S530ZZ
0S533ZZ
0S534ZZ
0S540ZZ
0S543ZZ
0S544ZZ
0S550ZZ
0S553ZZ
0S554ZZ
0S560ZZ
0S563ZZ
0S564ZZ
0S570ZZ
0S573ZZ
0S574ZZ
0S580ZZ
0S583ZZ
0S584ZZ
0S590ZZ
0S593ZZ
0S594ZZ
0S5B0ZZ
0S5B3ZZ
0S5B4ZZ
0S5C0ZZ
0S5C3ZZ
0S5C4ZZ
0S5D0ZZ
0S5D3ZZ
0S5D4ZZ
0S5F0ZZ
0S5F3ZZ
0S5F4ZZ
0S5G0ZZ
0S5G3ZZ
0S5G4ZZ
0S5H0ZZ
0S5H3ZZ
0S5H4ZZ
0S5J0ZZ
0S5J3ZZ
0S5J4ZZ
0S5K0ZZ
0S5K3ZZ
0S5K4ZZ
0S5L0ZZ
0S5L3ZZ
0S5L4ZZ
0S5M0ZZ
0S5M3ZZ
0S5M4ZZ
0S5N0ZZ
0S5N3ZZ
0S5N4ZZ
0S5P0ZZ
0S5P3ZZ
0S5P4ZZ
0S5Q0ZZ
0S5Q3ZZ
0S5Q4ZZ
0S9000Z
0S900ZX
0S900ZZ
0S9030Z
0S903ZX
0S903ZZ
0S9040Z
0S904ZX
0S904ZZ
0S9200Z
0S920ZX
0S920ZZ
0S9230Z
0S923ZX
0S923ZZ
0S9240Z
0S924ZX
0S924ZZ
0S9300Z
0S930ZX
0S930ZZ
0S9330Z
0S933ZX
0S933ZZ
0S9340Z
0S934ZX
0S934ZZ
0S9400Z
0S940ZX
0S940ZZ
0S9430Z
0S943ZX
0S943ZZ
0S9440Z
0S944ZX
0S944ZZ
0S9500Z
0S950ZX
0S950ZZ
0S9530Z
0S953ZX
0S953ZZ
0S9540Z
0S954ZX
0S954ZZ
0S9600Z
0S960ZX
0S960ZZ
0S9630Z
0S963ZX
0S963ZZ
0S9640Z
0S964ZX
0S964ZZ
0S9700Z
0S970ZX
0S970ZZ
0S9730Z
0S973ZX
0S973ZZ
0S9740Z
0S974ZX
0S974ZZ
0S9800Z
0S980ZX
0S980ZZ
0S9830Z
0S983ZX
0S983ZZ
0S9840Z
0S984ZX
0S984ZZ
0S9900Z
0S990ZX
0S990ZZ
0S9930Z
0S993ZX
0S993ZZ
0S9940Z
0S994ZX
0S994ZZ
0S9B00Z
0S9B0ZX
0S9B0ZZ
0S9B30Z
0S9B3ZX
0S9B3ZZ
0S9B40Z
0S9B4ZX
0S9B4ZZ
0S9C00Z
0S9C0ZX
0S9C0ZZ
0S9C30Z
0S9C3ZX
0S9C3ZZ
0S9C40Z
0S9C4ZX
0S9C4ZZ
0S9D00Z
0S9D0ZX
0S9D0ZZ
0S9D30Z
0S9D3ZX
0S9D3ZZ
0S9D40Z
0S9D4ZX
0S9D4ZZ
0S9F00Z
0S9F0ZX
0S9F0ZZ
0S9F30Z
0S9F3ZX
0S9F3ZZ
0S9F40Z
0S9F4ZX
0S9F4ZZ
0S9G00Z
0S9G0ZX
0S9G0ZZ
0S9G30Z
0S9G3ZX
0S9G3ZZ
0S9G40Z
0S9G4ZX
0S9G4ZZ
0S9H00Z
0S9H0ZX
0S9H0ZZ
0S9H30Z
0S9H3ZX
0S9H3ZZ
0S9H40Z
0S9H4ZX
0S9H4ZZ
0S9J00Z
0S9J0ZX
0S9J0ZZ
0S9J30Z
0S9J3ZX
0S9J3ZZ
0S9J40Z
0S9J4ZX
0S9J4ZZ
0S9K00Z
0S9K0ZX
0S9K0ZZ
0S9K30Z
0S9K3ZX
0S9K3ZZ
0S9K40Z
0S9K4ZX
0S9K4ZZ
0S9L00Z
0S9L0ZX
0S9L0ZZ
0S9L30Z
0S9L3ZX
0S9L3ZZ
0S9L40Z
0S9L4ZX
0S9L4ZZ
0S9M00Z
0S9M0ZX
0S9M0ZZ
0S9M30Z
0S9M3ZX
0S9M3ZZ
0S9M40Z
0S9M4ZX
0S9M4ZZ
0S9N00Z
0S9N0ZX
0S9N0ZZ
0S9N30Z
0S9N3ZX
0S9N3ZZ
0S9N40Z
0S9N4ZX
0S9N4ZZ
0S9P00Z
0S9P0ZX
0S9P0ZZ
0S9P30Z
0S9P3ZX
0S9P3ZZ
0S9P40Z
0S9P4ZX
0S9P4ZZ
0S9Q00Z
0S9Q0ZX
0S9Q0ZZ
0S9Q30Z
0S9Q3ZX
0S9Q3ZZ
0S9Q40Z
0S9Q4ZX
0S9Q4ZZ
0SB00ZX
0SB00ZZ
0SB03ZX
0SB03ZZ
0SB04ZX
0SB04ZZ
0SB20ZX
0SB20ZZ
0SB23ZX
0SB23ZZ
0SB24ZX
0SB24ZZ
0SB30ZX
0SB30ZZ
0SB33ZX
0SB33ZZ
0SB34ZX
0SB34ZZ
0SB40ZX
0SB40ZZ
0SB43ZX
0SB43ZZ
0SB44ZX
0SB44ZZ
0SB50ZX
0SB50ZZ
0SB53ZX
0SB53ZZ
0SB54ZX
0SB54ZZ
0SB60ZX
0SB60ZZ
0SB63ZX
0SB63ZZ
0SB64ZX
0SB64ZZ
0SB70ZX
0SB70ZZ
0SB73ZX
0SB73ZZ
0SB74ZX
0SB74ZZ
0SB80ZX
0SB80ZZ
0SB83ZX
0SB83ZZ
0SB84ZX
0SB84ZZ
0SB90ZX
0SB90ZZ
0SB93ZX
0SB93ZZ
0SB94ZX
0SB94ZZ
0SBB0ZX
0SBB0ZZ
0SBB3ZX
0SBB3ZZ
0SBB4ZX
0SBB4ZZ
0SBC0ZX
0SBC0ZZ
0SBC3ZX
0SBC3ZZ
0SBC4ZX
0SBC4ZZ
0SBD0ZX
0SBD0ZZ
0SBD3ZX
0SBD3ZZ
0SBD4ZX
0SBD4ZZ
0SBF0ZX
0SBF0ZZ
0SBF3ZX
0SBF3ZZ
0SBF4ZX
0SBF4ZZ
0SBG0ZX
0SBG0ZZ
0SBG3ZX
0SBG3ZZ
0SBG4ZX
0SBG4ZZ
0SBH0ZX
0SBH0ZZ
0SBH3ZX
0SBH3ZZ
0SBH4ZX
0SBH4ZZ
0SBJ0ZX
0SBJ0ZZ
0SBJ3ZX
0SBJ3ZZ
0SBJ4ZX
0SBJ4ZZ
0SBK0ZX
0SBK0ZZ
0SBK3ZX
0SBK3ZZ
0SBK4ZX
0SBK4ZZ
0SBL0ZX
0SBL0ZZ
0SBL3ZX
0SBL3ZZ
0SBL4ZX
0SBM0ZX
0SBM3ZX
0SBM4ZX
0SBN0ZX
0SBN3ZX
0SBN4ZX
0SBP0ZX
0SBP3ZX
0SBP4ZX
0SBQ0ZX
0SBQ3ZX
0SBQ4ZX
0SG1070
0SG1071
0SG107J
0SG10A0
0SG10AJ
0SG10J0
0SG10J1
0SG10JJ
0SG10K0
0SG10K1
0SG10KJ
0SG1370
0SG1371
0SG137J
0SG13A0
0SG13AJ
0SG13J0
0SG13J1
0SG13JJ
0SG13K0
0SG13K1
0SG13KJ
0SG1470
0SG1471
0SG147J
0SG14A0
0SG14AJ
0SG14J0
0SG14J1
0SG14JJ
0SG14K0
0SG14K1
0SG14KJ
0SG3070
0SG3071
0SG307J
0SG30A0
0SG30AJ
0SG30J0
0SG30J1
0SG30JJ
0SG30K0
0SG30K1
0SG30KJ
0SG3370
0SG3371
0SG337J
0SG33A0
0SG33AJ
0SG33J0
0SG33J1
0SG33JJ
0SG33K0
0SG33K1
0SG33KJ
0SG3470
0SG3471
0SG347J
0SG34A0
0SG34AJ
0SG34J0
0SG34J1
0SG34JJ
0SG34K0
0SG34K1
0SG34KJ
0SG504Z
0SG507Z
0SG50JZ
0SG50KZ
0SG534Z
0SG537Z
0SG53JZ
0SG53KZ
0SG544Z
0SG547Z
0SG54JZ
0SG54KZ
0SG604Z
0SG607Z
0SG60JZ
0SG60KZ
0SG634Z
0SG637Z
0SG63JZ
0SG63KZ
0SG644Z
0SG647Z
0SG64JZ
0SG64KZ
0SG704Z
0SG707Z
0SG70JZ
0SG70KZ
0SG734Z
0SG737Z
0SG73JZ
0SG73KZ
0SG744Z
0SG747Z
0SG74JZ
0SG74KZ
0SG804Z
0SG807Z
0SG80JZ
0SG80KZ
0SG834Z
0SG837Z
0SG83JZ
0SG83KZ
0SGH0KZ
0SGH34Z
0SGH35Z
0SGH37Z
0SGH3JZ
0SGH3KZ
0SGH44Z
0SGH45Z
0SGH47Z
0SGH4JZ
0SGH4KZ
0SGJ04Z
0SGJ05Z
0SGJ07Z
0SGJ0JZ
0SGJ0KZ
0SGJ34Z
0SGJ35Z
0SGJ37Z
0SGJ3JZ
0SGJ3KZ
0SGJ44Z
0SGJ45Z
0SGJ47Z
0SGJ4JZ
0SGJ4KZ
0SGK04Z
0SGK05Z
0SGK07Z
0SGK0JZ
0SGK0KZ
0SGK34Z
0SGK35Z
0SGK37Z
0SGK3JZ
0SGK3KZ
0SGK44Z
0SGK45Z
0SGK47Z
0SGK4JZ
0SGK4KZ
0SGL04Z
0SGL05Z
0SGL07Z
0SGL0JZ
0SGL0KZ
0SGL34Z
0SGL35Z
0SGL37Z
0SGL3JZ
0SGL3KZ
0SGL44Z
0SGL45Z
0SGL47Z
0SGL4JZ
0SGL4KZ
0SGM04Z
0SGM05Z
0SGM07Z
0SGM0JZ
0SGM0KZ
0SGM34Z
0SGM35Z
0SGM37Z
0SGM3JZ
0SGM3KZ
0SGM44Z
0SGM45Z
0SGM47Z
0SGM4JZ
0SGM4KZ
0SGN04Z
0SGN05Z
0SGN07Z
0SGN0JZ
0SGN0KZ
0SGN34Z
0SGN35Z
0SGN37Z
0SGN3JZ
0SGN3KZ
0SGN44Z
0SGN45Z
0SGN47Z
0SGN4JZ
0SGN4KZ
0SGP04Z
0SGP05Z
0SGP07Z
0SGP0JZ
0SGP0KZ
0SGP34Z
0SGP35Z
0SGP37Z
0SGP3JZ
0SGP3KZ
0SGP44Z
0SGP45Z
0SGP47Z
0SGP4JZ
0SGP4KZ
0SGQ04Z
0SGQ05Z
0SGQ07Z
0SGQ0JZ
0SGQ0KZ
0SGQ34Z
0SGQ35Z
0SGQ37Z
0SGQ3JZ
0SGQ3KZ
0SGQ44Z
0SGQ45Z
0SGQ47Z
0SGQ4JZ
0SGQ4KZ
0SH003Z
0SH004Z
0SH008Z
0SH00BZ
0SH00CZ
0SH00DZ
0SH033Z
0SH034Z
0SH038Z
0SH03BZ
0SH03CZ
0SH03DZ
0SH043Z
0SH044Z
0SH048Z
0SH04BZ
0SH04CZ
0SH04DZ
0SH203Z
0SH208Z
0SH233Z
0SH238Z
0SH243Z
0SH248Z
0SH303Z
0SH304Z
0SH308Z
0SH30BZ
0SH30CZ
0SH30DZ
0SH333Z
0SH334Z
0SH338Z
0SH33BZ
0SH33CZ
0SH33DZ
0SH343Z
0SH344Z
0SH348Z
0SH34BZ
0SH34CZ
0SH34DZ
0SH403Z
0SH408Z
0SH433Z
0SH438Z
0SH443Z
0SH448Z
0SH503Z
0SH504Z
0SH508Z
0SH533Z
0SH534Z
0SH538Z
0SH543Z
0SH544Z
0SH548Z
0SH603Z
0SH604Z
0SH608Z
0SH633Z
0SH634Z
0SH638Z
0SH643Z

0SH644Z
0SH648Z
0SH703Z
0SH704Z
0SH708Z
0SH733Z
0SH734Z
0SH738Z
0SH743Z
0SH744Z
0SH748Z
0SH803Z
0SH804Z
0SH808Z
0SH833Z
0SH834Z
0SH838Z
0SH843Z
0SH844Z
0SH848Z
0SH903Z
0SH904Z
0SH905Z
0SH908Z
0SH933Z
0SH934Z
0SH935Z
0SH938Z
0SH943Z
0SH944Z
0SH945Z
0SH948Z
0SHB03Z
0SHB04Z
0SHB05Z
0SHB08Z
0SHB33Z
0SHB34Z
0SHB35Z
0SHB38Z
0SHB43Z
0SHB44Z
0SHB45Z
0SHB48Z
0SHC03Z
0SHC04Z
0SHC05Z
0SHC08Z
0SHC33Z
0SHC34Z
0SHC35Z
0SHC38Z
0SHC43Z
0SHC44Z
0SHC45Z
0SHC48Z
0SHD03Z
0SHD04Z
0SHD05Z
0SHD08Z
0SHD33Z
0SHD34Z
0SHD35Z
0SHD38Z
0SHD43Z
0SHD44Z
0SHD45Z
0SHD48Z
0SHF03Z
0SHF04Z
0SHF05Z
0SHF08Z
0SHF33Z
0SHF34Z
0SHF35Z
0SHF38Z
0SHF43Z
0SHF44Z
0SHF45Z
0SHF48Z
0SHG03Z
0SHG04Z
0SHG05Z
0SHG08Z
0SHG33Z
0SHG34Z
0SHG35Z
0SHG38Z
0SHG43Z
0SHG44Z
0SHG45Z
0SHG48Z
0SHH03Z
0SHH04Z
0SHH05Z
0SHH08Z
0SHH33Z
0SHH34Z
0SHH35Z
0SHH38Z
0SHH43Z
0SHH44Z
0SHH45Z
0SHH48Z
0SHJ03Z
0SHJ04Z
0SHJ05Z
0SHJ08Z
0SHJ33Z
0SHJ34Z
0SHJ35Z
0SHJ38Z
0SHJ43Z
0SHJ44Z
0SHJ45Z
0SHJ48Z
0SHK03Z
0SHK04Z
0SHK05Z
0SHK08Z
0SHK33Z
0SHK34Z
0SHK35Z
0SHK38Z
0SHK43Z
0SHK44Z
0SHK45Z
0SHK48Z
0SHL03Z
0SHL04Z
0SHL05Z
0SHL08Z
0SHL33Z
0SHL34Z
0SHL35Z
0SHL38Z
0SHL43Z
0SHL44Z
0SHL45Z
0SHL48Z
0SHM03Z
0SHM04Z
0SHM05Z
0SHM08Z
0SHM33Z
0SHM34Z
0SHM35Z
0SHM38Z
0SHM43Z
0SHM44Z
0SHM45Z
0SHM48Z
0SHN03Z
0SHN04Z
0SHN05Z
0SHN08Z
0SHN33Z
0SHN34Z
0SHN35Z
0SHN38Z
0SHN43Z
0SHN44Z
0SHN45Z
0SHN48Z
0SHP03Z
0SHP04Z
0SHP05Z
0SHP08Z
0SHP33Z
0SHP34Z
0SHP35Z
0SHP38Z
0SHP43Z
0SHP44Z
0SHP45Z
0SHP48Z
0SHQ03Z
0SHQ04Z
0SHQ05Z
0SHQ08Z
0SHQ33Z
0SHQ34Z
0SHQ35Z
0SHQ38Z
0SHQ43Z
0SHQ44Z
0SHQ45Z
0SHQ48Z
0SJ00ZZ
0SJ03ZZ
0SJ04ZZ
0SJ0XZZ
0SJ20ZZ
0SJ23ZZ
0SJ24ZZ
0SJ2XZZ
0SJ30ZZ
0SJ33ZZ
0SJ34ZZ
0SJ3XZZ
0SJ40ZZ
0SJ43ZZ
0SJ44ZZ
0SJ4XZZ
0SJ50ZZ
0SJ53ZZ
0SJ54ZZ
0SJ5XZZ
0SJ60ZZ
0SJ63ZZ
0SJ64ZZ
0SJ6XZZ
0SJ70ZZ
0SJ73ZZ
0SJ74ZZ
0SJ7XZZ
0SJ80ZZ
0SJ83ZZ
0SJ84ZZ
0SJ8XZZ
0SJ90ZZ
0SJ93ZZ
0SJ94ZZ
0SJ9XZZ
0SJB0ZZ
0SJB3ZZ
0SJB4ZZ
0SJBXZZ
0SJC0ZZ
0SJC3ZZ
0SJC4ZZ
0SJCXZZ
0SJD0ZZ
0SJD3ZZ
0SJD4ZZ
0SJDXZZ
0SJF0ZZ
0SJF3ZZ
0SJF4ZZ
0SJFXZZ
0SJG0ZZ
0SJG3ZZ
0SJG4ZZ
0SJGXZZ
0SJH0ZZ
0SJH3ZZ
0SJH4ZZ
0SJHXZZ
0SJJ0ZZ
0SJJ3ZZ
0SJJ4ZZ
0SJJXZZ
0SJK0ZZ
0SJK3ZZ
0SJK4ZZ
0SJKXZZ
0SJL0ZZ
0SJL3ZZ
0SJL4ZZ
0SJLXZZ
0SJM0ZZ
0SJM3ZZ
0SJM4ZZ
0SJMXZZ
0SJN0ZZ
0SJN3ZZ
0SJN4ZZ
0SJNXZZ
0SJP0ZZ
0SJP3ZZ
0SJP4ZZ
0SJPXZZ
0SJQ0ZZ
0SJQ3ZZ
0SJQ4ZZ
0SJQXZZ
0SN00ZZ
0SN03ZZ
0SN04ZZ
0SN0XZZ
0SN20ZZ
0SN23ZZ
0SN24ZZ
0SN2XZZ
0SN30ZZ
0SN33ZZ
0SN34ZZ
0SN3XZZ
0SN40ZZ
0SN43ZZ
0SN44ZZ
0SN4XZZ
0SN50ZZ
0SN53ZZ
0SN54ZZ
0SN5XZZ
0SN60ZZ
0SN63ZZ
0SN64ZZ
0SN6XZZ
0SN70ZZ
0SN73ZZ
0SN74ZZ
0SN7XZZ
0SN80ZZ
0SN83ZZ
0SN84ZZ
0SN8XZZ
0SN90ZZ
0SN93ZZ
0SN94ZZ
0SN9XZZ
0SNB0ZZ
0SNB3ZZ
0SNB4ZZ
0SNBXZZ
0SNC0ZZ
0SNC3ZZ
0SNC4ZZ
0SNCXZZ
0SND0ZZ
0SND3ZZ
0SND4ZZ
0SNDXZZ
0SNF0ZZ
0SNF3ZZ
0SNF4ZZ
0SNFXZZ
0SNG0ZZ
0SNGXZZ
0SNHXZZ
0SNJXZZ
0SNKXZZ
0SNLXZZ
0SNMXZZ
0SNNXZZ
0SNPXZZ
0SNQXZZ
0SP008Z
0SP030Z
0SP033Z
0SP038Z
0SP048Z
0SP0X0Z
0SP0X3Z
0SP0X4Z
0SP230Z
0SP233Z
0SP2X0Z
0SP2X3Z
0SP308Z
0SP330Z
0SP333Z
0SP338Z
0SP348Z
0SP3X0Z
0SP3X3Z
0SP3X4Z
0SP430Z
0SP433Z
0SP4X0Z
0SP4X3Z
0SP508Z
0SP530Z
0SP533Z
0SP538Z
0SP548Z
0SP5X0Z
0SP5X3Z
0SP5X4Z
0SP608Z
0SP630Z
0SP633Z
0SP638Z
0SP648Z
0SP6X0Z
0SP6X3Z
0SP6X4Z
0SP708Z
0SP730Z
0SP733Z
0SP738Z
0SP748Z
0SP7X0Z
0SP7X3Z
0SP7X4Z
0SP808Z
0SP830Z
0SP833Z
0SP838Z
0SP848Z
0SP8X0Z
0SP8X3Z
0SP8X4Z
0SP908Z
0SP909Z
0SP90BZ
0SP90EZ
0SP90JZ
0SP930Z
0SP933Z
0SP938Z
0SP948Z
0SP94JZ
0SP9X0Z
0SP9X3Z
0SP9X4Z
0SP9X5Z
0SPA0JZ
0SPA4JZ
0SPB08Z
0SPB09Z
0SPB0BZ
0SPB0EZ
0SPB0JZ
0SPB30Z
0SPB33Z
0SPB38Z
0SPB48Z
0SPB4JZ
0SPBX0Z
0SPBX3Z
0SPBX4Z
0SPBX5Z
0SPC08Z
0SPC09Z
0SPC0EZ
0SPC0JC
0SPC0JZ
0SPC0LZ
0SPC0MZ
0SPC0NZ
0SPC30Z
0SPC33Z
0SPC38Z
0SPC3LZ
0SPC3MZ
0SPC3NZ
0SPC43Z
0SPC44Z
0SPC45Z
0SPC47Z
0SPC48Z
0SPC4JC
0SPC4JZ
0SPC4KZ
0SPC4LZ
0SPC4MZ
0SPC4NZ
0SPCX0Z
0SPCX3Z
0SPCX4Z
0SPCX5Z
0SPD00Z
0SPD03Z
0SPD04Z
0SPD05Z
0SPD07Z
0SPD08Z
0SPD09Z
0SPD0EZ
0SPD0JC
0SPD0JZ
0SPD0KZ
0SPD0LZ
0SPD0MZ
0SPD0NZ
0SPD30Z
0SPD33Z
0SPD34Z
0SPD35Z
0SPD37Z
0SPD38Z
0SPD3JC
0SPD3JZ
0SPD3KZ
0SPD3LZ
0SPD3MZ
0SPD3NZ
0SPD40Z
0SPD43Z
0SPD44Z
0SPD45Z
0SPD47Z
0SPD48Z
0SPD4JC
0SPD4JZ
0SPD4KZ
0SPD4LZ
0SPD4MZ
0SPD4NZ
0SPDX0Z
0SPDX3Z
0SPDX4Z
0SPDX5Z
0SPE0JZ
0SPE3JZ
0SPE4JZ
0SPF00Z
0SPF03Z
0SPF04Z
0SPF05Z
0SPF07Z
0SPF08Z
0SPF0JZ
0SPF0KZ
0SPF30Z
0SPF33Z
0SPF34Z
0SPF35Z
0SPF37Z
0SPF38Z
0SPF3JZ
0SPF3KZ
0SPF40Z
0SPF43Z
0SPF44Z
0SPF45Z
0SPF47Z
0SPF48Z
0SPF4JZ
0SPF4KZ
0SPFX0Z
0SPFX3Z
0SPFX4Z
0SPFX5Z
0SPG00Z
0SPG03Z
0SPG04Z
0SPG05Z
0SPG07Z
0SPG08Z
0SPG0JZ
0SPG0KZ
0SPG30Z
0SPG33Z
0SPG34Z
0SPG35Z
0SPG37Z
0SPG38Z
0SPG3JZ
0SPG3KZ
0SPG40Z
0SPG43Z
0SPG44Z
0SPG45Z
0SPG47Z
0SPG48Z
0SPG4JZ
0SPG4KZ
0SPGX0Z
0SPGX3Z
0SPGX4Z
0SPGX5Z
0SPH00Z
0SPH03Z
0SPH04Z
0SPH05Z
0SPH07Z
0SPH08Z
0SPH0JZ
0SPH0KZ
0SPH30Z
0SPH33Z
0SPH34Z
0SPH35Z
0SPH37Z
0SPH38Z
0SPH3JZ
0SPH3KZ
0SPH40Z
0SPH43Z
0SPH44Z
0SPH45Z
0SPH47Z
0SPH48Z
0SPH4JZ
0SPH4KZ
0SPHX0Z
0SPHX3Z
0SPHX4Z
0SPHX5Z
0SPJ00Z
0SPJ03Z
0SPJ04Z
0SPJ05Z
0SPJ07Z
0SPJ08Z
0SPJ0JZ
0SPJ0KZ
0SPJ30Z
0SPJ33Z
0SPJ34Z
0SPJ35Z
0SPJ37Z
0SPJ38Z
0SPJ3JZ
0SPJ3KZ
0SPJ40Z
0SPJ43Z
0SPJ44Z
0SPJ45Z
0SPJ47Z
0SPJ48Z
0SPJ4JZ
0SPJ4KZ
0SPJX0Z
0SPJX3Z
0SPJX4Z
0SPJX5Z
0SPK00Z
0SPK03Z
0SPK04Z
0SPK05Z
0SPK07Z
0SPK08Z
0SPK0JZ
0SPK0KZ
0SPK30Z
0SPK33Z
0SPK34Z
0SPK35Z
0SPK37Z
0SPK38Z
0SPK3JZ
0SPK3KZ
0SPK40Z
0SPK43Z
0SPK44Z
0SPK45Z
0SPK47Z
0SPK48Z
0SPK4JZ
0SPK4KZ
0SPKX0Z
0SPKX3Z
0SPKX4Z
0SPKX5Z
0SPL00Z
0SPL03Z
0SPL04Z
0SPL05Z
0SPL07Z
0SPL08Z
0SPL0JZ
0SPL0KZ
0SPL30Z
0SPL33Z
0SPL34Z
0SPL35Z
0SPL37Z
0SPL38Z
0SPL3JZ
0SPL3KZ
0SPL40Z
0SPL43Z
0SPL44Z
0SPL45Z
0SPL47Z
0SPL48Z
0SPL4JZ
0SPL4KZ
0SPLX0Z
0SPLX3Z
0SPLX4Z
0SPLX5Z
0SPM00Z
0SPM03Z
0SPM04Z
0SPM05Z
0SPM07Z
0SPM08Z
0SPM0JZ
0SPM0KZ
0SPM30Z
0SPM33Z
0SPM34Z
0SPM35Z
0SPM37Z
0SPM38Z
0SPM3JZ
0SPM3KZ
0SPM40Z
0SPM43Z
0SPM44Z
0SPM45Z
0SPM47Z
0SPM48Z
0SPM4JZ
0SPM4KZ
0SPMX0Z
0SPMX3Z
0SPMX4Z
0SPMX5Z
0SPN00Z
0SPN03Z
0SPN04Z
0SPN05Z
0SPN07Z
0SPN08Z
0SPN0JZ
0SPN0KZ
0SPN30Z
0SPN33Z
0SPN34Z
0SPN35Z
0SPN37Z
0SPN38Z
0SPN3JZ
0SPN3KZ
0SPN40Z
0SPN43Z
0SPN44Z
0SPN45Z
0SPN47Z
0SPN48Z
0SPN4JZ
0SPN4KZ
0SPNX0Z
0SPNX3Z
0SPNX4Z
0SPNX5Z
0SPP00Z
0SPP03Z
0SPP04Z
0SPP05Z

0SPP07Z
0SPP08Z
0SPP0JZ
0SPP0KZ
0SPP30Z
0SPP33Z
0SPP34Z
0SPP35Z
0SPP37Z
0SPP38Z
0SPP3JZ
0SPP3KZ
0SPP40Z
0SPP43Z
0SPP44Z
0SPP45Z
0SPP47Z
0SPP48Z
0SPP4JZ
0SPP4KZ
0SPPX0Z
0SPPX3Z
0SPPX4Z
0SPPX5Z
0SPQ00Z
0SPQ03Z
0SPQ04Z
0SPQ05Z
0SPQ07Z
0SPQ08Z
0SPQ0JZ
0SPQ0KZ
0SPQ30Z
0SPQ33Z
0SPQ34Z
0SPQ35Z
0SPQ37Z
0SPQ38Z
0SPQ3JZ
0SPQ3KZ
0SPQ40Z
0SPQ43Z
0SPQ44Z
0SPQ45Z
0SPQ47Z
0SPQ48Z
0SPQ4JZ
0SPQ4KZ
0SPQX0Z
0SPQX3Z
0SPQX4Z
0SPQX5Z
0SPR0JZ
0SPR3JZ
0SPR4JZ
0SPS0JZ
0SPS3JZ
0SPS4JZ
0SPT0JZ
0SPT3JZ
0SPT4JZ
0SPU0JZ
0SPU3JZ
0SPU4JZ
0SPV0JZ
0SPV3JZ
0SPV4JZ
0SPW0JZ
0SPW3JZ
0SPW4JZ
0SQ00ZZ
0SQ03ZZ
0SQ04ZZ
0SQ0XZZ
0SQ20ZZ
0SQ23ZZ
0SQ24ZZ
0SQ2XZZ
0SQ30ZZ
0SQ33ZZ
0SQ34ZZ
0SQ3XZZ
0SQ40ZZ
0SQ43ZZ
0SQ44ZZ
0SQ4XZZ
0SQ50ZZ
0SQ53ZZ
0SQ54ZZ
0SQ5XZZ
0SQ60ZZ
0SQ63ZZ
0SQ64ZZ
0SQ6XZZ
0SQ70ZZ
0SQ73ZZ
0SQ74ZZ
0SQ7XZZ
0SQ80ZZ
0SQ83ZZ
0SQ84ZZ
0SQ8XZZ
0SQ90ZZ
0SQ93ZZ
0SQ94ZZ
0SQ9XZZ
0SQB0ZZ
0SQB3ZZ
0SQB4ZZ
0SQBXZZ
0SQC0ZZ
0SQC3ZZ
0SQC4ZZ
0SQCXZZ
0SQD0ZZ
0SQD3ZZ
0SQD4ZZ
0SQDXZZ
0SQF0ZZ
0SQF3ZZ
0SQF4ZZ
0SQFXZZ
0SQG0ZZ
0SQG3ZZ
0SQG4ZZ
0SQGXZZ
0SQH0ZZ
0SQH3ZZ
0SQH4ZZ
0SQHXZZ
0SQJ0ZZ
0SQJ3ZZ
0SQJ4ZZ
0SQJXZZ
0SQK0ZZ
0SQK3ZZ
0SQK4ZZ
0SQKXZZ
0SQL0ZZ
0SQL3ZZ
0SQL4ZZ
0SQLXZZ
0SQM0ZZ
0SQM3ZZ
0SQM4ZZ
0SQMXZZ
0SQN0ZZ
0SQN3ZZ
0SQN4ZZ
0SQNXZZ
0SQP0ZZ
0SQP3ZZ
0SQP4ZZ
0SQPXZZ
0SQQ0ZZ
0SQQ3ZZ
0SQQ4ZZ
0SQQXZZ
0SR007Z
0SR00JZ
0SR00KZ
0SR207Z
0SR20JZ
0SR20KZ
0SR307Z
0SR30JZ
0SR30KZ
0SR407Z
0SR40JZ
0SR40KZ
0SR507Z
0SR50JZ
0SR50KZ
0SR607Z
0SR60JZ
0SR60KZ
0SR707Z
0SR70JZ
0SR70KZ
0SR807Z
0SR80JZ
0SR80KZ
0SR9019
0SR901A
0SR901Z
0SR9029
0SR902A
0SR902Z
0SR9039
0SR903A
0SR903Z
0SR9049
0SR904A
0SR904Z
0SR9069
0SR906A
0SR906Z
0SR907Z
0SR90EZ
0SR90J9
0SR90JA
0SR90JZ
0SR90KZ
0SRA009
0SRA00A
0SRA00Z
0SRA019
0SRA01A
0SRA01Z
0SRA039
0SRA03A
0SRA03Z
0SRA0J9
0SRA0JA
0SRA0JZ
0SRB019
0SRB01A
0SRB01Z
0SRB029
0SRB02A
0SRB02Z
0SRB039
0SRB03A
0SRB03Z
0SRB049
0SRB04A
0SRB04Z
0SRB069
0SRB06A
0SRB06Z
0SRB0EZ
0SRB0J9
0SRB0JA
0SRB0JZ
0SRC069
0SRC06A
0SRC06Z
0SRC0EZ
0SRC0J9
0SRC0JA
0SRC0JZ
0SRC0L9
0SRC0LA
0SRC0LZ
0SRC0M9
0SRC0MA
0SRC0MZ
0SRC0N9
0SRC0NA
0SRC0NZ
0SRD069
0SRD06A
0SRD06Z
0SRD0EZ
0SRD0J9
0SRD0JA
0SRD0JZ
0SRD0L9
0SRD0LA
0SRD0LZ
0SRD0M9
0SRD0MA
0SRD0MZ
0SRD0N9
0SRD0NA
0SRD0NZ
0SRE009
0SRE00A
0SRE00Z
0SRE019
0SRE01A
0SRE01Z
0SRE039
0SRE03A
0SRE03Z
0SRE0J9
0SRE0JA
0SRE0JZ
0SRR019
0SRR01A
0SRR01Z
0SRR039
0SRR03A
0SRR03Z
0SRR07Z
0SRR0J9
0SRR0JA
0SRR0JZ
0SRR0KZ
0SRS019
0SRS01A
0SRS01Z
0SRS039
0SRS03A
0SRS03Z
0SRS07Z
0SRS0J9
0SRS0JA
0SRS0JZ
0SRS0KZ
0SRT07Z
0SRT0J9
0SRT0JA
0SRT0JZ
0SRT0KZ
0SRU07Z
0SRU0J9
0SRU0JA
0SRU0JZ
0SRU0KZ
0SRV07Z
0SRV0J9
0SRV0JA
0SRV0JZ
0SRV0KZ
0SRW07Z
0SRW0J9
0SRW0JA
0SRW0JZ
0SRW0KZ
0SS004Z
0SS00ZZ
0SS034Z
0SS03ZZ
0SS044Z
0SS04ZZ
0SS0X4Z
0SS0XZZ
0SS304Z
0SS30ZZ
0SS334Z
0SS33ZZ
0SS344Z
0SS34ZZ
0SS3X4Z
0SS3XZZ
0SS504Z
0SS50ZZ
0SS534Z
0SS53ZZ
0SS544Z
0SS54ZZ
0SS5X4Z
0SS5XZZ
0SS604Z
0SS60ZZ
0SS634Z
0SS63ZZ
0SS644Z
0SS64ZZ
0SS6X4Z
0SS6XZZ
0SS704Z
0SS70ZZ
0SS734Z
0SS73ZZ
0SS744Z
0SS74ZZ
0SS7X4Z
0SS7XZZ
0SS804Z
0SS80ZZ
0SS834Z
0SS83ZZ
0SS844Z
0SS84ZZ
0SS8X4Z
0SS8XZZ
0SS904Z
0SS905Z
0SS90ZZ
0SS934Z
0SS935Z
0SS93ZZ
0SS944Z
0SS945Z
0SS94ZZ
0SS9X4Z
0SS9X5Z
0SS9XZZ
0SSB04Z
0SSB05Z
0SSB0ZZ
0SSB34Z
0SSB35Z
0SSB3ZZ
0SSB44Z
0SSB45Z
0SSB4ZZ
0SSBX4Z
0SSBX5Z
0SSBXZZ
0SSC04Z
0SSC05Z
0SSC0ZZ
0SSC34Z
0SSC35Z
0SSC3ZZ
0SSC44Z
0SSC45Z
0SSC4ZZ
0SSCX4Z
0SSCX5Z
0SSCXZZ
0SSD04Z
0SSD05Z
0SSD0ZZ
0SSD34Z
0SSD35Z
0SSD3ZZ
0SSD44Z
0SSD45Z
0SSD4ZZ
0SSDX4Z
0SSDX5Z
0SSDXZZ
0SSF04Z
0SSF05Z
0SSF0ZZ
0SSF34Z
0SSF35Z
0SSF3ZZ
0SSF44Z
0SSF45Z
0SSF4ZZ
0SSFX4Z
0SSFX5Z
0SSFXZZ
0SSG04Z
0SSG05Z
0SSG0ZZ
0SSG34Z
0SSG35Z
0SSG3ZZ
0SSG44Z
0SSG45Z
0SSG4ZZ
0SSGX4Z
0SSGX5Z
0SSGXZZ
0SSH04Z
0SSH05Z
0SSH0ZZ
0SSH34Z
0SSH35Z
0SSH3ZZ
0SSH44Z
0SSH45Z
0SSH4ZZ
0SSHX4Z
0SSHX5Z
0SSHXZZ
0SSJ04Z
0SSJ05Z
0SSJ0ZZ
0SSJ34Z
0SSJ35Z
0SSJ3ZZ
0SSJ44Z
0SSJ45Z
0SSJ4ZZ
0SSJX4Z
0SSJX5Z
0SSJXZZ
0SSK04Z
0SSK05Z
0SSK0ZZ
0SSK34Z
0SSK35Z
0SSK3ZZ
0SSK44Z
0SSK45Z
0SSK4ZZ
0SSKX4Z
0SSKX5Z
0SSKXZZ
0SSL04Z
0SSL05Z
0SSL0ZZ
0SSL34Z
0SSL35Z
0SSL3ZZ
0SSL44Z
0SSL45Z
0SSL4ZZ
0SSLX4Z
0SSLX5Z
0SSLXZZ
0SSM04Z
0SSM05Z
0SSM0ZZ
0SSM34Z
0SSM35Z
0SSM3ZZ
0SSM44Z
0SSM45Z
0SSM4ZZ
0SSMX4Z
0SSMX5Z
0SSMXZZ
0SSN04Z
0SSN05Z
0SSN0ZZ
0SSN34Z
0SSN35Z
0SSN3ZZ
0SSN44Z
0SSN45Z
0SSN4ZZ
0SSNX4Z
0SSNX5Z
0SSNXZZ
0SSP04Z
0SSP05Z
0SSP0ZZ
0SSP34Z
0SSP35Z
0SSP3ZZ
0SSP44Z
0SSP45Z
0SSP4ZZ
0SSPX4Z
0SSPX5Z
0SSPXZZ
0SSQ04Z
0SSQ05Z
0SSQ0ZZ
0SSQ34Z
0SSQ35Z
0SSQ3ZZ
0SSQ44Z
0SSQ45Z
0SSQ4ZZ
0SSQX4Z
0SSQX5Z
0SSQXZZ
0ST20ZZ
0ST40ZZ
0ST50ZZ
0ST60ZZ
0ST70ZZ
0ST80ZZ
0ST90ZZ
0STB0ZZ
0STC0ZZ
0STD0ZZ
0STF0ZZ
0STG0ZZ
0STH0ZZ
0STJ0ZZ
0STK0ZZ
0STL0ZZ
0STM0ZZ
0STN0ZZ
0STP0ZZ
0STQ0ZZ
0SU007Z
0SU00JZ
0SU00KZ
0SU037Z
0SU03JZ
0SU03KZ
0SU047Z
0SU04JZ
0SU04KZ
0SU207Z
0SU20JZ
0SU20KZ
0SU237Z
0SU23JZ
0SU23KZ
0SU247Z
0SU24JZ
0SU24KZ
0SU307Z
0SU30JZ
0SU30KZ
0SU337Z
0SU33JZ
0SU33KZ
0SU347Z
0SU34JZ
0SU34KZ
0SU407Z
0SU40JZ
0SU40KZ
0SU437Z
0SU43JZ
0SU43KZ
0SU447Z
0SU44JZ
0SU44KZ
0SU507Z
0SU50JZ
0SU50KZ
0SU537Z
0SU53JZ
0SU53KZ
0SU547Z
0SU54JZ
0SU54KZ
0SU607Z
0SU60JZ
0SU60KZ
0SU637Z
0SU63JZ
0SU63KZ
0SU647Z
0SU64JZ
0SU64KZ
0SU707Z
0SU70JZ
0SU70KZ
0SU737Z
0SU73JZ
0SU73KZ
0SU747Z
0SU74JZ
0SU74KZ
0SU807Z
0SU80JZ
0SU80KZ
0SU837Z
0SU83JZ
0SU83KZ
0SU847Z
0SU84JZ
0SU84KZ
0SU907Z
0SU909Z
0SU90BZ
0SU90JZ
0SU90KZ
0SU937Z
0SU93JZ
0SU93KZ
0SU947Z
0SU94JZ
0SU94KZ
0SUA09Z
0SUA0BZ
0SUB07Z
0SUB09Z
0SUB0BZ
0SUB0JZ
0SUB0KZ
0SUB37Z
0SUB3JZ
0SUB3KZ
0SUB47Z
0SUB4JZ
0SUB4KZ
0SUC07Z
0SUC09C
0SUC09Z
0SUC0JZ
0SUC0KZ
0SUC37Z
0SUC3JZ
0SUC3KZ
0SUC47Z
0SUC4JZ
0SUC4KZ
0SUD07Z
0SUD09C
0SUD09Z
0SUD0JZ
0SUD0KZ
0SUD37Z
0SUD3JZ
0SUD3KZ
0SUD47Z
0SUD4JZ
0SUD4KZ
0SUE09Z
0SUE0BZ
0SUF07Z
0SUF0JZ
0SUF0KZ
0SUF37Z
0SUF3JZ
0SUF3KZ
0SUF47Z
0SUF4JZ
0SUF4KZ
0SUG07Z
0SUG0JZ
0SUG0KZ
0SUG37Z
0SUG3JZ
0SUG3KZ
0SUG47Z
0SUG4JZ
0SUG4KZ
0SUH07Z
0SUH0JZ
0SUH0KZ
0SUH37Z
0SUH3JZ
0SUH3KZ
0SUH47Z
0SUH4JZ
0SUH4KZ
0SUJ07Z
0SUJ0JZ
0SUJ0KZ
0SUJ37Z
0SUJ3JZ
0SUJ3KZ
0SUJ47Z
0SUJ4JZ
0SUJ4KZ
0SUK07Z
0SUK0JZ
0SUK0KZ
0SUK37Z
0SUK3JZ
0SUK3KZ
0SUK47Z
0SUK4JZ
0SUK4KZ
0SUL07Z
0SUL0JZ
0SUL0KZ
0SUL37Z
0SUL3JZ

0SUL3KZ
0SUL47Z
0SUL4JZ
0SUL4KZ
0SUM07Z
0SUM0JZ
0SUM0KZ
0SUM37Z
0SUM3JZ
0SUM3KZ
0SUM47Z
0SUM4JZ
0SUM4KZ
0SUN07Z
0SUN0JZ
0SUN0KZ
0SUN37Z
0SUN3JZ
0SUN3KZ
0SUN47Z
0SUN4JZ
0SUN4KZ
0SUP07Z
0SUP0JZ
0SUP0KZ
0SUP37Z
0SUP3JZ
0SUP3KZ
0SUP47Z
0SUP4JZ
0SUP4KZ
0SUQ07Z
0SUQ0JZ
0SUQ0KZ
0SUQ37Z
0SUQ3JZ
0SUQ3KZ
0SUQ47Z
0SUQ4JZ
0SUQ4KZ
0SUR09Z
0SUR0BZ
0SUS09Z
0SUS0BZ
0SUT09Z
0SUU09Z
0SUV09Z
0SUW09Z
0SW000Z
0SW003Z
0SW004Z
0SW007Z
0SW008Z
0SW0X0Z
0SW0X3Z
0SW0X4Z
0SW0X7Z
0SW0X8Z
0SW0XAZ
0SW0XJZ
0SW0XKZ
0SW2X0Z
0SW2X3Z
0SW2X7Z
0SW2XJZ
0SW2XKZ
0SW3X0Z
0SW3X3Z
0SW3X4Z
0SW3X7Z
0SW3X8Z
0SW3XAZ
0SW3XJZ
0SW3XKZ
0SW4X0Z
0SW4X3Z
0SW4X7Z
0SW4XJZ
0SW4XKZ
0SW5X0Z
0SW5X3Z
0SW5X4Z
0SW5X7Z
0SW5X8Z
0SW5XJZ
0SW5XKZ
0SW6X0Z
0SW6X3Z
0SW6X4Z
0SW6X7Z
0SW6X8Z
0SW6XJZ
0SW6XKZ
0SW7X0Z
0SW7X3Z
0SW7X4Z
0SW7X7Z
0SW7X8Z
0SW7XJZ
0SW7XKZ
0SW8X0Z
0SW8X3Z
0SW8X4Z
0SW8X7Z
0SW8X8Z
0SW8XJZ
0SW8XKZ
0SW9X0Z
0SW9X3Z
0SW9X4Z
0SW9X5Z
0SW9X7Z
0SW9X8Z
0SW9XJZ
0SW9XKZ
0SWAXJZ
0SWBX0Z
0SWBX3Z
0SWBX4Z
0SWBX5Z
0SWBX7Z
0SWBX8Z
0SWBXJZ
0SWBXKZ
0SWCX0Z
0SWCX3Z
0SWCX4Z
0SWCX5Z
0SWCX7Z
0SWCX8Z
0SWCXJC
0SWCXJZ
0SWCXKZ
0SWD0JC
0SWD0JZ
0SWD0KZ
0SWD30Z
0SWD33Z
0SWD34Z
0SWD35Z
0SWD37Z
0SWD38Z
0SWD3JC
0SWD3JZ
0SWD3KZ
0SWD40Z
0SWD43Z
0SWD44Z
0SWD45Z
0SWD47Z
0SWD48Z
0SWD4JC
0SWD4JZ
0SWD4KZ
0SWDX0Z
0SWDX3Z
0SWDX4Z
0SWDX5Z
0SWDX7Z
0SWDX8Z
0SWDXJC
0SWDXJZ
0SWDXKZ
0SWE0JZ
0SWE3JZ
0SWE4JZ
0SWEXJZ
0SWF00Z
0SWF03Z
0SWF04Z
0SWF05Z
0SWF07Z
0SWF08Z
0SWF0JZ
0SWF0KZ
0SWF30Z
0SWF33Z
0SWF34Z
0SWF35Z
0SWF37Z
0SWF38Z
0SWF3JZ
0SWF3KZ
0SWF40Z
0SWF43Z
0SWF44Z
0SWF45Z
0SWF47Z
0SWF48Z
0SWF4JZ
0SWF4KZ
0SWFX0Z
0SWFX3Z
0SWFX4Z
0SWFX5Z
0SWFX7Z
0SWFX8Z
0SWFXJZ
0SWFXKZ
0SWG00Z
0SWG03Z
0SWG04Z
0SWG05Z
0SWG07Z
0SWG08Z
0SWG0JZ
0SWG0KZ
0SWG30Z
0SWG33Z
0SWG34Z
0SWG35Z
0SWG37Z
0SWG38Z
0SWG3JZ
0SWG3KZ
0SWG40Z
0SWG43Z
0SWG44Z
0SWG45Z
0SWG47Z
0SWG48Z
0SWG4JZ
0SWG4KZ
0SWGX0Z
0SWGX3Z
0SWGX4Z
0SWGX5Z
0SWGX7Z
0SWGX8Z
0SWGXJZ
0SWGXKZ
0SWH00Z
0SWH03Z
0SWH04Z
0SWH05Z
0SWH07Z
0SWH08Z
0SWH0JZ
0SWH0KZ
0SWH30Z
0SWH33Z
0SWH34Z
0SWH35Z
0SWH37Z
0SWH38Z
0SWH3JZ
0SWH3KZ
0SWH40Z
0SWH43Z
0SWH44Z
0SWH45Z
0SWH47Z
0SWH48Z
0SWH4JZ
0SWH4KZ
0SWHX0Z
0SWHX3Z
0SWHX4Z
0SWHX5Z
0SWHX7Z
0SWHX8Z
0SWHXJZ
0SWHXKZ
0SWJ00Z
0SWJ03Z
0SWJ04Z
0SWJ05Z
0SWJ07Z
0SWJ08Z
0SWJ0JZ
0SWJ0KZ
0SWJ30Z
0SWJ33Z
0SWJ34Z
0SWJ35Z
0SWJ37Z
0SWJ38Z
0SWJ3JZ
0SWJ3KZ
0SWJ40Z
0SWJ43Z
0SWJ44Z
0SWJ45Z
0SWJ47Z
0SWJ48Z
0SWJ4JZ
0SWJ4KZ
0SWJX0Z
0SWJX3Z
0SWJX4Z
0SWJX5Z
0SWJX7Z
0SWJX8Z
0SWJXJZ
0SWJXKZ
0SWK00Z
0SWK03Z
0SWK04Z
0SWK05Z
0SWK07Z
0SWK08Z
0SWK0JZ
0SWK0KZ
0SWK30Z
0SWK33Z
0SWK34Z
0SWK35Z
0SWK37Z
0SWK38Z
0SWK3JZ
0SWK3KZ
0SWK40Z
0SWK43Z
0SWK44Z
0SWK45Z
0SWK47Z
0SWK48Z
0SWK4JZ
0SWK4KZ
0SWKX0Z
0SWKX3Z
0SWKX4Z
0SWKX5Z
0SWKX7Z
0SWKX8Z
0SWKXJZ
0SWKXKZ
0SWL00Z
0SWL03Z
0SWL04Z
0SWL05Z
0SWL07Z
0SWL08Z
0SWL0JZ
0SWL0KZ
0SWL30Z
0SWL33Z
0SWL34Z
0SWL35Z
0SWL37Z
0SWL38Z
0SWL3JZ
0SWL3KZ
0SWL40Z
0SWL43Z
0SWL44Z
0SWL45Z
0SWL47Z
0SWL48Z
0SWL4JZ
0SWL4KZ
0SWLX0Z
0SWLX3Z
0SWLX4Z
0SWLX5Z
0SWLX7Z
0SWLX8Z
0SWLXJZ
0SWLXKZ
0SWM00Z
0SWM03Z
0SWM04Z
0SWM05Z
0SWM07Z
0SWM08Z
0SWM0JZ
0SWM0KZ
0SWM30Z
0SWM33Z
0SWM34Z
0SWM35Z
0SWM37Z
0SWM38Z
0SWM3JZ
0SWM3KZ
0SWM40Z
0SWM43Z
0SWM44Z
0SWM45Z
0SWM47Z
0SWM48Z
0SWM4JZ
0SWM4KZ
0SWMX0Z
0SWMX3Z
0SWMX4Z
0SWMX5Z
0SWMX7Z
0SWMX8Z
0SWMXJZ
0SWMXKZ
0SWN00Z
0SWN03Z
0SWN04Z
0SWN05Z
0SWN07Z
0SWN08Z
0SWN0JZ
0SWN0KZ
0SWN30Z
0SWN33Z
0SWN34Z
0SWN35Z
0SWN37Z
0SWN38Z
0SWN3JZ
0SWN3KZ
0SWN40Z
0SWN43Z
0SWN44Z
0SWN45Z
0SWN47Z
0SWN48Z
0SWN4JZ
0SWN4KZ
0SWNX0Z
0SWNX3Z
0SWNX4Z
0SWNX5Z
0SWNX7Z
0SWNX8Z
0SWNXJZ
0SWNXKZ
0SWP00Z
0SWP03Z
0SWP04Z
0SWP05Z
0SWP07Z
0SWP08Z
0SWP0JZ
0SWP0KZ
0SWP30Z
0SWP33Z
0SWP34Z
0SWP35Z
0SWP37Z
0SWP38Z
0SWP3JZ
0SWP3KZ
0SWP40Z
0SWP43Z
0SWP44Z
0SWP45Z
0SWP47Z
0SWP48Z
0SWP4JZ
0SWP4KZ
0SWPX0Z
0SWPX3Z
0SWPX4Z
0SWPX5Z
0SWPX7Z
0SWPX8Z
0SWPXJZ
0SWPXKZ
0SWQ00Z
0SWQ03Z
0SWQ04Z
0SWQ05Z
0SWQ07Z
0SWQ08Z
0SWQ0JZ
0SWQ0KZ
0SWQ30Z
0SWQ33Z
0SWQ34Z
0SWQ35Z
0SWQ37Z
0SWQ38Z
0SWQ3JZ
0SWQ3KZ
0SWQ40Z
0SWQ43Z
0SWQ44Z
0SWQ45Z
0SWQ47Z
0SWQ48Z
0SWQ4JZ
0SWQ4KZ
0SWQX0Z
0SWQX3Z
0SWQX4Z
0SWQX5Z
0SWQX7Z
0SWQX8Z
0SWQXJZ
0SWQXKZ
0SWR0JZ
0SWR3JZ
0SWR4JZ
0SWRXJZ
0SWS0JZ
0SWS3JZ
0SWS4JZ
0SWSXJZ
0SWT0JZ
0SWT3JZ
0SWT4JZ
0SWTXJZ
0SWU0JZ
0SWU3JZ
0SWU4JZ
0SWUXJZ
0SWV0JZ
0SWV3JZ
0SWV4JZ
0SWVXJZ
0SWW0JZ
0SWW3JZ
0SWW4JZ
0SWWXJZ
0T13073
0T13074
0T13076
0T13077
0T13078
0T13079
0T1307A
0T1307B
0T1307C
0T1307D
0T130J3
0T130J4
0T130J6
0T130J7
0T130J8
0T130J9
0T130JA
0T130JB
0T130JC
0T130JD
0T130K3
0T130K4
0T130K6
0T130K7
0T130K8
0T130K9
0T130KA
0T130KB
0T130KC
0T130KD
0T130Z3
0T130Z4
0T130Z6
0T130Z7
0T130Z8
0T130Z9
0T130ZA
0T130ZB
0T130ZC
0T130ZD
0T133JD
0T13473
0T13474
0T13476
0T13477
0T13478
0T13479
0T1347A
0T1347B
0T1347C
0T1347D
0T134J3
0T134J4
0T134J6
0T134J7
0T134J8
0T134J9
0T134JA
0T134JB
0T134JC
0T134JD
0T134K3
0T134K4
0T134K6
0T134K7
0T134K8
0T134K9
0T134KA
0T134KB
0T134KC
0T134KD
0T134Z3
0T134Z4
0T134Z6
0T134Z7
0T134Z8
0T134Z9
0T134ZA
0T134ZB
0T134ZC
0T134ZD
0T14073
0T14074
0T14076
0T14077
0T14078
0T14079
0T1407A
0T1407B
0T1407C
0T1407D
0T140J3
0T140J4
0T140J6
0T140J7
0T140J8
0T140J9
0T140JA
0T140JB
0T140JC
0T140JD
0T140K3
0T140K4
0T140K6
0T140K7
0T140K8
0T140K9
0T140KA
0T140KB
0T164K6
0T164K7
0T164K8
0T164K9
0T164KA
0T164KB
0T164KC
0T164KD
0T164Z6
0T164Z7
0T164Z8
0T164Z9
0T164ZA
0T164ZB
0T164ZC
0T164ZD
0T17076
0T17077
0T17078
0T17079
0T1707A
0T1707B
0T1707C
0T1707D
0T170J6
0T170J7
0T170J8
0T170J9
0T170JA
0T170JB
0T170JC
0T170JD
0T170K6
0T170K7
0T170K8
0T170K9
0T170KA
0T170KB
0T170KC
0T170KD
0T170Z6
0T170Z7
0T170Z8
0T170Z9
0T170ZA
0T170ZB
0T170ZC
0T170ZD
0T173JD
0T17476
0T17477
0T17478
0T17479
0T1747A
0T1747B
0T1747C
0T1747D
0T174J6
0T174J7
0T174J8
0T174J9
0T174JA
0T174JB
0T174JC
0T174JD
0T174K6
0T174K7
0T174K8
0T174K9
0T174KA
0T174KB
0T174KC
0T174KD
0T174Z6
0T174Z7
0T174Z8
0T174Z9
0T174ZA
0T174ZB
0T174ZC
0T174ZD
0T18076
0T18077
0T18078
0T18079
0T1807A
0T1807B
0T1807C
0T1807D
0T180J6
0T180J7
0T180J8
0T180J9
0T180JA
0T180JB
0T180JC
0T180JD
0T180K6
0T180K7
0T180K8
0T180K9
0T180KA
0T180KB
0T180KC
0T180KD
0T180Z6

0T180Z7
0T180Z8
0T180Z9
0T180ZA
0T180ZB
0T180ZC
0T180ZD
0T183JD
0T18476
0T18477
0T18478
0T18479
0T1847A
0T1847B
0T1847C
0T1847D
0T184J6
0T184J7
0T25X0Z
0T25XYZ
0T29X0Z
0T29XYZ
0T2BX0Z
0T2BXYZ
0T2DX0Z
0T2DXYZ
0T5D0ZZ
0T5D3ZZ
0T5D4ZZ
0T5D7ZZ
0T5D8ZZ
0T5DXZZ
0T760DZ
0T763DZ
0T764DZ
0T767DZ
0T767ZZ
0T768DZ
0T770DZ
0T773DZ
0T774DZ
0T777DZ
0T777ZZ
0T778DZ
0T780DZ
0T783DZ
0T783ZZ
0T784DZ
0T784ZZ
0T787DZ
0T787ZZ
0T788DZ
0T788ZZ
0T7B0DZ
0T7B0ZZ
0T7B3DZ
0T7B3ZZ
0T7B4DZ
0T7B4ZZ
0T7B7DZ
0T7B7ZZ
0T7B8DZ
0T7B8ZZ
0T7C0DZ
0T7C0ZZ
0T7C3DZ
0T7C3ZZ
0T7C4DZ
0T7C4ZZ
0T7C7DZ
0T7C7ZZ
0T7C8DZ
0T7C8ZZ
0T7D0DZ
0T7D0ZZ
0T7D3DZ
0T7D3ZZ
0T7D4DZ
0T7D4ZZ
0T7D7DZ
0T7D7ZZ
0T7D8DZ
0T7D8ZZ
0T820ZZ
0T823ZZ
0T824ZZ
0T8C0ZZ
0T8C3ZZ
0T8C4ZZ
0T9000Z
0T900ZX
0T900ZZ
0T9030Z
0T903ZX
0T903ZZ
0T9040Z
0T904ZX
0T904ZZ
0T9070Z
0T907ZX
0T907ZZ
0T9080Z
0T908ZX
0T908ZZ
0T9100Z
0T910ZX
0T910ZZ
0T9130Z
0T913ZX
0T913ZZ
0T9140Z
0T914ZX
0T914ZZ
0T9170Z
0T917ZX
0T917ZZ
0T9180Z
0T918ZX
0T918ZZ
0T9300Z
0T930ZX
0T930ZZ
0T9330Z
0T933ZX
0T933ZZ
0T9340Z
0T934ZX
0T934ZZ
0T9370Z
0T937ZX
0T937ZZ
0T9380Z
0T938ZX
0T938ZZ
0T9400Z
0T940ZX
0T940ZZ
0T9430Z
0T943ZX
0T943ZZ
0T9440Z
0T944ZX
0T944ZZ
0T9470Z
0T947ZX
0T947ZZ
0T9480Z
0T948ZX
0T948ZZ
0T9600Z
0T960ZX
0T960ZZ
0T9630Z
0T963ZX
0T963ZZ
0T9640Z
0T964ZX
0T964ZZ
0T9670Z
0T967ZX
0T967ZZ
0T9680Z
0T968ZX
0T968ZZ
0T9700Z
0T970ZX
0T970ZZ
0T9730Z
0T973ZX
0T973ZZ
0T9740Z
0T974ZX
0T974ZZ
0T9770Z
0T977ZX
0T977ZZ
0T9780Z
0T978ZX
0T978ZZ
0T9800Z
0T980ZX
0T980ZZ
0T9830Z
0T983ZX
0T983ZZ
0T9840Z
0T984ZX
0T984ZZ
0T9870Z
0T987ZX
0T987ZZ
0T9880Z
0T988ZX
0T988ZZ
0T9B00Z
0T9B0ZX
0T9B0ZZ
0T9B30Z
0T9B3ZX
0T9B3ZZ
0T9B40Z
0T9B4ZX
0T9B4ZZ
0T9B70Z
0T9B7ZX
0T9B7ZZ
0T9B80Z
0T9B8ZX
0T9B8ZZ
0T9C00Z
0T9C0ZX
0T9C0ZZ
0T9C30Z
0T9C3ZX
0T9C3ZZ
0T9C40Z
0T9C4ZX
0T9C4ZZ
0T9C70Z
0T9C7ZX
0T9C7ZZ
0T9C80Z
0T9C8ZX
0T9C8ZZ
0T9D00Z
0T9D0ZX
0T9D0ZZ
0T9D30Z
0T9D3ZX
0T9D3ZZ
0T9D40Z
0T9D4ZX
0T9D4ZZ
0T9D70Z
0T9D7ZX
0T9D7ZZ
0T9D80Z
0T9D8ZX
0T9D8ZZ
0T9DX0Z
0T9DXZX
0T9DXZZ
0TB00ZX
0TB00ZZ
0TB03ZX
0TB03ZZ
0TB04ZX
0TB04ZZ
0TB07ZX
0TB07ZZ
0TB08ZX
0TB08ZZ
0TB10ZX
0TB10ZZ
0TB13ZX
0TB13ZZ
0TB14ZX
0TB14ZZ
0TB17ZX
0TB17ZZ
0TB18ZX
0TB18ZZ
0TB30ZX
0TB30ZZ
0TB33ZX
0TB33ZZ
0TB34ZX
0TB34ZZ
0TB37ZX
0TB37ZZ
0TB38ZX
0TB38ZZ
0TB40ZX
0TB40ZZ
0TB43ZX
0TB43ZZ
0TB44ZX
0TB44ZZ
0TB47ZX
0TB47ZZ
0TB48ZX
0TB48ZZ
0TB60ZX
0TB60ZZ
0TB63ZX
0TB63ZZ
0TB64ZX
0TB64ZZ
0TB67ZX
0TB67ZZ
0TB68ZX
0TB68ZZ
0TB70ZX
0TB70ZZ
0TB73ZX
0TB73ZZ
0TB74ZX
0TB74ZZ
0TB77ZX
0TB77ZZ
0TB78ZX
0TB78ZZ
0TBB0ZX
0TBB0ZZ
0TBB3ZX
0TBB3ZZ
0TBB4ZX
0TBB4ZZ
0TBB7ZX
0TBB7ZZ
0TBB8ZX
0TBB8ZZ
0TBC0ZX
0TBC0ZZ
0TBC3ZX
0TBC3ZZ
0TBC4ZX
0TBC4ZZ
0TBC7ZX
0TBC7ZZ
0TBC8ZX
0TBC8ZZ
0TBD0ZX
0TBD0ZZ
0TBD3ZX
0TBD3ZZ
0TBD4ZX
0TBD4ZZ
0TBD7ZX
0TBD7ZZ
0TBD8ZX
0TBD8ZZ
0TBDXZX
0TBDXZZ
0TC00ZZ
0TC03ZZ
0TC04ZZ
0TC07ZZ
0TC08ZZ
0TC10ZZ
0TC13ZZ
0TC14ZZ
0TC17ZZ
0TC18ZZ
0TC30ZZ
0TC33ZZ
0TC34ZZ
0TC37ZZ
0TC38ZZ
0TC40ZZ
0TC43ZZ
0TC44ZZ
0TC47ZZ
0TC48ZZ
0TC60ZZ
0TC63ZZ
0TC64ZZ
0TC67ZZ
0TC68ZZ
0TC70ZZ
0TC73ZZ
0TC74ZZ
0TC77ZZ
0TC78ZZ
0TCB0ZZ
0TCB3ZZ
0TCB4ZZ
0TCB7ZZ
0TCB8ZZ
0TCC0ZZ
0TCC3ZZ
0TCC4ZZ
0TCC7ZZ
0TCC8ZZ
0TCD0ZZ
0TCD3ZZ
0TCD4ZZ
0TCD7ZZ
0TCD8ZZ
0TCDXZZ
0TD00ZZ
0TD03ZZ
0TD04ZZ
0TD10ZZ
0TD13ZZ
0TD14ZZ
0TF30ZZ
0TF33ZZ
0TF34ZZ
0TF37ZZ
0TF38ZZ
0TF3XZZ
0TF40ZZ
0TF43ZZ
0TF44ZZ
0TF47ZZ
0TF48ZZ
0TF4XZZ
0TF60ZZ
0TF63ZZ
0TF64ZZ
0TF67ZZ
0TF68ZZ
0TF6XZZ
0TF70ZZ
0TF73ZZ
0TF74ZZ
0TF77ZZ
0TF78ZZ
0TF7XZZ
0TFB0ZZ
0TFB3ZZ
0TFB4ZZ
0TFB7ZZ
0TFB8ZZ
0TFBXZZ
0TFC0ZZ
0TFC3ZZ
0TFC4ZZ
0TFC7ZZ
0TFC8ZZ
0TFCXZZ
0TFD0ZZ
0TFD3ZZ
0TFD4ZZ
0TFD7ZZ
0TFD8ZZ
0TFDXZZ
0TH502Z
0TH503Z
0TH50YZ
0TH532Z
0TH533Z
0TH53YZ
0TH542Z
0TH543Z
0TH54YZ
0TH572Z
0TH573Z
0TH57YZ
0TH582Z
0TH583Z
0TH58YZ
0TH902Z
0TH903Z
0TH90MZ
0TH90YZ
0TH932Z
0TH933Z
0TH93MZ
0TH93YZ
0TH942Z
0TH943Z
0TH94MZ
0TH94YZ
0TH972Z
0TH973Z
0TH97MZ
0TH97YZ
0TH982Z
0TH983Z
0TH98MZ
0TH98YZ
0THB02Z
0THB03Z
0THB0LZ
0THB0MZ
0THB0YZ
0THB32Z
0THB33Z
0THB3LZ
0THB3MZ
0THB3YZ
0THB42Z
0THB43Z
0THB4LZ
0THB4MZ
0THB4YZ
0THB72Z
0THB73Z
0THB7LZ
0THB7MZ
0THB7YZ
0THB82Z
0THB83Z
0THB8LZ
0THB8MZ
0THB8YZ
0THC0LZ
0THC3LZ
0THC4LZ
0THC7LZ
0THC8LZ
0THD02Z
0THD03Z
0THD0LZ
0THD0YZ
0THD32Z
0THD33Z
0THD3LZ
0THD3YZ
0THD42Z
0THD43Z
0THD4LZ
0THD4YZ
0THD72Z
0THD73Z
0THD7LZ
0THD7YZ
0THD82Z
0THD83Z
0THD8LZ
0THD8YZ
0THDX2Z
0THDX3Z
0THDXLZ
0TJ50ZZ
0TJ53ZZ
0TJ54ZZ
0TJ57ZZ
0TJ58ZZ
0TJ5XZZ
0TJ90ZZ
0TJ93ZZ
0TJ94ZZ
0TJ97ZZ
0TJ98ZZ
0TJ9XZZ
0TJB0ZZ
0TJB3ZZ
0TJB4ZZ
0TJB7ZZ
0TJB8ZZ
0TJBXZZ
0TJD0ZZ
0TJD3ZZ
0TJD4ZZ
0TJD7ZZ
0TJD8ZZ
0TJDXZZ
0TL30CZ
0TL30DZ
0TL30ZZ
0TL33CZ
0TL33DZ
0TL33ZZ
0TL34CZ
0TL34DZ
0TL34ZZ
0TL37DZ
0TL37ZZ
0TL38DZ
0TL38ZZ
0TL40CZ
0TL40DZ
0TL40ZZ
0TL43CZ
0TL43DZ
0TL43ZZ
0TN47ZZ
0TN48ZZ
0TN60ZZ
0TN63ZZ
0TN64ZZ
0TN67ZZ
0TN68ZZ
0TN70ZZ
0TN73ZZ
0TN74ZZ
0TN77ZZ
0TN78ZZ
0TNB0ZZ
0TNB3ZZ
0TNB4ZZ
0TNB7ZZ
0TNB8ZZ
0TNC0ZZ
0TNC3ZZ
0TNC4ZZ
0TNC7ZZ
0TNC8ZZ
0TND0ZZ
0TND3ZZ
0TND4ZZ
0TND7ZZ
0TND8ZZ
0TNDXZZ
0TP500Z
0TP502Z
0TP503Z
0TP507Z
0TP50CZ
0TP50DZ
0TP50JZ
0TP50KZ
0TP50YZ
0TP530Z
0TP532Z
0TP533Z
0TP537Z
0TP53CZ
0TP53DZ
0TP53JZ
0TP53KZ
0TP53YZ
0TP540Z
0TP542Z
0TP543Z
0TP547Z
0TP54CZ
0TP54DZ
0TP54JZ
0TP54KZ
0TP54YZ
0TP570Z
0TP572Z
0TP573Z
0TP577Z
0TP57CZ
0TP57DZ
0TP57JZ
0TP57KZ
0TP57YZ
0TP580Z
0TP582Z
0TP583Z
0TP587Z
0TP58CZ
0TP58DZ
0TP58JZ
0TP58KZ
0TP58YZ
0TP5X0Z
0TP5X2Z
0TP5X3Z
0TP5XDZ
0TP900Z
0TP902Z
0TP903Z
0TP907Z
0TP90CZ
0TP90DZ
0TP90JZ
0TP90KZ
0TP90MZ
0TP90YZ
0TP930Z
0TP932Z
0TP933Z
0TP937Z
0TP93CZ
0TP93DZ
0TP93JZ
0TP93KZ
0TP93MZ
0TP93YZ
0TP940Z
0TP942Z
0TP943Z
0TP947Z
0TP94CZ
0TP94DZ
0TP94JZ
0TP94KZ
0TP94MZ
0TP94YZ
0TP970Z
0TP972Z
0TP973Z
0TP977Z
0TP97CZ
0TP97DZ
0TP97JZ
0TP97KZ
0TP97MZ
0TP97YZ
0TP980Z
0TP982Z
0TP983Z
0TP987Z
0TP98CZ
0TP98DZ
0TP98JZ
0TP98KZ
0TP98MZ
0TP98YZ
0TP9X0Z
0TP9X2Z
0TP9X3Z
0TP9XDZ
0TP9XMZ
0TPB00Z
0TPB02Z
0TPB03Z
0TPB07Z
0TPB0CZ
0TPB0DZ
0TPB0JZ
0TPB0KZ
0TPB0LZ
0TPB0MZ
0TPB0YZ
0TPB30Z
0TPB32Z
0TPB33Z
0TPB37Z
0TPB3CZ
0TPB3DZ
0TPB3JZ
0TPB3KZ
0TPB3LZ
0TPB3MZ
0TPB3YZ
0TPB40Z
0TPB42Z
0TPB43Z
0TPB47Z
0TPB4CZ
0TPB4DZ
0TPB4JZ
0TPB4KZ
0TPB4LZ
0TPB4MZ
0TPB4YZ
0TPB70Z
0TPB72Z

0TPB73Z
0TPB77Z
0TPB7CZ
0TPB7DZ
0TPB7JZ
0TPB7KZ
0TPB7LZ
0TPB7MZ
0TPB7YZ
0TPB80Z
0TPB82Z
0TPB83Z
0TPB87Z
0TPB8CZ
0TPB8DZ
0TPB8JZ
0TPB8KZ
0TPB8LZ
0TPB8MZ
0TPB8YZ
0TPBX0Z
0TPBX2Z
0TPBX3Z
0TPBXDZ
0TPBXLZ
0TPBXMZ
0TPD00Z
0TPD02Z
0TPD03Z
0TPD07Z
0TPD0CZ
0TPD0DZ
0TPD0JZ
0TPD0KZ
0TPD0LZ
0TPD0YZ
0TPD30Z
0TPD32Z
0TPD33Z
0TPD37Z
0TPD3CZ
0TPD3DZ
0TPD3JZ
0TPD3KZ
0TPD3LZ
0TPD3YZ
0TPD40Z
0TPD42Z
0TPD43Z
0TPD47Z
0TPD4CZ
0TPD4DZ
0TPD4JZ
0TPD4KZ
0TPD4LZ
0TPD4YZ
0TPD70Z
0TPD72Z
0TPD73Z
0TPD77Z
0TPD7CZ
0TPD7DZ
0TPD7JZ
0TPD7KZ
0TPD7LZ
0TPD7YZ
0TPD80Z
0TPD82Z
0TPD83Z
0TPD87Z
0TPD8CZ
0TPD8DZ
0TPD8JZ
0TPD8KZ
0TPD8LZ
0TPD8YZ
0TPDX0Z
0TPDX2Z
0TPDX3Z
0TPDXDZ
0TPDXLZ
0TQ00ZZ
0TQ03ZZ
0TQ04ZZ
0TQ07ZZ
0TQ08ZZ
0TQ10ZZ
0TQ13ZZ
0TQ14ZZ
0TQ17ZZ
0TQ18ZZ
0TQ30ZZ
0TQ33ZZ
0TQ34ZZ
0TQ37ZZ
0TQ38ZZ
0TQ40ZZ
0TQ43ZZ
0TQ44ZZ
0TQ47ZZ
0TQ48ZZ
0TQ60ZZ
0TQ63ZZ
0TQ64ZZ
0TQ67ZZ
0TQ68ZZ
0TQ70ZZ
0TQ73ZZ
0TQ74ZZ
0TQ77ZZ
0TQ78ZZ
0TQB0ZZ
0TQB3ZZ
0TQB4ZZ
0TQB7ZZ
0TQB8ZZ
0TQC0ZZ
0TQC3ZZ
0TQC4ZZ
0TQC7ZZ
0TQC8ZZ
0TQD0ZZ
0TQD3ZZ
0TQD4ZZ
0TQD7ZZ
0TQD8ZZ
0TQDXZZ
0TR307Z
0TR30JZ
0TR30KZ
0TR347Z
0TR34JZ
0TR34KZ
0TR377Z
0TR37JZ
0TR37KZ
0TR387Z
0TR38JZ
0TR38KZ
0TR407Z
0TR40JZ
0TR40KZ
0TR447Z
0TR44JZ
0TR44KZ
0TR477Z
0TR47JZ
0TR47KZ
0TR487Z
0TR48JZ
0TR48KZ
0TR607Z
0TR60JZ
0TR60KZ
0TR647Z
0TR64JZ
0TR64KZ
0TR677Z
0TR67JZ
0TR67KZ
0TR687Z
0TR68JZ
0TR68KZ
0TR707Z
0TR70JZ
0TR70KZ
0TR747Z
0TR74JZ
0TR74KZ
0TR777Z
0TR77JZ
0TR77KZ
0TR787Z
0TR78JZ
0TR78KZ
0TRB07Z
0TRB0JZ
0TRB0KZ
0TRB47Z
0TRB4JZ
0TRB4KZ
0TRB77Z
0TRB7JZ
0TRB7KZ
0TRB87Z
0TRB8JZ
0TRB8KZ
0TRC07Z
0TRC0JZ
0TRC0KZ
0TRC47Z
0TRC4JZ
0TRC4KZ
0TRC77Z
0TRC7JZ
0TTB0ZZ
0TTD0ZZ
0TTD4ZZ
0TTD7ZZ
0TTD8ZZ
0TUD47Z
0TUD4JZ
0TUD4KZ
0TUD77Z
0TUD7JZ
0TUD7KZ
0TUD87Z
0TUD8JZ
0TUD8KZ
0TUDX7Z
0TUDXJZ
0TUDXKZ
0TV30CZ
0TV30DZ
0TV30ZZ
0TV33CZ
0TV33DZ
0TV33ZZ
0TV34CZ
0TV34DZ
0TV34ZZ
0TV37DZ
0TV37ZZ
0TV38DZ
0TV38ZZ
0TV40CZ
0TV40DZ
0TV40ZZ
0TV43CZ
0TV43DZ
0TV43ZZ
0TV44CZ
0TV44DZ
0TV44ZZ
0TV47DZ
0TV47ZZ
0TV48DZ
0TV48ZZ
0TV60CZ
0TV60DZ
0TV60ZZ
0TV63CZ
0TV63DZ
0TV63ZZ
0TV64CZ
0TV64DZ
0TV64ZZ
0TV67DZ
0TV67ZZ
0TV68DZ
0TV68ZZ
0TV70CZ
0TV70DZ
0TV70ZZ
0TV73CZ
0TV73DZ
0TV73ZZ
0TV74CZ
0TV74DZ
0TV74ZZ
0TV77DZ
0TV77ZZ
0TV78DZ
0TV78ZZ
0TVB0CZ
0TVB0DZ
0TVB0ZZ
0TVB3CZ
0TVB3DZ
0TVB3ZZ
0TVB4CZ
0TVB4DZ
0TVB4ZZ
0TVB7DZ
0TVB7ZZ
0TVB8DZ
0TVB8ZZ
0TVC0CZ
0TVC0DZ
0TVC0ZZ
0TVC3CZ
0TVC3DZ
0TVC3ZZ
0TVC4CZ
0TVC4DZ
0TVC4ZZ
0TVC7DZ
0TVC7ZZ
0TVC8DZ
0TVC8ZZ
0TVD0CZ
0TVD0DZ
0TVD0ZZ
0TVD3CZ
0TVD3DZ
0TVD3ZZ
0TVD4CZ
0TVD4DZ
0TVD4ZZ
0TVD7DZ
0TVD7ZZ
0TVD8DZ
0TVD8ZZ
0TVDXZZ
0TW500Z
0TW502Z
0TW503Z
0TW507Z
0TW50CZ
0TW50DZ
0TW50JZ
0TW50KZ
0TW50YZ
0TW530Z
0TW532Z
0TW533Z
0TW537Z
0TW53CZ
0TW53DZ
0TW53JZ
0TW53KZ
0TW53YZ
0TW540Z
0TW542Z
0TW543Z
0TW547Z
0TW54CZ
0TW54DZ
0TW54JZ
0TW54KZ
0TW54YZ
0TW570Z
0TW572Z
0TW573Z
0TW577Z
0TW57CZ
0TW57DZ
0TW57JZ
0TW57KZ
0TW57YZ
0TW580Z
0TW582Z
0TW583Z
0TW587Z
0TW58CZ
0TW58DZ
0TW58JZ
0TW58KZ
0TW58YZ
0TW5X0Z
0TW5X2Z
0TW5X3Z
0TW5X7Z
0TW5XCZ
0TW5XDZ
0TW5XJZ
0TW5XKZ
0TW900Z
0TW902Z
0TW903Z
0TW907Z
0TW90CZ
0TW90DZ
0TW90JZ
0TW90KZ
0TW90MZ
0TW90YZ
0TW930Z
0TW932Z
0TW933Z
0TW937Z
0TW93CZ
0TW93DZ
0TW93JZ
0TW93KZ
0TW93MZ
0TW93YZ
0TW940Z
0TW942Z
0TW943Z
0TW947Z
0TW94CZ
0TW94DZ
0TW94JZ
0TW94KZ
0TW94MZ
0TW94YZ
0TW970Z
0TW972Z
0TW973Z
0TW977Z
0TW97CZ
0TW97DZ
0TW97JZ
0TW97KZ
0TW97MZ
0TW97YZ
0TW980Z
0TW982Z
0TW983Z
0TW987Z
0TW98CZ
0TW98DZ
0TW98JZ
0TW98KZ
0TW98MZ
0TW98YZ
0TW9X0Z
0TW9X2Z
0TW9X3Z
0TW9X7Z
0TW9XCZ
0TW9XDZ
0TW9XJZ
0TW9XKZ
0TW9XMZ
0TWB00Z
0TWB02Z
0TWB03Z
0TWB07Z
0TWB0CZ
0TWB0DZ
0TWB0JZ
0TWB0KZ
0TWB0LZ
0TWB0MZ
0TWB0YZ
0TWB30Z
0TWB32Z
0TWB33Z
0TWB37Z
0TWB3CZ
0TWB3DZ
0TWB3JZ
0TWB3KZ
0TWB3LZ
0TWB3MZ
0TWB3YZ
0TWB40Z
0TWB42Z
0TWB43Z
0TWB47Z
0TWB4CZ
0TWB4DZ
0TWB4JZ
0TWB4KZ
0TWB4LZ
0TWB4MZ
0TWB4YZ
0TWB70Z
0TWB72Z
0TWB73Z
0TWB77Z
0TWB7CZ
0TWB7DZ
0TWB7JZ
0TWB7KZ
0TWB7LZ
0TWB7MZ
0TWB7YZ
0TWB80Z
0TWB82Z
0TWB83Z
0TWB87Z
0TWB8CZ
0TWB8DZ
0TWB8JZ
0TWB8KZ
0TWB8LZ
0TWB8MZ
0TWB8YZ
0TWBX0Z
0TWBX2Z
0TWBX3Z
0TWBX7Z
0TWBXCZ
0TWBXDZ
0TWBXJZ
0TWBXKZ
0TWBXLZ
0TWBXMZ
0TWD00Z
0TWD02Z
0TWD03Z
0TWD07Z
0TWD0CZ
0TWD0DZ
0TWD0JZ
0TWD0KZ
0TWD0LZ
0TWD0YZ
0TWD30Z
0TWD32Z
0TWD33Z
0TWD37Z
0TWD3CZ
0TWD3DZ
0TWD3JZ
0TWD3KZ
0TWD3LZ
0TWD3YZ
0TWD40Z
0TWD42Z
0TWD43Z
0TWD47Z
0TWD4CZ
0TWD4DZ
0TWD4JZ
0TWD4KZ
0TWD4LZ
0TWD4YZ
0TWD70Z
0TWD72Z
0TWD73Z
0TWD77Z
0TWD7CZ
0TWD7DZ
0TWD7JZ
0TWD7KZ
0TWD7LZ
0TWD7YZ
0TWD80Z
0TWD82Z
0TWD83Z
0TWD87Z
0TWD8CZ
0TWD8DZ
0TWD8JZ
0TWD8KZ
0TWD8LZ
0TWD8YZ
0TWDX0Z
0TWDX2Z
0TWDX3Z
0TWDX7Z
0TWDXCZ
0TWDXDZ
0TWDXJZ
0TWDXKZ
0TWDXLZ
0TY00Z0
0TY00Z1
0TY00Z2
0TY10Z0
0TY10Z1
0TY10Z2
0U15075
0U15076
0U15079
0U150J5
0U150J6
0U150J9
0U150K5
0U150K6
0U150K9
0U150Z5
0U150Z6
0U150Z9
0U15475
0U15476
0U15479
0U154J5
0U154J6
0U154J9
0U154K5
0U154K6
0U154K9
0U154Z5
0U154Z6
0U154Z9
0U16075
0U16076
0U16079
0U160J5
0U160J6
0U160J9
0U160K5
0U160K6
0U160K9
0U160Z5
0U160Z6
0U160Z9
0U16475
0U16476
0U16479
0U164J5
0U164J6
0U164J9
0U164K5
0U164K6
0U164K9
0U164Z5
0U164Z6
0U164Z9
0U23X0Z
0U23XYZ
0U28X0Z
0U28XYZ
0U2DX0Z
0U2DXHZ
0U2DXYZ
0U2HX0Z
0U2HXGZ
0U2HXYZ
0U2MX0Z
0U2MXYZ
0U500ZZ
0U503ZZ
0U504ZZ
0U508ZZ
0U510ZZ
0U513ZZ
0U514ZZ
0U518ZZ
0U520ZZ
0U523ZZ
0U524ZZ
0U528ZZ
0U540ZZ
0U543ZZ
0U544ZZ
0U548ZZ
0U550ZZ
0U553ZZ
0U554ZZ
0U557ZZ
0U558ZZ
0U560ZZ
0U563ZZ
0U564ZZ
0U567ZZ
0U568ZZ
0U570ZZ
0U573ZZ
0U574ZZ
0U577ZZ
0U578ZZ
0U590ZZ
0U593ZZ
0U594ZZ
0U7C0DZ
0U7C0ZZ
0U7C3DZ
0U7C3ZZ
0U7C4DZ
0U7C4ZZ
0U7C7DZ
0U7C7ZZ
0U7C8DZ
0U7C8ZZ
0U7G7DZ
0U7G7ZZ
0U7G8DZ
0U7G8ZZ
0U8K7ZZ
0U8K8ZZ
0U8KXZZ
0U9030Z
0U903ZZ
0U9080Z
0U908ZX
0U908ZZ
0U9130Z
0U913ZZ
0U9180Z
0U918ZX
0U918ZZ
0U9230Z
0U923ZZ
0U9280Z
0U928ZX
0U928ZZ
0U9430Z
0U943ZZ
0U9480Z
0U948ZX
0U948ZZ
0U9530Z
0U953ZZ
0U954ZZ
0U957ZZ
0U958ZZ
0U9630Z
0U963ZZ
0U964ZZ
0U967ZZ
0U968ZZ
0U9730Z
0U973ZZ
0U974ZZ
0U977ZZ
0U978ZZ
0U9930Z
0U993ZZ
0U994ZX
0U994ZZ
0U9970Z
0U997ZX
0U997ZZ
0U9980Z
0U998ZX
0U998ZZ
0U9C00Z
0U9C0ZX
0U9C0ZZ
0U9C30Z
0U9C3ZX
0U9C3ZZ
0U9C40Z
0U9C4ZX
0U9C4ZZ
0U9C70Z
0U9C7ZX
0U9C7ZZ
0U9C80Z
0U9C8ZX
0U9C8ZZ
0U9F00Z
0U9F0ZX
0U9F0ZZ
0U9F30Z
0U9F3ZX
0U9F3ZZ
0U9F40Z
0U9F4ZX
0U9F4ZZ

0U9F70Z
0U9F7ZX
0U9F7ZZ
0U9F80Z
0U9F8ZX
0U9F8ZZ
0U9G00Z
0U9G0ZX
0U9G0ZZ
0U9G30Z
0U9G3ZX
0U9G3ZZ
0U9G40Z
0U9G4ZX
0U9G4ZZ
0U9G70Z
0U9G7ZX
0U9G7ZZ
0U9G80Z
0U9G8ZX
0U9G8ZZ
0U9GX0Z
0U9GXZX
0U9GXZZ
0U9J00Z
0U9J0ZX
0U9J0ZZ
0U9JX0Z
0U9JXZX
0U9JXZZ
0U9K00Z
0U9K0ZX
0U9K0ZZ
0U9K30Z
0U9K3ZX
0U9K3ZZ
0U9K40Z
0U9K4ZX
0U9K4ZZ
0U9K70Z
0U9K7ZX
0U9K7ZZ
0U9K80Z
0U9K8ZX
0U9K8ZZ
0U9KX0Z
0U9KXZX
0U9KXZZ
0U9L00Z
0U9L0ZX
0U9L0ZZ
0U9LX0Z
0U9LXZX
0U9LXZZ
0U9M00Z
0U9M0ZX
0U9M0ZZ
0U9MX0Z
0U9MXZX
0U9MXZZ
0UB00ZX
0UB00ZZ
0UB03ZX
0UB03ZZ
0UB04ZX
0UB04ZZ
0UB07ZX
0UB07ZZ
0UB08ZX
0UB08ZZ
0UB10ZX
0UB10ZZ
0UB13ZX
0UB13ZZ
0UB14ZX
0UB14ZZ
0UB17ZX
0UB17ZZ
0UB18ZX
0UB18ZZ
0UB20ZX
0UB20ZZ
0UB23ZX
0UB23ZZ
0UB24ZX
0UB24ZZ
0UB27ZX
0UB27ZZ
0UB28ZX
0UB28ZZ
0UB40ZX
0UB40ZZ
0UB43ZX
0UB43ZZ
0UB44ZX
0UB44ZZ
0UB47ZX
0UB47ZZ
0UB48ZX
0UB48ZZ
0UB50ZX
0UB50ZZ
0UB53ZX
0UB53ZZ
0UB54ZX
0UB54ZZ
0UB57ZX
0UB57ZZ
0UB58ZX
0UB58ZZ
0UB60ZX
0UB60ZZ
0UB63ZX
0UB63ZZ
0UB64ZX
0UB64ZZ
0UB67ZX
0UB67ZZ
0UB68ZX
0UB68ZZ
0UB70ZX
0UB70ZZ
0UB73ZX
0UB73ZZ
0UB74ZX
0UB74ZZ
0UB77ZX
0UB77ZZ
0UB78ZX
0UB78ZZ
0UB90ZX
0UB90ZZ
0UB93ZX
0UB93ZZ
0UB94ZX
0UB94ZZ
0UB97ZX
0UB97ZZ
0UB98ZX
0UB98ZZ
0UBC0ZX
0UBC0ZZ
0UBC3ZX
0UBC3ZZ
0UBC4ZX
0UBC4ZZ
0UBC7ZX
0UBC7ZZ
0UBC8ZX
0UBC8ZZ
0UBF0ZX
0UBF0ZZ
0UBF3ZX
0UBF3ZZ
0UBF4ZX
0UBF4ZZ
0UBF7ZX
0UBF7ZZ
0UBF8ZX
0UBF8ZZ
0UBG0ZX
0UBG0ZZ
0UBG3ZX
0UBG3ZZ
0UBG4ZX
0UBG4ZZ
0UBG7ZX
0UBG7ZZ
0UBG8ZX
0UBG8ZZ
0UBGXZX
0UBGXZZ
0UBJ0ZX
0UBJ0ZZ
0UBJXZX
0UBJXZZ
0UBK0ZX
0UBK0ZZ
0UBK3ZX
0UBK3ZZ
0UBK4ZX
0UBK4ZZ
0UBK7ZX
0UBK7ZZ
0UBK8ZX
0UBK8ZZ
0UBKXZX
0UBKXZZ
0UBL0ZX
0UBL0ZZ
0UBLXZX
0UBLXZZ
0UBM0ZX
0UBM0ZZ
0UBMXZX
0UBMXZZ
0UC00ZZ
0UC03ZZ
0UC04ZZ
0UC08ZZ
0UC10ZZ
0UC13ZZ
0UC14ZZ
0UC18ZZ
0UC20ZZ
0UC23ZZ
0UC24ZZ
0UC28ZZ
0UC40ZZ
0UC43ZZ
0UC44ZZ
0UC48ZZ
0UC50ZZ
0UC53ZZ
0UC54ZZ
0UC57ZZ
0UC58ZZ
0UC60ZZ
0UC63ZZ
0UC64ZZ
0UC67ZZ
0UC68ZZ
0UC70ZZ
0UC73ZZ
0UC74ZZ
0UC77ZZ
0UC78ZZ
0UC90ZZ
0UC93ZZ
0UC94ZZ
0UC97ZZ
0UC98ZZ
0UCB0ZZ
0UCB3ZZ
0UCB4ZZ
0UCB7ZZ
0UCB8ZZ
0UCC0ZZ
0UCC3ZZ
0UCC4ZZ
0UCC7ZZ
0UCC8ZZ
0UCF0ZZ
0UCF3ZZ
0UCF4ZZ
0UCF7ZZ
0UCF8ZZ
0UCG0ZZ
0UCG3ZZ
0UCG4ZZ
0UCG7ZZ
0UCG8ZZ
0UCGXZZ
0UCJ0ZZ
0UCJXZZ
0UCK0ZZ
0UCK3ZZ
0UCK4ZZ
0UCK7ZZ
0UCK8ZZ
0UCKXZZ
0UCL0ZZ
0UCLXZZ
0UCM0ZZ
0UCMXZZ
0UDB7ZX
0UDB7ZZ
0UDB8ZX
0UDB8ZZ
0UDN0ZZ
0UDN3ZZ
0UDN4ZZ
0UF50ZZ
0UF53ZZ
0UF54ZZ
0UF57ZZ
0UF58ZZ
0UF5XZZ
0UF60ZZ
0UF63ZZ
0UF64ZZ
0UF67ZZ
0UF68ZZ
0UF6XZZ
0UF70ZZ
0UF73ZZ
0UF74ZZ
0UF77ZZ
0UF78ZZ
0UF7XZZ
0UF90ZZ
0UF93ZZ
0UF94ZZ
0UF97ZZ
0UF98ZZ
0UF9XZZ
0UH303Z
0UH30YZ
0UH333Z
0UH33YZ
0UH343Z
0UH34YZ
0UH37YZ
0UH38YZ
0UH803Z
0UH80YZ
0UH833Z
0UH83YZ
0UH843Z
0UH84YZ
0UH873Z
0UH87YZ
0UH883Z
0UH88YZ
0UH90HZ
0UH97HZ
0UH98HZ
0UHC01Z
0UHC31Z
0UHC41Z
0UHC71Z
0UHC7HZ
0UHC81Z
0UHC8HZ
0UHD03Z
0UHD0YZ
0UHD33Z
0UHD3YZ
0UHD43Z
0UHD4YZ
0UHD73Z
0UHD7YZ
0UHD83Z
0UHD8YZ
0UHF7GZ
0UHF8GZ
0UHG01Z
0UHG31Z
0UHG41Z
0UHG71Z
0UHG7GZ
0UHG81Z
0UHG8GZ
0UHGX1Z
0UHH03Z
0UHH0YZ
0UHH33Z
0UHH3YZ
0UHH43Z
0UHH4YZ
0UHH73Z
0UHH7YZ
0UHH83Z
0UHH8YZ
0UJ30ZZ
0UJ33ZZ
0UJ34ZZ
0UJ38ZZ
0UJ3XZZ
0UJ80ZZ
0UJ83ZZ
0UJ84ZZ
0UJ87ZZ
0UJ88ZZ
0UJ8XZZ
0UJD0ZZ
0UJD3ZZ
0UJD4ZZ
0UJD7ZZ
0UJD8ZZ
0UJDXZZ
0UJH0ZZ
0UJH3ZZ
0UJH4ZZ
0UJH7ZZ
0UJH8ZZ
0UJHXZZ
0UJM0ZZ
0UJMXZZ
0UL50CZ
0UL50DZ
0UL50ZZ
0UL53CZ
0UL53DZ
0UL53ZZ
0UL54CZ
0UL54DZ
0UL54ZZ
0UL57DZ
0UL57ZZ
0UL58DZ
0UL58ZZ
0UL60CZ
0UL60DZ
0UL60ZZ
0UL63CZ
0UL63DZ
0UL63ZZ
0UL64CZ
0UL64DZ
0UL64ZZ
0UL67DZ
0UL67ZZ
0UL68DZ
0UL68ZZ
0UL70CZ
0UL70DZ
0UP33YZ
0UP34YZ
0UP37YZ
0UP38YZ
0UP3X0Z
0UP3X3Z
0UP83YZ
0UP84YZ
0UP870Z
0UP873Z
0UP87DZ
0UP87YZ
0UP880Z
0UP883Z
0UP88DZ
0UP88YZ
0UP8X0Z
0UP8X3Z
0UP8XDZ
0UPD0YZ
0UPD30Z
0UPD31Z
0UPD33Z
0UPD37Z
0UPD3CZ
0UPD3DZ
0UPD3HZ
0UPD3JZ
0UPD3KZ
0UPD3YZ
0UPD40Z
0UPD41Z
0UPD43Z
0UPD47Z
0UPD4CZ
0UPD4DZ
0UPD4HZ
0UPD4JZ
0UPD4KZ
0UPD4YZ
0UPD70Z
0UPD71Z
0UPD73Z
0UPD77Z
0UPD7CZ
0UPD7DZ
0UPD7HZ
0UPD7JZ
0UPD7KZ
0UPD7YZ
0UPD80Z
0UPD81Z
0UPD83Z
0UPD87Z
0UPD8CZ
0UPD8DZ
0UPD8HZ
0UPD8JZ
0UPD8KZ
0UPD8YZ
0UPDX0Z
0UPDX3Z
0UPDXDZ
0UPDXHZ
0UPH00Z
0UPH01Z
0UPH03Z
0UPH07Z
0UPH0DZ
0UPH0JZ
0UPH0KZ
0UPH0YZ
0UPH30Z
0UPH31Z
0UPH33Z
0UPH37Z
0UPH3DZ
0UPH3JZ
0UPH3KZ
0UPH3YZ
0UPH40Z
0UPH41Z
0UPH43Z
0UPH47Z
0UPH4DZ
0UPH4JZ
0UPH4KZ
0UPH4YZ
0UPH70Z
0UPH71Z
0UPH73Z
0UPH77Z
0UPH7DZ
0UPH7JZ
0UPH7KZ
0UPH7YZ
0UPH80Z
0UPH81Z
0UPH83Z
0UPH87Z
0UPH8DZ
0UPH8JZ
0UPH8KZ
0UPH8YZ
0UPHX0Z
0UPHX1Z
0UPHX3Z
0UPHXDZ
0UPM00Z
0UPM07Z
0UPM0JZ
0UPM0KZ
0UPMX0Z
0UQ00ZZ
0UQ03ZZ
0UQ04ZZ
0UQ08ZZ
0UQ10ZZ
0UQ13ZZ
0UQ14ZZ
0UQ18ZZ
0UQ20ZZ
0UQ23ZZ
0UQ24ZZ
0UQ28ZZ
0UQ40ZZ
0UQ43ZZ
0UQ44ZZ
0UQ48ZZ
0UQ50ZZ
0UQ53ZZ
0UQ54ZZ
0UQ57ZZ
0UQ58ZZ
0UQ60ZZ
0UQ63ZZ
0UQ64ZZ
0UQ67ZZ
0UQ68ZZ
0UQ70ZZ
0UQ73ZZ
0UQ74ZZ
0UQ77ZZ
0UQ78ZZ
0UQ90ZZ
0UQ93ZZ
0UQ94ZZ
0UQ97ZZ
0UQ98ZZ
0UQC0ZZ
0UQC3ZZ
0UQC4ZZ
0UQC7ZZ
0UQC8ZZ
0UQF0ZZ
0UQF3ZZ
0UQF4ZZ
0UQF7ZZ
0UQF8ZZ
0UQG0ZZ
0UQG3ZZ
0UQG4ZZ
0UQG7ZZ
0UQG8ZZ
0UQGXZZ
0UQJ0ZZ
0UQJXZZ
0UQK0ZZ
0UQK3ZZ
0UQK4ZZ
0UQK7ZZ
0UQK8ZZ
0UQKXZZ
0UQL0ZZ
0UQLXZZ
0UQM0ZZ
0UQMXZZ
0US00ZZ
0US04ZZ
0US08ZZ
0US10ZZ
0US14ZZ
0US18ZZ
0US20ZZ
0US24ZZ
0US28ZZ
0US40ZZ
0US44ZZ
0US48ZZ
0US50ZZ
0US54ZZ
0US58ZZ
0US60ZZ
0US64ZZ
0US68ZZ
0US70ZZ
0US74ZZ
0US78ZZ
0US90ZZ
0US94ZZ
0US97ZZ
0US98ZZ
0US9XZZ
0USC0ZZ
0USC4ZZ
0USC8ZZ
0USF0ZZ
0USF4ZZ
0USF8ZZ
0USG0ZZ
0USG4ZZ
0USG7ZZ
0USG8ZZ
0USGXZZ
0UT00ZZ
0UT04ZZ
0UT07ZZ
0UT08ZZ
0UT0FZZ
0UT10ZZ
0UT14ZZ
0UT17ZZ
0UT18ZZ
0UT1FZZ
0UT20ZZ
0UT24ZZ
0UT27ZZ
0UT28ZZ
0UT2FZZ
0UT40ZZ
0UT44ZZ
0UT47ZZ
0UT48ZZ
0UT50ZZ
0UT54ZZ
0UT57ZZ
0UT58ZZ
0UT5FZZ
0UT60ZZ
0UT64ZZ
0UT67ZZ
0UT68ZZ
0UT6FZZ
0UT70ZZ
0UT74ZZ
0UT77ZZ
0UT78ZZ
0UT7FZZ
0UT90ZL
0UT90ZZ
0UT94ZL
0UT94ZZ
0UT97ZL
0UT97ZZ
0UT98ZL
0UT98ZZ
0UT9FZL
0UT9FZZ
0UTC0ZZ
0UTC4ZZ
0UTC7ZZ
0UTC8ZZ
0UTF0ZZ
0UTF4ZZ
0UTF7ZZ
0UTF8ZZ
0UTG0ZZ
0UTG4ZZ
0UTG7ZZ
0UTG8ZZ
0UTJ0ZZ
0UTJXZZ
0UTK0ZZ
0UTK4ZZ
0UTK7ZZ
0UTK8ZZ
0UTKXZZ
0UTL0ZZ
0UTLXZZ
0UTM0ZZ
0UTMXZZ
0UU407Z
0UU40JZ
0UU40KZ
0UU447Z
0UU44JZ
0UU44KZ
0UU507Z
0UU50JZ
0UU50KZ
0UU547Z
0UU54JZ
0UU54KZ
0UU577Z
0UU57JZ
0UU57KZ
0UU587Z
0UU58JZ
0UU58KZ
0UU607Z
0UU60JZ
0UU60KZ
0UU647Z
0UU64JZ
0UU64KZ
0UU677Z
0UU67JZ
0UU67KZ
0UU687Z
0UU68JZ
0UU68KZ
0UU707Z
0UU70JZ
0UU70KZ
0UU747Z
0UU74JZ
0UU74KZ
0UW33YZ
0UW34YZ

0UW37YZ
0UW38YZ
0UW3X0Z
0UW3X3Z
0UW83YZ
0UW84YZ
0UW87YZ
0UW88YZ
0UW8X0Z
0UW8X3Z
0UW8X7Z
0UW8XCZ
0UW8XDZ
0UW8XJZ
0UW8XKZ
0UWD3YZ
0UWD4YZ
0UWD73Z
0UWD77Z
0UWD7CZ
0UWD7DZ
0UWD7HZ
0UWD7JZ
0UWD7KZ
0UWD7YZ
0UWD80Z
0UWD81Z
0UWD83Z
0UWD87Z
0UWD8CZ
0UWD8DZ
0UWD8HZ
0UWD8JZ
0UWD8KZ
0UWD8YZ
0UWDX0Z
0UWDX3Z
0UWDX7Z
0UWDXCZ
0UWDXDZ
0UWDXHZ
0UWDXJZ
0UWDXKZ
0UWH00Z
0UWH01Z
0UWH03Z
0UWH07Z
0UWH0DZ
0UWH0JZ
0UWH0KZ
0UWH0YZ
0UWH30Z
0UWH31Z
0UWH33Z
0UWH37Z
0UWH3DZ
0UWH3JZ
0UWH3KZ
0UWH3YZ
0UWH40Z
0UWH41Z
0UWH43Z
0UWH47Z
0UWH4DZ
0UWH4JZ
0UWH4KZ
0UWH4YZ
0UWH70Z
0UWH71Z
0UWH73Z
0UWH77Z
0UWH7DZ
0UWH7JZ
0UWH7KZ
0UWH7YZ
0UWH80Z
0UWH81Z
0UWH83Z
0UWH87Z
0UWH8DZ
0UWH8JZ
0UWH8KZ
0UWH8YZ
0UWHX0Z
0UWHX3Z
0UWHX7Z
0UWHXDZ
0UWHXJZ
0UWHXKZ
0UWM00Z
0UWM07Z
0UWM0JZ
0UWM0KZ
0UWMX0Z
0UWMX7Z
0UWMXJZ
0UWMXKZ
0UY00Z0
0UY00Z1
0UY00Z2
0UY10Z0
0UY10Z1
0UY10Z2
0UY90Z0
0UY90Z1
0UY90Z2
0V1N07J
0V1N07K
0V1N07N
0V1N07P
0V1N0JJ
0V1N0JK
0V1N0JN
0V1N0JP
0V1N0KJ
0V1N0KK
0V1N0KN
0V1N0KP
0V1N0ZJ
0V1N0ZK
0V1N0ZN
0V1N0ZP
0V1N47J
0V1N47K
0V1N47N
0V1N47P
0V1N4JJ
0V1N4JK
0V1N4JN
0V1N4JP
0V1N4KJ
0V1N4KK
0V1N4KN
0V1N4KP
0V1N4ZJ
0V1N4ZK
0V1N4ZN
0V1N4ZP
0V1P07J
0V1P07K
0V1P07N
0V1P07P
0V1P0JJ
0V1P0JK
0V1P0JN
0V1P0JP
0V1P0KJ
0V1P0KK
0V1P0KN
0V1P0KP
0V1P0ZJ
0V1P0ZK
0V1P0ZN
0V1P0ZP
0V1P47J
0V1P47K
0V1P47N
0V1P47P
0V1P4JJ
0V1P4JK
0V1P4JN
0V1P4JP
0V1P4KJ
0V1P4KK
0V1P4KN
0V1P4KP
0V1P4ZJ
0V1P4ZK
0V1P4ZN
0V1P4ZP
0V1Q07J
0V1Q07K
0V1Q07N
0V1Q07P
0V1Q0JJ
0V1Q0JK
0V1Q0JN
0V1Q0JP
0V1Q0KJ
0V1Q0KK
0V1Q0KN
0V1Q0KP
0V1Q0ZJ
0V1Q0ZK
0V1Q0ZN
0V1Q0ZP
0V1Q47J
0V1Q47K
0V1Q47N
0V1Q47P
0V1Q4JJ
0V1Q4JK
0V1Q4JN
0V1Q4JP
0V1Q4KJ
0V1Q4KK
0V1Q4KN
0V1Q4KP
0V1Q4ZJ
0V1Q4ZK
0V1Q4ZN
0V1Q4ZP
0V24X0Z
0V24XYZ
0V28X0Z
0V28XYZ
0V2DX0Z
0V2DXYZ
0V2MX0Z
0V2MXYZ
0V2RX0Z
0V2RXYZ
0V2SX0Z
0V2SXYZ
0V500ZZ
0V503ZZ
0V504ZZ
0V507ZZ
0V508ZZ
0V510ZZ
0V513ZZ
0V514ZZ
0V520ZZ
0V523ZZ
0V524ZZ
0V530ZZ
0V533ZZ
0V534ZZ
0V550ZZ
0V553ZZ
0V554ZZ
0V55XZZ
0V560ZZ
0V563ZZ
0V564ZZ
0V570ZZ
0V573ZZ
0V574ZZ
0V590ZZ
0V593ZZ
0V594ZZ
0V5B0ZZ
0V5B3ZZ
0V5B4ZZ
0V5C0ZZ
0V5C3ZZ
0V5C4ZZ
0V5F0ZZ
0V5F3ZZ
0V5F4ZZ
0V5F8ZZ
0V5G0ZZ
0V5G3ZZ
0V5G4ZZ
0V5G8ZZ
0V5H0ZZ
0V5H3ZZ
0V5H4ZZ
0V5H8ZZ
0V5J0ZZ
0V5J3ZZ
0V5J4ZZ
0V5J8ZZ
0V5K0ZZ
0V5K3ZZ
0V5K4ZZ
0V5K8ZZ
0V5L0ZZ
0V5L3ZZ
0V5L4ZZ
0V5L8ZZ
0V5N0ZZ
0V5N3ZZ
0V5N4ZZ
0V5N8ZZ
0V5P0ZZ
0V5P3ZZ
0V5P4ZZ
0V5P8ZZ
0V5Q0ZZ
0V5Q3ZZ
0V5Q4ZZ
0V5Q8ZZ
0V5S0ZZ
0V5S3ZZ
0V5S4ZZ
0V5SXZZ
0V5T0ZZ
0V5T3ZZ
0V5T4ZZ
0V5TXZZ
0V7N0DZ
0V7N0ZZ
0V7N3DZ
0V7N3ZZ
0V7N4DZ
0V7N4ZZ
0V7P0DZ
0V7P0ZZ
0V7P3DZ
0V7P3ZZ
0V7P4DZ
0V7P4ZZ
0V7Q0DZ
0V7Q0ZZ
0V7Q3DZ
0V7Q3ZZ
0V7Q4DZ
0V7Q4ZZ
0V9000Z
0V900ZX
0V900ZZ
0V9030Z
0V903ZX
0V903ZZ
0V9040Z
0V904ZX
0V904ZZ
0V9070Z
0V907ZX
0V907ZZ
0V9080Z
0V908ZX
0V908ZZ
0V9100Z
0V910ZX
0V910ZZ
0V9130Z
0V913ZX
0V913ZZ
0V9140Z
0V914ZX
0V914ZZ
0V9200Z
0V920ZX
0V920ZZ
0V9230Z
0V923ZX
0V923ZZ
0V9240Z
0V924ZX
0V924ZZ
0V9300Z
0V930ZX
0V930ZZ
0V9330Z
0V933ZX
0V933ZZ
0V9340Z
0V934ZX
0V934ZZ
0V9500Z
0V950ZX
0V950ZZ
0V9530Z
0V953ZX
0V953ZZ
0V9540Z
0V954ZX
0V954ZZ
0V95X0Z
0V95XZX
0V95XZZ
0V9600Z
0V960ZX
0V960ZZ
0V9630Z
0V963ZX
0V963ZZ
0V9640Z
0V964ZX
0V964ZZ
0V9700Z
0V970ZX
0V970ZZ
0V9730Z
0V973ZX
0V973ZZ
0V9740Z
0V974ZX
0V974ZZ
0V9900Z
0V990ZX
0V990ZZ
0V9930Z
0V993ZX
0V993ZZ
0V9940Z
0V994ZX
0V994ZZ
0V9B00Z
0V9B0ZX
0V9B0ZZ
0V9B30Z
0V9B3ZX
0V9B3ZZ
0V9B40Z
0V9B4ZX
0V9B4ZZ
0V9C00Z
0V9C0ZX
0V9C0ZZ
0V9C30Z
0V9C3ZX
0V9C3ZZ
0V9C40Z
0V9C4ZX
0V9C4ZZ
0V9F00Z
0V9F0ZX
0V9F0ZZ
0V9F30Z
0V9F3ZX
0V9F3ZZ
0V9F40Z
0V9F4ZX
0V9F4ZZ
0V9G00Z
0V9G0ZX
0V9G0ZZ
0V9G30Z
0V9G3ZX
0V9G3ZZ
0V9G40Z
0V9G4ZX
0V9G4ZZ
0V9H00Z
0V9H0ZX
0V9H0ZZ
0V9H30Z
0V9H3ZX
0V9H3ZZ
0V9H40Z
0V9H4ZX
0V9H4ZZ
0V9J00Z
0V9J0ZX
0V9J0ZZ
0V9J30Z
0V9J3ZX
0V9J3ZZ
0V9J40Z
0V9J4ZX
0V9J4ZZ
0V9K00Z
0V9K0ZX
0V9K0ZZ
0V9K30Z
0V9K3ZX
0V9K3ZZ
0V9K40Z
0V9K4ZX
0V9K4ZZ
0V9L00Z
0V9L0ZX
0V9L0ZZ
0V9L30Z
0V9L3ZX
0V9L3ZZ
0V9L40Z
0V9L4ZX
0V9L4ZZ
0V9N00Z
0V9N0ZX
0V9N0ZZ
0V9N30Z
0V9N3ZX
0V9N3ZZ
0V9N40Z
0V9N4ZX
0V9N4ZZ
0V9P00Z
0V9P0ZX
0V9P0ZZ
0V9P30Z
0V9P3ZX
0V9P3ZZ
0V9P40Z
0V9P4ZX
0V9P4ZZ
0V9Q00Z
0V9Q0ZX
0V9Q0ZZ
0V9Q30Z
0V9Q3ZX
0V9Q3ZZ
0V9Q40Z
0V9Q4ZX
0V9Q4ZZ
0V9S00Z
0V9S0ZX
0V9S0ZZ
0V9S30Z
0V9S3ZX
0V9S3ZZ
0V9S40Z
0V9S4ZX
0V9S4ZZ
0V9SX0Z
0V9SXZX
0V9SXZZ
0V9T00Z
0V9T0ZX
0V9T0ZZ
0V9T30Z
0V9T3ZX
0V9T3ZZ
0V9T40Z
0V9T4ZX
0V9T4ZZ
0V9TX0Z
0V9TXZX
0V9TXZZ
0VB00ZX
0VB00ZZ
0VB03ZX
0VB03ZZ
0VB04ZX
0VB04ZZ
0VB07ZX
0VB07ZZ
0VB08ZX
0VB08ZZ
0VB10ZX
0VB10ZZ
0VB13ZX
0VB13ZZ
0VB14ZX
0VB14ZZ
0VB20ZX
0VB20ZZ
0VB23ZX
0VB23ZZ
0VB24ZX
0VB24ZZ
0VB30ZX
0VB30ZZ
0VB33ZX
0VB33ZZ
0VB34ZX
0VB34ZZ
0VB50ZX
0VB50ZZ
0VB53ZX
0VB53ZZ
0VB54ZX
0VB54ZZ
0VB5XZX
0VB5XZZ
0VB60ZX
0VB60ZZ
0VB63ZX
0VB63ZZ
0VB64ZX
0VB64ZZ
0VB70ZX
0VB70ZZ
0VB73ZX
0VB73ZZ
0VB74ZX
0VB74ZZ
0VB90ZX
0VB90ZZ
0VB93ZX
0VB93ZZ
0VB94ZX
0VB94ZZ
0VBB0ZX
0VBB0ZZ
0VBB3ZX
0VBB3ZZ
0VBB4ZX
0VBB4ZZ
0VBC0ZX
0VBC0ZZ
0VBC3ZX
0VBC3ZZ
0VBC4ZX
0VBC4ZZ
0VBF0ZX
0VBF0ZZ
0VBF3ZX
0VBF3ZZ
0VBF4ZX
0VBF4ZZ
0VBF8ZX
0VBF8ZZ
0VBG0ZX
0VBG0ZZ
0VBG3ZX
0VBG3ZZ
0VBG4ZX
0VBG4ZZ
0VBG8ZX
0VBG8ZZ
0VBH0ZX
0VBH0ZZ
0VBH3ZX
0VBH3ZZ
0VBH4ZX
0VBH4ZZ
0VBH8ZX
0VBH8ZZ
0VBJ0ZX
0VBJ0ZZ
0VBJ3ZX
0VBJ3ZZ
0VBJ4ZX
0VBJ4ZZ
0VBJ8ZX
0VBJ8ZZ
0VBK0ZX
0VBK0ZZ
0VBK3ZX
0VBK3ZZ
0VBK4ZX
0VBK4ZZ
0VBK8ZX
0VBK8ZZ
0VBL0ZX
0VBL0ZZ
0VBL3ZX
0VBL3ZZ
0VBL4ZX
0VBL4ZZ
0VBL8ZX
0VBL8ZZ
0VBN0ZX
0VBN0ZZ
0VBN3ZX
0VBN3ZZ
0VBN4ZX
0VBN4ZZ
0VBN8ZX
0VBN8ZZ
0VBP0ZX
0VBP0ZZ
0VBP3ZX
0VBP3ZZ
0VBP4ZX
0VBP4ZZ
0VBP8ZX
0VBP8ZZ
0VBQ0ZX
0VBQ0ZZ
0VBQ3ZX
0VBQ3ZZ
0VBQ4ZX
0VBQ4ZZ
0VBQ8ZX
0VBQ8ZZ
0VBS0ZX
0VBS0ZZ
0VBS3ZX
0VBS3ZZ
0VBS4ZX
0VBS4ZZ
0VBSXZX
0VBSXZZ
0VBT0ZX
0VBT0ZZ
0VBT3ZX
0VBT3ZZ
0VBT4ZX
0VBT4ZZ
0VBTXZX
0VBTXZZ
0VC00ZZ
0VC03ZZ
0VC04ZZ
0VC07ZZ
0VC08ZZ
0VC10ZZ
0VC13ZZ
0VC14ZZ
0VC20ZZ
0VC23ZZ
0VC24ZZ
0VC30ZZ
0VC33ZZ
0VC34ZZ
0VC50ZZ
0VC53ZZ
0VC54ZZ
0VC5XZZ
0VC60ZZ
0VC63ZZ
0VC64ZZ
0VC70ZZ
0VC73ZZ
0VC74ZZ
0VC90ZZ
0VC93ZZ
0VC94ZZ
0VCB0ZZ
0VCB3ZZ
0VCB4ZZ
0VCC0ZZ
0VCC3ZZ
0VCC4ZZ
0VCF0ZZ
0VCF3ZZ
0VCF4ZZ
0VCG0ZZ
0VCG3ZZ
0VCG4ZZ
0VCH0ZZ
0VCH3ZZ
0VCH4ZZ
0VCJ0ZZ
0VCJ3ZZ
0VCJ4ZZ
0VCK0ZZ
0VCK3ZZ
0VCK4ZZ
0VCL0ZZ
0VCL3ZZ
0VCL4ZZ
0VCN0ZZ
0VCN3ZZ
0VCN4ZZ
0VCP0ZZ
0VCP3ZZ
0VCP4ZZ
0VCQ0ZZ
0VCQ3ZZ

0VCQ4ZZ
0VCS0ZZ
0VCS3ZZ
0VCS4ZZ
0VCSXZZ
0VCT0ZZ
0VCT3ZZ
0VCT4ZZ
0VCTXZZ
0VH001Z
0VH031Z
0VH041Z
0VH071Z
0VH081Z
0VH403Z
0VH40YZ
0VH433Z
0VH43YZ
0VH443Z
0VH44YZ
0VH473Z
0VH47YZ
0VH483Z
0VH48YZ
0VH803Z
0VH80YZ
0VH833Z
0VH83YZ
0VH843Z
0VH84YZ
0VH873Z
0VH87YZ
0VH883Z
0VH88YZ
0VHD03Z
0VHD0YZ
0VHD33Z
0VHD3YZ
0VHD43Z
0VHD4YZ
0VHD73Z
0VHD7YZ
0VHD83Z
0VHD8YZ
0VHM03Z
0VHM0YZ
0VHM33Z
0VHM3YZ
0VHM43Z
0VHM4YZ
0VHM73Z
0VHM7YZ
0VHM83Z
0VHM8YZ
0VHR03Z
0VHR0YZ
0VHR33Z
0VHR3YZ
0VHR43Z
0VHR4YZ
0VHR73Z
0VHR7YZ
0VHR83Z
0VHR8YZ
0VHS03Z
0VHS0YZ
0VHS33Z
0VHS3YZ
0VHS43Z
0VHS4YZ
0VHS7YZ
0VHS8YZ
0VHSX3Z
0VJ40ZZ
0VJ43ZZ
0VJ44ZZ
0VJ4XZZ
0VJ80ZZ
0VJ83ZZ
0VJ84ZZ
0VJ8XZZ
0VJD0ZZ
0VJD3ZZ
0VJD4ZZ
0VJDXZZ
0VJM0ZZ
0VJM3ZZ
0VJM4ZZ
0VJMXZZ
0VJR0ZZ
0VJR3ZZ
0VJR4ZZ
0VJRXZZ
0VJS0ZZ
0VJS3ZZ
0VJS4ZZ
0VJSXZZ
0VLF0CZ
0VLF0DZ
0VLF0ZZ
0VLF3CZ
0VLF3DZ
0VLF3ZZ
0VLF4CZ
0VLF4DZ
0VLF4ZZ
0VLF8CZ
0VLF8DZ
0VLF8ZZ
0VLG0CZ
0VLG0DZ
0VLG0ZZ
0VLG3CZ
0VLG3DZ
0VLG3ZZ
0VLG4CZ
0VLG4DZ
0VLG4ZZ
0VLG8CZ
0VLG8DZ
0VLG8ZZ
0VLH0CZ
0VLH0DZ
0VLH0ZZ
0VLH3CZ
0VLH3DZ
0VLH3ZZ
0VLH4CZ
0VLH4DZ
0VLH4ZZ
0VLH8CZ
0VLH8DZ
0VLH8ZZ
0VLN0CZ
0VLN0DZ
0VLN0ZZ
0VLN3CZ
0VLN3DZ
0VLN3ZZ
0VLN4CZ
0VLN4DZ
0VLN4ZZ
0VLN8CZ
0VLN8DZ
0VLN8ZZ
0VLP0CZ
0VLP0DZ
0VLP0ZZ
0VLP3CZ
0VLP3DZ
0VLP3ZZ
0VLP4CZ
0VLP4DZ
0VLP4ZZ
0VLP8CZ
0VLP8DZ
0VLP8ZZ
0VLQ0CZ
0VLQ0DZ
0VLQ0ZZ
0VLQ3CZ
0VLQ3DZ
0VLQ3ZZ
0VLQ4CZ
0VLQ4DZ
0VLQ4ZZ
0VLQ8CZ
0VLQ8DZ
0VLQ8ZZ
0VM5XZZ
0VM60ZZ
0VM64ZZ
0VM70ZZ
0VM74ZZ
0VM90ZZ
0VM94ZZ
0VMB0ZZ
0VMB4ZZ
0VMC0ZZ
0VMC4ZZ
0VMF0ZZ
0VMF4ZZ
0VMG0ZZ
0VMG4ZZ
0VMH0ZZ
0VMH4ZZ
0VMSXZZ
0VN00ZZ
0VN03ZZ
0VN04ZZ
0VN07ZZ
0VN08ZZ
0VN10ZZ
0VN13ZZ
0VN14ZZ
0VN20ZZ
0VN23ZZ
0VN24ZZ
0VN30ZZ
0VN33ZZ
0VN34ZZ
0VN50ZZ
0VN53ZZ
0VN54ZZ
0VN5XZZ
0VN60ZZ
0VN63ZZ
0VN64ZZ
0VN70ZZ
0VN73ZZ
0VN74ZZ
0VN90ZZ
0VN93ZZ
0VN94ZZ
0VNB0ZZ
0VNB3ZZ
0VNB4ZZ
0VNC0ZZ
0VNC3ZZ
0VNC4ZZ
0VNF0ZZ
0VNF3ZZ
0VNF4ZZ
0VNT0ZZ
0VNT3ZZ
0VNT4ZZ
0VNTXZZ
0VP43YZ
0VP44YZ
0VP470Z
0VP473Z
0VP47YZ
0VP480Z
0VP483Z
0VP48YZ
0VP4X0Z
0VP4X1Z
0VP4X3Z
0VP800Z
0VP803Z
0VP807Z
0VP80JZ
0VP80KZ
0VP80YZ
0VP830Z
0VP833Z
0VP837Z
0VP83JZ
0VP83KZ
0VP83YZ
0VP840Z
0VP843Z
0VP847Z
0VP84JZ
0VP84KZ
0VP84YZ
0VP870Z
0VP873Z
0VP877Z
0VP87JZ
0VP87KZ
0VP87YZ
0VP880Z
0VP883Z
0VP887Z
0VP88JZ
0VP88KZ
0VP88YZ
0VP8X0Z
0VP8X3Z
0VPD3YZ
0VPD4YZ
0VPD70Z
0VPD73Z
0VPD7YZ
0VPD80Z
0VPD83Z
0VPD8YZ
0VPDX0Z
0VPDX3Z
0VPM3YZ
0VPM4YZ
0VPM70Z
0VPM73Z
0VPM7YZ
0VPM80Z
0VPM83Z
0VPM8YZ
0VPMX0Z
0VPMX3Z
0VPR00Z
0VPR03Z
0VPR07Z
0VPR0CZ
0VPR0JZ
0VPR0KZ
0VPR0YZ
0VPR30Z
0VPR33Z
0VPR37Z
0VPR3CZ
0VPR3JZ
0VPR3KZ
0VPR3YZ
0VPR40Z
0VPR43Z
0VPR47Z
0VPR4CZ
0VPR4JZ
0VPR4KZ
0VPR4YZ
0VPR70Z
0VPR73Z
0VPR77Z
0VPR7CZ
0VPR7DZ
0VPR7JZ
0VPR7KZ
0VPR7YZ
0VPR80Z
0VPR83Z
0VPR87Z
0VPR8CZ
0VPR8DZ
0VPR8JZ
0VPR8KZ
0VPR8YZ
0VPRX0Z
0VPRX3Z
0VPRXDZ
0VPS3YZ
0VPS4YZ
0VPS70Z
0VPS73Z
0VPS7YZ
0VPS80Z
0VPS83Z
0VPS8YZ
0VPSX0Z
0VPSX3Z
0VQ50ZZ
0VQ53ZZ
0VQ54ZZ
0VQ5XZZ
0VQ60ZZ
0VQ63ZZ
0VQ64ZZ
0VQ70ZZ
0VQ73ZZ
0VQ74ZZ
0VQQ3ZZ
0VQQ4ZZ
0VQQ8ZZ
0VQS0ZZ
0VQS3ZZ
0VQS4ZZ
0VQSXZZ
0VQT0ZZ
0VQT3ZZ
0VQT4ZZ
0VQTXZZ
0VR90JZ
0VRB0JZ
0VRC0JZ
0VS90ZZ
0VS93ZZ
0VS94ZZ
0VS98ZZ
0VSB0ZZ
0VSB3ZZ
0VSB4ZZ
0VSB8ZZ
0VSC0ZZ
0VSC3ZZ
0VSC4ZZ
0VSC8ZZ
0VSF0ZZ
0VSF3ZZ
0VSF4ZZ
0VSF8ZZ
0VSG0ZZ
0VSG3ZZ
0VSG4ZZ
0VSG8ZZ
0VSH0ZZ
0VSH3ZZ
0VSH4ZZ
0VSH8ZZ
0VT00ZZ
0VT04ZZ
0VT07ZZ
0VT08ZZ
0VT10ZZ
0VT14ZZ
0VT20ZZ
0VT24ZZ
0VT30ZZ
0VT34ZZ
0VT50ZZ
0VT54ZZ
0VT5XZZ
0VT60ZZ
0VT64ZZ
0VT70ZZ
0VT74ZZ
0VT90ZZ
0VT94ZZ
0VTB0ZZ
0VTB4ZZ
0VTC0ZZ
0VTC4ZZ
0VTF0ZZ
0VTF4ZZ
0VTG0ZZ
0VTG4ZZ
0VTH0ZZ
0VTH4ZZ
0VTJ0ZZ
0VTJ4ZZ
0VTK0ZZ
0VTK4ZZ
0VTL0ZZ
0VTL4ZZ
0VTN0ZZ
0VTN4ZZ
0VTP0ZZ
0VTP4ZZ
0VTQ0ZZ
0VTQ4ZZ
0VTS0ZZ
0VTS4ZZ
0VTSXZZ
0VTT0ZZ
0VTT4ZZ
0VTTXZZ
0VU107Z
0VU10JZ
0VU10KZ
0VU147Z
0VU14JZ
0VU14KZ
0VU187Z
0VU18JZ
0VU18KZ
0VU207Z
0VU20JZ
0VU20KZ
0VU247Z
0VU24JZ
0VU24KZ
0VU287Z
0VU28JZ
0VU28KZ
0VU307Z
0VU30JZ
0VU30KZ
0VU347Z
0VU34JZ
0VU34KZ
0VU387Z
0VU38JZ
0VU38KZ
0VU507Z
0VU50JZ
0VU50KZ
0VU547Z
0VU54JZ
0VU54KZ
0VU5X7Z
0VU5XJZ
0VU5XKZ
0VU607Z
0VU60JZ
0VU60KZ
0VU647Z
0VU64JZ
0VU64KZ
0VU687Z
0VU68JZ
0VU68KZ
0VU707Z
0VU70JZ
0VU70KZ
0VU747Z
0VU74JZ
0VU74KZ
0VU787Z
0VU78JZ
0VU78KZ
0VU907Z
0VU90JZ
0VU90KZ
0VUB07Z
0VUB0JZ
0VUB0KZ
0VUC07Z
0VUC0JZ
0VUC0KZ
0VUF07Z
0VUF0JZ
0VUF0KZ
0VUF47Z
0VUF4JZ
0VUF4KZ
0VUF87Z
0VUF8JZ
0VUF8KZ
0VUG07Z
0VUG0JZ
0VUG0KZ
0VUG47Z
0VUG4JZ
0VUG4KZ
0VUG87Z
0VUG8JZ
0VUG8KZ
0VUH07Z
0VUH0JZ
0VUH0KZ
0VUH47Z
0VUH4JZ
0VUH4KZ
0VUH87Z
0VUH8JZ
0VUH8KZ
0VUJ07Z
0VUJ0JZ
0VUJ0KZ
0VUJ47Z
0VUJ4JZ
0VUJ4KZ
0VUJ87Z
0VUJ8JZ
0VUJ8KZ
0VUK07Z
0VUK0JZ
0VUK0KZ
0VUK47Z
0VUK4JZ
0VUK4KZ
0VUK87Z
0VUK8JZ
0VUK8KZ
0VUL07Z
0VUL0JZ
0VUL0KZ
0VUL47Z
0VUL4JZ
0VUL4KZ
0VUL87Z
0VUL8JZ
0VUL8KZ
0VUN07Z
0VUN0JZ
0VUN0KZ
0VUN47Z
0VUN4JZ
0VUN4KZ
0VUN87Z
0VUN8JZ
0VUN8KZ
0VUP07Z
0VUP0JZ
0VUP0KZ
0VUP47Z
0VUP4JZ
0VUP4KZ
0VUP87Z
0VUP8JZ
0VUP8KZ
0VUQ07Z
0VUQ0JZ
0VUQ0KZ
0VUQ47Z
0VUQ4JZ
0VUQ4KZ
0VUQ87Z
0VUQ8JZ
0VUQ8KZ
0VUS07Z
0VUS0JZ
0VUS0KZ
0VUS47Z
0VUS4JZ
0VUS4KZ
0VUSX7Z
0VUSXJZ
0VUSXKZ
0VUT07Z
0VUT0JZ
0VUT0KZ
0VUT47Z
0VUT4JZ
0VUT4KZ
0VUTX7Z
0VUTXJZ
0VUTXKZ
0VW400Z
0VW403Z
0VW407Z
0VW40JZ
0VW40KZ
0VW40YZ
0VW430Z
0VW433Z
0VW437Z
0VW43JZ
0VW43KZ
0VW43YZ
0VW440Z
0VW443Z
0VW447Z
0VW44JZ
0VW44KZ
0VW44YZ
0VW470Z
0VW473Z
0VW477Z
0VW47JZ
0VW47KZ
0VW47YZ
0VW480Z
0VW483Z
0VW487Z
0VW48JZ
0VW48KZ
0VW48YZ
0VW4X0Z
0VW4X3Z
0VW4X7Z
0VW4XJZ
0VW4XKZ
0VW800Z
0VW803Z
0VW807Z
0VW80JZ
0VW80KZ
0VW80YZ
0VW830Z
0VW833Z
0VW837Z
0VW83JZ
0VW83KZ
0VW83YZ
0VW840Z
0VW843Z
0VW847Z
0VW84JZ
0VW84KZ
0VW84YZ
0VW870Z
0VW873Z
0VW877Z
0VW87JZ
0VW87KZ
0VW87YZ
0VW880Z
0VW883Z
0VW887Z
0VW88JZ
0VW88KZ
0VW88YZ
0VW8X0Z
0VW8X3Z
0VW8X7Z
0VW8XJZ
0VW8XKZ
0VWD00Z
0VWD03Z
0VWD07Z
0VWD0JZ
0VWD0KZ
0VWD0YZ
0VWD30Z
0VWD33Z
0VWD37Z
0VWD3JZ
0VWD3KZ
0VWD3YZ
0VWD40Z
0VWD43Z
0VWD47Z
0VWD4JZ
0VWD4KZ
0VWD4YZ
0VWD70Z
0VWD73Z
0VWD77Z
0VWD7JZ
0VWD7KZ
0VWD7YZ
0VWD80Z
0VWD83Z
0VWD87Z
0VWD8JZ
0VWD8KZ
0VWD8YZ
0VWDX0Z
0VWDX3Z
0VWDX7Z
0VWDXJZ
0VWDXKZ
0VWM00Z
0VWM03Z
0VWM07Z
0VWM0CZ
0VWM0JZ
0VWM0KZ
0VWM0YZ
0VWM30Z
0VWM33Z
0VWM37Z
0VWM3CZ
0VWM3JZ
0VWM3KZ
0VWM3YZ
0VWM40Z
0VWM43Z
0VWM47Z
0VWM4CZ
0VWM4JZ
0VWM4KZ
0VWM4YZ
0VWM70Z
0VWM73Z
0VWM77Z

0VWM7CZ
0VWM7JZ
0VWM7KZ
0VWM7YZ
0VWM80Z
0VWM83Z
0VWM87Z
0VWM8CZ
0VWM8JZ
0VWM8KZ
0VWM8YZ
0VWMX0Z
0VWMX3Z
0VWMX7Z
0VWMXCZ
0VWMXJZ
0VWMXKZ
0VWR00Z
0VWR03Z
0VWR07Z
0VWR0CZ
0VWR0DZ
0VWR0JZ
0VWR0KZ
0VWR0YZ
0VWR30Z
0VWR33Z
0VWR37Z
0VWR3CZ
0VWR3DZ
0VWR3JZ
0VWR3KZ
0VWR3YZ
0VWR40Z
0VWR43Z
0VWR47Z
0VWR4CZ
0VWR4DZ
0VWR4JZ
0VWR4KZ
0VWR4YZ
0VWR70Z
0VWR73Z
0VWR77Z
0VWR7CZ
0VWR7DZ
0VWR7JZ
0VWR7KZ
0VWR7YZ
0VWR80Z
0VWR83Z
0VWR87Z
0VWR8CZ
0VWR8DZ
0VWR8JZ
0VWR8KZ
0VWR8YZ
0VWRX0Z
0VWRX3Z
0VWRX7Z
0VWRXCZ
0VWRXDZ
0VWRXJZ
0VWRXKZ
0VWS00Z
0VWS03Z
0VWS07Z
0VWS0JZ
0VWS0KZ
0VWS0YZ
0VWS30Z
0VWS33Z
0VWS37Z
0VWS3JZ
0VWS3KZ
0VWS3YZ
0VWS40Z
0VWS43Z
0VWS47Z
0VWS4JZ
0VWS4KZ
0VWS4YZ
0VWS70Z
0VWS73Z
0VWS77Z
0VWS7JZ
0VWS7KZ
0VWS7YZ
0VWS80Z
0VWS83Z
0VWS87Z
0VWS8JZ
0VWS8KZ
0VWS8YZ
0VWSX0Z
0VWSX3Z
0VWSX7Z
0VWSXJZ
0VWSXKZ
0VXT0ZD
0VXT0ZS
0VXTXZD
0VXTXZS
0W0007Z
0W000JZ
0W000KZ
0W000ZZ
0W0037Z
0W003JZ
0W003KZ
0W003ZZ
0W0047Z
0W004JZ
0W004KZ
0W004ZZ
0W0207Z
0W020JZ
0W020KZ
0W020ZZ
0W0237Z
0W023JZ
0W023KZ
0W023ZZ
0W0247Z
0W024JZ
0W024KZ
0W190J4
0W190JG
0W190JW
0W190JY
0W193J4
0W193J9
0W193JB
0W193JG
0W193JJ
0W193JW
0W193JY
0W194J4
0W194JG
0W194JW
0W194JY
0W1B0J4
0W1B0JG
0W1B0JW
0W1B0JY
0W1B3J4
0W1B3J9
0W1B3JB
0W1B3JG
0W1B3JJ
0W1B3JW
0W1B3JY
0W1B4J4
0W1B4JG
0W1B4JW
0W1B4JY
0W1G0J9
0W1G0JB
0W1G0JG
0W1G0JJ
0W1G0JW
0W1G3J9
0W1G3JB
0W1G3JG
0W1G3JJ
0W1G3JW
0W1G3JY
0W1G4J4
0W1G4J9
0W1G4JB
0W1G4JG
0W1G4JJ
0W1G4JW
0W1G4JY
0W1J0J4
0W1J0J9
0W1J0JB
0W1J0JG
0W1J0JJ
0W1J0JW
0W1J0JY
0W1J3J4
0W1J3J9
0W1J3JB
0W1J3JG
0W1J3JJ
0W1J3JW
0W1J3JY
0W1J4J4
0W1J4J9
0W1J4JB
0W1J4JG
0W1J4JJ
0W1J4JW
0W1J4JY
0W20X0Z
0W20XYZ
0W21X0Z
0W21XYZ
0W22X0Z
0W22XYZ
0W24X0Z
0W24XYZ
0W25X0Z
0W25XYZ
0W26X0Z
0W26XYZ
0W28X0Z
0W28XYZ
0W29X0Z
0W29XYZ
0W2BX0Z
0W2BXYZ
0W2CX0Z
0W2CXYZ
0W2DX0Z
0W2DXYZ
0W2FX0Z
0W2FXYZ
0W2GX0Z
0W2GXYZ
0W2HX0Z
0W2HXYZ
0W2JX0Z
0W2JXYZ
0W2KX0Z
0W2KXYZ
0W2LX0Z
0W2LXYZ
0W2MX0Z
0W2MXYZ
0W2NX0Z
0W2NXYZ
0W300ZZ
0W303ZZ
0W304ZZ
0W310ZZ
0W313ZZ
0W314ZZ
0W320ZZ
0W323ZZ
0W324ZZ
0W330ZZ
0W333ZZ
0W334ZZ
0W337ZZ
0W338ZZ
0W33XZZ
0W340ZZ
0W343ZZ
0W344ZZ
0W350ZZ
0W353ZZ
0W354ZZ
0W360ZZ
0W363ZZ
0W364ZZ
0W380ZZ
0W383ZZ
0W384ZZ
0W390ZZ
0W393ZZ
0W394ZZ
0W3B0ZZ
0W3B3ZZ
0W3B4ZZ
0W3C0ZZ
0W3C3ZZ
0W3C4ZZ
0W3D0ZZ
0W3D3ZZ
0W3D4ZZ
0W3F0ZZ
0W3F3ZZ
0W3F4ZZ
0W3G0ZZ
0W3G3ZZ
0W3G4ZZ
0W3H0ZZ
0W3H3ZZ
0W3H4ZZ
0W3J0ZZ
0W3J3ZZ
0W3J4ZZ
0W3K0ZZ
0W3K3ZZ
0W3K4ZZ
0W3L0ZZ
0W3L3ZZ
0W3L4ZZ
0W3M0ZZ
0W3M3ZZ
0W3M4ZZ
0W3N0ZZ
0W3N3ZZ
0W3N4ZZ
0W3P0ZZ
0W3P3ZZ
0W3P4ZZ
0W3P7ZZ
0W3P8ZZ
0W3Q0ZZ
0W3Q3ZZ
0W3Q4ZZ
0W3Q7ZZ
0W3Q8ZZ
0W3R0ZZ
0W3R3ZZ
0W3R4ZZ
0W3R7ZZ
0W3R8ZZ
0W4M070
0W4M0J0
0W4M0K0
0W4N071
0W4N0J1
0W4N0K1
0W8NXZZ
0W9000Z
0W900ZX
0W900ZZ
0W9030Z
0W903ZX
0W903ZZ
0W9040Z
0W904ZX
0W904ZZ
0W9100Z
0W910ZX
0W910ZZ
0W9130Z
0W913ZX
0W913ZZ
0W9140Z
0W914ZX
0W914ZZ
0W9200Z
0W920ZX
0W920ZZ
0W9230Z
0W923ZX
0W923ZZ
0W9240Z
0W924ZX
0W924ZZ
0W9300Z
0W930ZX
0W930ZZ
0W9330Z
0W933ZX
0W933ZZ
0W9340Z
0W934ZX
0W934ZZ
0W9400Z
0W940ZX
0W940ZZ
0W9430Z
0W943ZX
0W943ZZ
0W9440Z
0W944ZX
0W944ZZ
0W9500Z
0W950ZX
0W950ZZ
0W9530Z
0W953ZX
0W953ZZ
0W9540Z
0W954ZX
0W954ZZ
0W9600Z
0W960ZX
0W960ZZ
0W9630Z
0W963ZX
0W963ZZ
0W9640Z
0W964ZX
0W964ZZ
0W9800Z
0W980ZX
0W980ZZ
0W9830Z
0W983ZX
0W983ZZ
0W9840Z
0W984ZX
0W984ZZ
0W9900Z
0W990ZX
0W990ZZ
0W9930Z
0W993ZX
0W993ZZ
0W9940Z
0W994ZX
0W994ZZ
0W9B00Z
0W9B0ZX
0W9B0ZZ
0W9B30Z
0W9B3ZX
0W9B3ZZ
0W9B40Z
0W9B4ZX
0W9B4ZZ
0W9C00Z
0W9C0ZX
0W9C0ZZ
0W9C30Z
0W9C3ZX
0W9C3ZZ
0W9C40Z
0W9C4ZX
0W9C4ZZ
0W9D00Z
0W9D0ZX
0W9D0ZZ
0W9D30Z
0W9D3ZX
0W9D3ZZ
0W9D40Z
0W9D4ZX
0W9D4ZZ
0W9F00Z
0W9F0ZX
0W9F0ZZ
0W9F30Z
0W9F3ZX
0W9F3ZZ
0W9F40Z
0W9F4ZX
0W9F4ZZ
0W9G00Z
0W9G0ZX
0W9G0ZZ
0W9G30Z
0W9G3ZX
0W9G3ZZ
0W9G40Z
0W9G4ZX
0W9G4ZZ
0W9H00Z
0W9H0ZX
0W9H30Z
0W9H3ZZ
0W9J30Z
0W9J3ZZ
0W9K00Z
0W9K0ZX
0W9K0ZZ
0W9K30Z
0W9K3ZX
0W9K3ZZ
0W9K40Z
0W9K4ZX
0W9K4ZZ
0W9L00Z
0W9L0ZX
0W9L0ZZ
0W9L30Z
0W9L3ZX
0W9L3ZZ
0W9L40Z
0W9L4ZX
0W9L4ZZ
0W9M00Z
0W9M0ZX
0W9M0ZZ
0W9M30Z
0W9M3ZX
0W9M3ZZ
0W9M40Z
0W9M4ZX
0W9M4ZZ
0W9N0ZX
0W9N30Z
0W9N3ZX
0W9N3ZZ
0W9N4ZX
0WB00ZX
0WB03ZX
0WB04ZX
0WB0XZX
0WB20ZX
0WB23ZX
0WB24ZX
0WB2XZX
0WB40ZX
0WB43ZX
0WB44ZX
0WB4XZX
0WB50ZX
0WB53ZX
0WB54ZX
0WB5XZX
0WB60ZX
0WB63ZX
0WB64ZX
0WB6XZX
0WB80ZX
0WB83ZX
0WB84ZX
0WB8XZX
0WBC3ZX
0WBC4ZX
0WBH3ZX
0WBH4ZX
0WBK0ZX
0WBK3ZX
0WBK4ZX
0WBKXZX
0WBKXZZ
0WBL0ZX
0WBL0ZZ
0WBL3ZX
0WBL3ZZ
0WBL4ZX
0WBL4ZZ
0WBLXZX
0WBLXZZ
0WBM0ZX
0WBM0ZZ
0WBM3ZX
0WBM3ZZ
0WBM4ZX
0WBM4ZZ
0WBMXZX
0WBMXZZ
0WBN0ZX
0WBN0ZZ
0WBN3ZX
0WBN3ZZ
0WBN4ZX
0WBN4ZZ
0WBNXZX
0WBNXZZ
0WC10ZZ
0WC13ZZ
0WC14ZZ
0WC1XZZ
0WC30ZZ
0WC33ZZ
0WC34ZZ
0WC3XZZ
0WC90ZZ
0WC93ZZ
0WC94ZZ
0WC9XZZ
0WCB0ZZ
0WCB3ZZ
0WCB4ZZ
0WCBXZZ
0WCC0ZZ
0WCC3ZZ
0WCC4ZZ
0WCCXZZ
0WCD0ZZ
0WCD3ZZ
0WCD4ZZ
0WCDXZZ
0WCG0ZZ
0WCG3ZZ
0WCG4ZZ
0WCGXZZ
0WCH0ZZ
0WCH3ZZ
0WCH4ZZ
0WCHXZZ
0WCJ0ZZ
0WCJ3ZZ
0WCJ4ZZ
0WCJXZZ
0WCP0ZZ
0WCP3ZZ
0WCP4ZZ
0WCP7ZZ
0WCP8ZZ
0WCPXZZ
0WCQ0ZZ
0WCQ3ZZ
0WCQ4ZZ
0WCQ7ZZ
0WCQ8ZZ
0WCQXZZ
0WCR0ZZ
0WCR3ZZ
0WCR4ZZ
0WCR7ZZ
0WCR8ZZ
0WCRXZZ
0WF10ZZ
0WF13ZZ
0WF14ZZ
0WF1XZZ
0WF30ZZ
0WF33ZZ
0WF34ZZ
0WF3XZZ
0WF90ZZ
0WF93ZZ
0WF94ZZ
0WF9XZZ
0WFB0ZZ
0WFB3ZZ
0WFB4ZZ
0WFBXZZ
0WFC0ZZ
0WFC3ZZ
0WFC4ZZ
0WFCXZZ
0WFD0ZZ
0WFD3ZZ
0WFD4ZZ
0WFDXZZ
0WFG0ZZ
0WFG3ZZ
0WFG4ZZ
0WFGXZZ
0WFJ0ZZ
0WFJ3ZZ
0WFJ4ZZ
0WFJXZZ
0WFP0ZZ
0WFP3ZZ
0WFP4ZZ
0WFP7ZZ
0WFP8ZZ
0WFPXZZ
0WFQ0ZZ
0WFQ3ZZ
0WFQ4ZZ
0WFQ7ZZ
0WFQ8ZZ
0WFQXZZ
0WFR0ZZ
0WFR3ZZ
0WFR4ZZ
0WFR7ZZ
0WFR8ZZ
0WFRXZZ
0WH001Z
0WH003Z
0WH00YZ
0WH031Z
0WH033Z
0WH03YZ
0WH041Z
0WH043Z
0WH04YZ
0WH101Z
0WH103Z
0WH10YZ
0WH131Z
0WH133Z
0WH13YZ
0WH141Z
0WH143Z
0WH14YZ
0WH201Z
0WH203Z
0WH20YZ
0WH231Z
0WH233Z
0WH23YZ
0WH241Z
0WH243Z
0WH24YZ
0WH301Z
0WH303Z
0WH30YZ
0WH331Z
0WH333Z
0WH33YZ
0WH341Z
0WH343Z
0WH34YZ
0WH401Z
0WH403Z
0WH40YZ
0WH431Z
0WH433Z
0WH43YZ
0WH441Z
0WH443Z
0WH44YZ
0WH501Z
0WH503Z
0WH50YZ
0WH531Z
0WH533Z
0WH53YZ
0WH541Z
0WH543Z
0WH54YZ
0WH601Z
0WH603Z
0WH60YZ
0WH631Z
0WH633Z
0WH63YZ
0WH641Z
0WH643Z
0WH64YZ
0WH801Z
0WH803Z
0WH80YZ
0WH831Z
0WH833Z
0WH83YZ
0WH841Z
0WH843Z
0WH84YZ
0WH901Z
0WH903Z
0WH90YZ
0WH931Z
0WH933Z
0WH93YZ
0WH941Z
0WH943Z
0WH94YZ
0WHB01Z
0WHB03Z

0WHB0YZ-0WUL4JZ

0WHB0YZ
0WHB31Z
0WHB33Z
0WHB3YZ
0WHB41Z
0WHB43Z
0WHB4YZ
0WHC01Z
0WHC03Z
0WHC0YZ
0WHC31Z
0WHC33Z
0WHC3YZ
0WHC41Z
0WHC43Z
0WHC4YZ
0WHD01Z
0WHD03Z
0WHD0YZ
0WHD31Z
0WHD33Z
0WHD3YZ
0WHD41Z
0WHD43Z
0WHD4YZ
0WHF01Z
0WHF03Z
0WHF0YZ
0WHF31Z
0WHF33Z
0WHF3YZ
0WHF41Z
0WHF43Z
0WHF4YZ
0WHG01Z
0WHG03Z
0WHG0YZ
0WHG31Z
0WHG33Z
0WHG3YZ
0WHG41Z
0WHG43Z
0WHG4YZ
0WHH01Z
0WHH03Z
0WHH0YZ
0WHH31Z
0WHH33Z
0WHH3YZ
0WHH41Z
0WHH43Z
0WHH4YZ
0WHJ01Z
0WHJ03Z
0WHJ0YZ
0WHJ31Z
0WHJ33Z
0WHJ3YZ
0WHJ41Z
0WHJ43Z
0WHJ4YZ
0WHK01Z
0WHK03Z
0WHK0YZ
0WHK31Z
0WHK33Z
0WHK3YZ
0WHK41Z
0WHK43Z
0WHK4YZ
0WHL01Z
0WHL03Z
0WHL0YZ
0WHL31Z
0WHL33Z
0WHL3YZ
0WHL41Z
0WHL43Z
0WHL4YZ
0WHM01Z
0WHM03Z
0WHM0YZ
0WHM31Z
0WHM33Z
0WHM3YZ
0WHM41Z
0WHM43Z
0WHM4YZ
0WHN01Z
0WHN03Z
0WHN0YZ
0WHN31Z
0WHN33Z
0WHN3YZ
0WHN41Z
0WHN43Z
0WHN4YZ
0WHP01Z
0WHP03Z
0WHP0YZ
0WHP31Z
0WHP33Z
0WHP3YZ
0WHP41Z
0WHP43Z
0WHP4YZ
0WHP71Z
0WHP73Z
0WHP7YZ
0WHP81Z
0WHP83Z
0WHP8YZ
0WHQ01Z
0WHQ03Z
0WHQ0YZ
0WHQ31Z
0WHQ33Z
0WHQ3YZ
0WHQ41Z
0WHQ43Z
0WHQ4YZ
0WHQ71Z
0WHQ73Z
0WHQ7YZ
0WHQ81Z
0WHQ83Z
0WHQ8YZ
0WHR01Z
0WHR03Z
0WHR0YZ
0WHR31Z
0WHR33Z
0WHR3YZ
0WHR41Z
0WHR43Z
0WHR4YZ
0WHR71Z
0WHR73Z
0WHR7YZ
0WHR81Z
0WHR83Z
0WHR8YZ
0WJ00ZZ
0WJ03ZZ
0WJ04ZZ
0WJ0XZZ
0WJ10ZZ
0WJ13ZZ
0WJ14ZZ
0WJ20ZZ
0WJ23ZZ
0WJ24ZZ
0WJ2XZZ
0WJ30ZZ
0WJ33ZZ
0WJ34ZZ
0WJ3XZZ
0WJ40ZZ
0WJ43ZZ
0WJ44ZZ
0WJ4XZZ
0WJ50ZZ
0WJ53ZZ
0WJ54ZZ
0WJ5XZZ
0WJ60ZZ
0WJ63ZZ
0WJ64ZZ
0WJ6XZZ
0WJ80ZZ
0WJ83ZZ
0WJ84ZZ
0WJ8XZZ
0WJ90ZZ
0WJ93ZZ
0WJ94ZZ
0WJB0ZZ
0WJB3ZZ
0WJB4ZZ
0WJC0ZZ
0WJC3ZZ
0WJC4ZZ
0WJD0ZZ
0WJD3ZZ
0WJD4ZZ
0WJF0ZZ
0WJF3ZZ
0WJF4ZZ
0WJFXZZ
0WJG0ZZ
0WJG3ZZ
0WJG4ZZ
0WJH0ZZ
0WJH3ZZ
0WJJ3ZZ
0WJK3ZZ
0WJK4ZZ
0WJKXZZ
0WJL3ZZ
0WJL4ZZ
0WJLXZZ
0WJM3ZZ
0WJMXZZ
0WJN3ZZ
0WJNXZZ
0WJP3ZZ
0WJP7ZZ
0WJP8ZZ
0WJQ3ZZ
0WJQ7ZZ
0WJQ8ZZ
0WJR3ZZ
0WJR7ZZ
0WJR8ZZ
0WP000Z
0WP001Z
0WP003Z
0WP007Z
0WP00JZ
0WP00KZ
0WP00YZ
0WP030Z
0WP031Z
0WP033Z
0WP037Z
0WP03JZ
0WP03KZ
0WP03YZ
0WP040Z
0WP041Z
0WP043Z
0WP047Z
0WP04JZ
0WP04KZ
0WP04YZ
0WP0X0Z
0WP0X1Z
0WP0X3Z
0WP0X7Z
0WP0XJZ
0WP0XKZ
0WP0XYZ
0WP103Z
0WP133Z
0WP143Z
0WP1X0Z
0WP1X1Z
0WP1X3Z
0WP200Z
0WP201Z
0WP203Z
0WP207Z
0WP20JZ
0WP20KZ
0WP20YZ
0WP230Z
0WP231Z
0WP233Z
0WP237Z
0WP23JZ
0WP23KZ
0WP23YZ
0WP240Z
0WP241Z
0WP243Z
0WP247Z
0WP24JZ
0WP24KZ
0WP24YZ
0WP2X0Z
0WP2X1Z
0WP2X3Z
0WP2X7Z
0WP2XJZ
0WP2XKZ
0WP2XYZ
0WP400Z
0WP401Z
0WP403Z
0WP407Z
0WP40JZ
0WP40KZ
0WP40YZ
0WP430Z
0WP431Z
0WP433Z
0WP437Z
0WP43JZ
0WP43KZ
0WP43YZ
0WP440Z
0WP441Z
0WP443Z
0WP447Z
0WP44JZ
0WP44KZ
0WP44YZ
0WP4X0Z
0WP4X1Z
0WP4X3Z
0WP4X7Z
0WP4XJZ
0WP4XKZ
0WP4XYZ
0WP500Z
0WP501Z
0WP503Z
0WP507Z
0WP50JZ
0WP50KZ
0WP50YZ
0WP530Z
0WP531Z
0WP533Z
0WP537Z
0WP53JZ
0WP53KZ
0WP53YZ
0WP540Z
0WP541Z
0WP543Z
0WP547Z
0WP54JZ
0WP54KZ
0WP54YZ
0WP5X0Z
0WP5X1Z
0WP5X3Z
0WP5X7Z
0WP5XJZ
0WP5XKZ
0WP5XYZ
0WP600Z
0WP601Z
0WP603Z
0WP607Z
0WP60JZ
0WP60KZ
0WP60YZ
0WP630Z
0WP631Z
0WP633Z
0WP637Z
0WP63JZ
0WP63KZ
0WP63YZ
0WP640Z
0WP641Z
0WP643Z
0WP647Z
0WP64JZ
0WP64KZ
0WP64YZ
0WP6X0Z
0WP6X1Z
0WP6X3Z
0WP6X7Z
0WP6XJZ
0WP6XKZ
0WP6XYZ
0WP800Z
0WP801Z
0WP803Z
0WP807Z
0WP80JZ
0WP80KZ
0WP80YZ
0WP830Z
0WP831Z
0WP833Z
0WP837Z
0WP83JZ
0WP83KZ
0WP83YZ
0WP840Z
0WP841Z
0WP843Z
0WP847Z
0WP84JZ
0WP84KZ
0WP84YZ
0WP8X0Z
0WP8X1Z
0WP8X3Z
0WP8X7Z
0WP8XJZ
0WP8XKZ
0WP8XYZ
0WP900Z
0WP901Z
0WP903Z
0WP90JZ
0WP90YZ
0WP930Z
0WP931Z
0WP933Z
0WP93JZ
0WP93YZ
0WP940Z
0WP941Z
0WP943Z
0WP94JZ
0WP94YZ
0WP9X0Z
0WP9X1Z
0WP9X3Z
0WPB00Z
0WPB01Z
0WPB03Z
0WPB0JZ
0WPB0YZ
0WPB30Z
0WPB31Z
0WPB33Z
0WPB3JZ
0WPB3YZ
0WPB40Z
0WPB41Z
0WPB43Z
0WPB4JZ
0WPB4YZ
0WPBX0Z
0WPBX1Z
0WPBX3Z
0WPCX0Z
0WPCX1Z
0WPCX3Z
0WPCX7Z
0WPCXJZ
0WPCXKZ
0WPCXYZ
0WPDX0Z
0WPDX1Z
0WPDX3Z
0WPFX0Z
0WPFX1Z
0WPFX3Z
0WPFX7Z
0WPFXJZ
0WPFXKZ
0WPFXYZ
0WPGX0Z
0WPGX1Z
0WPGX3Z
0WPHX0Z
0WPHX1Z
0WPHX3Z
0WPJ00Z
0WPJ01Z
0WPJ03Z
0WPJ0JZ
0WPJ0YZ
0WPJ30Z
0WPJ31Z
0WPJ33Z
0WPJ3JZ
0WPJ3YZ
0WPJ40Z
0WPJ41Z
0WPJ43Z
0WPJ4JZ
0WPJ4YZ
0WPJX0Z
0WPJX1Z
0WPJX3Z
0WPK00Z
0WPK01Z
0WPK03Z
0WPK07Z
0WPK0JZ
0WPK0KZ
0WPK0YZ
0WPK30Z
0WPK31Z
0WPK33Z
0WPK37Z
0WPK3JZ
0WPK3KZ
0WPK3YZ
0WPK40Z
0WPK41Z
0WPK43Z
0WPK47Z
0WPK4JZ
0WPK4KZ
0WPK4YZ
0WPKX0Z
0WPKX1Z
0WPKX3Z
0WPKX7Z
0WPKXJZ
0WPKXKZ
0WPKXYZ
0WPL00Z
0WPL01Z
0WPL03Z
0WPL07Z
0WPL0JZ
0WPL0KZ
0WPL0YZ
0WPL30Z
0WPL31Z
0WPL33Z
0WPL37Z
0WPL3JZ
0WPL3KZ
0WPL3YZ
0WPL40Z
0WPL41Z
0WPL43Z
0WPL47Z
0WPL4JZ
0WPL4KZ
0WPL4YZ
0WPLX0Z
0WPLX1Z
0WPLX3Z
0WPLX7Z
0WPLXJZ
0WPLXKZ
0WPLXYZ
0WPM00Z
0WPM01Z
0WPM03Z
0WPM0JZ
0WPM0YZ
0WPM30Z
0WPM31Z
0WPM33Z
0WPM3JZ
0WPM3YZ
0WPM40Z
0WPM41Z
0WPM43Z
0WPM4JZ
0WPM4YZ
0WPMX0Z
0WPMX1Z
0WPMX3Z
0WPMXYZ
0WPN31Z
0WPN33Z
0WPN37Z
0WPN3JZ
0WPN3KZ
0WPN3YZ
0WPN40Z
0WPN41Z
0WPN43Z
0WPN47Z
0WPN4JZ
0WPN4KZ
0WPN4YZ
0WPNX0Z
0WPNX1Z
0WPNX3Z
0WPNX7Z
0WPNXJZ
0WPNXKZ
0WPNXYZ
0WPP01Z
0WPP03Z
0WPP0YZ
0WPP31Z
0WPP33Z
0WPP3YZ
0WPP41Z
0WPP43Z
0WPP4YZ
0WPP71Z
0WPP73Z
0WPP7YZ
0WPP81Z
0WPP83Z
0WPP8YZ
0WPPX1Z
0WPPX3Z
0WPPXYZ
0WPQ01Z
0WPQ03Z
0WPQ0YZ
0WPQ31Z
0WPQ33Z
0WPQ3YZ
0WPQ41Z
0WPQ43Z
0WPQ4YZ
0WPQ71Z
0WPQ73Z
0WPQ7YZ
0WPQ81Z
0WPQ83Z
0WPQ8YZ
0WPQX1Z
0WPQX3Z
0WPQXYZ
0WPR01Z
0WPR03Z
0WPR0YZ
0WPR31Z
0WPR33Z
0WPR3YZ
0WPR41Z
0WPR43Z
0WPR4YZ
0WPR71Z
0WPR73Z
0WPR7YZ
0WPR81Z
0WPR83Z
0WPR8YZ
0WPRX1Z
0WPRX3Z
0WPRXYZ
0WQ00ZZ
0WQ03ZZ
0WQ04ZZ
0WQ0XZZ
0WQ20ZZ
0WQ23ZZ
0WQ24ZZ
0WQ2XZZ
0WQ30ZZ
0WQ33ZZ
0WQ34ZZ
0WQ3XZZ
0WQ40ZZ
0WQ43ZZ
0WQ44ZZ
0WQ4XZZ
0WQ50ZZ
0WQ53ZZ
0WQ54ZZ
0WQ5XZZ
0WQ60ZZ
0WQ63ZZ
0WQ64ZZ
0WQ6XZ2
0WQ6XZZ
0WQ80ZZ
0WQ83ZZ
0WQ84ZZ
0WQ8XZZ
0WQC0ZZ
0WQC3ZZ
0WQC4ZZ
0WQF0ZZ
0WQF3ZZ
0WQF4ZZ
0WQFXZ2
0WQFXZZ
0WQK0ZZ
0WQK3ZZ
0WQK4ZZ
0WQKXZZ
0WQL0ZZ
0WQL3ZZ
0WQL4ZZ
0WQLXZZ
0WQM0ZZ
0WQM3ZZ
0WQM4ZZ
0WQMXZZ
0WQN0ZZ
0WQN3ZZ
0WQN4ZZ
0WQNXZZ
0WU007Z
0WU00JZ
0WU00KZ
0WU047Z
0WU04JZ
0WU04KZ
0WU207Z
0WU20JZ
0WU20KZ
0WU247Z
0WU24JZ
0WU24KZ
0WU407Z
0WU40JZ
0WU40KZ
0WU447Z
0WU44JZ
0WU44KZ
0WU507Z
0WU50JZ
0WU50KZ
0WU547Z
0WU54JZ
0WU54KZ
0WU607Z
0WU60JZ
0WU60KZ
0WU647Z
0WU64JZ
0WU64KZ
0WU807Z
0WU80JZ
0WU80KZ
0WU847Z
0WU84JZ
0WU84KZ
0WUC07Z
0WUC0JZ
0WUC0KZ
0WUC47Z
0WUC4JZ
0WUC4KZ
0WUF07Z
0WUF0JZ
0WUF0KZ
0WUF47Z
0WUF4JZ
0WUF4KZ
0WUK07Z
0WUK0JZ
0WUK0KZ
0WUK47Z
0WUK4JZ
0WUK4KZ
0WUL07Z
0WUL0JZ
0WUL0KZ
0WUL47Z
0WUL4JZ

0WUL4KZ
0WUM07Z
0WUM0JZ
0WUM0KZ
0WUM47Z
0WUM4JZ
0WUM4KZ
0WUN07Z
0WUN0JZ
0WUN0KZ
0WUN47Z
0WUN4JZ
0WUN4KZ
0WW000Z
0WW001Z
0WW003Z
0WW007Z
0WW00JZ
0WW00KZ
0WW00YZ
0WW030Z
0WW031Z
0WW033Z
0WW037Z
0WW03JZ
0WW03KZ
0WW03YZ
0WW040Z
0WW041Z
0WW043Z
0WW047Z
0WW04JZ
0WW04KZ
0WW04YZ
0WW0X0Z
0WW0X1Z
0WW0X3Z
0WW0X7Z
0WW0XJZ
0WW0XKZ
0WW0XYZ
0WW100Z
0WW101Z
0WW103Z
0WW10JZ
0WW10YZ
0WW130Z
0WW131Z
0WW133Z
0WW13JZ
0WW13YZ
0WW140Z
0WW141Z
0WW143Z
0WW14JZ
0WW14YZ
0WW1X0Z
0WW1X1Z
0WW1X3Z
0WW1XJZ
0WW1XYZ
0WW200Z
0WW201Z
0WW203Z
0WW207Z
0WW20JZ
0WW20KZ
0WW20YZ
0WW230Z
0WW231Z
0WW233Z
0WW237Z
0WW23JZ
0WW23KZ
0WW23YZ
0WW240Z
0WW241Z
0WW243Z
0WW247Z
0WW24JZ
0WW24KZ
0WW24YZ
0WW2X0Z
0WW2X1Z
0WW2X3Z
0WW2X7Z
0WW2XJZ
0WW2XKZ
0WW2XYZ
0WW400Z
0WW401Z
0WW403Z
0WW407Z
0WW40JZ
0WW40KZ
0WW40YZ
0WW430Z
0WW431Z
0WW433Z
0WW437Z
0WW43JZ
0WW43KZ
0WW43YZ
0WW440Z
0WW441Z
0WW443Z
0WW447Z
0WW44JZ
0WW44KZ
0WW44YZ
0WW4X0Z
0WW4X1Z
0WW4X3Z
0WW4X7Z
0WW4XJZ
0WW4XKZ
0WW4XYZ
0WW500Z
0WW501Z
0WW503Z
0WW507Z
0WW50JZ
0WW50KZ
0WW50YZ
0WW530Z
0WW531Z
0WW533Z
0WW537Z
0WW53JZ
0WW53KZ
0WW53YZ
0WW540Z
0WW541Z
0WW543Z
0WW547Z
0WW54JZ
0WW54KZ
0WW54YZ
0WW5X0Z
0WW5X1Z
0WW5X3Z
0WW5X7Z
0WW5XJZ
0WW5XKZ
0WW5XYZ
0WW600Z
0WW601Z
0WW603Z
0WW607Z
0WW60JZ
0WW60KZ
0WW60YZ
0WW630Z
0WW631Z
0WW633Z
0WW637Z
0WW63JZ
0WW63KZ
0WW63YZ
0WW640Z
0WW641Z
0WW643Z
0WW647Z
0WW64JZ
0WW64KZ
0WW64YZ
0WW6X0Z
0WW6X1Z
0WW6X3Z
0WW6X7Z
0WW6XJZ
0WW6XKZ
0WW6XYZ
0WW800Z
0WW801Z
0WW803Z
0WW807Z
0WW80JZ
0WW80KZ
0WW80YZ
0WW830Z
0WW831Z
0WW833Z
0WW837Z
0WW83JZ
0WW83KZ
0WW83YZ
0WW840Z
0WW841Z
0WW843Z
0WW847Z
0WW84JZ
0WW84KZ
0WW84YZ
0WW8X0Z
0WW8X1Z
0WW8X3Z
0WW8X7Z
0WW8XJZ
0WW8XKZ
0WW8XYZ
0WW900Z
0WW901Z
0WW903Z
0WW90JZ
0WW90YZ
0WW930Z
0WW931Z
0WW933Z
0WW93JZ
0WW93YZ
0WW940Z
0WW941Z
0WW943Z
0WW94JZ
0WW94YZ
0WW9X0Z
0WW9X1Z
0WW9X3Z
0WW9XJZ
0WW9XYZ
0WWB00Z
0WWB01Z
0WWB03Z
0WWB0JZ
0WWB0YZ
0WWB30Z
0WWB31Z
0WWB33Z
0WWB3JZ
0WWB3YZ
0WWB40Z
0WWB41Z
0WWB43Z
0WWB4JZ
0WWB4YZ
0WWBX0Z
0WWBX1Z
0WWBX3Z
0WWBXJZ
0WWBXYZ
0WWC00Z
0WWC01Z
0WWC03Z
0WWC07Z
0WWC0JZ
0WWC0KZ
0WWC0YZ
0WWC30Z
0WWC31Z
0WWC33Z
0WWC37Z
0WWC3JZ
0WWC3KZ
0WWC3YZ
0WWC40Z
0WWC41Z
0WWC43Z
0WWC47Z
0WWC4JZ
0WWC4KZ
0WWC4YZ
0WWCX0Z
0WWCX1Z
0WWCX3Z
0WWCX7Z
0WWCXJZ
0WWCXKZ
0WWCXYZ
0WWD00Z
0WWD01Z
0WWD03Z
0WWD0YZ
0WWD30Z
0WWD31Z
0WWD33Z
0WWD3YZ
0WWD40Z
0WWD41Z
0WWD43Z
0WWD4YZ
0WWDX0Z
0WWDX1Z
0WWDX3Z
0WWDXYZ
0WWF00Z
0WWF01Z
0WWF03Z
0WWF07Z
0WWF0JZ
0WWF0KZ
0WWF0YZ
0WWF30Z
0WWF31Z
0WWF33Z
0WWF37Z
0WWF3JZ
0WWF3KZ
0WWF3YZ
0WWF40Z
0WWF41Z
0WWF43Z
0WWF47Z
0WWF4JZ
0WWF4KZ
0WWFX0Z
0WWFX1Z
0WWFX3Z
0WWFX7Z
0WWFXJZ
0WWFXKZ
0WWFXYZ
0WWGX0Z
0WWGX1Z
0WWGX3Z
0WWGXJZ
0WWGXYZ
0WWHX0Z
0WWHX1Z
0WWHX3Z
0WWHXYZ
0WWJX0Z
0WWJX1Z
0WWJX3Z
0WWJXJZ
0WWJXYZ
0WWKX0Z
0WWKX1Z
0WWKX3Z
0WWKX7Z
0WWKXJZ
0WWKXKZ
0WWKXYZ
0WWLX0Z
0WWLX1Z
0WWLX3Z
0WWLX7Z
0WWLXJZ
0WWLXKZ
0WWLXYZ
0WWMX0Z
0WWMX1Z
0WWMX3Z
0WWMX7Z
0WWMXJZ
0WWMXKZ
0WWMXYZ
0WWNX0Z
0WWNX1Z
0WWNX3Z
0WWNX7Z
0WWNXJZ
0WWNXKZ
0WWNXYZ
0WWP31Z
0WWP33Z
0WWP3YZ
0WWP41Z
0WWP43Z
0WWP4YZ
0WWP71Z
0WWP73Z
0WWP7YZ
0WWP81Z
0WWP83Z
0WWP8YZ
0WWPX1Z
0WWPX3Z
0WWPXYZ
0WWQ01Z
0WWQ03Z
0WWQ0YZ
0WWQX1Z
0WWQX3Z
0WWQXYZ
0WWR01Z
0WWR03Z
0WWR0YZ
0WWR31Z
0WWR33Z
0WWR3YZ
0WWR41Z
0WWR43Z
0WWR4YZ
0WWR71Z
0WWR73Z
0WWR7YZ
0WWR81Z
0WWR83Z
0WWR8YZ
0WWRX1Z
0WWRX3Z
0WWRXYZ
0X094JZ
0X094KZ
0X094ZZ
0X0B07Z
0X0B0JZ
0X0B0KZ
0X0B0ZZ
0X0B37Z
0X0B3JZ
0X0B3KZ
0X0B3ZZ
0X0B47Z
0X0B4JZ
0X0B4KZ
0X0B4ZZ
0X0C07Z
0X0C0JZ
0X0C0KZ
0X0C0ZZ
0X0C37Z
0X0C3JZ
0X0C3KZ
0X0C3ZZ
0X0C47Z
0X0C4JZ
0X0C4KZ
0X0C4ZZ
0X0D07Z
0X0D0JZ
0X0D0KZ
0X0D0ZZ
0X0D37Z
0X0D3JZ
0X0D3KZ
0X0D3ZZ
0X0D47Z
0X0D4JZ
0X0D4KZ
0X0D4ZZ
0X0F07Z
0X0F0JZ
0X0F0KZ
0X0F0ZZ
0X0F37Z
0X0F3JZ
0X0F3KZ
0X0F3ZZ
0X0F47Z
0X0F4JZ
0X0F4KZ
0X0F4ZZ
0X0G07Z
0X0G0JZ
0X0G0KZ
0X0G0ZZ
0X0G37Z
0X0G3JZ
0X0G3KZ
0X0G3ZZ
0X0G47Z
0X0G4JZ
0X0G4KZ
0X0G4ZZ
0X0H07Z
0X0H0JZ
0X0H0KZ
0X0H0ZZ
0X0H37Z
0X0H3JZ
0X0H3KZ
0X0H3ZZ
0X0H47Z
0X0H4JZ
0X0H4KZ
0X0H4ZZ
0X26X0Z
0X26XYZ
0X27X0Z
0X27XYZ
0X320ZZ
0X323ZZ
0X324ZZ
0X330ZZ
0X333ZZ
0X334ZZ
0X340ZZ
0X343ZZ
0X344ZZ
0X350ZZ
0X353ZZ
0X354ZZ
0X360ZZ
0X363ZZ
0X364ZZ
0X370ZZ
0X373ZZ
0X374ZZ
0X380ZZ
0X383ZZ
0X384ZZ
0X390ZZ
0X393ZZ
0X394ZZ
0X3B0ZZ
0X3B3ZZ
0X3B4ZZ
0X3C0ZZ
0X3C3ZZ
0X3C4ZZ
0X3D0ZZ
0X3D3ZZ
0X3D4ZZ
0X3F0ZZ
0X3F3ZZ
0X3F4ZZ
0X3G0ZZ
0X3G3ZZ
0X3G4ZZ
0X3H0ZZ
0X3H3ZZ
0X3H4ZZ
0X3J0ZZ
0X3J3ZZ
0X3J4ZZ
0X3K0ZZ
0X3K3ZZ
0X3K4ZZ
0X600ZZ
0X610ZZ
0X620ZZ
0X630ZZ
0X680Z1
0X680Z2
0X680Z3
0X690Z1
0X690Z2
0X690Z3
0X6B0ZZ
0X6C0ZZ
0X6D0Z1
0X6D0Z2
0X6D0Z3
0X6F0Z1
0X6F0Z2
0X6F0Z3
0X6J0Z0
0X6J0Z4
0X6J0Z5
0X6J0Z6
0X6J0Z7
0X6J0Z8
0X6J0Z9
0X6J0ZB
0X6J0ZC
0X6J0ZD
0X6J0ZF
0X6K0Z0
0X6K0Z4
0X6K0Z5
0X6K0Z6
0X6K0Z7
0X6K0Z8
0X6K0Z9
0X6K0ZB
0X6K0ZC
0X6K0ZD
0X6K0ZF
0X6L0Z0
0X6L0Z1
0X6L0Z2
0X6L0Z3
0X6M0Z0
0X6M0Z1
0X6M0Z2
0X6M0Z3
0X6N0Z0
0X6N0Z1
0X6N0Z2
0X6N0Z3
0X6P0Z0
0X6P0Z1
0X6P0Z2
0X6P0Z3
0X6Q0Z0
0X6Q0Z1
0X6Q0Z2
0X6Q0Z3
0X6R0Z0
0X6R0Z1
0X6R0Z2
0X6R0Z3
0X9200Z
0X920ZX
0X920ZZ
0X9230Z
0X923ZX
0X923ZZ
0X9240Z
0X924ZX
0X924ZZ
0X9300Z
0X930ZX
0X930ZZ
0X9330Z
0X933ZX
0X933ZZ
0X9340Z
0X934ZX
0X934ZZ
0X9400Z
0X940ZX
0X940ZZ
0X9430Z
0X943ZX
0X943ZZ
0X9440Z
0X944ZX
0X944ZZ
0X9500Z
0X950ZX
0X950ZZ
0X9530Z
0X953ZX
0X953ZZ
0X9540Z
0X954ZX
0X954ZZ
0X9600Z
0X960ZX
0X960ZZ
0X9630Z
0X963ZX
0X963ZZ
0X9640Z
0X964ZX
0X964ZZ
0X9700Z
0X970ZX
0X970ZZ
0X9730Z
0X973ZX
0X973ZZ
0X9740Z
0X974ZX
0X974ZZ
0X9800Z
0X980ZX
0X980ZZ
0X9830Z
0X983ZX
0X983ZZ
0X9840Z
0X984ZX
0X984ZZ
0X9900Z
0X990ZX
0X990ZZ
0X9930Z
0X993ZX
0X993ZZ
0X9940Z
0X994ZX
0X994ZZ
0X9B00Z
0X9B0ZX
0X9B0ZZ
0X9B30Z
0X9B3ZX
0X9B3ZZ
0X9B40Z
0X9B4ZX
0X9B4ZZ
0X9C00Z
0X9C0ZX
0X9C0ZZ
0X9C30Z
0X9C3ZX
0X9C3ZZ
0X9C40Z
0X9C4ZX
0X9C4ZZ
0X9D00Z
0X9D0ZX
0X9D0ZZ
0X9D30Z
0X9D3ZX
0X9D3ZZ
0X9D40Z
0X9D4ZX
0X9D4ZZ
0X9F00Z
0X9F0ZX
0X9F0ZZ
0X9F30Z
0X9F3ZX
0X9F3ZZ
0X9F40Z
0X9F4ZX
0X9F4ZZ
0X9G00Z
0X9G0ZX
0X9G0ZZ
0X9G30Z
0X9G3ZX
0X9G3ZZ
0X9G40Z
0X9G4ZX
0X9G4ZZ
0X9H00Z
0X9H0ZX
0X9H0ZZ
0X9H30Z
0X9H3ZX
0X9H3ZZ
0X9H40Z
0X9H4ZX
0X9H4ZZ
0X9J00Z
0X9J0ZX
0X9J0ZZ
0X9J30Z
0X9J3ZX
0X9J3ZZ
0X9J40Z
0X9J4ZX
0X9J4ZZ
0X9K00Z
0X9K0ZX
0X9K0ZZ
0X9K30Z
0X9K3ZX
0X9K3ZZ
0X9K40Z

0X9K4ZX
0X9K4ZZ
0XB20ZX
0XB23ZX
0XB24ZX
0XB30ZX
0XB33ZX
0XB34ZX
0XB40ZX
0XB43ZX
0XB44ZX
0XB50ZX
0XB53ZX
0XB54ZX
0XB60ZX
0XB63ZX
0XB64ZX
0XB70ZX
0XB73ZX
0XB74ZX
0XB80ZX
0XB83ZX
0XB84ZX
0XB90ZX
0XB93ZX
0XB94ZX
0XBB0ZX
0XBB3ZX
0XBB4ZX
0XBC0ZX
0XBC3ZX
0XBC4ZX
0XBD0ZX
0XBD3ZX
0XBD4ZX
0XBF0ZX
0XBF3ZX
0XBF4ZX
0XBG0ZX
0XBG3ZX
0XBG4ZX
0XBH0ZX
0XBH3ZX
0XBH4ZX
0XBJ0ZX
0XBJ3ZX
0XBJ4ZX
0XBK0ZX
0XBK3ZX
0XBK4ZX
0XH541Z
0XH543Z
0XH54YZ
0XH601Z
0XH603Z
0XH60YZ
0XH631Z
0XH633Z
0XH63YZ
0XH641Z
0XH643Z
0XH64YZ
0XH701Z
0XH703Z
0XH70YZ
0XH731Z
0XH733Z
0XH73YZ
0XH741Z
0XH743Z
0XH74YZ
0XH801Z
0XH803Z
0XH80YZ
0XH831Z
0XH833Z
0XH83YZ
0XH841Z
0XH843Z
0XH84YZ
0XH901Z
0XH903Z
0XH90YZ
0XH931Z
0XH933Z
0XH93YZ
0XH941Z
0XH943Z
0XH94YZ
0XHB01Z
0XHB03Z
0XHB0YZ
0XHB31Z
0XHB33Z
0XHB3YZ
0XHB41Z
0XHB43Z
0XHB4YZ
0XHC01Z
0XHC03Z
0XHC0YZ
0XHC31Z
0XHC33Z
0XHC3YZ
0XHC41Z
0XHC43Z
0XHC4YZ
0XHD01Z
0XHD03Z
0XHD0YZ
0XHD31Z
0XHD33Z
0XHD3YZ
0XHD41Z
0XHD43Z
0XHD4YZ
0XHF01Z
0XHF03Z
0XHF0YZ
0XHF31Z
0XHF33Z
0XHF3YZ
0XHF41Z
0XHF43Z
0XHF4YZ
0XHG01Z
0XHG03Z
0XHG0YZ
0XHG31Z
0XHG33Z
0XHG3YZ
0XHG41Z
0XHG43Z
0XHG4YZ
0XHH01Z
0XHH03Z
0XHH0YZ
0XHH31Z
0XHH33Z
0XHH3YZ
0XHH41Z
0XHH43Z
0XHH4YZ
0XHJ01Z
0XHJ03Z
0XHJ0YZ
0XHJ31Z
0XHJ33Z
0XHJ3YZ
0XHJ41Z
0XHJ43Z
0XHJ4YZ
0XHK01Z
0XHK03Z
0XHK0YZ
0XHK31Z
0XHK33Z
0XHK3YZ
0XHK41Z
0XHK43Z
0XHK4YZ
0XJ20ZZ
0XJ23ZZ
0XJ24ZZ
0XJ2XZZ
0XJ30ZZ
0XJ33ZZ
0XJ34ZZ
0XJ3XZZ
0XJ40ZZ
0XJ43ZZ
0XJ44ZZ
0XJ4XZZ
0XJ50ZZ
0XJ53ZZ
0XJ54ZZ
0XJ5XZZ
0XJ60ZZ
0XJ63ZZ
0XJ64ZZ
0XJ6XZZ
0XJ70ZZ
0XJ73ZZ
0XJ74ZZ
0XJ7XZZ
0XJ80ZZ
0XJ83ZZ
0XJ84ZZ
0XJ8XZZ
0XJ90ZZ
0XJ93ZZ
0XJ94ZZ
0XJ9XZZ
0XJB0ZZ
0XJB3ZZ
0XJB4ZZ
0XJBXZZ
0XJC0ZZ
0XJC3ZZ
0XJC4ZZ
0XJCXZZ
0XJD0ZZ
0XJD3ZZ
0XJD4ZZ
0XJDXZZ
0XJF0ZZ
0XJF3ZZ
0XJF4ZZ
0XJFXZZ
0XJG0ZZ
0XJG3ZZ
0XJG4ZZ
0XJGXZZ
0XJH0ZZ
0XJH3ZZ
0XJH4ZZ
0XJHXZZ
0XJJ0ZZ
0XJJ3ZZ
0XJJ4ZZ
0XJJXZZ
0XJK0ZZ
0XJK3ZZ
0XJK4ZZ
0XJKXZZ
0XM00ZZ
0XM10ZZ
0XM20ZZ
0XM30ZZ
0XM40ZZ
0XM50ZZ
0XM60ZZ
0XM70ZZ
0XM80ZZ
0XM90ZZ
0XMB0ZZ
0XMC0ZZ
0XMD0ZZ
0XMF0ZZ
0XMG0ZZ
0XMH0ZZ
0XMJ0ZZ
0XMK0ZZ
0XML0ZZ
0XMM0ZZ
0XMN0ZZ
0XMP0ZZ
0XMQ0ZZ
0XMR0ZZ
0XMS0ZZ
0XMT0ZZ
0XMV0ZZ
0XMW0ZZ
0XP600Z
0XP601Z
0XP603Z
0XP607Z
0XP60JZ
0XP60KZ
0XP60YZ
0XP630Z
0XP631Z
0XP633Z
0XP637Z
0XP63JZ
0XP63KZ
0XP63YZ
0XP640Z
0XP641Z
0XP643Z
0XP647Z
0XP64JZ
0XP64KZ
0XP64YZ
0XP6X0Z
0XP6X1Z
0XP6X3Z
0XP6X7Z
0XP6XJZ
0XP6XKZ
0XP6XYZ
0XP700Z
0XP701Z
0XP703Z
0XP707Z
0XP70JZ
0XP70KZ
0XP70YZ
0XP730Z
0XP731Z
0XP733Z
0XP737Z
0XP73JZ
0XP73KZ
0XP73YZ
0XP740Z
0XP741Z
0XP743Z
0XP747Z
0XP74JZ
0XP74KZ
0XP74YZ
0XP7X0Z
0XP7X1Z
0XP7X3Z
0XP7X7Z
0XP7XJZ
0XP7XKZ
0XP7XYZ
0XQ20ZZ
0XQ23ZZ
0XQ24ZZ
0XQ2XZZ
0XQ30ZZ
0XQ33ZZ
0XQ34ZZ
0XQ3XZZ
0XQ40ZZ
0XQ43ZZ
0XQ44ZZ
0XQ4XZZ
0XQ50ZZ
0XQ53ZZ
0XQ54ZZ
0XQ5XZZ
0XQ60ZZ
0XQ63ZZ
0XQ64ZZ
0XQ6XZZ
0XQ70ZZ
0XQ73ZZ
0XQ74ZZ
0XQ7XZZ
0XQ80ZZ
0XQ83ZZ
0XQ84ZZ
0XQ8XZZ
0XQ90ZZ
0XQ93ZZ
0XQ94ZZ
0XQ9XZZ
0XQB0ZZ
0XQB3ZZ
0XQB4ZZ
0XQBXZZ
0XQC0ZZ
0XQC3ZZ
0XQC4ZZ
0XQCXZZ
0XQD0ZZ
0XQD3ZZ
0XQD4ZZ
0XQDXZZ
0XQF0ZZ
0XQF3ZZ
0XQF4ZZ
0XQFXZZ
0XQG0ZZ
0XQG3ZZ
0XQG4ZZ
0XQGXZZ
0XQH0ZZ
0XQH3ZZ
0XQH4ZZ
0XQHXZZ
0XQJ0ZZ
0XQJ3ZZ
0XQJ4ZZ
0XQJXZZ
0XQK0ZZ
0XQK3ZZ
0XQK4ZZ
0XQKXZZ
0XQL0ZZ
0XQL3ZZ
0XQL4ZZ
0XQLXZZ
0XQM0ZZ
0XQM3ZZ
0XQM4ZZ
0XQMXZZ
0XQN0ZZ
0XQN3ZZ
0XQN4ZZ
0XQNXZZ
0XQP0ZZ
0XQP3ZZ
0XQP4ZZ
0XQPXZZ
0XQQ0ZZ
0XQQ3ZZ
0XQQ4ZZ
0XQQXZZ
0XQR0ZZ
0XQR3ZZ
0XQR4ZZ
0XQRXZZ
0XQS0ZZ
0XQS3ZZ
0XQS4ZZ
0XQSXZZ
0XQT0ZZ
0XQT3ZZ
0XQT4ZZ
0XQTXZZ
0XQV0ZZ
0XQV3ZZ
0XQV4ZZ
0XQVXZZ
0XQW0ZZ
0XQW3ZZ
0XQW4ZZ
0XQWXZZ
0XRL07N
0XRL07P
0XRL47N
0XRL47P
0XRM07N
0XRM07P
0XRM47N
0XRM47P
0XU207Z
0XU20JZ
0XU20KZ
0XU247Z
0XU24JZ
0XU24KZ
0XU307Z
0XU30JZ
0XU30KZ
0XU347Z
0XU34JZ
0XU34KZ
0XU407Z
0XU40JZ
0XU40KZ
0XU447Z
0XU44JZ
0XU44KZ
0XU507Z
0XU50JZ
0XU50KZ
0XU547Z
0XU54JZ
0XU54KZ
0XU607Z
0XU60JZ
0XU60KZ
0XU647Z
0XU64JZ
0XU64KZ
0XU707Z
0XU70JZ
0XU70KZ
0XU747Z
0XU74JZ
0XU74KZ
0XU807Z
0XU80JZ
0XU80KZ
0XU847Z
0XU84JZ
0XU84KZ
0XU907Z
0XU90JZ
0XU90KZ
0XU947Z
0XU94JZ
0XU94KZ
0XUB07Z
0XUB0JZ
0XUB0KZ
0XUB47Z
0XUB4JZ
0XUB4KZ
0XUC07Z
0XUC0JZ
0XUC0KZ
0XUC47Z
0XUC4JZ
0XUC4KZ
0XUD07Z
0XUD0JZ
0XUD0KZ
0XUD47Z
0XUD4JZ
0XUD4KZ
0XUF07Z
0XUF0JZ
0XUF0KZ
0XUF47Z
0XUF4JZ
0XUF4KZ
0XUG07Z
0XUG0JZ
0XUG0KZ
0XUG47Z
0XUG4JZ
0XUG4KZ
0XUH07Z
0XUH0JZ
0XUH0KZ
0XUH47Z
0XUH4JZ
0XUH4KZ
0XUJ07Z
0XUJ0JZ
0XUJ0KZ
0XUJ47Z
0XUJ4JZ
0XUJ4KZ
0XUK07Z
0XUK0JZ
0XUK0KZ
0XUK47Z
0XUK4JZ
0XUK4KZ
0XUL07Z
0XUL0JZ
0XUL0KZ
0XUL47Z
0XUL4JZ
0XUL4KZ
0XUM07Z
0XUM0JZ
0XUM0KZ
0XUM47Z
0XUM4JZ
0XUM4KZ
0XUN07Z
0XUN0JZ
0XUN0KZ
0XW6X0Z
0XW6X3Z
0XW6X7Z
0XW6XJZ
0XW6XKZ
0XW6XYZ
0XW7X0Z
0XW7X3Z
0XW7X7Z
0XW7XJZ
0XW7XKZ
0XW7XYZ
0Y0F4ZZ
0Y0G07Z
0Y0G0JZ
0Y0G0KZ
0Y0G0ZZ
0Y0G37Z
0Y0G3JZ
0Y0G3KZ
0Y0G3ZZ
0Y0G47Z
0Y0G4JZ
0Y0G4KZ
0Y0G4ZZ
0Y0H07Z
0Y0H0JZ
0Y0H0KZ
0Y0H0ZZ
0Y0H37Z
0Y0H3JZ
0Y0H3KZ
0Y0H3ZZ
0Y0H47Z
0Y0H4JZ
0Y0H4KZ
0Y0H4ZZ
0Y0J07Z
0Y0J0JZ
0Y0J0KZ
0Y0J0ZZ
0Y0J37Z
0Y0J3JZ
0Y0J3KZ
0Y0J3ZZ
0Y0J47Z
0Y0J4JZ
0Y0J4KZ
0Y0J4ZZ
0Y0K07Z
0Y0K0JZ
0Y0K0KZ
0Y0K0ZZ
0Y0K37Z
0Y0K3JZ
0Y0K3KZ
0Y0K3ZZ
0Y0K47Z
0Y0K4JZ
0Y0K4KZ
0Y0K4ZZ
0Y0L07Z
0Y0L0JZ
0Y0L0KZ
0Y0L0ZZ
0Y0L37Z
0Y0L3JZ
0Y0L3KZ
0Y0L3ZZ
0Y0L47Z
0Y0L4JZ
0Y0L4KZ
0Y0L4ZZ
0Y29X0Z
0Y29XYZ
0Y2BX0Z
0Y2BXYZ
0Y300ZZ
0Y303ZZ
0Y304ZZ
0Y310ZZ
0Y313ZZ
0Y314ZZ
0Y350ZZ
0Y353ZZ
0Y354ZZ
0Y360ZZ
0Y363ZZ
0Y364ZZ
0Y370ZZ
0Y373ZZ
0Y374ZZ
0Y380ZZ
0Y383ZZ
0Y384ZZ
0Y390ZZ
0Y393ZZ
0Y394ZZ
0Y3B0ZZ
0Y3B3ZZ
0Y3B4ZZ
0Y3C0ZZ
0Y3C3ZZ
0Y3C4ZZ
0Y3D0ZZ
0Y3D3ZZ
0Y3D4ZZ
0Y3F0ZZ
0Y3F3ZZ
0Y3F4ZZ
0Y3G0ZZ
0Y3G3ZZ
0Y3G4ZZ
0Y3H0ZZ
0Y3H3ZZ
0Y3H4ZZ
0Y3J0ZZ
0Y3J3ZZ
0Y3J4ZZ
0Y3K0ZZ
0Y3K3ZZ
0Y3K4ZZ
0Y3L0ZZ
0Y3L3ZZ
0Y3L4ZZ
0Y3M0ZZ
0Y3M3ZZ
0Y3M4ZZ
0Y3N0ZZ
0Y3N3ZZ
0Y3N4ZZ
0Y620ZZ
0Y630ZZ
0Y640ZZ
0Y670ZZ
0Y680ZZ
0Y6C0Z1
0Y6C0Z2
0Y6C0Z3
0Y6D0Z1
0Y6D0Z2
0Y6D0Z3
0Y6F0ZZ
0Y6G0ZZ
0Y6H0Z1
0Y6H0Z2
0Y6H0Z3
0Y6J0Z1
0Y6J0Z2
0Y6J0Z3
0Y6M0Z0
0Y6M0Z4
0Y6M0Z5
0Y6M0Z6
0Y6M0Z7
0Y6M0Z8
0Y6M0Z9
0Y6M0ZB
0Y6M0ZC
0Y6M0ZD
0Y6M0ZF
0Y6N0Z0
0Y6N0Z4
0Y6N0Z5
0Y6N0Z6
0Y6N0Z7
0Y6N0Z8
0Y6N0Z9
0Y6N0ZB
0Y6N0ZC
0Y6N0ZD
0Y6N0ZF
0Y6P0Z0
0Y6P0Z1
0Y9000Z
0Y900ZX
0Y900ZZ
0Y9030Z
0Y903ZX
0Y903ZZ
0Y9040Z
0Y904ZX
0Y904ZZ
0Y9100Z
0Y910ZX
0Y910ZZ
0Y9130Z
0Y913ZX
0Y913ZZ
0Y9140Z
0Y914ZX
0Y914ZZ
0Y9530Z
0Y953ZZ

0Y9630Z
0Y963ZZ
0Y9700Z
0Y970ZX
0Y970ZZ
0Y9730Z
0Y973ZX
0Y973ZZ
0Y9740Z
0Y974ZX
0Y974ZZ
0Y9800Z
0Y980ZX
0Y980ZZ
0Y9830Z
0Y983ZX
0Y983ZZ
0Y9840Z
0Y984ZX
0Y984ZZ
0Y9900Z
0Y990ZX
0Y990ZZ
0Y9930Z
0Y993ZX
0Y993ZZ
0Y9940Z
0Y994ZX
0Y994ZZ
0Y9B00Z
0Y9B0ZX
0Y9B0ZZ
0Y9B30Z
0Y9B3ZX
0Y9B3ZZ
0Y9B40Z
0Y9B4ZX
0Y9B4ZZ
0Y9C00Z
0Y9C0ZX
0Y9C0ZZ
0Y9C30Z
0Y9C3ZX
0Y9C3ZZ
0Y9C40Z
0Y9C4ZX
0Y9C4ZZ
0Y9D00Z
0Y9D0ZX
0Y9D0ZZ
0Y9D30Z
0Y9D3ZX
0Y9D3ZZ
0Y9D40Z
0Y9D4ZX
0Y9D4ZZ
0Y9F00Z
0Y9F0ZX
0Y9F0ZZ
0Y9F30Z
0Y9F3ZX
0Y9F3ZZ
0Y9F40Z
0Y9F4ZX
0Y9F4ZZ
0Y9G00Z
0Y9G0ZX
0Y9G0ZZ
0Y9G30Z
0Y9G3ZX
0Y9G3ZZ
0Y9G40Z
0Y9G4ZX
0Y9G4ZZ
0Y9H00Z
0Y9H0ZX
0Y9H0ZZ
0Y9H30Z
0Y9H3ZX
0Y9H3ZZ
0Y9H40Z
0Y9H4ZX
0Y9H4ZZ
0Y9J00Z
0Y9J0ZX
0Y9J0ZZ
0Y9J30Z
0Y9J3ZX
0Y9J3ZZ
0Y9J40Z
0Y9J4ZX
0Y9J4ZZ
0Y9K00Z
0Y9K0ZX
0Y9K0ZZ
0Y9K30Z
0Y9K3ZX
0Y9K3ZZ
0Y9K40Z
0Y9K4ZX
0Y9K4ZZ
0Y9L00Z
0Y9L0ZX
0Y9L0ZZ
0Y9L30Z
0Y9L3ZX
0Y9L3ZZ
0Y9L40Z
0Y9L4ZX
0Y9L4ZZ
0Y9M00Z
0Y9M0ZX
0Y9M0ZZ
0Y9M30Z
0Y9M3ZX
0Y9M3ZZ
0Y9M40Z
0Y9M4ZX
0Y9M4ZZ
0Y9N00Z
0Y9N0ZX
0Y9N0ZZ
0Y9N30Z
0Y9N3ZX
0Y9N3ZZ
0Y9N40Z
0Y9N4ZX
0Y9N4ZZ
0YB00ZX
0YB03ZX
0YB04ZX
0YB10ZX
0YB13ZX
0YB13ZZ
0YB14ZX
0YB14ZZ
0YB50ZX
0YB50ZZ
0YB53ZX
0YB53ZZ
0YB54ZX
0YB54ZZ
0YB60ZX
0YB60ZZ
0YB63ZX
0YB63ZZ
0YB64ZX
0YB64ZZ
0YB70ZX
0YB70ZZ
0YB73ZX
0YB73ZZ
0YB74ZX
0YB74ZZ
0YB80ZX
0YB80ZZ
0YB83ZX
0YB83ZZ
0YB84ZX
0YB84ZZ
0YB90ZX
0YB90ZZ
0YB93ZX
0YB93ZZ
0YB94ZX
0YB94ZZ
0YBB0ZX
0YBB0ZZ
0YBB3ZX
0YBB3ZZ
0YBB4ZX
0YBB4ZZ
0YBC0ZX
0YBC0ZZ
0YBC3ZX
0YBC3ZZ
0YBC4ZX
0YBC4ZZ
0YBD0ZX
0YBD0ZZ
0YBD3ZX
0YBD3ZZ
0YBD4ZX
0YBD4ZZ
0YBF0ZX
0YBF0ZZ
0YBF3ZX
0YBF3ZZ
0YBF4ZX
0YBF4ZZ
0YBG0ZX
0YBG0ZZ
0YBG3ZX
0YBG3ZZ
0YBG4ZX
0YBG4ZZ
0YBH0ZX
0YBH0ZZ
0YBH3ZX
0YBH3ZZ
0YBH4ZX
0YBH4ZZ
0YBJ0ZX
0YBJ0ZZ
0YBJ3ZX
0YBJ3ZZ
0YBJ4ZX
0YBJ4ZZ
0YBK0ZX
0YBK0ZZ
0YBK3ZX
0YBK3ZZ
0YBK4ZX
0YBK4ZZ
0YBL0ZX
0YBL0ZZ
0YBL3ZX
0YBL3ZZ
0YBL4ZX
0YBL4ZZ
0YBM0ZX
0YBM0ZZ
0YBM3ZX
0YBM3ZZ
0YBM4ZX
0YBM4ZZ
0YBN0ZX
0YBN0ZZ
0YBN3ZX
0YBN3ZZ
0YBN4ZX
0YBN4ZZ
0YH001Z
0YH003Z
0YH00YZ
0YH031Z
0YH033Z
0YH03YZ
0YH041Z
0YH043Z
0YH04YZ
0YH101Z
0YH103Z
0YH10YZ
0YH131Z
0YH133Z
0YH13YZ
0YH141Z
0YH143Z
0YH14YZ
0YH501Z
0YH503Z
0YH50YZ
0YH531Z
0YH533Z
0YH53YZ
0YH541Z
0YH543Z
0YH54YZ
0YH601Z
0YH603Z
0YH60YZ
0YH631Z
0YH633Z
0YH63YZ
0YH641Z
0YH643Z
0YH64YZ
0YH701Z
0YH703Z
0YH70YZ
0YH731Z
0YH733Z
0YH73YZ
0YH741Z
0YH743Z
0YH74YZ
0YH801Z
0YH803Z
0YH80YZ
0YH831Z
0YH833Z
0YH83YZ
0YH841Z
0YH843Z
0YH84YZ
0YH901Z
0YH903Z
0YH90YZ
0YH931Z
0YH933Z
0YH93YZ
0YH941Z
0YH943Z
0YH94YZ
0YHB01Z
0YHB03Z
0YHB0YZ
0YHB31Z
0YHB33Z
0YHB3YZ
0YHB41Z
0YHB43Z
0YHB4YZ
0YHC01Z
0YHC03Z
0YHC0YZ
0YHC31Z
0YHC33Z
0YHC3YZ
0YHC41Z
0YHC43Z
0YHC4YZ
0YHD01Z
0YHD03Z
0YHD0YZ
0YHD31Z
0YHD33Z
0YHD3YZ
0YHD41Z
0YHD43Z
0YHD4YZ
0YHF01Z
0YHF03Z
0YHF0YZ
0YHF31Z
0YHF33Z
0YHF3YZ
0YHF41Z
0YHF43Z
0YHF4YZ
0YHG01Z
0YHG03Z
0YHG0YZ
0YHG31Z
0YHG33Z
0YHG3YZ
0YHG41Z
0YHG43Z
0YHG4YZ
0YHH01Z
0YHH03Z
0YHH0YZ
0YHH31Z
0YHH33Z
0YHH3YZ
0YHH41Z
0YHH43Z
0YHH4YZ
0YHJ01Z
0YHJ03Z
0YHJ0YZ
0YHJ31Z
0YHJ33Z
0YHJ3YZ
0YHJ41Z
0YHJ43Z
0YHJ4YZ
0YHK01Z
0YHK03Z
0YHK0YZ
0YHK31Z
0YHK33Z
0YHK3YZ
0YHK41Z
0YHK43Z
0YHK4YZ
0YHL01Z
0YHL03Z
0YHL0YZ
0YHL31Z
0YHL33Z
0YHL3YZ
0YHL41Z
0YHL43Z
0YHL4YZ
0YHM01Z
0YHM03Z
0YHM0YZ
0YHM31Z
0YHM33Z
0YHM3YZ
0YHM41Z
0YHM43Z
0YHM4YZ
0YHN01Z
0YHN03Z
0YHN0YZ
0YHN31Z
0YHN33Z
0YHN3YZ
0YHN41Z
0YHN43Z
0YHN4YZ
0YJ00ZZ
0YJ03ZZ
0YJ04ZZ
0YJ0XZZ
0YJ10ZZ
0YJ13ZZ
0YJ14ZZ
0YJ1XZZ
0YJ50ZZ
0YJ53ZZ
0YJ54ZZ
0YJ5XZZ
0YJ60ZZ
0YJ63ZZ
0YJ64ZZ
0YJ6XZZ
0YJ70ZZ
0YJ73ZZ
0YJ74ZZ
0YJ7XZZ
0YJ80ZZ
0YJ83ZZ
0YJ84ZZ
0YJ8XZZ
0YJ90ZZ
0YJ93ZZ
0YJ94ZZ
0YJ9XZZ
0YJA0ZZ
0YJA3ZZ
0YJA4ZZ
0YJAXZZ
0YJB0ZZ
0YJB3ZZ
0YJB4ZZ
0YJBXZZ
0YJC0ZZ
0YJC3ZZ
0YJC4ZZ
0YJCXZZ
0YJD0ZZ
0YJD3ZZ
0YJD4ZZ
0YJDXZZ
0YJE0ZZ
0YJE3ZZ
0YJE4ZZ
0YJEXZZ
0YJF0ZZ
0YJF3ZZ
0YJF4ZZ
0YJFXZZ
0YJG0ZZ
0YJG3ZZ
0YJG4ZZ
0YJGXZZ
0YJH0ZZ
0YJH3ZZ
0YJH4ZZ
0YJHXZZ
0YJJ0ZZ
0YJJ3ZZ
0YJJ4ZZ
0YJJXZZ
0YJK0ZZ
0YJK3ZZ
0YJK4ZZ
0YJKXZZ
0YJL0ZZ
0YJL3ZZ
0YJL4ZZ
0YJLXZZ
0YJM0ZZ
0YJM3ZZ
0YJM4ZZ
0YJMXZZ
0YJN0ZZ
0YJN3ZZ
0YJN4ZZ
0YJNXZZ
0YM00ZZ
0YM10ZZ
0YM20ZZ
0YM30ZZ
0YM40ZZ
0YM50ZZ
0YM60ZZ
0YM70ZZ
0YM80ZZ
0YM90ZZ
0YMB0ZZ
0YMC0ZZ
0YMD0ZZ
0YMF0ZZ
0YMG0ZZ
0YMH0ZZ
0YMJ0ZZ
0YMK0ZZ
0YML0ZZ
0YMM0ZZ
0YMN0ZZ
0YMP0ZZ
0YMQ0ZZ
0YMR0ZZ
0YMS0ZZ
0YMT0ZZ
0YMU0ZZ
0YMV0ZZ
0YMW0ZZ
0YMX0ZZ
0YMY0ZZ
0YP900Z
0YP901Z
0YP903Z
0YP907Z
0YP90JZ
0YP90KZ
0YP90YZ
0YP930Z
0YP931Z
0YP933Z
0YP937Z
0YP93JZ
0YP93KZ
0YP93YZ
0YP940Z
0YP941Z
0YP943Z
0YP947Z
0YP94JZ
0YP94KZ
0YP94YZ
0YP9X0Z
0YP9X1Z
0YP9X3Z
0YP9X7Z
0YP9XJZ
0YP9XKZ
0YP9XYZ
0YPB00Z
0YPB01Z
0YPB03Z
0YPB07Z
0YPB0JZ
0YPB0KZ
0YPB0YZ
0YPB30Z
0YPB31Z
0YPB33Z
0YPB37Z
0YPB3JZ
0YPB3KZ
0YPB3YZ
0YPB40Z
0YPB41Z
0YPB43Z
0YPB47Z
0YPB4JZ
0YPB4KZ
0YPB4YZ
0YPBX0Z
0YPBX1Z
0YPBX3Z
0YPBX7Z
0YPBXJZ
0YPBXKZ
0YPBXYZ
0YQ00ZZ
0YQ03ZZ
0YQ04ZZ
0YQ0XZZ
0YQ10ZZ
0YQ13ZZ
0YQ14ZZ
0YQ1XZZ
0YQ50ZZ
0YQ53ZZ
0YQ54ZZ
0YQ5XZZ
0YQ60ZZ
0YQ63ZZ
0YQ64ZZ
0YQ6XZZ
0YQ70ZZ
0YQ73ZZ
0YQ74ZZ
0YQ7XZZ
0YQ80ZZ
0YQ83ZZ
0YQ84ZZ
0YQ8XZZ
0YQ90ZZ
0YQ93ZZ
0YQ94ZZ
0YQ9XZZ
0YQA0ZZ
0YQA3ZZ
0YQA4ZZ
0YQAXZZ
0YQB0ZZ
0YQB3ZZ
0YQB4ZZ
0YQBXZZ
0YQC0ZZ
0YQC3ZZ
0YQC4ZZ
0YQEXZZ
0YUS0KZ
0YUS47Z
0YUS4JZ
0YUS4KZ
0YUT07Z
0YUT0JZ
0YUT0KZ
0YUT47Z
0YUT4JZ
0YUT4KZ
0YUU07Z
0YUU0JZ
0YUU0KZ
0YUU47Z
0YUU4JZ
0YUU4KZ
0YUV07Z
0YUV0JZ
0YUV0KZ
0YUV47Z
0YUV4JZ
0YUV4KZ
0YUW07Z
0YUW0JZ
0YUW0KZ
0YUW47Z
0YUW4JZ
0YUW4KZ
0YUX07Z
0YUX0JZ
0YUX0KZ
0YUX47Z
0YUX4JZ
0YUX4KZ
0YUY07Z
0YUY0JZ
0YUY0KZ
0YUY47Z
0YUY4JZ
0YUY4KZ
0YW900Z
0YW903Z
0YW907Z
0YW90JZ
0YW90KZ
0YW90YZ
0YW930Z
0YW933Z
0YW937Z
0YW93JZ
0YW93KZ
0YW93YZ
0YW940Z
0YW943Z
0YW947Z
0YW94JZ
0YW94KZ
0YW94YZ
0YW9X0Z
0YW9X3Z
0YW9X7Z
0YW9XJZ
0YW9XKZ
0YW9XYZ
0YWB00Z
0YWB03Z
0YWB07Z
0YWB0JZ
0YWB0KZ
0YWB0YZ
0YWB30Z
0YWB33Z
0YWB37Z
0YWB3JZ
0YWB3KZ
0YWB3YZ
0YWB40Z
0YWB43Z
0YWB47Z
0YWB4JZ
0YWB4KZ
0YWB4YZ
0YWBX0Z
0YWBX3Z
0YWBX7Z
0YWBXJZ
0YWBXKZ
0YWBXYZ
102073Z
10207YZ
10900Z9
10900ZA
10900ZB
10900ZC
10900ZD
10900ZU
10903Z9
10903ZA
10903ZB
10903ZC
10903ZD
10903ZU
10904Z9
10904ZA
10904ZB
10904ZC
10904ZD
10904ZU
10907Z9
10907ZA
10907ZB
10907ZC
10907ZD
10907ZU
10908Z9
10908ZA
10908ZB
10908ZC
10908ZD
10908ZU
10A00ZZ
10A03ZZ
10A04ZZ
10A07Z6
10A07ZW

10A07ZX
10A07ZZ
10A08ZZ
10D00Z0
10D00Z1
10D00Z2
10D07Z3
10D07Z4
10D07Z5
10D07Z6
10D07Z7
10D07Z8
10D17Z9
10D17ZZ
10D18Z9
10D18ZZ
10D27ZZ
10D28ZZ
10E0XZZ
10H003Z
10H00YZ
10H073Z
10H07YZ
10J00ZZ
10J03ZZ
10J04ZZ
10J07ZZ
10J08ZZ
10J0XZZ
10J10ZZ
10J13ZZ
10J14ZZ
10J17ZZ
10J18ZZ
10J1XZZ
10J20ZZ
10J23ZZ
10J24ZZ
10J27ZZ
10J28ZZ
10J2XZZ
10P003Z
10P00YZ
10P073Z
10P07YZ
10Q00YE
10Q00YF
10Q00YG
10Q00YH
10Q00YJ
10Q00YK
10Q00YL
10Q00YM
10Q00YN
10Q00YP
10Q00YQ
10Q00YR
10Q00YS
10Q00YT
10Q00YV
10Q00YY
10Q00ZE
10Q00ZF
10Q00ZG
10Q00ZH
10Q00ZJ
10Q00ZK
10Q00ZL
10Q00ZM
10Q00ZN
10Q00ZP
10Q00ZQ
10Q00ZR
10Q00ZS
10Q00ZT
10Q00ZV
10Q00ZY
10Q03YE
10Q03YF
10Q03YG
10Q03YH
10Q03YJ
10Q03YK
10Q03YL
10Q03YM
10Q03YN
10Q03YP
10Q03YQ
10Q03YR
10Q03YS
10Q03YT
10Q03YV
10Q03YY
10Q03ZE
10Q03ZF
10Q03ZG
10Q03ZH
10Q03ZJ
10Q03ZK
10Q03ZL
10Q03ZM
10Q03ZN
10Q03ZP
10Q03ZQ
10Q03ZR
10Q03ZS
10Q03ZT
10Q03ZV
10Q03ZY
10Q04YE
10Q04YF
10Q04YG
10Q04YH
10Q04YJ
10Q04YK
10Q04YL
10Q04YM
10Q04YN
10Q04YP
10Q04YQ
10Q04YR
10Q04YS
10Q04YT
10Q04YV
10Q04YY
10Q04ZE
10Q04ZF
10Q04ZG
10Q04ZH
10Q04ZJ
10Q04ZK
10Q04ZL
10Q04ZM
10Q04ZN
10Q04ZP
10Q04ZQ
10Q04ZR
10Q04ZS
10Q04ZT
10Q04ZV
10Q04ZY
10Q07YE
10Q07YF
10Q07YG
10Q07YH
10Q07YJ
10Q07YK
10Q07YL
10Q07YM
10Q07YN
10Q07YP
10Q07YQ
10Q07YR
10Q07YS
10Q07YT
10Q07YV
10Q07YY
10Q07ZE
10Q07ZF
10Q07ZG
10Q07ZH
10Q07ZJ
10Q07ZK
10Q07ZL
10Q07ZM
10Q07ZN
10Q07ZP
10Q07ZQ
10Q07ZR
10Q07ZS
10Q07ZT
10Q07ZV
10Q07ZY
10Q08YE
10Q08YF
10Q08YG
10Q08YH
10Q08YJ
10Q08YK
10Q08YL
10Q08YM
10Q08YN
10Q08YP
10Q08YQ
10Q08YR
10Q08YS
10Q08YT
10Q08YV
10Q08YY
10Q08ZE
10Q08ZF
10Q08ZG
10Q08ZH
10Q08ZJ
10Q08ZK
10Q08ZL
10Q08ZM
10Q08ZN
10Q08ZP
10Q08ZQ
10Q08ZR
10Q08ZS
10Q08ZT
10Q08ZV
10Q08ZY
10S07ZZ
10S0XZZ
10S20ZZ
10S23ZZ
10S24ZZ
10S27ZZ
10S28ZZ
10T20ZZ
10T23ZZ
10T24ZZ
10T27ZZ
10T28ZZ
10Y03ZE
10Y03ZF
10Y03ZG
10Y03ZH
10Y03ZJ
10Y03ZK
10Y03ZL
10Y03ZM
10Y03ZN
10Y03ZP
10Y03ZQ
10Y03ZR
10Y03ZS
10Y03ZT
10Y03ZV
10Y03ZY
10Y04ZE
10Y04ZF
10Y04ZG
10Y04ZH
10Y04ZJ
10Y04ZK
10Y04ZL
10Y04ZM
10Y04ZN
10Y04ZP
10Y04ZQ
10Y04ZR
10Y04ZS
10Y04ZT
10Y04ZV
10Y04ZY
10Y07ZE
10Y07ZF
10Y07ZG
10Y07ZH
10Y07ZJ
10Y07ZK
10Y07ZL
10Y07ZM
10Y07ZN
10Y07ZP
10Y07ZQ
10Y07ZR
10Y07ZS
10Y07ZT
10Y07ZV
10Y07ZY
2W00X0Z
2W00X1Z
2W00X2Z
2W00X3Z
2W00X4Z
2W00X5Z
2W00X6Z
2W00X7Z
2W00XYZ
2W01X0Z
2W01X1Z
2W01X2Z
2W01X3Z
2W01X4Z
2W01X5Z
2W01X6Z
2W01X7Z
2W01X9Z
2W01XYZ
2W02X0Z
2W02X1Z
2W02X2Z
2W02X3Z
2W02X4Z
2W02X5Z
2W02X6Z
2W02X7Z
2W02XYZ
2W03X0Z
2W03X1Z
2W03X2Z
2W03X3Z
2W03X4Z
2W03X5Z
2W03X6Z
2W03X7Z
2W03XYZ
2W04X0Z
2W04X1Z
2W04X2Z
2W04X3Z
2W04X4Z
2W04X5Z
2W04X6Z
2W04X7Z
2W04XYZ
2W05X0Z
2W05X1Z
2W05X2Z
2W05X3Z
2W05X4Z
2W05X5Z
2W05X6Z
2W05X7Z
2W05XYZ
2W06X0Z
2W06X1Z
2W06X2Z
2W06X3Z
2W06X4Z
2W06X5Z
2W06X6Z
2W06X7Z
2W06XYZ
2W07X0Z
2W07X1Z
2W07X2Z
2W07X3Z
2W07X4Z
2W07X5Z
2W07X6Z
2W07X7Z
2W07XYZ
2W08X0Z
2W08X1Z
2W08X2Z
2W08X3Z
2W08X4Z
2W08X5Z
2W08X6Z
2W08X7Z
2W08XYZ
2W09X0Z
2W09X1Z
2W09X2Z
2W09X3Z
2W09X4Z
2W09X5Z
2W09X6Z
2W09X7Z
2W09XYZ
2W0AX0Z
2W0AX1Z
2W0AX2Z
2W0AX3Z
2W0AX4Z
2W0AX5Z
2W0AX6Z
2W0AX7Z
2W0AXYZ
2W0BX0Z
2W0BX1Z
2W0BX2Z
2W0BX3Z
2W0BX4Z
2W0BX5Z
2W0BX6Z
2W0BX7Z
2W0BXYZ
2W0CX0Z
2W0CX1Z
2W0CX2Z
2W0CX3Z
2W0CX4Z
2W0CX5Z
2W0CX6Z
2W0CX7Z
2W0CXYZ
2W0DX0Z
2W0DX1Z
2W0DX2Z
2W0DX3Z
2W0DX4Z
2W0DX5Z
2W0DX6Z
2W0DX7Z
2W0DXYZ
2W0EX0Z
2W0EX1Z
2W0EX2Z
2W0EX3Z
2W0EX4Z
2W0EX5Z
2W0EX6Z
2W0EX7Z
2W0EXYZ
2W0FX0Z
2W0FX1Z
2W0FX2Z
2W0FX3Z
2W0FX4Z
2W0FX5Z
2W0FX6Z
2W0FX7Z
2W0FXYZ
2W0GX0Z
2W0GX1Z
2W0GX2Z
2W0GX3Z
2W0GX4Z
2W0GX5Z
2W0GX6Z
2W0GX7Z
2W0GXYZ
2W0HX0Z
2W0HX1Z
2W0HX2Z
2W0HX3Z
2W0HX4Z
2W0HX5Z
2W0HX6Z
2W0HX7Z
2W0HXYZ
2W0JX0Z
2W0JX1Z
2W0JX2Z
2W0JX3Z
2W0JX4Z
2W0JX5Z
2W0JX6Z
2W0JX7Z
2W0JXYZ
2W0KX0Z
2W0KX1Z
2W0KX2Z
2W0KX3Z
2W0KX4Z
2W0KX5Z
2W0KX6Z
2W0KX7Z
2W0KXYZ
2W0LX0Z
2W0LX1Z
2W0LX2Z
2W0LX3Z
2W0LX4Z
2W0LX5Z
2W0LX6Z
2W0LX7Z
2W0LXYZ
2W0MX0Z
2W0MX1Z
2W0MX2Z
2W0MX3Z
2W0MX4Z
2W0MX5Z
2W0MX6Z
2W0MX7Z
2W0MXYZ
2W0NX0Z
2W0NX1Z
2W0NX2Z
2W0NX3Z
2W0NX4Z
2W0NX5Z
2W0NX6Z
2W0NX7Z
2W0NXYZ
2W0PX0Z
2W0PX1Z
2W0PX2Z
2W0PX3Z
2W0PX4Z
2W0PX5Z
2W0PX6Z
2W0PX7Z
2W0PXYZ
2W0QX0Z
2W0QX1Z
2W0QX2Z
2W0QX3Z
2W0QX4Z
2W0QX5Z
2W0QX6Z
2W0QX7Z
2W0QXYZ
2W0RX0Z
2W0RX1Z
2W0RX2Z
2W0RX3Z
2W0RX4Z
2W0RX5Z
2W0RX6Z
2W0RX7Z
2W0RXYZ
2W0SX0Z
2W0SX1Z
2W0SX2Z
2W0SX3Z
2W0SX4Z
2W0SX5Z
2W0SX6Z
2W0SX7Z
2W0SXYZ
2W0TX0Z
2W0TX1Z
2W0TX2Z
2W0TX3Z
2W0TX4Z
2W0TX5Z
2W0TX6Z
2W0TX7Z
2W0TXYZ
2W0UX0Z
2W0UX1Z
2W0UX2Z
2W0UX3Z
2W0UX4Z
2W0UX5Z
2W0UX6Z
2W0UX7Z
2W0UXYZ
2W0VX0Z
2W0VX1Z
2W0VX2Z
2W0VX3Z
2W0VX4Z
2W0VX5Z
2W0VX6Z
2W0VX7Z
2W0VXYZ
2W10X6Z
2W10X7Z
2W11X6Z
2W11X7Z
2W12X6Z
2W12X7Z
2W13X6Z
2W13X7Z
2W14X6Z
2W14X7Z
2W15X6Z
2W15X7Z
2W16X6Z
2W16X7Z
2W17X6Z
2W17X7Z
2W18X6Z
2W18X7Z
2W19X6Z
2W19X7Z
2W1AX6Z
2W1AX7Z
2W1BX6Z
2W1BX7Z
2W1CX6Z
2W1CX7Z
2W1DX6Z
2W1DX7Z
2W1EX6Z
2W1EX7Z
2W1FX6Z
2W1FX7Z
2W1GX6Z
2W1GX7Z
2W1HX6Z
2W1HX7Z
2W1JX6Z
2W1JX7Z
2W1KX6Z
2W1KX7Z
2W1LX6Z
2W1LX7Z
2W1MX6Z
2W1MX7Z
2W1NX6Z
2W1NX7Z
2W1PX6Z
2W1PX7Z
2W1QX6Z
2W1QX7Z
2W1RX6Z
2W1RX7Z
2W1SX6Z
2W1SX7Z
2W1TX6Z
2W1TX7Z
2W1UX6Z
2W1UX7Z
2W1VX6Z
2W1VX7Z
2W20X4Z
2W21X4Z
2W22X4Z
2W23X4Z
2W24X4Z
2W25X4Z
2W26X4Z
2W27X4Z
2W28X4Z
2W29X4Z
2W2AX4Z
2W2BX4Z
2W2CX4Z
2W2DX4Z
2W2EX4Z
2W2FX4Z
2W2GX4Z
2W2HX4Z
2W2JX4Z
2W2KX4Z
2W2LX4Z
2W2MX4Z
2W2NX4Z
2W2PX4Z
2W2QX4Z
2W2RX4Z
2W2SX4Z
2W2TX4Z
2W2UX4Z
2W2VX4Z
2W30X1Z
2W30X2Z
2W30X3Z
2W30XYZ
2W31X1Z
2W31X2Z
2W31X3Z
2W31X9Z
2W31XYZ
2W32X1Z
2W32X2Z
2W32X3Z
2W32XYZ
2W33X1Z
2W33X2Z
2W33X3Z
2W33XYZ
2W34X1Z
2W34X2Z
2W34X3Z
2W34XYZ
2W35X1Z
2W35X2Z
2W35X3Z
2W35XYZ
2W36X1Z
2W36X2Z
2W36X3Z
2W36XYZ
2W37X1Z
2W37X2Z
2W37X3Z
2W37XYZ
2W38X1Z
2W38X2Z
2W38X3Z
2W38XYZ
2W39X1Z
2W39X2Z
2W39X3Z
2W39XYZ
2W3AX1Z
2W3AX2Z
2W3AX3Z
2W3AXYZ
2W3BX1Z
2W3BX2Z
2W3BX3Z
2W3BXYZ
2W3CX1Z
2W3CX2Z
2W3CX3Z
2W3CXYZ
2W3DX1Z
2W3DX2Z
2W3DX3Z
2W3DXYZ
2W3EX1Z
2W3EX2Z
2W3EX3Z
2W3EXYZ
2W3FX1Z
2W3FX2Z
2W3FX3Z
2W3FXYZ
2W3GX1Z
2W3GX2Z
2W3GX3Z
2W3GXYZ
2W3HX1Z
2W3HX2Z
2W3HX3Z
2W3HXYZ
2W3JX1Z
2W3JX2Z
2W3JX3Z
2W3JXYZ
2W3KX1Z
2W3KX2Z
2W3KX3Z
2W3KXYZ
2W3LX1Z
2W3LX2Z
2W3LX3Z
2W3LXYZ
2W3MX1Z
2W3MX2Z
2W3MX3Z
2W3MXYZ
2W3NX1Z
2W3NX2Z
2W3NX3Z
2W3NXYZ
2W3PX1Z
2W3PX2Z
2W3PX3Z
2W3PXYZ
2W3QX1Z
2W3QX2Z
2W3QX3Z

2W3QXYZ
2W3RX1Z
2W3RX2Z
2W3RX3Z
2W3RXYZ
2W3SX1Z
2W3SX2Z
2W3SX3Z
2W3SXYZ
2W3TX1Z
2W3TX2Z
2W3TX3Z
2W3TXYZ
2W3UX1Z
2W3UX2Z
2W3UX3Z
2W3UXYZ
2W3VX1Z
2W3VX2Z
2W3VX3Z
2W3VXYZ
2W40X5Z
2W41X5Z
2W42X5Z
2W43X5Z
2W44X5Z
2W45X5Z
2W46X5Z
2W47X5Z
2W48X5Z
2W49X5Z
2W4AX5Z
2W4BX5Z
2W4CX5Z
2W4DX5Z
2W4EX5Z
2W4FX5Z
2W4GX5Z
2W4HX5Z
2W4JX5Z
2W4KX5Z
2W4LX5Z
2W4MX5Z
2W4NX5Z
2W4PX5Z
2W4QX5Z
2W4RX5Z
2W4SX5Z
2W4TX5Z
2W4UX5Z
2W4VX5Z
2W50X0Z
2W50X1Z
2W50X2Z
2W50X3Z
2W50X4Z
2W50X5Z
2W50X6Z
2W50X7Z
2W50XYZ
2W51X0Z
2W51X1Z
2W51X2Z
2W51X3Z
2W51X4Z
2W51X5Z
2W51X6Z
2W51X7Z
2W51X9Z
2W51XYZ
2W52X0Z
2W52X1Z
2W52X2Z
2W52X3Z
2W52X4Z
2W52X5Z
2W52X6Z
2W52X7Z
2W52XYZ
2W53X0Z
2W53X1Z
2W53X2Z
2W53X3Z
2W53X4Z
2W53X5Z
2W53X6Z
2W53X7Z
2W53XYZ
2W54X0Z
2W54X1Z
2W54X2Z
2W54X3Z
2W54X4Z
2W54X5Z
2W54X6Z
2W54X7Z
2W54XYZ
2W55X0Z
2W55X1Z
2W55X2Z
2W55X3Z
2W55X4Z
2W55X5Z
2W55X6Z
2W55X7Z
2W55XYZ
2W56X0Z
2W56X1Z
2W56X2Z
2W56X3Z
2W56X4Z
2W56X5Z
2W56X6Z
2W56X7Z
2W56XYZ
2W57X0Z
2W57X1Z
2W57X2Z
2W57X3Z
2W57X4Z
2W57X5Z
2W57X6Z
2W57X7Z
2W57XYZ
2W58X0Z
2W58X1Z
2W58X2Z
2W58X3Z
2W58X4Z
2W58X5Z
2W58X6Z
2W58X7Z
2W58XYZ
2W59X0Z
2W59X1Z
2W59X2Z
2W59X3Z
2W59X4Z
2W59X5Z
2W59X6Z
2W59X7Z
2W59XYZ
2W5AX0Z
2W5AX1Z
2W5AX2Z
2W5AX3Z
2W5AX4Z
2W5AX5Z
2W5AX6Z
2W5AX7Z
2W5AXYZ
2W5BX0Z
2W5BX1Z
2W5BX2Z
2W5BX3Z
2W5BX4Z
2W5BX5Z
2W5BX6Z
2W5BX7Z
2W5BXYZ
2W5CX0Z
2W5CX1Z
2W5CX2Z
2W5CX3Z
2W5CX4Z
2W5CX5Z
2W5CX6Z
2W5CX7Z
2W5CXYZ
2W5DX0Z
2W5DX1Z
2W5DX2Z
2W5DX3Z
2W5DX4Z
2W5DX5Z
2W5DX6Z
2W5DX7Z
2W5DXYZ
2W5EX0Z
2W5EX1Z
2W5EX2Z
2W5EX3Z
2W5EX4Z
2W5EX5Z
2W5EX6Z
2W5EX7Z
2W5EXYZ
2W5FX0Z
2W5FX1Z
2W5FX2Z
2W5FX3Z
2W5FX4Z
2W5FX5Z
2W5FX6Z
2W5FX7Z
2W5FXYZ
2W5GX0Z
2W5GX1Z
2W5GX2Z
2W5GX3Z
2W5GX4Z
2W5GX5Z
2W5GX6Z
2W5GX7Z
2W5GXYZ
2W5HX0Z
2W5HX1Z
2W5HX2Z
2W5HX3Z
2W5HX4Z
2W5HX5Z
2W5HX6Z
2W5HX7Z
2W5HXYZ
2W5JX0Z
2W5JX1Z
2W5JX2Z
2W5JX3Z
2W5JX4Z
2W5JX5Z
2W5JX6Z
2W5JX7Z
2W5JXYZ
2W5KX0Z
2W5KX1Z
2W5KX2Z
2W5KX3Z
2W5KX4Z
2W5KX5Z
2W5KX6Z
2W5KX7Z
2W5KXYZ
2W5LX0Z
2W5LX1Z
2W5LX2Z
2W5LX3Z
2W5LX4Z
2W5LX5Z
2W5LX6Z
2W5LX7Z
2W5LXYZ
2W5MX0Z
2W5MX1Z
2W5MX2Z
2W5MX3Z
2W5MX4Z
2W5MX5Z
2W5MX6Z
2W5MX7Z
2W5MXYZ
2W5NX0Z
2W5NX1Z
2W5NX2Z
2W5NX3Z
2W5NX4Z
2W5NX5Z
2W5NX6Z
2W5NX7Z
2W5NXYZ
2W5PX0Z
2W5PX1Z
2W5PX2Z
2W5PX3Z
2W5PX4Z
2W5PX5Z
2W5PX6Z
2W5PX7Z
2W5PXYZ
2W5QX0Z
2W5QX1Z
2W5QX2Z
2W5QX3Z
2W5QX4Z
2W5QX5Z
2W5QX6Z
2W5QX7Z
2W5QXYZ
2W5RX0Z
2W5RX1Z
2W5RX2Z
2W5RX3Z
2W5RX4Z
2W5RX5Z
2W5RX6Z
2W5RX7Z
2W5RXYZ
2W5SX0Z
2W5SX1Z
2W5SX2Z
2W5SX3Z
2W5SX4Z
2W5SX5Z
2W5SX6Z
2W5SX7Z
2W5SXYZ
2W5TX0Z
2W5TX1Z
2W5TX2Z
2W5TX3Z
2W5TX4Z
2W5TX5Z
2W5TX6Z
2W5TX7Z
2W5TXYZ
2W5UX0Z
2W5UX1Z
2W5UX2Z
2W5UX3Z
2W5UX4Z
2W5UX5Z
2W5UX6Z
2W5UX7Z
2W5UXYZ
2W5VX0Z
2W5VX1Z
2W5VX2Z
2W5VX3Z
2W5VX4Z
2W5VX5Z
2W5VX6Z
2W5VX7Z
2W5VXYZ
2W60X0Z
2W60XZZ
2W61X0Z
2W61XZZ
2W62X0Z
2W62XZZ
2W63X0Z
2W63XZZ
2W64X0Z
2W64XZZ
2W65X0Z
2W65XZZ
2W66X0Z
2W66XZZ
2W67X0Z
2W67XZZ
2W68X0Z
2W68XZZ
2W69X0Z
2W69XZZ
2W6AX0Z
2W6AXZZ
2W6BX0Z
2W6BXZZ
2W6CX0Z
2W6CXZZ
2W6DX0Z
2W6DXZZ
2W6EX0Z
2W6EXZZ
2W6FX0Z
2W6FXZZ
2W6GX0Z
2W6GXZZ
2W6HX0Z
2W6HXZZ
2W6JX0Z
2W6JXZZ
2W6KX0Z
2W6KXZZ
2W6LX0Z
2W6LXZZ
2W6MX0Z
2W6MXZZ
2W6NX0Z
2W6NXZZ
2W6PX0Z
2W6PXZZ
2W6QX0Z
2W6QXZZ
2W6RX0Z
2W6RXZZ
2W6SX0Z
2W6SXZZ
2W6TX0Z
2W6TXZZ
2W6UX0Z
2W6UXZZ
2W6VX0Z
2W6VXZZ
2Y00X5Z
2Y01X5Z
2Y02X5Z
2Y03X5Z
2Y04X5Z
2Y05X5Z
2Y40X5Z
2Y41X5Z
2Y42X5Z
2Y43X5Z
2Y44X5Z
2Y45X5Z
2Y50X5Z
2Y51X5Z
2Y52X5Z
2Y53X5Z
2Y54X5Z
2Y55X5Z
30230AZ
30230G0
30230G2
30230G3
30230G4
30230H0
30230H1
30230J0
30230J1
30230K0
30230K1
30230L0
30230L1
30230M0
30230M1
30230N0
30230N1
30230P0
30230P1
30230Q0
30230Q1
30230R0
30230R1
30230S0
30230S1
30230T0
30230T1
30230V0
30230V1
30230W0
30230W1
30230X0
30230X2
30230X3
30230X4
30230Y0
30230Y2
30230Y3
30230Y4
30233AZ
30233G0
30233G2
30233G3
30233G4
30233H0
30233H1
30233J0
30233J1
30233K0
30233K1
30233L0
30233L1
30233M0
30233M1
30233N0
30233N1
30233P0
30233P1
30233Q0
30233Q1
30233R0
30233R1
30233S0
30233S1
30233T0
30233T1
30233V0
30233V1
30233W0
30233W1
30233X0
30233X2
30233X3
30233X4
30233Y0
30233Y2
30233Y3
30233Y4
30240AZ
30240G0
30240G2
30240G3
30240G4
30240H0
30240H1
30240J0
30240J1
30240K0
30240K1
30240L0
30240L1
30240M0
30240M1
30240N0
30240N1
30240P0
30240P1
30240Q0
30240Q1
30240R0
30240R1
30240S0
30240S1
30240T0
30240T1
30240V0
30240V1
30240W0
30240W1
30240X0
30240X2
30240X3
30240X4
30240Y0
30240Y2
30240Y3
30240Y4
30243AZ
30243G0
30243G2
30243G3
30243G4
30243H0
30243H1
30243J0
30243J1
30243K0
30243K1
30243L0
30243L1
30243M0
30243M1
30243N0
30243N1
30243P0
30243P1
30243Q0
30243Q1
30243R0
30243R1
30243S0
30243S1
30243T0
30243T1
30243V0
30243V1
30243W0
30243W1
30243X0
30243X2
30243X3
30243X4
30243Y0
30243Y2
30243Y3
30243Y4
30250G0
30250G1
30250H0
30250H1
30250J0
30250J1
30250K0
30250K1
30250L0
30250L1
30250M0
30250M1
30250N0
30250N1
30250P0
30250P1
30250Q0
30250Q1
30250R0
30250R1
30250S0
30250S1
30250T0
30250T1
30250V0
30250V1
30250W0
30250W1
30250X0
30250X1
30250Y0
30250Y1
30253G0
30253G1
30253H0
30253H1
30253J0
30253J1
30253K0
30253K1
30253L0
30253L1
30253M0
30253M1
30253N0
30253N1
30253P0
30253P1
30253Q0
30253Q1
30253R0
30253R1
30253S0
30253S1
30253T0
30253T1
30253V0
30253V1
30253W0
30253W1
30253X0
30253X1
30253Y0
30253Y1
30260G0
30260G1
30260H0
30260H1
30260J0
30260J1
30260K0
30260K1
30260L0
30260L1
30260M0
30260M1
30260N0
30260N1
30260P0
30260P1
30260Q0
30260Q1
30260R0
30260R1
30260S0
30260S1
30260T0
30260T1
30260V0
30260V1
30260W0
30260W1
30260X0
30260X1
30260Y0
30260Y1
30263G0
30263G1
30263H0
30263H1
30263J0
30263J1
30263K0
30263K1
30263L0
30263L1
30263M0
30263M1
30263N0
30263N1
30263P0
30263P1
30263Q0
30263Q1
30263R0
30263R1
30263S0
30263S1
30263T0
30263T1
30263V0
30263V1
30263W0
30263W1
30263X0
30263X1
30263Y0
30263Y1
30273H1
30273J1
30273K1
30273L1
30273M1
30273N1
30273P1
30273Q1
30273R1
30273S1
30273T1
30273V1
30273W1
30277H1
30277J1
30277K1
30277L1
30277M1
30277N1
30277P1
30277Q1
30277R1
30277S1
30277T1
30277V1
30277W1
30280B1
30283B1
3C1ZX8Z
3E00X05
3E00X0M
3E00X28
3E00X29
3E00X3Z
3E00X4Z
3E00XBZ
3E00XGC
3E00XKZ
3E00XMZ
3E00XNZ
3E00XTZ
3E0102A

3E01305
3E0130M
3E01328
3E01329
3E0132A
3E0133Z
3E01340
3E0134Z
3E0136Z
3E0137Z
3E013BZ
3E013GC
3E013HZ
3E013KZ
3E013NZ
3E013TZ
3E013VG
3E013VJ
3E02305
3E0230M
3E02328
3E02329
3E0233Z
3E02340
3E0234Z
3E0236Z
3E0237Z
3E023BZ
3E023GC
3E023HZ
3E023KZ
3E023NZ
3E023TZ
3E03002
3E03003
3E03005
3E0300M
3E0300P
3E03016
3E03017
3E03028
3E03029
3E0303Z
3E0304Z
3E0306Z
3E0307Z
3E030FZ
3E030GC
3E030GN
3E030HZ
3E030KZ
3E030NZ
3E030PZ
3E030RZ
3E030TZ
3E030U0
3E030U1
3E030VG
3E030VH
3E030VJ
3E030WK
3E030WL
3E030XZ
3E03302
3E03303
3E03305
3E0330M
3E0330P
3E03316
3E03317
3E03328
3E03329
3E0333Z
3E0334Z
3E0336Z
3E0337Z
3E033FZ
3E033GC
3E033GN
3E033GQ
3E033HZ
3E033KZ
3E033NZ
3E033PZ
3E033RZ
3E033TZ
3E033U0
3E033U1
3E033VG
3E033VH
3E033VJ
3E033WK
3E033WL
3E033XZ
3E04002
3E04003
3E04005
3E0400M
3E0400P
3E04016
3E04017
3E04028
3E04029
3E0403Z
3E0404Z
3E0406Z
3E0407Z
3E040FZ
3E040GC
3E040GN
3E040HZ
3E040KZ
3E040NZ
3E040PZ
3E040RZ
3E040TZ
3E040VG
3E040VH
3E040VJ
3E040WK
3E040WL
3E040XZ
3E04302
3E04303
3E04305
3E0430M
3E0430P
3E04316
3E04317
3E04328
3E04329
3E0433Z
3E0434Z
3E0436Z
3E0437Z
3E043FZ
3E043GC
3E043GN
3E043GQ
3E043HZ
3E043KZ
3E043NZ
3E043PZ
3E043RZ
3E043TZ
3E043VG
3E043VH
3E043VJ
3E043WK
3E043WL
3E043XZ
3E05002
3E05003
3E05005
3E0500M
3E0500P
3E05016
3E05017
3E05028
3E05029
3E0503Z
3E0504Z
3E0506Z
3E0507Z
3E050FZ
3E050GC
3E050GN
3E050HZ
3E050KZ
3E050NZ
3E050PZ
3E050RZ
3E050TZ
3E050VG
3E050VH
3E050VJ
3E050WK
3E050WL
3E050XZ
3E05302
3E05303
3E05305
3E0530M
3E0530P
3E05316
3E05317
3E05328
3E05329
3E0533Z
3E0534Z
3E0536Z
3E0537Z
3E053FZ
3E053GC
3E053GN
3E053HZ
3E053KZ
3E053NZ
3E053PZ
3E053RZ
3E053TZ
3E053VG
3E053VH
3E053VJ
3E053WK
3E053WL
3E053XZ
3E06002
3E06003
3E06005
3E0600M
3E0600P
3E06016
3E06017
3E06028
3E06029
3E0603Z
3E0604Z
3E0606Z
3E0607Z
3E060FZ
3E060GC
3E060GN
3E060HZ
3E060KZ
3E060NZ
3E060PZ
3E060RZ
3E060TZ
3E060VG
3E060VH
3E060VJ
3E060WK
3E060WL
3E060XZ
3E06302
3E06303
3E06305
3E0630M
3E0630P
3E06316
3E06317
3E06328
3E06329
3E0633Z
3E0634Z
3E0636Z
3E0637Z
3E063FZ
3E063GC
3E063GN
3E063HZ
3E063KZ
3E063NZ
3E063PZ
3E063RZ
3E063TZ
3E063VG
3E063VH
3E063VJ
3E063WK
3E063WL
3E063XZ
3E07016
3E07017
3E070GC
3E070KZ
3E070PZ
3E07316
3E07317
3E073GC
3E073KZ
3E073PZ
3E074GC
3E08016
3E08017
3E080GC
3E080KZ
3E080PZ
3E08316
3E08317
3E083GC
3E083KZ
3E083PZ
3E084GC
3E09305
3E0930M
3E09328
3E09329
3E0933Z
3E0934Z
3E093BZ
3E093GC
3E093HZ
3E093KZ
3E093NZ
3E093TZ
3E09705
3E0970M
3E09728
3E09729
3E0973Z
3E0974Z
3E097BZ
3E097GC
3E097HZ
3E097KZ
3E097NZ
3E097TZ
3E09X05
3E09X0M
3E09X28
3E09X29
3E09X3Z
3E09X4Z
3E09XBZ
3E09XGC
3E09XHZ
3E09XKZ
3E09XNZ
3E09XTZ
3E0A305
3E0A30M
3E0A3GC
3E0B304
3E0B305
3E0B30M
3E0B328
3E0B329
3E0B33Z
3E0B3BZ
3E0B3GC
3E0B3HZ
3E0B3KZ
3E0B3NZ
3E0B3TZ
3E0B704
3E0B705
3E0B70M
3E0B728
3E0B729
3E0B73Z
3E0B7BZ
3E0B7GC
3E0B7HZ
3E0B7KZ
3E0B7NZ
3E0B7TZ
3E0BX04
3E0BX05
3E0BX0M
3E0BX28
3E0BX29
3E0BX3Z
3E0BXBZ
3E0BXGC
3E0BXHZ
3E0BXKZ
3E0BXNZ
3E0BXTZ
3E0C304
3E0C305
3E0C30M
3E0C328
3E0C329
3E0C33Z
3E0C3BZ
3E0C3GC
3E0C3HZ
3E0C3KZ
3E0C3MZ
3E0C3NZ
3E0C3SF
3E0C3TZ
3E0C704
3E0C705
3E0C70M
3E0C728
3E0C729
3E0C73Z
3E0C7BZ
3E0C7GC
3E0C7HZ
3E0C7KZ
3E0C7MZ
3E0C7NZ
3E0C7SF
3E0C7TZ
3E0CX04
3E0CX05
3E0CX0M
3E0CX28
3E0CX29
3E0CX3Z
3E0CXBZ
3E0CXGC
3E0CXHZ
3E0CXKZ
3E0CXMZ
3E0CXNZ
3E0CXSF
3E0CXTZ
3E0D304
3E0D305
3E0D30M
3E0D328
3E0D329
3E0D33Z
3E0D34Z
3E0D36Z
3E0D37Z
3E0D3BZ
3E0D3GC
3E0D3HZ
3E0D3KZ
3E0D3NZ
3E0D3RZ
3E0D3TZ
3E0D704
3E0D705
3E0D70M
3E0D728
3E0D729
3E0D73Z
3E0D74Z
3E0D76Z
3E0D77Z
3E0D7BZ
3E0D7GC
3E0D7HZ
3E0D7KZ
3E0D7NZ
3E0D7RZ
3E0D7TZ
3E0DX04
3E0DX05
3E0DX0M
3E0DX28
3E0DX29
3E0DX3Z
3E0DX4Z
3E0DX6Z
3E0DX7Z
3E0DXBZ
3E0DXGC
3E0DXHZ
3E0DXKZ
3E0DXNZ
3E0DXRZ
3E0DXTZ
3E0E304
3E0E305
3E0E30M
3E0E328
3E0E329
3E0E33Z
3E0E36Z
3E0E37Z
3E0E3BZ
3E0E3GC
3E0E3HZ
3E0E3KZ
3E0E3NZ
3E0E3SF
3E0E3TZ
3E0E4GC
3E0E704
3E0E705
3E0E70M
3E0E728
3E0E729
3E0E73Z
3E0E76Z
3E0E77Z
3E0E7BZ
3E0E7GC
3E0E7HZ
3E0E7KZ
3E0E7NZ
3E0E7SF
3E0E7TZ
3E0E804
3E0E805
3E0E80M
3E0E828
3E0E829
3E0E83Z
3E0E86Z
3E0E87Z
3E0E8BZ
3E0E8GC
3E0E8HZ
3E0E8KZ
3E0E8NZ
3E0E8SF
3E0E8TZ
3E0F304
3E0F305
3E0F30M
3E0F328
3E0F329
3E0F33Z
3E0F36Z
3E0F37Z
3E0F3BZ
3E0F3GC
3E0F3HZ
3E0F3KZ
3E0F3NZ
3E0F3SD
3E0F3SF
3E0F3TZ
3E0F4GC
3E0F704
3E0F705
3E0F70M
3E0F728
3E0F729
3E0F73Z
3E0F76Z
3E0F77Z
3E0F7BZ
3E0F7GC
3E0F7HZ
3E0F7KZ
3E0F7NZ
3E0F7SD
3E0F7SF
3E0F7TZ
3E0F804
3E0F805
3E0F80M
3E0F828
3E0F829
3E0F83Z
3E0F86Z
3E0F87Z
3E0F8BZ
3E0F8GC
3E0F8HZ
3E0F8KZ
3E0F8NZ
3E0F8SD
3E0F8SF
3E0F8TZ
3E0G304
3E0G305
3E0G30M
3E0G328
3E0G329
3E0G33Z
3E0G36Z
3E0G37Z
3E0G3BZ
3E0G3GC
3E0G3HZ
3E0G3KZ
3E0G3NZ
3E0G3SF
3E0G3TZ
3E0G4GC
3E0G704
3E0G705
3E0G70M
3E0G728
3E0G729
3E0G73Z
3E0G76Z
3E0G77Z
3E0G7BZ
3E0G7GC
3E0G7HZ
3E0G7KZ
3E0G7NZ
3E0G7SF
3E0G7TZ
3E0G804
3E0G805
3E0G80M
3E0G828
3E0G829
3E0G83Z
3E0G86Z
3E0G87Z
3E0G8BZ
3E0G8GC
3E0G8HZ
3E0G8KZ
3E0G8NZ
3E0G8SF
3E0G8TZ
3E0H304
3E0H305
3E0H30M
3E0H328
3E0H329
3E0H33Z
3E0H36Z
3E0H37Z
3E0H3BZ
3E0H3GC
3E0H3HZ
3E0H3KZ
3E0H3NZ
3E0H3SF
3E0H3TZ
3E0H4GC
3E0H704
3E0H705
3E0H70M
3E0H728
3E0H729
3E0H73Z
3E0H76Z
3E0H77Z
3E0H7BZ
3E0H7GC
3E0H7HZ
3E0H7KZ
3E0H7NZ
3E0H7SF
3E0H7TZ
3E0H804
3E0H805
3E0H80M
3E0H828
3E0H829
3E0H83Z
3E0H86Z
3E0H87Z
3E0H8BZ
3E0H8GC
3E0H8HZ
3E0H8KZ
3E0H8NZ
3E0H8SF
3E0H8TZ
3E0J304
3E0J305
3E0J30M
3E0J328
3E0J329
3E0J33Z
3E0J36Z
3E0J37Z
3E0J3BZ
3E0J3GC
3E0J3HZ
3E0J3KZ
3E0J3NZ
3E0J3SF
3E0J3TZ
3E0J3U0
3E0J3U1
3E0J4GC
3E0J704
3E0J705
3E0J70M
3E0J728
3E0J729
3E0J73Z
3E0J76Z
3E0J77Z
3E0J7BZ
3E0J7GC
3E0J7HZ
3E0J7KZ
3E0J7NZ
3E0J7SF
3E0J7TZ
3E0J7U0
3E0J7U1
3E0J804
3E0J805
3E0J80M
3E0J828
3E0J829
3E0J83Z
3E0J86Z
3E0J87Z
3E0J8BZ
3E0J8GC
3E0J8HZ
3E0J8KZ
3E0J8NZ
3E0J8SF
3E0J8TZ
3E0J8U0
3E0J8U1
3E0K304
3E0K305
3E0K30M
3E0K328
3E0K329
3E0K33Z
3E0K36Z
3E0K37Z
3E0K3BZ
3E0K3GC
3E0K3HZ
3E0K3KZ
3E0K3NZ
3E0K3SF
3E0K3TZ
3E0K4GC
3E0K704
3E0K705
3E0K70M
3E0K728
3E0K729
3E0K73Z
3E0K76Z
3E0K77Z
3E0K7BZ
3E0K7GC
3E0K7HZ
3E0K7KZ
3E0K7NZ
3E0K7SF
3E0K7TZ
3E0K804
3E0K805
3E0K80M
3E0K828
3E0K829
3E0K83Z

3E0K86Z
3E0K87Z
3E0K8BZ
3E0K8GC
3E0K8HZ
3E0K8KZ
3E0K8NZ
3E0K8SF
3E0K8TZ
3E0L05Z
3E0L304
3E0L305
3E0L30M
3E0L328
3E0L329
3E0L33Z
3E0L35Z
3E0L36Z
3E0L37Z
3E0L3BZ
3E0L3GC
3E0L3HZ
3E0L3KZ
3E0L3NZ
3E0L3SF
3E0L3TZ
3E0L45Z
3E0L4GC
3E0L704
3E0L705
3E0L70M
3E0L7SF
3E0M05Z
3E0M304
3E0M305
3E0M30M
3E0M328
3E0M329
3E0M33Z
3E0M35Z
3E0M36Z
3E0M37Z
3E0M3BZ
3E0M3GC
3E0M3HZ
3E0M3KZ
3E0M3NZ
3E0M3SF
3E0M3TZ
3E0M45Z
3E0M4GC
3E0M704
3E0M705
3E0M70M
3E0M7SF
3E0N304
3E0N305
3E0N30M
3E0N328
3E0N329
3E0N33Z
3E0N36Z
3E0N37Z
3E0N3BZ
3E0N3GC
3E0N3HZ
3E0N3KZ
3E0N3NZ
3E0N3SF
3E0N3TZ
3E0N4GC
3E0N704
3E0N705
3E0N70M
3E0N728
3E0N729
3E0N73Z
3E0N76Z
3E0N77Z
3E0N7BZ
3E0N7GC
3E0N7HZ
3E0N7KZ
3E0N7NZ
3E0N7SF
3E0N7TZ
3E0N804
3E0N805
3E0N80M
3E0N828
3E0N829
3E0N83Z
3E0N86Z
3E0N87Z
3E0N8BZ
3E0N8GC
3E0N8HZ
3E0N8KZ
3E0N8NZ
3E0N8SF
3E0N8TZ
3E0P05Z
3E0P304
3E0P305
3E0P30M
3E0P328
3E0P329
3E0P33Z
3E0P35Z
3E0P36Z
3E0P37Z
3E0P3BZ
3E0P3GC
3E0P3HZ
3E0P3KZ
3E0P3LZ
3E0P3NZ
3E0P3Q0
3E0P3Q1
3E0P3SF
3E0P3TZ
3E0P3VZ
3E0P45Z
3E0P4GC
3E0P704
3E0P705
3E0P70M
3E0P728
3E0P729
3E0P73Z
3E0P76Z
3E0P77Z
3E0P7BZ
3E0P7GC
3E0P7HZ
3E0P7KZ
3E0P7LZ
3E0P7NZ
3E0P7Q0
3E0P7Q1
3E0P7SF
3E0P7TZ
3E0P7VZ
3E0P804
3E0P805
3E0P80M
3E0P828
3E0P829
3E0P83Z
3E0P86Z
3E0P87Z
3E0P8BZ
3E0P8GC
3E0P8HZ
3E0P8KZ
3E0P8NZ
3E0P8SF
3E0P8TZ
3E0Q004
3E0Q005
3E0Q00M
3E0Q028
3E0Q029
3E0Q03Z
3E0Q06Z
3E0Q07Z
3E0Q0AZ
3E0Q0BZ
3E0Q0E0
3E0Q0E1
3E0Q0GC
3E0Q0HZ
3E0Q0KZ
3E0Q0NZ
3E0Q0SF
3E0Q0TZ
3E0Q304
3E0Q305
3E0Q30M
3E0Q328
3E0Q329
3E0Q33Z
3E0Q36Z
3E0Q37Z
3E0Q3AZ
3E0Q3BZ
3E0Q3E0
3E0Q3E1
3E0Q3GC
3E0Q3HZ
3E0Q3KZ
3E0Q3NZ
3E0Q3SF
3E0Q3TZ
3E0Q704
3E0Q705
3E0Q70M
3E0Q7SF
3E0R0AZ
3E0R0E0
3E0R0E1
3E0R302
3E0R303
3E0R304
3E0R305
3E0R30M
3E0R328
3E0R329
3E0R33Z
3E0R36Z
3E0R37Z
3E0R3AZ
3E0R3BZ
3E0R3E0
3E0R3E1
3E0R3GC
3E0R3HZ
3E0R3KZ
3E0R3NZ
3E0R3SF
3E0R3TZ
3E0R7SF
3E0S302
3E0S303
3E0S304
3E0S305
3E0S30M
3E0S328
3E0S329
3E0S33Z
3E0S36Z
3E0S37Z
3E0S3BZ
3E0S3GC
3E0S3HZ
3E0S3KZ
3E0S3NZ
3E0S3SF
3E0S3TZ
3E0S7SF
3E0T33Z
3E0T3BZ
3E0T3GC
3E0T3TZ
3E0U028
3E0U029
3E0U0GB
3E0U304
3E0U305
3E0U30M
3E0U328
3E0U329
3E0U33Z
3E0U36Z
3E0U37Z
3E0U3BZ
3E0U3GB
3E0U3GC
3E0U3HZ
3E0U3KZ
3E0U3NZ
3E0U3SF
3E0U3TZ
3E0U4GC
3E0V0GB
3E0V305
3E0V30M
3E0V328
3E0V329
3E0V33Z
3E0V36Z
3E0V37Z
3E0V3BZ
3E0V3GB
3E0V3GC
3E0V3HZ
3E0V3KZ
3E0V3NZ
3E0V3TZ
3E0W305
3E0W30M
3E0W328
3E0W329
3E0W33Z
3E0W36Z
3E0W37Z
3E0W3BZ
3E0W3GC
3E0W3HZ
3E0W3KZ
3E0W3NZ
3E0W3TZ
3E0X33Z
3E0X3BZ
3E0X3GC
3E0X3TZ
3E0Y304
3E0Y305
3E0Y30M
3E0Y328
3E0Y329
3E0Y33Z
3E0Y36Z
3E0Y37Z
3E0Y3BZ
3E0Y3GC
3E0Y3HZ
3E0Y3KZ
3E0Y3NZ
3E0Y3SF
3E0Y3TZ
3E0Y4GC
3E0Y704
3E0Y705
3E0Y70M
3E0Y7SF
3E1038X
3E1038Z
3E10X8X
3E10X8Z
3E1938X
3E1938Z
3E1978X
3E1978Z
3E1988X
3E1988Z
3E1B38X
3E1B38Z
3E1B78X
3E1B78Z
3E1B88X
3E1B88Z
3E1C38X
3E1C38Z
3E1CX8X
3E1CX8Z
3E1F38X
3E1F38Z
3E1F78X
3E1F78Z
3E1F88X
3E1F88Z
3E1G38X
3E1G38Z
3E1G78X
3E1G78Z
3E1G88X
3E1G88Z
3E1H38X
3E1H38Z
3E1H78X
3E1H78Z
3E1H88X
3E1H88Z
3E1J38X
3E1J38Z
3E1J78X
3E1J78Z
3E1J88X
3E1J88Z
3E1K38X
3E1K38Z
3E1K78X
3E1K78Z
3E1K88X
3E1K88Z
3E1L38X
3E1L38Z
3E1M38X
3E1M38Z
3E1M39Z
3E1N38X
3E1N38Z
3E1N78X
3E1N78Z
3E1N88X
3E1N88Z
3E1P38X
3E1P38Z
3E1P78X
3E1P78Z
3E1P88X
3E1P88Z
3E1Q38X
3E1Q38Z
3E1R38X
3E1R38Z
3E1S38X
3E1S38Z
3E1U38X
3E1U38Z
3E1Y38X
3E1Y38Z
4A0002Z
4A0004Z
4A000BZ
4A0034Z
4A003BD
4A003KD
4A003RD
4A0074Z
4A007BD
4A007KD
4A007RD
4A0084Z
4A008BD
4A008KD
4A008RD
4A00X2Z
4A00X4Z
4A01029
4A0102B
4A0104Z
4A01329
4A0132B
4A0134Z
4A01729
4A0172B
4A0174Z
4A01829
4A0182B
4A0184Z
4A01X29
4A01X2B
4A01X4Z
4A0204Z
4A0209Z
4A020CZ
4A020FZ
4A020HZ
4A020N6
4A020N7
4A020N8
4A020PZ
4A0234Z
4A0239Z
4A023CZ
4A023FZ
4A023HZ
4A023N6
4A023N7
4A023N8
4A023PZ
4A0274Z
4A0279Z
4A027CZ
4A027FZ
4A027HZ
4A027N6
4A027N7
4A027N8
4A027PZ
4A0284Z
4A0289Z
4A028CZ
4A028FZ
4A028HZ
4A028N6
4A028N7
4A028N8
4A028PZ
4A02X4A
4A02X4Z
4A02X9Z
4A02XCZ
4A02XFZ
4A02XHZ
4A02XM4
4A02XPZ
4A03051
4A03053
4A0305C
4A030B1
4A030B3
4A030BC
4A030BF
4A030H1
4A030J1
4A030J3
4A030JC
4A030R1
4A03351
4A03353
4A0335C
4A033B1
4A033B3
4A033BC
4A033BF
4A033H1
4A033J1
4A033J3
4A033JC
4A033R1
4A03X51
4A03XB1
4A03XH1
4A03XJ1
4A03XR1
4A04050
4A04051
4A04052
4A04053
4A040B0
4A040B1
4A040B2
4A040B3
4A040J0
4A040J1
4A040J2
4A040J3
4A040R1
4A04350
4A04351
4A04352
4A04353
4A043B0
4A043B1
4A043B2
4A043B3
4A043J0
4A043J1
4A043J2
4A043J3
4A043R1
4A04X51
4A04XB1
4A04XJ1
4A04XR1
4A05XLZ
4A0605Z
4A060BZ
4A0635Z
4A063BZ
4A0675Z
4A067BZ
4A0685Z
4A068BZ
4A07X0Z
4A07X7Z
4A07XBZ
4A08X0Z
4A0971Z
4A0975Z
4A097CZ
4A097DZ
4A097LZ
4A097MZ
4A0981Z
4A0985Z
4A098CZ
4A098DZ
4A098LZ
4A098MZ
4A09X1Z
4A09X5Z
4A09XCZ
4A09XDZ
4A09XLZ
4A09XMZ
4A0B78Z
4A0B7BZ
4A0B7GZ
4A0B88Z
4A0B8BZ
4A0B8GZ
4A0C35Z
4A0C3BZ
4A0C45Z
4A0C4BZ
4A0C75Z
4A0C7BZ
4A0C85Z
4A0C8BZ
4A0D73Z
4A0D75Z
4A0D7BZ
4A0D7DZ
4A0D7LZ
4A0D83Z
4A0D85Z
4A0D8BZ
4A0D8DZ
4A0D8LZ
4A0F33Z
4A0FX3Z
4A0H74Z
4A0H7CZ
4A0H7FZ
4A0H7HZ
4A0H84Z
4A0H8CZ
4A0H8FZ
4A0H8HZ
4A0HX4Z
4A0HXCZ
4A0HXFZ
4A0HXHZ
4A0J72Z
4A0J74Z
4A0J7BZ
4A0J82Z
4A0J84Z
4A0J8BZ
4A0JX2Z
4A0JX4Z
4A0JXBZ
4A0Z76Z
4A0Z7KZ
4A0ZX6Z
4A0ZXKZ
4A0ZXQZ
4A1002Z
4A1004G
4A1004Z
4A100BZ
4A1034G
4A1034Z
4A103BD
4A103KD
4A103RD
4A1074G
4A1074Z
4A107BD
4A107KD
4A107RD
4A1084G
4A1084Z
4A108BD
4A108KD
4A108RD
4A10X2Z
4A10X4G
4A10X4Z
4A11029
4A1102B
4A1104G
4A1104Z
4A11329
4A1132B
4A1134G
4A1134Z
4A11729
4A1172B
4A1174G
4A1174Z
4A11829
4A1182B
4A1184G
4A1184Z
4A11X29
4A11X2B
4A11X4G
4A11X4Z
4A1204Z
4A1209Z
4A120CZ
4A120FZ
4A120HZ
4A1234Z
4A1239Z
4A123CZ
4A123FZ
4A123HZ
4A1274Z
4A1279Z
4A127CZ
4A127FZ
4A127HZ
4A1284Z
4A1289Z
4A128CZ
4A128FZ
4A128HZ
4A12X45
4A12X4Z
4A12X9Z
4A12XCZ
4A12XFZ
4A12XHZ
4A12XM4
4A12XSH
4A13051
4A13053
4A1305C
4A130B1
4A130B3
4A130BC
4A130H1
4A130J1
4A130J3
4A130JC
4A130R1
4A13351
4A13353
4A1335C
4A133B1
4A133B3
4A133BC
4A133H1
4A133J1
4A133J3
4A133JC
4A133R1
4A13X51
4A13XB1
4A13XH1
4A13XJ1
4A13XR1
4A14050
4A14051
4A14052
4A14053
4A140B0
4A140B1
4A140B2
4A140B3
4A140J0
4A140J1
4A140J2
4A140J3
4A140R0
4A140R2
4A140R3
4A14350
4A14351
4A14352

4A14353
4A143B0
4A143B1
4A143B2
4A143B3
4A143J0
4A143J1
4A143J2
4A143J3
4A143R0
4A143R2
4A143R3
4A14X51
4A14XB1
4A14XJ1
4A1605Z
4A160BZ
4A1635Z
4A163BZ
4A1675Z
4A167BZ
4A1685Z
4A168BZ
4A1971Z
4A1975Z
4A197CZ
4A197DZ
4A197LZ
4A19X1Z
4A19X5Z
4A19XCZ
4A19XDZ
4A19XLZ
4A1B78Z
4A1B7BZ
4A1B7GZ
4A1B88Z
4A1B8BZ
4A1B8GZ
4A1BXSH
4A1D73Z
4A1D75Z
4A1D7BZ
4A1D7DZ
4A1D7LZ
4A1D83Z
4A1D85Z
4A1D8BZ
4A1D8DZ
4A1D8LZ
4A1GXSH
4A1H74Z
4A1H7CZ
4A1H7FZ
4A1H7HZ
4A1H84Z
4A1H8CZ
4A1H8FZ
4A1H8HZ
4A1HX4Z
4A1HXCZ
4A1HXFZ
4A1HXHZ
4A1J72Z
4A1J74Z
4A1J7BZ
4A1J82Z
4A1J84Z
4A1J8BZ
4A1JX2Z
4A1JX4Z
4A1JXBZ
4A1Z7KZ
4A1ZXKZ
4A1ZXQZ
4B00XVZ
4B01XVZ
4B02XSZ
4B02XTZ
4B09XSZ
4B0FXVZ
5A02110
5A02115
5A02116
5A0211D
5A02210
5A02215
5A02216
5A0221D
5A05121
5A0512C
5A05221
5A0522C
5A0920Z
5A09357
5A09358
5A09359
5A0935B
5A0935Z
5A09457
5A09458
5A09459
5A0945B
5A0945Z
5A09557
5A09558
5A09559
5A0955B
5A0955Z
5A12012
5A1213Z
5A1221Z
5A1223Z
5A1522F
5A1522G
5A1522H
5A19054
5A1935Z
5A1945Z
5A1955Z
5A1C00Z
5A1C60Z
5A1D70Z
5A1D80Z
5A1D90Z
5A2204Z
6A0Z0ZZ
6A0Z1ZZ
6A150ZZ
6A151ZZ
6A210ZZ
6A211ZZ
6A220ZZ
6A221ZZ
6A3Z0ZZ
6A3Z1ZZ
6A4Z0ZZ
6A4Z1ZZ
6A550Z0
6A550Z1
6A550Z2
6A550Z3
6A550ZT
6A550ZV
6A551Z0
6A551Z1
6A551Z2
6A551Z3
6A551ZT
6A551ZV
6A600ZZ
6A601ZZ
6A650ZZ
6A651ZZ
6A750Z4
6A750Z5
6A750Z6
6A750Z7
6A750ZZ
6A751Z4
6A751Z5
6A751Z6
6A751Z7
6A751ZZ
6A800ZZ
6A801ZZ
6A930ZZ
6A931ZZ
6AB50BZ
6ABB0BZ
6ABF0BZ
6ABT0BZ
7W00X0Z
7W00X1Z
7W00X2Z
7W00X3Z
7W00X4Z
7W00X5Z
7W00X6Z
7W00X7Z
7W00X8Z
7W00X9Z
7W01X0Z
7W01X1Z
7W01X2Z
7W01X3Z
7W01X4Z
7W01X5Z
7W01X6Z
7W01X7Z
7W01X8Z
7W01X9Z
7W02X0Z
7W02X1Z
7W02X2Z
7W02X3Z
7W02X4Z
7W02X5Z
7W02X6Z
7W02X7Z
7W02X8Z
7W02X9Z
7W03X0Z
7W03X1Z
7W03X2Z
7W03X3Z
7W03X4Z
7W03X5Z
7W03X6Z
7W03X7Z
7W03X8Z
7W03X9Z
7W04X0Z
7W04X1Z
7W04X2Z
7W04X3Z
7W04X4Z
7W04X5Z
7W04X6Z
7W04X7Z
7W04X8Z
7W04X9Z
7W05X0Z
7W05X1Z
7W05X2Z
7W05X3Z
7W05X4Z
7W05X5Z
7W05X6Z
7W05X7Z
7W05X8Z
7W05X9Z
7W06X0Z
7W06X1Z
7W06X2Z
7W06X3Z
7W06X4Z
7W06X5Z
7W06X6Z
7W06X7Z
7W06X8Z
7W06X9Z
7W07X0Z
7W07X1Z
7W07X2Z
7W07X3Z
7W07X4Z
7W07X5Z
7W07X6Z
7W07X7Z
7W07X8Z
7W07X9Z
7W08X0Z
7W08X1Z
7W08X2Z
7W08X3Z
7W08X4Z
7W08X5Z
7W08X6Z
7W08X7Z
7W08X8Z
7W08X9Z
7W09X0Z
7W09X1Z
7W09X2Z
7W09X3Z
7W09X4Z
7W09X5Z
7W09X6Z
7W09X7Z
7W09X8Z
7W09X9Z
8C01X6J
8C01X6L
8C02X6K
8C02X6L
8E01XY7
8E023DZ
8E090CZ
8E093CZ
8E094CZ
8E097CZ
8E098CZ
8E09XBF
8E09XBG
8E09XBH
8E09XBZ
8E09XCZ
8E09XY8
8E0H300
8E0H30Z
8E0HX62
8E0HXY9
8E0KX1Z
8E0KXY7
8E0UXY7
8E0VX1C
8E0VX1D
8E0VX63
8E0W0CZ
8E0W3CZ
8E0W4CZ
8E0W7CZ
8E0W8CZ
8E0WXBF
8E0WXBG
8E0WXBH
8E0WXBZ
8E0WXCZ
8E0WXY8
8E0X0CZ
8E0X3CZ
8E0X4CZ
8E0XXBF
8E0XXBG
8E0XXBH
8E0XXBZ
8E0XXCZ
8E0XXY8
8E0Y0CZ
8E0Y3CZ
8E0Y4CZ
8E0YXBF
8E0YXBG
8E0YXBH
8E0YXBZ
8E0YXCZ
8E0YXY8
8E0ZXY1
8E0ZXY4
8E0ZXY5
8E0ZXY6
9WB0XBZ
9WB0XCZ
9WB0XDZ
9WB0XFZ
9WB0XGZ
9WB0XHZ
9WB0XJZ
9WB0XKZ
9WB0XLZ
9WB1XBZ
9WB1XCZ
9WB1XDZ
9WB1XFZ
9WB1XGZ
9WB1XHZ
9WB1XJZ
9WB1XKZ
9WB1XLZ
9WB2XBZ
9WB2XCZ
9WB2XDZ
9WB2XFZ
9WB2XGZ
9WB2XHZ
9WB2XJZ
9WB2XKZ
9WB2XLZ
9WB3XBZ
9WB3XCZ
9WB3XDZ
9WB3XFZ
9WB3XGZ
9WB3XHZ
9WB3XJZ
9WB3XKZ
9WB3XLZ
9WB4XBZ
9WB4XCZ
9WB4XDZ
9WB4XFZ
9WB4XGZ
9WB4XHZ
9WB4XJZ
9WB4XKZ
9WB4XLZ
9WB5XBZ
9WB5XCZ
9WB5XDZ
9WB5XFZ
9WB5XGZ
9WB5XHZ
9WB5XJZ
9WB5XKZ
9WB5XLZ
9WB6XBZ
9WB6XCZ
9WB6XDZ
9WB6XFZ
9WB6XGZ
9WB6XHZ
9WB6XJZ
9WB6XKZ
9WB6XLZ
9WB7XBZ
9WB7XCZ
9WB7XDZ
9WB7XFZ
9WB7XGZ
9WB7XHZ
9WB7XJZ
9WB7XKZ
9WB7XLZ
9WB8XBZ
9WB8XCZ
9WB8XDZ
9WB8XFZ
9WB8XGZ
9WB8XHZ
9WB8XJZ
9WB8XKZ
9WB8XLZ
9WB9XBZ
9WB9XCZ
9WB9XDZ
9WB9XFZ
9WB9XGZ
9WB9XHZ
9WB9XJZ
9WB9XKZ
9WB9XLZ
B00B0ZZ
B00B1ZZ
B00BYZZ
B00BZZZ
B01B0ZZ
B01B1ZZ
B01BYZZ
B01BZZZ
B02000Z
B0200ZZ
B02010Z
B0201ZZ
B020Y0Z
B020YZZ
B020ZZZ
B02700Z
B0270ZZ
B02710Z
B0271ZZ
B027Y0Z
B027YZZ
B027ZZZ
B02800Z
B0280ZZ
B02810Z
B0281ZZ
B028Y0Z
B028YZZ
B028ZZZ
B02900Z
B0290ZZ
B02910Z
B0291ZZ
B029Y0Z
B029YZZ
B029ZZZ
B02B00Z
B02B0ZZ
B02B10Z
B02B1ZZ
B02BY0Z
B02BYZZ
B02BZZZ
B030Y0Z
B030YZZ
B030ZZZ
B039Y0Z
B039YZZ
B039ZZZ
B03BY0Z
B03BYZZ
B03BZZZ
B03CY0Z
B03CYZZ
B03CZZZ
B040ZZZ
B04BZZZ
B2000ZZ
B2001ZZ
B200YZZ
B2010ZZ
B2011ZZ
B201YZZ
B2020ZZ
B2021ZZ
B202YZZ
B2030ZZ
B2031ZZ
B203YZZ
B2040ZZ
B2041ZZ
B204YZZ
B2050ZZ
B2051ZZ
B205YZZ
B2060ZZ
B2061ZZ
B206YZZ
B2070ZZ
B2071ZZ
B207YZZ
B2080ZZ
B2081ZZ
B208YZZ
B20F0ZZ
B20F1ZZ
B20FYZZ
B210010
B2100ZZ
B210110
B2101ZZ
B210Y10
B210YZZ
B211010
B2110ZZ
B211110
B2111ZZ
B211Y10
B211YZZ
B212010
B2120ZZ
B212110
B2121ZZ
B212Y10
B212YZZ
B213010
B2130ZZ
B213110
B2131ZZ
B213Y10
B213YZZ
B2140ZZ
B2141ZZ
B214YZZ
B2150ZZ
B2151ZZ
B215YZZ
B2160ZZ
B2161ZZ
B216YZZ
B2170ZZ
B2171ZZ
B22100Z
B2210ZZ
B22110Z
B2211ZZ
B221Y0Z
B221YZZ
B221Z2Z
B221ZZZ
B22300Z
B2230ZZ
B22310Z
B2231ZZ
B223Y0Z
B223YZZ
B223Z2Z
B223ZZZ
B22600Z
B2260ZZ
B22610Z
B2261ZZ
B226Y0Z
B226YZZ
B226Z2Z
B226ZZZ
B231Y0Z
B231YZZ
B231ZZZ
B233Y0Z
B233YZZ
B233ZZZ
B236Y0Z
B236YZZ
B236ZZZ
B240YZZ
B240ZZ3
B240ZZ4
B240ZZZ
B241YZZ
B241ZZ3
B241ZZ4
B241ZZZ
B244YZZ
B244ZZ3
B244ZZ4
B244ZZZ
B245YZZ
B245ZZ3
B245ZZ4
B245ZZZ
B246YZZ
B246ZZ3
B246ZZ4
B246ZZZ
B24BYZZ
B24BZZ3
B24BZZ4
B24BZZZ
B24CYZZ
B24CZZ3
B24CZZ4
B24CZZZ
B24DYZZ
B24DZZ3
B24DZZ4
B24DZZZ
B3000ZZ
B3001ZZ
B300YZZ
B300ZZZ
B3010ZZ
B3011ZZ
B301YZZ
B301ZZZ
B3020ZZ
B3021ZZ
B302YZZ
B302ZZZ
B3030ZZ
B3031ZZ
B303YZZ
B303ZZZ
B3040ZZ
B3041ZZ
B304YZZ
B304ZZZ
B3050ZZ
B3051ZZ
B305YZZ
B305ZZZ
B3060ZZ
B3061ZZ
B306YZZ
B306ZZZ
B3070ZZ
B3071ZZ
B307YZZ
B307ZZZ
B3080ZZ
B3081ZZ
B308YZZ
B308ZZZ
B3090ZZ
B3091ZZ
B309YZZ
B309ZZZ
B30B0ZZ
B30B1ZZ
B30BYZZ
B30BZZZ
B30C0ZZ
B30C1ZZ
B30CYZZ
B30CZZZ
B30D0ZZ
B30D1ZZ
B30DYZZ
B30DZZZ
B30F0ZZ
B30F1ZZ
B30FYZZ
B30FZZZ
B30G0ZZ
B30G1ZZ
B30GYZZ
B30GZZZ
B30H0ZZ
B30H1ZZ
B30HYZZ
B30HZZZ
B30J0ZZ
B30J1ZZ
B30JYZZ
B30JZZZ
B30K0ZZ
B30K1ZZ
B30KYZZ
B30KZZZ
B30L0ZZ
B30L1ZZ
B30LYZZ
B30LZZZ
B30M0ZZ
B30M1ZZ
B30MYZZ
B30MZZZ
B30N0ZZ
B30N1ZZ
B30NYZZ
B30NZZZ
B30P0ZZ
B30P1ZZ
B30PYZZ
B30PZZZ
B30Q0ZZ
B30Q1ZZ
B30QYZZ
B30QZZZ
B30R0ZZ
B30R1ZZ
B30RYZZ
B30RZZZ
B30S0ZZ
B30S1ZZ
B30SYZZ
B30SZZZ
B30T0ZZ
B30T1ZZ
B30TYZZ
B30TZZZ
B310010
B3100ZZ
B310110
B3101ZZ
B310Y10
B310YZZ
B310ZZZ
B311010
B3110ZZ
B311110
B3111ZZ
B311Y10
B311YZZ

B311ZZZ
B312010
B3120ZZ
B312110
B3121ZZ
B312Y10
B312YZZ
B312ZZZ
B313010
B3130ZZ
B313110
B3131ZZ
B313Y10
B313YZZ
B313ZZZ
B314010
B3140ZZ
B314110
B3141ZZ
B314Y10
B314YZZ
B314ZZZ
B315010
B3150ZZ
B315110
B3151ZZ
B315Y10
B315YZZ
B315ZZZ
B316010
B3160ZZ
B316110
B3161ZZ
B316Y10
B316YZZ
B316ZZZ
B317010
B3170ZZ
B317110
B3171ZZ
B317Y10
B317YZZ
B317ZZZ
B318010
B3180ZZ
B318110
B3181ZZ
B318Y10
B318YZZ
B318ZZZ
B319010
B3190ZZ
B319110
B3191ZZ
B319Y10
B319YZZ
B319ZZZ
B31B010
B31B0ZZ
B31B110
B31B1ZZ
B31BY10
B31BYZZ
B31BZZZ
B31C010
B31C0ZZ
B31C110
B31C1ZZ
B31CY10
B31CYZZ
B31CZZZ
B31D010
B31D0ZZ
B31D110
B31D1ZZ
B31DY10
B31DYZZ
B31DZZZ
B31F010
B31F0ZZ
B31F110
B31F1ZZ
B31FY10
B31FYZZ
B31FZZZ
B31G010
B31G0ZZ
B31G110
B31G1ZZ
B31GY10
B31GYZZ
B31GZZZ
B31H010
B31H0ZZ
B31H110
B31H1ZZ
B31HY10
B31HYZZ
B31HZZZ
B31J010
B31J0ZZ
B31J110
B31J1ZZ
B31JY10
B31JYZZ
B31JZZZ
B31K010
B31K0ZZ
B31K110
B31K1ZZ
B31KY10
B31KYZZ
B31KZZZ
B31L010
B31L0ZZ
B31L110
B31L1ZZ
B31LY10
B31LYZZ
B31LZZZ
B31M010
B31M0ZZ
B31M110
B31M1ZZ
B31MY10
B31MYZZ
B31MZZZ
B31N010
B31N0ZZ
B31N110
B31N1ZZ
B31NY10
B31NYZZ
B31NZZZ
B31P010
B31P0ZZ
B31P110
B31P1ZZ
B31PY10
B31PYZZ
B31PZZZ
B31Q010
B31Q0ZZ
B31Q110
B31Q1ZZ
B31QY10
B31QYZZ
B31QZZZ
B31R010
B31R0ZZ
B31R110
B31R1ZZ
B31RY10
B31RYZZ
B31RZZZ
B31S010
B31S0ZZ
B31S110
B31S1ZZ
B31SY10
B31SYZZ
B31SZZZ
B31T010
B31T0ZZ
B31T110
B31T1ZZ
B31TY10
B31TYZZ
B31TZZZ
B31U010
B31U0ZZ
B31U110
B31U1ZZ
B31UY10
B31UYZZ
B31UZZZ
B3200ZZ
B3201ZZ
B320YZZ
B320Z2Z
B320ZZZ
B3250ZZ
B3251ZZ
B325YZZ
B325Z2Z
B325ZZZ
B3280ZZ
B3281ZZ
B328YZZ
B328Z2Z
B328ZZZ
B32G0ZZ
B32G1ZZ
B32GYZZ
B32GZ2Z
B32GZZZ
B32R0ZZ
B32R1ZZ
B32RYZZ
B32RZ2Z
B32RZZZ
B32S0ZZ
B32S1ZZ
B32SYZZ
B32SZ2Z
B32SZZZ
B32T0ZZ
B32T1ZZ
B32TYZZ
B32TZ2Z
B32TZZZ
B330Y0Z
B330YZZ
B330ZZZ
B335Y0Z
B335YZZ
B335ZZZ
B338Y0Z
B338YZZ
B338ZZZ
B33GY0Z
B33GYZZ
B33GZZZ
B33HY0Z
B33HYZZ
B33HZZZ
B33JY0Z
B33JYZZ
B33JZZZ
B33KY0Z
B33KYZZ
B33KZZZ
B33MY0Z
B33MYZZ
B33MZZZ
B33QY0Z
B33QYZZ
B33QZZZ
B33RY0Z
B33RYZZ
B33RZZZ
B340ZZ3
B340ZZZ
B341ZZ3
B341ZZZ
B342ZZ3
B342ZZZ
B343ZZ3
B343ZZZ
B344ZZ3
B344ZZZ
B345ZZ3
B345ZZZ
B346ZZ3
B346ZZZ
B347ZZ3
B347ZZZ
B348ZZ3
B348ZZZ
B34HZZ3
B34HZZZ
B34JZZ3
B34JZZZ
B34KZZ3
B34KZZZ
B34RZZ3
B34RZZZ
B34SZZ3
B34SZZZ
B34TZZ3
B34TZZZ
B34VZZ3
B34VZZZ
B4000ZZ
B4001ZZ
B400YZZ
B4020ZZ
B4021ZZ
B402YZZ
B4030ZZ
B4031ZZ
B403YZZ
B4040ZZ
B4041ZZ
B404YZZ
B4050ZZ
B4051ZZ
B405YZZ
B4060ZZ
B4061ZZ
B406YZZ
B4070ZZ
B4071ZZ
B407YZZ
B4080ZZ
B4081ZZ
B408YZZ
B4090ZZ
B4091ZZ
B409YZZ
B40B0ZZ
B40B1ZZ
B40BYZZ
B40C0ZZ
B40C1ZZ
B40CYZZ
B40D0ZZ
B40D1ZZ
B40DYZZ
B40F0ZZ
B40F1ZZ
B40FYZZ
B40G0ZZ
B40G1ZZ
B40GYZZ
B40J0ZZ
B40J1ZZ
B40JYZZ
B40M0ZZ
B40M1ZZ
B40MYZZ
B410010
B4100ZZ
B410110
B4101ZZ
B410Y10
B410YZZ
B410ZZZ
B412010
B4120ZZ
B412110
B4121ZZ
B412Y10
B412YZZ
B412ZZZ
B413010
B4130ZZ
B413110
B4131ZZ
B413Y10
B413YZZ
B413ZZZ
B414010
B4140ZZ
B414110
B4141ZZ
B414Y10
B414YZZ
B414ZZZ
B415010
B4150ZZ
B415110
B4151ZZ
B415Y10
B415YZZ
B415ZZZ
B416010
B4160ZZ
B416110
B4161ZZ
B416Y10
B416YZZ
B416ZZZ
B417010
B4170ZZ
B417110
B4171ZZ
B417Y10
B417YZZ
B417ZZZ
B418010
B4180ZZ
B418110
B4181ZZ
B418Y10
B418YZZ
B418ZZZ
B419010
B4190ZZ
B419110
B4191ZZ
B419Y10
B419YZZ
B419ZZZ
B41B010
B41B0ZZ
B41B110
B41B1ZZ
B41BY10
B41BYZZ
B41BZZZ
B41C010
B41C0ZZ
B41C110
B41C1ZZ
B41CY10
B41CYZZ
B41CZZZ
B41D010
B41D0ZZ
B41D110
B41D1ZZ
B41DY10
B41DYZZ
B41DZZZ
B41F010
B41F0ZZ
B41F110
B41F1ZZ
B41FY10
B41FYZZ
B41FZZZ
B41G010
B41G0ZZ
B41G110
B41G1ZZ
B41GY10
B41GYZZ
B41GZZZ
B41J010
B41J0ZZ
B41J110
B41J1ZZ
B41JY10
B41JYZZ
B41JZZZ
B4200ZZ
B4201ZZ
B420YZZ
B420Z2Z
B420ZZZ
B4210ZZ
B4211ZZ
B421YZZ
B421Z2Z
B421ZZZ
B4240ZZ
B4241ZZ
B424YZZ
B424Z2Z
B424ZZZ
B4280ZZ
B4281ZZ
B428YZZ
B428Z2Z
B428ZZZ
B42C0ZZ
B42C1ZZ
B42CYZZ
B42CZ2Z
B42CZZZ
B42F0ZZ
B42F1ZZ
B42FYZZ
B42FZ2Z
B42FZZZ
B42G0ZZ
B42G1ZZ
B42GYZZ
B42GZ2Z
B42GZZZ
B42H0ZZ
B42H1ZZ
B42HYZZ
B42HZ2Z
B42HZZZ
B42M0ZZ
B42M1ZZ
B42MYZZ
B42MZ2Z
B42MZZZ
B430Y0Z
B430YZZ
B430ZZZ
B431Y0Z
B431YZZ
B431ZZZ
B434Y0Z
B434YZZ
B434ZZZ
B438Y0Z
B438YZZ
B438ZZZ
B43CY0Z
B43CYZZ
B43CZZZ
B43FY0Z
B43FYZZ
B43FZZZ
B43GY0Z
B43GYZZ
B43GZZZ
B43HY0Z
B43HYZZ
B43HZZZ
B440ZZ3
B440ZZZ
B444ZZ3
B444ZZZ
B445ZZ3
B445ZZZ
B446ZZ3
B446ZZZ
B447ZZ3
B447ZZZ
B448ZZ3
B448ZZZ
B44BZZ3
B44BZZZ
B44FZZ3
B44FZZZ
B44GZZ3
B44GZZZ
B44HZZ3
B44HZZZ
B44KZZ3
B44KZZZ
B44LZZ3
B44LZZZ
B44NZZ3
B44NZZZ
B5000ZZ
B5001ZZ
B500YZZ
B5010ZZ
B5011ZZ
B501YZZ
B5020ZZ
B5021ZZ
B502YZZ
B5030ZZ
B5031ZZ
B503YZZ
B5040ZZ
B5041ZZ
B504YZZ
B5050ZZ
B5051ZZ
B505YZZ
B5060ZZ
B5061ZZ
B506YZZ
B5070ZZ
B5071ZZ
B507YZZ
B5080ZZ
B5081ZZ
B508YZZ
B5090ZZ
B5091ZZ
B509YZZ
B50B0ZZ
B50B1ZZ
B50BYZZ
B50C0ZZ
B50C1ZZ
B50CYZZ
B50D0ZZ
B50D1ZZ
B50DYZZ
B50F0ZZ
B50F1ZZ
B50FYZZ
B50G0ZZ
B50G1ZZ
B50GYZZ
B50H0ZZ
B50H1ZZ
B50HYZZ
B50J0ZZ
B50J1ZZ
B50JYZZ
B50K0ZZ
B50K1ZZ
B50KYZZ
B50L0ZZ
B50L1ZZ
B50LYZZ
B50M0ZZ
B50M1ZZ
B50MYZZ
B50N0ZZ
B50N1ZZ
B50NYZZ
B50P0ZZ
B50P1ZZ
B50PYZZ
B50Q0ZZ
B50Q1ZZ
B50QYZZ
B50R0ZZ
B50R1ZZ
B50RYZZ
B50S0ZZ
B50S1ZZ
B50SYZZ
B50T0ZZ
B50T1ZZ
B50TYZZ
B50V0ZZ
B50V1ZZ
B50VYZZ
B50W0ZZ
B50W1ZZ
B50WYZZ
B5100ZA
B5100ZZ
B5101ZA
B5101ZZ
B510YZA
B510YZZ
B510ZZA
B510ZZZ
B5110ZA
B5110ZZ
B5111ZA
B5111ZZ
B511YZA
B511YZZ
B511ZZA
B511ZZZ
B5120ZA
B5120ZZ
B5121ZA
B5121ZZ
B512YZA
B512YZZ
B512ZZA
B512ZZZ
B5130ZA
B5130ZZ
B5131ZA
B5131ZZ
B513YZA
B513YZZ
B513ZZA
B513ZZZ
B5140ZA
B5140ZZ
B5141ZA
B5141ZZ
B514YZA
B514YZZ
B514ZZA
B514ZZZ
B5150ZA
B5150ZZ
B5151ZA
B5151ZZ
B515YZA
B515YZZ
B515ZZA
B515ZZZ
B5160ZA
B5160ZZ
B5161ZA
B5161ZZ
B516YZA
B516YZZ
B516ZZA
B516ZZZ
B5170ZA
B5170ZZ
B5171ZA
B5171ZZ
B517YZA
B517YZZ
B517ZZA
B517ZZZ
B5180ZA
B5180ZZ
B5181ZA
B5181ZZ
B518YZA
B518YZZ
B518ZZA
B518ZZZ
B5190ZA
B5190ZZ
B5191ZA
B5191ZZ
B519YZA
B519YZZ
B519ZZA
B519ZZZ
B51B0ZA
B51B0ZZ
B51B1ZA
B51B1ZZ
B51BYZA
B51BYZZ
B51BZZA
B51BZZZ
B51C0ZA
B51C0ZZ
B51C1ZA
B51C1ZZ
B51CYZA
B51CYZZ
B51CZZA
B51CZZZ
B51D0ZA
B51D0ZZ
B51D1ZA
B51D1ZZ
B51DYZA
B51DYZZ
B51DZZA
B51DZZZ
B51F0ZA
B51F0ZZ
B51F1ZA
B51F1ZZ
B51FYZA
B51FYZZ
B51FZZA
B51FZZZ
B51G0ZA
B51G0ZZ
B51G1ZA
B51G1ZZ
B51GYZA
B51GYZZ
B51GZZA
B51GZZZ
B51H0ZA

B51H0ZZ
B51H1ZA
B51H1ZZ
B51HYZA
B51HYZZ
B51HZZA
B51HZZZ
B51J0ZA
B51J0ZZ
B51J1ZA
B51J1ZZ
B51JYZA
B51JYZZ
B51JZZA
B51JZZZ
B51K0ZA
B51K0ZZ
B51K1ZA
B51K1ZZ
B51KYZA
B51KYZZ
B51KZZA
B51KZZZ
B51L0ZA
B51L0ZZ
B51L1ZA
B51L1ZZ
B51LYZA
B51LYZZ
B51LZZA
B51LZZZ
B51M0ZA
B51M0ZZ
B51M1ZA
B51M1ZZ
B51MYZA
B51MYZZ
B51MZZA
B51MZZZ
B51N0ZA
B51N0ZZ
B51N1ZA
B51N1ZZ
B51NYZA
B51NYZZ
B51NZZA
B51NZZZ
B51P0ZA
B51P0ZZ
B51P1ZA
B51P1ZZ
B51PYZA
B51PYZZ
B51PZZA
B51PZZZ
B51Q0ZA
B51Q0ZZ
B51Q1ZA
B51Q1ZZ
B51QYZA
B51QYZZ
B51QZZA
B51QZZZ
B51R0ZA
B51R0ZZ
B51R1ZA
B51R1ZZ
B51RYZA
B51RYZZ
B51RZZA
B51RZZZ
B51S0ZA
B51S0ZZ
B51S1ZA
B51S1ZZ
B51SYZA
B51SYZZ
B51SZZA
B51SZZZ
B51T0ZA
B51T0ZZ
B51T1ZA
B51T1ZZ
B51TYZA
B51TYZZ
B51TZZA
B51TZZZ
B51V0ZA
B51V0ZZ
B51V1ZA
B51V1ZZ
B51VYZA
B51VYZZ
B51VZZA
B51VZZZ
B51W0ZA
B51W0ZZ
B51W1ZA
B51W1ZZ
B51WYZA
B51WYZZ
B51WZZA
B51WZZZ
B52200Z
B5220ZZ
B52210Z
B5221ZZ
B522Y0Z
B522YZZ
B522Z2Z
B522ZZZ
B52800Z
B5280ZZ
B52810Z
B5281ZZ
B528Y0Z
B528YZZ
B528Z2Z
B528ZZZ
B52900Z
B5290ZZ
B52910Z
B5291ZZ
B529Y0Z
B529YZZ
B529Z2Z
B529ZZZ
B52F00Z
B52F0ZZ
B52F10Z
B52F1ZZ
B52FY0Z
B52FYZZ
B52FZ2Z
B52FZZZ
B52G00Z
B52G0ZZ
B52G10Z
B52G1ZZ
B52GY0Z
B52GYZZ
B52GZ2Z
B52GZZZ
B52H00Z
B52H0ZZ
B52H10Z
B52H1ZZ
B52HY0Z
B52HYZZ
B52HZ2Z
B52HZZZ
B52J00Z
B52J0ZZ
B52J10Z
B52J1ZZ
B52JY0Z
B52JYZZ
B52JZ2Z
B52JZZZ
B52K00Z
B52K0ZZ
B52K10Z
B52K1ZZ
B52KY0Z
B52KYZZ
B52KZ2Z
B52KZZZ
B52L00Z
B52L0ZZ
B52L10Z
B52L1ZZ
B52LY0Z
B52LYZZ
B52LZ2Z
B52LZZZ
B52Q00Z
B52Q0ZZ
B52Q10Z
B52Q1ZZ
B52QY0Z
B52QYZZ
B52QZ2Z
B52QZZZ
B52R00Z
B52R0ZZ
B52R10Z
B52R1ZZ
B52RY0Z
B52RYZZ
B52RZ2Z
B52RZZZ
B52S00Z
B52S0ZZ
B52S10Z
B52S1ZZ
B52SY0Z
B52SYZZ
B52SZ2Z
B52SZZZ
B52T00Z
B52T0ZZ
B52T10Z
B52T1ZZ
B52TY0Z
B52TYZZ
B52TZ2Z
B52TZZZ
B531Y0Z
B531YZZ
B531ZZZ
B532Y0Z
B532YZZ
B532ZZZ
B535Y0Z
B535YZZ
B535ZZZ
B538Y0Z
B538YZZ
B538ZZZ
B539Y0Z
B539YZZ
B539ZZZ
B53BY0Z
B53BYZZ
B53BZZZ
B53CY0Z
B53CYZZ
B53CZZZ
B53DY0Z
B53DYZZ
B53DZZZ
B53HY0Z
B53HYZZ
B53HZZZ
B53LY0Z
B53LYZZ
B53LZZZ
B53MY0Z
B53MYZZ
B53MZZZ
B53NY0Z
B53NYZZ
B53NZZZ
B53PY0Z
B53PYZZ
B53PZZZ
B53SY0Z
B53SYZZ
B53SZZZ
B53TY0Z
B53TYZZ
B53TZZZ
B53VY0Z
B53VYZZ
B53VZZZ
B543ZZ3
B543ZZA
B543ZZZ
B544ZZ3
B544ZZA
B544ZZZ
B546ZZ3
B546ZZA
B546ZZZ
B547ZZ3
B547ZZA
B547ZZZ
B548ZZ3
B548ZZA
B548ZZZ
B549ZZ3
B549ZZA
B549ZZZ
B54BZZ3
B54BZZA
B54BZZZ
B54CZZ3
B54CZZA
B54CZZZ
B54DZZ3
B54DZZA
B54DZZZ
B54JZZ3
B54JZZA
B54JZZZ
B54KZZ3
B54KZZA
B54KZZZ
B54LZZ3
B54LZZA
B54LZZZ
B54MZZ3
B54MZZA
B54MZZZ
B54NZZ3
B54NZZA
B54NZZZ
B54PZZ3
B54PZZA
B54PZZZ
B54TZZ3
B54TZZA
B54TZZZ
B7000ZZ
B7001ZZ
B700YZZ
B7010ZZ
B7011ZZ
B701YZZ
B7040ZZ
B7041ZZ
B704YZZ
B7050ZZ
B7051ZZ
B705YZZ
B7060ZZ
B7061ZZ
B706YZZ
B7070ZZ
B7071ZZ
B707YZZ
B7080ZZ
B7081ZZ
B708YZZ
B7090ZZ
B7091ZZ
B709YZZ
B70B0ZZ
B70B1ZZ
B70BYZZ
B70C0ZZ
B70C1ZZ
B70CYZZ
B8000ZZ
B8001ZZ
B800YZZ
B8010ZZ
B8011ZZ
B801YZZ
B8020ZZ
B8021ZZ
B802YZZ
B803ZZZ
B804ZZZ
B805ZZZ
B806ZZZ
B807ZZZ
B82500Z
B8250ZZ
B82510Z
B8251ZZ
B825Y0Z
B825YZZ
B825ZZZ
B82600Z
B8260ZZ
B82610Z
B8261ZZ
B826Y0Z
B826YZZ
B826ZZZ
B82700Z
B8270ZZ
B82710Z
B8271ZZ
B827Y0Z
B827YZZ
B827ZZZ
B835Y0Z
B835YZZ
B835ZZZ
B836Y0Z
B836YZZ
B836ZZZ
B837Y0Z
B837YZZ
B837ZZZ
B845ZZZ
B846ZZZ
B847ZZZ
B902ZZZ
B9040ZZ
B9041ZZ
B904YZZ
B9050ZZ
B9051ZZ
B905YZZ
B9060ZZ
B9061ZZ
B906YZZ
B9070ZZ
B9071ZZ
B907YZZ
B9080ZZ
B9081ZZ
B908YZZ
B9090ZZ
B9091ZZ
B909YZZ
B90B0ZZ
B90B1ZZ
B90BYZZ
B90C0ZZ
B90C1ZZ
B90CYZZ
B90D0ZZ
B90D1ZZ
B90DYZZ
B90FZZZ
B90HZZZ
B91GYZZ
B91GZZZ
B91JYZZ
B91JZZZ
B92000Z
B9200ZZ
B92010Z
B9201ZZ
B920Y0Z
B920YZZ
B920ZZZ
B92200Z
B9220ZZ
B92210Z
B9221ZZ
B922Y0Z
B922YZZ
B922ZZZ
B92600Z
B9260ZZ
B92610Z
B9261ZZ
B926Y0Z
B926YZZ
B926ZZZ
B92900Z
B9290ZZ
B92910Z
B9291ZZ
B929Y0Z
B929YZZ
B929ZZZ
B92D00Z
B92D0ZZ
B92D10Z
B92D1ZZ
B92DY0Z
B92DYZZ
B92DZZZ
B92F00Z
B92F0ZZ
B92F10Z
B92F1ZZ
B92FY0Z
B92FYZZ
B92FZZZ
B92J00Z
B92J0ZZ
B92J10Z
B92J1ZZ
B92JY0Z
B92JYZZ
B92JZZZ
B930Y0Z
B930YZZ
B930ZZZ
B932Y0Z
B932YZZ
B932ZZZ
B936Y0Z
B936YZZ
B936ZZZ
B939Y0Z
B939YZZ
B939ZZZ
B93DY0Z
B93DYZZ
B93DZZZ
B93FY0Z
B93FYZZ
B93FZZZ
B93JY0Z
B93JYZZ
B93JZZZ
BB07YZZ
BB08YZZ
BB09YZZ
BB0DZZZ
BB12ZZZ
BB13ZZZ
BB14ZZZ
BB16ZZZ
BB17YZZ
BB18YZZ
BB19YZZ
BB1CZZZ
BB1DZZZ
BB2400Z
BB240ZZ
BB2410Z
BB241ZZ
BB24Y0Z
BB24YZZ
BB24ZZZ
BB2700Z
BB270ZZ
BB2710Z
BB271ZZ
BB27Y0Z
BB27YZZ
BB27ZZZ
BB2800Z
BB280ZZ
BB2810Z
BB281ZZ
BB28Y0Z
BB28YZZ
BB28ZZZ
BB2900Z
BB290ZZ
BB2910Z
BB291ZZ
BB29Y0Z
BB29YZZ
BB29ZZZ
BB2F00Z
BB2F0ZZ
BB2F10Z
BB2F1ZZ
BB2FY0Z
BB2FYZZ
BB2FZZZ
BB3GY0Z
BB3GYZZ
BB3GZZZ
BB4BZZZ
BB4CZZZ
BD11YZZ
BD11ZZZ
BD12YZZ
BD12ZZZ
BD13YZZ
BD13ZZZ
BD14YZZ
BD14ZZZ
BD15YZZ
BD15ZZZ
BD16YZZ
BD16ZZZ
BD19YZZ
BD19ZZZ
BD1BYZZ
BD1BZZZ
BD2400Z
BD240ZZ
BD2410Z
BD241ZZ
BD24Y0Z
BD24YZZ
BD24ZZZ
BD41ZZZ
BD42ZZZ
BD47ZZZ
BD48ZZZ
BD49ZZZ
BD4CZZZ
BF000ZZ
BF001ZZ
BF00YZZ
BF030ZZ
BF031ZZ
BF03YZZ
BF0C0ZZ
BF0C1ZZ
BF0CYZZ
BF100ZZ
BF101ZZ
BF10YZZ
BF110ZZ
BF111ZZ
BF11YZZ
BF120ZZ
BF121ZZ
BF12YZZ
BF130ZZ
BF131ZZ
BF13YZZ
BF140ZZ
BF141ZZ
BF14YZZ
BF180ZZ
BF181ZZ
BF18YZZ
BF2500Z
BF250ZZ
BF2510Z
BF251ZZ
BF25Y0Z
BF25YZZ
BF25ZZZ
BF2600Z
BF260ZZ
BF2610Z
BF261ZZ
BF26Y0Z
BF26YZZ
BF26ZZZ
BF2700Z
BF270ZZ
BF2710Z
BF271ZZ
BF27Y0Z
BF27YZZ
BF27ZZZ
BF2C00Z
BF2C0ZZ
BF2C10Z
BF2C1ZZ
BF2CY0Z
BF2CYZZ
BF2CZZZ
BF35Y0Z
BF35YZZ
BF35ZZZ
BF36Y0Z
BF36YZZ
BF36ZZZ
BF37Y0Z
BF37YZZ
BF37ZZZ
BF40ZZZ
BF42ZZZ
BF43ZZZ
BF45ZZZ
BF46ZZZ
BF47ZZZ
BF4CZZZ
BG2200Z
BG220ZZ
BG2210Z
BG221ZZ
BG22Y0Z
BG22YZZ
BG22ZZZ
BG2300Z
BG230ZZ
BG2310Z
BG231ZZ
BG23Y0Z
BG23YZZ
BG23ZZZ
BG2400Z
BG240ZZ
BG2410Z
BG241ZZ
BG24Y0Z
BG24YZZ
BG24ZZZ
BG32Y0Z
BG32YZZ
BG32ZZZ
BG33Y0Z
BG33YZZ
BG33ZZZ
BG34Y0Z
BG34YZZ
BG34ZZZ
BG40ZZZ
BG41ZZZ
BG42ZZZ
BG43ZZZ
BG44ZZZ
BH00ZZZ
BH01ZZZ
BH02ZZZ
BH030ZZ
BH031ZZ
BH03YZZ
BH03ZZZ
BH040ZZ
BH041ZZ
BH04YZZ
BH04ZZZ
BH050ZZ
BH051ZZ
BH05YZZ
BH05ZZZ
BH060ZZ
BH061ZZ
BH06YZZ
BH06ZZZ
BH30Y0Z
BH30YZZ
BH30ZZZ
BH31Y0Z
BH31YZZ
BH31ZZZ
BH32Y0Z
BH32YZZ
BH32ZZZ
BH3DY0Z
BH3DYZZ
BH3DZZZ
BH3FY0Z
BH3FYZZ
BH3FZZZ
BH3GY0Z
BH3GYZZ
BH3GZZZ
BH3HY0Z
BH3HYZZ
BH3HZZZ
BH3JY0Z
BH3JYZZ
BH3JZZZ
BH40ZZZ
BH41ZZZ
BH42ZZZ
BH47ZZZ
BH48ZZZ
BH49ZZZ
BH4BZZZ
BH4CZZZ
BL30Y0Z
BL30YZZ
BL30ZZZ

BL31Y0Z
BL31YZZ
BL31ZZZ
BL32Y0Z
BL32YZZ
BL32ZZZ
BL33Y0Z
BL33YZZ
BL33ZZZ
BL40ZZZ
BL41ZZZ
BL42ZZZ
BL43ZZZ
BN00ZZZ
BN01ZZZ
BN02ZZZ
BN03ZZZ
BN04ZZZ
BN05ZZZ
BN06ZZZ
BN070ZZ
BN071ZZ
BN07YZZ
BN07ZZZ
BN080ZZ
BN081ZZ
BN08YZZ
BN08ZZZ
BN090ZZ
BN091ZZ
BN09YZZ
BN09ZZZ
BN0BZZZ
BN0CZZZ
BN0DZZZ
BN0GZZZ
BN0HZZZ
BN0JZZZ
BN170ZZ
BN171ZZ
BN17YZZ
BN17ZZZ
BN180ZZ
BN181ZZ
BN18YZZ
BN18ZZZ
BN190ZZ
BN191ZZ
BN19YZZ
BN19ZZZ
BN200ZZ
BN201ZZ
BN20YZZ
BN20ZZZ
BN230ZZ
BN231ZZ
BN23YZZ
BN23ZZZ
BN250ZZ
BN251ZZ
BN25YZZ
BN25ZZZ
BN260ZZ
BN261ZZ
BN26YZZ
BN26ZZZ
BN290ZZ
BN291ZZ
BN29YZZ
BN29ZZZ
BN2F0ZZ
BN2F1ZZ
BN2FYZZ
BN2FZZZ
BN39YZZ
BN39ZZZ
BP00ZZZ
BP01ZZZ
BP02ZZZ
BP03ZZZ
BP04ZZZ
BP05ZZZ
BP06ZZZ
BP07ZZZ
BP080ZZ
BP081ZZ
BP08YZZ
BP08ZZZ
BP090ZZ
BP091ZZ
BP09YZZ
BP09ZZZ
BP0AZZZ
BP0BZZZ
BP0C0ZZ
BP0C1ZZ
BP0CYZZ
BP0CZZZ
BP0D0ZZ
BP0D1ZZ
BP0DYZZ
BP0DZZZ
BP0EZZZ
BP0FZZZ
BP0G0ZZ
BP0G1ZZ
BP0GYZZ
BP0GZZZ
BP0H0ZZ
BP0H1ZZ
BP0HYZZ
BP0HZZZ
BP0JZZZ
BP0KZZZ
BP0L0ZZ
BP0L1ZZ
BP0LYZZ
BP0LZZZ
BP0M0ZZ
BP0M1ZZ
BP0MYZZ
BP0MZZZ
BP0NZZZ
BP0PZZZ
BP0RZZZ
BP0SZZZ
BP0XZZZ
BP0YZZZ
BP10ZZZ
BP11ZZZ
BP12ZZZ
BP13ZZZ
BP14ZZZ
BP15ZZZ
BP16ZZZ
BP17ZZZ
BP180ZZ
BP181ZZ
BP18YZZ
BP18ZZZ
BP190ZZ
BP191ZZ
BP19YZZ
BP19ZZZ
BP1AZZZ
BP1BZZZ
BP1C0ZZ
BP1C1ZZ
BP1CYZZ
BP1D0ZZ
BP1D1ZZ
BP1DYZZ
BP1EZZZ
BP1FZZZ
BP1G0ZZ
BP1G1ZZ
BP1GYZZ
BP1H0ZZ
BP1H1ZZ
BP1HYZZ
BP1JZZZ
BP1KZZZ
BP1L0ZZ
BP1L1ZZ
BP1LYZZ
BP1LZZZ
BP1M0ZZ
BP1M1ZZ
BP1MYZZ
BP1MZZZ
BP1NZZZ
BP1PZZZ
BP1RZZZ
BP1SZZZ
BP1XZZZ
BP1YZZZ
BP200ZZ
BP201ZZ
BP20YZZ
BP210ZZ
BP211ZZ
BP21YZZ
BP220ZZ
BP221ZZ
BP22YZZ
BP22ZZZ
BP230ZZ
BP231ZZ
BP23YZZ
BP23ZZZ
BP240ZZ
BP241ZZ
BP24YZZ
BP24ZZZ
BP250ZZ
BP251ZZ
BP25YZZ
BP25ZZZ
BP260ZZ
BP261ZZ
BP26YZZ
BP26ZZZ
BP270ZZ
BP271ZZ
BP27YZZ
BP27ZZZ
BP280ZZ
BP281ZZ
BP28YZZ
BP28ZZZ
BP290ZZ
BP291ZZ
BP29YZZ
BP29ZZZ
BP2A0ZZ
BP2A1ZZ
BP2AYZZ
BP2AZZZ
BP2B0ZZ
BP2B1ZZ
BP2BYZZ
BP2BZZZ
BP2CZZZ
BP2DZZZ
BP2E0ZZ
BP2E1ZZ
BP2EYZZ
BP2EZZZ
BP2F0ZZ
BP2F1ZZ
BP2FYZZ
BP2FZZZ
BP2G0ZZ
BP2G1ZZ
BP2GYZZ
BP2GZZZ
BP2H0ZZ
BP2H1ZZ
BP2HYZZ
BP2HZZZ
BP2J0ZZ
BP2J1ZZ
BP2JYZZ
BP2JZZZ
BP2K0ZZ
BP2K1ZZ
BP2KYZZ
BP2KZZZ
BP2L0ZZ
BP2L1ZZ
BP2LYZZ
BP2LZZZ
BP2M0ZZ
BP2M1ZZ
BP2MYZZ
BP2MZZZ
BP2N0ZZ
BP2N1ZZ
BP2NYZZ
BP2NZZZ
BP2P0ZZ
BP2P1ZZ
BP2PYZZ
BP2PZZZ
BP2Q0ZZ
BP2Q1ZZ
BP2QYZZ
BP2QZZZ
BP2R0ZZ
BP2R1ZZ
BP2RYZZ
BP2RZZZ
BP2S0ZZ
BP2S1ZZ
BP2SYZZ
BP2SZZZ
BP2T0ZZ
BP2T1ZZ
BP2TYZZ
BP2TZZZ
BP2U0ZZ
BP2U1ZZ
BP2UYZZ
BP2UZZZ
BP2V0ZZ
BP2V1ZZ
BP2VYZZ
BP2VZZZ
BP2W0ZZ
BP2W1ZZ
BP2WYZZ
BP2X0ZZ
BP2X1ZZ
BP2XYZZ
BP2XZZZ
BP2Y0ZZ
BP2Y1ZZ
BP2YYZZ
BP2YZZZ
BP38Y0Z
BP38YZZ
BP38ZZZ
BP39Y0Z
BP39YZZ
BP39ZZZ
BP3CY0Z
BP3CYZZ
BP3CZZZ
BP3DY0Z
BP3DYZZ
BP3DZZZ
BP3EY0Z
BP3EYZZ
BP3EZZZ
BP3FY0Z
BP3FYZZ
BP3FZZZ
BP3GY0Z
BP3GYZZ
BP3GZZZ
BP3HY0Z
BP3HYZZ
BP3HZZZ
BP3JY0Z
BP3JYZZ
BP3JZZZ
BP3KY0Z
BP3KYZZ
BP3KZZZ
BP3LY0Z
BP3LYZZ
BP3LZZZ
BP3MY0Z
BP3MYZZ
BP3MZZZ
BP48ZZ1
BP48ZZZ
BP49ZZ1
BP49ZZZ
BP4GZZ1
BP4GZZZ
BP4HZZ1
BP4HZZZ
BP4LZZ1
BP4LZZZ
BP4MZZ1
BP4MZZZ
BP4NZZ1
BP4NZZZ
BP4PZZ1
BP4PZZZ
BQ000ZZ
BQ001ZZ
BQ00YZZ
BQ00ZZ1
BQ00ZZZ
BQ010ZZ
BQ011ZZ
BQ01YZZ
BQ01ZZ1
BQ01ZZZ
BQ03ZZ1
BQ03ZZZ
BQ04ZZ1
BQ04ZZZ
BQ070ZZ
BQ071ZZ
BQ07YZZ
BQ07ZZZ
BQ080ZZ
BQ081ZZ
BQ08YZZ
BQ08ZZZ
BQ0DZZZ
BQ0FZZZ
BQ0G0ZZ
BQ0G1ZZ
BQ0GYZZ
BQ0GZZZ
BQ0H0ZZ
BQ0H1ZZ
BQ0HYZZ
BQ0HZZZ
BQ0JZZZ
BQ0KZZZ
BQ0LZZZ
BQ0MZZZ
BQ0PZZZ
BQ0QZZZ
BQ0VZZZ
BQ0WZZZ
BQ0X0ZZ
BQ0X1ZZ
BQ0XYZZ
BQ0Y0ZZ
BQ0Y1ZZ
BQ0YYZZ
BQ100ZZ
BQ101ZZ
BQ10YZZ
BQ10ZZZ
BQ110ZZ
BQ111ZZ
BQ11YZZ
BQ11ZZZ
BQ13ZZZ
BQ14ZZZ
BQ170ZZ
BQ171ZZ
BQ17YZZ
BQ17ZZZ
BQ180ZZ
BQ181ZZ
BQ18YZZ
BQ18ZZZ
BQ1DZZZ
BQ1FZZZ
BQ1G0ZZ
BQ1G1ZZ
BQ1GYZZ
BQ1GZZZ
BQ1H0ZZ
BQ1H1ZZ
BQ1HYZZ
BQ1HZZZ
BQ1JZZZ
BQ1KZZZ
BQ1LZZZ
BQ1MZZZ
BQ1PZZZ
BQ1QZZZ
BQ1VZZZ
BQ1WZZZ
BQ1X0ZZ
BQ1X1ZZ
BQ1XYZZ
BQ1XZZZ
BQ1Y0ZZ
BQ1Y1ZZ
BQ1YYZZ
BQ1YZZZ
BQ200ZZ
BQ201ZZ
BQ20YZZ
BQ20ZZZ
BQ210ZZ
BQ211ZZ
BQ21YZZ
BQ21ZZZ
BQ230ZZ
BQ231ZZ
BQ23YZZ
BQ23ZZZ
BQ240ZZ
BQ241ZZ
BQ24YZZ
BQ24ZZZ
BQ270ZZ
BQ271ZZ
BQ27YZZ
BQ27ZZZ
BQ280ZZ
BQ281ZZ
BQ28YZZ
BQ28ZZZ
BQ2B0ZZ
BQ2B1ZZ
BQ2BYZZ
BQ2C0ZZ
BQ2C1ZZ
BQ2CYZZ
BQ2D0ZZ
BQ2D1ZZ
BQ2DYZZ
BQ2DZZZ
BQ2F0ZZ
BQ2F1ZZ
BQ2FYZZ
BQ2FZZZ
BQ2G0ZZ
BQ2G1ZZ
BQ2GYZZ
BQ2GZZZ
BQ2H0ZZ
BQ2H1ZZ
BQ2HYZZ
BQ2HZZZ
BQ2J0ZZ
BQ2J1ZZ
BQ2JYZZ
BQ2JZZZ
BQ2K0ZZ
BQ2K1ZZ
BQ2KYZZ
BQ2KZZZ
BQ2L0ZZ
BQ2L1ZZ
BQ2LYZZ
BQ2LZZZ
BQ2M0ZZ
BQ2M1ZZ
BQ2MYZZ
BQ2MZZZ
BQ2P0ZZ
BQ2P1ZZ
BQ2PYZZ
BQ2PZZZ
BQ2Q0ZZ
BQ2Q1ZZ
BQ2QYZZ
BQ2QZZZ
BQ2R0ZZ
BQ2R1ZZ
BQ2RYZZ
BQ2RZZZ
BQ2S0ZZ
BQ2S1ZZ
BQ2SYZZ
BQ2SZZZ
BQ2V0ZZ
BQ2V1ZZ
BQ2VYZZ
BQ2VZZZ
BQ2W0ZZ
BQ2W1ZZ
BQ2WYZZ
BQ2WZZZ
BQ2X0ZZ
BQ2X1ZZ
BQ2XYZZ
BQ2XZZZ
BQ2Y0ZZ
BQ2Y1ZZ
BQ2YYZZ
BQ2YZZZ
BQ30Y0Z
BQ30YZZ
BQ30ZZZ
BQ31Y0Z
BQ31YZZ
BQ31ZZZ
BQ33Y0Z
BQ33YZZ
BQ33ZZZ
BQ34Y0Z
BQ34YZZ
BQ34ZZZ
BQ37Y0Z
BQ37YZZ
BQ37ZZZ
BQ38Y0Z
BQ38YZZ
BQ38ZZZ
BQ3DY0Z
BQ3DYZZ
BQ3DZZZ
BQ3FY0Z
BQ3FYZZ
BQ3FZZZ
BQ3GY0Z
BQ3GYZZ
BQ3GZZZ
BQ3HY0Z
BQ3HYZZ
BQ3HZZZ
BQ3JY0Z
BQ3JYZZ
BQ3JZZZ
BQ3KY0Z
BQ3KYZZ
BQ3KZZZ
BQ3LY0Z
BQ3LYZZ
BQ3LZZZ
BQ3MY0Z
BQ3MYZZ
BQ3MZZZ
BQ3PY0Z
BQ3PYZZ
BQ3PZZZ
BQ3QY0Z
BQ3QYZZ
BQ3QZZZ
BQ3VY0Z
BQ3VYZZ
BQ3VZZZ
BQ3WY0Z
BQ3WYZZ
BQ3WZZZ
BQ40ZZZ
BQ41ZZZ
BQ42ZZZ
BQ47ZZZ
BQ48ZZZ
BQ49ZZZ
BR00ZZ1
BR00ZZZ
BR010ZZ
BR011ZZ
BR01YZZ
BR01ZZZ
BR020ZZ
BR021ZZ
BR02YZZ
BR02ZZZ
BR030ZZ
BR031ZZ
BR03YZZ
BR03ZZZ
BR040ZZ
BR041ZZ
BR04YZZ
BR04ZZZ
BR050ZZ
BR051ZZ
BR05YZZ
BR05ZZZ
BR060ZZ
BR061ZZ
BR06YZZ
BR06ZZZ
BR07ZZ1
BR07ZZZ
BR08ZZZ
BR09ZZ1
BR09ZZZ
BR0BZZZ
BR0CZZZ
BR0D0ZZ
BR0D1ZZ
BR0DYZZ
BR0DZZZ
BR0FZZZ
BR0GZZ1
BR0GZZZ
BR0HZZZ
BR100ZZ
BR101ZZ
BR10YZZ
BR10ZZZ
BR110ZZ
BR111ZZ
BR11YZZ
BR11ZZZ
BR120ZZ
BR121ZZ
BR12YZZ
BR12ZZZ
BR130ZZ
BR131ZZ
BR13YZZ
BR13ZZZ
BR140ZZ
BR141ZZ
BR14YZZ
BR14ZZZ
BR150ZZ
BR151ZZ
BR15YZZ
BR15ZZZ
BR160ZZ
BR161ZZ
BR16YZZ
BR16ZZZ
BR170ZZ
BR171ZZ
BR17YZZ
BR17ZZZ
BR180ZZ
BR181ZZ
BR18YZZ
BR18ZZZ
BR190ZZ
BR191ZZ
BR19YZZ
BR19ZZZ
BR1B0ZZ
BR1B1ZZ
BR1BYZZ
BR1BZZZ
BR1C0ZZ
BR1C1ZZ
BR1CYZZ
BR1CZZZ
BR1D0ZZ
BR1D1ZZ
BR1DYZZ
BR1DZZZ
BR1F0ZZ
BR1F1ZZ
BR1FYZZ
BR1FZZZ
BR1G0ZZ
BR1G1ZZ
BR1GYZZ
BR1GZZZ
BR1H0ZZ
BR1H1ZZ
BR1HYZZ
BR1HZZZ
BR200ZZ
BR201ZZ
BR20YZZ
BR20ZZZ
BR270ZZ
BR271ZZ
BR27YZZ
BR27ZZZ
BR290ZZ
BR291ZZ
BR29YZZ
BR29ZZZ
BR2C0ZZ
BR2C1ZZ
BR2CYZZ
BR2CZZZ
BR2D0ZZ
BR2D1ZZ
BR2DYZZ
BR2DZZZ
BR2F0ZZ
BR2F1ZZ
BR2FYZZ
BR2FZZZ
BR30Y0Z
BR30YZZ

BL31Y0Z-BR30YZZ

APPENDIX H: NON-OR NOT AFFECTING MS-DRG ASSIGNMENT

BR30ZZZ
BR31Y0Z
BR31YZZ
BR31ZZZ
BR32Y0Z
BR32YZZ
BR32ZZZ
BR33Y0Z
BR33YZZ
BR33ZZZ
BR37Y0Z
BR37YZZ
BR37ZZZ
BR39Y0Z
BR39YZZ
BR39ZZZ
BR3CY0Z
BR3CYZZ
BR3CZZZ
BR3FY0Z
BR3FYZZ
BR3FZZZ
BR40ZZZ
BR47ZZZ
BR49ZZZ
BR4FZZZ
BT000ZZ
BT001ZZ
BT00YZZ
BT00ZZZ
BT010ZZ
BT011ZZ
BT01YZZ
BT01ZZZ
BT020ZZ
BT021ZZ
BT02YZZ
BT02ZZZ
BT030ZZ
BT031ZZ
BT03YZZ
BT03ZZZ
BT040ZZ
BT041ZZ
BT04YZZ
BT04ZZZ
BT050ZZ
BT051ZZ
BT05YZZ
BT05ZZZ
BT060ZZ
BT061ZZ
BT06YZZ
BT06ZZZ
BT070ZZ
BT071ZZ
BT07YZZ
BT07ZZZ
BT080ZZ
BT081ZZ
BT08YZZ
BT08ZZZ
BT0B0ZZ
BT0B1ZZ
BT0BYZZ
BT0BZZZ
BT0C0ZZ
BT0C1ZZ
BT0CYZZ
BT0CZZZ
BT100ZZ
BT101ZZ
BT10YZZ
BT10ZZZ
BT110ZZ
BT111ZZ
BT11YZZ
BT11ZZZ
BT120ZZ
BT121ZZ
BT12YZZ
BT12ZZZ
BT130ZZ
BT131ZZ
BT13YZZ
BT13ZZZ
BT140ZZ
BT141ZZ
BT14YZZ
BT14ZZZ
BT150ZZ
BT151ZZ
BT15YZZ
BT15ZZZ
BT160ZZ
BT161ZZ
BT16YZZ
BT16ZZZ
BT170ZZ
BT171ZZ
BT17YZZ
BT17ZZZ
BT1B0ZZ
BT1B1ZZ
BT1BYZZ
BT1BZZZ
BT1C0ZZ
BT1C1ZZ
BT1CYZZ
BT1CZZZ
BT1D0ZZ
BT1D1ZZ
BT1DYZZ
BT1DZZZ
BT1F0ZZ
BT1F1ZZ
BT1FYZZ
BT1FZZZ
BT1G0ZZ
BT1G1ZZ
BT1GYZZ
BT1GZZZ
BT2000Z
BT200ZZ
BT2010Z
BT201ZZ
BT20Y0Z
BT20YZZ
BT20ZZZ
BT2100Z
BT210ZZ
BT2110Z
BT211ZZ
BT21Y0Z
BT21YZZ
BT21ZZZ
BT2200Z
BT220ZZ
BT2210Z
BT221ZZ
BT22Y0Z
BT22YZZ
BT22ZZZ
BT2300Z
BT230ZZ
BT2310Z
BT231ZZ
BT23Y0Z
BT23YZZ
BT23ZZZ
BT2900Z
BT290ZZ
BT2910Z
BT291ZZ
BT29Y0Z
BT29YZZ
BT29ZZZ
BT30Y0Z
BT30YZZ
BT30ZZZ
BT31Y0Z
BT31YZZ
BT31ZZZ
BT32Y0Z
BT32YZZ
BT32ZZZ
BT33Y0Z
BT33YZZ
BT33ZZZ
BT39Y0Z
BT39YZZ
BT39ZZZ
BT40ZZZ
BT41ZZZ
BT42ZZZ
BT43ZZZ
BT45ZZZ
BT46ZZZ
BT47ZZZ
BT48ZZZ
BT49ZZZ
BT4JZZZ
BU000ZZ
BU001ZZ
BU00YZZ
BU010ZZ
BU011ZZ
BU01YZZ
BU020ZZ
BU021ZZ
BU02YZZ
BU060ZZ
BU061ZZ
BU06YZZ
BU080ZZ
BU081ZZ
BU08YZZ
BU090ZZ
BU091ZZ
BU09YZZ
BU100ZZ
BU101ZZ
BU10YZZ
BU10ZZZ
BU110ZZ
BU111ZZ
BU11YZZ
BU11ZZZ
BU120ZZ
BU121ZZ
BU12YZZ
BU12ZZZ
BU160ZZ
BU161ZZ
BU16YZZ
BU16ZZZ
BU180ZZ
BU181ZZ
BU18YZZ
BU18ZZZ
BU190ZZ
BU191ZZ
BU19YZZ
BU19ZZZ
BU33Y0Z
BU33YZZ
BU33ZZZ
BU34Y0Z
BU34YZZ
BU34ZZZ
BU35Y0Z
BU35YZZ
BU35ZZZ
BU36Y0Z
BU36YZZ
BU36ZZZ
BU39Y0Z
BU39YZZ
BU39ZZZ
BU3BY0Z
BU3BYZZ
BU3BZZZ
BU3CY0Z
BU3CYZZ
BU3CZZZ
BU40YZZ
BU40ZZZ
BU41YZZ
BU41ZZZ
BU42YZZ
BU42ZZZ
BU43YZZ
BU43ZZZ
BU44YZZ
BU44ZZZ
BU45YZZ
BU45ZZZ
BU46YZZ
BU46ZZZ
BU4CYZZ
BU4CZZZ
BV000ZZ
BV001ZZ
BV00YZZ
BV010ZZ
BV011ZZ
BV01YZZ
BV020ZZ
BV021ZZ
BV02YZZ
BV030ZZ
BV031ZZ
BV03YZZ
BV050ZZ
BV051ZZ
BV05YZZ
BV060ZZ
BV061ZZ
BV06YZZ
BV080ZZ
BV081ZZ
BV08YZZ
BV100ZZ
BV101ZZ
BV10YZZ
BV10ZZZ
BV180ZZ
BV181ZZ
BV18YZZ
BV18ZZZ
BV2300Z
BV230ZZ
BV2310Z
BV231ZZ
BV23Y0Z
BV23YZZ
BV23ZZZ
BV30Y0Z
BV30YZZ
BV30ZZZ
BV33Y0Z
BV33YZZ
BV33ZZZ
BV34Y0Z
BV34YZZ
BV34ZZZ
BV35Y0Z
BV35YZZ
BV35ZZZ
BV36Y0Z
BV36YZZ
BV36ZZZ
BV37Y0Z
BV37YZZ
BV37ZZZ
BV44ZZZ
BV49ZZZ
BV4BZZZ
BW00ZZZ
BW01ZZZ
BW03ZZZ
BW0BZZZ
BW0CZZZ
BW0JZZZ
BW0KZZZ
BW0LZZZ
BW0MZZZ
BW110ZZ
BW111ZZ
BW11YZZ
BW11ZZZ
BW190ZZ
BW191ZZ
BW19YZZ
BW19ZZZ
BW1C0ZZ
BW1C1ZZ
BW1CYZZ
BW1CZZZ
BW1J0ZZ
BW1J1ZZ
BW1JYZZ
BW1JZZZ
BW2000Z
BW200ZZ
BW2010Z
BW201ZZ
BW20Y0Z
BW20YZZ
BW20ZZZ
BW2100Z
BW210ZZ
BW2110Z
BW211ZZ
BW21Y0Z
BW21YZZ
BW21ZZZ
BW2400Z
BW240ZZ
BW2410Z
BW241ZZ
BW24Y0Z
BW24YZZ
BW24ZZZ
BW2500Z
BW250ZZ
BW2510Z
BW251ZZ
BW25Y0Z
BW25YZZ
BW25ZZZ
BW2800Z
BW280ZZ
BW2810Z
BW281ZZ
BW28Y0Z
BW28YZZ
BW28ZZZ
BW2900Z
BW290ZZ
BW2910Z
BW291ZZ
BW29Y0Z
BW29YZZ
BW29ZZZ
BW2F00Z
BW2F0ZZ
BW2F10Z
BW2F1ZZ
BW2FY0Z
BW2FYZZ
BW2FZZZ
BW2G00Z
BW2G0ZZ
BW2G10Z
BW2G1ZZ
BW2GY0Z
BW2GYZZ
BW2GZZZ
BW30Y0Z
BW30YZZ
BW30ZZZ
BW33Y0Z
BW33YZZ
BW38Y0Z
BW38YZZ
BW38ZZZ
BW3FY0Z
BW3FYZZ
BW3FZZZ
BW3GY0Z
BW3GYZZ
BW3GZZZ
BW3HY0Z
BW3HYZZ
BW3HZZZ
BW3PY0Z
BW3PYZZ
BW3PZZZ
BW40ZZZ
BW41ZZZ
BW4FZZZ
BW4GZZZ
BY30Y0Z
BY30YZZ
BY30ZZZ
BY31Y0Z
BY31YZZ
BY31ZZZ
BY32Y0Z
BY32YZZ
BY32ZZZ
BY33Y0Z
BY33YZZ
BY33ZZZ
BY34Y0Z
BY34YZZ
BY34ZZZ
BY35Y0Z
BY35YZZ
BY35ZZZ
BY36Y0Z
BY36YZZ
BY36ZZZ
BY47ZZZ
BY48ZZZ
BY49ZZZ
BY4BZZZ
BY4CZZZ
BY4DZZZ
BY4FZZZ
BY4GZZZ
C0101ZZ
C010YZZ
C015DZZ
C015YZZ
C01YYZZ
C0201ZZ
C020FZZ
C020SZZ
C020YZZ
C025DZZ
C025YZZ
C02YYZZ
C030BZZ
C030KZZ
C030MZZ
C030YZZ
C03YYZZ
C050VZZ
C050YZZ
C05YYZZ
C2161ZZ
C216YZZ
C21G1ZZ
C21GDZZ
C21GSZZ
C21GYZZ
C21GZZZ
C21YYZZ
C2261ZZ
C226YZZ
C22G1ZZ
C22GDZZ
C22GKZZ
C22GSZZ
C22GYZZ
C22GZZZ
C22YYZZ
C23GKZZ
C23GMZZ
C23GQZZ
C23GRZZ
C23GYZZ
C23YYZZ
C2561ZZ
C256YZZ
C25YYZZ
C51B1ZZ
C51BYZZ
C51C1ZZ
C51CYZZ
C51D1ZZ
C51DYZZ
C51N1ZZ
C51NYZZ
C51P1ZZ
C51PYZZ
C51Q1ZZ
C51QYZZ
C51R1ZZ
C51RYZZ
C51YYZZ
C7101ZZ
C710DZZ
C710YZZ
C7121ZZ
C712YZZ
C713DZZ
C713YZZ
C7151ZZ
C715YZZ
C71D1ZZ
C71DYZZ
C71J1ZZ
C71JYZZ
C71K1ZZ
C71KYZZ
C71L1ZZ
C71LYZZ
C71M1ZZ
C71MYZZ
C71N1ZZ
C71NYZZ
C71P1ZZ
C71PYZZ
C71YYZZ
C7221ZZ
C722YZZ
C72YYZZ
C7551ZZ
C755YZZ
C75D1ZZ
C75DYZZ
C75J1ZZ
C75JYZZ
C75K1ZZ
C75KYZZ
C75L1ZZ
C75LYZZ
C75M1ZZ
C75MYZZ
C75N1ZZ
C75NYZZ
C75P1ZZ
C75PYZZ
C75YYZZ
C7631ZZ
C7637ZZ
C763CZZ
C763DZZ
C763HZZ
C763WZZ
C763YZZ
C76YYZZ
C8191ZZ
C819YZZ
C81YYZZ
C91B1ZZ
C91BYZZ
C91YYZZ
CB121ZZ
CB129ZZ
CB12TZZ
CB12VZZ
CB12YZZ
CB1YYZZ
CB221ZZ
CB229ZZ
CB22YZZ
CB2YYZZ
CB32KZZ
CB32YZZ
CB3YYZZ
CD151ZZ
CD15DZZ
CD15YZZ
CD171ZZ
CD17DZZ
CD17YZZ
CD1YYZZ
CD271ZZ
CD27DZZ
CD27YZZ
CD2YYZZ
CF141ZZ
CF14YZZ
CF151ZZ
CF15YZZ
CF161ZZ
CF16YZZ
CF1C1ZZ
CF1CYZZ
CF1YYZZ
CF241ZZ
CF24YZZ
CF251ZZ
CF25YZZ
CF261ZZ
CF26YZZ
CF2YYZZ
CG111ZZ
CG11SZZ
CG11YZZ
CG121ZZ
CG12FZZ
CG12GZZ
CG12YZZ
CG14GZZ
CG14YZZ
CG1YYZZ
CG211ZZ
CG21SZZ
CG21YZZ
CG2YYZZ
CG421ZZ
CG42FZZ
CG42GZZ
CG42YZZ
CG4YYZZ
CH101ZZ
CH10SZZ
CH10YZZ
CH111ZZ
CH11SZZ
CH11YZZ
CH121ZZ
CH12SZZ
CH12YZZ
CH1YYZZ
CH201ZZ
CH20SZZ
CH20YZZ
CH211ZZ
CH21SZZ
CH21YZZ
CH221ZZ
CH22SZZ
CH22YZZ
CH2YYZZ
CP111ZZ
CP11YZZ
CP141ZZ
CP14YZZ
CP151ZZ
CP15YZZ
CP161ZZ
CP16YZZ
CP171ZZ
CP17YZZ
CP181ZZ
CP18YZZ
CP191ZZ
CP19YZZ
CP1B1ZZ
CP1BYZZ
CP1C1ZZ
CP1CYZZ
CP1D1ZZ
CP1DYZZ
CP1F1ZZ
CP1FYZZ
CP1YYZZ
CP1Z1ZZ
CP1ZYZZ
CP211ZZ
CP21YZZ
CP221ZZ
CP22YZZ
CP231ZZ
CP23YZZ
CP241ZZ
CP24YZZ
CP261ZZ
CP26YZZ
CP271ZZ
CP27YZZ
CP281ZZ
CP28YZZ
CP291ZZ
CP29YZZ
CP2B1ZZ
CP2BYZZ
CP2C1ZZ
CP2CYZZ
CP2D1ZZ
CP2DYZZ
CP2F1ZZ
CP2FYZZ
CP2G1ZZ
CP2GYZZ
CP2H1ZZ
CP2HYZZ
CP2J1ZZ
CP2JYZZ
CP2YYZZ
CP55ZZZ
CP5NZZZ
CP5PZZZ
CP5YYZZ
CT131ZZ
CT13FZZ
CT13GZZ
CT13YZZ
CT1H1ZZ
CT1HYZZ
CT1YYZZ
CT231ZZ
CT23YZZ
CT2YYZZ
CT631ZZ
CT63FZZ
CT63GZZ
CT63HZZ
CT63YZZ
CT6YYZZ

CV191ZZ
CV19YZZ
CV1YYZZ
CW101ZZ
CW10DZZ
CW10FZZ
CW10GZZ
CW10LZZ
CW10SZZ
CW10YZZ
CW111ZZ
CW11DZZ
CW11FZZ
CW11GZZ
CW11LZZ
CW11SZZ
CW11YZZ
CW131ZZ
CW13DZZ
CW13FZZ
CW13GZZ
CW13KZZ
CW13LZZ
CW13SZZ
CW13YZZ
CW141ZZ
CW14DZZ
CW14FZZ
CW14GZZ
CW14LZZ
CW14SZZ
CW14YZZ
CW161ZZ
CW16DZZ
CW16FZZ
CW16GZZ
CW16LZZ
CW16SZZ
CW16YZZ
CW1B1ZZ
CW1BDZZ
CW1BFZZ
CW1BGZZ
CW1BLZZ
CW1BSZZ
CW1BYZZ
CW1D1ZZ
CW1DDZZ
CW1DFZZ
CW1DGZZ
CW1DLZZ
CW1DSZZ
CW1DYZZ
CW1J1ZZ
CW1JDZZ
CW1JFZZ
CW1JGZZ
CW1JLZZ
CW1JSZZ
CW1JYZZ
CW1M1ZZ
CW1MDZZ
CW1MFZZ
CW1MGZZ
CW1MLZZ
CW1MSZZ
CW1MYZZ
CW1N1ZZ
CW1NDZZ
CW1NFZZ
CW1NGZZ
CW1NLZZ
CW1NSZZ
CW1NYZZ
CW1YYZZ
CW1ZZZZ
CW201ZZ
CW20DZZ
CW20FZZ
CW20GZZ
CW20KZZ
CW20LZZ
CW20SZZ
CW20YZZ
CW211ZZ
CW21DZZ
CW21FZZ
CW21GZZ
CW21KZZ
CW21LZZ
CW21SZZ
CW21YZZ
CW231ZZ
CW23DZZ
CW23FZZ
CW23GZZ
CW23KZZ
CW23LZZ
CW23SZZ
CW23YZZ
CW241ZZ
CW24DZZ
CW24FZZ
CW24GZZ
CW24KZZ
CW24LZZ
CW24SZZ
CW24YZZ
CW261ZZ
CW26DZZ
CW26FZZ
CW26GZZ
CW26KZZ
CW26LZZ
CW26SZZ
CW26YZZ
CW2B1ZZ
CW2BDZZ
CW2BFZZ
CW2BGZZ
CW2BKZZ
CW2BLZZ
CW2BSZZ
CW2BYZZ
CW2D1ZZ
CW2DDZZ
CW2DFZZ
CW2DGZZ
CW2DKZZ
CW2DLZZ
CW2DSZZ
CW2DYZZ
CW2J1ZZ
CW2JDZZ
CW2JFZZ
CW2JGZZ
CW2JKZZ
CW2JLZZ
CW2JSZZ
CW2JYZZ
CW2M1ZZ
CW2MDZZ
CW2MFZZ
CW2MGZZ
CW2MKZZ
CW2MLZZ
CW2MSZZ
CW2MYZZ
CW2YYZZ
CW3NYZZ
CW501ZZ
CW50DZZ
CW50YZZ
CW511ZZ
CW51DZZ
CW51YZZ
CW531ZZ
CW53DZZ
CW53YZZ
CW541ZZ
CW54DZZ
CW54YZZ
CW561ZZ
CW56DZZ
CW56YZZ
CW5B1ZZ
CW5BDZZ
CW5BYZZ
CW5D1ZZ
CW5DDZZ
CW5DYZZ
CW5J1ZZ
CW5JDZZ
CW5JYZZ
CW5M1ZZ
CW5MDZZ
CW5MYZZ
CW70NZZ
CW70YZZ
CW73NZZ
CW73YZZ
CW7GGZZ
CW7GYZZ
CW7N8ZZ
CW7NGZZ
CW7NNZZ
CW7NPZZ
CW7NYZZ
CW7YYZZ
D0000ZZ
D0001ZZ
D0002ZZ
D0003Z0
D0003ZZ
D0004ZZ
D0005ZZ
D0006ZZ
D0010ZZ
D0011ZZ
D0012ZZ
D0013Z0
D0013ZZ
D0014ZZ
D0015ZZ
D0016ZZ
D0060ZZ
D0061ZZ
D0062ZZ
D0063Z0
D0063ZZ
D0064ZZ
D0065ZZ
D0066ZZ
D0070ZZ
D0071ZZ
D0072ZZ
D0073Z0
D0073ZZ
D0074ZZ
D0075ZZ
D0076ZZ
D01097Z
D01098Z
D01099Z
D0109BZ
D0109CZ
D0109YZ
D010B7Z
D010B8Z
D010B9Z
D010BBZ
D010BCZ
D010BYZ
D01197Z
D01198Z
D01199Z
D0119BZ
D0119CZ
D0119YZ
D011B7Z
D011B8Z
D011B9Z
D011BBZ
D011BCZ
D011BYZ
D01697Z
D01698Z
D01699Z
D0169BZ
D0169CZ
D0169YZ
D016B7Z
D016B8Z
D016B9Z
D016BBZ
D016BCZ
D016BYZ
D01797Z
D01798Z
D01799Z
D0179BZ
D0179CZ
D0179YZ
D017B7Z
D017B8Z
D017B9Z
D017BBZ
D017BCZ
D017BYZ
D0Y07ZZ
D0Y08ZZ
D0Y0FZZ
D0Y0KZZ
D0Y17ZZ
D0Y18ZZ
D0Y1FZZ
D0Y1KZZ
D0Y67ZZ
D0Y68ZZ
D0Y6FZZ
D0Y6KZZ
D0Y77ZZ
D0Y78ZZ
D0Y7FZZ
D0Y7KZZ
D7000ZZ
D7001ZZ
D7002ZZ
D7003Z0
D7003ZZ
D7004ZZ
D7005ZZ
D7006ZZ
D7010ZZ
D7011ZZ
D7012ZZ
D7013Z0
D7013ZZ
D7014ZZ
D7015ZZ
D7016ZZ
D7020ZZ
D7021ZZ
D7022ZZ
D7023Z0
D7023ZZ
D7024ZZ
D7025ZZ
D7026ZZ
D7030ZZ
D7031ZZ
D7032ZZ
D7033Z0
D7033ZZ
D7034ZZ
D7035ZZ
D7036ZZ
D7040ZZ
D7041ZZ
D7042ZZ
D7043Z0
D7043ZZ
D7044ZZ
D7045ZZ
D7046ZZ
D7050ZZ
D7051ZZ
D7052ZZ
D7053Z0
D7053ZZ
D7054ZZ
D7055ZZ
D7056ZZ
D7060ZZ
D7061ZZ
D7062ZZ
D7063Z0
D7063ZZ
D7064ZZ
D7065ZZ
D7066ZZ
D7070ZZ
D7071ZZ
D7072ZZ
D7073Z0
D7073ZZ
D7074ZZ
D7075ZZ
D7076ZZ
D7080ZZ
D7081ZZ
D7082ZZ
D7083Z0
D7083ZZ
D7084ZZ
D7085ZZ
D7086ZZ
D71097Z
D71098Z
D71099Z
D7109BZ
D7109CZ
D7109YZ
D710B7Z
D710B8Z
D710B9Z
D710BBZ
D710BCZ
D710BYZ
D71197Z
D71198Z
D71199Z
D7119BZ
D7119CZ
D7119YZ
D711B7Z
D711B8Z
D711B9Z
D711BBZ
D711BCZ
D711BYZ
D71297Z
D71298Z
D71299Z
D7129BZ
D7129CZ
D7129YZ
D712B7Z
D712B8Z
D712B9Z
D712BBZ
D712BCZ
D712BYZ
D71397Z
D71398Z
D71399Z
D7139BZ
D7139CZ
D7139YZ
D713B7Z
D713B8Z
D713B9Z
D713BBZ
D713BCZ
D713BYZ
D71497Z
D71498Z
D71499Z
D7149BZ
D7149CZ
D7149YZ
D714B7Z
D714B8Z
D714B9Z
D714BBZ
D714BCZ
D714BYZ
D71597Z
D71598Z
D71599Z
D7159BZ
D7159CZ
D7159YZ
D715B7Z
D715B8Z
D715B9Z
D715BBZ
D715BCZ
D715BYZ
D71697Z
D71698Z
D71699Z
D7169BZ
D7169CZ
D7169YZ
D716B7Z
D716B8Z
D716B9Z
D716BBZ
D716BCZ
D716BYZ
D71797Z
D71798Z
D71799Z
D7179BZ
D7179CZ
D7179YZ
D717B7Z
D717B8Z
D717B9Z
D717BBZ
D717BCZ
D717BYZ
D71897Z
D71898Z
D71899Z
D7189BZ
D7189CZ
D7189YZ
D718B7Z
D718B8Z
D718B9Z
D718BBZ
D718BCZ
D718BYZ
D7Y08ZZ
D7Y0FZZ
D7Y18ZZ
D7Y1FZZ
D7Y28ZZ
D7Y2FZZ
D7Y38ZZ
D7Y3FZZ
D7Y48ZZ
D7Y4FZZ
D7Y58ZZ
D7Y5FZZ
D7Y68ZZ
D7Y6FZZ
D7Y78ZZ
D7Y7FZZ
D7Y88ZZ
D7Y8FZZ
D8000ZZ
D8001ZZ
D8002ZZ
D8003Z0
D8003ZZ
D8004ZZ
D8005ZZ
D8006ZZ
D81097Z
D81098Z
D81099Z
D8109BZ
D8109CZ
D8109YZ
D810B7Z
D810B8Z
D810B9Z
D810BBZ
D810BCZ
D810BYZ
D8Y07ZZ
D8Y08ZZ
D8Y0FZZ
D9000ZZ
D9001ZZ
D9002ZZ
D9003Z0
D9003ZZ
D9004ZZ
D9005ZZ
D9006ZZ
D9010ZZ
D9011ZZ
D9012ZZ
D9013Z0
D9013ZZ
D9014ZZ
D9015ZZ
D9016ZZ
D9030ZZ
D9031ZZ
D9032ZZ
D9033Z0
D9033ZZ
D9034ZZ
D9035ZZ
D9036ZZ
D9040ZZ
D9041ZZ
D9042ZZ
D9043Z0
D9043ZZ
D9044ZZ
D9045ZZ
D9046ZZ
D9050ZZ
D9051ZZ
D9052ZZ
D9053Z0
D9053ZZ
D9054ZZ
D9055ZZ
D9056ZZ
D9060ZZ
D9061ZZ
D9062ZZ
D9063Z0
D9063ZZ
D9064ZZ
D9065ZZ
D9066ZZ
D9070ZZ
D9071ZZ
D9072ZZ
D9073Z0
D9073ZZ
D9074ZZ
D9075ZZ
D9076ZZ
D9080ZZ
D9081ZZ
D9082ZZ
D9083Z0
D9083ZZ
D9084ZZ
D9085ZZ
D9086ZZ
D9090ZZ
D9091ZZ
D9092ZZ
D9093Z0
D9093ZZ
D9094ZZ
D9095ZZ
D9096ZZ
D90B0ZZ
D90B1ZZ
D90B2ZZ
D90B3Z0
D90B3ZZ
D90B4ZZ
D90B5ZZ
D90B6ZZ
D90D0ZZ
D90D1ZZ
D90D2ZZ
D90D3Z0
D90D3ZZ
D90D4ZZ
D90D5ZZ
D90D6ZZ
D90F0ZZ
D90F1ZZ
D90F2ZZ
D90F3Z0
D90F3ZZ
D90F4ZZ
D90F5ZZ
D90F6ZZ
D91097Z
D91098Z
D91099Z
D9109BZ
D9109CZ
D9109YZ
D910B7Z
D910B8Z
D910B9Z
D910BBZ
D910BCZ
D910BYZ
D91197Z
D91198Z
D91199Z
D9119BZ
D9119CZ
D9119YZ
D911B7Z
D911B8Z
D911B9Z
D911BBZ
D911BCZ
D911BYZ
D91397Z
D91398Z
D91399Z
D9139BZ
D9139CZ
D9139YZ
D913B7Z
D913B8Z
D913B9Z
D913BBZ
D913BCZ
D913BYZ
D91497Z
D91498Z
D91499Z
D9149BZ
D9149CZ
D9149YZ
D914B7Z
D914B8Z
D914B9Z
D914BBZ
D914BCZ
D914BYZ
D91597Z
D91598Z
D91599Z
D9159BZ
D9159CZ
D9159YZ
D915B7Z
D915B8Z
D915B9Z
D915BBZ
D915BCZ
D915BYZ
D91697Z
D91698Z
D91699Z
D9169BZ
D9169CZ
D9169YZ
D916B7Z
D916B8Z
D916B9Z
D916BBZ
D916BCZ
D916BYZ
D91797Z
D91798Z
D91799Z
D9179BZ
D9179CZ
D9179YZ
D917B7Z
D917B8Z
D917B9Z
D917BBZ
D917BCZ
D917BYZ
D91897Z
D91898Z
D91899Z
D9189BZ
D9189CZ
D9189YZ
D918B7Z
D918B8Z
D918B9Z
D918BBZ
D918BCZ
D918BYZ
D91997Z
D91998Z
D91999Z
D9199BZ
D9199CZ
D9199YZ
D919B7Z
D919B8Z
D919B9Z
D919BBZ
D919BCZ
D919BYZ
D91B97Z
D91B98Z
D91B99Z
D91B9BZ
D91B9CZ
D91B9YZ
D91BB7Z
D91BB8Z
D91BB9Z
D91BBBZ
D91BBCZ
D91BBYZ
D91D97Z
D91D98Z
D91D99Z
D91D9BZ

D91D9CZ
D91D9YZ
D91DB7Z
D91DB8Z
D91DB9Z
D91DBBZ
D91DBCZ
D91DBYZ
D91F97Z
D91F98Z
D91F99Z
D91F9BZ
D91F9CZ
D91F9YZ
D91FB7Z
D91FB8Z
D91FB9Z
D91FBBZ
D91FBCZ
D91FBYZ
D9Y07ZZ
D9Y08ZZ
D9Y0FZZ
D9Y17ZZ
D9Y18ZZ
D9Y1FZZ
D9Y37ZZ
D9Y38ZZ
D9Y47ZZ
D9Y48ZZ
D9Y4CZZ
D9Y4FZZ
D9Y57ZZ
D9Y58ZZ
D9Y5FZZ
D9Y67ZZ
D9Y68ZZ
D9Y6FZZ
D9Y77ZZ
D9Y78ZZ
D9Y7FZZ
D9Y87ZZ
D9Y88ZZ
D9Y8FZZ
D9Y97ZZ
D9Y98ZZ
D9Y9FZZ
D9YB7ZZ
D9YB8ZZ
D9YBCZZ
D9YBFZZ
D9YCCZZ
D9YCFZZ
D9YD7ZZ
D9YD8ZZ
D9YDCZZ
D9YDFZZ
D9YF7ZZ
D9YF8ZZ
DB000ZZ
DB001ZZ
DB002ZZ
DB003Z0
DB003ZZ
DB004ZZ
DB005ZZ
DB006ZZ
DB010ZZ
DB011ZZ
DB012ZZ
DB013Z0
DB013ZZ
DB014ZZ
DB015ZZ
DB016ZZ
DB020ZZ
DB021ZZ
DB022ZZ
DB023Z0
DB023ZZ
DB024ZZ
DB025ZZ
DB026ZZ
DB050ZZ
DB051ZZ
DB052ZZ
DB053Z0
DB053ZZ
DB054ZZ
DB055ZZ
DB056ZZ
DB060ZZ
DB061ZZ
DB062ZZ
DB063Z0
DB063ZZ
DB064ZZ
DB065ZZ
DB066ZZ
DB070ZZ
DB071ZZ
DB072ZZ
DB073Z0
DB073ZZ
DB074ZZ
DB075ZZ
DB076ZZ
DB080ZZ
DB081ZZ
DB082ZZ
DB083Z0
DB083ZZ
DB084ZZ
DB085ZZ
DB086ZZ
DB1097Z
DB1098Z
DB1099Z
DB109BZ
DB109CZ
DB109YZ
DB10B7Z
DB10B8Z
DB10B9Z
DB10BBZ
DB10BCZ
DB10BYZ
DB1197Z
DB1198Z
DB1199Z
DB119BZ
DB119CZ
DB119YZ
DB11B7Z
DB11B8Z
DB11B9Z
DB11BBZ
DB11BCZ
DB11BYZ
DB1297Z
DB1298Z
DB1299Z
DB129BZ
DB129CZ
DB129YZ
DB12B7Z
DB12B8Z
DB12B9Z
DB12BBZ
DB12BCZ
DB12BYZ
DB1597Z
DB1598Z
DB1599Z
DB159BZ
DB159CZ
DB159YZ
DB15B7Z
DB15B8Z
DB15B9Z
DB15BBZ
DB15BCZ
DB15BYZ
DB1697Z
DB1698Z
DB1699Z
DB169BZ
DB169CZ
DB169YZ
DB16B7Z
DB16B8Z
DB16B9Z
DB16BBZ
DB16BCZ
DB16BYZ
DB1797Z
DB1798Z
DB1799Z
DB179BZ
DB179CZ
DB179YZ
DB17B7Z
DB17B8Z
DB17B9Z
DB17BBZ
DB17BCZ
DB17BYZ
DB1897Z
DB1898Z
DB1899Z
DB189BZ
DB189CZ
DB189YZ
DB18B7Z
DB18B8Z
DB18B9Z
DB18BBZ
DB18BCZ
DB18BYZ
DB27HZZ
DB27JZZ
DB28DZZ
DB28HZZ
DB28JZZ
DBY07ZZ
DBY08ZZ
DBY0FZZ
DBY0KZZ
DBY17ZZ
DBY18ZZ
DBY1FZZ
DBY1KZZ
DBY27ZZ
DBY28ZZ
DBY2FZZ
DBY2KZZ
DBY57ZZ
DBY58ZZ
DBY5FZZ
DBY5KZZ
DBY67ZZ
DBY68ZZ
DBY6FZZ
DBY6KZZ
DBY77ZZ
DBY78ZZ
DBY7FZZ
DBY7KZZ
DBY87ZZ
DBY88ZZ
DBY8FZZ
DBY8KZZ
DD000ZZ
DD001ZZ
DD002ZZ
DD003Z0
DD003ZZ
DD004ZZ
DD005ZZ
DD006ZZ
DD010ZZ
DD011ZZ
DD012ZZ
DD013Z0
DD013ZZ
DD014ZZ
DD015ZZ
DD016ZZ
DD020ZZ
DD021ZZ
DD022ZZ
DD023Z0
DD023ZZ
DD024ZZ
DD025ZZ
DD026ZZ
DD030ZZ
DD031ZZ
DD032ZZ
DD033Z0
DD033ZZ
DD034ZZ
DD035ZZ
DD036ZZ
DD040ZZ
DD041ZZ
DD042ZZ
DD043Z0
DD043ZZ
DD044ZZ
DD045ZZ
DD046ZZ
DD050ZZ
DD051ZZ
DD052ZZ
DD053Z0
DD053ZZ
DD054ZZ
DD055ZZ
DD056ZZ
DD070ZZ
DD071ZZ
DD072ZZ
DD073Z0
DD073ZZ
DD074ZZ
DD075ZZ
DD076ZZ
DD1097Z
DD1098Z
DD1099Z
DD109BZ
DD109CZ
DD109YZ
DD10B7Z
DD10B8Z
DD10B9Z
DD10BBZ
DD10BCZ
DD10BYZ
DD1197Z
DD1198Z
DD1199Z
DD119BZ
DD119CZ
DD119YZ
DD11B7Z
DD11B8Z
DD11B9Z
DD11BBZ
DD11BCZ
DD11BYZ
DD1297Z
DD1298Z
DD1299Z
DD129BZ
DD129CZ
DD129YZ
DD12B7Z
DD12B8Z
DD12B9Z
DD12BBZ
DD12BCZ
DD12BYZ
DD1397Z
DD1398Z
DD1399Z
DD139BZ
DD139CZ
DD139YZ
DD13B7Z
DD13B8Z
DD13B9Z
DD13BBZ
DD13BCZ
DD13BYZ
DD1497Z
DD1498Z
DD1499Z
DD149BZ
DD149CZ
DD149YZ
DD14B7Z
DD14B8Z
DD14B9Z
DD14BBZ
DD14BCZ
DD14BYZ
DD1597Z
DD1598Z
DD1599Z
DD159BZ
DD159CZ
DD159YZ
DD15B7Z
DD15B8Z
DD15B9Z
DD15BBZ
DD15BCZ
DD15BYZ
DD1797Z
DD1798Z
DD1799Z
DD179BZ
DD179CZ
DD179YZ
DD17B7Z
DD17B8Z
DD17B9Z
DD17BBZ
DD17BCZ
DD17BYZ
DD20DZZ
DD20HZZ
DD20JZZ
DD21DZZ
DD21HZZ
DD21JZZ
DD22DZZ
DD22HZZ
DD22JZZ
DD23DZZ
DD23HZZ
DD23JZZ
DD24DZZ
DD24HZZ
DD24JZZ
DD25DZZ
DD25HZZ
DD25JZZ
DD27DZZ
DD27HZZ
DD27JZZ
DDY07ZZ
DDY08ZZ
DDY0FZZ
DDY0KZZ
DDY17ZZ
DDY18ZZ
DDY1CZZ
DDY1FZZ
DDY1KZZ
DDY27ZZ
DDY28ZZ
DDY2CZZ
DDY2FZZ
DDY2KZZ
DDY37ZZ
DDY38ZZ
DDY3CZZ
DDY3FZZ
DDY3KZZ
DDY47ZZ
DDY48ZZ
DDY4CZZ
DDY4FZZ
DDY4KZZ
DDY57ZZ
DDY58ZZ
DDY5CZZ
DDY5FZZ
DDY5KZZ
DDY77ZZ
DDY78ZZ
DDY7CZZ
DDY7FZZ
DDY7KZZ
DDY8CZZ
DDY8FZZ
DDY8KZZ
DF000ZZ
DF001ZZ
DF002ZZ
DF003Z0
DF003ZZ
DF004ZZ
DF005ZZ
DF006ZZ
DF010ZZ
DF011ZZ
DF012ZZ
DF013Z0
DF013ZZ
DF014ZZ
DF015ZZ
DF016ZZ
DF020ZZ
DF021ZZ
DF022ZZ
DF023Z0
DF023ZZ
DF024ZZ
DF025ZZ
DF026ZZ
DF030ZZ
DF031ZZ
DF032ZZ
DF033Z0
DF033ZZ
DF034ZZ
DF035ZZ
DF036ZZ
DF1097Z
DF1098Z
DF1099Z
DF109BZ
DF109CZ
DF109YZ
DF10B7Z
DF10B8Z
DF10B9Z
DF10BBZ
DF10BCZ
DF10BYZ
DF1197Z
DF1198Z
DF1199Z
DF119BZ
DF119CZ
DF119YZ
DF11B7Z
DF11B8Z
DF11B9Z
DF11BBZ
DF11BCZ
DF11BYZ
DF1297Z
DF1298Z
DF1299Z
DF129BZ
DF129CZ
DF129YZ
DF12B7Z
DF12B8Z
DF12B9Z
DF12BBZ
DF12BCZ
DF12BYZ
DF1397Z
DF1398Z
DF1399Z
DF139BZ
DF139CZ
DF139YZ
DF13B7Z
DF13B8Z
DF13B9Z
DF13BBZ
DF13BCZ
DF13BYZ
DF20DZZ
DF20HZZ
DF20JZZ
DF21DZZ
DF21HZZ
DF21JZZ
DF22DZZ
DF22HZZ
DF22JZZ
DF23DZZ
DF23HZZ
DF23JZZ
DFY07ZZ
DFY08ZZ
DFY0CZZ
DFY0FZZ
DFY0KZZ
DFY17ZZ
DFY18ZZ
DFY1CZZ
DFY1FZZ
DFY1KZZ
DFY27ZZ
DFY28ZZ
DFY2CZZ
DFY2FZZ
DFY2KZZ
DFY37ZZ
DFY38ZZ
DFY3CZZ
DFY3FZZ
DFY3KZZ
DG000ZZ
DG001ZZ
DG002ZZ
DG003Z0
DG003ZZ
DG005ZZ
DG006ZZ
DG010ZZ
DG011ZZ
DG012ZZ
DG013Z0
DG013ZZ
DG015ZZ
DG016ZZ
DG020ZZ
DG021ZZ
DG022ZZ
DG023Z0
DG023ZZ
DG025ZZ
DG026ZZ
DG040ZZ
DG041ZZ
DG042ZZ
DG043Z0
DG043ZZ
DG045ZZ
DG046ZZ
DG050ZZ
DG051ZZ
DG052ZZ
DG053Z0
DG053ZZ
DG055ZZ
DG056ZZ
DG1097Z
DG1098Z
DG1099Z
DG109BZ
DG109CZ
DG109YZ
DG10B7Z
DG10B8Z
DG10B9Z
DG10BBZ
DG10BCZ
DG10BYZ
DG1197Z
DG1198Z
DG1199Z
DG119BZ
DG119CZ
DG119YZ
DG11B7Z
DG11B8Z
DG11B9Z
DG11BBZ
DG11BCZ
DG11BYZ
DG1297Z
DG1298Z
DG1299Z
DG129BZ
DG129CZ
DG129YZ
DG12B7Z
DG12B8Z
DG12B9Z
DG12BBZ
DG12BCZ
DG12BYZ
DG1497Z
DG1498Z
DG1499Z
DG149BZ
DG149CZ
DG149YZ
DG14B7Z
DG14B8Z
DG14B9Z
DG14BBZ
DG14BCZ
DG14BYZ
DG1597Z
DG1598Z
DG1599Z
DG159BZ
DG159CZ
DG159YZ
DG15B7Z
DG15B8Z
DG15B9Z
DG15BBZ
DG15BCZ
DG15BYZ
DG20DZZ
DG20HZZ
DG20JZZ
DG21DZZ
DG21HZZ
DG21JZZ
DG22DZZ
DG22HZZ
DG22JZZ
DG24DZZ
DG24HZZ
DG24JZZ
DG25DZZ
DG25HZZ
DG25JZZ
DGY07ZZ
DGY08ZZ
DGY0FZZ
DGY0KZZ
DGY17ZZ
DGY18ZZ
DGY1FZZ
DGY1KZZ
DGY27ZZ
DGY28ZZ
DGY2FZZ
DGY2KZZ
DGY47ZZ
DGY48ZZ
DGY4FZZ
DGY4KZZ
DGY57ZZ
DGY58ZZ
DGY5FZZ
DGY5KZZ
DH020ZZ
DH021ZZ
DH022ZZ
DH023Z0
DH023ZZ
DH024ZZ
DH025ZZ
DH026ZZ
DH030ZZ
DH031ZZ
DH032ZZ
DH033Z0
DH033ZZ
DH034ZZ
DH035ZZ
DH036ZZ
DH040ZZ
DH041ZZ
DH042ZZ
DH043Z0
DH043ZZ
DH044ZZ
DH045ZZ
DH046ZZ
DH060ZZ
DH061ZZ
DH062ZZ
DH063Z0
DH063ZZ
DH064ZZ
DH065ZZ
DH066ZZ
DH070ZZ
DH071ZZ
DH072ZZ
DH073Z0
DH073ZZ
DH074ZZ
DH075ZZ
DH076ZZ
DH080ZZ
DH081ZZ
DH082ZZ
DH083Z0
DH083ZZ
DH084ZZ
DH085ZZ
DH086ZZ
DH090ZZ
DH091ZZ
DH092ZZ
DH093Z0
DH093ZZ
DH094ZZ

DH095ZZ
DH096ZZ
DH0B0ZZ
DH0B1ZZ
DH0B2ZZ
DH0B3Z0
DH0B3ZZ
DH0B4ZZ
DH0B5ZZ
DH0B6ZZ
DHY27ZZ
DHY28ZZ
DHY2FZZ
DHY37ZZ
DHY38ZZ
DHY3FZZ
DHY47ZZ
DHY48ZZ
DHY4FZZ
DHY5FZZ
DHY67ZZ
DHY68ZZ
DHY6FZZ
DHY77ZZ
DHY78ZZ
DHY7FZZ
DHY87ZZ
DHY88ZZ
DHY8FZZ
DHY97ZZ
DHY98ZZ
DHY9FZZ
DHYB7ZZ
DHYB8ZZ
DHYBFZZ
DHYCFZZ
DM000ZZ
DM001ZZ
DM002ZZ
DM003Z0
DM003ZZ
DM004ZZ
DM005ZZ
DM006ZZ
DM010ZZ
DM011ZZ
DM012ZZ
DM013Z0
DM013ZZ
DM014ZZ
DM015ZZ
DM016ZZ
DM1097Z
DM1098Z
DM1099Z
DM109BZ
DM109CZ
DM109YZ
DM10B7Z
DM10B8Z
DM10B9Z
DM10BBZ
DM10BCZ
DM10BYZ
DM1197Z
DM1198Z
DM1199Z
DM119BZ
DM119CZ
DM119YZ
DM11B7Z
DM11B8Z
DM11B9Z
DM11BBZ
DM11BCZ
DM11BYZ
DM20DZZ
DM20HZZ
DM20JZZ
DM21DZZ
DM21HZZ
DM21JZZ
DMY07ZZ
DMY08ZZ
DMY0FZZ
DMY0KZZ
DMY17ZZ
DMY18ZZ
DMY1FZZ
DMY1KZZ
DP000ZZ
DP001ZZ
DP002ZZ
DP003Z0
DP003ZZ
DP004ZZ
DP005ZZ
DP006ZZ
DP020ZZ
DP021ZZ
DP022ZZ
DP023Z0
DP023ZZ
DP024ZZ
DP025ZZ
DP026ZZ
DP030ZZ
DP031ZZ
DP032ZZ
DP033Z0
DP033ZZ
DP034ZZ
DP035ZZ
DP036ZZ
DP040ZZ
DP041ZZ
DP042ZZ
DP043Z0
DP043ZZ
DP044ZZ
DP045ZZ
DP046ZZ
DP050ZZ
DP051ZZ
DP052ZZ
DP053Z0
DP053ZZ
DP054ZZ
DP055ZZ
DP056ZZ
DP060ZZ
DP061ZZ
DP062ZZ
DP063Z0
DP063ZZ
DP064ZZ
DP065ZZ
DP066ZZ
DP070ZZ
DP071ZZ
DP072ZZ
DP073Z0
DP073ZZ
DP074ZZ
DP075ZZ
DP076ZZ
DP080ZZ
DP081ZZ
DP082ZZ
DP083Z0
DP083ZZ
DP084ZZ
DP085ZZ
DP086ZZ
DP090ZZ
DP091ZZ
DP092ZZ
DP093Z0
DP093ZZ
DP094ZZ
DP095ZZ
DP096ZZ
DP0B0ZZ
DP0B1ZZ
DP0B2ZZ
DP0B3Z0
DP0B3ZZ
DP0B4ZZ
DP0B5ZZ
DP0B6ZZ
DP0C0ZZ
DP0C1ZZ
DP0C2ZZ
DP0C3Z0
DP0C3ZZ
DP0C4ZZ
DP0C5ZZ
DP0C6ZZ
DPY07ZZ
DPY08ZZ
DPY0FZZ
DPY27ZZ
DPY28ZZ
DPY2FZZ
DPY37ZZ
DPY38ZZ
DPY3FZZ
DPY47ZZ
DPY48ZZ
DPY4FZZ
DPY57ZZ
DPY58ZZ
DPY5FZZ
DPY67ZZ
DPY68ZZ
DPY6FZZ
DPY77ZZ
DPY78ZZ
DPY7FZZ
DPY87ZZ
DPY88ZZ
DPY8FZZ
DPY97ZZ
DPY98ZZ
DPY9FZZ
DPYB7ZZ
DPYB8ZZ
DPYBFZZ
DPYC7ZZ
DPYC8ZZ
DPYCFZZ
DT000ZZ
DT001ZZ
DT002ZZ
DT003Z0
DT003ZZ
DT004ZZ
DT005ZZ
DT006ZZ
DT010ZZ
DT011ZZ
DT012ZZ
DT013Z0
DT013ZZ
DT014ZZ
DT015ZZ
DT016ZZ
DT020ZZ
DT021ZZ
DT022ZZ
DT023Z0
DT023ZZ
DT024ZZ
DT025ZZ
DT026ZZ
DT030ZZ
DT031ZZ
DT032ZZ
DT033Z0
DT033ZZ
DT034ZZ
DT035ZZ
DT036ZZ
DT1097Z
DT1098Z
DT1099Z
DT109BZ
DT109CZ
DT109YZ
DT10B7Z
DT10B8Z
DT10B9Z
DT10BBZ
DT10BCZ
DT10BYZ
DT1197Z
DT1198Z
DT1199Z
DT119BZ
DT119CZ
DT119YZ
DT11B7Z
DT11B8Z
DT11B9Z
DT11BBZ
DT11BCZ
DT11BYZ
DT1297Z
DT1298Z
DT1299Z
DT129BZ
DT129CZ
DT129YZ
DT12B7Z
DT12B8Z
DT12B9Z
DT12BBZ
DT12BCZ
DT12BYZ
DT1397Z
DT1398Z
DT1399Z
DT139BZ
DT139CZ
DT139YZ
DT13B7Z
DT13B8Z
DT13B9Z
DT13BBZ
DT13BCZ
DT13BYZ
DT20DZZ
DT20HZZ
DT20JZZ
DT21DZZ
DT21HZZ
DT21JZZ
DT22DZZ
DT22HZZ
DT22JZZ
DT23DZZ
DT23HZZ
DT23JZZ
DTY07ZZ
DTY08ZZ
DTY0CZZ
DTY0FZZ
DTY17ZZ
DTY18ZZ
DTY1CZZ
DTY1FZZ
DTY27ZZ
DTY28ZZ
DTY2CZZ
DTY2FZZ
DTY37ZZ
DTY38ZZ
DTY3CZZ
DTY3FZZ
DU000ZZ
DU001ZZ
DU002ZZ
DU003Z0
DU003ZZ
DU004ZZ
DU005ZZ
DU006ZZ
DU010ZZ
DU011ZZ
DU012ZZ
DU013Z0
DU013ZZ
DU014ZZ
DU015ZZ
DU016ZZ
DU020ZZ
DU021ZZ
DU022ZZ
DU023Z0
DU023ZZ
DU024ZZ
DU025ZZ
DU026ZZ
DU1097Z
DU1098Z
DU1099Z
DU109BZ
DU109CZ
DU109YZ
DU10B7Z
DU10B8Z
DU10B9Z
DU10BBZ
DU10BCZ
DU10BYZ
DU1197Z
DU1198Z
DU1199Z
DU119BZ
DU119CZ
DU119YZ
DU11B7Z
DU11B8Z
DU11B9Z
DU11BBZ
DU11BCZ
DU11BYZ
DU1297Z
DU1298Z
DU1299Z
DU129BZ
DU129CZ
DU129YZ
DU12B7Z
DU12B8Z
DU12B9Z
DU12BBZ
DU12BCZ
DU12BYZ
DU20DZZ
DU20HZZ
DU20JZZ
DU21DZZ
DU21HZZ
DU21JZZ
DU22DZZ
DU22HZZ
DU22JZZ
DUY07ZZ
DUY08ZZ
DUY0CZZ
DUY0FZZ
DUY17ZZ
DUY18ZZ
DUY1CZZ
DUY1FZZ
DUY27ZZ
DUY28ZZ
DUY2CZZ
DUY2FZZ
DV000ZZ
DV001ZZ
DV002ZZ
DV003Z0
DV003ZZ
DV004ZZ
DV005ZZ
DV006ZZ
DV010ZZ
DV011ZZ
DV012ZZ
DV013Z0
DV013ZZ
DV014ZZ
DV015ZZ
DV016ZZ
DV1097Z
DV1098Z
DV1099Z
DV109BZ
DV109CZ
DV109YZ
DV10B7Z
DV10B8Z
DV10B9Z
DV10BBZ
DV10BCZ
DV10BYZ
DV1197Z
DV1198Z
DV1199Z
DV119BZ
DV119CZ
DV119YZ
DV11B7Z
DV11B8Z
DV11B9Z
DV11BBZ
DV11BCZ
DV11BYZ
DV20DZZ
DV20HZZ
DV20JZZ
DV21DZZ
DV21HZZ
DV21JZZ
DVY07ZZ
DVY08ZZ
DVY0CZZ
DVY0FZZ
DVY0KZZ
DVY17ZZ
DVY18ZZ
DVY1FZZ
DW010ZZ
DW011ZZ
DW012ZZ
DW013Z0
DW013ZZ
DW014ZZ
DW015ZZ
DW016ZZ
DW020ZZ
DW021ZZ
DW022ZZ
DW023Z0
DW023ZZ
DW024ZZ
DW025ZZ
DW026ZZ
DW030ZZ
DW031ZZ
DW032ZZ
DW033Z0
DW033ZZ
DW034ZZ
DW035ZZ
DW036ZZ
DW040ZZ
DW041ZZ
DW042ZZ
DW043Z0
DW043ZZ
DW044ZZ
DW045ZZ
DW046ZZ
DW050ZZ
DW051ZZ
DW052ZZ
DW053Z0
DW053ZZ
DW054ZZ
DW055ZZ
DW056ZZ
DW060ZZ
DW061ZZ
DW062ZZ
DW063Z0
DW063ZZ
DW064ZZ
DW065ZZ
DW066ZZ
DW1197Z
DW1198Z
DW1199Z
DW119BZ
DW119CZ
DW119YZ
DW11B7Z
DW11B8Z
DW11B9Z
DW11BBZ
DW11BCZ
DW11BYZ
DW1297Z
DW1298Z
DW1299Z
DW129BZ
DW129CZ
DW129YZ
DW12B7Z
DW12B8Z
DW12B9Z
DW12BBZ
DW12BCZ
DW12BYZ
DW1397Z
DW1398Z
DW1399Z
DW139BZ
DW139CZ
DW139YZ
DW13B7Z
DW13B8Z
DW13B9Z
DW13BBZ
DW13BCZ
DW13BYZ
DW1697Z
DW1698Z
DW1699Z
DW169BZ
DW169CZ
DW169YZ
DW16B7Z
DW16B8Z
DW16B9Z
DW16BBZ
DW16BCZ
DW16BYZ
DW21DZZ
DW21HZZ
DW21JZZ
DW22DZZ
DW22HZZ
DW22JZZ
DW23DZZ
DW23HZZ
DW23JZZ
DW26DZZ
DW26HZZ
DW26JZZ
DWY17ZZ
DWY18ZZ
DWY1FZZ
DWY27ZZ
DWY28ZZ
DWY2FZZ
DWY37ZZ
DWY38ZZ
DWY3FZZ
DWY47ZZ
DWY48ZZ
DWY4FZZ
DWY57ZZ
DWY58ZZ
DWY5FZZ
DWY5GDZ
DWY5GFZ
DWY5GGZ
DWY5GHZ
DWY5GYZ
DWY67ZZ
DWY68ZZ
DWY6FZZ
F003GKZ
F003GMZ
F003GPZ
F003GYZ
F003GZZ
F00Z01Z
F00Z02Z
F00Z0KZ
F00Z0ZZ
F00Z11Z
F00Z12Z
F00Z19Z
F00Z1KZ
F00Z1ZZ
F00Z21Z
F00Z22Z
F00Z29Z
F00Z2KZ
F00Z2ZZ
F00Z31Z
F00Z32Z
F00Z3KZ
F00Z3ZZ
F00Z41Z
F00Z42Z
F00Z4ZZ
F00Z51Z
F00Z52Z
F00Z59Z
F00Z5KZ
F00Z6KZ
F00Z6MZ
F00Z6PZ
F00Z6YZ
F00Z6ZZ
F00Z7KZ
F00Z7MZ
F00Z7PZ
F00Z7YZ
F00Z7ZZ
F00Z8KZ
F00Z8MZ
F00Z8PZ
F00Z8YZ
F00Z8ZZ
F00Z9KZ
F00Z9PZ
F00Z9QZ
F00Z9YZ
F00Z9ZZ
F00ZBKZ
F00ZBNZ
F00ZBPZ
F00ZBQZ
F00ZBTZ
F00ZBYZ
F00ZBZZ
F00ZCKZ
F00ZCMZ
F00ZCPZ
F00ZCYZ
F00ZCZZ
F00ZDKZ
F00ZDNZ
F00ZDPZ
F00ZDQZ
F00ZDSZ
F00ZDTZ
F00ZDYZ
F00ZDZZ
F00ZFKZ
F00ZFNZ
F00ZFPZ
F00ZFSZ
F00ZFTZ
F00ZFYZ
F00ZFZZ
F00ZGKZ
F00ZGMZ
F00ZGPZ
F00ZGYZ
F00ZGZZ
F00ZHYZ
F00ZHZZ
F00ZJTZ
F00ZJWZ
F00ZJYZ
F00ZKKZ
F00ZKPZ
F00ZKYZ
F00ZKZZ
F00ZLKZ
F00ZLMZ
F00ZLPZ
F00ZLYZ
F00ZLZZ
F00ZMKZ
F00ZMPZ
F00ZMSZ
F00ZMVZ
F00ZMYZ
F00ZMZZ
F00ZNNZ
F00ZNPZ
F00ZNQZ
F00ZNSZ
F00ZNTZ
F00ZNYZ
F00ZPYZ
F00ZPZZ
F00ZQ1Z
F00ZQ2Z
F00ZQKZ
F00ZQZZ
F00ZR1Z
F00ZR2Z
F00ZRKZ
F00ZRZZ
F00ZS1Z
F00ZS2Z
F00ZSKZ
F00ZSZZ
F00ZT1Z
F00ZT2Z
F00ZTKZ
F00ZTZZ
F00ZV1Z
F00ZV2Z
F00ZVKZ
F00ZVZZ
F00ZW1Z
F00ZW2Z
F00ZWKZ
F00ZWZZ
F00ZXZZ
F0100EZ
F0100FZ
F0100UZ
F0100YZ
F0100ZZ
F0101ZZ

F0103ZZ
F0104ZZ
F0105YZ
F0105ZZ
F0106YZ
F0106ZZ
F010GZZ
F0110EZ
F0110FZ
F0110UZ
F0110YZ
F0110ZZ
F0111ZZ
F0113ZZ
F0114ZZ
F0115YZ
F0115ZZ
F0116YZ
F0116ZZ
F011GZZ
F0120EZ
F0120FZ
F0120UZ
F0120YZ
F0120ZZ
F0121ZZ
F0123ZZ
F0124ZZ
F0125YZ
F0125ZZ
F0126YZ
F0126ZZ
F012GZZ
F0130EZ
F0130FZ
F0130UZ
F0130YZ
F0130ZZ
F0131ZZ
F0133ZZ
F0134ZZ
F0135YZ
F0135ZZ
F0136YZ
F0136ZZ
F013GZZ
F01D0EZ
F01D0FZ
F01D0UZ
F01D0YZ
F01D0ZZ
F01D1ZZ
F01D5YZ
F01D5ZZ
F01D6YZ
F01D6ZZ
F01F0EZ
F01F0FZ
F01F0UZ
F01F0YZ
F01F0ZZ
F01F1ZZ
F01F5YZ
F01F5ZZ
F01F6YZ
F01F6ZZ
F01G0EZ
F01G0FZ
F01G0UZ
F01G0YZ
F01G0ZZ
F01G1ZZ
F01G5YZ
F01G5ZZ
F01G6YZ
F01G6ZZ
F01H0EZ
F01H0FZ
F01H0UZ
F01H0YZ
F01H0ZZ
F01H1ZZ
F01H5YZ
F01H5ZZ
F01H6YZ
F01H6ZZ
F01J0EZ
F01J0FZ
F01J0UZ
F01J0YZ
F01J0ZZ
F01J1ZZ
F01J5YZ
F01J5ZZ
F01J6YZ
F01J6ZZ
F01K0EZ
F01K0FZ
F01K0UZ
F01K0YZ
F01K0ZZ
F01K1ZZ
F01K5YZ
F01K5ZZ
F01K6YZ
F01K6ZZ
F01L0EZ
F01L0FZ
F01L0UZ
F01L0YZ
F01L0ZZ
F01L1ZZ
F01L5YZ
F01L5ZZ
F01L6YZ
F01L6ZZ
F01M0EZ
F01M0FZ
F01M0UZ
F01M0YZ
F01M0ZZ
F01M1ZZ
F01M5YZ
F01M5ZZ
F01M6YZ
F01M6ZZ
F01N0EZ
F01N0FZ
F01N0UZ
F01N0YZ
F01N0ZZ
F01Z2KZ
F01Z2MZ
F01Z2NZ
F01Z2PZ
F01Z2QZ
F01Z2SZ
F01Z2YZ
F01Z2ZZ
F01Z77Z
F01Z9JZ
F01ZBEZ
F01ZBFZ
F01ZBUZ
F01ZBZZ
F01ZCEZ
F01ZCFZ
F01ZCUZ
F01ZCZZ
F01ZDEZ
F01ZDFZ
F01ZDUZ
F01ZDYZ
F01ZDZZ
F01ZFEZ
F01ZFFZ
F01ZFUZ
F01ZFZZ
F0209YZ
F07D6CZ
F07D6DZ
F07D6EZ
F07D6FZ
F07D6GZ
F07D6HZ
F07D6UZ
F07D6YZ
F07D6ZZ
F07D7ZZ
F07F0EZ
F07F0FZ
F07F0UZ
F07F0YZ
F07F0ZZ
F07F1EZ
F07F1FZ
F07F1UZ
F07F1YZ
F07F1ZZ
F07F2EZ
F07F2FZ
F07F2UZ
F07F2YZ
F07F2ZZ
F07F3EZ
F07F3FZ
F07F3UZ
F07F3YZ
F07F3ZZ
F07F6BZ
F07F6CZ
F07F6DZ
F07F6EZ
F07F6FZ
F07F6GZ
F07F6HZ
F07F6UZ
F07F6YZ
F07F6ZZ
F07F7ZZ
F07G0EZ
F07G0FZ
F07G0UZ
F07G0YZ
F07G0ZZ
F07G1EZ
F07G1FZ
F07G1UZ
F07G1YZ
F07G1ZZ
F07G2EZ
F07G2FZ
F07G2UZ
F07G2YZ
F07G2ZZ
F07G3EZ
F07G3FZ
F07G3UZ
F07G3YZ
F07G3ZZ
F07G6BZ
F07G6CZ
F07G6DZ
F07G6EZ
F07G6FZ
F07G6GZ
F07G6HZ
F07G6UZ
F07G6YZ
F07G6ZZ
F07G7ZZ
F07H0EZ
F07H0FZ
F07H0UZ
F07H0YZ
F07H0ZZ
F07H1EZ
F07H1FZ
F07H1UZ
F07H1YZ
F07H1ZZ
F07H2EZ
F07H2FZ
F07H2UZ
F07H2YZ
F07H2ZZ
F07H3EZ
F07H3FZ
F07H3UZ
F07H3YZ
F07H3ZZ
F07H6BZ
F07H6CZ
F07H6DZ
F07H6EZ
F07H6FZ
F07H6GZ
F07H6HZ
F07H6UZ
F07H6YZ
F07H6ZZ
F07H7ZZ
F07J0EZ
F07J0FZ
F07J0UZ
F07J0YZ
F07J0ZZ
F07J1EZ
F07J1FZ
F07J1UZ
F07J1YZ
F07J1ZZ
F07J2EZ
F07J2FZ
F07J2UZ
F07J2YZ
F07J2ZZ
F07J3EZ
F07J3FZ
F07J3UZ
F07J3YZ
F07J3ZZ
F07J6BZ
F07J6CZ
F07J6DZ
F07J6EZ
F07J6FZ
F07J6GZ
F07J6HZ
F07J6UZ
F07J6YZ
F07J6ZZ
F07J7ZZ
F07K0EZ
F07K0FZ
F07K0UZ
F07K0YZ
F07K0ZZ
F07K1EZ
F07K1FZ
F07K1UZ
F07K1YZ
F07K1ZZ
F07K2EZ
F07K2FZ
F07K2UZ
F07K2YZ
F07K2ZZ
F07K3EZ
F07K3FZ
F07K3UZ
F07K3YZ
F07K3ZZ
F07K6BZ
F07K6CZ
F07K6DZ
F07K6EZ
F07K6FZ
F07K6GZ
F07K6HZ
F07K6UZ
F07K6YZ
F07K6ZZ
F07K7ZZ
F07L0EZ
F07L0FZ
F07L0UZ
F07L0YZ
F07L0ZZ
F07L1EZ
F07L1FZ
F07L1UZ
F07L1YZ
F07L1ZZ
F07L2EZ
F07L2FZ
F07L2UZ
F07L2YZ
F07L2ZZ
F07L3EZ
F07L3FZ
F07L3UZ
F07L3YZ
F07L3ZZ
F07L6BZ
F07L6CZ
F07L6DZ
F07L6EZ
F07L6FZ
F07L6GZ
F07L6HZ
F07L6UZ
F07L6YZ
F07L6ZZ
F07L7ZZ
F07M0EZ
F07M0FZ
F07M0UZ
F07M0YZ
F07M0ZZ
F07M1EZ
F07M1FZ
F07M1UZ
F07M1YZ
F07M1ZZ
F07M2EZ
F07M2FZ
F07M2UZ
F07M2YZ
F07M2ZZ
F07M3EZ
F07M3FZ
F07M3UZ
F07M3YZ
F07M3ZZ
F07M6BZ
F07M6CZ
F07M6DZ
F07M6EZ
F07M6FZ
F07M6GZ
F07M6HZ
F07M6UZ
F07M6YZ
F07M6ZZ
F07M7ZZ
F07N1EZ
F07N1FZ
F07N1UZ
F07N1YZ
F07N1ZZ
F07N6BZ
F07N6CZ
F07N6DZ
F07N6EZ
F07N6FZ
F07N6GZ
F07N6HZ
F07N6UZ
F07N6YZ
F07N6ZZ
F07Z4DZ
F07Z4EZ
F07Z4FZ
F07Z4UZ
F07Z4YZ
F07Z4ZZ
F07Z5CZ
F07Z5EZ
F07Z5FZ
F07Z5UZ
F07Z5YZ
F07Z5ZZ
F07Z8CZ
F07Z8DZ
F07Z8EZ
F07Z8FZ
F07Z8UZ
F07Z8YZ
F07Z8ZZ
F07Z9CZ
F07Z9DZ
F07Z9EZ
F07Z9FZ
F07Z9GZ
F07Z9UZ
F07Z9YZ
F07Z9ZZ
F08D5BZ
F08D5CZ
F08D5DZ
F08D5EZ
F08D5FZ
F08D5UZ
F08D5YZ
F08D5ZZ
F08F5BZ
F08F5CZ
F08F5DZ
F08F5EZ
F08F5FZ
F08F5UZ
F08F5YZ
F08F5ZZ
F08G5BZ
F08G5CZ
F08G5DZ
F08G5EZ
F08G5FZ
F08G5UZ
F08G5YZ
F08G5ZZ
F08H5BZ
F08H5CZ
F08H5DZ
F08H5EZ
F08H5FZ
F08H5UZ
F08H5YZ
F08H5ZZ
F08J5BZ
F08J5CZ
F08J5DZ
F08J5EZ
F08J5FZ
F08J5UZ
F08J5YZ
F08J5ZZ
F08K5BZ
F08K5CZ
F08K5DZ
F08K5EZ
F08K5FZ
F08K5UZ
F08K5YZ
F08K5ZZ
F08L5BZ
F08L5CZ
F08L5DZ
F08L5EZ
F08L5FZ
F08L5UZ
F08L5YZ
F08L5ZZ
F08M5BZ
F08M5CZ
F08M5DZ
F08M5EZ
F08M5FZ
F08M5UZ
F08M5YZ
F08M5ZZ
F08Z0EZ
F08Z0FZ
F08Z0UZ
F08Z0YZ
F08Z0ZZ
F08Z1EZ
F08Z1FZ
F08Z1UZ
F08Z1YZ
F08Z1ZZ
F08Z2EZ
F08Z2FZ
F08Z2UZ
F08Z2YZ
F08Z2ZZ
F08Z3CZ
F08Z3DZ
F08Z3EZ
F08Z3FZ
F08Z3UZ
F08Z3YZ
F08Z3ZZ
F08Z4DZ
F08Z4EZ
F08Z4FZ
F08Z4UZ
F08Z4YZ
F08Z4ZZ
F08Z6ZZ
F08Z7BZ
F08Z7CZ
F08Z7DZ
F08Z7EZ
F08Z7FZ
F08Z7GZ
F08Z7UZ
F08Z7YZ
F08Z7ZZ
F09Z0KZ
F09Z0ZZ
F09Z1KZ
F09Z1ZZ
F09Z2KZ
F09Z2LZ
F09Z2PZ
F09Z2YZ
F09Z2ZZ
F09Z3XZ
F09Z3ZZ
F0BZ01Z
F0BZ02Z
F0BZ09Z
F0BZ0KZ
F0BZ0PZ
F0BZ0YZ
F0C33EZ
F0C33FZ
F0C33UZ
F0C33YZ
F0C33ZZ
F0CH3EZ
F0CH3FZ
F0CH3UZ
F0CH3YZ
F0CH3ZZ
F0CM3EZ
F0CM3FZ
F0CM3UZ
F0CM3YZ
F0CM3ZZ
F0CZ08Z
F0CZ0ZZ
F0CZ1KZ
F0CZ1LZ
F0CZ1NZ
F0CZ1PZ
F0CZ1QZ
F0CZ1SZ
F0CZ1TZ
F0CZ1YZ
F0CZ1ZZ
F0CZ2KZ
F0CZ2LZ
F0CZ2NZ
F0CZ2PZ
F0CZ2QZ
F0CZ2SZ
F0CZ2TZ
F0CZ2YZ
F0CZ2ZZ
F0DZ05Z
F0DZ0ZZ
F0DZ11Z
F0DZ12Z
F0DZ15Z
F0DZ1KZ
F0DZ1LZ
F0DZ1ZZ
F0DZ21Z
F0DZ22Z
F0DZ25Z
F0DZ2KZ
F0DZ2LZ
F0DZ2ZZ
F0DZ3MZ
F0DZ4SZ
F0DZ4VZ
F0DZ51Z
F0DZ52Z
F0DZ55Z
F0DZ5KZ
F0DZ5LZ
F0DZ5ZZ
F0DZ6EZ
F0DZ6FZ
F0DZ6UZ
F0DZ6ZZ
F0DZ7EZ
F0DZ7FZ
F0DZ7UZ
F0DZ7ZZ
F0DZ8EZ
F0DZ8FZ
F0DZ8UZ
F0DZ8ZZ
F0DZ9EZ
F0DZ9FZ
F0DZ9UZ
F0DZ9ZZ
F0FZ0EZ
F0FZ0FZ
F0FZ0UZ
F0FZ0ZZ
F0FZ1EZ
F0FZ1FZ
F0FZ1UZ
F0FZ1ZZ
F0FZ2EZ
F0FZ2FZ
F0FZ2UZ
F0FZ2ZZ
F0FZ3EZ
F0FZ3FZ
F0FZ3UZ
F0FZ3ZZ
F0FZ4EZ
F0FZ4FZ
F0FZ4UZ
F0FZ4ZZ
F0FZ5EZ
F0FZ5FZ
F0FZ5UZ
F0FZ5ZZ
F0FZ6EZ
F0FZ6FZ
F0FZ6UZ
F0FZ6ZZ
F0FZ7EZ
F0FZ7FZ
F0FZ7UZ
F0FZ7ZZ
F0FZ8EZ
F0FZ8FZ
F0FZ8UZ
F0FZ8ZZ
F0FZ9EZ
F0FZ9FZ
F0FZ9UZ
F0FZ9ZZ
F0FZBEZ
F0FZBFZ
F0FZBUZ
F0FZBZZ
F0FZCEZ
F0FZCFZ
F0FZCUZ
F0FZCZZ
F0FZDEZ
F0FZDFZ
F0FZDUZ
F0FZDZZ
F0FZFEZ
F0FZFFZ
F0FZFUZ
F0FZFZZ
F0FZGEZ
F0FZGFZ
F0FZGUZ
F0FZGZZ
F0FZHEZ
F0FZHFZ
F0FZHUZ
F0FZHZZ
F0FZJKZ
F0FZJLZ
F0FZJMZ
F0FZJPZ
F0FZJZZ
F13Z00Z
F13Z01Z
F13Z02Z
F13Z03Z
F13Z08Z
F13Z09Z
F13Z0ZZ
F13Z10Z
F13Z11Z
F13Z12Z
F13Z1ZZ
F13Z20Z
F13Z21Z
F13Z22Z
F13Z2ZZ
F13Z31Z
F13Z32Z
F13Z3ZZ
F13Z41Z
F13Z42Z
F13Z4KZ
F13Z4ZZ
F13Z51Z
F13Z52Z
F13Z5KZ
F13Z5ZZ
F13Z61Z
F13Z62Z
F13Z6ZZ
F13Z71Z
F13Z7KZ
F13Z7ZZ
F13Z83Z
F13Z84Z
F13Z8ZZ
F13Z91Z

F13Z92Z
F13Z9ZZ
F13ZB1Z
F13ZB2Z
F13ZBZZ
F13ZC1Z
F13ZC2Z
F13ZCZZ
F13ZD3Z
F13ZD4Z
F13ZDZZ
F13ZF3Z
F13ZF4Z
F13ZFZZ
F13ZG3Z
F13ZG4Z
F13ZGZZ
F13ZH3Z
F13ZH4Z
F13ZHZZ
F13ZJ3Z
F13ZJ4Z
F13ZJZZ
F13ZK7Z
F13ZKZZ
F13ZL7Z
F13ZLZZ
F13ZM6Z
F13ZMZZ
F13ZN6Z
F13ZNZZ
F13ZP1Z
F13ZP2Z
F13ZP4Z
F13ZP9Z
F13ZPKZ
F13ZPLZ
F13ZPPZ
F13ZPZZ
F13ZQKZ
F13ZQPZ
F13ZQYZ
F13ZQZZ
F14Z01Z
F14Z02Z
F14Z03Z
F14Z04Z
F14Z05Z
F14Z07Z
F14Z09Z
F14Z0KZ
F14Z0LZ
F14Z0PZ
F14Z0YZ
F14Z0ZZ
F14Z15Z
F14Z1ZZ
F14Z21Z
F14Z22Z
F14Z23Z
F14Z24Z
F14Z25Z
F14Z2KZ
F14Z2LZ
F14Z2PZ
F14Z2ZZ
F14Z31Z
F14Z32Z
F14Z33Z
F14Z34Z
F14Z35Z
F14Z3KZ
F14Z3LZ
F14Z3PZ
F14Z3ZZ
F14Z41Z
F14Z42Z
F14Z43Z
F14Z44Z
F14Z4KZ
F14Z4LZ
F14Z4ZZ
F14Z51Z
F14Z52Z
F14Z53Z
F14Z54Z
F14Z55Z
F14Z5KZ
F14Z5LZ
F14Z5ZZ
F14Z65Z
F14Z6ZZ
F14Z70Z
F14Z7ZZ
F14Z85Z
F14Z8ZZ
F15Z08Z
F15Z0ZZ
F15Z18Z
F15Z1ZZ
F15Z28Z
F15Z2ZZ
F15Z38Z
F15Z3ZZ
F15Z48Z
F15Z4ZZ
F15Z58Z
F15Z5ZZ
F15Z68Z
F15Z6ZZ
F15Z75Z
F15Z7ZZ
GZ10ZZZ
GZ11ZZZ
GZ12ZZZ
GZ13ZZZ
GZ14ZZZ
GZ2ZZZZ
GZ3ZZZZ
GZ50ZZZ
GZ51ZZZ
GZ52ZZZ
GZ53ZZZ
GZ54ZZZ
GZ55ZZZ
GZ56ZZZ
GZ58ZZZ
GZ59ZZZ
GZ60ZZZ
GZ61ZZZ
GZ63ZZZ
GZ72ZZZ
GZB0ZZZ
GZB1ZZZ
GZB2ZZZ
GZB3ZZZ
GZB4ZZZ
GZC9ZZZ
GZFZZZZ
GZGZZZZ
GZHZZZZ
GZJZZZZ
HZ2ZZZZ
HZ30ZZZ
HZ31ZZZ
HZ32ZZZ
HZ33ZZZ
HZ34ZZZ
HZ35ZZZ
HZ36ZZZ
HZ37ZZZ
HZ38ZZZ
HZ39ZZZ
HZ3BZZZ
HZ3CZZZ
HZ40ZZZ
HZ41ZZZ
HZ42ZZZ
HZ43ZZZ
HZ44ZZZ
HZ45ZZZ
HZ46ZZZ
HZ47ZZZ
HZ48ZZZ
HZ49ZZZ
HZ4BZZZ
HZ4CZZZ
HZ50ZZZ
HZ51ZZZ
HZ52ZZZ
HZ53ZZZ
HZ54ZZZ
HZ55ZZZ
HZ56ZZZ
HZ57ZZZ
HZ58ZZZ
HZ59ZZZ
HZ5BZZZ
HZ5CZZZ
HZ5DZZZ
HZ63ZZZ
HZ80ZZZ
HZ81ZZZ
HZ82ZZZ
HZ83ZZZ
HZ84ZZZ
HZ85ZZZ
HZ86ZZZ
HZ87ZZZ
HZ88ZZZ
HZ89ZZZ
HZ90ZZZ
HZ91ZZZ
HZ92ZZZ
HZ93ZZZ
HZ94ZZZ
HZ95ZZZ
HZ96ZZZ
HZ97ZZZ
HZ98ZZZ
HZ99ZZZ
X2A5312
X2C0361
X2C1361
X2C2361
X2C3361
X2RF032
X2RF332
X2RF432
XHRPXL2
XK02303
XNS0032
XNS0332
XNS3032
XNS3332
XNS4032
XNS4332
XR2G021
XR2H021
XRG0092
XRG00F3
XRG1092
XRG10F3
XRG2092
XRG20F3
XRG4092
XRG40F3
XRG6092
XRG60F3
XRG7092
XRG70F3
XRG8092
XRG80F3
XRGA092
XRGA0F3
XRGB092
XRGB0F3
XRGC092
XRGC0F3
XRGD092
XRGD0F3
XV508A4
XW03321
XW03331
XW03341
XW03351
XW03372
XW03392
XW033A3
XW033B3
XW033C3
XW033F3
XW033G4
XW033H4
XW04321
XW04331
XW04341
XW04351
XW04372
XW04392
XW043A3
XW043B3
XW043C3
XW043F3
XW043G4
XW043H4
XW0DX82
XY0VX83

2019 HCPCS Level II Advisor

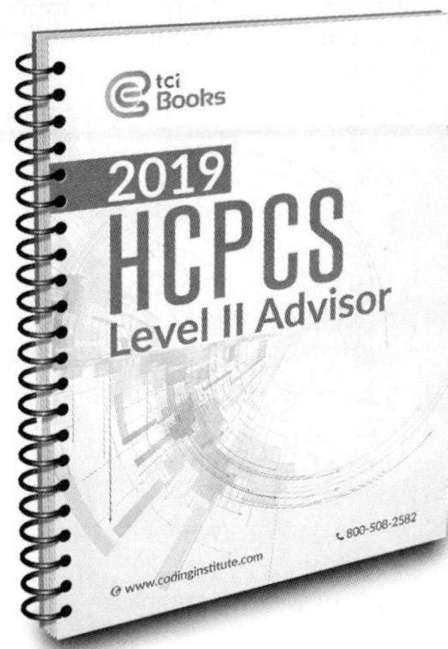
tci Books
2019
HCPCS
Level II Advisor
800-508-2582
www.codinginstitute.com

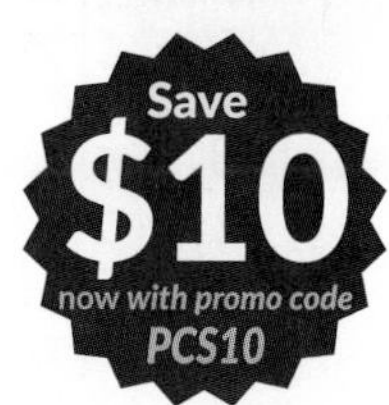
Save
$10
now with promo code
PCS10

Jumpstart your workflow with easy access to the latest code updates to bill supplies, equipment, and drugs to Medicare and other payers.

TCI's **HCPCS Level II Advisor 2019**, jam-packed with everything you need for quick and accurate HCPCS coding, including expert guidance and best-in-class tips on code selection—as well as 2019 HCPCS code updates. And navigation couldn't be easier!

Conquer accurate HCPCS coding and reap the reimbursement you've earned:

- New, revised, and deleted HCPCS codes for 2019 (with a deleted codes crosswalk)
- **NEW!** Enhanced and detailed illustrations
- **NEW!** Certification exam prep advice
- **NEW!** More colored symbols for quick code searches
- **NEW!** Coding tips and definitions throughout the Tabular List
- **NEW!** MACRA updates
- **NEW!** Expanded stick-on tabs
- Comprehensive Alphabetic Index with hundreds of additional entries
- **5,000+** HCPCS codes with complete code descriptors
- CPT® crosswalk codes under each G code
- Table of Drugs and Biologicals, **including more brand-name drugs and generic drugs**
- Pub 100 references
- CCI edits (Column 1 and Column 2)
- Dictionary-style headers and color-coded bleed tabs

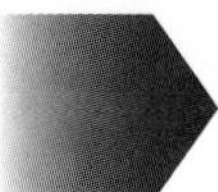

Ensure your practice gets full reimbursement for supplies, drugs, and DME with the **HCPCS Level II Advisor 2019**.

Expedite your coding with at-a-glance alerts in vibrant eye-catching colors:

- New and revised codes
- MIPS code
- Carrier judgment
- Special coverage instructions apply
- Not payable by Medicare
- Non-covered by Medicare
- Non-covered by Medicare statute
- ASC Payment Indicator
- APC Status Indicator
- ASC Approved Procedure
- Service not separately priced by Part B
- Other carrier priced
- Reasonable charge
- Price established using national RVUs
- Price subject to national limitation amount
- Price established by carriers
- Statute references
- BETOS code and descriptor
- Paid under the DME fee schedule
- DME Modifier
- AHA Coding Clinic®

PRE-ORDER ONLINE or call **1-800-508-2582** today to get your copy
or visit https://www.codinginstitute.com/books/hcpcs-level-ii-advisor.html?year=2019.

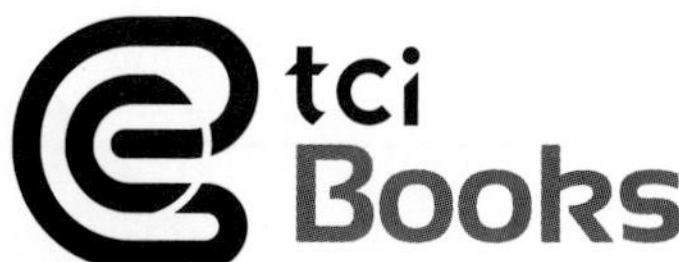
tci
Books

Call us: 800-508-2582 | www.codinginstitute.com
The Coding Institute LLC
2222 Sedwick Road Durham, NC 27713

CPT® is a registered trademark of the American Medical Association

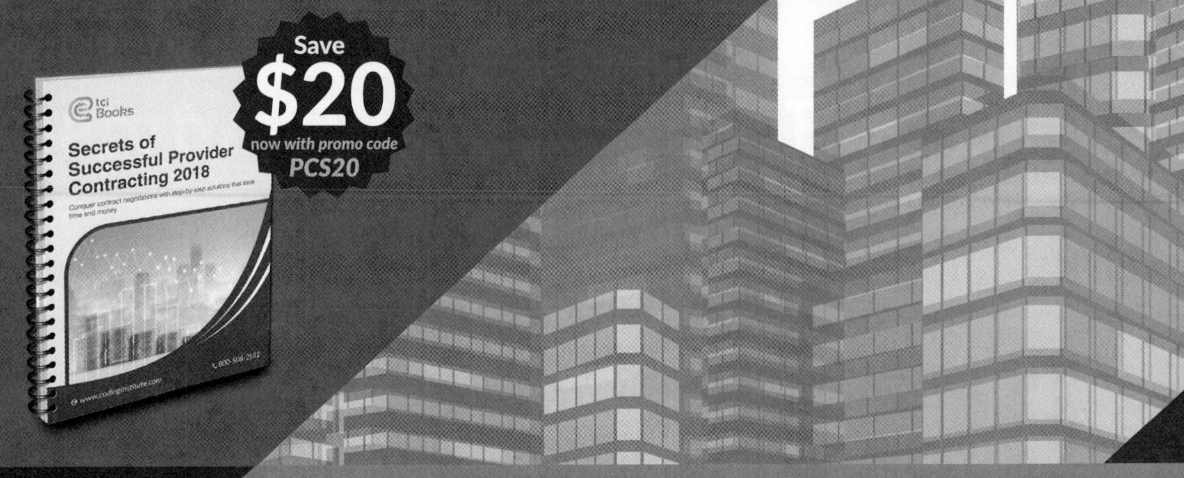

Save
$20
now with promo code
PCS20
tci Books
Secrets of Successful Provider Contracting 2018

tci Books

Secrets of Successful Provider Contracting 2018

When it comes to hammering out the details of provider contracts, don't go to the table without the hammer.

Team up with TCI and negotiate like a pro. The **Secrets of Successful Provider Contracting 2018** will transform how you view contracts and approach negotiations.

Get the revenue you deserve with step-by-step solutions to both physician contracting and private exchange provider contracting. Master high-impact negotiation strategies, learn the ins and outs of recognizing opportunities for provider contracting, and be equipped to meet 2018 Stark exception and compliance regulations.

Lock in revenue with best-in-class tactics and insider know-how:

- ✓ 5 critical terms that are negotiable in provider contracts
- ✓ Top compliance concerns for physician contracts
- ✓ Distinguish between private and public exchanges and how payment terms differ.
- ✓ Know if you're automatically included in private exchanges under existing contracts.
- ✓ Learn how to perform due diligence before joining a private exchange network.
- ✓ Use this checklist for a payer contract that protects your profits.
- ✓ Know what to include in a contract termination notice.
- ✓ Avoid liability with waiver via instructions.
- ✓ Identify problematic POS billing.
- ✓ Get your overpayment refund (PPACA).
- ✓ Monitor anticipated payments so you know how much money to expect.
- ✓ Ask these strategic questions as part of a comprehensive physician payment program.
- ✓ Develop your physician payment monitoring program with a step-by-step guide.
- ✓ Ask these questions about each payment to ensure compliance.
- ✓ Know the red flags and early warning signs of compliance issues.
- ✓ Look for these key "takeaways" to ensure a more compliant contracting process.
- ✓ Identify hidden information, such as silent PPOs, that could affect the contract.
- ✓ Understand alternative contract negotiations, including patient education to discover a win-win.
- ✓ Get to know tracking reports to monitor insurance payments.
- ✓ 5 sure-fire ways to ace payer contract negotiation
- ✓ Learn how to avoid common payer contract negotiation mistakes.
- ✓ **And so much more!**

To order the ***Secrets of Successful Provider Contracting 2018***, call **1-800-508-2582** or visit https://www.codinginstitute.com/books/secrets-of-successful-provider-contracting.html.

Call us: 800-508-2582 | www.codinginstitute.com

The Coding Institute LLC
2222 Sedwick Road Durham, NC 27713

NOTES

NOTES

NOTES

NOTES

NOTES

NOTES